2nd edition

comprehensive pharmacy review

2nd edition

comprehensive pharmacy review

EDITOR
Leon Shargel, Ph.D., R.Ph.

ASSOCIATE EDITORS
Alan H. Mutnick, Pharm.D., R.Ph.
Paul F. Souney, M.S., R.Ph.
David C. Kosegarten, Ph.D., R.Ph.
Sunil Jambhekar, Ph.D.
Edward F. LaSala, Ph.D., R.Ph.
Douglas J. Pisano, M.S., R.Ph.
Larry N. Swanson, Pharm.D., R.Ph.

SANS TACHE

Harwal Publishing

Philadelphia • Baltimore • Hong Kong • London • Munich • Sydney • Tokyo

A Waverly Company

Harwal

The authors and publisher have made a conscientious effort to ensure that the drug information and recommended dosages in this book are accurate and in accord with accepted standards at the time of publication. However, pharmacology is a rapidly changing science, so readers are advised, before administering any drug, to check the package insert provided by the manufacturer for the recommended dose, for contraindications for administration, and for added warnings and precautions. This recommendation is especially important for new, infrequently used, or highly toxic drugs.

Library of Congress Cataloging-in Publication Data

Comprehensive pharmacy review / editor, Leon Shargel ; associate editors, Alan H. Mutnick . . .[et al.]. — 2nd ed.
p. cm.
Rev. ed. of: Pharmacy review. 1992.
Includes index.
ISBN 0-683-06253-0
1. Pharmacy—Examinations, questions, etc. 2. Pharmacy—Outlines, syllabi, etc. I. Shargel, Leon, 1941– . II. Mutnick, Alan H. III. Pharmacy review. IV. Series.
[DNLM: 1. Pharmacy—examination questions. 2. Pharmacy—outlines. QV 18 P53751 1993]
RS97.P49 1993
615'.1'076—dc20
DNLM/DLC
for Library of Congress 92-48560
CIP

10 9 8 7 6 5

Contents

Contributors

Anton H. Amann, Ph.D.
Senior Vice President
Scientific Operations
Apotex USA, Inc.
New York, New York

Ernest R. Anderson, Jr., M.S.
Director of Pharmacy
Lahey Clinic
Burlington, Massachusetts

Connie Lee Barnes, Pharm.D.
Assistant Professor of Pharmacy Practice
Campbell University School of Pharmacy
Buies Creek, North Carolina

Lyndon Braun, Pharm.D., M.B.A.
Assistant Director of Pharmacy
California Pacific Medical Center
San Francisco Medical Center
San Francisco, California

Todd A. Brown, R.Ph.
Clinical Assistant Professor of Pharmacy Practice
Bouve College of Pharmacy and Health Sciences
Northeastern University
Boston, Massachusetts

Ronald J. Callahan, Ph.D., B.C.N.P.
Assistant Professor of Radiology
Harvard Medical School
Adjunct Associate Professor of Radiopharmaceutics
Massachusetts College of Pharmacy and Allied Health Sciences
Director of Nuclear Pharmacy
Massachusetts General Hospital
Boston, Massachusetts

Ronnie Chapman, Pharm.D.
Assistant Professor of Pharmacy Practice
Campbell University School of Pharmacy
Buies Creek, North Carolina
Clinical Pharmacist
Veterans Administration Medical Center
Durham, North Carolina

Louise Glassner Cohen, Pharm.D., R.Ph.
Associate Professor of Clinical Pharmacy
Massachusetts College of Pharmacy and Allied Health Sciences
Clinical Pharmacy Coordinator
Infectious Disease Section
Massachusetts General Hospital
Boston, Massachusetts

Michael J. DeFelice, M.S., R.Ph.
Assistant Professor of Pharmacy Practice
Massachusetts College of Pharmacy and Allied Health Sciences
Boston, Massachusetts

Stephen L. DePietro, B.S., R.Ph.
Instructor of Pharmacy Practice
Massachusetts College of Pharmacy and Allied Health Sciences
Boston, Massachusetts

Stephen C. Dragotakes, R.Ph., B.C.N.P.
Instructor in Radiopharmaceutics
Massachusetts College of Pharmacy and Allied Health Sciences
Division of Nuclear Medicine
Department of Radiology
Massachusetts General Hospital
Boston, Massachusetts

Helen L. Figge, Pharm.D., R.Ph.
Research Associate, Department of Pathology
Albany Medical College
Albany, New York

Constance McKenzie Fleming, Pharm.D.
Assistant Professor of Pharmacy Practice
Director of Experiential Programs
Campbell University School of Pharmacy
Buies Creek, North Carolina

Stephen Fuller, Pharm.D.
Assistant Professor of Pharmacy Practice
Campbell University School of Pharmacy
Buies Creek, North Carolina
Department Head
Department of Pharmacy Education
Fayetteville Health Education Center
Fayetteville, North Carolina

Steven Grossman, B.S., R.Ph.
Pierce Apothecary
Boston, Massachusetts

Sunil Jambhekar, Ph.D.
Associate Professor and Interim Chairman
Department of Pharmaceutics and Industrial Pharmacy
Massachusetts College of Pharmacy and Allied Health Sciences
Boston, Massachusetts

John E. Janosik, Pharm.D., R.Ph.
Manager
Regional Drug Information
Kaiser Permanente
Brooklyn Heights, Ohio

Jerome P. Janousek, M.S.
Director of Pharmacy
Beth Israel Hospital
Boston, Massachusetts

Kevin P. Keating, M.D.
Assistant Professor of Surgery
Associate Director
Surgery Critical Care
Director
Nutritional Support Services
Hartford Hospital
Hartford, Connecticut

David C. Kosegarten, Ph.D., R.Ph.
Associate Professor of Pharmacology and Toxicology
Massachusetts College of Pharmacy and Allied Health Sciences
Boston, Massachusetts

Edward F. LaSala, Ph.D., R.Ph.
Emeritus Professor of Chemistry (retired)
Massachusetts College of Pharmacy and Allied Health Sciences
Boston, Massachusetts

Suellen O'Neill, M.S., Pharm.D.
Associate Professor of Clinical Practice
Massachusetts College of Pharmacy and Allied Health Sciences
Boston, Massachusetts

Joseph F. Palumbo, M.S., R.Ph.
Professor Emeritus (retired)
Bouve College of Pharmacy and Health Sciences
Northeastern University
Boston, Massachusetts

Douglas J. Pisano, M.S., R.Ph.
Assistant Professor of Pharmacy Practice
Massachusetts College of Pharmacy and Allied Health Sciences
Boston, Massachusetts

David Platt, Pharm.D.
Associate Director
Department of Pharmacy Screening
Hartford Hospital
Hartford, Connecticut

Kim Poinsett-Holmes, Pharm.D.
Senior Drug Information Associate
Drug Information and Medical Services
Glaxo Research Institute
Research Triangle Park, North Carolina

Robert A. Quercia, M.S., R.Ph.
Associate Clinical Professor
University of Connecticut School of Pharmacy
Storrs, Connecticut
Supervisor
Drug Information Service
Director
Total Parenteral Nutrition Service
Department of Pharmacy
Hartford Hospital
Hartford, Connecticut

John D. Leary, Ph.D., R.Ph.
Professor of Biochemistry
Massachusetts College of Pharmacy and Allied Health Sciences
Boston, Massachusetts

Vincent C. Lopresti, Ph.D.
Associate Professor of Science
Wheelock College
Boston, Massachusetts

Dennis G. Lyons, R.Ph.
Senior Drug Policy Advisor
Massachusetts Department of Public Health
Division of Food and Drugs
Jamaica Plain, Massachusetts

Louise Mallet, Pharm.D.
Centre Hospitalier Mont Joli
Mont Joli, Québec

William W. McCloskey, Pharm.D.
Associate Professor of Clinical Pharmacy
Massachusetts College of Pharmacy and Allied Health Sciences
Boston, Massachusetts

H. William McGhee, Pharm.D.
Clinical Pharmacy Coordinator
Children's Hospital of Pittsburgh
Pittsburgh, Pennsylvania

Alan H. Mutnick, Pharm.D., R.Ph.
Senior Assistant Director, Clinical Practice
The University of Iowa Hospitals and Clinics
Adjunct Associate Professor of Clinical Practice
University of Iowa College of Pharmacy
Iowa City, Iowa

Azita Razzaghi, Pharm.D.
Coordinator
Medical Surveillance
Procter & Gamble Pharmaceuticals
Norwich, New York

Joseph M. Sceppa, M.S.
Director of Pharmacy
Children's Hospital Medical Center
Boston, Massachusetts

Gerald E. Schumacher, Pharm.D., Ph.D.
Professor of Pharmacy
Bouve College of Pharmacy and Health Sciences
Northeastern University
Boston, Massachusetts

Leon Shargel, Ph.D., R.Ph.
Vice President
Pharmakinetics Laboratories, Inc.
Baltimore, Maryland

Brian F. Shea, Pharm.D.
Director
Drug Information Center
Department of Pharmacy Services
Brigham and Women's Hospital
Boston, Massachusetts

Lisa P. Shopper, Pharm.D.
Adjunct Clinical Assistant Professor
University of Missouri-Kansas City
Kansas City, Missouri

Paul F. Souney, M.S., R.Ph.
Information Scientist
Astra/Merck
Sharon, Massachusetts

Larry N. Swanson, Pharm.D., R.Ph.
Professor and Chairman
Department of Pharmacy Practice
Campbell University School of Pharmacy
Buies Creek, North Carolina

Cheryl A. Stoukides, Pharm.D., R.Ph.
Clinical Assistant Professor
University of Rhode Island College of Pharmacy
Director
University of Rhode Island Drug Information Center
Providence, Rhode Island

Barbara Szymusiak-Mutnick, M.H.P., R.Ph.
Clinical Pharmacist
The University of Iowa Hospitals and Clinics
Iowa City, Iowa

F. Randy Vogenberg, M.Ed., R.Ph., F.A.S.C.P.
Assistant Professor of Pharmacy Practice
Massachusetts College of Pharmacy and Allied Health Sciences
Boston, Massachusetts

Andrew L. Wilson, Pharm.D.
Director of Pharmacy Services
St. Louis University Hospital
St. Louis, Missouri

Preface

The profession of pharmacy has changed significantly during the last 3 decades. Pharmacy has evolved from the practice of preparing, preserving, compounding, and dispensing drugs to a patient-oriented practice, in which the pharmacist not only must understand the biologic and chemical nature of drugs but also must be a knowledgeable health professional. The formal education of the pharmacist has reflected these changes by an increase in the required years of education and by an increase in the emphasis on both behavioral and clinical sciences.

Our initial plan for *Comprehensive Pharmacy Review* was modest enough—to produce a comprehensive study guide for pharmacy students who are preparing for the NABPLEX®. Accordingly, we set out to develop outlines and practice questions for the subjects in the pharmacy school curriculum. These, along with the separate booklet of simulated NABPLEX® exams that supplements this review, would provide both guidance and test practice for NABPLEX® candidates.

What actually materialized is something more ambitious. While the principal market for *Comprehensive Pharmacy Review* remains NABPLEX® candidates, the book is also intended for a broader audience of pharmacy undergraduates and professionals who seek detailed summaries of pharmacy subjects. Encompassed by the review is a range of topics central to the study of pharmacy—chemistry, pharmaceutics, pharmacology, pharmacy practice, clinical pharmacy—organized to parallel the pharmacy curriculum and presented in outline form for easy use. It can therefore be used as a quick review (or preview) of essential topics by a diverse group of readers, including:

- Matriculating pharmacy students. The organization and topical coverage of *Comprehensive Pharmacy Review* is such that many pharmacy students will want to purchase it in their freshman year and use it throughout their undergraduate training to prepare for course examinations.

- Instructors and preceptors. *Comprehensive Pharmacy Review* also functions as an instructor's manual and a reference for teachers and tutors in pharmacy schools. Chapter outlines can be used to organize courses and to plan specific lectures.

- Professional pharmacists. *Comprehensive Pharmacy Review* offers practitioners a convenient handbook of pharmacy facts. It can be used as a course refresher and as a source of recent information on pharmacy practice. The appendices include prescription dispensing information, common prescription drugs, and general pharmacy references.

This volume represents the contributions of nearly 2 dozen specialists, each delivering a current summary of his or her field to a review guide that is not only accurate and up-to-date, but also comprehensible to students, teachers, and practitioners alike. If you have any suggestions on how we might improve *Comprehensive Pharmacy Review,* please write us at Harwal Publishing Company, 200 Chester Field Parkway, Malvern, PA 19355.

Introduction to the NABPLEX®

In 1975, the Study Commission on Pharmacy presented its report to the American Association of Colleges of Pharmacy.* This study commission, chaired by John S. Millis, evaluated the state of pharmacy practice and pharmaceutical education of pharmacists, recognizing the changes that have occurred in medical knowledge and public expectation of health care. The study commission's report stimulated changes in the scope of pharmaceutical education and pharmacy practice.

According to the Study Commission report, pharmacy should be conceived as a "knowledge system" in which the pharmacist generates knowledge about drugs; acquires relevant knowledge from the biological, chemical, physical, and behavioral sciences; and tests, organizes, and applies that knowledge. Included in the report was a suggestion that the curricula of the schools of pharmacy should be based on competencies desired for their graduates rather than on the basis of knowledge available in the several relevant sciences.

After graduating from an accredited pharmacy program, the prospective pharmacist must demonstrate that he or she has the competency to practice pharmacy. Currently, every state and the District of Columbia require that the graduate pass an examination for licensure to practice pharmacy. Most states use the National Association of Boards of Pharmacy Licensure Examination (NABPLEX®), which is administered three times each year (January, June, and September) by the National Association of Boards of Pharmacy (NABP®).

The standards of competence for the practice of pharmacy are set by each state board. The NABPLEX® is not a competitive examination; however, it is the principal instrument used by the state boards of pharmacy to assess the knowledge and proficiency necessary for a candidate to practice pharmacy. All NABPLEX® questions are based on competency statements, which are reviewed and revised periodically. The competency statements summarize the knowledge that the candidate is expected to have acquired and to be able to demonstrate.

The NABPLEX® was introduced to state boards in 1976 and was composed of five subtests: pharmacy, mathematics, chemistry, pharmacology, and pharmacy practice. These tests examined basic skills and knowledge without regard to geographic or practice setting. Because of the evolution of pharmacy practice, the current NABPLEX® has an integrated format, focusing on patient profiles and practice situations. According to NABP®, the intent of the test is to approximate practice conditions as closely as possible and to examine the basic skills and knowledge that a pharmacist needs.

---

*Study Commission on Pharmacy: *Pharmacists for the Future.* Ann Arbor, Health Administration Press, 1975.

NABPLEX® Competency Statements

The questions in the NABPLEX® are based on the NABPLEX® competency statements and are published annually.* According to the National Association of the Boards of Pharmacy (NABP®), the competency statements were "developed to reflect the skills and knowledge important to an entry-level pharmacist and to form the foundation of the NABPLEX® examination." Those candidates planning to take the NABPLEX® should review the competency statements published in the latest edition of the *NABPLEX® Candidates Review Guide.*

Essentially, the NABPLEX® competency statements cover five major areas of pharmacy practice, and a percentage of the test covers the practice component. In addition, for each major competency statement, a subset of statements details individual competencies.

The major competency headings stated in the *NABPLEX® Candidates Review Guide* are the following:

1. Interpreting and Dispensing Prescriptions/Medication Orders
2. Assessing Prescriptions/Medication Orders and the Drugs Used in Dispensing Them
3. Compounding and Calculation Involved in the Extemporaneous Preparation of Prescription/Medication Orders
4. Monitoring Drug Therapy
5. Counseling Patients and Health Professionals

**NABPLEX® Candidates Review Guide*. National Association of Boards of Pharmacy, O'Hare Corporate Center, 1300 Higgins Road, Suite 103, Park Ridge, IL 60068.

Part I
Pharmaceutics and Biopharmaceutics

Leon Shargel
Sunil Jambhekar

1

Drug Product Development in the Pharmaceutical Industry

Anton H. Amann
Leon Shargel

I. INTRODUCTION. Different drug product development approaches are generally used to produce new chemical entities, product line extensions, generic products, and specialty products.

A. New chemical entities are drug substances with unknown clinical, toxicologic, physical, and chemical properties. The following phases of product development proceed sequentially:

1. **Preclinical stage.** Animal pharmacology and toxicology data are obtained to determine some degree of safety and efficacy of the drug. An **investigational new drug (IND) application** for human testing is submitted to the Food and Drug Administration (FDA). Since it is highly probable that the product will not reach the marketplace at this stage, no attempt is made to develop a final formulation.

2. **Phase I**
   - **a.** Clinical testing takes place after submission of the IND application.
   - **b.** Healthy volunteers are used in phase I clinical studies to determine the tolerance and toxicity of the drug.

3. **Phase II**
   - **a.** A limited number of patients with the disease for which the drug was developed are treated under close supervision.
   - **b.** Dose-response studies are performed to determine the optimum dosage regimen for treating the disease.
   - **c.** Safety is measured by attempting to determine the **therapeutic index** (ratio of toxic dose to effective dose).
   - **d.** A final drug formulation is developed, which is a bioequivalent to the dosage form used in the initial clinical studies.

4. **Phase III**
   - **a.** Large scale, multicenter studies are performed, using the final dosage form developed in phase II, to determine the safety and efficacy of the drug product in a large patient population with the disease for which the drug was developed.
   - **b.** Side effects are critically monitored. In a large population, new toxic effects may occur that were not evident in previous clinical trials.

5. **Submission of a new drug application (NDA).** When all clinical trials are completed to the satisfaction of the medical community and the drug product is found to be efficacious by all parameters, an NDA is submitted to the FDA for review and approval.

6. **Phase IV**
   - **a.** After the NDA is submitted and prior to approval by the FDA to market the product, manufacturing scale-up* activities occur.
   - **b.** Slight modifications of the drug formulation may occur as a result of data obtained during manufacturing scale-up and validation.

7. **Phase V**
   - **a.** After market approval of the drug, product development may continue.

---

*Scale-up is the increase in the batch size from the clinical batch, the pilot batch, or both up to several hundred thousand dose units to the full-scale production batch size, using the finished, marketed product (> million dose units).

b. Improvements in the drug product may be performed as a result of equipment, regulatory, supply, or market demands.

B. **Product line extensions** are dosage forms in which the physical form or strength of the products change—not the use and indication. Product line extension development is usually performed during phases III, IV, or V of drug product development.

C. **Generic drug products**

1. After **patent expiration** of the brand drug product, a generic drug product, containing the same amount of the drug in the same type of dosage form (i.e., tablets, capsules, liquids, semisolids, injectables), may be developed.
2. Generic drug products must be bioequivalents (i.e., have the same rate and extent of drug absorption) to the brand drug product and are, therefore, expected to give the same clinical response (see Chapter 6). These studies are generally done in healthy human volunteers.
3. The generic drug product may differ from the brand product in the amount and type of excipients and in the physical appearance (i.e., size, color, shape, taste) of the dosage form.
4. Prior to marketing, the manufacturer must submit an **abbreviated new drug application (ANDA)** to the FDA for approval. Since preclinical safety and efficacy studies have already been performed for the NDA-approved brand product, only bioequivalence studies are required for the ANDA.

D. **Specialty drug products** are existing products that are developed in a new delivery system or for a new therapeutic indication. The safety and efficacy of the drug have been established in an NDA-approved dosage form. For example, the nitroglycerin transdermal delivery system (patch) was developed after experience with the nitroglycerin sublingual tablets.

II. PRODUCT DEVELOPMENT.

For each drug, various activities and information are required to develop a safe, effective, stable, and pharmaceutically elegant dosage form.

A. **New chemical entities**

1. **Preformulation** is the characterization of all the physical and chemical properties of the active drug substance, such as the therapeutic use of the drug, the type of drug delivery system (e.g., immediate release, controlled release, suppository), and the route of administration (e.g., oral, parenteral, topical, transdermal).
   a. Preformulation activities are usually performed during the preclinical stage, although these activities may continue into phases I and II.
   b. Information obtained during preformulation includes:
      (1) **General characteristics.** Particle size, particle shape, crystalline morphology, density, surface area, hygroscopicity, and powder flow
      (2) **Solubility characteristics.** Intrinsic dissolution, pH solubility profile, and general solubility characteristics in various solvents
      (3) **Chemical characteristics.** Surface energy, pH stability profile, pK_a, temperature stability (dry or under various humidity conditions), and excipient interactions
      (4) **Analytical methods development.** Developing analytical, stability, and cleaning methods, and identification of impurities
2. **Formulation development** is an ongoing activity. Initial drug formulations are developed for early clinical studies. Once the submission of an NDA is considered, an attempt to develop the final dosage form is made. The route of administration is important in determining the modifications needed.
   a. **Injectable drug product**
      (1) A final injectable drug product is usually developed at the preclinical phase.
      (2) A major concern is the stability of the drug in solution.
      (3) Very few excipients are allowed in injectable products, forcing the formulator to choose a final product early.
      (4) If changes in the formulation are made, bioavailability studies are not required for intravenous injections since the product is injected directly into the body.
      (5) Formulation changes may require acute toxicity studies.

b. **Topical drug products for local application** include antibacterials, antifungals, corticosteroids, and local anesthetics.
   (1) The final dosage form for a topical drug product is usually developed during phase I since any major formulation changes may require further clinical trials.
   (2) The release of the drug from the matrix is measured in vitro using various diffusion cell models.
   (3) Local irritation and systemic drug absorption are of great concern.

c. **Topical drug products for systemic drug absorption** include drug delivery through skin (transdermal), mucous membranes (intranasal), and rectal mucosa.
   (1) A prototype formulation is developed for phase I.
   (2) A final topical drug product is developed during phase III after consideration of the technology available and the desired systemic levels.

d. **Oral drug products**
   (1) Prototype dosage forms are often developed during the preclinical phase to assure that the drug is optimally available and the product dissolves in the gastrointestinal tract.
   (2) In early product development, capsule dosage forms are often developed for phase I clinical trials. If the drug shows efficacy, the same drug formulation may be used in phase II studies.
   (3) Final product development begins if the drug is to proceed to phase III clinical studies.

3. Final drug product. Considerations in the development of a final dosage form include:
   a. Color, shape, size, taste, flavor, viscosity, sensitivity, skin feel, and physical appearance of the dosage form
   b. Size and shape of the package container
   c. Production equipment
   d. Production site
   e. Country of origin
   f. Country in which to market the drug

B. Product line extensions are drug products containing an NDA-approved drug in a different dosage strength or in a different dosage form (e.g., modified release).

1. Solid oral product line extensions
   a. The simplest dosage form to develop is a different dosage strength of a given drug in a tablet or capsule in which only bioequivalence studies are needed.
   b. It is more difficult to develop a modified-release dosage form when only an instant-release dosage form exists. Under these conditions, clinical trials are generally required.
   c. Considerations in developing these dosage forms are similar to those under final drug product (II A 3).
   d. Marketing has a role in the choice of this particular dosage form.
   e. Because the original drug product (brand) has contributed to the body of knowledge about this drug, no preformulation is needed. All other factors considered for the original product are similar. If the relationship between in vitro dissolution and in vivo bioavailability is known, the innovator can progress to a finished dosage form relatively quickly.
   f. **Regulatory approval** is based on the following major documents:
      (1) Stability information
      (2) Analytical and manufacturing controls
      (3) Bioequivalence studies
      (4) Clinical trials in the case of modified-release dosage forms
   g. A new therapeutic indication for the drug requires new efficacy studies and NDA.

2. Liquid product line extensions
   a. If the current marketed product is a liquid preparation, then the considerations for the solid oral dosage forms are needed.
   b. If the marketed product is a solid oral dosage form, and the product line extension is a liquid, product development must proceed with caution, since the rate and extent of absorption for a liquid and solid dosage form may not be the same.
   c. **Regulatory approval** is based on the following:
      (1) Bioequivalence studies
      (2) Stability
      (3) Analytical and manufacturing controls
      (4) Safety studies (e.g., local irritation depending on the drug substance)

(5) Clinical efficacy studies must be performed if the product line extension is not bioequivalent to the originally marketed drug product.

3. **Topical product line extensions**
   a. Topical drug products include creams, ointments, lotions, gels, aerosols, sprays, foams, and solutions.
   b. Considerations in formulation development are:
      (1) Local irritation
      (2) Application site
      (3) Cosmetic elegance
      (4) Formulation excipients as possible sensitizers
      (5) Drug release from vehicle
      (6) Systemic drug absorption
   c. **Regulatory approval** is generally based on the following:
      (1) Stability studies
      (2) Analytical and manufacturing controls
      (3) Clinical efficacy studies
      (4) Safety studies—topical irritation and sensitization

4. **Injectable product line extensions** include drug products given by injection (syringe) or infusion. They include intravenous, intramuscular, intraperitoneal, and subcutaneous administration.
   a. Injectable drug products are classified into **small volume** (less than 100 ml) and **large volume** (greater than 100 ml) **parenteral products.**
      (1) Small volume parenterals generally contain a drug substance for a specific disease.
      (2) Large volume parenteral products usually do not contain an active drug substance and are generally used for volume and nutrition replacement (e.g., isotonic saline, 5% dextrose).
      (3) Many small volume parenterals are mixed with large volume parenteral products prior to intravenous administration of the drug. They can also be used to infuse drug products.
   b. The assurance of sterility and lack of pyrogenicity in manufacturing is a major consideration with injectable products.
   c. Containers for parenteral drug products may include:
      (1) Glass ampules and vials
      (2) Plastic and glass containers
      (3) Syringes and cartridges
   d. If the drug is in solution or if the product is a large volume parenteral, regulatory approval consists of:
      (1) Stability
      (2) Analytical and manufacturing controls
   e. If the drug is in a suspension for intraperitoneal, subcutaneous, and intramuscular administration, regulatory approval also requires bioavailability studies.

C. Oral generic drug products

1. **Preformulation** of generic drug products includes:
   a. **Literature review** for pharmacokinetic and physiochemical data
   b. **Patent review and exclusivity status**
   c. **Evaluation of the brand product,** including:
      (1) **Formulation characteristics,** including physical appearance, color, shape, and odor
      (2) **Physical characteristics**
         (a) **Tablets and capsules.** Disintegration, hardness, thickness, and friability
         (b) **Liquids.** Color, pH, odor, taste, and viscosity
         (c) **Semisolids.** Skin feel, viscosity, skin sensitivity, and pH
      (3) **Chemical characteristics** such as potency, uniformity, dissolution (for solid dosage forms) release of drug from semisolid products, and degradation products
   d. **Characterization of the active drug substance**
      (1) **Physical characteristics** such as particle size and shape, crystalline morphology, density, and surface area, which are important for solid dosage forms and suspensions, but not as important for solutions
      (2) **Solubility characteristics**

(3) **Chemical characteristics** such as impurities and related compounds, degradation products, and excipient interactions
(4) **Analytical methods development,** including validation of methods for release, stability, dissolution, and cleaning
(5) **Evaluation of reproducibility** in at least three batches

2. **Formulation development.** Generic drug products must be **bioequivalent to the brand,** not better. The steps in formulation development consist of:
   a. **Development of a discriminating dissolution method** for comparison of the oral generic product with the brand product. Decisions in the formulation development are then based on the in vitro studies.
   b. **Comparisons of the formulations under different physical conditions,** such as pH, temperature, and light
   c. **Stability studies** on both the generic product and the brand product
   d. **Evaluation of the manufacturing processes and equipment**
   e. **Evaluation of raw materials and excipients**

3. **Regulatory approval** is based on the following:
   a. Stability information
   b. Analytical and manufacturing information
   c. Bioavailability and bioequivalence studies

D. **Injectable generic drug products** generally follow the procedures described under product line extensions (see II B).

E. **Specialty products**

1. **Examples** of such dosage forms are:
   a. Liposomal formulations for intravenous administration
   b. Microspheres for intravenous administration
   c. Aerosol products
   d. Transdermal patches

2. **Development efforts** for any of these products can be as a product line extension or as a generic drug, depending on the use, indication, and demonstration of bioequivalence.

3. **Regulatory approval** may consist of any of the following items, depending on the development approach.
   a. Stability information (for all)
   b. Analytical and manufacturing information (for all)
   c. Bioavailability studies (if bioequivalent to the original dosage form or brand)
   d. Clinical trials, which are needed for products that are to be given for a new indication, use, or route of administration or do not demonstrate bioequivalence to the original product or brand

STUDY QUESTIONS

Directions: Each question below contains three suggested answers of which **one or more** is correct. Choose the answer

A if **I only** is correct
B if **III only** is correct
C if **I and II** are correct
D if **II and III** are correct
E if **I, II, and III** are correct

1. Healthy human volunteers are used in drug development for

I. phase I testing after the submission of an investigational new drug (IND) application
II. generic drug development for an abbreviated new drug application (ANDA) submission
III. phase III testing just prior to the submission of a new drug application (NDA)

2. The required information contained in a new drug application (NDA) that is NOT included in the abbreviated new drug application (ANDA) consists of

I. preclinical animal toxicity studies
II. clinical efficacy studies
III. human safety and tolerance studies

3. A product line extension contains the new drug application (NDA)-approved drug in a

I. new dosage form
II. new dosage strength
III. new therapeutic indication

1-C
2-E
3-C

ANSWERS AND EXPLANATIONS

1. The answer is C (I, II) *[I A 2, C].*
Phase I testing entails the first human studies performed during new drug development. The purpose of the phase I studies is to establish the tolerance and toxicity of the drug in humans. Clinical studies for generic drug development are most often performed in healthy human volunteers. The objective of generic drug studies is to establish the bioequivalence of the generic drug product against the brand name drug product. Phase III testing entails large scale, multicentered clinical studies performed in patients with the disease to be treated. The objectives of the phase III studies are to determine the safety and efficacy of the drug in a large patient population.

2. The answer is E (all) *[I A].*
The development of a new drug requires very extensive toxicity and efficacy testing in animals and humans. The new drug application (NDA) documents all the studies performed on the drug. The abbreviated new drug application (ANDA) is used for generic drug product submissions. The generic drug product is similar to the original, brand drug product that has already been marketed. Since the efficacy, safety, and toxicity of this drug product have been well studied and documented, further studies of this nature are unnecessary.

3. The answer is C (I, II) *[II B].*
Product line extensions are developed after further studies with the original new drug application (NDA)-approved drug product. From these studies, the manufacturer may choose to develop a new dosage form (e.g., controlled-release product) or a new dosage strength. A new therapeutic indication requires an NDA (new drug application).

2
Pharmaceutical Calculations

Sunil Jambhekar

I. FUNDAMENTALS OF MEASUREMENT AND CALCULATION

A. Numbers and numerals

1. A **number** is a total quantity or amount of units.
2. A **numeral** is a word, sign, or group of words and signs representing a number. For example, the numeral 2 represents the number that is two times the unit 1.

B. Arabic numerals—a zero and nine digits—are a form of notation based on a **decimal system,** in which values assigned to digits depend on the place they occupy in a row.

1. The **value of a digit increases tenfold** each time it moves one place to the **left** of the decimal point; the **value decreases tenfold** each time it moves one place to the **right**.
2. A **zero** marks any place not occupied by a digit.
3. The **total value** of any number expressed by Arabic numerals is the sum of the values of its digits as determined by their position.

C. Roman numerals.

In contrast to Arabic numerals, Roman numerals express numbers by use of a few letters of the alphabet. **They are customarily used to designate quantities on prescriptions** when ingredients are measured by the apothecaries' system.

1. The **position** of a Roman numeral **indicates whether to add or subtract the numeral from a succession of bases,** ranging from values of 1–1000. These eight fixed values (bases) are used:
   - **a.** **ss** = ½
   - **b.** **I** (or **i**) = 1
   - **c.** **V** (or **v**) = 5
   - **d.** **X** (or **x**) = 10
   - **e.** **L** (or **l**) = 50
   - **f.** **C** (or **c**) = 100
   - **g.** **D** (or **d**) = 500
   - **h.** **M** (or **m**) = 1000
2. **Combining these letters** (Table 2-1) expresses other quantities.

II. CONVERSIONS—translations of measurements made in one system into equivalent values in another system—are frequently required in pharmacy. **Practical equivalents** are discussed below.

A. The **metric, avoirdupois** (weight), **U.S. liquid measure** (volume), and **apothecaries' system** (volume and weight) all differ and require conversion when quantities must be compared; that is, **all quantities must be converted to a single system** (Table 2-2).

B. The **accuracy of conversion factors for pharmacy** has not been satisfactorily established. The *United States Pharmacopeia* (USP) permits the pharmacist to dispense prepared dosage forms (e.g., tablets and capsules) in approximate equivalents; that is, for a prepared drug prescribed in metric values, an approximate equivalent in apothecaries' values may be dispensed, and vice versa.

1. **Equivalent values** are listed in the USP Table of Metric–Apothecaries' Approximate Dose Equivalents. Table 2-3 provides conversions sufficient for all practical purposes.

Table 2-1. Guidelines for the Use of Roman Numeral Designations of Pharmaceutical Quantities

Rule

Two or more letters express a quantity that is the **sum of their values** if they are **successively equal or smaller in value.**

Examples

ii = 2	xxii = 22	ci = 101	mx = 1010
iii = 3	li = 51	cl = 150	mc = 1100
vi = 6	lv = 55	cc = 200	md = 1500
xi = 11	lx = 60	dv = 505	mdclxvi = 1666
xv = 15	lxxvii = 77	dc = 600	mm = 2000
xx = 20			

Rule

Two or more letters express a quantity that is the **sum of the values remaining after the value of each smaller letter is subtracted from the value of a following greater letter.**

Examples

iv = 4	xxiv = 24	xcix = 99	cm = 900
ix = 9	xl = 40	cd = 400	cmxcix = 999
xiv = 14	xliv = 44	cdxl = 440	mcdxcii = 1492
xix = 19	xc = 90	cdxliv = 444	

2. **Exact equivalents** must be used for conversion of specific quantities when converting formulas; exact equivalents rounded to three significant figures must be used for compounding prescriptions.

III. RATIOS, PROPORTIONS, AND PERCENTAGES

A. **Ratios.** A ratio is the **relation of two like quantities expressed as a common fraction** (e.g., 10/5 represents the ratio of 10 and 5). When a fraction is to be interpreted as a ratio, it is written **10:5** and always read as "10 to 5." The rules governing common fractions apply to ratios.

1. If the two terms of a ratio are **multiplied or divided by the same number,** the **value of the ratio is unchanged**. For example, the ratio of 15:3 (or 15/3) has a value of 5. If both terms are multiplied by 2, the ratio becomes 30:6 (or 30/6) and still has the value of 5.

2. **Ratios having the same values are equivalent.** Their **cross products are equal** (the product of the numerator of one and the denominator of the other always equals the product of the denominator of one and the numerator of the other). Their **reciprocals are also equal**.

Table 2-2. Common Conversion Equivalents

Length

1 meter (m) = 39.37 inches (in)
1 in = 2.54 centimeters (cm)

Volume

1 milliliter (ml) = 16.23 minims (♍)
1 ♍ = 0.06 ml
1 fluidram (*f* ʒ) = 3.696 ml
1 fluidounce (*f* ℥) = 29.573 ml
1 pint (pt) = 473 ml
1 gallon U.S. (gal) = 3785 ml

Weight

1 gram (g) = 15.432 grains (gr)
1 kilogram (kg) = 2.20 pounds avoirdupois (lb avoir)
1 gr = 0.065 g [65 milligrams (mg)]
1 ounce avoirdupois (oz avoir) = 28.35 g = 437.5 gr
1 ounce apothecaries' (℥) = 31.103 g = 480 gr
1 lb avoir = 454 g
1 pound apothecaries' (lb apoth) = 373.2 g

Table 2-3. Apothecaries' System and Metric Equivalents

Apothecaries' System	Metric Equivalent
Fluid measure	
1 minim (♏)	0.062 milliliters (ml)
60 ♏ = 1 fluidram (fluidrachm) [*f* ʒ]	3.696 ml
8 *f* ʒ, or 480 ♏ = 1 fluidounce (*f* ℥)	29.573 ml
16 *f* ℥ = 1 pint (pt or O)	473 ml, or 0.473 liter (L)
2 pt, or 32 *f* ℥, = 1 quart (qt)	946 ml, or 0.946 L
4 qt, or 8 pt, = 1 gallon (gal or C)	3785 ml, or 3.785 L
Weight	
1 grain (gr)	0.065 gram (g)
20 gr = 1 scruple (℈)	1.295 g
3 ℈, or 60 gr, = 1 ʒ	3.887 g
8 ʒ, or 480 gr, = 1 ℥	31.103 g
12 ℥, or 5760 gr, = 1 pound (lb apoth)	373 g, or 0.373 kilogram (kg)

B. Proportions

1. **The equality of two ratios is expressed by a proportion.** These standard forms may all be used to express proportions:
   a. a:b = c:d
   b. a:b :: c:d
   c. a/b = c/d

2. The terms of a proportion are designated as the **extremes** (the outer members, or **a** and **d** in the examples above) and the **means** (the middle members, or **b** and **c** in the examples above).

3. In any proportion, the **product of the extremes equals the product of the means,** allowing determination of any missing term when the other three terms are known. For example, if a/b = c/d, then:
   a. a = bc/d
   b. b = ad/c
   c. c = ad/b
   d. d = bc/a

4. **Many pharmaceutical calculations can be solved directly by using proportions.** For example, suppose one has the information that 15 tablets contain 75 grains (gr) of aspirin, and one needs to know how many grains 4 tablets contain. Proportions provide the answer as follows:

$$\frac{15 \text{ tablets}}{4 \text{ tablets}} = \frac{75 \text{ gr}}{x \text{ gr}}$$

$$x = \frac{75 \times 4}{15}, \text{ or } 20 \text{ gr}$$

C. Percentages play an important role in pharmaceutical calculations. Often, they are used to express the **concentration of a solute in solution, the amount of active material in a drug or preparation,** or **the quantity of an active ingredient in a dosage form**.

1. Percentage indicates the **rate per hundred** expressed by a number and a percent sign (%). A percentage may also be expressed as a **ratio,** given as a common or decimal fraction; that is, 25% indicates 25 parts of 100 parts and may also be expressed as 25/100 or 0.25.

2. For computational purposes, percents are generally changed to **equivalent decimal fractions** by dropping the percent sign and dividing the numerator by 100. Thus, 15% = 15/100, or 0.15; and 0.01% = 0.01/100, or 0.0001.

3. **Percent concentrations** are expressed in a variety of ways.
   a. Percent weight-in-volume (% w/v) expresses the number of grams (g) of constituent in 1 decaliter (dl), which is 100 milliliters (ml), of solution or liquid preparation.
      (1) Metric system. The required number of milliliters are multiplied by the percentage strength (expressed as a decimal) to determine the number of grams of solute or constituent in the liquid preparation. (The volume in milliliters represents the weight in

grams of the solution or liquid preparation as if it were pure water). For example, if a pharmacist needs to know how many grams of dextrose are required to prepare 3000 ml of 4% solution, then the following calculation is used: Given that 3000 ml = 3000 g of solution, and 4% = 4/100 = 0.04, then

$$3000 \text{ g} \times 0.04 = 120 \text{ g}.$$

(2) **Apothecaries' system.** The weight of a fluidounce (*f* ℥) of water (455 gr) must be multiplied by the required number of fluidounces of solution and by the percentage strength to determine the number of grains of solute in the liquid preparation. (Volume in fluidounces multiplied by 455 gr represents the weight in grains of the solution.) For example, if the pharmacist needs to know how many grains of atropine sulfate are required to prepare ½ *f* ℥ of a 2.5% solution, then the following calculation is used: Given that ½ *f* ℥ × 455 gr/*f* ℥ = 227.5 gr of solution, and 2.5% = 0.025, then

$$227.5 \text{ gr} \times 0.025 = 5.687 \text{ gr}.$$

b. **Percent volume-in-volume** (% v/v) expresses the number of milliliters of a constituent in 1 dl of solution or liquid preparation. For example, if the pharmacist needs to find the % v/v of liquified phenol in 300 ml of a lotion containing 6 ml of liquified phenol, then the following calculation is used:

$$\frac{300 \text{ ml}}{6 \text{ ml}} = \frac{100\%}{x\%}, \text{ and } x\% = 2\% \text{ v/v}.$$

c. **Percent weight-in-weight** (% w/w) expresses the number of grams of a constituent in 100 gr of solution or mixture. Because liquids are not customarily measured by weight, weight-in-weight solutions or liquid preparations should be designated as such (e.g., 8% w/w).

(1) A specified volume of a solution or liquid preparation of given % w/w strength is often impossible to prepare because the volume displaced by the active component is unknown. However, if the **specific gravity of the solvent** is known, the weight of the active component may be calculated. For example, if the pharmacist needs to know how to prepare 200 ml of a 3% w/w solution of a substance in a solvent having a specific gravity of 1.25, then this calculation is used: Given that 200 ml × 1.25 specific gravity = 250 g (weight of solvent), and 3% w/w = 3 g of drug + 97 g of solvent in 100 g of solution, then

$$\frac{97 \text{ g of solvent}}{250 \text{ g of solvent}} = \frac{3\%}{x\%}, \text{ and}$$

$x\%$ = 7.73 g of drug to be dissolved in 250 g (or 200 ml) of solvent.

(2) If the **specific gravity of the solvent is not known,** other data, such as the weight of solvent and solute, or the volume and specific gravity of the finished solution, must be given to complete the computation. For example, if the pharmacist needs to know the percentage strength (% w/w) of a solution of 10 g of boric acid dissolved in 1 dl of water, then this calculation is used: Given that 100 ml of water = 100 g of water, and 100 g of water + 10 g of boric acid (H_3BO_3) = 110 g of solution, then

$$\frac{110 \text{ g}}{10 \text{ g}} = \frac{100\%}{x\%}, \text{ and } x\% = 9.09\% \text{ w/w}.$$

4. The percent sign (%) used without qualification has the following meanings in **pharmacy practice:**
   a. **Mixtures of solids and semisolids:** % = % (w/w).
   b. **Solutions or suspensions of solids in liquids:** % = % (w/v). For example, a 2% solution is prepared by dissolving 2 g of solid, or 2 ml of liquid, in sufficient solvent to make 1 dl of solution.

5. **Additional terms** are sometimes used to express concentrations.
   a. **Milligrams percent** (mg %) expresses the number of **milligrams of substance per 1 dl of liquid** and is used to express the concentration of a drug or natural substance in a biologic fluid, such as blood. The equivalent term **mg/dl** is preferred.
   b. **Concentration of very dilute solutions** may be expressed in **parts per million (ppm)**. For example, 6 ppm corresponds to 0.0006%.

IV. CALCULATION OF MILLIEQUIVALENTS

A. Electrolytes

1. **Electrolyte ions in plasma** include the cations sodium (Na^+), potassium (K^+), calcium (Ca^{2+}), and magnesium (Mg^{2+}); the anions chloride (Cl^-), bicarbonate (HCO_3^-), and sulfate (SO_4^{2-}); organic acid; and protein. They play an important role in the maintenance of acid–base balance, regulation of body metabolism, and control of body water volume.
2. **Electrolyte solutions** are liquid preparations used to treat electrolyte disturbances of body fluids. The concentrations of these solutions are almost always expressed in chemical units known as **milliequivalents (mEq)**.
   a. A **milliequivalent unit** is related to the total number of **ionic charges** in solution and also takes into account the **valence of the ions**. Thus, **it measures the amount of chemical activity of an electrolyte.**
   b. Under normal circumstances, **plasma** contains 155 mEq of cations and 155 mEq of anions. The total concentration of cations always equals the total concentration of anions.

B. Calculating milliequivalents

1. A milliequivalent represents the **amount of solute** (in milligrams) equal to 1/1000 of its gram equivalent weight. For example, given that the molecular weight (mol wt) of potassium chloride (KCl) = 74.5, and the equivalent weight of KCl = 74.5 g, then

$$1 \text{ mEq of KCl} = 1/1000 \times 74.5 \text{ g} = 0.0745 \text{ g } (74.5 \text{ mg}).$$

2. The **equivalent weight** of a bivalent compound is obtained by dividing the molecular weight by the total valence of the positive or negative radical. For example, given that the mol wt of calcium chloride ($CaCl_2$) $\times$ $2H_2O$ = 147, and the equivalent weight of $CaCl_2 \times 2H_2O$ = 147/2 = 73.5 g, then

$$1 \text{ mEq } CaCl_2 \times 2H_2O = 1/1000 \times 73.5 \text{ g} = 0.0735 \text{ g } (73.5 \text{ mg}).$$

3. The mEq value for a **cation present in a solution** can be computed similarly. For example, for a solution containing 15 mg/dl of Ca^{2+}, where the mol wt of Ca^{2+} = 40, and the equivalent weight of Ca^{2+} = 40/2 = 20 g, then

$$1 \text{ mEq of } Ca^{2+} = 1/1000 \times 20 \text{ g} = 0.02 \text{ g } (20 \text{ mg}).$$

   Thus, a solution containing 15 mg/dl of Ca^{2+} = 150 mg Ca^{2+}/L or

$$\frac{150 \text{ mg/L}}{20 \text{ mg/mEq}} = 7.5 \text{ mEq/L}$$

4. **Milliequivalent weights of important ions** are given in Table 2-4.

V. CALCULATION OF MILLIOSMOLES

A. Osmotic pressure. Electrolytes help **control body water volumes** by establishing **osmotic pressure.** This pressure is proportional to the total number of particles of solution and is expressed in units of **milliosmoles (mOsmol).**

B. Calculating milliosmoles

1. For **nonelectrolytes** (e.g., dextrose), 1 millimole (mmol) [1 formula weight in milligrams] represents 1 mOsmol.
2. For **electrolytes,** this relationship does not hold, because the total number of particles in solution depends on the degree of dissociation of a substance. For example, 1 mmol of KCl (completely dissociated) represents 2 mOsmol of total particles ($K^+ + Cl^-$). Similarly, 1 mmol of $CaCl_2$ represents 3 mOsmol of total particles ($Ca^+ + Cl^- + Cl^-$).
3. The **milliosmolar value of the separate ions of an electrolyte** may be obtained by dividing the concentration of the ions in milligrams per liter (mg/L) by the ions' atomic weight. The **milliosmolar value of the complete electrolyte in solution** equals the sum of the milliosmolar

Table 2-4. Valences, Atomic Weights, and Milliequivalent Weights of Selected Ions

Ion	Formula	Valence	Atomic or Formula Weight	Milliequivalent Weight (mg)
Ammonium	NH_4^+	1	18	18
Lithium	Li^+	1	7	7
Potassium	K^+	1	39	39
Sodium	Na^+	1	23	23
Calcium	Ca^{2+}	2	40	20
Magnesium	Mg^{2+}	2	24	12
Acetate	$C_2H_3O_2^-$	1	59	59
Bicarbonate	HCO_3^-	1	61	61
Chloride	Cl^-	1	35.5	35.5
Gluconate	$C_6H_{11}O_7^-$	1	195	195
Lactate	$C_3H_5O_3^-$	1	89	89
Carbonate	CO_3^{2-}	2	60	30
Phosphate	$H_2PO_4^-$	1	97	97
	HPO_4^{2-}	2	96	48
Sulfate	SO_4^{2-}	2	96	48
Citrate	$C_6H_5O_7^{3-}$	3	189	63

values of the separate ions. For example, to determine how many milliosmoles are represented in 2 L of 0.9% sodium chloride (NaCl) solution, the following calculation is used:

1 mmol of NaCl = 2 mOsmol of total particles ($Na^+ + Cl^-$)
Mol wt of NaCl = 58.5
1 mmol of NaCl = 58.5 mg = 2 mOsmol
2000 ml (2 L) × 0.009 g/ml (0.9% solution) = 18 g (18,000 mg) NaCl
18,000 mg/58.5 mg = 307.69 mOsmol for each ion
Total mOsmol = 307.69 × 2 ($Na^+ + Cl^-$) = 615 mOsmol

VI. ISOTONIC SOLUTIONS

A. Definitions

1. **Isosmotic** describes solutions that have the same osmotic pressure. Solutions intended to be mixed with body fluid should have the same osmotic pressure.
2. **Isotonic** describes solutions that have the same osmotic pressure (tonicity) as a body fluid.
3. **Hypotonic** describes solutions with a lower osmotic pressure than a body fluid.
4. **Hypertonic** describes solutions with a higher osmotic pressure than a body fluid.

B. Preparation of isotonic solutions. In preparing isotonic solutions, calculations are made in terms of the colligative properties of solutions. Theoretically, any one of these properties may be used for computing tonicity, but comparison of freezing points is most commonly used. The freezing point of blood serum and lacrimal fluid is −52°C.

1. When 1 g mol wt of any **nonelectrolyte** is dissolved in 1000 g of water, the freezing point of the solution is about −1.86°C. By simple proportion, the weight of any nonelectrolyte needed to make the solution isotonic with the body fluid may be calculated.
   a. Boric acid (H_3BO_3) has a mol wt of 61.8 g. Thus, 61.8 g of H_3BO_3 in 1000 g of water should produce a freezing point of −1.86°C. Therefore,

   $$-1.86°C/-0.52°C = 61.8\ g/x\ g, \text{ and } x = 17.3\ g.$$

   b. **Thus, 17.3 g of H_3BO_3 in 1000 g of water provide a solution that is isotonic.**
2. With **electrolytes,** however, the **degree of dissociation** must be taken into account. Since osmotic pressure depends upon the number of particles, the greater the dissociation, the smaller the quantity required to produce any given osmotic pressure.
   a. For example, NaCl in weak solution is about 80% dissociated. Therefore, each 100 molecules yield 180 particles, or 1.8 times as many particles as are yielded by 100 molecules

of a nonelectrolyte. This dissociation factor, *i*, must be included in the calculations to determine the strength of an isotonic solution of NaCl (mol wt = 58.5 g):

$$-1.86°C \times 1.8/-0.52°C = 58.5 \text{ g}/x \text{ g, and } x = 9.09 \text{ g}.$$

b. Hence, 9.09 g of NaCl in 1000 g of water (0.9% w/v) should make a solution isotonic with body fluids.

c. A simple isotonic solution may, thus, be calculated by the following general formula:

$$0.52 \times \text{mol wt}/1.86 \times \text{dissociation factor } (i) = \text{g solute}/1000 \text{ g of water}.$$

d. A special problem arises when a prescription requires an isotonic solution by adding the proper amount of a substance other than the active ingredients. For instance, the amount of NaCl required in preparing 100 ml (1% w/v) of solution of atropine sulfate, which is to be made isotonic with lacrimal fluid, will depend upon how much NaCl is in effect represented by the atropine sulfate.

3. The **tonic effect of two substances** is the quantity of one substance that is equivalent in tonic effects to the quantity of the other substance in a specified quantity of solvent.

a. For example, earlier it was demonstrated that both 17.3 g of H_3BO_3 and 9.09 g of NaCl/1000 g of water produce an aqueous isotonic solution. Hence, 17.3 g of H_3BO_3 are equivalent in tonicity to 9.09 g of NaCl. Therefore, 1 g of H_3BO_3 must be equivalent to 0.52 g of NaCl (9.09 g/17.3 g). Likewise, 1 g of NaCl must be equivalent in tonicity to 1.9 g of H_3BO_3 (17.3 g/0.09 g).

b. Theoretically, for every substance there is one quantity that should have a constant tonic effect if dissolved in 1000 g of water. This is 1 g mol wt of the substance divided by its *i*, or dissociation value. Hence, the relative quantity of NaCl that is equivalent to H_3BO_3 in tonicity effects is determined as follows:

$$\frac{\text{mol wt of NaCl}/i \text{ value}}{\text{mol wt of } H_3BO_3/i \text{ value}} = \frac{58.5/1.8}{61.8/1.0}$$

c. Using this approach and recalling problems involving 1 g of atropine sulfate in 1000 ml of solution, the mol wt of NaCl and the mol wt of atropine sulfate are 58.5 and 695 g, respectively, and their *i* values are 1.8 and 2.6, respectively. Hence,

$$695 \times 1.8/58.5 \times 2.6 = 1 \text{ g}/x \text{ g, where}$$

$x = 0.12$ g NaCl are represented by 1 g of atropine sulfate. Since an isotonic solution should contain the equivalent of 0.9 g of NaCl in each 100 ml of solution, the addition of NaCl required in this example is 0.9 g − 0.12 g = 0.78 g. Table 2-5 provides the NaCl equivalents of various drugs.

Table 2-5. Sodium Chloride (NaCl) Equivalents

Substance	Molecular Weight	Ions	*i*	Equivalent NaCl
Antazoline phosphate	363	2	1.8	0.16
Antipyrine	188	1	1.0	0.17
Atropine sulfate•H_2O	695	3	2.6	0.12
Benzalkonium chloride	360	2	1.8	0.16
Benzyl alcohol	108	1	1.0	0.30
Boric acid	61.8	1	1.0	0.52
Carbachol (carbamylcholine chloride)	183	2	1.8	0.33
Chloramphenicol	323	1	1.0	0.10
Chlorobutanol	177	1	1.0	0.18
Chlortetracycline hydrochloride	515	2	1.8	0.11
Cocaine hydrochloride	340	2	1.8	0.17
Cyclopentolate hydrochloride	328	2	1.8	0.18
Dextrose (anhydrous)	180	1	1.0	0.18
Dextrose•H_2O	198	1	1.0	0.16
Dibucaine hydrochloride	380	2	1.8	0.15
Ephedrine hydrochloride	202	2	1.8	0.29

(continued on next page)

Table 2-5. Continued

Substance	Molecular Weight	Ions	*i*	Equivalent NaCl
Ephedrine sulfate	429	3	2.6	0.20
Epinephrine bitartrate	333	2	1.8	0.18
Epinephrine hydrochloride	220	2	1.8	0.27
Ethylmorphine hydrochloride•$2H_2O$	386	2	1.8	0.15
Eucatropine hydrochloride	328	2	1.8	0.22
Fluorescein sodium	376	3	2.6	0.22
Glycerin	92.1	1	1.0	0.36
Homatropine hydrobromide	356	2	1.8	0.16
Hydroxyamphetamine hydrobromide	232	2	1.8	0.25
Lidocaine hydrochloride	289	2	1.8	0.22
Morphine hydrochloride•$3H_2O$	376	2	1.8	0.16
Morphine sulfate•$5H_2O$	759	3	2.6	0.11
Naphazoline hydrochloride	247	2	1.8	0.27
Oxytetracycline hydrochloride	497	2	1.8	0.12
Phenacaine hydrochloride	353	2	1.8	0.17
Phenylephrine hydrochloride	204	2	1.8	0.29
Physostigmine salicylate	413	2	1.8	0.14
Physostigmine sulfate	649	3	2.6	0.13
Pilocarpine hydrochloride	245	2	1.8	0.24
Pilocarpine nitrate	271	2	1.8	0.22
Piperocaine hydrochloride	298	2	1.8	0.20
Potassium biphosphate	136	2	1.8	0.43
Potassium chloride	74.6	2	1.8	0.78
Potassium iodide	166	2	1.8	0.35
Potassium nitrate	101	2	1.8	0.58
Potassium penicillin G	372	2	1.8	0.16
Procaine hydrochloride	273	2	1.8	0.21
Proparacaine hydrochloride	331	2	1.8	0.18
Scopolamine hydrobromide•$3H_2O$ (hyoscine hydrobromide)	438	2	1.8	0.13
Scopolamine hydrochloride•$2H_2O$ (hyoscine hydrochloride)	376	2	1.8	0.16
Silver nitrate	170	2	1.8	0.34
Sodium bicarbonate	84	2	1.8	0.70
Sodium bisulfite	104	3	2.6	0.81
Sodium borate•$10H_2O$ (borax)	381	5	4.2	0.36
Sodium carbonate	106	3	2.6	0.80
Sodium carbonate•H_2O	124	3	2.6	0.68
Sodium chloride	58	2	1.8	1.00
Sodium citrate•$2H_2O$	294	4	3.4	0.38
Sodium iodide	150	2	1.8	0.39
Sodium lactate	112	2	1.8	0.52
Sodium nitrate	85	2	1.8	0.69
Sodium phosphate, dibasic, anhydrous	142	3	2.6	0.53
Sodium phosphate, dibasic•$7H_2O$	268	3	2.6	0.31
Sodium phosphate, monobasic, anhydrous	120	2	1.8	0.49
Sodium phosphate, monobasic•H_2O	138	2	1.8	0.42
Sodium sulfite	126	3	2.6	0.64
Tetracaine hydrochloride	301	2	1.8	0.19
Tetracycline hydrochloride	481	2	1.8	0.12
Tetrahydrozoline hydrochloride	237	2	1.8	0.25
Urea	60.1	1	1.0	0.54
Zinc chloride	136	3	2.6	0.62
Zinc sulfate•$7H_2O$	288	2	1.4	0.16

STUDY QUESTIONS

Directions: Each of the numbered items or incomplete statements in this section is followed by answers or by completions of the statement. Select the **one** lettered answer or completion that is **best** in each case.

1. A physician requests ½ kg of bacitracin ointment containing 250 units of bacitracin per gram. How many grams of bacitracin ointment (500 units/g) must be used to make this ointment?

(A) 100
(B) 250
(C) 280
(D) 300
(E) 400

2. How many grains of benzocaine are needed to prepare the following prescription?

Rx

Benzocaine	1% w/w
Glycerin	2.5%
Hydrophilic ointment q.s. ii℥	
sig: Apply as needed	

(A) 1.2
(B) 6.0
(C) 9.6
(D) 10.0
(E) 10.5

3. How many 8- *f* ℥ bottles can be packaged from a 2-gal bottle of cough syrup?

(A) 10
(B) 15
(C) 20
(D) 28
(E) 32

4. A solution contains 2.5 mEq calcium (Ca^{2+}) per 50 ml. Express the solution strength of Ca^{2+} in terms of mg/L. (The atomic weight of Ca^{2+} is 40.)

(A) 250
(B) 350
(C) 500
(D) 1000
(E) 1500

5. How many grams of potassium chloride (KCl) are used in making 500 ml of a solution containing 3 mEq of K^+ per teaspoonful? (The atomic weight of K^+ = 39 and Cl^- = 35.5.)

(A) 5
(B) 10
(C) 15
(D) 22.35
(E) 32.62

6. How many grams of water are needed to make 150 g of a 4% w/w solution of potassium acetate?

(A) 100
(B) 130
(C) 135
(D) 144
(E) 156

1-B 4-D
2-C 5-D
3-E 6-D

ANSWERS AND EXPLANATIONS

1. The answer is B *[II B; Tables 2-2, 2-3].*
Given that ½ kg = 500 g, then

$$\frac{1\text{ g}}{500\text{ g}} = \frac{250\text{ units}}{x\text{ units}}\text{, and}$$

$$x = 125{,}000\text{ units.}$$

$$\text{Thus, } \frac{500\text{ units}}{125{,}000\text{ units}} = \frac{1\text{ g}}{x\text{ g}}\text{, and}$$

$$x = 250\text{ g.}$$

2. The answer is C *[III C 3 a (2)].*
Given that ii ℥ = 960 gr, then

$$\frac{100\text{ gr}}{960\text{ gr}} = \frac{1\text{ gr}}{x\text{ gr}}\text{, and}$$

$$x = 9.6\text{ gr.}$$

3. The answer is E *[II B; Table 2-3].*
Given that 2 gal = 256 *f* ℥, then

$$\frac{8\ f\ ℥}{256\ f\ ℥} = \frac{1\text{ bottle}}{x\text{ bottles}}\text{, and}$$

$$x = 32\text{ bottles.}$$

4. The answer is D *[IV B; Table 2-4].*
The valence of calcium (Ca^{2+}) is +2; hence,

$$1\text{ mEq} = \frac{40\text{ mg}}{2} = 20\text{ mg, and}$$

1 mEq = 20 mg of Ca^{2+}. Therefore, 2.5 mEq = 50 mg, thus

$$\frac{50\text{ ml}}{1000\text{ ml}} = \frac{50\text{ mg}}{x\text{ mg}}\text{, and}$$

$$x = 1000\text{ mg.}$$

5. The answer is D *[IV B; Table 2-4].*
The atomic weight and equivalent weight of potassium chloride (KCl) = 74.5 g; 1 mEq = 74.5 mg of KCl. Thus,

$$\frac{1\text{ mEq}}{3\text{ mEq}} = \frac{74.5\text{ mg}}{x\text{ mg}}\text{, and}$$

$$x = 223.5\text{ mg.}$$

Given that 1 tbls = 5 ml; hence,

$$\frac{5\text{ml}}{500\text{ ml}} = \frac{223.5\text{ mg}}{x\text{ mg}}\text{, and}$$

$$x = 22{,}350\text{ mg} = 22.35\text{ g of KCl.}$$

6. The answer is D *[III C 3 c].*
Given that 4% w/w is 4 g of potassium acetate in 100 g of solution; therefore, 100 g − 4 g of potassium acetate = 96 g of water. Thus,

$$\frac{100\text{ g}}{150\text{ g}} = \frac{96\text{ g}}{x\text{ g}}, \text{ and}$$

$$x = 144\text{ g of water.}$$

3
Drug Solution Chemistry

Sunil Jambhekar

I. INTRODUCTION

A. Solutions are defined as homogeneous substances that have, within certain limits, continuously variable compositions. Their properties and composition are uniform at a nonmolecular level. A variety of drugs exist in this form, requiring an understanding of the basic properties of solutions.

B. Solutes and solvents. The **components** of a solution may be defined as the **solvent** (usually the component present in greatest quantity) and the **solutes** (other components dissolved in the solvent). Solutes may be nonelectrolytes or electrolytes.

1. **Nonelectrolytes** are substances that **do not form ions** when dissolved in water and, thus, do not conduct an electric current through the solution. Examples include sucrose, glucose, glycerin, and urea.
2. **Electrolytes** are substances that **do form ions** in solution and, thus, can conduct an electric current through the solution. Examples include sodium chloride (NaCl), hydrochloric acid (HCl), and ephedrine. Electrolytes include strong electrolytes and weak electrolytes.
   a. **Strong electrolytes are completely ionized** in water at all concentrations, as with HCl and NaCl.
   b. **Weak electrolytes are partially ionized** in water at most concentrations, as with aspirin and ephedrine.

C. Concentration of a solution may be expressed in terms of the **quantity of solute in a definite volume of solution** or as the **quantity of solute in a definite mass of solvent or solution.**

D. Colligative properties of a solution are those properties that are **dependent on the number of particles of solute in the solution** and **independent of the chemical nature of the solute.**

II. CONCENTRATION EXPRESSIONS

A. Molarity. The molarity **(M)** of a solution is the number of moles **(mol)** of solute in 1 liter **(L)** of solution.

1. **All solutions of the same molarity contain the same number of solute molecules** in a definite volume of solution.
2. When a solution contains **more than one solute,** it may have **different molarities for each solute**. For example, a solution may be 0.001 M for phenobarbital and 0.1 M for NaCl. One liter of such a solution is prepared by adding 0.001 mol of phenobarbital (0.001 mol × 232.32 g/mol = 0.2323 g) [g = gram] and 0.1 mol of NaCl (0.1 mol × 48.45 g/mol = 4.845 g) to sufficient water to make 1 L of solution.
3. A solution containing only **one solute** may have **different molarities for the various ionic components of the solute**. For example, a molar solution of NaCl is 1 M for both sodium (Na^+) and chloride (Cl^-) ions, whereas a molar solution of sodium carbonate (Na_2CO_3) is 1 M for the CO_3 and 2 M for the Na^+ (each mole of this salt contains 2 mol of Na^+).
4. Molarity **changes value with temperature** because of the contraction and expansion of liquids. It should not be used when the properties of the solution are to be studied at various temperatures.

B. Normality. The normality **(N)** of a solution is the number of gram-equivalent weights of solute in 1 L of solution.

1. The **equivalent weight** of any material is the weight that would react with, or be produced by, its reaction with 7.999 g of oxygen (O_2) or 1.008 g of hydrogen (H) [see III for details].

2. A molar solution of NaCl is also 1 N for both its ions. However, a molar solution of Na_2CO_3 is 2 N for both its ions.

3. Normality provides a convenient unit of measurement for certain quantitative analyses. However, like molarity, it **changes value with temperature**.

C. Molality. The molality **(m)** of a solution is the number of moles of solute in 1000 g of solvent.

1. Molality is used more frequently than molarity or normality, because molal solutions are **prepared in units of weight** and **do not change with temperature**.

2. Molal solutions are prepared by adding the proper weight of solvent to the carefully weighed amount of solute.

3. Molality may be **converted to molarity or normality** if the final volume of the solution is known or if the density is determined. In dilute aqueous solutions (< 0.1 M), **molarity and molality may be assumed to be equivalent for practical purposes.**

D. Mole fraction. The mole fraction **(x)** provides a measure of the ratio of the moles of one component of a solution to the total moles of all components.

1. For a **two-component system** (solvent and solute), the mole fraction is expressed as:

$$x_1 = \frac{n_1}{n_1 + n_2} \quad \text{and} \quad x_2 = \frac{n_2}{n_1 + n_2}$$

where x_1 is the mole fraction of component 1 (usually the solvent), x_2 is the mole fraction of component 2 (usually the solute), and n_1 and n_2 are the number of moles of components in the solution.

2. The **sum of the mole fractions for a solution** (x_1 and x_2 in the example above) **must be equal to 1**.

3. **Mole percent** (the number of moles in 100 mol of solution) is obtained by multiplying the mole fraction by 100.

E. Percent expressions. Percent expressions are commonly used to express the concentrations of pharmaceutical solutions. These include **percent weight-in-weight (% w/w), percent volume-in-volume (% v/v), percent weight-in-volume (% w/v),** and **milligrams percent (mg %, or mg/dl).** For details, see and Chapter 2 III C.

III. EQUIVALENT WEIGHTS

A. Gram atoms

1. As stated above, the **equivalent weight** of any material is the weight that would react with, or be produced by, its reaction with 7.999 g of O_2 or 1.008 g of H.

2. A **gram atom of H** weighs 1.008 g and consists of 6×10^{23} (Avogadro's number) of H atoms. This amount of H combines with other atoms in proportions that depend on the **valence** of the atoms.

3. One gram atom of H (1.008 g) combines with 19 g of fluorine (F) [atomic weight of 19]; however, it combines with only 8 g of O_2 (atomic weight of 16). The **quantity of an element combining with 1.008 g of H** is referred to as the **equivalent weight** of the combining element.

B. Calculation of equivalent weight

1. One equivalent weight of F (19 g) is identical to its atomic weight; however, one equivalent weight of O_2 (8 g) is half its atomic weight. This equation relates equivalent weight (g/Eq) and atomic weight:

$$\text{Equivalent weight} = \frac{\text{atomic weight}}{\text{number of equivalents/atomic weight (valence)}}$$

2. The **number of equivalents/atomic weight** (e.g., 1 for F and 2 for O_2) indicates the common valence of an element.

3. Equivalent weights may be calculated for **molecules** as well as atoms.
   a. For example, the **equivalent weight of NaCl** is identical to its molecular weight (58.5) and is the **sum of the equivalent weights of Na (23 g/Eq) and Cl (35.5 g/Eq)**. Both Na and Cl have a valence of 1.
   b. In contrast, the **equivalent weight of Na_2CO_3** is 53 g/Eq, or half its molecular weight of 106. Two atoms of Na are present, each with an atomic weight of 23 (2 × 23 = 46); these have a **total valence of 2** and an equivalent weight of 23 g/Eq. One CO_3 group has a molecular weight of 60 and a **valence of 2,** for an equivalent weight of 30 (23 + 30 = 53 g/Eq). This equation shows the relation of equivalent weight to molecular weight:

$$\text{Equivalent weight} = \frac{\text{molecular weight (g/mol)}}{\text{equivalents/mol}}.$$

4. In **hospital situations,** solutions containing various electrolytes may be administered to correct serious electrolyte imbalances. Concentrations of these solutions are usually expressed as **equivalents/liter** (Eq/L) or as **milliequivalents/liter** (mEq/L) [see Chapter 2 IV]. For example, normal Na^+ concentration in human plasma is about 142 mEq/L. These equations are used to calculate the quantity of an electrolyte needed to prepare an electrolyte solution:

$$\text{Equivalent weight (g/Eq)} = \frac{\text{g/L}}{\text{Eq/L}}, \text{ and equivalent weight (mg/Eq)} = \frac{\text{mg/L}}{\text{mEq/L}}$$

IV. COLLIGATIVE PROPERTIES

A. Lowering of vapor pressure. A solute lowers the vapor pressure of a solution in an amount dependent on the mole fraction of the solute.

B. Elevation of boiling point. The boiling point is the temperature at which the vapor pressure of a liquid equals an external pressure of 760 millimeters of mercury (mm Hg). The boiling point of a solution of a nonvolatile solute is higher than that of the pure solvent because the solute lowers the vapor pressure of the solvent. The amount of elevation of the boiling point depends on the mole fraction of the solute.

C. Depression of freezing point. The freezing point (or melting point) of a pure compound is the temperature at which the solid and liquid phases are in equilibrium under a pressure of 1 atmosphere (atm). The freezing point of a solution is the temperature at which the solid phase of the pure solvent and the liquid phase of the solution are in equilibrium under a pressure of 1 atm. The amount of depression of the freezing point depends on the molality of the solution.

D. Osmotic pressure

1. **Osmosis** is the process by which solvent molecules pass through a **semipermeable membrane** (a barrier through which only solvent molecules may pass) from a region of dilute solution to one of more concentrated solution.

2. The pressure that must be applied to the more concentrated solution to prevent the flow of pure solvent into the solution is known as the **osmotic pressure**.

3. Solvent molecules move from a region where their **escape tendency is high** to one where their **escape tendency is low**. The presence of dissolved solute lowers the escape tendency of the solvent in proportion to solute concentration.

V. ELECTROLYTE SOLUTIONS AND IONIC EQUILIBRIA

A. Acid–base equilibria

1. **Arrhenius ionic dissociation theory.** According to this theory, an **acid** is a substance that liberates H^+ in aqueous solution, and a **base** is a substance that liberates hydroxyl ions (OH^-) in aqueous solution. This definition applies only under aqueous conditions, however.

2. **Lowry-Bronsted theory.** This is a more powerful concept that applies in both aqueous and nonaqueous systems; however, it is most commonly used for pharmaceutical and biologic systems because these are primarily aqueous systems.
   a. According to this definition, an **acid** is a substance (charged or uncharged) capable of **donating a proton,** and a **base** is a substance (charged or uncharged) capable of **accepting a proton from an acid.**
   b. The **dissociation of an acid** (HA) always produces a base (A^-) according to this formula:

$$HA \rightleftharpoons H^+ + A^-$$

   c. HA and A^- are referred to as **conjugate acid–base pair** (an acid and a base that differ in their structure by a proton and exist in equilibrium). The proton of an acid does not exist free in solution but combines with the solvent. [In water, this hydrated proton is known as a **hydronium ion** (H_3O^+).]
   d. The **relative strengths** of acids and bases are determined by their ability to donate or accept protons.
      (1) For example, in water, HCl donates a proton more readily than does acetic acid. Thus, it is a stronger acid.
      (2) Acid strength is also determined by the **affinity of the solvent for protons**. For example, HCl may dissociate completely in liquid ammonia but only very slightly in glacial acetic acid. Thus, HCl is a strong acid in liquid ammonia and a weak acid in glacial acetic acid.
3. **Lewis theory.** This theory extends the acid–base concept to reactions in which protons are not involved. It defines an **acid** as **a molecule or ion that accepts an electron pair** from some other atom and a **base** as a **substance that donates an electron pair** to be shared with an atom.

B. H^+ concentration values are very small and are, thus, expressed in **exponential notation as pH.**

1. The pH is defined as the **logarithm of the reciprocal of the H^+ concentration,**

$$pH = \log \frac{1}{[H^+]}$$

   where $[H^+]$ indicates the molar concentration of H.

2. Since the logarithm of a reciprocal equals the **negative logarithm** of the number, this equation may be rewritten as:

$$pH = -\log [H^+] \text{ or } [H^+] = 10^{-pH}$$

3. The pH value may, thus, be defined as the **negative logarithm of the H^+ value.**
   a. For example, if the H^+ concentration of a solution is 5×10^{-6}, the pH value may be calculated as follows:

$$\begin{aligned} pH &= -\log[5 \times 10^{-6}] \\ \log 5 &= 0.6990 \quad \text{or} \quad \log 10^{-6} = -6.0 \\ pH &= -[-6 + 0.7] \\ &= -[-5.3] \\ &= 5.3 \end{aligned}$$

   b. **As pH decreases, H^+ concentration increases exponentially.**
      (1) When the pH decreases from 6 to 5, the H^+ concentration increases from 10^{-6} to 10^{-5}, or 10 times its original value.
      (2) When the pH falls from 5 to 4.7, the H^+ concentration increases from 1×10^{-5} to 2×10^{-5}, doubling its initial value.

C. Dissociation constants

1. **Ionization** refers to the complete separation of the ions in a crystal lattice when the salt is dissolved.

2. **Dissociation** refers to the separation of ions in solution when the ions are associated by interionic attraction.
   a. For **weak electrolytes,** the dissociation is a reversible process. The equilibrium of this process may be expressed by the **law of mass action,** which states that the rate of the chemical reaction is proportional to the product of the concentration of the reacting substances, each raised to a power equal to the number of moles of the substance in solution.

b. For **weak acids,** dissociation in water is expressed as:

$$HA \rightleftharpoons H^+ + A^-$$

(1) The **dynamic equilibrium** between the simultaneous forward and reverse reactions is indicated by the arrows. By the law of mass action:

$$\text{Rate of forward reaction} = K_1[HA]$$
$$\text{Rate of reverse reaction} = K_2[H^+][A^-]$$

(2) At equilibrium, the **rates are equal**. Therefore,

$$K_1[HA] = K_2[H^+][A^-]$$

(3) Thus, the **equilibrium expression for the dissociation of a weak acid** may be written as:

$$K_a = \frac{K_1}{K_2} = \frac{[H^+][A^-]}{[HA]}$$

where K_a represents the acid dissociation constant.

(4) For a weak acid, the **acid dissociation constant** is conventionally expressed as **pK_a**, as follows:

$$pK_a = -\log[K_a]$$

(5) For example, the K_a of acetic acid at 25°C is 1.75×10^{-5}. The pK_a may be calculated as follows:

$$pK_a = -\log[1.75 \times 10^{-5}]$$
$$\log 1.75 = 0.2430 \text{ or } \log 10^{-5} = -5$$
$$pK_a = -[0.2430 - 5]$$
$$= -[4.75]$$
$$= -4.75$$

c. For **weak bases,** dissociation may be expressed using the K_a expression for the **conjugate acid of the base** (the acid formed when a proton reacts with the base). For a base that does not contain a hydroxyl group,

$$BH^+ \rightleftharpoons H^+ + B$$

(1) The **dissociation constant** for this reaction can be expressed as:

$$K_a = \frac{[H^+][B]}{[BH^+]}$$

(2) However, a **base dissociation constant** has traditionally been defined for the reaction of a weak base, using this expression:

$$B + H_2O \rightleftharpoons OH^- + BH$$

$$K_b = \frac{[OH^-][BH^+]}{[B]}$$

where K_b represents the dissociation constant of a weak base.

(3) This **dissociation constant** can be expressed as pK_b, as follows:

$$pK_b = -\log[K_b]$$

d. Certain compounds (acids or bases) may accept or donate more than one proton and consequently have **more than one dissociation constant**.

D. Henderson-Hasselbalch equations describe the relationship between ionized and nonionized species.

1. For **weak acids,** the equation is obtained from the equation in section V C 2 b as follows:

$$\frac{1}{[H^+]} = \frac{1}{K_a} \times \frac{[A^-]}{[HA]}$$

a. The **logarithm** of this equation is:

$$-\log[H^+] = -\log[K_a] + \log \frac{[A^-]}{[HA]}$$

b. Since $-\log[H^+] = pH$, and $-\log[K_a] = pK_a$, this equation may be expressed as:

$$pH = pK_a + \log \frac{[base]}{[acid]}$$

c. For practical purposes, the anion $[A^-]$ is assumed to be coming from the highly dissociated salt. Thus, the **Henderson-Hasselbalch equation for a weak acid** can be written as:

$$pH = pK_a + \log \frac{[salt]}{[acid]}$$

2. For **weak bases,** the Henderson-Hasselbalch equation is obtained from the equation in section V C 2 c (1) as follows:

$$\frac{1}{[H^+]} = \frac{1}{K_a} \times \frac{[B]}{[BH]}$$

a. The **logarithm** of this equation is:

$$-\log[H^+] = -\log[K_a] + \log \frac{[B]}{[BH]}$$

b. Since $-\log[H^+] = pH$, and $-\log[K_a] = pK_a$, this equation may be expressed as:

$$pH = pK_a + \log \frac{[B]}{[BH]}$$

c. For practical purposes, the conjugate acid [BH] is assumed to be coming from the highly dissociated salt. Thus, the **Henderson-Hasselbalch equation for a weak base** can be written as:

$$pH = pK_a + \log \frac{[base]}{[salt]}$$

E. Degree of ionization (α) is the fraction of a weak electrolyte ionized in solution. Because gastrointestinal membranes act like a lipoid barrier, the **nonionized form** of an acidic or basic drug is **preferentially absorbed** by passive routes. Thus, the **greater the fraction of drug in the nonionized form at an absorption site, the faster the absorption**. The value of α **increases** the more the drug is ionized.

1. For a **weak electrolyte,** α can be calculated as follows:

$$\alpha = \frac{I}{T}$$

where I represents the ionized species, and T represents the total species, or ionized (I) plus nonionized (U).

a. The equation above can thus be represented as:

$$\alpha = \frac{I}{I + U}$$

or

$$\frac{1}{\alpha} = \frac{I + U}{I} = 1 + \frac{U}{I}$$

or

$$\frac{1}{\alpha} - 1 = \frac{U}{I}$$

b. Therefore,

$$\frac{1 - \alpha}{\alpha} = \frac{U}{I}$$

or

$$\frac{I}{U} = \frac{\alpha}{1 - \alpha} = \frac{[ionized]}{[nonionized]}$$

2. For a **weak acid,** the **Henderson-Hasselbalch equation** is:

$$pH = pK_a + \log \frac{[\text{ionized}]}{[\text{nonionized}]}$$

a. By substituting the equation in V E 1 b into the Henderson-Hasselbalch equation, this equation is obtained:

$$pH = pK_a + \log \frac{[\alpha]}{[1 - \alpha]}$$

b. It is apparent from this that the ratio of ionized to nonionized species depends solely upon pH and pK_a. For a **weak acid,** the **degree of ionization increases as pH increases**. For example, when the pH of a weakly acidic drug is equal to the pK_a, 50% of the drug is ionized. When pH is one unit higher than pK_a, approximately 90% of the drug is ionized. When pH is two units higher than pK_a, approximately 99% of the drug is ionized.

3. For a **weak base,** the equation expressing the degree of ionization is:

$$pH = pK_a + \log \frac{[1 - \alpha]}{[\alpha]}$$

a. For a **weak base,** the **degree of ionization decreases as pH increases.**
b. When the pH of a weakly basic drug is equal to the pK_a, 50% of the drug is ionized, as with a weak acid. However, when pH is one unit higher than pK_a, approximately 90% of the drug remains in the nonionized form; when pH is two units higher than pK_a, approximately 99% of the drug remains in the nonionized form.

F. Solubility of a weak acid or base varies considerably as a function of pH. As a result, the dissolution rate of the drugs differs in various regions of the gastrointestinal tract.

1. For a **weak acid,** the total solubility (C_s) is given by this expression:

$$C_s = [HA] + [A^-]$$

where [HA] is the intrinsic solubility of the nonionized acid (denoted as C_O) and $[A^-]$ is the concentration of its anion.

a. The **anion concentration** can be expressed in terms of the dissociation constant (K_a) and C_O, giving this equation:

$$C_s = C_O + \frac{K_a C_O}{[H^+]}$$

b. This equation indicates that the **solubility of a weak acid increases with increasing pH** (i.e., with decreasing H^+ concentration). Solubility is optimal at higher pH.

2. For a **weak base,** the total solubility is given by this expression, which indicates that the **solubility of a weak base decreases with increasing pH** (i.e., is optimal at lower pH):

$$C_s = C_O + \frac{C_O [H^+]}{K_a}$$

G. Buffers and buffer capacity

1. A **buffer** is a compound or mixture of compounds that, by its presence in solution, resists changes in pH upon addition of small quantities of acid or base. A buffer may be a **combination of a weak acid and its conjugate base** or a **combination of a weak base and its conjugate acid**. However, buffer solutions are **more commonly prepared from weak acids and their salts**. They are not ordinarily prepared from weak bases and their salts, because of the instability and volatility of weak bases and because their pH depends on the dissociation constant of water (pK_w), which is affected by temperature changes.

a. For a **weak acid and its salt,** the buffer equation below is satisfactory for calculations within the pH range of 4–10 and is important in the preparation of buffered pharmaceutical solutions:

$$pH = pK_a + \log \frac{[\text{salt}]}{[\text{acid}]}$$

b. For a **weak base and its salt,** the buffer equation is similar but also depends on the dissociation constant of water (pK_w). The equation becomes:

$$pH = pK_w - pK_b + \log \frac{[base]}{[salt]}$$

2. Buffer action is the resistance to a change in pH.

3. Buffer capacity is the ability of a buffer solution to resist changes in pH. The **smaller the pH change** caused by addition of a given amount of acid or base, the **greater the buffer capacity** of the solution.

a. Buffer capacity may be defined as the **number of gram equivalents in an acid or base that changes the pH of a liter of buffer solution by one unit.**

b. Buffer capacity is **influenced by the concentration of the buffer constituents** because a higher concentration of these provides a greater acid or base reserve. Buffer capacity (β) is related to the total concentration (C) as follows:

$$\beta = 2.3\,C \frac{K_a[H^+]}{[K_a + (H^+)]^2}$$

where C represents the molar concentrations of the acid and the salt.

c. Thus, **buffer capacity depends on the value of the ratio of the salt to the acid form**. It increases as the ratio approaches unity; maximum buffer capacity occurs when $pH = pK_a$ and is represented by $\beta = 0.576\ C$.

VI. CHEMICAL KINETICS AND DRUG STABILITY

A. Introduction. The **stability of a drug's active component** is a major criterion in the rational design and evaluation of dosage forms for a drug. **Stability problems** may determine the acceptance or rejection of a given formulation.

1. Extensive chemical degradation of the active ingredient may cause **substantial loss of active ingredient from the dosage form.**

2. Chemical degradation may produce a **toxic product with undesirable side effects**.

3. Instability of the drug product may result in **decreased bioavailability,** which can lead to a substantial reduction in the therapeutic efficacy of the dosage form.

B. Rates and orders of reactions

1. Rate of a reaction (or degradation rate) is the velocity with which it occurs, expressed as dC/dt (the change in concentration, or C, within a given time interval, or dt).

a. Reaction rates depend on such conditions as **reactant concentration, temperature, pH,** and **presence of solvents or additives**. Radiation and catalytic agents such as polyvalent cations also have an effect.

b. The effective study of reaction rates requires application of **pharmacokinetic principles** (see Chapter 6 V A).

2. Order of a reaction refers to the way in which the concentration of the drug or reactant in a chemical reaction influences the rate. The study of reaction orders also requires application of pharmacokinetic principles (see Chapter 6 V). For the most part, **pharmaceutical degradation** can be treated as a **zero-order** or a **first-order reaction,** as summarized below.

a. Zero-order reaction is one in which the **rate is independent of the concentration of the reactants** (see Chapter 6 V A 1 b for details). Other factors, such as absorption of light in certain photochemical reactions, determine the rate.

(1) A **zero-order reaction** can be expressed as:

$$C = -k_0t + C_0$$

where C is the drug concentration, k_0 is the zero-order rate constant in units of concentration/time, t is the time, and C_0 is the initial concentration.

(2) When this equation is plotted with C on the vertical axis (ordinate) against t on the horizontal axis (abcissa), the **slope of the line is equal to $-k_0$** (Figure 3-1). The negative sign indicates that the slope is decreasing.

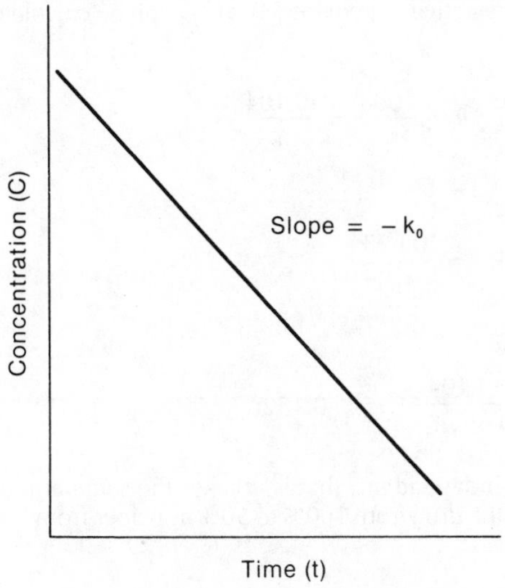

Figure 3-1. Linear plot of concentration (*C*) versus time (*t*) for a zero-order reaction. The slope of the line is equal to the zero-order rate constant, $-k_o$.

b. First-order reaction is one in which the **rate depends on the first power of the concentration of a single reactant.**

(1) The **reaction rate** is directly proportional to the concentration of the reacting substance, according to this equation:

$$C = C_0 e^{-kt}$$

where C is the concentration of the reacting material, C_0 is the initial concentration, k is the first-order rate constant in units of reciprocal time, and t is time.

(2) In a first-order reaction, **concentration decreases exponentially with time**. A plot of the logarithm of concentration against time produces a straight line with a slope of $-k/2.303$ (Figure 3-2).

(3) The **half-life** of a reaction is the period of time required for the concentration of a drug to decrease by one-half ($t_{1/2}$). For a first-order reaction, this is expressed by:

$$t_{1/2} = \frac{0.693}{k}$$

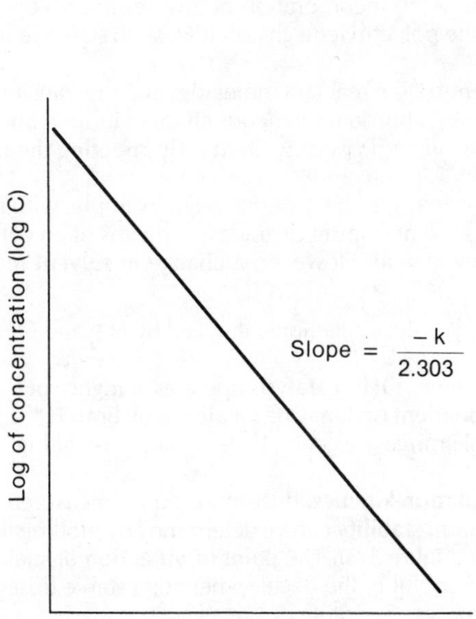

Figure 3-2. Linear plot of the logarithm of concentration (*log C*) versus time (*t*) for a first-order reaction. The slope of the line is equal to $-k/2.303$.

(4) The **time required for 10% of a drug to degrade** ($t_{10\%}$) is also important, as it represents a reasonable limit of degradation for the active ingredients. The $t_{10\%}$ can be calculated as:

$$t_{10\%} = \frac{2.303}{k} \log \frac{100}{90} = \frac{0.104}{k}$$

(a) Since

$$k = \frac{0.693}{t_{1/2}}$$

(b) Then

$$t_{10\%} = \frac{0.104}{0.693/t_{1/2}} = 0.152t_{1/2}$$

(5) Both $t_{1/2}$ and $t_{10\%}$ are **concentration-independent;** that is, it takes the same amount of time to reduce the concentration of the drug from 100% to 50% as it does from 50% to 25%.

C. Factors affecting reaction rates. Factors other than concentration may affect a drug's reaction rate and stability. Among these are temperature, the presence of a solvent, pH, and the presence of additives.

1. **Temperature.** An **increase in temperature** causes an increase in reaction rate, as expressed in the equation first suggested by Arrhenius:

$$k = Ae^{-Ea/RT} \text{ or } \log k = \log A - \frac{Ea}{2.303} \times \frac{1}{RT}$$

where k is the specific reaction rate constant, A is a constant known as the frequency factor, Ea is the energy of activation, R is the gas constant (0.987 cal/degree × mole), and T is the absolute temperature.

a. The **constants A and Ea** may be obtained by determining k at several temperatures and then plotting log k against 1/T. The slope of the resulting line equals −Ea/2.303R, and the intercept on the vertical axis equals log A.

b. The activation energy (Ea) is the amount of energy required to put the molecules in an **activated state**—molecules must be activated to react. As **temperature increases,** more molecules are activated and the **reaction rate increases**.

2. **Presence of solvent.** Many dosage forms require the incorporation of a water-miscible solvent [low molecular-weight alcohols, such as the polyethylene glycols (PEGs)] to stabilize the drug.

a. In addition to **altering the activity coefficients** of the reactant molecules and the transition state, a change in the solvent system may bring about simultaneous changes in such physicochemical parameters as pK_a, surface tension, and viscosity, **indirectly affecting the reaction rate**.

b. In some cases, **additional reaction pathways** may also be generated. For example, with an increasing concentration of ethanol in the solvent, aspirin degrades by means of an extra route, forming the ethyl ester of acetylsalicylic acid. However, a **change in solvent may also stabilize the drug**.

3. **Change in pH.** The magnitude of the rate of a hydrolytic reaction catalyzed by H^+ and OH^- can vary considerably with pH.

a. **H^+ catalysis** predominates at **lower pH,** whereas **OH^- catalysis** operates at **higher pH**. At **intermediate pH,** the rate may be **pH-independent** or it may be catalyzed by **both H^+ and OH^-**. (Rate constants in the intermediate pH range are generally less than those at higher or lower pH values, however.)

b. To determine the **influence of pH on degradation kinetics,** decomposition is measured at several H^+ concentrations. The **pH of optimum stability** can be determined by plotting the logarithm of the rate constant (k) versus pH (Figure 3-3). The **point of inflection** of such a plot represents the pH of optimum stability, useful in the development of a stable dosage formulation.

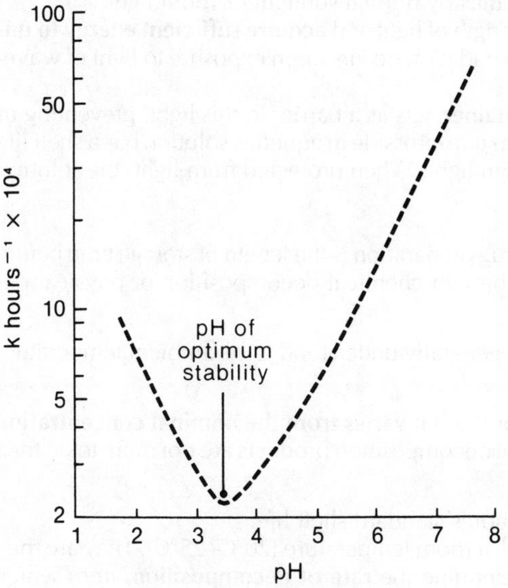

Figure 3-3. A plot of the logarithm of the rate constant (*k*) versus *pH,* used to determine the pH of optimum stability.

4. Presence of additives

a. Buffer salts must be added to many drug solutions to maintain the formulation at optimum pH. These salts **may affect the rate of degradation,** primarily from salt effect results of the increasing ionic strength.

(1) Increasing salt concentrations (particularly from polyelectrolytes such as citrate and phosphate) can **substantially affect the magnitude of pK_a,** causing a change in the rate constant.

(2) Buffer salts can also **promote drug degradation** through general acid or base catalysis.

b. Addition of surfactant agents may accelerate or decelerate drug degradation.

(1) Acceleration of degradation is frequently observed because micellar catalysis may provide a model for enzyme reactions.

(2) Stabilization of a drug through addition of a surfactant is less frequently observed.

c. Complexing agents may improve drug stability. Aromatic esters such as benzocaine, procaine, hydrochloride, and tetracaine **increase in half-life** in the presence of caffeine. This increased stability appears to result from the formation of a less reactive complex between the aromatic ester and caffeine.

D. Modes of pharmaceutical degradation. The decomposition of active ingredients in a dosage form can occur through several pathways (e.g., hydrolysis, oxidation, photolysis). (For details, see Chapter 11, II A.)

1. Hydrolysis is the most frequent type of degradation because many medicinal compounds are esters, amides, or lactams.

a. H^+ and OH^- are the most common catalysts of hydrolytic degradation in solution.

b. Esters most frequently undergo hydrolytic reactions that result in drug instability. Because esters are rapidly degraded in aqueous solution, formulators are reluctant to incorporate drugs having ester functional groups into liquid dosage forms.

2. Oxidation is usually mediated through reaction with atmospheric oxygen under ambient conditions (auto-oxidation).

a. Medicinal compounds that undergo auto-oxidation at room temperature are affected by **oxygen dissolved in the solvent and in the void space of their packages**. These compounds should be packed under an **inert atmosphere** (e.g., nitrogen, carbon dioxide) to exclude air from their containers.

b. Most oxidation reactions involve a **free radical mechanism** and a **chain reaction**. (Free radicals tend to take electrons from other compounds.)

(1) Antioxidants in the formulation react with the free radicals by providing electrons and easily available hydrogen atoms, thus preventing the propagation of chain reactions.

(2) Commonly used antioxidants include ascorbic acid, butylated hydroxyanisole (BHA), butylated hydroxytoluene (BHT), propyl gallate, sodium bisulfite, sodium sulfite, and the tocopherols.

3. **Photolysis** is the degradation of drug molecules by normal sunlight or room light.
   a. Molecules may absorb the proper wavelength of light and **acquire sufficient energy to undergo reaction**. Generally, photolytic degradation occurs upon exposure to light of wavelengths less than 40 μm.
   b. An **amber glass bottle** or an **opaque container** acts as a barrier to this light, preventing or retarding photolysis. For example, sodium nitroprusside in aqueous solution has a shelf life of only 4 hours if exposed to normal room light. When protected from light, the solution is stable for at least 1 year.

E. **Determination of shelf life.** The shelf life of a drug preparation is the length of storage time before the preparation becomes unfit for use, either through chemical decomposition or physical deterioration.

1. **Storage temperature** affects shelf life and is generally understood to be ambient temperature unless special storage conditions are given.

2. In general, a preparation is considered fit for use if it **varies from the nominal concentration or dose by no more than ± 5%,** provided the decomposition products are not more toxic than the original material.

3. **Shelf testing** aids in determining a formulation's standard shelf life.
   a. Samples are stored at about 3°C–5°C and at room temperature (20°C–25°C). They are then analyzed at various time intervals to determine the **rate of decomposition,** from which shelf life may be calculated.
   b. Because storage time at these temperatures may result in an extended testing time, **accelerated testing** is generally conducted as well, using a range of higher temperatures. The **rate constants** obtained from these samples are used to predict shelf life at ambient or refrigeration temperatures.
   c. **Prediction of stability at room temperature** can be obtained from accelerated testing data by the Arrhenius equation:

$$\log \frac{k_2}{k_1} = \frac{Ea(T_2 - T_1)}{2.303\, RT_2T_1}$$

where k_2 and k_1 are the rate constants at the absolute temperatures T_2 and T_1, respectively, R is the gas constant, and Ea is the energy of activation.

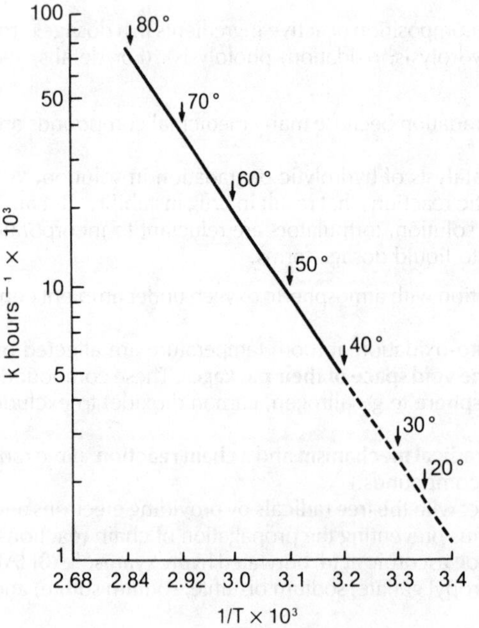

Figure 3-4. A plot of the logarithm of the rate constant (*k*) versus the reciprocal of absolute temperature (*1/T*), showing the temperature dependency of degradation rates.

d. As an **alternate method,** an expression of concentration can be plotted as a linear function of time. Rate constants (k) for degradation at several temperatures are obtained; the logarithm of the rate constant (log k) is then plotted against the reciprocal of absolute temperature (1/T) to obtain, by extrapolation, the rate constant for degradation at room temperature (Figure 3-4).

e. The **length of time the drug will maintain its required potency** can also be predicted by calculation of the drug's $t_{10\%}$ [see VI B 2 b (4)]. This method applies to chemical reactions with activation energies in the range of 10–30 kcal/mol, which is the magnitude of the activation energy for many pharmaceutical degradations occurring in solution.

STUDY QUESTIONS

Directions: Each of the numbered items or incomplete statements in this section is followed by answers or by completions of the statement. Select the **one** lettered answer or completion that is **best** in each case.

1. Molarity is defined as

(A) gram molecular weight of solute in 1 L of solution
(B) gram equivalent weight of solute in 1 L of solution
(C) saturated solution of a solute in 1 L of solution
(D) milliliters of solvent required to dissolve 10 g of solute
(E) supersaturated solution of a solute

2. Which of the following substances is classified as a weak electrolyte?

(A) Glucose
(B) Urea
(C) Ephedrine
(D) Sodium chloride (NaCl)
(E) Sucrose

3. The pH value is calculated mathematically as the

(A) log of the hydroxyl ion (OH^-) concentration
(B) negative log of the OH^- concentration
(C) log of the hydrogen ion (H^+) concentration
(D) negative log of the H^+ concentration
(E) ratio of H^+/OH^- concentration

4. Which of the following properties is classified as a colligative property?

(A) Solubility of a solute
(B) Osmotic pressure
(C) Hydrogen ion (H^+) concentration
(D) Dissociation of a solute
(E) Miscibility of the liquids

5. The colligative properties of a solution are related to the

(A) pH of the solution
(B) number of ions in the solution
(C) total number of solute particles in the solution
(D) number of nonionized molecules in the solution
(E) pK_a of the solution

6. The pH of a buffer system can be calculated by using the

(A) Noyes-Whitney equation
(B) Henderson-Hasselbalch equation
(C) Michaelis-Menten equation
(D) Yong equation
(E) Stokes equation

7. Which of the following mechanisms is most frequently responsible for chemical degradation?

(A) Racemization
(B) Photolysis
(C) Hydrolysis
(D) Decarboxylation
(E) Oxidation

8. Which of the following equations is used to predict the stability of a drug product at room temperature from experiments at accelerated temperatures?

(A) Stokes equation
(B) Yong equation
(C) Arrhenius equation
(D) Michaelis-Menten equation
(E) Hixson-Crowell equation

9. Based on the relationship between the degree of ionization and the solubility of a weak acid, the drug aspirin (pK_a 3.49) will be most soluble at

(A) pH 1.0
(B) pH 2.0
(C) pH 3.0
(D) pH 4.0
(E) pH 6.0

1-A	4-B	7-C
2-C	5-C	8-C
3-D	6-B	9-E

10. All of the following statements concerning chemical degradation are true EXCEPT

(A) as temperature increases, degradation decreases
(B) most drugs degrade by a first-order process
(C) chemical degradation may produce a toxic product
(D) chemical degradation may result in a loss of active ingredients
(E) chemical degradation may affect the therapeutic activity of a drug

11. All of the following statements concerning zero-order degradation are true EXCEPT

(A) its rate is independent of the concentration
(B) a plot of concentration versus time yields a straight line on rectilinear paper
(C) its half-life is a changing parameter
(D) its concentration remains unchanged with respect to time
(E) the slope of a plot of concentration versus time yields a rate constant

12. All of the following statements concerning first-order degradation are true EXCEPT

(A) its rate is dependent on the concentration
(B) its half-life is a changing parameter
(C) a plot of the logarithm of concentration versus time yields a straight line
(D) its $t_{10\%}$ is independent of the concentration
(E) a plot of the logarithm of concentration versus time allows determination of the rate constant

---

10-A
11-D
12-B

ANSWERS AND EXPLANATIONS

1. The answer is A *[II A].*
Molarity is the number of moles (gram molecular weights) of solute in 1 L of solution. Molarity is the expression of concentration commonly used in analytical work. All solutions of the same molarity contain the same number of solute molecules in a definite volume of solution. When a solution contains more than one solute, it may have different molar concentrations with respect to the various solutes.

2. The answer is C *[I B 2 b].*
Glucose, urea, and sucrose are nonelectrolytes, while sodium chloride (NaCl) is an example of a strong electrolyte. Electrolytes are substances that form ions when dissolved in water and, thus, can conduct an electric current through the solution. Ions are particles that bear electrical charges: Cations are positively charged ions, and anions are negatively charged. Strong electrolytes are completely ionized in water at all concentrations; weak electrolytes (e.g., ephedrine) are only partially ionized at most concentrations. Nonelectrolytes do not form ions when in solution and, thus, are nonconductors.

3. The answer is D *[V B].*
The pH is a measure of the acidity or alkalinity of an aqueous solution. The pH is the logarithm of the reciprocal of the hydrogen ion (H^+) concentration expressed in moles per liter. Since the logarithm of a reciprocal equals the negative logarithm of the number, the pH is the negative logarithm of the H^+ concentration. A pH of 7.0 indicates neutrality; as the pH decreases, the acidity increases. The pH of arterial blood is 7.35 to 7.45; of urine, 5 to 8; of gastric juice, about 1.4; of cerebrospinal fluid, 7.35 to 7.40. The concept of pH was introduced by Sörensen in the early 1900s.

4. The answer is B *[IV].*
Osmotic pressure is an example of a colligative property. The osmotic pressure is the amount of pressure needed to stop osmosis across a semipermeable membrane between a solution and pure solvent. Colligative properties depend upon the number of solute particles and are independent of the chemical nature of the solute. Other colligative properties of solutes are the reduction in vapor pressure of a solution, elevation of its boiling point, and depression of its freezing point.

5. The answer is C *[IV].*
The colligative properties of a solution are related to the total number of solute particles in a solution. Examples of colligative properties are osmotic pressure, lowering of vapor pressure, elevation of the boiling point, and depression of the freezing (or melting) point.

6. The answer is B *[V D].*
The Henderson-Hasselbalch equation for a weak acid and its salt is represented as:

$$pH = pK_a + \log \frac{[salt]}{[acid]}$$

where pK_a is the negative log of the dissociation constant of a weak acid, and [salt]/[acid] is the ratio of the molar concentration of salt and acid used to prepare a buffer.

7. The answer is C *[VI D].*
Although it is true that all of the mechanisms listed in the question can be responsible, the chemical degradation of medicinal compounds is most frequently due to hydrolysis. This is especially true of esters in liquid formulations, and drugs having ester functional groups are, therefore, formulated in dry form whenever possible. Oxidation, another common mode of degradation, is minimized by including antioxidants, such as ascorbic acid, in drug formulations. Photolysis is reduced by packaging susceptible products in amber or opaque containers. Decarboxylation, the removal of COOH groups, affects carboxylic acid compounds. Racemization neutralizes the effects of an optically active compound by converting half its molecules into the mirror-image configuration, so that the dextro- and levorotatory forms cancel one another out. This form of degradation affects only drugs characterized by optical isomerism.

8. The answer is C *[VI E 3; Figure 3-4].*
Testing of a drug formulation to determine its shelf life can be accelerated by applying the Arrhenius equation to data obtained at higher temperatures. The method involves the determination of rate constant (k) values for the degradation of a drug at various elevated temperatures. The log of k is then plotted against the reciprocal of the absolute temperature, and the k value for degradation at room temperature is obtained by extrapolation.

9. The answer is E *[V E 2 b, F].*
The solubility of a weak acid varies as a function of pH. Since pH and pK_a (the dissociation constant) are related, solubility is also related to the degree of ionization. The drug aspirin is a weak acid and will be completely ionized at pH that is 2 units above its pK_a. Therefore, it will be most soluble at pH 6.0.

10. The answer is A *[VI B 1, 2, C 1; Figures 3-1, 3-2].*
A number of factors may affect the reaction velocity, or degradation rate, of a pharmaceutical product. Among these are temperature, solvents, and light. The degradation increases two to three times with each 10° increase in temperature. The effect of temperature on reaction rate is given by the Arrhenius equation:

$$k = Ae^{-Ea/RT}$$

where k is the reaction rate constant, A is the frequency factor, Ea is the energy of activation, R is the gas constant, and T is the absolute temperature.

11. The answer is D *[VI B 2 a; Figure 3-1].*
In zero-order degradation, the concentration of a drug decreases over time; it is the *change* of concentration with respect to time that is unchanged. In the equation:

$$\frac{-dC}{dt} = k$$

the fact that dC/dt is negative signifies that the concentration is decreasing; however, the *velocity* of concentration change is seen to be constant.

12. The answer is B *[VI B 2 b; Figure 3-2].*
The half-life ($t_{1/2}$) is the time required for the concentration of a drug to decrease by one-half. For a first-order degradation,

$$t_{1/2} = \frac{0.693}{k}$$

Since both k and 0.693 are constants, then $t_{1/2}$ is a constant.

4 Pharmaceutical Drug Forms

Sunil Jambhekar

I. SOLUTIONS

A. Introduction. Drugs in solution are more homogeneous and easier to swallow than drugs in solid form. For drugs with a slow dissolution rate, onset of action and bioavailability are also improved. However, drugs in solution are bulkier, degrade more rapidly, and are more likely to interact with constituents than those in solid form. **Water** is the **most commonly used vehicle** for drug solutions. The ***United States Pharmacopeia (USP)*** recognizes four standards of water for the preparation of dosage forms.

1. **Purified water USP** is water obtained by distillation or by ion exchange treatment. It may not contain more than 10 parts per million (ppm) of total solid and should have a pH between 5 and 7. Purified water is issued in prescriptions and finished manufactured products except parenteral and ophthalmic products.

2. **Water for injection USP** conforms to the standards of purified water but is also free of pyrogen. It is used as a solvent for the preparation of parenteral solutions.

3. **Sterile water for injection USP** is water for injection that has been sterilized and packaged in single-dose containers of type I and II glass that do not exceed a capacity of 1 L. The limitations for total solids depend upon the size of the container.

4. **Bacteriostatic water for injection USP** is sterile water for injection that contains one or more suitable bacteriostatic agents. It is also packaged in a single- or multiple-dose container of type I or II glass that does not exceed the capacity of 30 ml.

B. Aromatic waters are **saturated aqueous solutions of volatile oils** or other aromatic or volatile substances.

1. **Uses.** An aromatic water may be used as a pleasantly flavored vehicle for a water-soluble drug or as an aqueous phase in an emulsion or suspension.
   a. If a large amount of water-soluble drug is added to an aromatic water, an insoluble layer may form at the top.
   b. This "salting out" is a competitive process in which the molecules of water-soluble drugs have more attraction for the solvent molecules of water than the volatile oil molecules. The associated water molecules are pulled away from the volatile oil molecules, which are no longer held in solution.

2. **Storage.** Aromatic waters should be stored in tight, light-resistant bottles to reduce volatization and degradation from sunlight.

3. **Preparation.** Aromatic waters may be prepared by any of the following three methods:
   a. **Distillation** is a universal method but is not practical or economical for most products; however, it is the only method of preparing strong rose water and orange flower water.
   b. **Solution method.** For this method, 2 ml or 2 g of the volatile substance are agitated for 15 minutes with sufficient water to make 1000 ml of solution, set aside for 12 hours, and filtered through wet filter paper to prevent the passage of excess oil into the filtrate and to eliminate adsorption of the dissolved aromatics.
   c. **Alternate solution method.** This method is the most expedient way to produce aromatic waters.
      (1) The volatile substance is thoroughly mixed with an inert adsorptive agent (e.g., talc,

purified siliceous earth). Then, 1 L of purified water is added and agitated for 10 minutes. The solution is filtered until a clear filtrate is obtained.

(2) The volatile substance is adsorbed on the inert agent, increasing the total area of volatile substance exposed to the water, thus facilitating the formation of a saturated solution. The inert agent also acts as a clarifier in filtration, as the undissolved material remains adsorbed and does not pass through the filter.

C. Syrups. A syrup is a **concentrated or nearly saturated aqueous solution of sugar**. Syrup NF contains 850 g of sucrose and sufficient purified water (450 ml) to make 1 L of syrup; however, it is not saturated. It is an 85% weight-in-volume (w/v) or approximately 65% weight-in-weight (w/w) solution with a specific gravity of 1.30. The high sugar content provides a moderately high viscosity and high specific gravity.

1. Uses. The sweet taste of syrups makes them useful vehicles for orally administered drugs.

a. Flavoring syrups (e.g., cherry syrup, cocoa syrup, tolu balsam syrup) are those that contain no medicinal agent. The choice of a syrup as a masking and flavoring vehicle must be determined by a taste panel. Traditionally, **aromatic eriodictyon syrup** or **glycyrrhiza syrup** are thought to **mask the bitter taste** of alkaloids; **cherry** or **raspberry syrup,** the **saline taste** of certain other drugs.

b. Medicinal syrups (e.g., chlorpheniramine maleate syrup, ephedrine sulfate syrup, piperazine citrate syrup) are those that contain therapeutically active compounds.

2. Preparation. Syrups may be prepared by any one of the following three methods

a. Agitation of sucrose and water produces an odorless, colorless syrup. As the sugar dissolves and saturation is approached, the dissolution rate and the concentration gradient decrease. Thus, agitation is a slow process.

b. Agitation with heat often produces a syrup with a pale yellow color. A solution of sucrose undergoes hydrolysis to dextrose and fructose in the presence of heat; with excessive heat, the sweet taste is destroyed, and a dark brown liquid results. This method cannot be used to prepare a syrup containing a thermolabile or a volatile ingredient.

c. Percolation is an extraction process in which the desired constituents are dissolved from a granulated or powdered drug by the descent at a controlled rate of suitable solvent through a column of the drug.

3. Characteristics

a. Syrups have a **low solvent capacity for water-soluble drugs** because the hydrogen bonding between sucrose and water is very strong. For this reason, it may be difficult or impossible to dissolve a drug in a syrup; often the drug is best dissolved in a small quantity of water to which the flavoring syrup is then added.

b. The **sucrose concentration** of syrup plays a critical role in the control of microorganic growth.

(1) Dilute sucrose solutions are excellent media for microorganisms.

(2) As the concentration of sucrose approaches saturation, the syrup becomes self-preserved. However, a saturated solution is undesirable because the temperature fluctuations may cause crystallization. **Syrup USP** is a self-preserved solution with a minimal chance of crystallization.

D. Solutions are **liquid preparations that contain one or more solutes but are not, by their method of preparation or ingredients, classified within another category**. Nasal, ophthalmic, and parenteral solutions are physically solutions; however, they are classified separately because of their specific use and method of preparation.

1. Mouthwashes are solutions used for cleansing the mouth or treating diseased conditions of the oral mucous membrane. They frequently contain alcohol or glycerin to aid in dissolving the volatile ingredients and are more often used cosmetically than therapeutically.

2. Astringents are locally applied solutions that precipitate protein, reducing cell permeability without injury.

a. Astringents cause **constriction** with wrinkling of the skin and blanching.

b. Because astringents **reduce secretions,** they may be used as antiperspirants.

c. Aluminum acetate solution and **aluminum subacetate solution** are used as wet dressings in contact dermatitis. The precipitation is minimized by the addition of boric acid.

d. Calcium hydroxide solution is a mild astringent employed in lotions as a reactant and an alkalizer.

3. **Antibacterial topical solutions** (e.g., benzalkonium chloride solution, strong iodine solution, methylrosaniline chloride solutions) kill bacteria when applied to the skin or mucous membrane in the proper strength and under appropriate conditions.

E. Elixirs are **pleasantly flavored hydroalcoholic solutions** intended for oral use. The presence of sugar and alcohol distinguishes the elixir from other categories. Elixirs that contain therapeutically active compounds are known as **medicated elixirs** (e.g., phenobarbital elixir).

1. **Alcohol content**
   - **a.** The alcohol content of elixirs varies from 5%–40%. Sufficient alcohol is used to maintain the drug in solution. Most elixirs become turbid when moderately diluted by aqueous liquids.
   - **b.** An **iso-alcoholic elixir** is a vehicle for various drugs that require solvents of different alcoholic concentrations. It consists of a low-alcoholic elixir (8%–10% alcohol) and a high-alcoholic elixir (75%–78% alcohol). By mixing appropriate volumes of the two elixirs, an alcoholic content sufficient to dissolve the drugs can be obtained.
2. **Preparation.** Elixirs are prepared by dissolving the ingredients in the appropriate solvent. Usually, the alcohol-soluble substances are dissolved in the alcohol and water-soluble substances in water. The aqueous solution is then added to the alcoholic solution and stirred.
3. **Uses.** Elixirs are not the preferred vehicle for salts as alcohol accentuates a saline taste. Salts also have limited solubility in alcohol; therefore, the alcoholic content of salt-containing elixirs must be low.

F. Spirits (also called **essences**) are **alcoholic or hydroalcoholic solutions of volatile substances** containing 50%–90% alcohol. This **high alcoholic content** maintains the water-insoluble volatile oils in solution. If water is added to a spirit, the oils separate.

1. **Uses.** Some spirits are **medicinal spirits** (e.g., aromatic ammonia spirit), and many spirits (e.g., compound orange spirit, compound cardamom spirit) are used as **flavoring agents**.
2. **Storage.** Spirits should be stored in tight containers to reduce loss by evaporation.

G. Tinctures are **alcoholic or hydroalcoholic solutions of chemicals or soluble constituents of crude drugs**. Although tinctures vary in drug concentration (up to 50%), those prepared from potent drugs are usually 10% in strength (i.e., 100 ml of tincture has the activity of 10 g of the drug).

1. **Alcohol content.** Generally, tinctures are considered to be stable preparations. The alcohol content among the official tinctures varies from 17% to 21% with opium tincture USP and from 77% to 83% in tolu balsam tincture NF.
2. **Preparation.** Most tinctures are prepared by an extraction process of maceration or percolation. The selection of a solvent (also known as menstruum) is based on the solubility of the active and inert constituents of the crude drugs.
   - **a.** Ideally, only the active ingredient should be extracted by the solvent. However, frequently some unwanted material also gets extracted.
   - **b.** If any extracted material is detrimental to the product, it can be removed by additional processes.
3. **Storage**
   - **a.** Tinctures may precipitate inactive constituents upon aging. Glycerin may be added to the hydroalcoholic solvent (as with aromatic rhubarb) to increase the solubility of the active constituent and to reduce precipitation upon storage.
   - **b.** Tinctures must be tightly stoppered and kept from excessive temperatures. Because many of the constituents found in tinctures undergo a photochemical change upon exposure to light, they must be stored in light-resistant containers.

H. Fluid extracts are **liquid extracts of vegetable drugs containing alcohol as a solvent, preservative, or both**.

1. **Preparation.** Tinctures are prepared by percolation so that each milliliter contains the therapeutic constituents of 1 g of the standard drug.
2. **Potency**
   - **a.** Because of high alcohol content, fluid extracts are sometimes referred to as "100% tinctures." Fluid extracts of potent drugs are usually 10 times as concentrated (or potent) as the

corresponding tincture (e.g., the usual dose of tincture belladonna is 0.6 ml; the equivalent dose of more potent fluid extract would be 0.06 ml).

b. Many fluid extracts are considered too potent for self-administration by patients so they are almost never prescribed. In addition, many fluid extracts are simply too bitter. Today, therefore, most fluid extracts are either modified by flavoring or sweetening agents.

II. SUSPENSIONS

A. Introduction. A suspension is a two-phase system composed of a **solid material dispersed in a liquid**. The particle size of the dispersed solid is usually greater than 0.5 μm; the liquid can be oily or aqueous. However, most suspensions of pharmaceutical interest are aqueous. **Lotions, magmas** (i.e., suspensions of finely divided material in a small amount of water), and **mixtures** are all suspensions that have had official formulas for some time (e.g., calamine lotion USP, kaolin mixture with pectin NF). Official formulas are given in the USP and the NF.

1. A **complete formula** and a **detailed method of preparation** are available for some official suspensions, while **only the concentration of active ingredients is given** for others, allowing the manufacturer considerable latitude in formulation.

2. Some drugs are provided in a package in a **dry form** to circumvent the instability of aqueous dispersions. Water is added at the time of dispensing to complete the suspension.

B. Purposes of suspension

1. **Sustaining effect.** For a sustained-release preparation, suspension introduces a dissolution or diffusion step as the drug goes from solid form to solution form to final absorption.

2. **Stability.** Drug degradation in suspension or solid dosage forms occurs much more slowly than degradation in solution form.

3. **Taste.** A bad-tasting material can be converted into an insoluble form and then prepared as a suspension, obviating the taste problem.

4. **Basic solubility.** When suitable solvents are not available, the suspension provides an alternative. For example, only water can be used as a solvent for ophthalmic preparations because of the possibility of corneal damage. Ophthalmic suspensions provide an alternative.

C. Suspension parameters

1. **Properties of an ideal suspension**
   a. **Uniform particle size.** All particles behave alike and produce consistent behavior for the suspension as a whole.
   b. **No particle–particle interaction.** Each particle remains discrete with no aggregation or clumping (such a suspension is known as a **monodispersed suspension**).
   c. **No sedimentation.** Drug particles are either stationary or move randomly throughout the dispersion medium, so the drug is always uniformly distributed.

2. **Controlling fundamental parameters.** The ideal properties of a suspension, which are not usually realized, can be approximated.
   a. **Particle size** should be as **small as possible**. A small particle size favors a slower sedimentation rate, according to Stoke's law:

$$\text{Sedimentation rate} = \frac{d^2(\rho - \rho_0)g}{18\eta},$$

   where d is the particle diameter, ρ is the density of the solid, ρ_0 is the density of the sedimentation medium, g is the acceleration due to gravity, and η is the viscosity of the dispersion medium.
   b. **High concentrations of solids** increase the possibility of particle–particle collisions, thus promoting particle–particle interactions. However, the concentrations of solids are usually fixed in a given formula, so this parameter can seldom be changed.
   c. **Particle–particle interactions** should be avoided. With aggregation, the resulting clumps behave like larger particles and settle at a faster rate.
      (1) **Aggregations can be prevented** if the **particles have a similar electrical charge**. A solid dispersed in an aqueous system always has some charge, resulting from ionization of

chemical groups on the solid surface, adsorption of surfactant molecules on the solid surface, or adsorption of electrolytes from solution.

(2) The **sign of the charge can usually be predicted** if it results from **adsorption of an ionic surfactant**. For example, sodium lauryl sulfate used as a dispersing agent yields a negative charge to solid particles. In contrast, the **sign of the charge can rarely be predicted** if it results from **adsorption of an electrolyte.**

(3) The **magnitude of the charge** is the difference in electrical potential between the charged solid surface and the bulk of the liquid. Most important is the **zeta potential,** determined from the fixed layers of ions on the particle surface (Figure 4-1). This layer of ions is tightly bound and is considered part of the particle for practical purposes.

(4) To maintain a **monodispersed system,** the zeta potential must be great enough for particles to repel each other (**critical zeta potential**). This value is specific for each given suspension.

d. **Density and viscosity** can be manipulated to reduce sedimentation. According to **Stoke's law:**

(1) **The sedimentation rate equals zero when the densities of the solid and the dispersion medium are equal.** However, it is difficult to prepare aqueous solutions with a density sufficient to match that of the solids commonly used in suspensions. In addition, solution density also changes with temperature.

(2) **The sedimentation rate is inversely proportional to the viscosity of the dispersion medium.** However, an increase in viscosity only slows the sedimentation rate and cannot stop it completely.

D. Suspending agents include hydrophilic colloids, clays, and a few other agents. Some of these are also used as **emulsifying agents** (see III).

1. **Hydrophilic colloids** increase the viscosity of water by binding water molecules, thus limiting their mobility or fluidity. Viscosity is proportional to the concentration of the colloid. These agents **support the growth of microorganisms** and require a preservative. They are **anionic** (with the exception of methylcellulose) and, thus, incompatible with quaternary antibacterial agents and other positively charged drugs. Most are **insoluble in alcoholic solutions.**

a. **Acacia** is usually used as the mucilage (35% dispersion in water). Viscosity is greatest between pH 5 and pH 9. It is susceptible to microbial decomposition.

b. **Tragacanth** is usually used as a 6% dispersion in water (mucilage) and has an advantage over acacia in that less is needed. Also, tragacanth does not contain the oxidase present in acacia, which catalyzes the decomposition of organic chemicals. Its viscosity is greatest at pH 5.

c. **Methylcellulose** is a polymer that is nonionic and stable to heat and light. It is available in

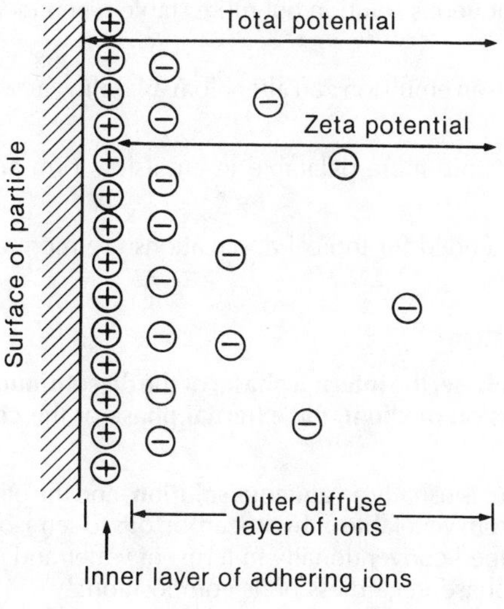

Figure 4-1. Schematic representation of the zeta potential of a particle in a suspension. The zeta potential is determined from the difference in the charge between the fixed layer of ions adhering to the particle surface and the bulk of the liquid.

several viscosity grades. Because it is soluble in cold water but not in hot water, dispersions are prepared by adding the material to boiling water and then cooling the preparation until the material dissolves.

d. **Carboxymethylcellulose** is an anionic material that is soluble in water and available in three viscosity grades. Prolonged exposure to heat causes loss of viscosity.

2. **Clays** (e.g., bentonite, Veegum) are silicates that are anionic in aqueous dispersions. Strongly hydrated, they exhibit **thixotropy** (the property of forming a gel-like structure on standing and becoming fluid on agitation).
   a. **Bentonite's** official form is as the 5% magma.
   b. **Veegum** is hydrated to a greater degree than bentonite and, thus, is more viscous at the same concentration.

3. **Other agents** include agar, chondrus (carrageenan), gelatin, pectin, and gelatinized starch. The use of all of these is limited by their susceptibility to bacterial attack, their incompatibilities, and their cost.

E. Preparation

1. **Solids are wetted initially** to separate individual particles and coat them with a layer of dispersion medium. Wetting may be accomplished by **levigation** (i.e., the addition of a suitable nonsolvent, or **levigating agent,** to the solid material, followed by blending to form a paste), using a glass mortar and pestle; or a **surfactant** may be employed.

2. **Suspending agents** are **then added** as dry powder along with the active ingredient. For best results, however, the suspending agent should be added in the form of its **aqueous dispersion**.
   a. This dispersion may be added to the solid (or the levigated solid) by way of **geometric dilution** to ensure proper dispersion.
   b. The preparation is then brought to the desired volume by stirring in the appropriate vehicle.

III. EMULSIONS

A. Introduction. An emulsion is a heterogeneous system, consisting of at least **one immiscible liquid intimately dispersed in another in the form of droplets** (droplet diameter usually exceeds 0.1 μm). Emulsions are **inherently unstable** because the droplets of the dispersed liquid tend to coalesce to form large droplets until all of the dispersed droplets have coalesced. An **emulsifying agent,** the third component of the system, is used to prevent the coalescence and maintain the integrity of the individual droplets of dispersed liquid.

B. Purposes of emulsions

1. **Increase solubility.** Many drugs have limited solubility but have the maximum activity in solution form.

2. **Increase stability.** Many drugs are unstable in aqueous solution but more stable when incorporated into an emulsion.

3. **Prolong drug action.** Incorporation of a drug into an emulsion can alter bioavailability, as with certain intramuscular injection preparations.

4. **Improve taste.** Objectionable medicinal agents are more palatable in emulsion form and, thus, more conveniently administered.

5. **Improve appearance.** Oleaginous materials intended for topical applications are more appealing in an emulsified form.

C. Phases of emulsions. Emulsions are **two-phase systems**.

1. The **liquid** or **droplet** is known as the **dispersed phase,** the **internal phase,** or the **discontinuous phase**. The other liquid is known as the **dispersion medium,** the **external phase** or the **continuous phase**.

2. In pharmaceutical applications, one of the phases is usually an **aqueous solution,** and the other phase is **lipid** or **oily** in nature. The lipids range from vegetable or hydrocarbon oils to semisolid hydrocarbons and waxes. Emulsions are described conventionally in terms of water and oil, where oil represents the lipid or nonaqueous phase, regardless of its composition.

a. If **water** is the **internal phase,** the emulsion is classified as a **water-in-oil (w/o)** type.
b. If **water** is the **external phase,** the emulsion is classified as an **oil-in-water (o/w)** type.

3. The **type of emulsion** formed is primarily determined by the **relative phase volumes** and the **emulsifying agent** used.
   a. For an ideal emulsion, the maximum concentration of internal phase is 74% (i.e., an o/w emulsion can theoretically be prepared containing up to but not more than 74% oil).
   b. Choice of an emulsifying agent is perhaps more important in determining the final emulsion type. Most agents preferentially form one type of emulsion or the other if the phase volume permits.

D. Factors affecting emulsification

1. **Interfacial tension.** The **internal phase** (oil or water) must be reduced to small droplets. This can be done only if necessary energy in the form of work is applied to create small droplets. The amount of work required depends on the **interfacial tension** (the tension between the two phases of the system). The addition of an emulsifying agent reduces interfacial tension, thereby reducing the amount of energy needed to produce an emulsion.

2. **Surface free energy.** The energy or work can also be interpreted as surface free energy or excess potential energy, which makes an emulsion unstable.
   a. Surface free energy, however small, promotes coalescence and emulsion instability.
   b. Emulsifying agents provide a mechanical barrier to coalescence that counterbalances the surface free energy. Three mechanisms are thought to provide this barrier.
      (1) Some emulsifying agents function by forming a strong pliable film around the dispersed droplets.
      (2) **Charge repulsion** can cause the droplets to repel each other and prevent the coalescence. For example, the oil droplets in an aqueous phase usually possess an electrical charge, due to the nature of the emulsifying agent or resulting from absorption of ions from solution.
      (3) **Steric repulsion** occurs when the long hydrocarbon chains of the surfactant or emulsifying agent prevent water droplets in an oily phase from contacting each other. Thus, a more hydrophilic emulsifying agent tends to produce an o/w emulsion, whereas a more hydrophobic agent forms a w/o emulsion.

E. Emulsifying agents. Any compound that lowers the interfacial tension and forms a film at an interface can potentially function as an emulsifying agent. The effectiveness of the emulsifying agent depends on its chemical structure, concentration, solubility, pH, physical properties, and electrostatic effect. **True emulsifying agents** (primary agents) are capable of forming and stabilizing emulsions by themselves. **Stabilizers** (auxiliary agents) do not form acceptable emulsions when used alone but do assist primary agents in stabilizing the product (e.g., they may increase viscosity). Emulsifying agents may be **natural** or **synthetic**.

1. **Natural emulsifying agents:**
   a. **Acacia** forms a good stable emulsion of low viscosity that tends to cream easily, is acidic, and is stable at a pH range of 2–10. Like other gums, it is negatively charged, dehydrates easily, and generally requires a preservative. It is incompatible with Peruvian balsam, bismuth salts, and carbonates.
   b. **Tragacanth** forms a stable emulsion that is coarser than acacia emulsion. It is anionic, difficult to hydrate, and used mainly for its viscosity effects. Less than 1/10 of the amount used for acacia is needed.
   c. **Agar** is an anionic gum used primarily to increase viscosity. Its stability is affected by heating, dehydration, and destruction of charge. It is also susceptible to microbial degradation.
   d. **Pectin** is a quasi-emulsifier that is used in the same proportion as tragacanth.
   e. **Gelatin** provides good emulsion stabilization in the concentration range of 0.5%–1.0%. It may be anionic or cationic, depending upon isoelectric point. Type A gelatin (+) is used in acid media; type B gelatin (−), in basic media.
   f. **Methylcellulose** is nonionic and induces viscosity. It is used as a primary emulsifier with mineral oil or cod liver oil and yields an o/w emulsion. It is usually used in 2% concentration and forms a continuous film.
   g. **Carboxymethylcellulose** is anionic and usually used to increase viscosity. It tolerates alcohol up to 40%. It forms a basic solution and precipitates in the presence of free acids.

2. **Synthetic emulsifying agents** may be anionic, cationic, or nonionic
   a. **Anionic synthetic agents** include **sulfuric acid esters** (e.g., sodium lauryl sulfate), **sulfonic acid derivatives** (e.g., dioctyl sodium sulfosuccinate), and **soaps**. Soaps are for external use. They have a high pH and, therefore, are sensitive to the addition of acids and electrolytes.
      (1) **Alkali soaps** are hydrophilic and form o/w emulsion.
      (2) **Metallic soaps** are water insoluble and form w/o emulsion.
      (3) **Monovalent soaps** form o/w emulsion.
      (4) **Polyvalent soaps** form w/o emulsion.
   b. **Cationic synthetic agents** (e.g., benzalkonium chloride) are used as surface-active agents in 1% concentration. They are incompatible with soaps.
   c. **Nonionic synthetic agents** are resistant to the addition of acids and electrolytes.
      (1) The **sorbitan esters** known as **spans** are hydrophobic in nature and form w/o emulsion. They have low hydrophilic–lipophilic balance (HLB) values (1–9).
      (2) The **polysorbates** known as **tweens** are hydrophilic in nature and form o/w emulsion. They may form complexes with phenolic compounds. They have high HLB values (11–20).

F. Rating emulsifying agents

1. The **HLB system** provides a means by which to rate an emulsifying agent's balance between hydrophilic and lipophilic solution tendencies. As an emulsifying agent becomes more hydrophilic, its solubility in water increases, favoring formation of an o/w emulsion. Conversely, more lipophilic agents favor formation of w/o emulsions. Thus, the type of emulsion formed is related to the balance between hydrophilic and lipophilic solution tendencies of the surface-active emulsifying agent. (**Surface-active agents** or **surfactants** are amphiphiles in which the molecules or ions contain both hydrophilic and lipophilic portions.)
2. The **HLB scale** is a numerical scale extending from 1 to approximately 50 based on the balance between these two opposing tendencies.
   a. More hydrophilic surfactants have high HLB numbers (> 10).
   b. More lipophilic surfactants have low HLB numbers (1–10).
   c. HLB values help determine a surfactant's application (Tables 4-1 and 4-2).
   d. Tweens and spans with their widely different HLB values are often used in combination to provide an effective emulsifying agent, usually a total concentration of approximately 2% w/v.

G. Preparation. Emulsions may be prepared by the following four methods:

1. **Wet gum method** (also called the English method). A primary emulsion of the fixed oil, water, and acacia (in a 4:2:1 ratio) is prepared as follows.
   a. Two parts of water are added all at once to one part of acacia, and the mixture is triturated until a smooth mucilage is formed.
   b. Oil is then added in small increments (1–5 ml) with continuous trituration until the primary emulsion is formed.
   c. The mixture (an o/w emulsion) is then triturated for another 5 minutes.
   d. The mixture (o/w) may then be brought to volume with water and mixing.
2. **Dry gum method** (also called the continental method). A primary emulsion of the fixed oil, water, and acacia (in a 4:2:1 ratio) is prepared as follows:
   a. Oil is added to the acacia, and the mixture is triturated until the powder is distributed uniformly throughout the oil. Water is then added all at once, followed by rapid trituration to form the primary emulsion.

Table 4-1. Hydrophilic-Lipophilic Balance (HLB) Values Affecting Surfactant Application

HLB Value Range	Surfactant Application
0–3	Antifoaming agents
4–6	Water-in-oil emulsifying agents
7–9	Wetting agents
8–18	Oil-in-water emulsifying agents
13–15	Detergents
10–18	Solubilizing agents

Table 4-2. Commonly Used Surfactants and Their Hydrophilic–Lipophilic Balance (HLB) Values

Agent	HLB Value
Sorbitan trioleate (Span 85, Arlacel 85)	1.8
Sorbitan tristearate (Span 65)	2.1
Propylene glycol monostearate (pure)	3.4
Sorbitan sesquioleate (Arlacel C)	3.7
Sorbitan monooleate (Span 80y)	4.3
Sorbitan monostearate (Arlacel 60)	4.7
Glyceryl monostearate (Aldo 28, Tegin)	5.5
Sorbitan monopalmitate (Span 40, Arlacel 40)	6.7
Sorbitan monolaurate (Span 20, Arlacel 20)	8.6
Gelatin	9.8
Triethanolamine oleate (Trolamine)	12.0
Polyoxyethylene alkyl phenol (Igepal CA-630)	12.8
Tragacanth	13.2
Polyoxyethylene sorbitan monolaurate (Tween 21)	13.3
Polyoxyethylene castor oil (Atlas G-1794)	13.3
Polyoxyethylene sorbitan monooleate (Tween 80)	15.0
Polyoxyethylene sorbitan monopalmitate (Tween 40)	15.6
Polyoxyethylene sorbitan monolaurate (Tween 20)	16.7
Polyoxyethylene lauryl ether (Brij 35)	16.9
Polyoxyethylene monostearate (Myrj 52)	16.9
Sodium oleate	18.0
Sodium lauryl sulfate	40.0

b. Any remaining water and other ingredients are added to finish the product.

(1) Electrolytes in high concentration tend to crack an emulsion; thus, they should be added last in as dilute a form as possible.

(2) Alcoholic solutions, which tend to dehydrate and precipitate hydrocolloids, should be added in as dilute a form as possible.

3. Bottle method (a variation of the dry gum method used for volatile oils). Oil is added to the acacia in a bottle. The ratio of oil, water, and acacia should be 3:2:1 or 2:1:1, as the low viscosity of the volatile oil requires a higher proportion of acacia.

4. Nascent soap method. A soap is formed by mixing relatively equal volumes of an oil and an aqueous solution containing a sufficient amount of alkali. The soap thus formed acts as an emulsifying agent.

a. This method can be used for forming an o/w or w/o emulsion, depending on the soap formed. For example, olive oil, which contains oleic acid, and lime water are mixed during the preparation of calamine lotion to calcium oleate, an emulsifying agent.

b. A 50:50 ratio of oil to water ensures sufficient formation of emulsifying agent, provided the oil contains an adequate amount of free fatty acid. (Olive oil usually does; cottonseed oil, peanut oil, and some other vegetable oils do not.)

c. The addition of an acid destroys the emulsifying soap, causing separation of the emulsion.

H. Incorporation of medicinal agents. Medicinal agents may be incorporated into an emulsion either during the formation of the emulsion or after the emulsion is formed.

1. Addition of a drug during emulsion formation. Generally, it is best to incorporate a drug into a vehicle during emulsion formation when it can be incorporated in molecular form. Soluble drugs should be dissolved in the appropriate phase (e.g., drugs soluble in the external phase of the emulsion should be added as a solution to the primary emulsion).

2. Addition of a drug to a preformed emulsion may present some difficulty, which can be overcome by keeping in mind the type of emulsion and the nature of the emulsifier (Table 4-3).

a. Addition of oleaginous materials to a w/o emulsion presents no problem because of the miscibility of the additive with the external phase, but **addition of oleaginous materials to an o/w emulsion** may be difficult after emulsion formation.

(1) Occasionally, a small amount of oily material may be added, if some excess emulsifier was used in the original formation.

Table 4-3. Selected Commercial Emulsion Bases: Emulsion Type and Emulsifier Used

Commercial Base	Emulsion Type	Emulsifier Used
Allercreme Skin Lotion	o/w	Triethanolamine stearate
Almay Emulsion Base	o/w	Fatty acid glycol esters
Cetaphil	o/w	Sodium lauryl sulfate
Dermovan	o/w	Fatty acid amides
Eucerin	w/o	Wool wax alcohols
HEB Base	o/w	Sodium lauryl sulfate
Keri Lotion	o/w	Nonionic emulsifiers
Lubriderm	o/w	Triethanolamine stearate
Neobase	o/w	Polyhydric alcohol esters
Neutrogena Lotion	o/w	Triethanolamine lactate
Nivea Cream	w/o	Wool wax alcohols
pHorsix	o/w	Polyoxyethylene emulsifiers
Polysorb Hydrate	w/o	Sorbitan sesquioleate
Velvachol	o/w	Sodium lauryl sulfate

w/o = water-in-oil.
o/w = oil-in-water.

(2) A small quantity of an oil-soluble drug may also be added if it is dissolved in a very small quantity of oil by using geometric dilution techniques.

b. **Addition of water or aqueous material to a w/o emulsion** is extremely difficult, unless enough emulsifier has been incorporated into the emulsion, but **addition of aqueous materials to an o/w emulsion** usually presents no problems if the added material does not interact with the emulsifying agent. Potential interactions should be expected with cationic compounds and salts of weak bases.

c. **Addition of small quantities of alcoholic solutions to an o/w emulsion** is possible, provided the solute is compatible or dispersible in the aqueous phase of the emulsion. If acacia or other gum is used as the emulsifying agent, the alcoholic solution should be diluted with water before addition. Some commercial emulsion bases and their general composition are included in Table 4-3.

d. **Addition of crystalline drugs to a w/o emulsion** occurs more easily if they are dissolved in a small quantity of oil before addition.

I. Emulsion stability. Creaming and coalescence may affect emulsion stability

1. **Creaming** occurs when suspended particles or droplets tend to rise or sediment, a process that depends on the specific gravities of the phases.
   a. Large particles cream much more rapidly than small particles; thus, formation of large aggregates by coalescence accelerates creaming.
   b. If creaming takes place without any aggregation, the emulsion can be reconstituted by mixing or shaking.

2. **Coalescence** is a process by which the emulsified particles merge with each other to form large particles. The major factor that prevents coalescence in the emulsion is the mechanical strength of the interfacial barrier. This is particularly true in o/w systems containing nonionic surfactants and w/o emulsion systems in which electrical effects are negligible. Thus, it is clear that the formation of thick interfacial film is essential in minimal coalescence.

IV. OINTMENTS

A. Introduction. Ointments are **semisolid preparations intended for external use**. They are easily spread; their plastic viscosity may be controlled by modification of the formulation. Ointments are typically used as:

1. **Emollients,** which make the skin more pliable
2. **Protective barriers,** which prevent harmful substances from coming in contact with the skin
3. **Vehicles** in which to incorporate medication

B. Ointment bases

1. **Oleaginous bases** are anhydrous and insoluble in water; they cannot absorb or contain water and are not washable in water.
   a. **Petrolatum** is a good base for oil-insoluble ingredients. It forms an occlusive film on the skin, absorbs less than 5% water under normal conditions, and does not become rancid. Wax may be incorporated to stiffen the base.
   b. **Synthetic esters** are used as oleaginous base constituents, including glyceryl monostearate, isopropyl myristate, isopropyl palmitate, butyl stearate, and butyl palmitate. Long-chain alcohols, such as cetyl alcohol, steryl alcohol and polyethylene glycol (PEG), may also be used.
   c. **Lanolin derivatives** are commonly used in topical and cosmetic preparations. Examples include lanolin oil (Lantrol) and hydrogenated lanolin.

2. **Absorption bases** are anhydrous, water-insoluble, and, therefore, not washable in water; however, these bases can absorb water. They permit the inclusion of water-soluble medicaments through prior solution and uptake of the solution as the internal phase.
   a. **Wool fat** (anhydrous lanolin) contains a high percent of cholesterol as well as esters and alcohol containing fatty acids. It absorbs twice its weight in water and melts between 36° C and 42° C.
   b. **Hydrophilic petrolatum** is a white petrolatum combined with 8% white beeswax, 3% stearyl alcohol, and 3% cholesterol, which are added to a w/o emulsifier.
      (1) Prepared forms include Aquaphor, which employs wool alcohol to render white petrolatum emulsifiable; Polysorb, which uses sorbitan sesquioleate, and Arlacel A as the emulsifiers (Kessolin).
      (2) Kessolin appears to be superior to the USP base. Aquaphor is superior in its ability to absorb water.

3. **Emulsion bases** may be w/o emulsions, which are water-insoluble and not washable in water but can absorb water because of their aqueous internal phase, or o/w emulsions, which are water-insoluble but washable in water and able to absorb water in their aqueous external phase.
   a. **Hydrous wool fat** (lanolin) is a w/o emulsion containing about 25% water. It acts as an emollient and forms occlusive films on the skin, effectively preventing epidermal water loss.
   b. **Cold cream** is a w/o emulsion prepared by melting white wax, spermaceti, and expressed almond oil together, adding hot aqueous solution of sodium borate, and stirring until cool.
      (1) Use of mineral oil rather than almond oil makes a more stable cold cream; however, cold cream prepared with almond oil makes a better emollient base.
      (2) This ointment should be freshly prepared.
   c. **Hydrophilic ointment** is an o/w emulsion employing sodium lauryl sulfate as an emulsifying agent. It absorbs about 30%–50% w/w without losing consistency. It is readily miscible with water and, thus, can be removed from the skin easily.
   d. **Vanishing cream** is an o/w emulsion, which contains a large percentage of water as well as humectant (e.g., glycerin, propylene glycol), which retards surface evaporation of the product. An excess of stearic acid in the formula helps to form a thin film when the water evaporates.
   e. **Other emulsion bases** include Dermovan, a hypoallergenic, greaseless emulsion base, and Unibase, a nongreasy emulsion base that absorbs about 30% of its weight in water and has a pH close to that of skin.

C. Water-soluble bases may be anhydrous or may contain some water. They are washable in water and absorb water to the point of solubility

1. **PEG ointment** consists of a blend of water-soluble polymeric glycols that form a semisolid base capable of solubilizing water-soluble drugs and some water-insoluble drugs. It is compatible with a wide range of drugs.
   a. This base contains 40% PEG 4000 and 60% PEG 400 and is prepared by the fusion method (see IV D 2).
   b. Only a small amount of liquid ($< 5\%$) can be incorporated without loss of viscosity. This base can be made stiffer by increasing the amount of PEG 4000 up to 60%.

2. **Propylene glycol** and **propylene glycol-ethanol** form a clear gel when mixed with 2% hydroxypropyl cellulose. This base has become popular as a dermatologic vehicle.

D. Incorporation of medicinal agents. Substances may be incorporated into an ointment base by **levigation** or by the **fusion method**. Insoluble substances should be first reduced to the finest possible form and levigated before incorporation, by levigating with a small amount of a compatible levigating agent or with the base itself.

1. **Levigation.** The substance is incorporated into the ointment by levigation on an ointment slab.
   a. Stainless steel spatulas with long flexible broad blades should be used for levigating. If interaction with a metal spatula is possible (as when incorporating iodine and mercuric salts), a hard rubber spatula may be used.
   b. Insoluble substances should be powdered finely in a mortar and then may be mixed with an equal quantity of base until a smooth grit-free mixture is obtained. The rest of the base is added in increments.
   c. Levigation of powder into a small portion of base may be facilitated by using a melted base or by using a small quantity of compatible levigation aid, such as mineral oil or glycerin.
   d. Water-soluble salts may be incorporated by dissolving them in the smallest possible amount of water and then incorporating the aqueous solution directly into the base, if the base is compatible.
      (1) Usually organic solvents such as ether, chloroform, or alcohol should not be used for dissolving the drug because the drug may crystallize as the solvent evaporates.
      (2) Solvents should be used as levigating aids only if the solid is going to become a fine powder, following the evaporation of the solvent.

2. **Fusion method.** This method may be used when the base contains solids with higher melting points, such as waxes, cetyl alcohol, and glyceryl monostearate. This method is also useful for solid medicaments, which are readily soluble in the melted base.
   a. The oil phase should be melted separately, starting with materials with the highest melting point. All other oil-soluble ingredients are then added in a decreasing order of melting point.
   b. The ingredients in the water phase are combined and heated separately to a temperature equal to, or several degrees above, that of the melted oil phase.
   c. The two phases are then combined. If a w/o system is desired, the hot aqueous phase is incorporated into the hot oil phase with agitation. If an o/w system is preferred, the hot oil phase is incorporated into the hot aqueous phase.
   d. Volatile materials (e.g., menthol, camphor, iodine, alcohol, perfumes) should be added after the melted mixture has cooled to about 40° C or less.

V. SUPPOSITORIES

A. Introduction. A suppository is a **solid or semisolid mass intended to be inserted into a body orifice** (e.g., the rectum, vagina, urethra) to provide either a local or systemic therapeutic effect. Once inserted, a suppository either melts at body temperature or dissolves (or disintegrates) into the cavity's aqueous secretions.

1. Suppositories are frequently used for local effects such as relief of hemorrhoids or infection in the rectum, vagina, or urethra.

2. Suppositories can provide systemic medication when used rectally. The absorption of drug from a suppository through a rectal mucosa into the circulation involves two steps:
   a. Release of the drug from a vehicle, followed by diffusion of the drug through the mucosa.
   b. The drug is then transported via veins or lymph vessels into the blood circulation. Since the rectal veins bypass the liver, the first-pass effect is avoided.

3. Rectal suppositories are useful when oral administration is inappropriate, as with infants; debilitated individuals; comatose patients; and patients with nausea, vomiting, and gastrointestinal disturbances. Some drugs may cause irritation to the gastrointestinal tract.

B. Types of suppositories

1. **Rectal suppositories** are usually cylindrical and tapered to a point, forming a bullet-like shape. Contraction of the rectum causes a suppository of this shape to move inward rather than outward. The adult suppository weighs about 2 g; suppositories for infants or children are smaller.

2. **Vaginal suppositories** are oval and typically weigh about 5 g. Drugs administered by this route are intended to have a local effect, but systemic absorption can occur. Antiseptics, contraceptive agents, and drugs used to treat trichomonal, monilial, or bacterial infections are commonly formulated into suppositories.

3. **Urethral suppositories** are long and tapered, having a length of about 60 mm and a diameter of 4–5 mm. Drugs administered by this route (usually anti-infectives) have local action only. The only urethral suppository in common use is the nitrofurazone (Furacin) urethral insert.

C. Suppository bases

1. **Criteria for satisfactory suppository bases.** Suppository bases should:
   a. Remain firm at room temperature for insertion. (Preferably, it should not soften below 30° C to avoid premature melting during storage)
   b. Have a narrow (or sharp) melting range
   c. Yield a clear melt just below body temperature or dissolve or disintegrate rapidly in the cavity fluid
   d. Be inert and compatible with a variety of drugs
   e. Be nonirritating and nonsensitizing
   f. Have wetting and emulsifying properties
   g. If the base is fatty, it should have an acid value below 0.2, a saponification value in the range of 200–245, and an iodine value less than 7

2. **Selecting a suppository base.** The lipid–water solubility must be considered because of its relationship to the rate of drug release.
   a. If an oil-soluble drug is incorporated into an oily base, the rate of absorption is somewhat less than that achieved with a water-soluble base. The lipid-soluble drug tends to remain dissolved in the oily pool from the suppository and has less tendency to escape into mucous secretions from which it is ultimately absorbed.
   b. Conversely, a water-soluble drug tends to pass more rapidly from the oil phase to the aqueous phase. Therefore, if rapid onset of action is desired, the water-soluble drug should be incorporated into the oily base.

3. **Bases that melt** include **cocoa butter,** other **combinations of fats and waxes,** the **witepsol bases,** and **wecobee bases** (Table 4-4)
   a. **Cocoa butter** (theobroma oil) is the most widely used suppository base. It is firm and solid up to a temperature of 32° C at which point it begins to soften. At 34–35° C, it melts to produce a thin, bland, oily liquid.
      (1) Cocoa butter is a good base for a **rectal suppository** but is less than ideal for a vaginal or urethral suppository.
      (2) A mixture of triglycerides, cocoa butter exhibits polymorphism. Depending upon the fusion temperature, it may crystallize into any one of the four crystal forms.
      (3) **Major limitations of cocoa butter.** Because of the following limitations, many combinations of fats and waxes are used as substitutes (see Table 4-4).
         (a) An inability to absorb aqueous solutions. The addition of nonionic surfactants to the base ameliorates this problem to some extent; however, the resultant suppositories exhibit poor stability and may turn rancid rapidly.
         (b) The lowering of the melting point produced by certain drugs (e.g., chloral hydrate)

Table 4-4. Composition, Melting Range, and Congealing Range of Selected Bases That Melt

Base	Composition	Melting Range (° C)	Congealing Range (° C)
Cocoa butter	Mixed triglycerides of oleic, palmitic, and stearic acids	34–35	28 or less
Cotmar	Partially hydrogenated cottonseed oil	34–75	. . .
Dehydag	Hydrogenated fatty alcohols and esters		
Base I		33–36	32–33
Base II		37–39	36–37
Base III		9 ranges	9 ranges
Wecobee R	Glycerides of saturated fatty acids C_{12}–C_{18}	33–35	31–32
Wecobee SS	Triglycerides derived from coconut oil	40–43	33–35
Witepsol	Triglycerides of saturated fatty acids C_{12}–C_{18},		
H-12	with varied portions of the corresponding	32–33	29–31
H-15	partial glycerides	33–35	32–34
H-85		42–44	36–38

b. **Witepsol bases** contain natural saturated fatty acid chains between C_{12} and C_{18} with lauric acid being the major component. All 12 bases of this series are colorless and almost odorless. Witepsol H15 has drug-release characteristics similar to those of cocoa butter.
   (1) Unlike cocoa butter, witepsol bases do not exhibit polymorphism when heated and cooled.
   (2) The interval between softening and melting temperature is very small. Because witepsol bases solidify rapidly in the mold, lubrication of the mold is not necessary.
c. **Wecobee bases** are derived from coconut oil and appear similar in action to witepsol bases. Incorporation of glyceryl monostearate and propylene glycol monostearate make these bases emulsifiable.

4. **Bases that dissolve** include PEG polymers in the molecular weight range of 400–6000.
   a. At room temperature, PEG 400 is a liquid, PEG 1000 is a semisolid, PEG 1500 and 1540 are fairly firm semisolids, and PEG 4000 and 6000 are firm, wax-like solids.
   b. These bases are water-soluble; however, the dissolution process is very slow. In the rectum and the vagina, where the amount of fluid is very small, they dissolve very slowly, but they soften and spread.
   c. Several drugs complex with PEG, which influences drug release and absorption.
   d. Mixtures of PEG polymers in varying proportions provide a base of different properties (Table 4-5).

D. Preparation. Suppositories may be prepared by the following three methods:

1. **Hand-rolling** involves molding the suppository with the fingers after the formation of a plastic mass.
   a. A finely powdered drug is mixed with the grated base in a mortar and pestle, using levigation and geometric dilution techniques. A small quantity of fixed oil may be added to facilitate the preparation of the mass.
   b. The uniformly mixed semiplastic mass is kneaded further and then rolled into a cylinder.

2. **Compression** is generally employed when cocoa butter is used as a base.
   a. A uniform mixture of drug and base is prepared as for the hand-rolling method.
   b. The mixture is then placed into a chamber mold, and the mold is cooled.
   c. This procedure generally produces a 2-g suppository; however, the volume of the active ingredients may affect the amount of cocoa butter required for an individual formula, if the active ingredient is present in a relatively large amount.
      (1) The amount of cocoa butter needed may be determined by calculating the total amount of active ingredient to be used, dividing this number by the cocoa butter density factor (Table 4-6) and subtracting the resulting number from the total amount of cocoa butter required for the desired number of suppositories.
      (2) For example, suppose 12 suppositories, each containing 300 mg of aspirin, are required. The mold has a 2-g capacity. For 13 suppositories (calculated to provide one extra), 3.9 g of aspirin (13×0.3 g = 3.9 g) is required. This is divided by the density factor of aspirin (1.1) [see Table 4-6]. Thus, 3.9 g of aspirin replaces 3.55 g of cocoa butter. The total amount of cocoa butter needed for 13 suppositories of 2 g each equals 26 g; with aspirin needed, the amount of cocoa butter required is 26 g − 3.55 g, or 22.45 g.

Table 4-5. Mixtures of Polyethylene Glycol (PEG) Bases Providing Satisfactory Room Temperature Stability and Dissolution Characteristics

Base	Comments	Components	Proportion (%)
1	Provides a good general-purpose, water-soluble suppository base	PEG 6000	50
		PEG 1540	30
		PEG 400	20
2	Provides a good general-purpose base that is slightly softer than base 1 and dissolves more readily	PEG 4000	60
		PEG 1000	30
		PEG 400	10
3	Has a higher melting point than the other bases, which is usually sufficient to compensate for the melting-point lowering effect of such drugs as chloral hydrate and camphor	PEG 6000	30
		PEG 1540	70

Table 4-6. Cocoa Butter Density Factors of Drugs Commonly Used in Suppositories

Drug	Cocoa Butter Density Factor	Drug	Cocoa Butter Density Factor
Aloin	1.3	Dimenhydrinate	1.3
Aminophylline	1.1	Diphenhydramine hydrochloride	1.3
Aminopyrine	1.3	Gallic acid	2.0
Aspirin	1.1	Morphine hydrochloride	1.6
Barbital sodium	1.2	Pentobarbital	1.2
Belladonna extract	1.3	Phenobarbital sodium	1.2
Bismuth subgallate	2.7	Salicylic acid	1.3
Chloral hydrate	1.3	Secobarbital sodium	1.2
Codeine phosphate	1.1	Tannic acid	1.6
Digitalis leaf	1.6		

3. **The fusion method** is the principal way of making suppositories commercially and is primarily used when cocoa butter, PEG, and glycerin–gelatin bases are used. Molds made of aluminum, brass, or nickel–copper alloys are employed, which can make from 6–50 suppositories.
   a. **Capacity of the molds** is determined by melting a sufficient quantity of base over a steam bath, pouring it into the molds, and allowing it to congeal. The sample suppositories are then trimmed, removed, and weighed. Once the weight is known, the suppositories can be prepared.
      (1) To prepare suppositories, the drug is reduced to a fine powder, and a small amount of grated cocoa butter is liquified in a suitable container placed in a water bath at 33° C or less.
      (2) The finely powdered drug is mixed with melted cocoa butter with continuous stirring.
      (3) The remainder of the grated cocoa butter is added with stirring, while maintaining the temperature at 33° C or below. The liquid should appear creamy rather than clear.
      (4) The creamy melt is poured into the mold at room temperature. The mold must be very lightly lubricated with mineral oil; the melt should be poured continuously to avoid layering.
      (5) The suppositories are allowed to congeal and then are placed in a refrigerator for 30 minutes to harden. Then they can be removed from the refrigerator, trimmed, and unmolded.
   b. The fusion process should be used carefully with **thermolabile drugs** and **insoluble powders**.
      (1) **Insoluble powders** in the liquid may settle during pouring, collecting at the top of the suppository and causing a nonuniform drug distribution.
      (2) **Hard crystalline materials** (e.g., iodine, merbromin) can be incorporated by dissolving the crystals in a minimum volume of suitable solvent prior to incorporation into the base.
      (3) **Vegetable extract** can be incorporated by moistening with a few drops of alcohol and levigating with a small amount of melted cocoa butter.

VI. POWDERS

A. **Introduction.** A pharmaceutical powder is a **mixture of finely divided drugs or chemicals in dry form** meant for internal or external use.

1. **Advantages of powder**
   a. Flexibility of compounding
   b. Good chemical stability
   c. Rapid dispersion of ingredients (because of the small particle size)

2. **Disadvantages of powder**
   a. Time-consuming preparation
   b. Inaccuracy of dose
   c. Unsuitability for many unpleasant tasting, hygroscopic, and deliquescent drugs

3. **Milling** is the mechanical process of reducing the particle size of solids (**comminution**) before incorporation into a final product (Tables 4-7 and 4-8). The particle size of a given powder is related to the proportion of the powder that can pass through the opening of standard sieves of varying dimensions in a specified time period. (**Micrometrics** is the study of particle size.) After milling, various substances are mixed as needed.
   a. **Advantages of milling**
      (1) Increases the surface area, which may increase dissolution rate and bioavailability (e.g., griseofulvin)
      (2) Increases extraction or leaching from animal glands (such as the liver and pancreas) and from crude vegetable extracts
      (3) Facilitates drying of wet masses by increasing surface area and reducing the distance moisture must travel to reach the outer surface; micronization and subsequent drying, in turn, increase stability as occluded solvent is removed.
      (4) Improves mixing or blending of several solid ingredients if they are reduced to approximately the same size; minimizes segregation and provides greater dose uniformity
      (5) Permits uniform distribution of coloring agents in artificially colored solid pharmaceuticals
      (6) Improves the function of lubricants used in compressed tablets and capsules to coat the surface of the granulation or powder
      (7) Improves the texture, appearance, and physical stability of ointments, creams, and pastes
   b. **Disadvantages of milling**
      (1) May change the polymorphic form of the active ingredient, rendering it less active
      (2) May degrade the drug as a result of heat buildup during milling, oxidation, or adsorption of unwanted moisture (due to increased surface area)
      (3) Decreases the bulk density of the active compound and excipients, causing flow problems and segregation
      (4) Decreases raw material particle size, possibly creating static charge problems that may cause particle aggregation and decreased dissolution rate
      (5) Increases surface area, which may promote air adsorption that may inhibit wettability of the drug
   c. **Comminution techniques.** On a large scale, various mills and pulverizers (e.g., rotary cutter, hammer, roller, fluid energy mill) may be used during manufacturing. On a small scale, the pharmacist usually uses one of the following comminution techniques:
      (1) **Trituration.** The substance is reduced to small particles by rubbing it in a mortar with a pestle. The term is also used to designate the process by which fine powders are intimately mixed in a mortar.
      (2) **Pulverization by intervention.** Substances are reduced and subdivided with an additional material (i.e., solvent) that can be removed easily after pulverization is complete. The technique is often used with substances that are gummy and tend to reagglomerate or tend to resist grinding; for example, camphor can be reduced readily after the addition of a small amount of alcohol or other volatile solvent, which is then permitted to evaporate.
      (3) **Levigation.** The substance is reduced in particle size by adding a suitable nonsolvent (levigating agent) to form a paste and then rubbing the paste in a mortar and pestle or using an ointment slab and spatula. This method is often used to incorporate solids into dermatologic or ophthalmic ointments and suspensions, to prevent a gritty feel. Mineral oil is a common levigating agent.

Table 4-7. *United States Pharmacopeia (USP)* Standards for Powders of Animal and Vegetable Drugs

Type of Powder	Sieve Size All Particles Pass Through	Sieve Size Percentage of Particles Pass Through
Very coarse (#8)	#20 sieve	20% through a #60 sieve
Coarse (#20)	#20 sieve	40% through a #60 sieve
Moderately coarse (#40)	#40 sieve	40% through a #80 sieve
Fine (#60)	#60 sieve	40% through a #100 sieve
Very fine (#80)	#80 sieve	No limit

Table 4-8. *United States Pharmacopeia (USP)* Standards for Powders of Chemicals

Type of Powder	Sieve Size All Particles Pass Through	Sieve Size Percentage of Particles Pass Through
Coarse (#20)	#20 sieve	60% through a #40 sieve
Moderately coarse (#40)	#40 sieve	60% through a #60 sieve
Fine (#80)	#80 sieve	No limit
Very fine (#120)	#120 sieve	No limit

B. Mixing powders. Powders may be mixed (blended) by the following five methods:

1. **Spatulation.** Small amounts of powders are blended by the movement of a spatula through the powders on a sheet of paper or a pill tile.
   - **a.** This method is not suitable for large quantities of powders or for powders containing one or more potent substances because homogeneous blending may not occur.
   - **b.** It is particularly useful for solid substances that liquify or form **eutectic mixtures** (mixtures that melt at lower temperature than any of their ingredients) when in close and prolonged contact with one another since very little compression or compaction results.
     - **(1)** Such substances include phenol, camphor, menthol, thymol, aspirin, phenylsalicylate, phenacetin, and other similar chemicals.
     - **(2)** To diminish contact, powders prepared from such substances are commonly mixed in the presence of an inert diluent such as light magnesium oxide or magnesium carbonate, kaolin, starch, or bentonite.
     - **(3)** Silicic acid (about 20%) prevents eutexia with aspirin, phenylsalicylate, and other troublesome compounds.
2. **Trituration** is used both to comminute and to mix powders.
   - **a.** If comminution is desired, a porcelain or a Wedgwood mortar with a rough inner surface is preferred to a glass mortar with a smooth working surface.
   - **b.** A glass mortar may be preferred for chemicals that may stain a porcelain or Wedgwood surface and for simple admixture of substances without special need for comminution. A glass mortar cleans more readily after use.
3. **Geometric dilution** is employed when potent substances are to be mixed with a large amount of diluent.
   - **a.** The potent drug is placed upon an approximately equal volume of diluent in a mortar, and the substances are thoroughly mixed by trituration.
   - **b.** A second portion of diluent, equal in volume to the powder mixture in the mortar, is added, and the trituration is repeated. The process is continued, adding equal volumes of diluent to that powder present in the mortar until all the diluent is incorporated.
4. **Sifting.** Powders are mixed by passing them through sifters similar to those used to sift flour. This process results in a light, fluffy product and is generally not acceptable for incorporation of potent drugs into a diluent base.
5. **Tumbling** is the process of mixing powders in a large container rotated by a motorized process. These blenders are widely employed in industry, as are large-volume powder mixers, which use motorized blades to blend the powder contained in a large mixing vessel.

C. Use and packaging of powders. Depending upon their intended use, powders are packaged and dispensed by pharmacists as bulk powders or as divided powders.

1. **Bulk powders** are dispensed by the pharmacist in bulk containers: a **perforated or sifter can** for external dusting; an **aerosol container** for spraying onto skin; or a **wide-mouthed glass or pasteboard jar** that permits easy removal of a spoonful of powder.
   - **a. Powders commonly dispensed in bulk form**
     - **(1) Antacid powders** and **laxative powders,** used by mixing the directed amount of powder (usually a teaspoonful or so) in a portion of liquid, which is then drunk
     - **(2) Douche powders,** dissolved in warm water and applied vaginally
     - **(3) Medicated or nonmedicated powders for external use,** usually dispensed in a sifter to aid convenient application to the skin

(4) **Dentifrices** or **dental cleansing powders,** used for oral hygiene

(5) **Insufflations** (e.g., powders meant to be blown into body cavities such as the ear, nose, throat, tooth sockets, vagina) administered by means of insufflator (powder blower)

b. **Nonpotent substances** are generally dispensed in bulk powder form. Those intended for external use should bear a label indicating this.

c. **Hygroscopic, deliquescent, or volatile powders** should be packed in glass jars rather than pasteboard containers. Amber or green glass should be used if needed to prevent the light-sensitive components of the powder from decomposition. All powders should be stored in tightly closed containers.

2. **Divided powders** are dispensed in the form of individual doses, generally in properly folded papers (i.e., **chartulae**). However, they may also be dispensed in metal foil; small, heat-sealed plastic bags; or other containers.

a. After weighing, comminuting, and mixing ingredients, the powders must be accurately divided into the prescribed number of doses.

b. Depending upon the potency of the drug substance, the pharmacist decides whether to weigh each portion separately before packaging or to approximate portions by the block-and-divide method.

c. **Powder papers** may be of any convenient size that fits the required dose. There are four basic types of powder papers.

(1) **Vegetable parchment,** a thin semiopaque moisture-resistant paper

(2) **White bond,** an opaque paper with no moisture-resistant properties

(3) **Glassine,** a glazed, transparent moisture-resistant paper

(4) **Waxed paper,** a transparent waterproof paper

d. Hygroscopic drugs and volatile drugs can be protected best with waxed paper, double-wrapped with a bond paper to improve the appearance. Parchment and glassine papers are of limited use for these drugs.

D. Special problems. Volatile substances, eutectic mixtures, liquids, and hygroscopic or deliquescent substances present problems when mixing into powders that require special treatment.

1. **Volatile substances,** such as camphor, menthol, and essential oils, may be lost by volatilization after incorporation into powders. This process is prevented or retarded by use of heat-sealed plastic bags or by double wrapping with waxed or glassine paper inside white bond paper.

2. **Liquids** may be incorporated into divided powders in small amounts

a. Magnesium carbonate, starch, or lactose may be added to increase the absorbability of the powders by increasing surface area.

b. When the liquid is a solvent for a nonvolatile heat-stable compound, it may be evaporated gently in a water bath. Some fluidextracts and tinctures may be treated in this way.

3. **Hygroscopic and deliquescent substances** that become moist because of an affinity for moisture in the air may be prepared as divided powders by adding inert diluents. Double-wrapping is desirable for further protection.

4. **Eutectic mixtures.** See VI B 1 b.

VII. CAPSULES

A. Introduction. Capsules are **solid dosage forms in which one or more medicinal or inert substances are enclosed within a small gelatin shell**. Gelatin capsules may be hard or soft. Most are intended to be swallowed whole, but occasionally the contents may be removed from the gelatin shell and employed as a premeasured medicinal powder (e.g., Theo-Dur Sprinkle, an anhydrous theophylline preparation meant to be sprinkled on a small amount of soft food before ingestion).

B. Hard gelatin capsules

1. **Preparation** of filled hard capsules includes preparing the formulation, selecting the appropriate capsule, filling the capsule shells, and cleaning and polishing the filled capsules.

a. Empty hard capsule shells are manufactured from a mixture of gelatin, colorants, and sometimes an opacifying agent such as titanium dioxide; the *USP* also permits the addition of 0.15% sulfur dioxide to prevent decomposition of gelatin during manufacture.

b. **Gelatin USP** is obtained by the partial hydrolysis of collagen obtained from the skin, white connective tissue, and bones of animals. Type A and type B are obtained by acid and alkali processing, respectively.
c. Capsule shells are cast by dipping cold metallic molds or pins into gelatin solutions maintained at a uniform temperature and an exact degree of fluidity.
   (1) Variation in gelatin solution viscosity increases or decreases capsule wall thickness.
   (2) Once the pins have been withdrawn from the gelatin solution, they are rotated while being dried in kilns through which a strong blast of filtered air with controlled humidity is forced. Each capsule is then mechanically stripped, trimmed, and joined.

2. **Storage.** Hard capsules should be stored in tightly closed glass containers, protected from dust and extremes of humidity and temperature.
   a. These capsules contain 12%–16% water, varying with the storage conditions. When humidity is low, the capsules become brittle; if humidity is high, the capsules become flaccid and shapeless.
   b. Storage in high temperature areas also affects the quality of hard gelatin capsules.

3. **Sizes.** Hard capsules are available in a variety of sizes.
   a. Empty capsules are numbered from 000 (the largest size that can be swallowed) to 5 (the smallest size). Approximate capsule capacity ranges from 600 mg to 30 mg for capsules from 000 to 5, respectively; however, capacity varies because of varying densities of powdered drug materials and degree of pressure used in filling the capsules.
   b. Large sizes are available for veterinary medicine.
   c. **Selecting capsules.** Generally, hard gelatin capsules are used to encapsulate between 65 mg and 1 g of powdered material, including the drug and any diluents needed. Capsule size should be chosen carefully. A properly filled capsule should have its body filled with the drug mixture and its cap fully extended down the body. The cap is meant to enclose the powder, not to retain additional powder.
      (1) If the drug dose for a single capsule is inadequate to fill the capsule, a diluent, such as lactose must be added.
      (2) If the amount of drug representing a usual dose is too large to place in a single capsule, two or more capsules may be required to provide the particular dose.
      (3) Lubricants such as magnesium stearate (frequently less than 1%) are added to facilitate the flow of the powder when an automatic capsule filling machine is used.
      (4) Wetting agents such as lithium carbonate are added to capsule formulations to enhance drug dissolution.
   d. **Filling capsules.** Capsules are usually filled by the punch method.
      (1) The powder is placed on paper and flattened with a spatula so that the layer of powder is no more than about ⅓ the length of the capsule. The paper is held in the left hand, and the body of the capsule, held in the right hand, is pressed repeatedly into the powder until the body is filled. Then, the cap is replaced and the capsule weighed.
      (2) Granular material that does not lend itself well to the punch method may be poured into each capsule from the powder paper on which it was weighed.
      (3) Crystalline materials, especially materials consisting of a mass of filament-like crystals as with the quinine salts, will not fit into a capsule easily unless first powdered.
      (4) Once filled, capsules must be cleaned and polished.
         (a) On a small scale, capsules may be cleaned individually or in small numbers by rubbing them on a clean gauze or cloth.
         (b) On a large scale, many capsule-filling machines have a cleaning vacuum that removes any extraneous material from the capsules as they leave the machine.

C. Soft gelatin capsules

1. **Preparation**
   a. Soft gelatin capsules are prepared from gelatin shells to which glycerin or a polyhydric alcohol (e.g., sorbitol) has been added, rendering the shells elastic or plastic-like.
   b. These shells contain preservatives (e.g., methyl and propyl parabens, sorbic acid) to prevent the growth of fungi.

2. **Uses.** Soft gelatin shells, which are oblong, elliptical, or spherical in shape, may be used to contain liquids, suspensions, pasty materials, dry powders, or pelletized materials.
   a. Drugs commercially prepared in soft capsules include ethchlorvynol (Placidyl, Abbott),

demeclocycline hydrochloride (Declomycin, Lederle), chlorotrianisene (TACE, Merrell Dow), chloral hydrate (Noctec, Squibb), digoxin (Lanoxicaps, Burroughs Wellcome) vitamin A, and vitamin E.

b. Soft gelatin capsules are usually prepared by the plate process, using a rotary or reciprocating productive die.

D. Uniformity and disintegration

1. The uniformity of dosage forms can be demonstrated by either weight variation or content uniformity methods. The official compendia should be consulted for details of these procedures.
2. Disintegration tests are usually not required for capsules unless they have been treated to resist solution in gastric fluid (enteric-coated). In this case they must meet the requirements for disintegration of enteric-coated tablets.

VIII. TABLETS

A. Introduction

1. The **oral route** is the most important method of administering drugs when systemic effects are desired. Oral drugs may be given as solids or liquids.
   a. Advantages of solid dosage forms
   (1) Accurate dosage
   (2) Easy shipping and handling
   (3) Less shelf space needed per dose than for liquid
   (4) No preservation requirements
   (5) No taste-masking problem
   (6) Generally more stable than liquids with longer expiration dates
   b. Advantages of liquid dosage forms
   (1) The drug may be more effective in liquid than in solid form (e.g., adsorbents, antacids).
   (2) They may be useful for patients who have trouble swallowing solid dosage forms (e.g., pediatric and geriatric dosage forms).
2. **Tablets** are the **most commonly used solid dosage forms.**
   a. Advantages of tablets
   (1) Precision and low-content variability of the unit dose
   (2) Low manufacturing cost
   (3) Easy to package and ship
   (4) Simple to identify
   (5) Easy to swallow
   (6) Lend themselves to special-release forms
   (7) Best suited to large-scale production
   (8) Most stable of all oral dosage forms
   (9) Essentially tamperproof
   b. Disadvantages of tablets
   (1) Some drugs resist compression into tablets.
   (2) Some drugs (e.g., those with poor wetting, slow dissolution properties, intermediate to large doses, optimum absorption high in the gastrointestinal tract, or any combination of these features) may be difficult to formulate to provide adequate bioavailability.
   (3) Some drugs (e.g., bitter-tasting drugs, drugs with an objectionable odor, or those sensitive to oxygen or atmospheric moisture) may require encapsulation or entrapment prior to compression. A capsule form may be a better approach.

B. Tablet design and formulation

1. **Characteristics of ideal tablets**
   a. They should be free of defects, such as chips, cracks, discoloration, and contamination.
   b. They should have the strength to withstand the mechanical stresses of production.
   c. They should be chemically and physically stable over time.
   d. They should release the medicinal agents in a predictable and reproducible manner.

2. **Tablet excipients.** Tablets may be manufactured by **wet granulation, dry granulation,** or **direct compression**. Regardless of the method of manufacture, tablets for oral ingestion usually contain excipients, components added to the active ingredients that have special functions (Table 4-9).
   a. **Diluents** are fillers designed to make up the required bulk of the tablet when the drug dosage amount is inadequate. Diluents may also improve cohesion, permit use of direct compression, or promote flow.
      (1) **Common diluents** include kaolin, lactose, mannitol, starch, powdered sugar, and calcium phosphate.
      (2) **Selection of the diluent** is based partly on the experience of the manufacturer as well as on diluent cost and compatibility with the other tablet ingredients. For example, calcium salts cannot be employed as fillers for tetracycline products since calcium interferes with tetracycline's absorption from the gastrointestinal tract.
   b. **Binders and adhesives** are materials added in either dry or liquid form to promote the granulation process or to promote cohesive compacts during the direct compression process.
      (1) **Common binding agents** include a 10%–20% aqueous preparation of cornstarch; a 25%–50% solution of glucose; molasses; various natural gums, such as acacia; cellulose derivatives, such as methylcellulose, carboxymethylcellulose, and microcrystalline cellulose; gelatins; and povidone. The natural gums are variable in composition and usually contaminated with bacteria.
      (2) If the drug substance is adversely affected by an aqueous binder, a nonaqueous binder may be used, or the binder may be added dry. Generally, the binding action is more effective when binder is mixed in liquid form.
      (3) The amount of binder or adhesive used depends on the manufacturer's experience and on the other tablet ingredients. Overwetting usually results in granules that are too hard for proper tableting; underwetting usually results in the preparation of tablets that are too soft and tend to crumble.

Table 4-9. Common Tablet Excipients

Diluents	**Disintegrants**
Calcium phosphate dihydrate NF (dibasic)	Alginates
Calcium sulfate dihydrate NF	Cellulose
Cellulose NF (microcrystalline)	Cellulose derivatives
Cellulose derivatives	Clays
Dextrose	PVP (cross-linked)
Lactose USP	Starch
Lactose USP (anhydrous)	Starch derivatives
Lactose USP (spray-dried)	**Lubricants**
Mannitol USP	PEGs
Starches (directly compressible)	Stearic acid
Starches (hydrolyzed)	Stearic acid salts
Sorbitol	Stearic acid derivatives
Sucrose USP (powder)	Surfactants
Sucrose-based materials	Talc
	Waxes
Binders and adhesives	**Glidants**
Acacia	Cornstarch
Cellulose derivatives	Silica derivatives
Gelatin	Talc
Glucose	**Colors, flavors, and sweeteners**
PVP	FD&C and D&C dyes and lakes
Sodium alginate and alginate derivatives	Flavors are available in two forms:
Sorbitol	spray-dried and oils
Starch (paste)	Artificial sweeteners
Starch (pregelatinized)	Natural sweeteners
Tragacanth	

D&C = drugs and cosmetics; FD&C = food, drugs, and cosmetics; NF = National Formulary; PEG = polyethylene glycol; PVP = polyvinylpyrrolidone, more commonly called povidone.

c. **Disintegrants** are added to tablet formulations to facilitate tablet disintegration when it contacts water in the gastrointestinal tract. Disintegrants appear to function by drawing water into the tablet, swelling, and causing the tablet to burst.
   (1) Tablet disintegration may be critical to the subsequent dissolution of the drug and satisfactory drug bioavailability.
   (2) **Common disintegrants** include cornstarch and potato starch; starch derivatives, such as sodium starch glycolate; cellulose derivatives, such as sodium carboxymethylcellulose; clays, such as Veegum and bentonite; cation exchange resins; and others.
   (3) The total **amount of disintegrant** is not always added to the drug–diluent mixture. A portion may be added (with the lubricant) to the prepared granulation of the drug, causing double disintegration of the tablet. The portion of disintegrant added last causes the breakup of the tablets into small pieces or chunks; the portion added first breaks the pieces of tablet into fine particles.

d. **Lubricants, antiadherents, and glidants** have overlapping function.
   (1) **Lubricants** are intended to reduce the friction during tablet ejection between the walls of the tablet and the walls of the die cavity in which the tablet was formed. Talc, magnesium stearate, and calcium stearate are among those commonly used.
   (2) **Antiadherents** reduce sticking or adhesion of the tablet granulation or powder to the faces of the punches or to the die walls.
   (3) **Glidants** promote the flow of the tablet granulation or powder materials by reducing friction among particles.

e. **Colors and dyes** serve to disguise off color drugs, to provide product identification, and to produce a more elegant product. **Food, drug, and cosmetic dyes** and **drug and cosmetic dyes** are applied as solutions; **lakes** (dyes that have been absorbed on a hydrous oxide) are usually employed as dry powders.

f. **Flavoring agents** are usually limited to chewable tablets or tablets intended to dissolve in the mouth.
   (1) Generally, water-soluble flavors have poor stability; hence, flavor oils or dry powders are usually used.
   (2) Flavor oils may be added to tablet granulations in solvents, dispersed on clays and other adsorbents, or are emulsified in aqueous granulating agents. Usually, the maximum amount of oil that can be added to a granulation without influencing its tablet characteristics is 0.5%–0.75%.

g. **Artificial sweeteners,** like flavors, are usually used only with chewable tablets or tablets intended to dissolve in the mouth.
   (1) Some sweetness may come from the diluent (e.g., mannitol, lactose); agents such as saccharin and aspartame may also be added.
   (2) Saccharin has an unpleasant aftertaste
   (3) Aspartame is not stable in the presence of moisture.

h. **Adsorbents** (e.g., magnesium oxide, magnesium carbonate, bentonite, silicon dioxide) are substances capable of holding quantities of fluid in an apparently dry state.

C. **Tablet types and classes.** Tablets are classified by their route of administration, drug delivery system, and form and method of manufacture (Table 4-10).

1. **Tablets for oral ingestion** are designed to be swallowed intact with the exception of chewable tablets. They may be coated to mask the drug's taste, color, or odor; to control drug release;

Table 4-10. Tablet Types and Classes

Tablets for oral ingestion	Tablets used in the oral cavity
Compressed tablets	Buccal tablets
Multiple compressed tablets	Sublingual tablets
Layered tablets	Troches, lozenges, and dental cones
Compression-coated tablets	
Repeat-action tablets	**Tablets used to prepare solutions**
Delayed-action and enteric-coated tablets	Effervescent tablets
Sugar- and chocolate-coated tablets	Dispensing tablets
Film-coated tablets	Hypodermic tablets
Air suspension-coated tablets	Tablet triturates
Chewable tablets	

to protect the drug from the stomach's acid environment; to incorporate another drug, providing sequential release or avoiding incompatibilities; or to improve appearance.

a. **Compressed tablets** are formed by compression and have no special coating. They are made from powdered, crystalline, or granular materials, alone or in combination with such excipients as binders, disintegrants, diluents, and colorants.

b. **Multiple compressed tablets** may be layered or compression-coated.
   (1) **Layered tablets** are prepared by compressing an additional tablet granulation around a previously compressed granulation. The operation may be repeated to produce multiple layers.
   (2) **Compression-coated tablets** (also called **dry-coated tablets**) are prepared by feeding previously compressed tablets into a special tableting machine and compressing an outer shell around them. This process applies a thinner, more uniform coating than sugar-coating and can be used safely with drugs sensitive to moisture. It can be used to separate incompatible materials, to produce repeat-action or prolonged-action products, or to provide a multilayered appearance.

c. **Repeat-action tablets** are layered or compression-coated tablets in which the outer layer or shell provides an initial drug dose, rapidly disintegrating in the stomach [e.g., Repetabs (Schering) and Extentabs (Robins)]. The inner layer (or inner tablet) is comprised of components that are insoluble in gastric media but soluble in intestinal media.

d. **Delayed-action** and **enteric-coated tablets** delay the release of a drug from a dosage form to prevent drug destruction by gastric juices, to prevent stomach lining irritation by the drug, or to promote absorption, which may be better in the intestine than in the stomach.
   (1) Tablets coated so as to remain intact in the stomach but yield their ingredients in the intestines are said to be **enteric-coated**. [e.g., Enseals (Lilly) and Ecotrin (Smith Kline & French)] Enteric-coated tablets are a form of delayed-action tablet, but not all delayed-action tablets are enteric or intended to produce an enteric effect.
   (2) Among the agents used to enteric-coat tablets are fats, fatty acids, waxes, shellac, and cellulose acetate phthalate.

e. **Sugar-** and **chocolate-coated tablets** are compressed tablets coated to protect the drug from air and humidity, to provide a barrier to the drug's objectionable taste or smell, or to improve the tablet's appearance. Chocolate-coated tablets are rare today.
   (1) Sugar-coated tablets may be coated with a colored or an uncolored sugar. The process includes **seal coating** (waterproofing), **subcoating, syrup coating** (for smoothing and coloring), and **polishing,** all of which take place in a series of mechanically operated coating pans.
   (2) **Disadvantages of sugar-coating** include the time and expertise required for the process and the increase in tablet size and weight. Sugar-coated tablets may be 50% larger and heavier than the original tablets.

f. **Film-coated tablets** are compressed tablets coated with a thin layer of a water-insoluble or water-soluble polymer (e.g., hydroxypropyl methylcellulose, ethylcellulose, povidone, PEG).
   (1) The film is generally colored, and it is more durable, less bulky, and less time-consuming to apply than sugar-coating. It typically increases tablet weight by only 2%–3% and provides increased formulation efficiency, increased resistance to chipping, and increased output.
   (2) Film-coating solutions generally contain a film former, an alloying substance, a plasticizer, a surfactant, opacifiers, sweeteners, flavors, colors, glossants, and a volatile solvent.
   (3) The volatile solvents used in these solutions are expensive and potentially toxic when released into the atmosphere. Hence, manufacturers are exploring the development and use of **aqueous-based solutions**.

g. **Air suspension–coated tablets** are fed into a vertical cylinder and supported by a column of air that enters from the bottom of the cylinder. As the coating solution enters the system, it is rapidly applied to the suspended, rotating solids (**Wurster process**). Rounding coats can be applied in less than 1 hour with the assistance of warm air blasts released in the chamber.

h. **Chewable tablets** disintegrate smoothly and rapidly when chewed or allowed to dissolve in the mouth, yielding a creamy base (from specially colored and flavored mannitol).
   (1) These tablets are especially useful in formulations for children and are commonly used for multivitamin tablets.
   (2) They are also used for some antacids and antibiotics.

2. **Tablets used in the oral cavity** are allowed to dissolve in the mouth.
   a. **Buccal tablets** and **sublingual tablets** are absorbed through the oral mucosa after dissolving in the buccal pouch (buccal tablets) or below the tongue (sublingual tablets). These forms are useful for **drugs that are destroyed by gastric juice** or **poorly absorbed from the intestinal tract** such as sublingual nitroglycerin tablets, which dissolve very promptly to give rapid drug effects, and buccal progesterone tablets, which dissolve slowly.
   b. **Troches, lozenges,** and **dental cones** dissolve slowly in the mouth and provide primarily local effects.

3. **Tablets used to prepare solutions** are dissolved in water prior to administration.
   a. **Effervescent tablets** are prepared by compressing granular effervescent salts or other materials (e.g., citric acid, tartaric acid, sodium bicarbonate) that have the capacity to release carbon dioxide gas when in contact with water. Commercial alkalinizing analgesic tablets are frequently made to effervesce to encourage fast dissolution and absorption (e.g., Alka-Seltzer).
   b. **Other tablets** used to prepare solutions include dispensing tablets, hypodermic tablets, and tablet triturates.

D. Processing problems

1. **Capping** is the partial or complete separation of the top or bottom crowns of a tablet from the main body of the tablet. **Lamination** is separation of a tablet into two or more distinct layers. Both of these problems usually result from air entrapment during processing.

2. **Picking** is removal of a tablet's surface material by a punch. **Sticking** is adhesion of tablet material to a die wall. These problems may result from excessive moisture or substances with low melting temperatures in the formulation.

3. **Mottling** is an unequal color distribution on a tablet, with light or dark areas standing out on an otherwise uniform surface. This may result from use of a drug with a color different from that of the tablet excipients or from a drug with colored degradation products. Colorants may solve the problem but may also create other problems.

E. Tablet evaluation and control

1. **General appearance** of tablets is important for consumer acceptance, lot-to-lot uniformity, tablet-to-tablet uniformity, and monitoring of the manufacturing process. Tablet appearance includes visual identity and overall appearance. **Control of appearance** includes measurement of such attributes as size, shape, color, odor, taste, surface, texture, physical flaws, consistency, and legibility of any markings.

2. **Hardness** and **resistance to friability** are necessary for tablets to withstand the mechanical shocks of manufacture, packaging, and shipping, and to ensure consumer acceptance. Hardness relates to both tablet disintegration and to drug dissolution. Certain tablets intended to dissolve slowly are made hard, whereas others intended to dissolve rapidly are made soft. Friability relates to the tablet's tendency to crumble.
   a. **Tablet hardness testers** measure the degree of force required to break a tablet.
   b. **Friabilators** determine friability by allowing the tablet to roll and fall into a rotating tumbling apparatus. The tablets are weighed before and after a specified number of rotations, and the weight loss is determined.
      (1) **Resistance to weight loss** indicates the tablet's ability to withstand abrasion during handling, packaging, and shipping. Compressed tablets that lose less than 0.5%–1% of their weight are generally considered acceptable.
      (2) Some chewable tablets and most effervescent tablets are highly friable and require special unit packaging.

3. **Weight** of tablets is routinely measured to ensure that the tablet contains the proper amount of drug.
   a. The *USP* defines a **weight variation standard** to which tablets must conform.
   b. These standards are applicable for tablets containing 50 mg or more of drug substance in which the drug substance represents 50% or more (by weight) of the dosage form unit.

4. **Content uniformity** is evaluated to ensure that each tablet contains the amount of drug substance desired with little variation among contents within a batch. The *USP* defines content uniformity tests for tablets containing 50 mg or less of drug substance.

5. **Disintegration** is evaluated to ensure that the tablet's drug substance is fully available for absorption from the gastrointestinal tract.
   a. All *USP* tablets must pass an **official disintegration test** conducted in vitro with special equipment.
      (1) **Uncoated *USP* tablets** have disintegration times as low as 2 minutes (nitroglycerin) to 5 minutes (aspirin); the majority have a maximum disintegration time of 30 minutes.
      (2) **Buccal tablets** must disintegrate within 4 hours.
      (3) **Enteric-coated tablets** must show no evidence of disintegration after 1 hour in simulated gastric fluid. In simulated intestinal fluid, they should disintegrate in 2 hours plus the time specified.
   b. **Dissolution requirements** in the *USP* have replaced earlier disintegration requirements for many drugs.
6. **Dissolution characteristics** are tested to determine drug absorption and physiologic availability, which depend on the drug in its dissolved state.
   a. The *USP* gives **standards for tablet dissolution**.
   b. An increased emphasis on dissolution testing and determination of bioavailability has increased the use of sophisticated systems for the testing and analysis of tablet dissolution.

IX. CONTROLLED-RELEASE DOSAGE FORMS

A. **Introduction.** Controlled-release dosage forms (also known as delayed-release, sustained-action, prolonged-action, sustained-release, prolonged-release, timed-release, slow-release, extended-action, and extended-release forms) are **designed to release drug substance slowly for prolonged action in the body**. Controlled-release forms have the following **advantages**:
   1. Reduction of problems with patient compliance
   2. Employment of less total drug
   3. Minimization or elimination of local or systemic side effects
   4. Minimization of drug accumulation (with chronic dosage)
   5. Reduction of potentiation or loss of drug activity (with chronic use)
   6. Improvement in treatment efficiency
   7. Improvement in speed of control of condition
   8. Reduction in drug level fluctuation
   9. Improvement in bioavailability for some drugs
   10. Improvement in ability to provide special effects (e.g., morning relief of arthritis by bed-time dosing)
   11. Reduction in cost

B. **Sustained-release forms.** The variety of sustained-release forms available can be grouped by the pharmaceutical mechanism employed to provide controlled release.
   1. **Coated beads or granules** [e.g., Theo-Dur Sprinkle (Key), Spansules (Smith Kline & French), and Sequels (Lederle)] produce a blood-level profile similar to that obtained with multiple dosing.
      a. A solution of the drug substance in a nonaqueous solvent (e.g., alcohol) is coated onto small, inert beads or granules made of a combination of sugar and starch. (When the drug dose is large, the starting granules may be composed of the drug itself.)
      b. Some of the beads or granules are left uncoated to provide an immediate release of the drug.
      c. Coats of a lipid material (such as beeswax) or a cellulosic material (e.g., ethylcellulose) are applied to the remainder of the granules with some granules receiving few coats and some granules many. The various coating thicknesses produce a sustained-release effect.
   2. **Microencapsulation** is a process by which solids, liquids, or even gases are encapsulated into microscopic particles by formation of thin coatings of a "wall" material around the substance to be encapsulated. An **example** of a microencapsulated dosage form is Measurin (Winthrop).

a. **Coacervation,** which involves addition of a hydrophilic substance to a colloidal drug dispersion, is the most common method of microencapsulation.
b. **Hydrophilic substances,** which act as the coating material, are selected from a variety of natural and synthetic polymers, including shellacs, waxes, gelatin, starches, cellulose acetate phthalate, ethylcellulose, and others. Once the coating material dissolves, all the drug inside the microcapsule is immediately available for dissolution and absorption. Wall thickness can be varied from less than 1–200 μm by changing the amount of the coating material (3%–30% of total weight).

3. **Matrix devices** may employ insoluble plastics (e.g., polyethylene, polyvinyl acetate, polymethacrylate), hydrophilic polymers (e.g., methylcellulose, hydroxypropyl methylcellulose), or fatty compounds (e.g., various waxes, glyceryl tristearate). Examples include Gradumet (Abbott), Lonatabs (Geigy), Dospan (Merrell Dow), and Slow-K (Ciba).
   a. The most common method of preparation is **mixing of the drug with the matrix material** followed by **compression of the material into tablets.**
   b. The primary dose (the portion of the drug to be released immediately) is placed on the tablet as a layer or coat. The remainder of the dose is released slowly from the matrix.

4. **Osmotic systems** include the **Oros system,** an oral osmotic pump composed of a core tablet and a semipermeable coating with a 0.4-mm diameter hole (produced by a laser beam) for drug exit.
   a. This system requires only osmotic pressure to be effective and is essentially independent of pH changes in the environment.
   b. The drug-release rate can be changed by changing the surface area, the nature of the membrane, or the diameter of the drug-release hole.

5. **Ion-exchange resins** may be complexed to drugs by passage of a cationic drug solution through a column containing the resin. The drug is complexed to the resin by replacement of hydrogen atoms. Examples include Biphetamine capsules (Fisons; resin complexes of amphetamine and dextroamphetamine), Ionamin capsules (Fisons; resin complexes of phentermine), and the Pennkinetic system (Fisons), which incorporates a polymer barrier coating and bead technology in addition to the ion-exchange mechanism.
   a. After complexing, the **resin–drug complex** is washed and then tableted, encapsulated, or suspended in an aqueous vehicle.
   b. Drug release from the complex depends on the ionic environment within the gastrointestinal tract and on the resin's properties. Generally, release is greater in the highly acidic stomach than in the less acidic small intestine.

6. **Complex formation** may be used for certain drug substances that combine chemically with other agents. For example, hydroxypropyl-β-cyclodextrin forms a chemical complex that may be only slowly soluble from body fluids, depending on the pH of the environment.

7. **Hydrocolloid systems** (e.g., Valrelease, a slow-release form of diazepam) include a unique, **hydrodynamically balanced drug delivery system (HBS)** developed by Roche.
   a. The HBS consists of a matrix designed so that the dosage form, on contact with gastric fluid, demonstrates a bulk density less than one and, thus, remains buoyant.
   b. When in contact with gastric fluid, the outermost hydrocolloids swell to form a boundary layer, which prevents immediate penetration of fluid into the formulation.
   c. This outer hydrocolloid layer slowly erodes with subsequent formation of a new boundary layer.
   d. The process is continuous, with each new outer layer eroding slowly. The drug is released gradually through each layer as fluid slowly penetrates the matrix.

C. **Transdermal drug delivery systems (TDDS)** are designed to support the passage of drug substances from the skin surface, through the skin layers, and into the systemic circulation.

1. **Advantages of TDDS**
   a. Bypass of hepatic first-pass metabolism and gastrointestinal incompatibilities
   b. Improvement of patient compliance
   c. Ease of treatment termination (by removal of the TDDS)

2. **Microporous membranes** may be used as rate-controlling barriers in a TDDS. These membranes are a few millimeters thick and have varying pore sizes. They may be made from such materials as regenerated cellulose nitrate or acetate, polypropylene, and others.

3. **Examples** include the Transderm-Scōp (Ciba) and various systems for the delivery of nitroglycerin.
   a. The Transderm-Scōp system delivers scopolamine (to prevent and treat motion-induced nausea) without eliciting the side effects that normally accompany oral or intramuscular administration.
   b. TDDS nitroglycerin forms include Transderm-Nitro (Ciba), which employs a microporous membrane; Nitrodisc (Searle), which has the drug microsealed in a solid polymer; and Nitro-Dur (Key), which uses a 2% diffusion matrix.
      (1) These devices range from 5–20 cm^2 in surface area and are generally applied to the upper arm or chest. They release from 2.5–22.4 mg/24 hour, depending on the drug content and the surface area.
      (2) TDDS nitroglycerin offers a significant improvement in sustained-release therapy over sublingual nitroglycerin and nitroglycerin topical ointments.

X. DRUG PUBLICATIONS

A. *United States Pharmacopeia (USP)* and *The National Formulary (NF).* The *USP* and *NF* are the official compendia, legally recognized by the United States. Since 1975, both compendia are published as a single volume by the United States Pharmacopeial Convention, Inc., Rockville, Maryland. The *USP/NF* provides standards for drugs and chemicals used in the practice of medicine and pharmacy. The *USP* provides standards for drugs and their dosage forms and some medicinal devices; the *NF* provides standards for pharmaceutical ingredients, including excipients.

1. The monograph for each drug or dosage form establishes the following:
   a. Its official **title**
   b. A **definition** and **description** of the substance
   c. **Standards** for the following characteristics:
      (1) Identity
      (2) Quality
      (3) Strength
      (4) Purity
      (5) Packaging
      (6) Labeling
2. When feasible, the following information is also given:
   a. Standards for bioavailability and stability
   b. Proper handling and storage procedures
   c. Assay procedures
   d. Formulas for making the substance or dosage form
3. In addition, the *USP* provides a wealth of **general information** on such subjects as:
   a. Testing and assaying of products
   b. Controlled substances regulations
   c. Food and Drug Administration (FDA) requirements
   d. Good manufacturing practices
   e. Pharmaceutical dosage forms
   f. Factors affecting stability
   g. Sterilization
   h. Reagents and solutions used in tests and assays
   i. Container specifications for dispensing
   j. Molecular formulas and molecular weights

B. *United States Pharmacopeial Drug Information (USPDI).* The *USPDI System* is a three-volume (four-book) publication by the United States Pharmacopeial Convention, Inc., Rockville, Maryland, which is continually revised and provides drug information for the health care professional and the patient.

1. *Drug Information for the Health Care Professional* (volume I, parts IA and IB) includes information for prescribers, dispensers, and other health care professionals on categories of drug use.
2. *Advice for the Patient* (volume II) contains information for the patient. Monographs correspond directly to monographs in volume I and provide a coordinated approach to patient education, including patient consultation guidelines.

3. *Approved Drug Products and Legal Requirements* (volume III) includes information on bioequivalence and therapeutic equivalence relating to drug product selection available in the *FDA Orange Book*. In addition, this volume contains information on the federal Controlled Substances Act, Poison Prevention Packaging Act and Regulations, FD&C Act, Good Manufacturing Practices, and other legal information pertaining to pharmacy practice. Furthermore, a medicine chart, which is a drug product identification directory, is printed in color.

STUDY QUESTIONS

Directions: Each of the numbered items or incomplete statements in this section is followed by answers or by completions of the statement. Select the **one** lettered answer or completion that is **best** in each case.

1. All of the following statements concerning syrup NF are true EXCEPT

(A) it contains 850 g of sucrose
(B) it is made with purified water
(C) it has a specific gravity of 1.30
(D) it is a supersaturated solution
(E) it has a moderately high viscosity

2. All of the following preparations contain alcohol EXCEPT

(A) syrup USP
(B) terpin hydrate elixir USP
(C) aromatic ammonia spirit USP
(D) green soap tincture USP
(E) eriodictyon fluidextract NF

3. Which of the following solutions is used as an astringent?

(A) Strong iodine solution USP
(B) Aluminum acetate topical solution USP
(C) Acetic acid NF
(D) Aromatic ammonia spirit USP
(E) Benzalkonium chloride solution NF

4. The particle size of the dispersed solid in a suspension is usually greater than

(A) 0.5 μm
(B) 0.4 μm
(C) 0.3 μm
(D) 0.2 μm
(E) 0.1 μm

5. In the extemporaneous preparation of a suspension, levigation is used to

(A) reduce zeta potential
(B) avoid bacterial growth
(C) reduce particle size
(D) enhance viscosity
(E) reduce viscosity

6. Which of the following compounds is a natural emulsifying agent?

(A) Acacia
(B) Lactose
(C) Polysorbate 20
(D) Polysorbate 80
(E) Sorbitan monopalmitate

7. Vanishing cream is an ointment that may be classified as

(A) a water-soluble base
(B) an oleaginous base
(C) an absorption base
(D) an emulsion base
(E) an oleic base

8. Rectal suppositories intended for adult use usually weigh approximately

(A) 1 g
(B) 2 g
(C) 3 g
(D) 4 g
(E) 5 g

9. A satisfactory suppository base must meet all of the following criteria EXCEPT

(A) it should have a narrow melting range
(B) it should be nonirritating and nonsensitizing
(C) it should dissolve or disintegrate rapidly in the body cavity
(D) it should melt below 30° C
(E) it should be inert

10. Cocoa butter (theobroma oil) exhibits all of the following properties EXCEPT

(A) it melts at temperatures beween 33° C and 35° C
(B) it is a mixture of glycerides
(C) it is a polymorph
(D) it is useful in formulating rectal suppositories
(E) it is soluble in water

1-D 4-A 7-D 10-E
2-A 5-C 8-B
3-B 6-A 9-D

11. In the fusion method of making cocoa butter suppositories, which of the following substances is most likely to be used for lubricating the mold?

(A) Mineral oil
(B) Propylene glycol
(C) Cetyl alcohol
(D) Stearic acid
(E) Magnesium silicate

12. A very fine powdered chemical is defined as one that will

(A) completely pass through a #80 sieve
(B) completely pass through a #120 sieve
(C) completely pass through a #20 sieve
(D) pass through a #60 sieve and not more than 40% through a #100 sieve
(E) pass through a #40 sieve and not more than 60% through a #60 sieve

13. Camphor is usually milled by which of the following techniques?

(A) Trituration
(B) Levigation
(C) Pulverization by intervention
(D) Geometric dilution
(E) Attrition

14. The dispensing pharmacist usually accomplishes the blending of potent powders with a large amount of diluent by

(A) spatulation
(B) sifting
(C) trituration
(D) geometric dilution
(E) levigation

15. Which type of paper will best protect a divided hygroscopic powder?

(A) Waxed paper
(B) Glassine
(C) White bond
(D) Blue bond
(E) Vegetable parchment

16. Which of the following capsule sizes has the smallest capacity?

(A) 5
(B) 4
(C) 1
(D) 0
(E) 000

17. The shells of soft gelatin capsules may be made elastic or plastic-like by the addition of

(A) sorbitol
(B) povidone
(C) polyethylene glycol (PEG)
(D) lactose
(E) hydroxypropyl methylcellulose (HPMC)

18. *United States Pharmacopeia (USP)* tests for ensuring the quality of drug products in tablet form include all of the following EXCEPT

(A) disintegration
(B) dissolution
(C) hardness and friability
(D) content uniformity
(E) weight variation

19. The *United States Pharmacopeia (USP)* content uniformity test for tablets is used to ensure which of the following qualities?

(A) Bioequivalency
(B) Dissolution
(C) Potency
(D) Purity
(E) Toxicity

11-A	14-D	17-A
12-B	15-A	18-C
13-C	16-A	19-C

Directions: Each question below contains three suggested answers of which **one or more** is correct. Choose the answer

A if **I only** is correct
B if **III only** is correct
C if **I and II** are correct
D if **II and III** are correct
E if **I, II, and III** are correct

20. Forms of water that are suitable for use in parenteral preparations include which of the following?

I. Purified water USP
II. Water for injection USP
III. Sterile water for injection USP

21. The particles in an ideal suspension should satisfy which of the following criteria?

I. Their size should be uniform
II. They should be stationary or move randomly
III. They should remain discrete

22. The sedimentation of particles in a suspension can be minimized by

I. adding sodium benzoate
II. increasing the viscosity of the suspension
III. reducing the particle size of the active ingredient

23. Ingredients that may be used as suspending agents include

I. methylcellulose
II. acacia
III. talc

24. Mechanisms thought to provide stable emulsions include the

I. formation of interfacial film
II. lowering of interfacial tension
III. presence of charge on the ions

25. Nonionic surface-active agents used as synthetic emulsifiers include

I. tragacanth
II. sodium lauryl sulfate
III. sorbitan esters (spans)

26. Advantages of systemic drug administration by rectal suppositories include

I. avoidance of first-pass effects
II. suitability when the oral route is not feasible
III. predictable drug release and absorption

27. True statements concerning the milling of powders include

I. a fine particle size is essential if the lubricant is to function properly
II. an increased surface area may enhance the dissolution rate
III. milling may cause degradation of thermolabile drugs

28. Substances that may be used to insulate powder components that may liquify when mixed include

I. talc
II. kaolin
III. light magnesium oxide

29. A Wedgwood mortar may be preferable to a glass mortar when

I. a volatile oil is added to a powder mixture
II. colored substances (dyes) are mixed into a powder
III. comminution is desired in addition to mixing

30. Divided powders may be dispensed in

I. individual-dose packets
II. a bulk container
III. a perforated, sifter-type container

31. True statements about the function of excipients used in tablet formulations include

I. binders promote granulation during the wet granulation process
II. glidants help to promote the flow of the tablet granulation during manufacture
III. lubricants help the patient to swallow the tablets

20-D	23-C	26-C	29-B
21-E	24-E	27-E	30-A
22-D	25-B	28-D	31-C

SUMMARY OF DIRECTIONS

A	B	C	D	E
I only	III only	I, II only	II, III only	All are correct

32. Manufacturing variables that would be likely to affect the dissolution of a prednisone tablet in the body include

I. the amount and type of binder added
II. the amount and type of disintegrant added
III. the force of compression used during tableting

33. Agents that might be used to coat enteric-coated tablets include

I. hydroxypropyl methylcellullose (HPMC)
II. carboxymethylcellulose (CMC)
III. cellulose acetate phthalate (CAP)

34. The amount of nitroglycerin that a transdermal patch delivers within a 24-hour period depends on the

I. occlusive backing on the patch
II. diffusion rate of nitroglycerin from the patch
III. surface area of the patch

Directions: Each group of items in this section consists of lettered options followed by a set of numbered items. For each item, select the **one** lettered option that is most closely associated with it. Each lettered option may be selected once, more than once, or not at all.

Questions 35–38

For each of the tablet processing problems listed below, select the most likely reason for the condition.

(A) Excessive moisture in the granulation
(B) Entrapment of air
(C) Tablet friability
(D) Degraded drug
(E) Tablet hardness

35. Picking

36. Mottling

37. Capping

38. Sticking

Questions 39–41

For each description of a comminution procedure below, select the process that it best describes.

(A) Trituration
(B) Spatulation
(C) Levigation
(D) Pulverization by intervention
(E) Tumbling

39. Rubbing or grinding a substance in a mortar with a rough inner surface

40. Reducing and subdividing a substance by adding an easily removed solvent

41. Adding a suitable agent to form a paste and then rubbing or grinding the paste in a mortar

32-E	35-A	38-A	41-C
33-B	36-D	39-A	
34-E	37-B	40-D	

Questions 42–45

Match the drug product below with the type of controlled-release dosage form that it represents.

(A) Matrix device
(B) Ion-exchange resin complex
(C) Hydrocolloid system
(D) Osmotic system
(E) Coated granules

42. Biphetamine capsules
43. Thorazine Spansule capsules
44. Valrelease
45. Slow-K

42-B
43-E
44-C
45-A

ANSWERS AND EXPLANATIONS

1. The answer is D *[I C].*
Syrup NF is a nearly saturated aqueous solution containing in each liter of syrup 850 g of sucrose in about 450 ml of purified water. The high sugar content gives syrup a moderately high viscosity and a high specific gravity. The NF does not specify the addition of a preservative; this is perhaps due to the high sugar content of the syrup. Syrups are useful as flavoring vehicles for medicinal agents.

2. The answer is A *[I C, E–H].*
Syrups are concentrated aqueous sugar solutions; they do not contain alcohol. Elixirs, spirits, tinctures, and fluidextracts are all preparations containing various concentrations of alcohol.

3. The answer is B *[I D 2].*
Aluminum acetate and aluminum subacetate solutions are astringents used as wet dressings for contact dermatitis and as antiperspirants. Strong iodine solution and benzalkonium chloride are topical antibacterial solutions; acetic acid is added to products as an acidifier; and aromatic ammonia spirit is a respiratory stimulant.

4. The answer is A *[II A 1].*
A suspension is a two-phase system: It consists of a finely powdered solid dispersed in a liquid vehicle. The particle size of the suspended solid should be as small as possible to minimize sedimentation; however, the particle size is usually greater than 0.5 μm.

5. The answer is C *[II E 1].*
Levigation is the process of blending and grinding a substance to separate the particles, reduce their size, and form a paste. It is performed by adding a small amount of suitable levigating agent such as glycerin to the solid and then blending the mixture, using a mortar and pestle.

6. The answer is A *[III E 1 a].*
Acacia (gum arabic) is the exudate obtained from the stems and branches of various species of Acacia, a woody plant native to Africa. Acacia is a natural emulsifying agent that provides a good stable emulsion of low viscosity. Emulsions consist of droplets of one or more immiscible liquids dispersed in another liquid. Emulsions are inherently unstable: The droplets tend to coalesce into larger and larger drops. The purpose of an emulsifying agent is to keep the droplets dispersed and prevent them from coalescing. Polysorbate 20, polysorbate 80, and sorbitan monopalmitate are also emulsifiers but are synthetic, not natural, substances.

7. The answer is D *[IV A, B 3 d].*
Ointments are typically used as emollients to soften the skin, as protective barriers, or as vehicles for medication. To serve these functions, a variety of ointment bases are available. Vanishing cream, an emulsion type of ointment base, is an oil-in-water (o/w) emulsion that contains a high percentage of water. Stearic acid is present to create a thin film on the skin when the water evaporates.

8. The answer is B *[V B 1].*
By convention, a rectal suppository for an adult weighs about 2 g; suppositories for infants or children are smaller. Vaginal suppositories typically weigh about 5 g. Rectal suppositories are usually shaped like a rather elongated bullet, being cylindrical and tapered at one end. Vaginal suppositories are usually ovoid.

9. The answer is D *[V C 1].*
A satisfactory suppository base should remain firm at room temperature; preferably, it should not melt below 30° C to avoid premature softening during storage and insertion. A satisfactory suppository base should also be inert, nonsensitizing, nonirritating, and compatible with a variety of drugs. Moreover, it should melt just below body temperature and should dissolve or disintegrate rapidly in the fluid of the body cavity into which it is inserted.

10. The answer is E *[V C 3 a].*
Cocoa butter is a fat obtained from the seed of *Theobroma cacao*. Chemically, it is a mixture of stearin, palmitin, and other glycerides which are insoluble in water and freely soluble in ether and chloroform. Depending on the fusion temperature, cocoa butter may crystallize into any one of four crystal forms. Cocoa butter is a good base for rectal suppositories but is less than ideal for vaginal or urethral suppositories.

11. The answer is A *[V D 3 a (4)].*
In the fusion method of making suppositories, molds made of aluminum, brass, or nickel–copper alloys are used. A mixture of finely powdered drug in melted cocoa butter is poured into a mold that is lubricated very lightly with mineral oil.

12. The answer is B *[VI A 3; Tables 4-7 and 4-8].*
The *United States Pharmacopeia (USP)* definition of a very fine chemical powder is one that will completely pass through a standard #120 sieve (which has 125-μm openings). The *USP* classification for powdered vegetable and animal drugs differs from that for powdered chemicals. To be classified as very fine, powdered vegetable and animal drugs must pass completely through a #80 sieve (which has 180-μm openings).

13. The answer is C *[VI A 3 c (2)].*
Pulverization by intervention is the milling technique used for drug substances that are gummy and tend to reagglomerate or resist grinding (e.g., camphor, iodine). "Intervention" refers to the addition of a small amount of material that aids milling and that can be removed easily after pulverization is complete. For example, camphor can be reduced readily if a small amount of volatile solvent (e.g., alcohol) is added; the solvent is then allowed to evaporate.

14. The answer is D *[VI B 3].*
When mixing potent substances with a large amount of diluent, the pharmacist uses geometric dilution. The potent drug and an equal amount of diluent are first mixed in a mortar by trituration. A volume of diluent equal to the mixture in the mortar is then added, and the mix is again triturated. The procedure is repeated, each time adding diluent equal in volume to the mixture then in the mortar, until all the diluent has been incorporated.

15. The answer is A *[VI C 2 d].*
Hygroscopic and volatile drugs can be protected best by the use of waxed paper, which is waterproof. The packet may be double-wrapped with a bond paper to improve the appearance of the completed powder.

16. The answer is A *[VII B 3 a].*
Hard capsules are numbered from 000 (the largest size) to 5 (the smallest size). The approximate capsule capacity ranges from 600 mg to 30 mg; however, the capsule capacity depends on the density of the contents.

17. The answer is A *[VII C].*
The shells of soft gelatin capsules are plasticized by the addition of a polyhydric alcohol (polyol) such as glycerin or sorbitol. An antifungal preservative may also be added. Both hard and soft gelatin capsules may be filled with a powder or other dry substance; soft gelatin capsules also are useful dosage forms for liquids or semisolids.

18. The answer is C *[VIII E].*
To satisfy the *United States Pharmacopeia (USP)* standards, tablets are required to meet a weight variation test (if the active ingredient comprises the bulk of the tablet) or a content uniformity test (if the active ingredient comprises less than 50% of the tablet bulk or if the tablet is coated). Many tablets for oral administration are required to meet a disintegration test, with disintegration times specified in the individual monographs. A dissolution test may be required instead if the active component of the tablet has limited water-solubility. Hardness and friability would affect a tablet's disintegration and dissolution rates, but hardness and friability tests are in-house quality control tests, and are not official *USP* tests.

19. The answer is C *[VIII E 4].*
The content uniformity test, in effect, is a test of potency. To ensure that each tablet or capsule contains the amount of drug substance intended, the *United States Pharmacopeia (USP)* provides two tests: weight variation and content uniformity. The content uniformity test may be used for any dosage unit but is required for coated tablets, for tablets in which the active ingredient comprises less than 50% of the tablet bulk, for suspensions in single-unit containers or in soft capsules, and for many solids that contain added substances. The weight variation test may be used for liquid-filled soft capsules, for any dosage-form unit that contains at least 50 mg of a single drug if the drug comprises at least 50% of the bulk, for solids without added substances, and for freeze-dried solutions.

20. The answer is D (II, III) *[I A 1–4].*
Water for injection USP is water that has been purified by distillation or by reverse osmosis. It is used in preparing parenteral solutions that are subject to final sterilization. For parenteral solutions prepared aseptically and not subsequently sterilized, sterile water for injection USP is used. Sterile water for injection USP is water for injection USP that has been sterilized and suitably packaged; it meets the *USP* requirements for sterility. Bacteriostatic water for injection USP is sterile water for injection USP that contains one or more antimicrobial agents. It can be used in parenteral solutions if the antimicrobial additives are compatible with the other ingredients in the solution, but it cannot be used in newborn infants. Purified water USP is not used in parenteral preparations.

21. The answer is E (all) *[II C 1].*
An ideal suspension would have particles of uniform size, minimal sedimentation, and no interaction between particles. These ideal criteria are rarely realized, although they can be approximated by keeping the particle size as small as possible, keeping the densities of the solid and the dispersion medium as similar as possible, and keeping the dispersion medium as viscous as possible.

22. The answer is D (II, III) *[II C 2 a, d].*
As Stoke's law indicates, the sedimentation rate of a suspension is slowed by reducing its density, reducing the size of the suspended particles, or by increasing its viscosity (achieved by incorporating a thickening agent). Sodium benzoate is an antifungal agent and would not reduce the sedimentation rate of a suspension.

23. The answer is C (I, II) *[II D].*
Acacia and methylcellulose are both commonly used as suspending agents. Acacia is a natural product; methylcellulose is a synthetic polymer. By increasing the viscosity of the liquid, these agents enable particles to remain suspended for a longer period of time.

24. The answer is E (all) *[III D].*
Emulsifying agents provide a mechanical barrier to coalescence, reducing the natural tendency of the internal-phase (oil or water) droplets in the emulsion to coalesce. Three mechanisms appear to be involved: Some emulsifiers promote stability by forming strong, pliable interfacial films around the droplets. Emulsifying agents also reduce interfacial tension. An electrical charge on the ions in the emulsion can create charge repulsion that causes droplets to repel one another, thereby preventing coalescence.

25. The answer is B (III) *[III E 2 c].*
All of the substances listed in the question are emulsifying agents, but only sorbitan esters are nonionic synthetic agents. Tragacanth, like acacia, is a natural emulsifying agent, and sodium lauryl sulfate is an anionic surfactant. Sorbitan esters (known colloquially as spans by virtue of their trade names) are hydrophobic and form water-in-oil (w/o) emulsions. The polysorbates (known colloquially as tweens) are also nonionic, synthetic sorbitan derivatives, but they are hydrophilic and, therefore, form oil-in-water (o/w) emulsions. Sodium lauryl sulfate, as an alkali soap, is also hydrophilic and, thus, forms o/w emulsions.

26. The answer is C (I, II) *[V A 2, 3, C 2].*
Rectal suppositories are useful for delivering systemic medication under certain circumstances. Absorption of a drug from a rectal suppository involves release of the drug from the suppository vehicle, followed by diffusion of the drug through the rectal mucosa and transport to the circulation by way of the rectal veins. Because the rectal veins bypass the liver, rapid hepatic degradation of certain drugs (first-pass effect) is avoided. The rectal route is also useful when a drug cannot be given orally (e.g., because of vomiting). However, the extent of drug release and absorption is variable; it depends on the properties of the drug, the suppository base, and the environment in the rectum.

27. The answer is E (all) *[VI A 3 a, b].*
Milling is the process of mechanically reducing the particle size of solids before formulation into a final product. For a lubricant to work effectively, it must coat the surface of the granulation or powder. Hence, fine particle size is essential. Decreasing the particle size increases the surface area, and this may enhance the dissolution rate. Possible degradation of thermolabile drugs may occur as a result of heat buildup during milling.

28. The answer is D (II, III) *[VI B 1 b].*
Some solid substances (e.g., aspirin, phenylsalicylate, phenacetin, thymol, camphor) liquify or form eutectic mixtures when in close and prolonged contact with one another. Such substances are best insulated by the addition of light magnesium oxide or magnesium carbonate; other inert diluents that may be used are kaolin, starch, or bentonite.

29. The answer is B (III) *[VI B 2].*
In the mixing of powders, if comminution is especially desired, a porcelain or Wedgwood mortar having a rough inner surface is preferred over the smooth working surface of the glass mortar. A glass mortar cleans more easily after use and, therefore, may be preferable for chemicals that may stain a porcelain or Wedgwood mortar and for simple mixing of substances without the need for comminution.

30. The answer is A (I) *[VI C 2].*
Powders for oral use may be dispensed by the pharmacist in bulk form or divided into premeasured doses (divided powders). Divided powders are traditionally dispensed in folded paper packets (chartulae) made of parchment, bond paper, glassine, or waxed paper. However, if the powder needs greater protection from humidity or evaporation, the individual doses may be packaged in metal foil or small plastic bags.

31. The answer is C (I, II) *[VIII B 2 a–d].*
Tablets for oral ingestion usually contain excipients that are added to the formulation for their special functions. Binders and adhesives are added to promote granulation or compaction. Diluents are fillers added to make up the required tablet bulk; they may also aid in the manufacturing process. Disintegrants aid tablet disintegration in gastrointestinal fluids. Lubricants, antiadherents, and glidants aid in reducing friction or adhesion between particles or between the tablet and the die. For example, lubricants are used in tablet manufacture to reduce friction when the tablet is ejected from the die cavity in which it was formed. Lubricants are usually hydrophobic substances that can affect the dissolution rate of the active ingredient in a tablet.

32. The answer is E (all) *[VIII B 2 b, c, E 2, 5, 6].*
Disintegrants are added to tablet formulations to facilitate tablet disintegration in the gastrointestinal fluids. The tablet's disintegration in the body is critical to its dissolution and subsequent absorption and bioavailability. The binder and the compression force used during tablet manufacturing both affect a tablet's hardness, and this also affects tablet disintegration and drug dissolution.

33. The answer is B (III) *[VIII C 1 d].*
An enteric-coated tablet has a coating that remains intact in the stomach but dissolves in the intestines to yield the tablet's ingredients there. Enteric coatings include various fats, fatty acids, waxes, and shellacs. Cellulose acetate phthalate remains intact in the stomach because it dissolves only above pH 6. Other enteric-coating materials include povidone (polyvinylpyrrolidone; PVP), polyvinyl acetate phthalate (PVAP), and hydroxypropyl methylcellulose phthalate (HPMCP).

34. The answer is E (all) *[IX C 2, 3].*
The delivery of drugs through a transdermal drug delivery system (TDDS) depends on the microporous membranes that act as rate-controlling barriers, the mechanism by which the drug diffuses through these barriers (e.g., reservoir, matrix), and the surface area of the patch.

35–38. The answers are: 35-A, 36-D, 37-B, 38-A *[VIII D].*
Sticking refers to tablet material adhering to a die wall. Sticking may be due to excessive moisture or to ingredients with low melting temperatures. Mottling is uneven color distribution; it is most often due to poor mixing of the tablet granulation but may also result from a degraded drug that produces a colored metabolite. Capping is the separation of the top or bottom crown of a tablet from the main body of the tablet. Capping implies that compressed powder is not cohesive. Reasons for capping include excessive force of compression, use of insufficient binder, worn tablet tooling equipment, and air entrapment during processing. Picking refers to surface material from a tablet sticking to a punch. Picking may be caused by a granulation that is too damp, by a scratched punch, by static charges on the powder, and particularly by use of a punch tip with engraving or embossing.

39–41. The answers are: 39-A, 40-D, 41-C *[VI A 3 c].*
Comminution is the process of reducing the particle size of a powder to increase the powder's fineness. Several comminution techniques are suitable for small-scale use in a pharmacy. Trituration is used both to comminute and to mix dry powders; if comminution is desired, the substance is rubbed in a mortar

with a rough inner surface. Pulverization by intervention is often used for substances that tend to agglomerate or to resist grinding. A small amount of easily removed (e.g., volatile) solvent is added, and after the substance is pulverized, the solvent is allowed to evaporate or is otherwise removed. Levigation is often used to prepare pastes or ointments. The powder is reduced by adding a suitable nonsolvent (levigating agent) to form a paste and then rubbing the paste in a mortar, using a pestle, or on an ointment slab, using a spatula. Spatulation and tumbling are procedures for mixing or blending powders, not for reducing them. Spatulation is blending small amounts of powders together by stirring them with a spatula on a sheet of paper or a pill tile. Tumbling is the process of blending large amounts of powder in a large rotating container.

42–45. The answers are: 42-B, 43-E, 44-C, 45-A *[IX].*
Controlled-release dosage forms are designed to release a drug slowly for prolonged action in the body. A variety of pharmaceutical mechanisms are employed to provide the controlled release. Ion-exchange resins may be complexed to drugs (e.g., Biphentamine capsules) by passing a cationic drug solution through a column containing the resin. The drug is complexed to the resin by replacement of hydrogen atoms. Drug release from the complex depends on the ionic environment within the gastrointestinal tract and on the resin's properties. Coated beads or granules (e.g., Thorazine Spansule capsules) produce blood levels similar to those obtained with multiple dosing. The various coating thicknesses produce a sustained-release effect.

The hydrocolloid system (e.g., Valrelease, a slow-release form of diazepam) includes a unique hydrodynamically balanced drug-delivery system (HBS). Outermost hydrocolloids swell to form a boundary when in contact with gastric fluid, preventing penetration of fluid into the formulation. As outer layers erode new boundary layers form, allowing a gradual release of the drug.

Matrix devices may employ insoluble plastics, hydrophilic polymers, or fatty compounds, which are mixed with the drug and compressed into a tablet. The primary dose, the portion of the drug to be released immediately, is placed on the tablet as a layer or coat. The remainder of the dose is released slowly from the matrix.

5
Extemporaneous Prescription Compounding

Michael J. DeFelice
Steven Grossman
Leon Shargel

I. INTRODUCTION

A. Definitions

1. **Extemporaneous compounding** is the preparation, mixing, assembling, packaging, and labeling of a drug product based on a prescription order from a licensed practitioner for the individual patient.

2. **Manufacturing** is the mass production of compounded prescription products for resale to pharmacies and is regulated by the Food and Drug Administration (FDA).

B. Regulation

1. **Current good manufacturing practices (cGMP)** are the standards of practice used in the pharmaceutical industry and are regulated by the FDA. Community pharmacists must comply with cGMP but must also assure a quality product, which includes using proper materials, weighing equipment, a documented technique, and dispensing and storage instructions.

2. **Legal considerations**
   a. Extemporaneous compounding by the pharmacist of a prescription order from a licensed practitioner, as with the dispensing of any other prescription, is controlled by the state board of registration in pharmacy.
   b. The legal risk (liability) of compounding is no greater than filling a prescription for a manufactured product as the pharmacist must assure that the correct drug, dose, and directions are provided. The pharmacist is also responsible for preparing a quality pharmaceutical product, providing proper instructions regarding its storage, and advising the patient of any adverse effects.

II. REQUIREMENTS FOR COMPOUNDING

A. Sources for chemicals and drugs. Pharmacists must obtain small quantities of the appropriate chemicals or drugs from wholesalers. These wholesalers then act as consultants to the pharmacists by assuring them of their product's purity and quality.

B. Equipment. The correct equipment is also important when compounding. Many state boards of pharmacy have a required minimum list of equipment for compounding prescriptions. Suggested equipment, which varies according to the amount of material needed and the type of compounded prescription (e.g., parenteral), includes:

1. Class A prescription balance or electronic balance
2. Hot plate with magnetic stirrers
3. Electric mixer
4. Special containers for packaging (e.g., applicator tip bottles)
5. Graduated cylinders from 10 ml to 1000 ml
6. Glass, Wedgwood, and porcelain mortars and pestles of various sizes
7. Funnels of various sizes

8. Spatulas of various sizes, including several rubber spatulas
9. Weighing and filter papers
10. Stirring rods (glass)
11. Ointment/pill tile
12. Capsule filling machine
13. Ointment filling machine
14. Autoclave
15. Laminar flow clean bench
16. Special suppository molds
17. Record-keeping system (compounding log book)
18. Glass beakers from 50 ml to 1000 ml

C. Location of compounding area. Many pharmacies actively involved in compounding have dedicated a separate area in the pharmacy to this process. The ideal location is away from heavy foot traffic and is near a sink where there is enough space to work and store all chemicals and equipment.

D. Souces of information

1. Library at a college of pharmacy
2. Textbooks
   a. *Remington's Pharmaceutical Sciences*
   b. *Merck Manual*
   c. *United States Pharmacopeia (USP)* and *National Formulary (NF)*
3. Journals (e.g., *U.S. Pharmacist, Pharmacy Times, Hospital Pharmacy*)
4. Manufacturer's drug product information inserts

III. COMPOUNDING OF SOLUTIONS

A. Definition. *USP volume XXII,* defines a **solution** as a liquid preparation that contains one or more chemical substances dissolved in a suitable solvent or mixture of mutually miscible solvents. Although the uniformity of the dosage in a solution can be assumed, the stability, pH, solubility of the drug or chemicals, taste (for oral solutions), and packaging need to be considered.

B. Types of solutions

1. **Sterile parenteral and ophthalmic solutions.** These solutions require special consideration for their preparation, which is discussed in XI.
2. **Nonsterile solutions** include oral, topical, and otic solutions.

C. Preparation of solutions. Solutions are the easiest of the dosage forms to compound extemporaneously, as long as a few general rules are followed.

1. Each drug or chemical is dissolved in the solvent in which it is most soluble. Thus, the solubility characteristics of each drug or chemical must be known.
2. If an alcoholic solution is used, the aqueous solution is added to the alcoholic solution.
3. The salt form of the drug, and not the free-acid or base form, which both have poor solubility, is used.
4. Flavoring or sweetening agents are prepared ahead of time.
5. If the required chemical or drug is in bulk or powder form, then the particle size is reduced first, using a mortar and pestle, a sieve, or other suitable means.
6. The proper vehicle (e.g., syrup, elixir aromatic water, purified water) must be selected.

D. Examples

1. **Example 1**

   a. **Medication order**

   Phenobarbital 1 g
   Belladonna Tr* 5 ml
   Peppermint water qs 120 ml

   b. **Compounding procedure.** Sodium phenobarbital (equivalent to 1 g of phenobarbital) is dissolved in the aromatic water. This solution is then added slowly in divided portions to the tincture contained in a beaker and is stirred continuously or a magnetic stirrer is used.

2. **Example 2**

   a. **Medication order**

   Potassium chloride 500 mg/10 ml
   Aromatic elixir ad 60 ml

   b. **Compounding procedure.** Potassium chloride (3g) is dissolved with the smallest amount of purified water possible. A sufficient amount of aromatic elixir is added to bring the final volume up to 60 ml.

3. **Example 3**

   a. **Medication order**

   Salicylic acid 2%
   Lactic acid 6 ml
   Flexible collodion ad 30 ml

   b. **Compounding procedure.** Pharmacists must use caution when preparing this prescription because flexible collodion is extremely flammable. A 1-oz applicator tip bottle is calibrated, using ethanol, which is poured out and allowed to evaporate, resulting in a dry bottle. Salicylic acid (0.6 g) is added directly into the bottle, to which is added the 6 ml of lactic acid. The bottle is agitated or a glass stirring rod is used to dissolve the salicylic acid. Flexible collodion is added up to the calibrated 30-ml mark on the applicator tip bottle.

4. **Example 4**

   a. **Medication order**

   Iodine 2%
   Sodium iodide 2.4%
   Alcohol q.s. 30 ml

   b. **Compounding procedure.** Iodine (0.6 g) and sodium iodide (0.72 g) are dissolved in the alcohol, and the final solution is placed in an amber bottle. A **rubber spatula** is used because **iodine is corrosive**.

IV. COMPOUNDING OF SUSPENSIONS

A. Definition. Suspensions are defined by the *USP* as liquid preparations that consist of solid particles dispersed throughout a liquid phase in which the particles are not soluble.

B. General characteristics

1. All suspensions must contain an antimicrobial agent as a preservative.
2. Particles settle in all suspensions unless a suspending agent is added; thus, suspensions must be well shaken before use to ensure the distribution of particles for a uniform dose.
3. Tight containers are necessary to ensure the stability of the final product.
4. Principles to keep in mind when compounding include the following.

   a. Insoluble powders should be small and uniform in size to decrease settling.

*Abbreviations are listed in Appendix B.

b. The suspension should be viscous.
c. Topical suspensions should have a smooth impalpable texture.
d. Oral suspensions should have a pleasant odor and taste.

C. Formation of suspensions. Suspensions are easy to compound; however, physical stability after compounding the final product is problematic. The following steps may minimize stability problems.

1. The particle size of all powders used in the formulation must be reduced.
2. A thickening agent (suspending agent) must be used to increase viscosity. Common suspending agents include bentonite, Veegum, methylcellulose, and tragacanth.
3. A levigating agent may aid in the initial dispersion of insoluble particles. Common levigating agents include glycerin, propylene glycol, alcohol, syrups, and water.
4. Flavoring agents and preservatives should be selected and added if the product is intended for oral use. Common preservatives include methyl and propylparabens, benzoic acid, and sodium benzoate. Flavoring agents may be any flavored syrup (Table 5-1).
5. The source of the active ingredients (e.g., bulk powders versus tablets or capsules) must be considered.

D. Preparation of suspensions

1. The insoluble powders are triturated to a fine powder, using a Wedgwood mortar.
2. A small portion of liquid is used as a levigating agent, and the powders are triturated until a smooth paste is formed. The levigating agent is added slowly and mixed deliberately.
3. The vehicle containing the suspending agent is added in divided portions. A high-speed mixer greatly increases the dispersion.
4. The product is brought to the required volume using the vehicle.
5. The final mixture is transferred to a "tight" bottle for dispensing to the patient.
6. All suspensions are dispensed with a "shake well" label.
7. Suspensions are never filtered.
8. The water-soluble ingredients are mixed, including flavoring agents, in the vehicle before mixing with the insoluble ingredients.

Table 5-1. Selected Flavor Applications

Drug Category	Preferred Flavors
Antibiotics	Cherry, maple, pineapple, orange, raspberry, banana–pineapple, banana–vanilla, butterscotch–maple, coconut custard, strawberry, vanilla, lemon custard, cherry custard, fruit–cinnamon
Antihistamines	Apricot, black currant, cherry, cinnamon, custard, grape, honey, lime, loganberry, peach–orange, peach–rum, raspberry, root beer, wild cherry
Barbiturates	Banana–pineapple, banana–vanilla, black currant, cinnamon–peppermint, grenadine–strawberry, lime, orange, peach–orange, root beer
Decongestants and Expectorants	Anise, apricot, black currant, butterscotch, cherry, coconut custard, custard mint–strawberry, grenadine–peach, strawberry, lemon, gooseberry, loganberry, maple, orange, orange–lemon, coriander, orange–peach, pineapple, raspberry, strawberry, tangerine
Electrolyte solutions	Cherry, grape, lemon–lime, raspberry, wild cherry syrup, black currant, grenadine–strawberry, lime, port wine, sherry wine, root beer, wild strawberry

E. Examples

1. Example 1

a. Medication order

Propranolol HCl 4 mg/ml
Disp 30 ml
Sig: 1 ml p.o. t.i.d.

b. Calculations. Propranolol HCl, 4 mg/ml × 30 ml = 120 mg. Propranolol HCl is available in immediate-release and extended-release (long-acting) dosage forms. Only the immediate-release tablets are used for compounded prescriptions; therefore, some combination of propranolol HCl tablets, which yields 120 mg active drug (e.g., 3 × 40-mg tablets), is used.

c. Compounding procedure. The propranolol tablets are reduced to a fine powder in a Wedgwood mortar. The powder is levigated to a smooth paste, using a 2% methylcellulose solution. To this mixture, about 10 ml of a suitable flavoring agent are added. The mixture is transferred to a calibrated container and brought to the final volume with purified water. A "shake well" label is attached to the prescription container.

2. Example 2

a. Medication order

Zinc oxide 10
Ppt sulfur 10
Bentonite 3.6
Purified water ad 90 ml
Sig: Apply t.i.d.

b. Compounding procedure. The powders are reduced to a fine uniform mixture in a mortar. The powders are dissolved to a smooth paste using water and transferred to a calibrated bottle. The final volume is attained with purified water. A "shake well" label is attached to the prescription container.

3. Example 3

a. Medication order

Rifampin suspension 20 mg/ml
Disp 120 ml
Sig: U.D.

b. Calculations. Rifampin, 20 mg/ml × 120 ml = 2400 mg. Rifampin is available in 150-mg and 300-mg capsules. Hence, 8 capsules containing 300 mg of rifampin in each capsule or 16 capsules containing 150 mg of rifampin per capsule are needed.

c. Compounding procedure. The contents of the appropriate number of rifampin capsules are emptied into a 120-ml prescription bottle. This powder is levigated with a small amount of 1% methylcellulose solution. Twenty milliliters of simple syrup are added and shaken. The mixture is brought to the final volume with simple syrup. "Shake well" and "refrigerate" labels are attached to the prescription container.

V. EMULSIONS

A. Definition. Emulsions are produced by a two-phase system in which one liquid is dispersed throughout another liquid in the form of small droplets (see Chapter 4).

B. General characteristics. Emulsions can be used externally as lotions and creams or internally to mask the taste of oily medications.

1. The two liquids in an emulsion are immiscible and, like suspensions, require the use of an emulsifying agent.
2. Emulsions are classified as either **oil-in-water (o/w)** or **water-in-oil (w/o)**.
3. Emulsions are unstable, and the following steps must be taken to prevent the two phases of an emulsion from separating into two layers after preparation.
   a. The correct proportions of oil and water should be used during preparation. The internal phase should represent about 40%–60% of the total volume.
   b. An emulsifying agent is needed for emulsion formation.
   c. A hand homogenizer, which reduces the size of globules of the internal phase, may be used.

d. Preservatives should be added if the preparation is intended to last longer than a few days. Generally, a combination of methylparaben (0.2%) and propylparaben (0.02%) is employed.
e. A "shake well" label should be placed on the final product.
f. The product should be protected from light and excessive temperatures. Both freezing and heat may have an effect on stability.

C. Emulsifying agents

1. Gums, such as **acacia** and **tragacanth,** are used to form oil-in-water emulsions. These emulsifying agents are for general use, especially for emulsions intended for internal administration (Table 5-2).
   a. One gram of acacia powder is used for every 4 ml of fixed oil or 1 g to 2 ml for a volatile oil.
   b. If using tragacanth in place of acacia, 0.1 g of tragacanth is used for every 1 g of acacia.

Table 5-2. Agents Used in Prescription Compounding

	Ointments		
Oleaginous or hydrocarbon bases		**Hydrous emulsion bases (w/o)**	
Anhydrous		Hydrous	
Nonhydrophilic		Hydrophilic	
Insoluble in water		Insoluble in water	
Not water removable (occlusive)		Not water removable (occlusive)	
Good vehicles for antibiotics		**Examples**	
Example		Cold cream	
Petrolatum		Hydrous lanolin	
Absorption, or hydrophilic, bases		**Emulsion bases (o/w)**	
Anhydrous		Hydrous	
Hydrophilic		Hydrophilic	
Insoluble in water		Insoluble in water	
Not water removable (occlusive)		Water removable	
		Can absorb 30%–50% of weight	
Examples		**Examples**	
Hydrophilic petrolatum		Hydrophilic ointment USP	
Lanolin USP (anhydrous)		Acid mantle cream	
	Suspending Agents		
Acacia 10%		Sodium alginate 1%–2%	
Bentonite 6%		Tragacanth 1%–3%	
Carboxymethylcellulose 1%–3%		Veegum 6%	
Methylcellulose 1%–7%			
	Preservatives		
Methylparaben		Propylparaben 0.01%–0.04%	
	Emulsifying Agents		
Hydrophilic colloids		**Surfactant-hydrophilic–lipophilic balance**	
Acacia		Nonionic-polysorbate 80 (concentrations used, 1%–30%)	
Tragacanth			
Pectin	Favor o/w	Tweens	
Carboxymethylcellulose		Spans	
Methylcellulose			
		Soaps	
Proteins		Triethanolamine	
Gelatin		Stearic acid	
Egg whites	Favor o/w	**Others**	
Inorganic gels and magmas		Sodium lauryl sulfate	
Milk of magnesia		Dioctyl sodium sulfosuccinate	
Bentonite	Favor o/w	Cetyl pyridinium	

o/w = oil-in-water; w/o = water-in-oil.

2. **Methylcellulose** and **carboxymethylcellulose** are used for oil-in-water emulsions. The concentration of these agents vary, depending on the grade that is used. Methylcellulose is available in several viscosity grades, ranging from 15 to 4000 designated by a centipoise number, which is a unit of viscosity.
3. **Soaps** can be used to prepare oil-in-water or water-in-oil emulsions for external preparations.
4. **Nonionic emulsifying agents** can be used for oil-in-water and water-in-oil emulsions.

D. Formation and preparation of emulsions. The procedure for the preparation of an emulsion depends on the desired emulsifying agent in the formulation.

1. A **mortar and pestle** are frequently all the equipment that is needed.
   - **a.** A mortar with a rough surface (e.g., Wedgwood) should be used. This rough surface allows maximal dispersion of globules to produce a fine particle size.
   - **b.** A rapid motion is essential when triturating an emulsion using a mortar and pestle.
   - **c.** The mortar should be capable of holding at least three times the quantity being made. Trituration seldom requires more than 5 minutes to create the emulsion.
2. **Electric mixers** and **hand homogenizers** are useful for producing emulsions after the coarse emulsion is formed in the mortar.
3. The **order of mixing of ingredients** in an emulsion depends on the type of emulsion being prepared (i.e., o/w or w/o) as well as the emulsifying agent chosen. Methods used for compounding include the following.
   - **a. Dry gum (continental) method** is used in the formation of emulsions using natural emulsifying agents and requires a specific order of mixing.
   - **b. Wet gum (English) method** is used in the formation of emulsions using natural emulsifying agents and requires a specific order of mixing.
   - **c. Bottle method** is used in the formation of emulsions using natural emulsifying agents and requires a specific order of mixing.
   - **d. Beaker method** is used to prepare emulsions using synthetic emulsifying agents and produces a satisfactory product regardless of the order of mixing.
4. **Preservatives.** If the emulsion is kept for an extended period of time, refrigeration is usually sufficient. The product should not be frozen. If a preservative is used, it must be soluble in the water phase to have any effect.
5. **Flavoring agents.** If the addition of a flavor is needed to mask the taste of the oil phase, the flavor should be added to the oil before emulsification (Table 5-3).

E. Examples

1. **Example 1**
   - **a. Medication order**

     Mineral oil 18 ml
     Acacia q.s.
     distilled water q.s. ad 90.0 ml
     Sig: 1 tbsp q.d.

   - **b. Compounding procedure.** With the dry gum method, an initial emulsion (primary emulsion) is formed, using 4 parts of oil (18 ml), 2 parts (9 ml) of water, and 1 part (4.5 g) of powdered acacia. The mineral oil is triturated with the acacia in a Wedgwood mortar. The 9 ml of water are added all at once and, with rapid trituration, form the primary emulsion, which is triturated for about 5 minutes. The remaining water is incorporated in small amounts with trituration. The emulsion is transferred to a 90-ml prescription bottle, and a "shake well" label is attached to the container.

Table 5-3. Flavor Selection Guide

Taste	Masking Flavor
Salt	Butterscotch, maple
Bitter	Wild cherry, walnut, chocolate mint, licorice
Sweet	Fruit, berry, vanilla
Acid	Citrus

2. **Example 2**
   a. **Medication order**

      Zinc oxide 8 g
      Calamine 8 g
      Olive oil 30 ml
      Lime water 30 ml

   b. **Compounding procedure.** The olive oil is placed in a suitably sized beaker. Using an electric mixer, the zinc oxide, the calamine, and the lime water are added in that order. This yields a water-in-oil emulsion. This procedure is known as the **nascent soap method**. The olive oil reacts with the calcium hydroxide solution (lime water) and forms a soap. For this reaction to occur, fresh lime water is required.

3. **Example 3**
   a. **Medication order**

      Mineral oil 50 ml
      Water q.s. 100 ml
      Sig: 2.5 ml p.o. h.s.

   b. **Compounding procedure.** Using a combination of nonionic emulsifying agents, such as Span 40 and Tween 40, the correct hydrophilic–lipophilic balance (HLB) is obtained. Next, the mineral oil is warmed in a water bath to about 16°C, and the Span 40 is dissolved in the heated mineral oil. The water is warmed to about 18°C, and the Tween 40 is dissolved in the heated water. This mixture is added to the mineral oil and dissolved Span 40 and stirred until cooled. An "external use only" label is added to the container.

VI. POWDERED DOSAGE FORMS

A. Definition. Powders are dry mixtures of drugs or chemicals intended for internal or external use. The two major types are powder papers and bulk powders.

B. General characteristics

1. Powder dosage forms are used when drug stability or solubility is a concern. These dosage forms may also be used when the powders are too bulky to make into capsules and when the patient has difficulty swallowing a capsule.
2. Some **disadvantages** to powders include unpleasant-tasting medications and, occasionally, the rapid deterioration of powders.
3. Blending of powders may be accomplished by using trituration in a mortar, stirring with a spatula, and sifting. Geometric dilution should be used if needed. When heavy powders are mixed with lighter ones, the heavier powder should be placed on top of the lighter one and then blended. When mixing two or more powders, each powder should be pulverized separately to about the same particle size before blending together.
   a. The **mortar and pestle method** is preferred when pulverization and a thorough mixing of ingredients are desired (geometric dilution). A Wedgwood mortar is preferable, but glass or porcelain may also be used.
   b. Light powders are mixed best by using the **sifting method**. The sifting is repeated three to four times to insure thorough mixing of the powders.

C. Preparation of powder dosage forms

1. Bulk powders, which may be used internally or topically, include dusting powders, douche powders, laxatives, antacids, and insufflation powders.
2. After a bulk powder has been pulverized and blended, it should be dispensed in an appropriate container.
   a. Hygroscopic or effervescent salts should always be placed in a widemouthed jar.
   b. Dusting powders should be placed in a container with a sifter top.
3. Eutectic mixtures of powders can cause problems since they liquify. One remedy is to add an inert powder, such as magnesium oxide, to separate the eutectic materials.
4. **Powder papers** are also called divided powders.
   a. The entire powder is initially blended. Each dose is then individually weighed.

b. The dosage should be weighed, then transferred onto a powder paper and folded. This technique requires practice. Hygroscopic, deliquescent, and effervescent powders require the use of glassine paper as an inside lining. Plastic bags or envelopes with snap-and-seal closures offer a convenient alternative to powder papers.

c. The folded papers are dispensed in a powder box or other suitable container; however, these containers are not child-resistant.

D. Examples

1. Example 1

a. Medication order

Camphor 100 mg
Menthol 200 mg
Zinc oxide 800 mg
Talc 1900 mg
M foot powder
Sig: Apply to aa bid

b. Compounding procedure. The camphor and menthol are triturated together in a glass mortar, where a liquid eutectic is formed. The zinc oxide and talc are blended and mixed with the eutectic, using geometric dilution. This mixing results in a dry powder, which is passed through a wire mesh sieve. The final product is dispensed in a container with a sifter top.

2. Example 2

a. Medication order

Psyllium mucilloid 2 g
Citric acid
Sodium bicarbonate aa 0.25 g
M. Ft d.t.d. charts v
Sig: Empty the contents of one chart into glass
of water and take h.s.

b. Calculations. Calculate for one extra powder paper:

Psyllium mucilloid 2 g $\times$ 6 doses = 12 g
Citric acid 0.25 g $\times$ 6 doses = 1.5 g
Sodium bicarbonate 0.25 g $\times$ 6 doses = 1.5 g
Total weight = 15 g
15 g/6 doses = 2.5 g/dose

c. Compounding procedure. The ingredients are first pulverized and weighed. The citric acid and sodium bicarbonate are mixed together first; the psyllium mucilloid is then added, using geometric dilution. Each dose (2.5 g) of the resultant mixture is weighed and placed into a powder paper. This preparation is an effervescent powder. When dissolved in water, the citric acid and sodium bicarbonate react to form carbonic acid, which yields carbon dioxide, making the solution more palatable.

VII. CAPSULES

A. Definition. Capsules are solid dosage forms in which the drug is enclosed within a hard or soft soluble container or shell made from suitable gelatin. Hard gelatin capsules may be manually filled for extemporaneous compounding.

B. Capsule sizes

1. A list of capsule sizes and the approximate amount of powder that may be contained in the capsule usually appear on the side of the capsule box (Table 5-4).

2. Capsule sizes for oral administration in humans range from no. 5, the smallest, to no. 000, the largest.

3. No. 0 is usually the largest oral size suitable for patients.

4. Capsules for veterinarians are available in nos. 10, 11, and 12, containing approximately 30, 15, and 7.5 g respectively.

Table 5-4. Approximate Amount of Powder Contained in Capsules

Capsule Size	Range of Powder Capacity
No. 5	60–130 mg
No. 4	95–260 mg
No. 3	130–390 mg
No. 2	195–520 mg
No. 1	225–650 mg
No. 0	325–910 mg
No. 00	390–1300 mg
No. 000	650–2000 mg

C. Preparation of hard and soft capsules

1. As with the bulk powders, all ingredients are triturated and blended, using geometric dilution.
2. The correct size capsule must be determined by trying different capsule sizes, weighing them, and then choosing the appropriate size.
3. Prior to filling capsules with the medication, the body and cap of the capsule are separated. Filling is accomplished by using the "punch" method.
   a. The powder formulation is compressed with a spatula on a pill tile or paper sheet with a uniform depth of approximately half the length of the capsule body.
   b. The empty capsule body is repeatedly pressed into the powder until full.
   c. The capsule is then weighed to insure an accurate dose. An empty tare capsule of the same size is placed on the pan containing the weights.
   d. For a large number of capsules, capsule-filling machines can be used for small-scale use to save time.
4. The capsule is wiped clean of any powder or oil and dispensed in a suitable prescription vial.

D. Examples

1. **Example 1**
   a. **Medication order**

      Rifampin 100 mg
      dtd #50
      Sig: 1 cap p.o. q.d.

   b. **Calculations.** Calculate for at least one extra capsule.

$$51 \text{ caps} \times 100 \text{ mg/caps} = 5100 \text{ mg rifampin}$$
$$5100 \text{ mg rifampin} \div 300 \text{ mg/caps} = 17 \text{ caps}$$

   c. **Compounding procedure.** Seventeen rifampin capsules, each containing 300 mg rifampin, are used. The content of each capsule is emptied, and the powder is weighed. Enough lactose is added to make a total of 10.2 g of powder. The powders are combined, using geometric dilution, and 50 capsules can be punched out. Each capsule should weigh 10.2 g/51 caps or 200 mg,
2. **Example 2**
   a. **Medication order.** This order is for veterinary use only.

      Castor oil 8 ml
      Disp 12 caps
      Sig: 2 caps p.o. h.s.

   b. **Calculations.** No calculations are necessary.
   c. **Compounding procedure.** A no. 11 veterinary capsule is used. Using a calibrated dropper or a pipette, 8 ml of the oil are carefully added to the inside of each capsule body. Next, the lower inside portion of the cap is moistened, using a glass rod or brush. The cap and body are joined together, using a twisting motion, to form a tight seal. The capsules are placed on a piece of wetted filter paper and checked for signs of leakage. The capsules are dispensed in the appropriate size and type of prescription vial.

VIII. MOLDED TABLETS (TABLET TRITURATES)

A. Definition. Tablet triturates are molded tablets made of powders created by moistening the powder mixture with alcohol and water. They are used for compounding potent drugs in small doses.

B. Formulation and preparation of tablet triturates

1. Tablet triturates are made in special molds consisting of a pegboard and a corresponding perforated plate.
2. In addition to the mold, a diluent, usually a mixture of lactose and sucrose (80/20), and a moistening agent, usually a mixture of ethyl alcohol and water (60/40), are required.
3. The diluent is triturated with the active ingredients.
4. A paste is then made, using the alcohol and water mixture.
5. This paste is spread into the mold, allowed to dry, and then punched out of the mold.

C. Example

1. **Medication order**

   Atropine sulfate 0.4 mg
   Disp # 500 TT
   Sig. u.d.

2. **Calculations.** For 500 TT: 500 × 0.4 mg = 200 mg atropine sulfate.
3. **Compounding procedure.** The 200 mg of atropine sulfate, 7 g of sucrose, and 28 g of lactose are weighed and mixed by geometric dilution. The powder is wetted with a mixture of 40% purified water and 60% ethyl alcohol (95%). The paste that is formed is spread onto the tablet triturate mold and dried; the tablets are then punched out of the mold. This procedure is repeated until the required amount of tablet triturates has been prepared.

IX. OINTMENTS, CREAMS, PASTES, AND GELS

A. General characteristics. These dosage forms are semisolid preparations generally applied externally. Semisolid dosage forms may contain active drugs intended to:

1. Act solely on the surface of the skin to produce a local effect (e.g., antifungal agent)
2. Release the medication, which, in turn, penetrates into the skin (e.g., cortisol cream)
3. Release medication for systemic absorption through the skin (e.g., nitroglycerin)

B. Types of ointment bases

1. **Hydrophobic bases** feel greasy and contain mixtures of fats, oils, and waxes. Hydrophobic bases **cannot be washed off using water**.
2. **Hydrophilic bases** are nongreasy and are usually oil-in-water emulsions. They **can be washed off with water**.

C. Preparation of ointments, creams, pastes, and gels

1. Mixing can be done in a mortar or on an ointment slab.
2. Liquids are incorporated by gradually adding them to an absorption-type base, using levigation.
3. Insoluble powders are reduced to a fine powder and then added to the base, using geometric dilution.
4. Water-soluble substances are dissolved with water and then incorporated into the base.
5. The final product should be smooth (impalpable) and free of any abrasive particles.

D. Examples

1. **Example 1**
   a. **Medication order**

      Sulfur
      Salicyclic acid aa 600 mg
      White petrolatum ad 30 g
      Sig: Apply tid

   b. **Compounding procedure.** The particle sizes of the sulfur and salicylic acid are reduced separately in a Wedgwood mortar and then blended together. Using a pill tile, the powder mixture is levigated with the base. Using geometric dilution, the base and powders are blended to the final volume. A rubber spatula is used for weighing and levigating because of the corrosive action of salicylic acid. An ointment jar is used for dispensing, and an "external use only" label is placed on the jar.

2. **Example 2**
   a. **Medication order**

      Methylparaben 0.25 g
      Propylparaben 0.15 g
      Sodium lauryl sulfate 10 g
      Propylene glycol 120 g
      Stearyl alcohol 250 g
      White petrolatum 250 g
      Purified water 370 g
      Disp 60 g
      Sig: Apply UD

   b. **Compounding procedure.** The stearyl alcohol and the white petrolatum are melted on a steam bath and heated to about 75°C. The other ingredients, previously dissolved in purified water at about 78°C, are added. The mixture is stirred until it congeals. An ointment jar is used for dispensing, and an "external use only" label is placed on the jar.

X. SUPPOSITORIES

A. General characteristics

1. Suppositories are molded solid dosage forms intended for insertion into a body cavity. They are used to deliver drugs for their local or systemic effects.
2. Suppositories differ in size and shape and include:
   a. Rectal
   b. Vaginal
   c. Urethral
   d. Nasal

B. Common suppository bases

1. **Cocoa butter** (theobroma oil), which melts at body temperature, is a fat-soluble mixture of triglycerides, which is most often used for rectal suppositories. Witepsol is a synthetic triglyceride.
2. **Polyethylene glycol** (PEG, carbowax) **derivatives** are water-soluble bases suitable for vaginal and rectal suppositories.
3. **Glycerinated gelatin** is a water-miscible base often used in vaginal suppositories.

C. Suppository molds

1. Suppository molds can be made of rubber, plastic, brass, stainless steel, or other suitable material.
2. The formulation and volume of the base depends on the size of the mold used, less the displacement caused by the active ingredient.

D. Methods of preparation and dispensing suppositories

1. **Molded suppositories** are prepared by first melting the base and then incorporating the medications uniformly into the base. This mixture is then poured into the suppository mold (fusion method).
2. **Hand-rolled suppositories** require a special technique. With proper technique, it is possible to make a product equal in quality to the molded suppositories.
3. **Containers** for the suppositories are determined by the method and base used in preparation. Hand-rolled and molded suppositories should be dispensed in special boxes that prevent the suppositories from coming in contact with each other.
4. **Storage conditions.** If appropriate, a "refrigerate" label should appear on the container. Regardless of the base or medication used in the formulation, the patient should be instructed to store the suppositories in a cool dry place.

E. Examples

1. **Example 1**
   a. **Medication order**

      Naproxen suppository 500 mg
      Disp #12
      Sig: Insert UD into rectum

   b. **Calculations.** Each standard adult suppository should weigh 2 g.

      2 g (total weight) − 0.540 g (weight of each 500-mg tablet) naproxen per suppository
      = 1.46 g cocoa butter per suppository × 13 suppositories
      = 18.98 g cocoa butter

   c. **Compounding procedure.** The 13 naproxen 500-mg tablets are triturated to a fine powder, using a Wedgwood mortar. The 18.98-g cocoa butter base is melted in a beaker, using a water bath. The temperature of the water bath should not exceed 36°C. The powder is then added and stirred until mixed. The mixture is poured into an appropriate rectal suppository mold (about 2 g/suppository) and placed into a refrigerator until the suppositories congeal. Any excess is scraped from the top of the mold, and a suppository box is used for dispensing. A "refrigerate" label is placed on the box.

2. **Example 2**
   a. **Medication order**

      Progesterone 50 mg
      Disp #14
      Sig: 1 pv b.i.d. days 14–28 of cycle

   b. **Calculations.** Total weight of each vaginal suppository is 1.9 g.

      50 mg progesterone/suppository × 15 = 750 mg progesterone
      1.9 g (total weight) − 0.050 g progesterone
      = 1.85 g PEG × 15 suppositories
      = 27.75 g PEG total

   c. **Compounding procedure.** The PEG is melted to 50°C, and 700 mg progesterone is added. This mixture is poured into a vaginal suppository mold, allowed to cool, cleaned, and dispensed. PEG quantity is calculated using the vaginal mold volume.

XI. PARENTERAL PRODUCTS

A. General requirements. The extemporaneous compounding of sterile products is no longer confined only to the hospital environment; it now is done by community pharmacists engaged in home care practice. Minimum requirements include:

1. Proper equipment and supplies
2. Proper facilities, including a laminar flow clean bench
3. Proper documentation of all products made

4. Quality control, including batch sterility testing
5. Proper storage both at the facility and while the product is in transport to the patient's home
6. Proper labeling of the prescription product
7. Knowledge of product's stability and incompatibilities
8. Knowledge of all ancillary equipment involved in production or delivery of the medications

B. Preparation of parenteral products

1. Preparation of sterile products requires special skills and training. **Attempts to prepare parenteral products or provide this service without proper training should not be made.**
2. These products must be prepared in a clean room, using aseptic technique (i.e., working under controlled conditions to minimize contamination).
3. Dry powders of parenteral drugs for reconstitution are used for drug products that are unstable as solutions. It is important to know the correct diluents that can be used to yield a solution.
4. Solutions of drugs for parenteral administration may also be further diluted prior to administration. If further dilution is required, then the pharmacist must know the stability and compatibility of the drug in the diluent.

C. Reconstitution of a dry powder from a vial

1. Work takes place in a laminar flow clean bench, observing sterile technique.
2. The manufacturer's instructions should be checked to determine the required volume of diluent.
3. The appropriate needle size and syringe are chosen, keeping in mind that the capacity of the syringe should be slightly larger than the volume required for reconstitution.
4. Using the correct diluent, the surface of the container is cleaned, using an alcohol prep pad, after which the alcohol is permitted to evaporate.
5. The syringe is filled with the diluent to the proper volume.
6. The surface of the vial containing the sterile powder is cleaned, using an alcohol prep pad, after which it is permitted to dry. The diluent is injected into the vial containing the dry powder.
7. The vial is gently shaken or rolled, and the powder is allowed to dissolve.
8. After the powder has dissolved, the vial is inverted and the desired volume is withdrawn.
9. The vehicle is prepared by swabbing the medication port of the bag or bottle with an alcohol prep pad.
10. The solution in the syringe is injected into the vehicle. If a plastic container is used, care must be taken not to puncture the side walls of the container with the tip of the needle.
11. The container should be shaken to assure thorough mixing of the contents.
12. The contents of the container should be checked for particulate matter.
13. A sterile seal or cap is applied over the port of the container.
14. All needles and syringes should be properly discarded.
15. The bag is labeled.

D. Removing the fluid contents from an ampule

1. The ampule, is held upright to open it, and the top is tapped to remove any solution trapped in this area.
2. The neck of the ampule is swabbed with an alcohol swab.
3. The ampule is grasped on each side of the neck with the thumb and index finger of each hand and quickly snapped open.
4. A 5-μm filter needle is attached to a syringe of the appropriate size.

5. The ampule is tilted, and the needle is inserted.
6. The needle is positioned near the neck of the ampule, and the solution is withdrawn from the ampule.
7. If the solution is for an intravenous push (bolus injection), the filter needle is removed from the syringe and replaced with a cap.
8. If the solution is for an intravenous infusion, then the filter needle is removed and replaced with a new needle of the appropriate size. The drug is injected into the appropriate vehicle.
9. All materials should be discarded properly, and the final product should be labeled.

E. Removing drug solution from a vial

1. The tab around the rubber closure on the vial is removed, and this surface is swabbed with an alcohol prep pad.
2. An equivalent amount of air is injected into the vial to prevent the creation of a negative vacuum and to allow the removal of the drug.
3. Using the appropriate needle size and syringe, the needle is inserted into the rubber closure bevel at a 45° angle.
4. The plunger is pushed down, and air is released into the vial; when the plunger is pulled back, the solution is withdrawn.
5. The solution is then injected into the appropriate vehicle.

STUDY QUESTIONS

Directions: Each of the numbered items or incomplete statements in this section is followed by answers or by completions of the statement. Select the **one** lettered answer or completion that is **best** in each case.

Questions 1–3

The following medication order is given to the pharmacist by the physician:

Olive oil	60.0
ASA	0.6
Water	120.0
Sig:15 ml tid	

1. The final dosage form of this prescription will be

(A) a solution
(B) an elixir
(C) an emulsion
(D) a suspension
(E) a lotion

2. When preparing this prescription, the pharmacist needs to add

(A) Tween 80
(B) acacia
(C) glycerin
(D) alcohol
(E) propylene glycol (PEG)

3. Which of the following caution labels should the pharmacist affix to the container when dispensing this product?

(A) Do not refrigerate
(B) Shake well
(C) For external use only
(D) No preservatives added

Directions: Each item below contains three suggested answers of which **one or more** is correct. Choose the answer

A if **I only** is correct
B if **III only** is correct
C if **I and II** are correct
D if **II and III** are correct
E if **I, II, and III** are correct

4. Correct statements about the prescription below include which of the following?

Morphine 1 mg/ml
Flavored vehicle qs ad 120 ml
Sig: 5–20 mg po q 3–4 hours prn pain

I. The amount of morphine needed is 240 mg
II. Powdered morphine alkaloid should be used when compounding this prescription
III. The final dosage form of this prescription is a solution

5. When preparing the following prescription, the pharmacist should

Podophyllum 5%
Salicylic acid 10%
Acetone 20%
Flexible collodion ad 30 ml
Sig: Apply q hs

I. triturate 1.5 g of podophyllum with the 8 ml of acetone
II. add 3 g of salicylic acid to the collodion with trituration
III. affix an "external use only" label to the container

1-C
2-B
3-B
4-B
5-B

SUMMARY OF DIRECTIONS

A	B	C	D	E
I only	III only	I, II only	II, III only	All are correct

6. Correct statements about the prescription below include which of the following?

    Sulfur 6
    Purified water
    Camphor water aa qs ad 60

    I. Precipitated sulfur can be used to prepare this prescription
    II. The sulfur can be triturated with glycerin prior to mixing with other ingredients
    III. A "shake well" label should be affixed to the bottle

7. Correct statements about the prescription below include which of the following?

    Starch 10%
    Menthol 1%
    Camphor 2%
    Calamine qs ad 120.0

    I. The powders should be blended together in a mortar, using geometric dilution
    II. The prescription should be prepared by dissolving the camphor in a sufficient amount of 90% alcohol
    III. An eutectic mixture should be avoided

8. When preparing the following prescription, the pharmacist should

    Salicylic acid 3 g
    Sulfur Ppt 7 g
    Lanolin 10 g
    White petrolatum 10 g

    I. mix the powders, using geometric dilution in a mortar
    II. use a rubber spatula to weigh and levigate the salicylic acid
    III. place on an ointment tile and levigate the ingredients, using geometric dilution

9. An equal volume of air is injected when removing drug solutions from

    I. vials
    II. ampules
    III. syringes

6-E
7-A
8-E
9-A

ANSWERS AND EXPLANATIONS

1–3. The answers are: 1-C *[VI B 1],* **2-B** *[VI B 2, C 1],* **3-B** *[VI B 1, 3 d–f].*
Since olive oil and water are two immiscible liquids, their incorporation requires a two-phase system in which one liquid is dispersed throughout another liquid in the form of small droplets. To accomplish this, an emulsifying agent is necessary. Acacia is the most suitable emulsifying agent when forming an oil-in-water emulsion that is intended for internal use.

Emulsions are physically unstable. They must be protected against the effects of microbial contamination and physical separation. Shaking before use redistributes the two layers of an emulsion. Since light, air, and microorganisms also affect the stability of an emulsion, preservatives could be added.

4. The answer is B (III) *[III A, C 3].*
The concentration of morphine needed for the prescription described in the question is 1 mg/ml, and since 120 ml is the final volume, 120 mg of morphine is needed to compound this prescription. Morphine alkaloid has poor solubility; therefore, one of the salt forms should be used. Because morphine is dissolved in the vehicle, resulting in a liquid preparation, the final dosage form is a solution.

5. The answer is B (III) *[III C 1, 5, D 3 b].*
Calculating for the amount of each ingredient of the prescription in the question requires 1.5 g of podophyllum, 3 g of salicylic acid, and 6 ml of acetone. The correct procedure would be to triturate the podophyllum with the acetone, then add the triturated salicylic acid to a calibrated bottle containing the podophyllum and acetone. Flexible collodion is then added up to the 30 ml calibration. An "external use only" label should be affixed to the container.

6. The answer is E (all) *[IV B 2, C 5, D 1, 2].*
While precipitated sulfur can be used to prepare the prescription described in the question, it is difficult to triturate; therefore, it must first be levigated with a suitable levigating agent (e.g., glycerin). All suspensions, due to their instability, require shaking prior to use to redistribute the insoluble ingredients.

7. The answer is A (I) *[VI D 1].*
The proper procedure for compounding the prescription described in the question is to first form a liquid eutectic. This is done by triturating the menthol and camphor together in a mortar. This eutectic is then blended with the powdered starch and calamine, using geometric dilution.

8. The answer is E (all) *[IX C 1–3, D 1 b].*
The proper procedure for preparing the prescription given in the question is to reduce the particle size of each powder and mix them together, using geometric dilution. This ensures the proper blending of the powders. Next, this powdered mixture is incorporated, geometrically, with the petrolatum. Then, the lanolin is added geometrically. Since salicylic acid is corrosive, a rubber spatula should be used.

9. The answer is A (I) *[XI E 2].*
An equal volume of air must be injected when removing a drug solution from a vial. This is done to prevent the formation of a vacuum within the vial. This problem does not occur with ampules and syringes containing drug solutions; therefore, it is unnecessary to inject any air when removing them.

6 Biopharmaceutics and Pharmacokinetics

Leon Shargel

I. INTRODUCTION

A. Biopharmaceutics is the study of the relationship of a drug product's physical and chemical properties to its bioavailability.

1. A **drug product** is the finished dosage form (e.g., tablet, capsule, solution), which contains the active drug ingredient, usually in association with inactive ingredients.
2. **Bioavailability** is a measurement of the rate and extent (amount) of therapeutically active drug that reaches the systemic circulation.

B. Pharmacokinetics is the study of drug movement in the body over time during the drug's absorption, distribution, and elimination (excretion and biotransformation).

II. DRUG ABSORPTION

A. Transport of drugs across a cell membrane. The cell membrane is a semipermeable structure composed of lipids and proteins. Drugs may be transported by **passive diffusion** or **carrier-mediated transport**.

1. **General principles**
   a. Generally, proteins and drugs bound to proteins do not cross cell membranes.
   b. **Nonpolar lipid-soluble drugs** traverse cell membranes more easily than **ionic** or **polar water-soluble drugs**.
   c. **Small molecular weight drugs** diffuse across a cell membrane more easily than **large** or **high molecular weight drugs**.

2. **Passive diffusion**
   a. **Fick's law of diffusion.** Most drugs cross cell membranes by passive diffusion, **moving from an area of high concentration to an area of lower concentration** according to Fick's law of diffusion:

$$\frac{dQ}{dt} = \frac{DAK}{h}(C_a - C_p),$$

   where dQ/dt is the rate of drug diffusion, D is the diffusion constant, A is the surface area of the membrane, K is the oil/water partition coefficient of the drug, h is the thickness of the membrane, and $(C_a - C_p)$ is the difference between the drug concentration at the absorption site and in the plasma, respectively.
   b. **Ionization of a weak electrolyte drug** is influenced by the pH of the medium in which the drug is dissolved and the pK_a (see III A 4 b) of the drug. The nonionized species is more lipid soluble than the ionized species and diffuses more easily across the cell membrane by passive transport.

3. **Carrier-mediated transport**
   a. **Active transport** of drugs across a membrane is a carrier-mediated transport system with the following characteristics:
   (1) The drug moves against a concentration gradient.
   (2) The process requires energy.
   (3) The carrier may be selective for certain types of drugs resembling natural substrates or metabolites that are normally actively transported.

(4) The carrier system may be saturated at a high drug concentration.
(5) The process may be competitive (drugs with similar structures may compete for the same carrier).

b. **Facilitated diffusion** is also a carrier-mediated transport system. However, facilitated diffusion occurs with a concentration gradient and does not require energy.

B. Routes of drug administration. Drugs may be administered by **parenteral, enteral, inhalation,** intranasal, or **topical routes.**

1. Parenteral administration

a. **Intravenous bolus injection.** The drug is injected directly into the bloodstream. The drug rapidly distributes throughout the body and generally acts very rapidly. Any side effects, including an intense pharmacologic response, anaphylaxis, or overt toxicity, also occur rapidly.

b. **Intra-arterial injection.** The drug is injected into a specific artery to achieve a specific high tissue drug concentration before drug distribution throughout the body. Intra-arterial injection is used for diagnostic agents and occasionally for cancer chemotherapy.

c. **Intravenous infusion.** The drug is given intravenously at a constant input rate. Intravenous infusion maintains a relatively constant plasma drug concentration.

d. **Intramuscular injection.** The drug is injected into a muscular area, where the drug is promptly absorbed. The rate of drug absorption depends upon the vascularity of the muscle site, the drug's lipid solubility, and the vehicle in which the drug is contained.

e. **Subcutaneous injection.** The drug is injected beneath the skin. Because the subcutaneous area is less vascular than muscular areas, drug absorption may be less rapid. The factors that affect intramuscular absorption also affect subcutaneous absorption.

2. Enteral administration

a. **Buccal and sublingual administration.** A tablet or lozenge is placed under the tongue (sublingual) or in the cheek (buccal). This allows a nonpolar, lipid-soluble drug to be absorbed across the epithelial lining of the mouth. Drug absorption after buccal or sublingual administration is directly into the systemic circulation bypassing the liver and any first-pass effects.

b. **Oral drug administration** (the most common route). The drug is swallowed and is systemically absorbed from the gastrointestinal tract by way of the mesenteric circulation to the hepatic portal vein into the liver and then to the systemic circulation.

(1) The oral route is the most convenient and safest route of drug administration.
(2) The oral route has some **disadvantages.**
   (a) The drug may not be absorbed from the gastrointestinal tract consistently or completely.
   (b) The drug may be digested by gastrointestinal enzymes or decomposed by the acid pH of the stomach.
   (c) The drug may irritate mucosal epithelial cells or complex with gastrointestinal tract contents.
   (d) Some drugs may be incompletely absorbed due to first-pass effects or presystemic elimination (e.g., the drug is metabolized by the liver prior to systemic absorption).
   (e) The absorption rate may be erratic because of delayed gastric emptying or changes in intestinal motility.
(3) Most drugs are absorbed from the gastrointestinal tract by **passive diffusion. Carrier-mediated transport** plays a smaller role.
(4) The drug is absorbed throughout the gastrointestinal tract, but the **duodenal region,** which has a large surface area composed of villi and microvilli, is the primary site. The large blood supply provided by the mesenteric vessels allows the drug to be absorbed more efficiently by passive diffusion (see II A 2).
(5) **Delay in gastric emptying** delays the arrival of the drug in the duodenum for systemic absorption. Various factors affect gastric emptying time, including meal content, emotional factors, and anticholinergic drugs.
(6) **Normal intestinal motility** from peristalsis brings the drug in contact with the intestinal epithelial cells. A sufficient period of contact (**residence time**) is needed to allow for drug absorption across the cell membranes from the mucosal to the serosal surface.
(7) A few drugs, such as **cimetidine** and **acetaminophen,** when given in an immediate-release oral dosage form to fasted subjects produce a blood concentration curve consisting of two peaks; this **double peak phenomenon** has been attributed to variability in stomach emptying, variable intestinal motility, and enterohepatic cycling.

c. **Rectal administration.** The drug in solution (enema) or suppository form is inserted into the rectum. Drug diffuses from the solution or is released from the suppository and absorbed across the rectum's mucosal surface.

3. **Inhalation.** The drug is given as an aerosol (liquid or solid particles) into the respiratory tract. Smaller particles reach deeper into the small bronchioles than do larger particles. The drug enters the circulation by diffusion across the alveolar membranes. Nebulizers and metered-dose inhalers are commonly used for delivering drugs for inhalation.

4. **Intranasal administration.** The drug is contained in a solution or suspension and is administered to the nasal mucosa either as a spray or drops. The medication may be used for local activity (e.g., nasal decongestants, intranasal steroids) or for systemic effects.

5. **Topical (percutaneous) administration.** The drug (i.e., in a lotion, ointment, cream, patch) is placed on the skin, with or without an occlusive dressing. Lipid-soluble drugs, such as nitroglycerin, diffuse across the skin into the systemic circulation.

C. **Local drug activity versus systemic drug absorption.** The drug administration route, absorption site, and the bioavailability of the drug from the dosage form are major factors in the design of a drug product.

1. Drugs intended for **local activity,** such as topical antibiotics, anti-infectives, antifungal agents, and local anesthetics are formulated in dosage forms that minimize systemic drug absorption. The concentration of these drugs at the application site affects their activity.

2. When **systemic drug absorption** is desired, the bioavailability of the drug from the dosage form at the absorption site must be considered (e.g., a drug given intravenously is 100% bioavailable because all of the drug is placed directly into the systemic circulation). The amount (dose) of drug in the dosage form is based on the extent of drug absorption and on the desired systemic drug concentration. The type of dosage form (e.g., immediate release, controlled release) influences the rate of drug absorption.

III. BIOPHARMACEUTIC PRINCIPLES

A. Physicochemical drug properties

1. **Drug dissolution.** For most drugs with limited water solubility, the rate at which the solid drug enters into solution (dissolution) is often the rate-limiting step in the drug's bioavailability. The **Noyes Whitney equation** describes the rate of drug dissolution.

$$\text{Rate of dissolution} = \frac{dC}{dt} = \frac{DAK}{h}\,(C_s - C_b),$$

where D is the diffusion coefficient, A is the surface area of the drug, K is the partition coefficient (water/oil), h is the thickness of the stagnant layer, C_s, is the concentration of drug in the stagnant layer (a saturated solution around the solid drug particle), and C_b, is concentration of the drug in the bulk phase of the solvent.

2. **Drug solubility** is the maximum concentration of the drug solute dissolved in the solvent (usually water) under specified conditions of temperature, pH, and pressure. The drug's solubility in saturated solution is a static property; whereas the drug dissolution rate is a dynamic property that relates more closely to the rate of drug absorption.

3. **Particle size and surface area** are inversely related. As solid drug particle size decreases, the surface area of the particles increases.
   a. As described by the Noyes Whitney equation, the dissolution rate is **directly proportional to the surface area**. An increase in surface area allows for more contact between the solid drug particle and the aqueous solvent, resulting in a faster dissolution rate (see III A 1).
   b. With certain **hydrophobic drugs,** excessive particle size reduction does not always produce an increased dissolution rate. These small particles tend to reaggregate into larger particles to reduce the high surface free energy produced by particle size reduction.
   c. To prevent the formation of aggregates, small drug particles may be dispersed (**molecular dispersion**) in polyethylene glycol (PEG), polyvinylpyrrolidone (PVP; povidone), dextrose, or other agents. For example, a molecular dispersion of griseofulvin in a water-soluble carrier such as PEG 4000 (e.g., Gris-PEG) enhances the drug's dissolution and bioavailability.

4. **Partition coefficient and extent of ionization**
   a. **Partition coefficient** of a drug is the ratio of a drug's solubility at equilibrium in an aqueous solvent and a nonaqueous solvent. Hydrophilic drugs with higher water solubility have a faster dissolution rate than hydrophobic or lipophilic drugs, which have poor water solubility.
   b. **Extent of ionization.** Drugs that are weak electrolytes exist in both an ionized form and a nonionized (weak acid or weak base) form. The extent of ionization depends upon the pK_a, of the weak electrolyte and pH of the solvent. The drug's ionized form is more water soluble than its nonionized form. The **Henderson Hasselbalch equation** describes the relationship between ionized and nonionized forms.
      (1) For weak acids,

$$pH = pK_a + \log \frac{[\text{salt}]}{[\text{nonionized acid}]}$$

      (2) For weak bases,

$$pH = pK_a + \log \frac{[\text{nonionized base}]}{[\text{salt}]}$$

5. **Salt formation**
   a. The choice of salt form for a drug depends upon the drug's desired physical and chemical properties. Certain salts are designed to provide slower dissolution, slower bioavailability, and longer duration of activity. Other salts may be chosen for greater stability, less local irritation at the absorption site, or less systemic toxicity.
      (1) Some soluble salt forms are generally less stable than the nonionized form. For example, sodium aspirin is less stable than aspirin in the acid form.
      (2) A solid dosage form containing buffering agents may be formulated with the free acid form of the drug (e.g., buffered aspirin).
         (a) The buffering agent forms an alkaline medium within the gastrointestinal tract, and the drug dissolves in situ.
         (b) The dissolved salt form of the drug then diffuses into the bulk fluid of the gastrointestinal tract, forms a fine precipitate that redissolves rapidly, and becomes available for absorption.
   b. **Effervescent granules** or **tablets** containing the acid drug along with sodium bicarbonate, tartaric acid, citric acid, and other ingredients are added to water just before oral administration. The excess sodium bicarbonate forms an alkaline solution in which the drug dissolves. Carbon dioxide is also formed by the decomposition of carbonic acid.
   c. For weakly acidic drugs, potassium and sodium salts are more water soluble than divalent cation salts such as magnesium and aluminum.
   d. For weak bases, common water-soluble salts include the hydrochloride, sulfate, citrate, and gluconate salts. The napsylate, stearate, and estolate salts of weak bases are less water soluble.

6. **Polymorphism** is the ability of a drug to exist in more than one crystalline form.
   a. Different polymorphs have different physical properties, including melting points and dissolution rates.
   b. **Amorphous polymorphs** are nonrigid, **noncrystalline forms,** which have faster dissolution rates than crystalline forms of the same drug.

7. **Hydrates.** A drug may exist in a **hydrated (solvated) form** or as an **anhydrous molecule**. Dissolution rates differ for hydrated and anhydrated forms. For example, the anhydrous form of ampicillin dissolves faster and is more rapidly absorbed than the hydrated form.

8. **Complex formation in drug interaction.** A complex may be a reversible or irreversible interaction between a drug and another substance. For example, tetracycline and calcium (or some other divalent cation such as magnesium or aluminum) form a complex known as a **chelate**. Many drugs adsorb strongly on charcoal. Drugs may also bind proteins, such as albumin, to form a drug–protein complex.
   a. Complex formation usually alters the drug's physical and chemical characteristics. For example:
      (1) The chelate of tetracycline with calcium is less water soluble and is poorly absorbed.
      (2) Theophylline complexed with ethylene diamine to form aminophylline is more water soluble and is used for parenteral administration.

(3) Cyclodextrins have been used to form complexes with many different drugs to increase their water solubility.

b. Large drug complexes, such as drug–protein complexes, do not cross cell membranes easily. These complexes must first dissociate to free the drug for absorption at the absorption site, permitting diffusion across cell membranes into tissues or glomerular filtering prior to excretion into the urine.

B. Drug product formulation

1. General considerations

a. Design of the appropriate dosage form depends on the:
(1) Drug's physical and chemical properties
(2) Dose of the drug
(3) Administration route
(4) Type of drug product desired
(5) Desired therapeutic effect
(6) Bioavailability of the drug from the dosage form
(7) Pharmacokinetics and pharmacodynamics of the drug

b. Bioavailability. The more complicated the formulation of the finished drug product (e.g., a controlled-release tablet, enteric-coated tablet), the greater the potential for a bioavailability problem. The bioavailability of a drug from a solid dosage form depends on a succession of rate processes, including:
(1) **Disintegration** of the drug product and subsequent release of the drug
(2) **Dissolution** of the drug in an aqueous environment
(3) **Absorption** of the drug across cell membranes into the systemic circulation (Figure 6-1)

c. Rate-limiting step in the bioavailability of a drug from a drug product is the slowest rate in a series of kinetic processes.
(1) For most conventional solid drug products, such as tablets and capsules, the dissolution rate is the slowest, or rate-limiting step, for bioavailability.
(2) For a controlled-release or sustained-action drug product, the release of the drug from the dosage form is the rate-limiting step.

2. Solutions are homogeneous mixtures of one or more solutes dispersed molecularly in a dissolving medium (solvent).

a. Compared with other oral drug formulations, a drug dissolved in an aqueous solution is in the most bioavailable and consistent form. Because the drug is already dissolved, no dissolution step is necessary before systemic absorption. Oral drug solutions are often used as the reference preparation for solid oral formulations.

b. A drug dissolved in a hydroalcoholic solution (e.g., elixir) also has good bioavailability. Alcohol aids drug solubility. However, the drug may form a fine precipitate upon dilution

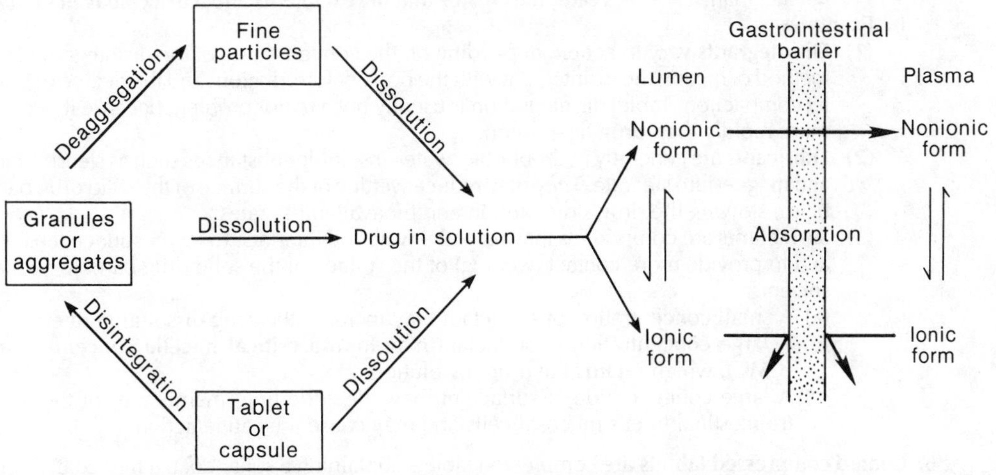

Figure 6-1. Diagrammatic representation of a drug's disintegration, dissolution, and absorption following oral administration in tablet or capsule form. (Adapted with permission from Blanchard J: Gastrointestinal absorption II. Formulation factors affecting bioavailability. *Am J Pharm* 150:132–151, 1978.)

in the bulk contents of the gastrointestinal tract. The precipitate's fine, solid drug particles are well dispersed, have a large surface area, and are rapidly re-dissolved before systemic absorption.

c. A highly viscous syrup may slow the drug's outward diffusion, slowing the rate of bioavailability.

3. Suspensions are pharmaceutical dispersions in which finely divided solid particles of a drug are dispersed in a liquid medium that is not a solvent for the drug.

a. Drug bioavailability of a well-prepared suspension may be similar to that of a solution because the small drug particles are dispersed and offer a large surface area for rapid dissolution. A slow drug dissolution rate of the suspension may decrease the rate of bioavailability.

b. Suspending agents (often a cellulose derivative or gum, such as methylcellulose or acacia) are added to suspensions to impart viscosity and prevent the drug particles from settling and agglomerating. Highly viscous suspensions with a large concentration of suspending agent prolong gastric emptying time, slow drug dissolution, and slow the rate of drug bioavailability.

4. Capsules are hard or soft gelatin shells in which drugs are contained. A capsule containing a drug is considered a solid dosage form. **Coating** the capsule's gelatin shell (or coating the drug particles within a capsule) can alter the drug's bioavailability.

a. Hard gelatin capsules are usually filled with a powder blend that contains the drug. Typically, the powder blend is simpler and less compacted than the blend in a compressed tablet. After ingestion, the gelatin softens, swells, and begins to dissolve in the gastrointestinal tract. The drug is released rapidly, disperses easily, and has good bioavailability. Hard gelatin capsules are the preferred dosage form for early clinical trials of a new drug.

b. Soft gelatin capsules may contain a nonaqueous solution, a powder, or a suspension of a drug. The vehicle may be water miscible, as with PEG. The cardiac glycoside, digoxin, dispersed in such a water-miscible vehicle (Lanoxicaps), has better bioavailability than a digoxin compressed tablet formulation (Lanoxin). However, a soft gelatin capsule that contains the drug dissolved in a **hydrophobic vehicle,** such as a vegetable oil, may have slower bioavailability than a compressed tablet formulation.

5. Compressed tablets are solid dosage forms in which high pressure is used to compress a powder blend or granulation, which contains the active drug and other ingredients or excipients, into a solid mass.

a. Excipients, including diluents (fillers), binders, disintegrants, lubricants, dye, and flavoring and sweetening agents have the following properties:

(1) They provide for the efficient manufacture of compressed tablets.

(2) They influence the tablets' physical and chemical characteristics.

(3) They affect the drug's bioavailability. **The higher the ratio of excipient to active drug** (greater than 5:1), the **greater the chance that the excipients affect drug bioavailability**.

b. Examples

(1) Disintegrants vary in action, depending on the concentration of the disintegrant, the method of mixing the disintegrant with the powder formulation, and the degree of tablet compaction. Tablet disintegration is usually not a major problem because it occurs more rapidly than drug dissolution.

(2) Lubricants are generally hydrophobic, water-insoluble substances such as stearic acid and magnesium stearate. They may reduce wetting of the surface of the solid drug particles, slowing the drug's dissolution and bioavailability rates.

(3) Surfactants are compounds that act at the water/oil interface to lower surface tension and to provide more contact (wetting) of the surface of the solid drug particle by the solvent.

(a) A small concentration of surfactant may increase the drug dissolution rate.

(b) A large concentration of surfactant may form a **critical micelle concentration (CMC),** which retards the drug dissolution rate.

(c) A large concentration of surfactant may affect the lipid membranes of the gastrointestinal tract's mucosal cells and may cause a laxative action.

6. Coated compressed tablets are compressed tablets containing a sugar coat, a film coat, or an enteric coat. The coating has the following properties:

a. It protects the drug from moisture, light, and air.

b. It masks the drug's taste or odor.

c. It improves the tablet's appearance.
d. It controls the drug's release rate.

7. **Modified-release dosage forms** are drug products designed to alter the rate or timing of drug release. Because modified-release dosage forms are more complex than conventional, immediate-release dosage forms, more stringent quality control and bioavailability tests are required. **Dose dumping**—the abrupt release of a large amount of a drug in an uncontrolled manner—can be a major problem.
   a. Extended-release dosage forms include such drug products as **controlled-release, sustained-action,** and **long-acting drug delivery systems**. These dosage forms allow at least a twofold reduction in dosing frequency compared to a conventional immediate-release drug product.
      (1) The extended, slow release of controlled-release drug products produces a relatively flat, sustained plasma drug concentration, which avoids toxicity from high-peak or low-trough concentration peaks.
      (2) Extended-release dosage forms may yield an immediate (initial) release of the drug, followed by a slower sustained release.
   b. Delayed-release dosage forms release the active drug at a time other than promptly after administration at a desired site or location in the gastrointestinal tract. For example, an enteric-coated drug product does not dissolve in the stomach's acid pH but dissolves in the more alkaline pH of the small intestine.

8. **Transdermal drug delivery systems**—often referred to as **patches**—are controlled-release devices containing drug for systemic absorption through the skin. Patches (e.g., nicotine, nitroglycerin, estradiol) are manufactured in a variety of proprietary patents. In some cases, the patch controls the drug absorption rate through the skin, and in other cases, the skin itself—particularly the stratum corneum—is the rate-controlling step.

9. **Site-specific carrier systems** refer to drug carrier systems that place the drug at or near the receptor site. **Targeted drug delivery** may be accomplished by:
   a. Delivery of the drug to the capillary bed of the active site
   b. Delivery of the drug to a special cell type (e.g., tumor cells) and not to normal cells
   c. Delivery of the drug to a specific organ or tissue by complexing the drug with a carrier that recognizes the target

IV. BIOAVAILABILITY AND BIOEQUIVALENCE

A. Bioavailability and therapeutic effect

1. **Pharmacologic responses** occur when drugs combine with **receptors** in the body. This drug–receptor interaction is usually reversible. As more drug molecules combine with the receptor, the intensity of the pharmacologic effect increases up to a maximum effect (Figure 6-2). The **time course of the pharmacologic response** depends on the rates of association and dissociation of the drug with the receptor and the drug concentration at the receptor site.
   a. Onset time. As drug is systemically absorbed, the drug concentration at the receptor rises to a **minimum effective concentration (MEC)** and a pharmacologic response is initiated. The time from drug administration to the MEC is known as the onset time.
   b. Duration of action. As long as the drug concentration remains above the MEC, pharmacologic activity is observed. The duration of action is the time for which the drug concentration remains above the MEC.
   c. Therapeutic window. As the drug concentration increases, other receptors may combine with the drug to exert a toxic or adverse response. This drug concentration is the **minimum toxic concentration (MTC)**. The drug concentration range between the MEC and the MTC is the therapeutic window.

2. **Measuring bioavailability**
   a. Plasma drug concentration versus time curve measures the bioavailability of a drug from a drug product (Figure 6-3).
      (1) Time for peak plasma drug concentration (T_{max}) relates to the rate constants for systemic drug absorption and elimination. If two oral drug products contain the same amount of active drug but different excipients, the dosage form that yields the faster rate of drug absorption has the shorter T_{max} since the elimination rate constant for the drug from both dosage forms is the same.

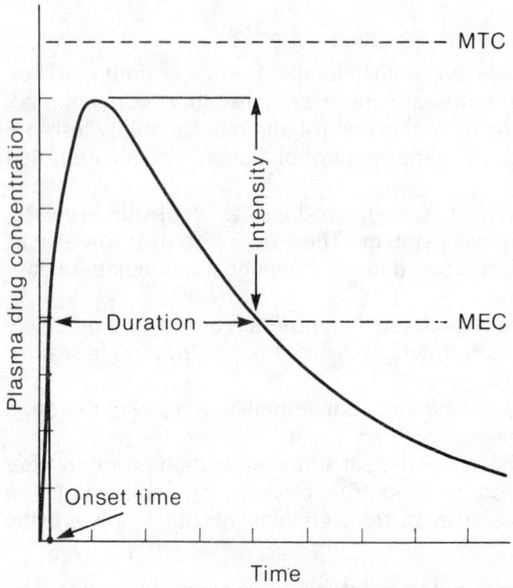

Figure 6-2. Generalized plasma drug concentration versus time curve after oral drug administration. *MEC* = minimum effective concentration; *MTC* = minimum toxic concentration. (Adapted with permission from Shargel L, Yu ABC: *Applied Biopharmaceutics and Pharmacokinetics,* 3rd ed. East Norwalk, CT, Appleton & Lange, 1993, p 34.)

(2) **Peak plasma drug concentration** (C_{max})—the plasma drug concentration at T_{max}—relates to the intensity of the pharmacologic response. Ideally, C_{max} should be within the therapeutic window.

(3) **Area under the plasma drug concentration versus time curve (AUC)** relates to the amount or extent of drug absorption. The amount of systemic drug absorption is directly related to the AUC. The AUC is usually calculated by the **trapezoidal rule** and is expressed in units of concentration multiplied by time (e.g., $\mu g \times hr/ml$).

b. Measurement of urinary drug excretion can determine bioavailability from a drug product. This method is most accurate if the active therapeutic moiety is excreted unchanged in significant quantity in the urine (Figure 6-4).

(1) The **cumulative amount** of active drug excreted in the urine (D_U^∞) is directly related to the extent of systemic drug absorption.

(2) The **rate of drug excretion** in the urine (dD_U/dt) is directly related to the rate of systemic drug absorption.

(3) The **time for the drug to be completely excreted (t^∞)** corresponds to the total time for the drug to be systemically absorbed and completely excreted after administration.

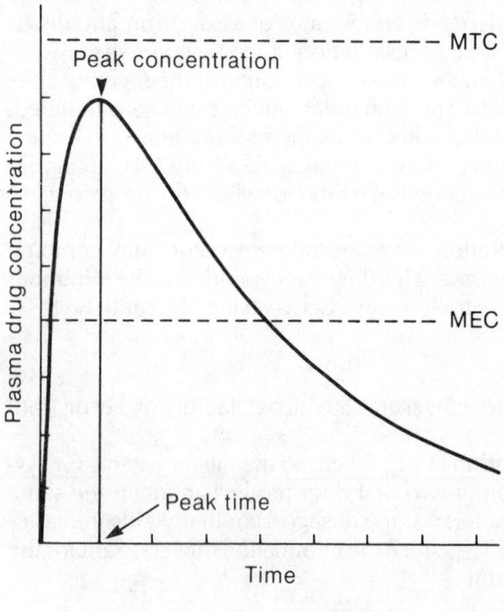

Figure 6-3. Generalized plasma drug concentration versus time curve, showing peak time and peak concentration. *MEC* = minimum effective concentration; *MTC* = minimum toxic concentration. (Adapted with permission from Shargel L, Yu ABC: *Applied Biopharmaceutics and Pharmacokinetics,* 3rd ed. East Norwalk, CT, Appleton & Lange, 1993, p 35.)

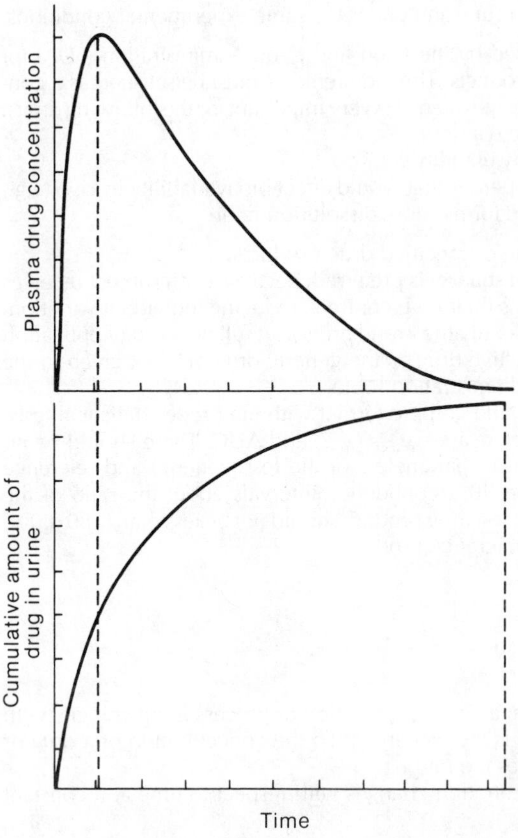

Figure 6-4. These corresponding plots show the relationship of the plasma drug concentration versus time curve to the cumulative amount of drug in the urine versus time curve. (Adapted with permission from Shargel L, Yu ABC: *Applied Biopharmaceutics and Pharmacokinetics,* 3rd ed. East Norwalk, CT, Appleton & Lange, 1993, p 201.)

c. **Acute pharmacologic effects,** such as changes in heart rate, blood pressure, electrocardiogram (ECG), or clotting time, can be used to measure bioavailability when no assay for drug concentration is available. Parameters for measuring an acute pharmacologic effect include onset time, duration of action, and intensity of the effect.
d. **Clinical (pharmacodynamic) responses to a drug** can be used to measure bioavailability quantitatively; however, they are less precise than other methods and highly variable because of individual differences in drug pharmacodynamics and subjective measurements.
e. **The rate of drug dissolution** in vitro for certain drugs correlates with drug bioavailability in vivo. When the dissolution test in vitro is considered statistically adequate to predict drug bioavailability, then dissolution may be used in place of an in vivo bioavailability study.

3. **Relative and absolute bioavailability**
   a. **Relative bioavailability**—the systemic availability of the drug from a dosage form as compared to a reference standard—is calculated as the ratio of the AUC for the dosage form to the AUC for the reference dosage form. A relative bioavailability of 1 (or 100%) implies that drug bioavailability from both dosage forms is the same but does not indicate the completeness of systemic drug absorption. The determination of relative bioavailability is very important in generic drug studies (e.g., bioequivalence studies).
   b. **Absolute bioavailability (F)**—the fraction of drug systemically absorbed and the availability of the drug from the dosage form as compared to the availability of the drug after intravenous administration—is usually calculated as the ratio of the AUC for the dosage form given orally to the AUC obtained after intravenous drug administration. An F value of 0.80 (or 80%) indicates that only 80% of the drug was systemically available from the dosage form.

B. **Bioequivalence.** A generic drug product is considered bioequivalent to the brand drug product if its rate and extent of systemic absorption (bioavailability) do not show a statistically significant difference when administered at the same dose of the active ingredient in the same chemical form, in a similar dosage form, by the same route, and under the same experimental conditions.

1. **Bioequivalence requirements** are imposed by the Food and Drug Administration (FDA) for bioequivalence testing of generic drug products. The requirements must be satisfied as a condition for marketing. Determination of bioequivalence is very important for the following drugs:
   a. Those that have a narrow therapeutic window
   b. Those that demonstrate variable bioavailability
   c. Those that have physicochemical properties that would affect bioavailability in vivo (e.g., poor aqueous solubility, polymorphic forms, slow dissolution rate)
2. **Bioequivalence studies** permit evaluation of specified drug products.
   a. Usually a **crossover design** (e.g., **Latin square**) is preferred, because each subject receives each dosage form. Subjects then act as their own controls, reducing individual variation.
   b. The **reference standard,** which is generally the brand drug with full new drug application (NDA) approval contains the same active drug as the generic drug product given in the same molar dose and by the same administration route.
   c. Data are presented in both tabulated and graphic format with the proper statistical tests.
   d. The important bioavailability parameters are C_{max}, T_{max}, and AUC. There should be no statistical differences between the mean parameters of the test (generic) and reference (brand) drug products. Moreover, the 90% confidence intervals about the ratio of the means for AUC and C_{max} values of the test drug product should not be less than 0.80 (80%) nor greater than 1.20 (120%) of the reference product.

V. PHARMACOKINETICS

A. Introduction

1. **Rates and orders of reactions.** The **rate** of a chemical reaction or process is the velocity with which it occurs. The **order** of a reaction is the way in which the concentration of a drug or reactant in a chemical reaction influences the rate.
   a. **Zero-order reaction.** The drug concentration changes with respect to time at a constant rate, according to this equation:

$$\frac{dC}{dt} = -k_0,$$

   where C is the drug concentration and k_0, is the zero-order rate constant given in units of concentration/time (e.g., mg/ml/hour). Integration of this equation yields the linear (straight-line) equation:

$$C = -k_0t + C_0,$$

   where k_0 is the slope of the line (see Chapter 3, Figure 3-1) and C_0, is the y intercept, or drug concentration, when time (t) is equal to zero. The negative sign indicates that the slope is decreasing.
   b. **First-order reaction.** The drug concentration changes with respect to time equal to the product of the rate constant and the concentration of drug remaining, according to this equation:

$$\frac{dC}{dt} = -kC,$$

   where k is the first-order rate constant, given in units of reciprocal time, or $time^{-1}$ (e.g., 1/hr or hr^{-1}).
   (1) Integration of the above equation yields the following mathematically equivalent equations:

$$C = C_0e^{-kt}$$
$$\ln C = -kt + \ln C_0$$
$$\log C = -\frac{kt}{2.3} + \log C^0$$

   (2) A graph of the above equation shown in Chapter 3, Figure 3-2, demonstrates the linear relationship of the log of the concentration versus time. In Figure 3-2, the slope of the line is equal to $-k/2.3$, and the y intercept is C_0. It should be noted that the values for C are plotted on logarithmic coordinates, and the values for t are on linear coordinates.

(3) The **half-life ($t_{1/2}$)** of a reaction is the time required for the concentration of a drug to decrease by one-half. For a first-order reaction, the half-life is a constant and is related to the first-order rate constant, according to this equation:

$$t_{1/2} = \frac{0.693}{k}$$

2. Models and compartments

a. A **model** is a mathematical description of a biologic system and is used as a concise way to express quantitative relationships.

b. A **compartment** is a group of tissues with similar blood flows and drug affinities. A compartment is not a real physiologic or anatomic region.

3. Drug distribution

a. Drugs distribute rapidly to tissues with high blood flow and more slowly to tissues with a low blood flow.

b. Drugs rapidly cross capillary membranes into tissues because of **passive diffusion** and **hydrostatic pressure**. **Drug permeability** across capillary membranes may vary.

(1) Generally, drugs easily cross the capillaries of the glomerulus of the kidney and the sinusoids of the liver.

(2) The brain's capillaries are surrounded by glial cells, creating a **blood–brain barrier** that acts as a thick lipid membrane, which polar and ionic hydrophilic drugs cross very slowly.

c. Drugs may accumulate in tissues as a result of their physicochemical characteristics or special affinity of the tissue for the drug.

(1) Lipid-soluble drugs may accumulate in adipose (fat) tissue from partitioning of the drug.

(2) Tetracycline may accumulate in bone from complex formation with calcium.

d. Plasma protein binding of drugs affects drug distribution.

(1) A drug bound to a protein forms a complex that is too large to cross cell membranes.

(2) **Albumin** is the major plasma protein involved in drug protein binding. **α_1-Glycoprotein,** also found in plasma, is important for the binding of such basic drugs as propranolol.

(3) Potent drugs such as phenytoin, which are highly bound (> 90%) to plasma proteins, may be displaced by other highly bound drugs. The displacement of the bound drug results in more free (nonbound) drug, which rapidly reaches the drug receptors and causes a more intense pharmacologic response.

B. One-compartment model

1. Intravenous bolus injection. The entire drug dose rapidly enters the body, and the rate of absorption is neglected in calculations (Figure 6-5). The entire body acts as a single compartment, and the drug rapidly equilibrates with all the tissues in the body.

a. Drug elimination is a first-order kinetic process, according to the equations in V A 1 b.

(1) The first-order elimination rate constant (k) represents the sum of all the rate constants for drug removal from the body, including the rate constants for renal excretion and metabolism (**biotransformation**) as described by this equation:

$$k = k_e + k_m,$$

where k_e is the rate constant for renal excretion, and k_m is the rate constant for metabolism. This equation assumes that all rates are first-order processes.

(2) The **elimination half-life ($t_{1/2}$)** is given by this equation:

$$t_{1/2} = \frac{0.693}{k}$$

b. Apparent volume of distribution (V_D) is the hypothetical volume of body fluid in which the drug is dissolved. This is not a true anatomic or physical volume.

(1) The V_D is needed to estimate the amount of drug in the body relative to the concentration of drug in the plasma, as shown in the following relationship:

$$V_D \times C_p = D_B,$$

where V_D is the apparent volume of distribution, C_p is the plasma drug concentration, and D_B is the amount of drug in the body.

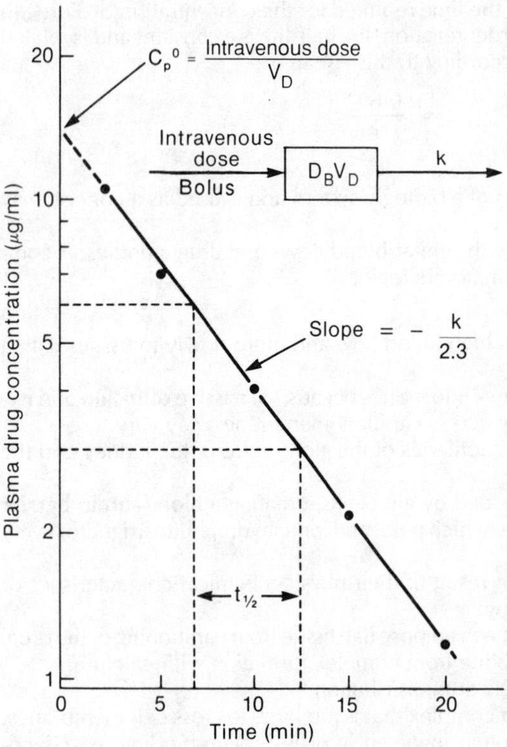

Figure 6-5. Generalized pharmacokinetic model for a drug administered by rapid intravenous bolus injection. $C_p{}^o$ = the extrapolated drug concentration; V_D = the apparent volume of distribution; D_B = the amount of drug in the body; k = the elimination rate constant; $t_{1/2}$ = the elimination half-life. (Adapted with permission from Gibaldi M, Perrier D: *Pharmacokinetics,* 2nd ed. New York, Marcel Dekker, 1982, p 4.)

(2) To calculate the V_D after an intravenous bolus injection, the equation above is rearranged to give:

$$V_D = \frac{D_B{}^o}{C_p{}^o},$$

where $D_B{}^o$ is the dose (D_o) of drug given by intravenous bolus, and $C_p{}^o$ is the extrapolated drug concentration at zero time on the y axis, after the drug has equilibrated.

(3) According to the above equation, V_D is larger when the drug is distributed more extravascularly into the tissues, and $C_p{}^o$ is, therefore, smaller. When more drug is contained in the vascular space or plasma, $C_p{}^o$ is larger, and V_D is smaller.

2. Single oral dose. If the drug is in a conventional dosage form (e.g., a tablet or capsule), the drug is rapidly absorbed by first-order kinetics. Elimination of the drug also follows first-order kinetics (Figure 6-6).

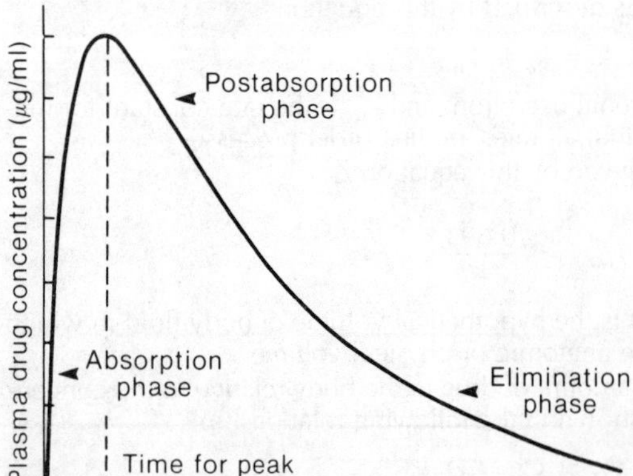

Figure 6-6. Generalized plot for a one-compartment model showing first-order drug absorption and first-order drug elimination. (Adapted with permission from Shargel L, Yu ABC: *Applied Biopharmaceutics and Pharmacokinetics,* 3rd ed. East Norwalk, CT, Appleton & Lange, 1993, p 170.)

a. This equation describes the pharmacokinetics of **first-order absorption and elimination:**

$$C_p = \frac{FD_o k_A}{V_D (k_A - k)} (e^{-kt} - e^{-kt})$$

where k_A is the first-order absorption rate constant, and F is the fraction of drug bioavailable. Changes in F, D_o, V_D, k_A, and k affect the plasma drug concentration.

b. The time for maximum or **peak drug absorption** is given by this equation:

$$T_{max} = \frac{2.3 \log (k_A/k)}{k_A - k}$$

T_{max} depends only on the rate constants k_A and k, not on F, D_o, or V_D

c. After T_{max} is obtained, the peak drug concentration (C_{max}) is calculated, using the equation in V B 2 a and substituting T_{max} for t

d. The AUC may be determined by integration of $\int_0^t C_p dt$, using the trapezoidal rule or by this equation:

$$\int_0^t C_p dt = AUC = \frac{FD_o}{V_D k},$$

where changes in F, D_o, k, and V_D affect the AUC. Small changes in k_A do not affect the AUC.

e. Lag time occurs just at the beginning of systemic drug absorption. For some individuals, systemic drug absorption is delayed after oral drug administration due to delayed stomach emptying or other factors.

3. Intravenous infusion. Zero-order absorption and first-order elimination occur (Figure 6-7).

a. A few oral controlled-release drug products release the drug by zero-order kinetics and have **zero-order systemic absorption.**

b. The plasma drug concentration at any time after the start of an intravenous infusion is given by this equation:

$$C_p = \frac{R}{V_D k} (1 - e^{-kt}),$$

where R is the zero-order rate of infusion given in units as mg/hr or mg/min.

c. If the intravenous infusion is stopped, the plasma drug concentration declines by a first-order process, and the elimination half-life or k may be obtained from the declining plasma drug concentration versus time curve.

d. As the drug is infused, the plasma drug concentration increases to a plateau, or **steady-state concentration.**

(1) Under steady-state conditions, the fraction of drug absorbed equals the fraction of drug eliminated from the body.

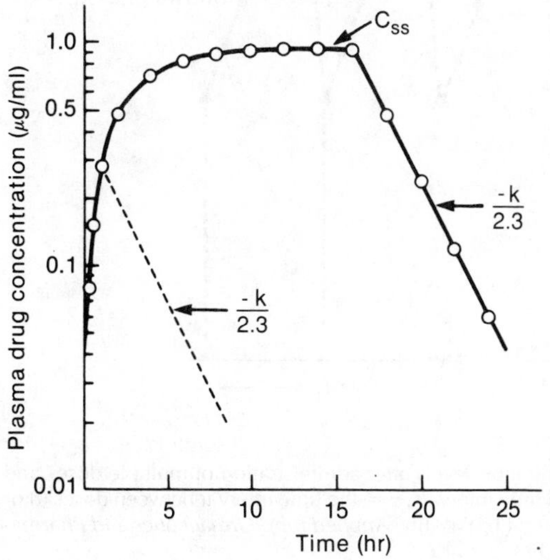

Figure 6-7. Generalized semilogarithmic plot for a drug showing zero-order absorption and first-order elimination. C_{ss} = the steady-state concentration; k = the elimination rate constant. (Adapted with permission from Gibaldi M, Perrier D: *Pharmacokinetics,* 2nd ed. New York, Marcel Dekker, 1982, p 30.)

(2) The plasma concentration at steady state (C_{ss}) is given by this equation:

$$C_{ss} = \frac{R}{V_D k}$$

(3) The **rate of drug infusion (R)** may be calculated from a rearrangement of the above equation, provided that the desired C_{ss}, the V_D, and the k are known. The values are often readily obtainable from the drug literature. To calculate the rate of infusion, use the rearranged equation:

$$R = C_{ss} V_D k,$$

where C_{ss} is the desired (target) plasma drug concentration. The product, $V_D k$ is also equal to total body clearance, Cl_T.

e. A **loading dose (D_L)** is given as an initial intravenous bolus injection of drug to produce the C_{ss} as rapidly as possible. The intravenous infusion is started at the same time.

(1) The **time to reach C_{ss}** depends on the drug's elimination half-life. To reach 95% or 99% of the C_{ss} without a D_L would take 4.32 or 6.65 half-lives, respectively.

(2) The D_L is the amount of drug that, when dissolved in the apparent V_D, produces the desired C_{ss}. Thus, D_L is calculated by the following equations:

$$D_L = C_{ss} V_D \text{ and } D_L = R/k.$$

f. For a drug with a narrow therapeutic window, an intravenous infusion provides a relatively constant plasma drug concentration that does not rise above the MTC or fall below the MEC.

4. Multiple doses. Many drugs are given intermittently in a multiple-dose regimen for continuous or prolonged therapeutic activity. This regimen is often used in the treatment of a chronic disease.

a. If drug doses are given at frequent intervals before complete elimination of the previous dose, then plasma drug concentrations accumulate and rise to a plateau or steady-state level.

b. At **steady state,** plasma drug concentration fluctuates between a maximum (C_{max}^{∞}) and a minimum (C_{min}^{∞}) [Figure 6-8].

c. When calculating a multiple-dose regimen, the **superposition principle** assumes that previous drug doses have no effect on the subsequent doses. Thus, the predicted plasma drug concentration is the total plasma drug concentration obtained by adding the residual drug concentrations found after each previous dose.

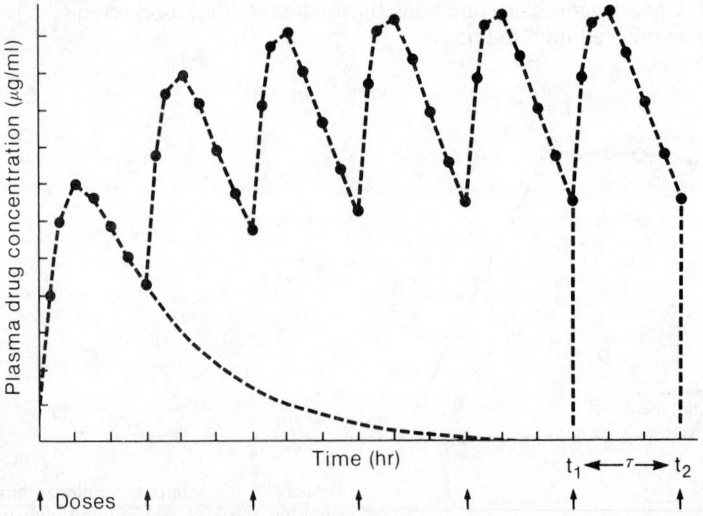

Figure 6-8. Generalized plot showing plasma drug concentration levels after administration of multiple doses and levels of accumulation when equal doses are given at equal time intervals. τ = the time interval between doses (*t*) or the frequency of dosing. (Adapted with permission from Shargel L, Yu ABC: *Applied Biopharmaceutics and Pharmacokinetics,* 3rd ed. East Norwalk, CT, Appleton & Lange, 1993, p 354.)

d. When designing a multiple-dose regimen, only the **dosing rate** (D_o/τ) can be easily adjusted.

(1) The dosing rate is based on the **size of the dose (D_o)** and the **time interval, τ, between doses,** or the **frequency of dosing**.

(2) The dosing rate is given by this equation:

$$\text{Dosing rate} = D_o/\tau$$

(3) As long as the dosing rate is the same, the expected **average drug concentration at steady state (C_{av}^{∞})** is the same.

(a) For example, if a 600-mg dose is given every 12 hours, the dosing rate is 600 mg/12 hr, or 50 mg/hr.

(b) A dose of 300 mg every 6 hours, or 200 mg every 4 hours, would also give the same dosing rate (50 mg/hr) with the same expected C_{av}^{∞}.

(c) For a larger dose given over a longer time interval (e.g., 600 mg every 12 hours), the C_{max}^{∞} is higher and the C_{min}^{∞} lower compared to a smaller dose given more frequently (e.g., 200 mg every 4 hours).

e. Certain antibiotics may be given by **multiple rapid intravenous bolus injections.**

(1) The peak or **maximum serum drug concentration** at steady state may be estimated by the following equation:

$$C_{max}^{\infty} = \frac{D_o/V_D}{1 - e^{-k\tau}}$$

(2) The **minimum serum drug concentration,** C_{min}^{∞} at steady state is the drug concentration after the drug declines one dosage interval. Thus, C_{min}^{∞} is determined by this equation:

$$C_{min}^{\infty} = C_{max}^{\infty}\, e^{-k\tau}$$

(3) The **average drug concentration,** C_{av}^{∞} at steady state may be estimated from the same equation as for multiple oral doses:

$$C_{av}^{\infty} = \frac{FD_o}{kV_D\tau},$$

for intravenous bolus injections, F = 1.

f. Orally administered drugs given in **immediate-release dosage forms,** such as solutions, conventional tablets, and capsules by multiple oral doses are generally rapidly absorbed and slowly eliminated, $k_A >> k$. C_{max}^{∞} and C_{min}^{∞}, for these drugs may be approximated by the equations in V B 4 e (1) (2).

(1) For more exact calculations of C_{min}^{∞} and C_{max}^{∞} after multiple oral doses, the following equations may be used:

$$C_{max}^{\infty} = \frac{FD_o}{V_D}\,\frac{1}{1 - e^{-k\tau}}, \text{ and}$$

$$C_{min}^{\infty} = \frac{FD_o k_A}{V_D\,(k_A - k)}\,\frac{1}{1 - e^{-k\tau}}\,e^{-k\tau}$$

(2) The calculation of C_{av}^{∞} is the same as for multiple intravenous bolus injections, using the equation in V B 4 e (3).

(3) The term $1/(1 - e^{-k\tau})$ is known as the **accumulation rate.**

(4) The fraction of drug remaining in the body (f) after a dosage interval is given by this equation:

$$f = e^{-k\tau}.$$

(5) An initial loading drug dose, D_L, may be given to obtain a therapeutic steady-state drug level quickly.

(a) For multiple oral doses, D_L may be calculated by:

$$D_L = D_M\,\frac{1}{1 - e^{-k\tau}},$$

where D_M is the maintenance dose.

(b) If D_M is given at a dosage interval equal to the drug's elimination half-life, then D_L will equal twice the maintenance dose.

C. Multicompartment models

1. **Introduction.** Drugs that exhibit multicompartment pharmacokinetics distribute into different tissue groups at different rates. Tissues with high blood flow equilibrate with a drug more rapidly than tissues with small blood flow. Drug concentration in various tissues depends on the drug's physical–chemical characteristics and the nature of the tissue. For example, highly lipid-soluble drugs accumulate slowly in fat (lipid) tissue.

2. **Two-compartment model (intravenous bolus injection)**
   - **a.** After an intravenous bolus injection, the drug distributes and equilibrates rapidly into highly perfused tissues (**central compartment**) and more slowly into peripheral tissues (**tissue compartment**) [Figure 6-9].
   - **b.** The initial rapid decline in plasma drug concentration is known as the **distribution phase**. The slower rate of decline in drug concentration after complete equilibration is known as the **elimination phase**.

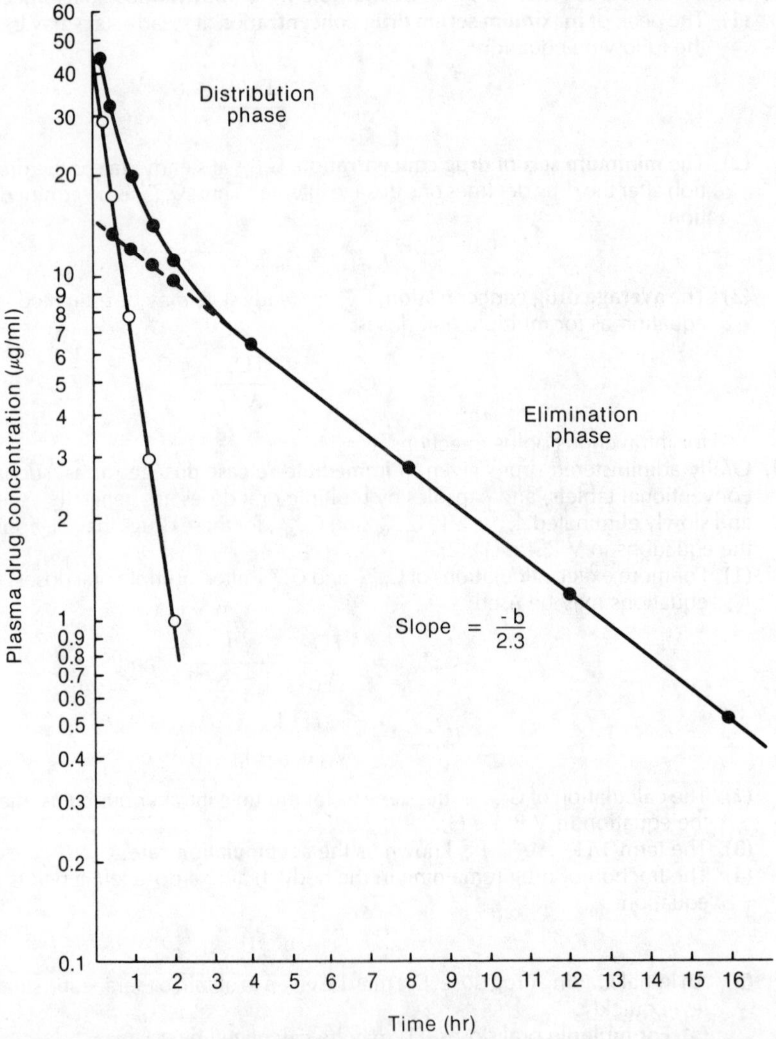

Figure 6-9. Generalized plot showing drug distribution and equilibration for a two-compartment model (intravenous bolus injection). The distribution phase represents the initial rapid decline in plasma drug concentration. The elimination phase represents the slower rate of decline after the drug's complete equilibration. (Adapted with permission from Shargel L, Yu ABC: *Applied Biopharmaceutics and Pharmacokinetics,* 3rd ed. East Norwalk, CT, Appleton & Lange, 1993, p 62.)

c. The **plasma drug concentration** at any time is the sum of two first-order processes, as given in this equation:

$$C_p = Ae^{-at} + Be^{-bt},$$

where a and b are hybrid first-order rate constants, and A and B are y intercepts.

(1) The **hybrid first-order rate constant b** is obtained from the slope of the elimination phase of the curve (Figure 6-9) and represents first-order elimination of drug from the body after the drug has equilibrated with all tissues.

(2) The **hybrid first-order rate constant a** is obtained from the slope of the residual line of the distribution phase after subtraction of the elimination phase.

d. The **apparent volume of distribution** depends on the type of pharmacokinetic calculation. Volumes of distribution include the volume of the central compartment (V_p), the volume of distribution at steady state (V_{ss}), and the volume of the tissue compartment (V_t).

3. Two-compartment model (oral drug administration)

a. A drug with a rapid distribution phase may not demonstrate two-compartment characteristics after oral administration. As the drug is absorbed, it equilibrates with the tissues so that the elimination half-life of the curve's elimination portion equals 0.693/b.

b. Two-compartment characteristics may be observed if the drug is rapidly absorbed and the distribution phase is slower.

4. Models with additional compartments

a. Addition of each new compartment to the model requires an additional first-order plot.

b. Addition of a third compartment implies that the drug slowly equilibrates into a deep tissue space. If the drug is given at frequent intervals, it begins to accumulate into the third compartment.

c. The terminal linear phase generally represents drug elimination from the body after equilibration. The rate constant from the elimination phase is generally used for dosage regimen calculations.

d. Adequate pharmacokinetic description of multicompartment models is often difficult and depends on proper plasma sampling and drug concentration determination.

D. Nonlinear pharmacokinetics. Also termed capacity-limited, dose-dependent, or saturation pharmacokinetics, nonlinear pharmacokinetics do not follow first-order kinetics as the dose is increased (Figure 6-10). Nonlinear pharmacokinetics result from saturation of an enzyme- or carrier-mediated system.

1. Characteristics of nonlinear pharmacokinetics:

a. AUC is not proportional to the dose.

b. Amount of drug excreted in the urine is not proportional to the dose.

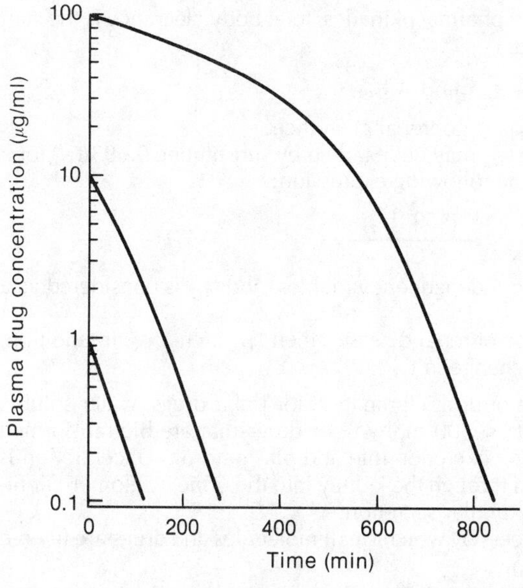

Figure 6-10. Generalized plot showing plasma drug concentration versus time for a drug with Michaelis-Menten (nonlinear) elimination kinetics. For this one-compartment model (intravenous injection), the doses are 1 mg, 10 mg, and 100 mg, and the apparent in vivo rate constant (k_M) = 10 mg. The maximum velocity of the reaction (V_{max}) = 0.2 mg/min. (Adapted with permission from Gibaldi M, Perrier D: *Pharmacokinetics*, 2nd ed. New York, Marcel Dekker, 1982, p 271.)

c. Elimination half-life may increase at high doses.
d. The ratio of metabolites formed changes with increased dose.

2. **Michaelis-Menten kinetics,** which describes the velocity of enzyme reactions, is often used to describe nonlinear pharmacokinetics.
a. The **Michaelis-Menten equation** describes the rate of change (velocity) of plasma drug concentration after an intravenous bolus injection, as follows:

$$-\frac{dC_p}{dt} = \frac{V_{max}\, C_p}{k_M + C_p},$$

where, V_{max} is the maximum velocity of the reaction, C_p is the substrate or plasma drug concentration, and k_M is the rate constant equal to the C_p at 0.5 V_{max}.
b. At very low C_p, where $k_M >> C_p$, the above equation reduces to a first-order rate equation since both k_M and V_{max} are constants.

$$-\frac{dC_p}{dt} = \frac{V_{max}\, C_p}{k_M} = k'Cp$$

c. At high C_p, where $C_p >> k_M$, the Michaelis-Menten equation becomes a zero-order rate equation:

$$-\frac{dC_p}{dt} = V_{max}$$

3. Drugs that follow nonlinear pharmacokinetics may demonstrate zero-order elimination rates at very high drug concentrations, a mix of zero- and first-order elimination rates at intermediate drug concentrations, and first-order elimination rates at very low drug concentrations (see Figure 6-10).

E. **Clearance** is a measurement of drug elimination from the body.

1. **Total body clearance (Cl_T)** may be defined as the drug elimination rate divided by the plasma drug concentration. The concept of clearance considers the body to contain an apparent volume of distribution in which the drug is dissolved. A constant portion of this volume is cleared (removed) from the body per unit time.
a. These equations express the measurement of total body clearance.

$$Cl_T = \frac{\text{drug elimination}}{\text{plasma drug concentration}} = \frac{dDe/dt}{C_p},$$

$$Cl_T = V_D k, \text{ and}$$

$$Cl_T = \frac{FD_o}{AUC}.$$

b. For drugs that follow first-order (linear) pharmacokinetics, total body clearance is the sum of all the clearances in the body. Thus,

$$Cl_T = Cl_R + Cl_{NR},$$

where Cl_R is renal clearance, and Cl_{NR} is nonrenal clearance.
c. The relationship between Cl_T and the $t_{1/2}$ may be obtained by substituting $0.693/t_{1/2}$ for k in the equation in V E 1 a to obtain the following expression:

$$t_{1/2} = \frac{0.693\, V_D}{Cl_T}$$

Generally, V_D and Cl_T are considered independent variables, and $t_{1/2}$ is considered as a dependent variable.
d. As clearance decreases (as in the case of renal disease), then $t_{1/2}$ increases. In addition, changes in V_D cause a proportional change in $t_{1/2}$.

2. **Renal drug excretion** is the major route of drug elimination for polar drugs, water-soluble drugs, drugs with low molecular weight (< 500 mol wt), or drugs that are biotransformed slowly. The relationship between the drug excretion rate and plasma drug concentration is shown in Figure 6-11. Drugs are excreted through the kidney into the urine by glomerular filtration, tubular reabsorption, and active tubular secretion.
a. **Glomerular filtration** is a passive process by which small molecules and drugs are filtered through the glomerulus of the nephron.

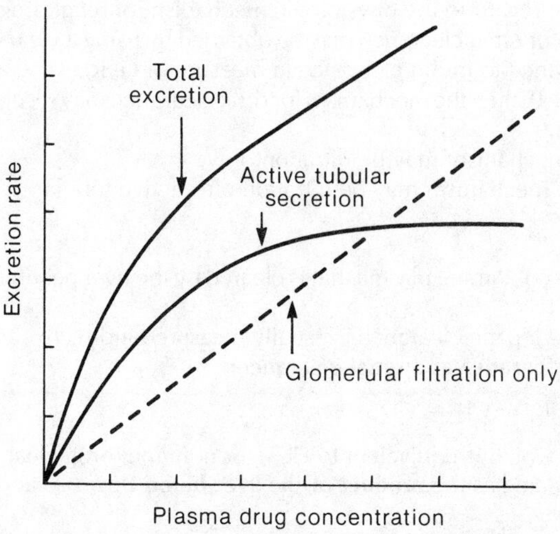

Figure 6-11. Generalized plot showing the excretion rate versus plasma drug concentration for a drug that demonstrates active tubular secretion and for one secreted by glomerular filtration only. (Adapted with permission from Shargel L, Yu ABC: *Applied Biopharmaceutics and Pharmacokinetics,* 3rd ed. East Norwalk, CT, Appleton & Lange, 1993, p 283.)

(1) Drugs bound to plasma proteins are too large to be filtered at the glomerulus.

(2) Drugs such as **creatinine** or **inulin,** which are not actively secreted or reabsorbed, are used to measure the **glomerular filtration rate (GFR)**.

b. Tubular reabsorption is a passive process that follows **Fick's law of diffusion.**

(1) Lipid-soluble drugs may be reabsorbed from the lumen of the nephron back into the systemic circulation.

(2) For weak electrolyte drugs, urine pH affects the ratio of nonionized and ionized drug.

(a) If the drug exists primarily in the nonionized or lipid-soluble form, then it is reabsorbed more easily from the lumen of the nephron.

(b) If the drug exists primarily in the ionized or water-soluble form, then it is excreted more easily in the urine.

(c) Depending upon the drug's pK_a, alteration of urine pH alters the ratio of ionized to nonionized drug, affecting the rate of drug excretion. For example, alkalinization of the urine by the administration of sodium bicarbonate increases the excretion of salicylates (weak acids).

(3) An increase in urine flow resulting from simultaneous administration of a diuretic decreases the time for drug reabsorption. Consequently, more drug is excreted.

c. Active tubular secretion is an active transport system that is carrier-mediated and requires energy.

(1) Two active tubular secretion pathways exist in the kidney—one system for weak acids and one system for weak bases.

(2) The active tubular secretion system demonstrates competition effects. For example, probenecid (a weak acid) competes for the same system as penicillin, decreasing the rate of penicillin excretion.

(3) The renal clearance of drugs such as **p-aminohippurate (PAH),** which are actively secreted, is used to measure **effective renal blood flow (ERBF)**.

3. Renal clearance is the volume of drug contained in the plasma that is removed by the kidney per unit time. **Units for renal clearance** are in volume per time (e.g., ml/min or L/hr).

a. Renal clearance may be measured by dividing the rate of drug excretion by the plasma drug concentration, as shown:

$$Cl_R = \frac{\text{Rate of drug excretion}}{C_p} = \frac{dD_U/dt}{C_p}$$

b. Measurement of renal clearance may also be expressed by these equations:

$$Cl_R = k_e V_D,$$

where k_e is the first-order renal excretion rate constant, and

$$Cl_R = \frac{D_U^\infty}{AUC},$$

where D_U^∞ is the total amount of parent (unchanged) drug excreted in the urine.

c. Renal clearance is measured without regard to the physiologic mechanism of renal drug excretion. The probable mechanism for renal clearance may be obtained by using a **clearance ratio,** which relates drug clearance to inulin clearance (a measure of GFR).

(1) If the clearance ratio is less than 1.0, then the mechanism for drug clearance may result from filtration plus reabsorption.

(2) If the ratio is equal to 1.0, the mechanism may be filtration only.

(3) If the ratio is more than 1.0, the mechanism may be filtration plus active tubular secretion.

4. Hepatic clearance is the volume of drug-containing plasma that is cleared by the liver per unit time.

a. Measurement of hepatic clearance. Hepatic clearance is usually measured indirectly, as the **difference between total body clearance and renal clearance:**

$$Cl_H = Cl_T - Cl_R,$$

where Cl_H is the hepatic clearance, which is equivalent to Cl_{NR}, or nonrenal drug clearance; however, it may also be calculated as the **product of the liver blood flow (Q)** and the **extraction ratio (ER):**

$$Cl_H = QER.$$

(1) The extraction ratio represents the fraction of drug that is irreversibly removed by an organ or tissue as the drug-containing plasma perfuses that tissue.

(2) The extraction ratio is obtained by measuring the plasma drug concentration entering the liver and the plasma drug exiting the liver:

$$ER = \frac{C_a - C_v}{C_a},$$

where C_a is the arterial plasma drug concentration entering the liver, and C_v is the venous plasma drug concentration exiting the liver.

(3) Values for ER may range from 0 to 1. For example, if ER equals 0.9, then 90% of the incoming drug is removed by the liver as the plasma perfuses this organ. If ER equals 0, then no drug is removed by the liver.

b. Blood flow, intrinsic clearance, and **protein binding** affect hepatic clearance.

(1) Blood flow to the liver is approximately 1.5 L/min and may be altered by exercise, food, disease, or drugs.

(a) Blood enters the liver by way of the hepatic portal vein and hepatic artery and leaves by way of the hepatic vein.

(b) After oral drug administration, the drug is absorbed from the gastrointestinal tract into the mesenteric vessels and proceeds to the hepatic portal vein, to the liver, and then to the systemic circulation.

(2) Intrinsic clearance describes the liver's ability to remove the drug independently of blood flow.

(a) The mechanism of intrinsic drug clearance is primarily the result of the inherent ability of the **biotransformation enzymes** (mixed function oxidases) to metabolize the drug as it enters the liver.

(b) Normally, basal mixed-function oxidase enzymes act to biotransform drugs. These enzymes may be increased by various drugs, such as phenobarbital, or by environmental agents, such as tobacco smoke. Moreover, these same enzymes may be inhibited by other drugs and environmental agents (e.g., cimetidine, acute lead poisoning).

(3) Protein binding. Drugs that are bound to protein are not easily cleared by the liver (or kidney) because only the free, or nonplasma protein-bound, drug crosses the cell membrane into the tissue.

(a) The **free drug** is available to the drug-metabolizing enzymes for biotransformation.

(b) A sudden increase in free-drug plasma concentration in the plasma results in more available drug at pharmacologic receptors, producing a more intense effect at organs (e.g., kidney, liver) involved in drug removal.

c. **Blood flow (Q), intrinsic clearance (Cl_{int}),** and the **free-plasma drug concentration** (f) are related to hepatic clearance by the following equation:

$$Cl_H = Q \frac{f\,Cl_{int}}{Q + Cl_{int}}$$

(1) The hepatic clearance of drugs, such as propranolol, which have high extraction ratios and high Cl_{int} values, is most affected by changes in blood flow and inhibitors of the drug metabolism enzymes.
(2) The hepatic clearance of drugs that have low extraction ratios and low Cl_{int} values (e.g., theophylline) is most affected by changes in Cl_{int} and is affected only slightly by changes in hepatic blood flow.
(3) Only drugs that are highly plasma protein-bound (i.e., $> 95\%$) and have a low intrinsic clearance (e.g., phenytoin) are affected by a sudden shift in protein binding, causing an increase in free-drug plasma concentration.

d. **Biliary drug excretion,** an active transport process, is also included in hepatic clearance. Separate active secretion systems exist for both weak acids and weak bases.
(1) Drugs excreted in the bile are usually high molecular weight compounds (i.e., > 500 mol wt) or polar drugs, such as reserpine, digoxin, and various glucuronide conjugates.
(2) Drugs may be recycled by means of the **enterohepatic circulation.**
(a) Some drugs are absorbed from the gastrointestinal tract by way of the mesenteric and hepatic portal vein, proceeding to the liver. The liver may secrete some of the drug (unchanged or as a glucuronide metabolite) into the bile.
(b) From the bile (stored in the gallbladder), the drug may empty into the gastrointestinal tract by way of the bile duct.
(c) If the drug is a **glucuronide metabolite,** bacteria in the gastrointestinal tract may hydrolyze the glucuronide moiety, allowing the released drug to be reabsorbed.

e. **First-pass effects (presystemic elimination)** may occur with drugs given orally. A portion of the drug is eliminated prior to systemic absorption.
(1) The mechanism of first-pass effects generally results from rapid drug biotransformation by the liver enzymes. Other mechanisms may include metabolism of the drug by the gastrointestinal mucosal cells or intestinal flora or biliary secretion.
(2) First-pass effects are usually observed by measuring the **absolute bioavailability** (F) for the drug. If F is less than 1, then some of the drug was eliminated prior to systemic absorption.
(3) Drugs that demonstrate a **high hepatic extraction ratio,** such as propranolol, demonstrate first-pass effects.
(4) If the drug's first-pass effect is extremely high (i.e., $> 90\%$), then either:
(a) The drug dose could be increased (e.g., propranolol, penicillin).
(b) The drug could be given by an alternate route of drug administration (e.g., nitroglycerin, insulin).
(c) The dosage form could be modified (e.g., mesalamine).

VI. CLINICAL PHARMACOKINETICS

VI. CLINICAL PHARMACOKINETICS is the application of pharmacokinetic principles for the rational design of an individualized dosage regimen. Two main objectives of clinical pharmacokinetics are **maintenance of an optimum drug concentration at the receptor site** to produce the desired therapeutic response for a specific time period and **minimization of any adverse or toxic effects** due to the drug.

A. Design factors for an individualized dosage regimen

1. Drug pharmacokinetics in the patient, including absorption, distribution, and an elimination profile

2. The patient's normal physiologic condition, including such characteristics as age, weight, gender, and nutritional status

3. Pathophysiologic conditions [e.g., renal disease, congestive heart failure (CHF), liver disease] that may affect drug pharmacokinetics in the patient

4. Other interventions such as diet, which may modify the drug's predicted therapeutic activity

5. Environmental factors, which may affect drug pharmacokinetics (e.g., smoking increases theophylline clearance)
6. Consideration of the drug's **target concentration** (i.e., the desired plasma or serum drug concentration for optimal therapeutic effect) and **therapeutic window** (i.e., the range of plasma drug concentration between the MTC and the MEC)
   a. Increased probability of an adverse response to the drug as the plasma drug concentration approaches the MTC
   b. Increased probability that the drug lacks efficacy (i.e., does not produce a therapeutic response) as plasma drug concentration approaches the MEC

B. Clinical pharmacist's responsibilities. The appropriate drug must be selected, usually in conjunction with the clinician, and the dosage regimen must be designed for the patient.

1. **Dosage regimen**
   a. **Target drug concentration** and **dosing rate** must be determined.
      (1) **Dosing rate (D_o/τ)** is the main parameter that the clinical pharmacist may adjust. This rate is based on knowledge of the target drug concentration, the therapeutic window, and the estimated clearance of the drug in the patient, as shown in these equations:

$$\text{Target drug concentration} = \text{dosing rate} \times \frac{1}{\text{clearance}}, \text{ and}$$

$$C_{av}^{\infty} = \frac{FD_o}{\tau} \times \frac{1}{Cl_T},$$

where F is the fraction of drug absorbed.
      (2) **Drug dose** should be adjusted to commercially available dosage forms and strengths. For example, if the drug is manufactured in 125-mg, 250-mg, and 500-mg tablets, then the calculated dose should be rounded to the nearest strength.
      (3) **Dosage interval** (τ) should be set at intervals convenient for the patient. For example, a dose given every 8 hours is more practical than a dose every 7.3 hours. When adjusting the dose and dosage interval, the C_{av}^{∞} is the same as long as the same dosing rate is maintained. However, the C_{min}^{∞} and C_{max}^{∞} will vary and should be checked.
      (4) With more drugs available as **extended-release drug products,** the clinical pharmacist should consider this form rather than an immediate-release dosage form, depending upon the patient's needs.
   b. **Nomograms** are often used to develop dosage regimens. These are based on average, or population, pharmacokinetic parameters. Although easy to use, nomograms may not apply to the patient's special needs.
2. The **patient's response** to the drug and dosage regimen must be evaluated.
3. **Serum or plasma drug concentrations** must be determined as needed.
   a. **Therapeutic drug monitoring (TDM)** can verify the adequacy of the dosage regimen, using plasma or drug concentrations.
   b. **Number of blood samples** and the **timing for blood sample collection** are important considerations for TDM.
   c. Drug levels in plasma or serum must be properly assayed.
   d. **Pharmacokinetic interpretation** of the serum drug concentration must be performed.
   e. The **dosage must be readjusted,** if necessary, according to the results obtained by TDM.
   f. Plasma drug concentrations must be further monitored.
   g. **Special recommendations** or **patient education** must be provided to ensure proper compliance to the dosage regimen. Patients should understand their drug dosage regimen in relation to meals, other drugs, their daily routines, and their sleep habits.

VII. PHARMACOKINETICS IN RENAL DISEASE

A. Overview. The patient with renal disease poses a special problem because of the kidneys' role in pharmacokinetics. The kidneys regulate body fluids, electrolyte balance, metabolite waste removal, and drug excretion. **Acute renal failure,** which alters kidney function, may result from a variety of causes, including disease, traumatic injury, and nephrotoxic agents.

1. Renal failure generally results in a **reduction in the GFR** and a decreased ability of the kidneys to remove metabolite wastes, such as urea and drugs.

2. Renal disease may also **decrease plasma drug-protein binding** due to competition for binding sites by accumulating metabolite wastes, including urea, the active drug, and its biotransformation products.

B. Measuring glomerular filtration rate (GFR)

1. **Criteria necessary for drugs used to measure GFR**
   a. The drug is filtered at the glomerulus.
   b. The drug must not be reabsorbed or actively secreted.
   c. The drug should not be metabolized.
   d. The drug should not be highly bound to plasma proteins.
   e. The drug should be nontoxic and should not affect renal function.
   f. The drug should be easily measured in plasma and urine.

2. **Inulin and creatinine**
   a. **Inulin,** a polysaccharide, meets most of the above criteria. However, inulin is an exogenous substance that must be administered in addition to any other drug therapy.
   b. **Creatinine,** an endogenous substance formed from creatinine phosphate during muscle metabolism, provides an alternative.
      (1) Creatinine production may vary with gender, age, and body weight.
      (2) Creatinine is filtered at the glomerulus and is not reabsorbed.
      (3) A small fraction may be actively secreted so that the creatinine clearance value for measurement of GFR may be slightly higher compared to the inulin clearance value.

3. **Creatinine clearance (Cl_{CR})** is the most common method for obtaining the GFR. Cl_{CR} may be estimated by using both urine and serum values or by using only serum creatinine concentration.
   a. Creatinine clearance measurement, using both urine and serum concentrations, is more accurate and is usually estimated by the following equation:

$$Cl_{CR} = \frac{C_U \dot{V}\, 100}{C_{CR}\, 1440},$$

   where C_{CR} is the creatinine serum concentration in mg/dl of the twelfth-hour serum, $\dot{V}$ is the 24-hour urine volume, C_U is the concentration of creatinine in the urine, and Cl_{CR} is the creatinine clearance in milliliters per minute.
   b. Creatinine clearance may be estimated from the serum creatinine concentration because there is usually an inverse relationship between serum creatinine concentration and GFR.
      (1) The **Siersback-Nielsen nomogram** may be used to obtain the creatinine clearance, using the serum creatinine concentration (mg/dl) and the patient's body weight and gender (Figure 6-12).
      (2) The **Cockcroft and Gault method,** which is also based on body weight, age, and gender, calculates creatinine clearance from serum creatinine, using the following relationship:
         (a) For males,

$$Cl_{CR} = \frac{(140 - \text{age in years})\ \text{body weight (kg)}}{72\ (C_{CR}\ \text{in mg/dl})} = \text{ml/min}.$$

         (b) For females, 0.85 of the Cl_{CR} obtained for males is used.
      (3) These methods assume stable renal functions; however, renal function may change, depending upon the progress of the renal disease, causing changes in Cl_{CR}.

C. Dosage adjustment

1. **Dosage adjustment for renal disease** is usually based on the following assumptions, which may not be valid for every patient:
   a. The desired plasma or serum drug concentration in a patient with renal disease is the same as that for a patient without renal disease. A major exception is digoxin; renal disease may alter normal serum potassium concentrations, thus altering the target digoxin serum concentration.
   b. Other pharmacokinetic parameters (e.g., V_D, plasma drug protein binding, nonrenal drug elimination or biotransformation) are not markedly altered in renal disease.
   c. Normal GFR is 100 ml/min or greater. Unless the GFR falls significantly below normal, dosage should not be adjusted for a patient with minor renal impairment.

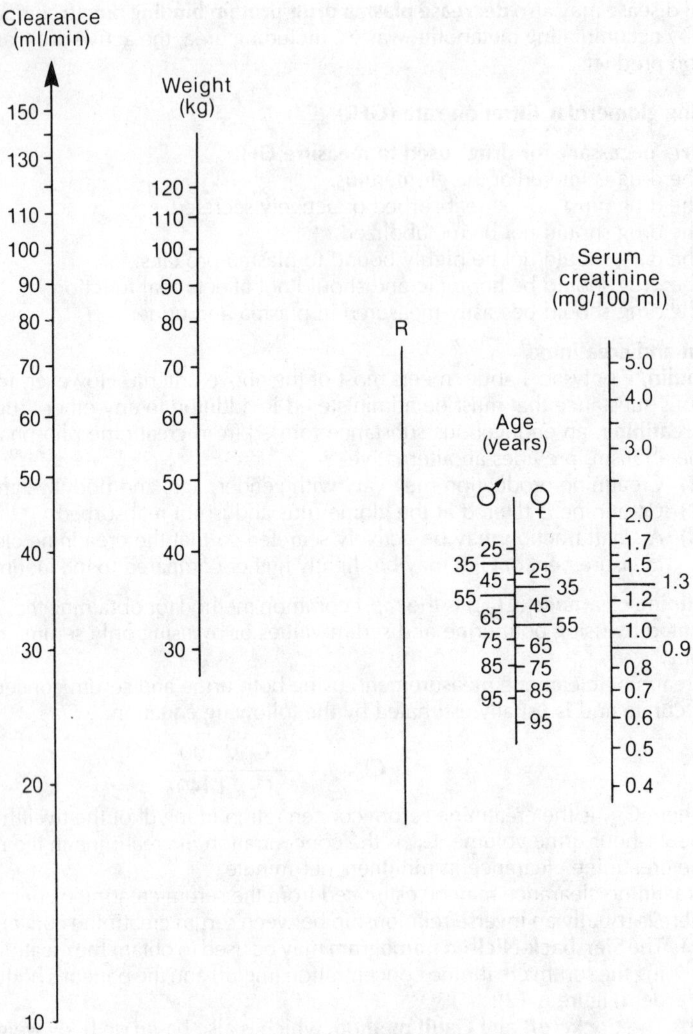

Figure 6-12. Nomogram for evaluation of endogenous creatinine clearance. To use the nomogram, connect with a ruler the patient's weight on the second line from the left with the patient's age on the fourth line. Note the point of intersection on *R* and keep the ruler there. Turn the right part of the ruler to the appropriate serum creatinine value, and the left side will indicate the clearance in milliliters per minute. (Reprinted with permission from Kampmann J, Siersback-Nielsen JM: Rapid evaluation of creatinine clearance. *Acta Med Scand* 196:517–520, 1974.)

d. Drugs such as gentamicin (primarily eliminated by renal excretion) are more affected by diminished renal function than drugs such as theophylline (primarily eliminated by biotransformation, which is more affected by nonrenal or hepatic clearance).

e. All drug elimination pathways follow first-order pharmacokinetics.

f. Whenever the dosage of a drug is adjusted for the patient with renal disease, therapeutic drug monitoring is important to help prevent adverse drug reactions and maintain proper drug therapy.

2. Dosage adjustment for the renally impaired patient attempts to estimate the fraction of total body drug clearance remaining.

a. Total body clearance is the sum of renal clearance and nonrenal clearance, as follows:

$$Cl_T = Cl_R + Cl_{NR}$$

b. Because V_D is assumed to be constant, then:

$$k = k_R + k_{NR}$$

c. As k_R decreases in renal disease, then k (i.e., the overall rate constant for drug elimination) also decreases.

3. The **Guisti and Hayton method** estimates the fraction of k remaining in the patient, using the following equation:

$$\frac{k_U}{k_N} = 1 - f_e\left(1 - \frac{Cl_{CR}^{\ U}}{Cl_{CR}^{\ N}}\right),$$

where k_U is the first-order elimination rate constant in the renally impaired (uremic) patient; k_N is the patient's normal elimination rate constant; f_e is the fraction of drug excreted unchanged in the urine; $Cl_{CR}^{\ N}$ is the normal creatinine clearance (GFR), assumed to be 100 ml/min; and $Cl_{CR}^{\ U}$ is the creatinine clearance in the renally impaired patient, usually estimated from the serum creatinine concentration.

a. The values for k, k_{NR}, and f_e are the standard population pharmacokinetic parameters obtained from the literature.

b. After the value for k_U/k_N is obtained, the dosage regimen may be calculated by either decreasing the normal dose, prolonging the dosage interval, or both.

(1) **To decrease the dose and maintain a constant dosage interval,** the following equation is used:

$$D_U^{\ 0} = \frac{k_U}{k_N} \times D_N^{\ 0},$$

where $D_U^{\ 0}$ is the dose in renal disease, $D_N^{\ 0}$ is the normal dose, and k_U/k_N is calculated.

(2) **To prolong the interval and maintain a constant dose,** the following equation is used:

$$T_U = \frac{k_N}{k_U} \times T_N,$$

where T_U is the dosage interval in renal disease, and T_N is the normal dosage interval.

4. **Loading dose.** Because V_D is assumed to be approximately the same in both the normal and renally impaired patient, the loading dose (D_L) is generally the same.

VIII. PHARMACOKINETICS IN HEPATIC DISEASE

A. Overview. Pharmacokinetic alterations in hepatic disease (e.g., cirrhosis, hepatitis) are much more difficult to predict quantitatively compared to renal disease. As yet, no reliable measurement of hepatic function is available to estimate the amount of hepatic drug clearance remaining in the patient.

B. Pharmacokinetic alterations due to hepatic disease:

1. **Decreased hepatic drug clearance**

a. Drugs that demonstrate significant first-pass effects, such as propranolol, have greater bioavailability.

b. The $t_{1/2}$ for drugs that are eliminated by hepatic clearance increases.

2. **Decreased plasma protein binding of drugs**

a. The liver is the main organ involved in the synthesis of albumin and other plasma proteins.

b. In hepatic disease, the plasma protein concentration may be quantitatively decreased, and proteins that are formed may be qualitatively altered—resulting in decreased plasma protein binding.

STUDY QUESTIONS

Directions: Each of the numbered items or incomplete statements in this section is followed by answers or by completions of the statement. Select the **one** lettered answer or completion that is **best** in each case.

1. The term bioavailability refers to the

(A) relationship between the physical and chemical properties of a drug and the systemic absorption of the drug
(B) measurement of the rate and amount of therapeutically active drug that reaches the systemic circulation
(C) movement of a drug into the body tissues over time
(D) dissolution of a drug in the gastrointestinal tract
(E) amount of drug destroyed by the liver prior to systemic absorption from the gastrointestinal tract

2. The route of drug administration that gives the most rapid onset of the pharmacologic effect is

(A) intramuscular injection
(B) intravenous injection
(C) intradermal injection
(D) oral administration
(E) subcutaneous injection

3. The route of drug administration that provides complete (100%) bioavailability is

(A) intramuscular injection
(B) intravenous injection
(C) intradermal injection
(D) oral administration
(E) subcutaneous injection

4. After oral administration, drugs generally are absorbed best from the

(A) buccal cavity
(B) stomach
(C) duodenum
(D) ileum
(E) rectum

5. All of the following are characteristics of an active transport process EXCEPT

(A) active transport moves drug molecules against a concentration gradient
(B) active transport follows Fick's law of diffusion
(C) active transport is a carrier-mediated transport system
(D) active transport requires energy
(E) active transport of drug molecules may be saturated at high drug concentrations

6. The passage of drug molecules across a cell membrane from a region of high drug concentration to a region of low drug concentration is known as

(A) active transport
(B) bioavailability
(C) biopharmaceutics
(D) passive diffusion
(E) pinocytosis

7. Creatinine clearance is used as a measurement of

(A) renal excretion rate
(B) glomerular filtration rate (GFR)
(C) active renal secretion
(D) passive renal absorption
(E) drug metabolism rate

1-B 4-C 7-B
2-B 5-B
3-B 6-D

Questions 8–11

A new cephalosporin antibiotic was given by a single intravenous bolus injection to an adult male patient (age, 58 years; weight, 75 kg) at a dose of 5 mg/kg. The antibiotic follows the pharmacokinetics of a one-compartment model and has an elimination half-life of 2 hours. The apparent volume of distribution is 0.28 L/kg, and the drug is 35% bound to plasma proteins.

8. What would be the initial plasma drug concentration (C_p^0) in this patient?

(A) 0.24 mg/L
(B) 1.80 mg/L
(C) 17.9 mg/L
(D) 56.0 mg/L

9. The predicted plasma drug concentration (C_p) at 8 hours after the dose would be

(A) 0.73 mg/L
(B) 1.11 mg/L
(C) 2.64 mg/L
(D) 4.02 mg/L
(E) 15.1 mg/L

10. The amount of drug in the patient's body (D_B) at 8 hours after the dose would be

(A) 15.3 mg
(B) 23.3 mg
(C) 84.4 mg
(D) 100.0 mg
(E) 112 mg

11. How long after the dose would exactly 75% of the drug be eliminated from the patient?

(A) 2 hours
(B) 4 hours
(C) 6 hours
(D) 8 hours
(E) 10 hours

12. The equation that describes the rate of drug dissolution from a tablet is known as

(A) Fick's law
(B) Henderson-Hasselbalch equation
(C) Law of mass action
(D) Michaelis-Menten equation
(E) Noyes Whitney equation

13. Which of the following conditions generally increases the rate of drug dissolution from a tablet?

(A) An increase in the particle size of the drug
(B) A decrease in the surface area of the drug
(C) Use of the free acid or free base form of the drug
(D) Use of the ionized or salt form of the drug
(E) Use of sugar coating around the tablet

14. Dose dumping is a problem in the formulation of

(A) compressed tablets
(B) modified-release drug products
(C) hard gelatin capsules
(D) soft gelatin capsules
(E) suppositories

15. The rate-limiting step in the bioavailability of a lipid-soluble drug formulated as an immediate-release compressed tablet is the rate of

(A) disintegration of the tablet and release of the drug
(B) dissolution of the drug
(C) transport of the drug molecules across the intestinal mucosal cells
(D) blood flow to the gastrointestinal tract
(E) biotransformation (metabolism) of the drug by the liver prior to systemic absorption

16. The extent of ionization of a weak electrolyte drug is dependent upon the

(A) pH of the media and pK_a of the drug
(B) oil/water partition coefficient of the drug
(C) particle size and surface area of the drug
(D) Noyes Whitney equation for the drug
(E) polymorphic form of the drug

8-C	11-B	14-B
9-B	12-E	15-B
10-B	13-D	16-A

Questions 17–22

A physician wishes to give an intravenous infusion of the antibiotic carbenicillin to a young adult male patient (age, 35 years; weight, 70 kg) with normal renal function. The desired steady-state plasma drug concentration is 15 mg/dl. The physician would like the antibiotic to be infused into the patient for 10 hours. Carbenicillin has an elimination half-life ($t_{1/2}$) of 1.0 hours and an apparent volume distribution (V_D) of 9 L in this patient.

17. Assuming no loading dose, what rate of intravenous infusion would you recommend for this patient?

(A) 93.6 mg/hr
(B) 135 mg/hr
(C) 468 mg/hr
(D) 936 mg/hr
(E) 1350 mg/hr

18. Assuming that no loading intravenous dose was given, how long after the start of the intravenous infusion would the plasma drug concentration reach 95% of the theoretical steady-state drug concentration?

(A) 1 hour
(B) 3.3 hours
(C) 4.3 hours
(D) 6.6 hours
(E) 10 hours

19. What loading dose would you recommend?

(A) 93.6 mg
(B) 135 mg
(C) 468 mg
(D) 936 mg
(E) 1350 mg

20. You would like to infuse the antibiotic as a solution containing 10 g of the drug in 500 ml of 5% dextrose. How many milliliters per hour of this solution would you infuse into the patient?

(A) 10 ml/hr
(B) 46.8 ml/hr
(C) 100 ml/hr
(D) 936 ml/hr
(E) 1141 ml/hr

21. What is the total body clearance rate for carbenicillin in this patient?

(A) 100 ml/hr
(B) 936 ml/hr
(C) 4862 ml/hr
(D) 6237 ml/hr
(E) 9000 ml/hr

22. Assuming that the patient's renal clearance for carbenicillin is 86 ml/min, what is the hepatic clearance for carbenicillin?

(A) 108 ml/hr
(B) 1077 ml/hr
(C) 3840 ml/hr
(D) 5160 ml/hr
(E) 6844 ml/hr

23. The earliest evidence that a drug is stored in a tissue is

(A) an increase in plasma protein binding
(B) a large apparent volume of distribution (V_D)
(C) a decrease in the rate of formation of metabolites by the liver
(D) an increase in the number of side effects produced by the drug
(E) a decrease in the amount of free drug excreted in the urine

24. The intensity of the pharmacologic action of a drug is most dependent upon the

(A) concentration of the drug at the receptor site
(B) elimination half-life ($t_{1/2}$) of the drug
(C) onset time of the drug after oral administration
(D) minimum toxic drug concentration (MTC) in the plasma
(E) minimum effective concentration (MEC) of the drug in the body

---

17-D	20-B	23-B
18-C	21-D	24-A
19-E	22-B	

25. Drugs that demonstrate nonlinear pharmacokinetics show which of the following properties?

(A) A constant ratio of drug metabolites is formed as the administered dose increases
(B) The elimination half-life ($t_{1/2}$) increases as the administered dose is increased
(C) The area under the plasma drug concentration versus time curve (AUC) increases in direct proportion to an increase in the administered dose
(D) Both low and high doses follow first-order elimination kinetics
(E) The steady-state drug concentration increases in direct proportion to the dosing rate

26. The loading dose (D_L) of a drug is generally based upon the

(A) total body clearance (Cl_T) of the drug
(B) percent of drug bound to plasma proteins
(C) fraction of drug excreted unchanged in the urine
(D) apparent volume of distribution (V_D) and the desired drug concentration in plasma
(E) area under the plasma drug concentration versus time curve (AUC)

27. The renal clearance of inulin is used as a measurement of

(A) effective renal blood flow
(B) rate of renal drug excretion
(C) intrinsic enzyme activity
(D) active renal secretion
(E) glomerular filtration rate (GFR)

28. All of the following statements are true for plasma protein binding of a drug EXCEPT

(A) displacement of a drug from plasma protein binding sites results in a transient enlarged volume of distribution (V_D)
(B) displacement of a drug from plasma protein binding sites makes more free drug available for glomerular filtration
(C) displacement of a potent drug that is normally more than 95% bound may result in an adverse toxicity
(D) albumin is the major protein involved in protein binding of drugs
(E) drugs highly bound to plasma proteins generally have a larger V_D compared to drugs highly bound to tissue proteins

29. The onset time for a drug given orally is the time for the

(A) drug to reach the peak plasma drug concentration
(B) drug to reach the minimum effective concentration (MEC)
(C) drug to reach the minimum toxic concentration (MTC)
(D) drug to begin to be eliminated from the body
(E) drug to begin to be absorbed from the small intestine

30. The initial distribution of a drug into the tissues is determined chiefly by the

(A) rate of blood flow to the tissue
(B) glomerular filtration rate (GFR)
(C) stomach emptying time
(D) drug affinity for the tissue
(E) plasma protein binding of the drug

31. Which of the following tissues has the greatest capacity to biotransform drugs?

(A) Brain
(B) Kidney
(C) Liver
(D) Lung
(E) Skin

32. The principle of superposition in designing multiple dosage regimens assumes that

(A) each dose affects the next subsequent dose, causing nonlinear elimination
(B) each dose of drug is eliminated by zero-order elimination
(C) steady-state plasma drug concentrations are reached at approximately 10 half-lives
(D) early doses of drug do not affect subsequent doses
(E) the fraction of drug absorbed is equal to the fraction of drug eliminated

33. The rate of drug bioavailability is most rapid when the drug is formulated as a

(A) controlled-release product
(B) hard gelatin capsule
(C) compressed tablet
(D) solution
(E) suspension

25-B	28-E	31-C
26-D	29-B	32-D
27-E	30-A	33-D

Questions 34–36

A new cardiac glycoside has been developed for oral and intravenous administration. The drug has an elimination half-life ($t_{1/2}$) of 24 hours and an apparent volume of distribution (V_D) of 3 L/kg. The effective drug concentration is 1.5 ng/ml. Toxic effects of the drug are observed at drug concentrations above 4 ng/ml. The drug is bound to plasma proteins at approximately 25%. The drug is 75% bioavailable after an oral dose.

34. What would an oral maintenance dose be if given once a day for a 65-kg man (age, 68 years) with congestive heart failure (CHF) and normal renal function?

(A) 0.125 mg
(B) 0.180 mg
(C) 0.203 mg
(D) 0.270 mg
(E) 0.333 mg

35. What would a loading dose (D_L) be for this patient?

(A) 0.270 mg
(B) 0.293 mg
(C) 0.450 mg
(D) 0.498 mg
(E) 0.540 mg

36. Assuming that the drug is available in tablets of 0.125 mg and 0.250 mg, what would this patient's plasma drug concentration be if the patient uses a dosage regimen of 0.125 mg every 12 hours?

(A) 1.39 ng/ml
(B) 1.85 ng/ml
(C) 2.78 ng/ml
(D) 3.18 ng/ml
(E) 6.94 ng/ml

Directions: The question below contains three suggested answers of which **one or more** is correct. Choose the answer

A if **I only** is correct
B if **III only** is correct
C if **I and II** are correct
D if **II and III** are correct
E if **I, II, and III** are correct

37. Which of the following equations is true for a zero-order reaction rate of a drug?

I. $\frac{dA}{dt} = -k$

II. $t_{1/2} = \frac{0.693}{k}$

III. $A = A_0e^{-kt}$

34-D
35-E
36-A
37-A

ANSWERS AND EXPLANATIONS

1. The answer is B *[I A 2].*
Bioavailability is the measurement of the rate and extent (amount) of therapeutically active drug that reaches the systemic circulation. The relationship of a drug's physical and chemical properties to its systemic absorption (i.e., to its bioavailability) refers to its biopharmaceutics. The movement of a drug into body tissues is an aspect of pharmacokinetics, which is the study of drug movement in the body over time. The dissolution of a drug in the gastrointestinal tract is a physicochemical property that affects the drug's bioavailability. Significant destruction of a drug by the liver before it is systemically absorbed (known as the first-pass effect because it occurs during the drug's first passage through the liver) markedly reduces the drug's bioavailability.

2. The answer is B *[II B 1 a].*
When the active form of the drug is given intravenously, it is placed directly into the systemic circulation. The drug is delivered rapidly to all tissues, including the drug receptor sites. For all other routes of drug administration (with the exception of intra-arterial injection), the drug must be systemically absorbed prior to distribution to the drug receptor sites, and therefore, the onset of pharmacologic effects is slower. If the drug is a prodrug, which must be converted to an active drug, then intravenous injection may not produce the most rapid onset of activity. For a prodrug, oral administration may produce the most rapid onset of activity if conversion to the active form takes place in the gastrointestinal tract or liver.

3. The answer is B *[II C 2].*
When a drug is given by intravenous injection, the entire dose is placed into the systemic circulation. With other routes of administration, drug may be lost prior to reaching the systemic circulation. For example, with first-pass effects, a portion of an orally administered drug is eliminated, usually through degradation by liver enzymes, before the drug reaches its receptor sites.

4. The answer is C *[II B 2 b (4)].*
Drugs given orally are well absorbed from the duodenum. The duodenum has a large surface area due to the presence of villi and microvilli. In addition, the duodenum is well perfused by the mesenteric blood vessels, which helps to maintain a concentration gradient between the lumen of the duodenum and the blood.

5. The answer is B *[II A 2, 3].*
Fick's law of diffusion describes passive diffusion of drug molecules moving from a high concentration to a low concentration. This process is not saturable and does not require energy.

6. The answer is D *[II A 2].*
The transport of a drug across a cell membrane by passive diffusion follows Fick's law of diffusion: the drug moves with a concentration gradient; that is, from an area of high concentration to an area of low concentration. In contrast, drugs that are actively transported move against a concentration gradient.

7. The answer is B *[VII B 3].*
A substance that is used to measure the glomerular filtration rate (GFR) must be filtered only and not reabsorbed or actively secreted. Although inulin clearance gives an accurate measurement of GFR, creatinine clearance is generally used, since no exogenous drug needs to be given. However, creatinine formation depends upon muscle mass and muscle metabolism, which may change with age and various disease conditions.

8–11. The answers are: 8-C *[V A 1 b],* **9-B** *[V B 1 a],* **10-B** *[V B 1 a],* **11-B** *[V A 1 b].*
Substituting the data for this patient in the equation for the initial plasma drug concentration ($C_p{}^0$), one obtains:

$$C_p{}^0 = \frac{D_0}{V_D} = \frac{5 \text{ mg/kg}}{0.28 \text{ kg}} = 17.9 \text{ mg/L}$$

To obtain the patient's plasma drug concentration (C_p) at 8 hours after the dose, the following calculation is performed:

$$C_p = C_p{}^0 e^{-kt},$$

$$k = \frac{0.693}{t_{1/2}} = \frac{0.693}{2} = 0.347 \text{ hr}^{-1},$$

$$C_p = 17.9 \, e^{-(0.347)(8)},$$

$$C_p = (17.9)(0.0623) = 1.11 \text{ mg/L}$$

The amount of drug in the patient's body at 8 hours would be calculated as follows:

$$D_B = C_pV_D = (1.11)\ (0.28)\ (75) = 23.3 \text{ mg}.$$

For any first-order elimination process, 50% of the initial amount of drug is eliminated at the end of the first half-life, and 50% of the remaining amount of drug (i.e., 75% of the original amount) is eliminated at the end of the second half-life. Since the drug in the present case has an elimination half-life ($t_{1/2}$) of 2 hours, 75% of the dose would be eliminated at two half-lives, or 4 hours.

12. The answer is E *[III A 1].*
The Noyes Whitney equation describes the rate at which a solid drug dissolves. Fick's law is similar to the Noyes Whitney equation in that both equations describe drug movement due to a concentration gradient. Fick's law generally refers to the passive diffusion or passive transport of drugs. The law of mass action concerns the rate of a chemical reaction; the Michaelis-Menten equation deals with enzyme kinetics; and the Henderson-Hasselbalch equation gives the pH of a buffer solution.

13. The answer is D *[III A 1–3].*
The ionized or salt form of a drug has a charge and is generally more water-soluble and, therefore, dissolves more rapidly than the nonionized (free acid or free base) form of the drug. The dissolution rate is directly proportional to the surface area and inversely proportional to the particle size. Therefore, an increase in the particle size or a decrease in the surface area slows the dissolution rate.

14. The answer is B *[III B 7].*
A modified-release, or controlled-release, drug product contains two or more conventional doses of the drug, and therefore, an abrupt release of the drug, known as dose dumping, may cause some degree of intoxication.

15. The answer is B *[III A 1, 4 a].*
For drugs that are lipid-soluble, the rate of dissolution is the slowest (i.e., rate-limiting) step in drug absorption and, thus, in the drug's bioavailability. The disintegration rate of an immediate-release or conventional compressed tablet is usually more rapid than the rate of drug dissolution. Since the cell membrane is a lipoprotein structure, transport of a lipid-soluble drug across the cell membrane is generally rapid.

16. The answer is A *[III A 4 b].*
The extent of ionization of a weak electrolyte is described by the Henderson-Hasselbalch equation, which relates the pH of the solvent to the pK_a of the drug.

17–22. The answers are: 17-D *[V B 3 d],* **18-C** *[V B 3 e],* **19-E** *[V B 3 e],* **20-B** *[V B 3],* **21-D** *[V E 2],* **22-B** *[V E 4 a].*
The equation for the plasma concentration at steady state (C_{ss}) provides the formula for calculating the rate of an intravenous infusion (R). The equation is:

$$C_{ss} = \frac{R}{kV_D},$$

where k is the first-order elimination rate constant, and V_D is the apparent volume of distribution. Rearranging the equation and plugging in the data for this patient gives the following calculations:

$$R = C_{ss}kV_D = \frac{15 \text{ mg}}{100 \text{ ml}} \times \frac{0.693}{1 \text{ hr}} \times 9000 \text{ ml},$$

$$R = 936 \text{ mg/hr}.$$

The time it takes for an infused drug to reach the C_{ss} depends upon the drug's elimination half-life. The time to reach 95% of the C_{ss} is equal to 4.3 times the half-life, whereas the time to reach 99% of the C_{ss} is equal to 6.6 times the half-life. Since the half-life in the present case is given as 1 hour, the time to reach 95% of the C_{ss} would be 4.3 × 1 hour, or 4.3 hours.

The proper loading dose (D_L) is calculated as follows:

$$D_L = C_{ss} V_D = \frac{15 \text{ mg}}{100 \text{ ml}} \times 9000 \text{ ml} = 1350 \text{ mg}.$$

The answer to question 17 shows that the infusion rate should be 936 mg/hr. Therefore, using a drug solution containing 10 g in 500 ml, the required infusion rate is:

$$\frac{936 \text{ mg}}{1 \text{ hr}} \times \frac{500 \text{ ml}}{10{,}000 \text{ mg}} = 46.8 \text{ ml/hr}.$$

The patient's total body clearance (Cl_T) is calculated as follows:

$$Cl_T = kV_D,$$

$$Cl_T = \frac{0.693}{1} \times 9000 \text{ ml} = 6237 \text{ ml/hr}.$$

The hepatic clearance (Cl_H) is the difference between total clearance (Cl_T) and renal clearance (Cl_R):

$$Cl_H = Cl_T - Cl_R$$

$$Cl_H = 6237 - (86 \text{ ml/min} \times 60 \text{ min/hr}) = 1077 \text{ ml/hr}.$$

23. The answer is B *[V B 1 b].*
A very large apparent volume of distribution (V_D) is an early sign that a drug is not concentrated in the plasma but is distributed widely in the tissues. An increase in plasma protein binding would signify that the drug is in the plasma rather than in the tissues. A decrease in hepatic metabolism, an increase in side effects, or a decrease in urinary excretion of free drug would be due to a decrease in drug elimination.

24. The answer is A *[IV A 1].*
As more drug is concentrated at the receptor site, more receptors interact with the drug to produce a pharmacologic effect. The intensity of the response increases up to a maximum response. When all the available receptors are occupied by drug molecules, any additional drug will not produce a more intense response.

25. The answer is B *[V D 1].*
Nonlinear pharmacokinetics is a term used to indicate that the elimination of a drug is not first-order at all drug concentrations. In the case of some drugs, such as phenytoin, as the plasma drug concentration increases, the elimination pathway for metabolism of the drug becomes saturated and the half-life increases. The area under the plasma drug concentration versus time curve (AUC) of such a drug is not proportional to the dose; neither is the rate of metabolite formation, and the metabolic rate would indeed be related to the effects of the drug.

26. The answer is D *[V B 3 e; 4 f (5)].*
A loading dose (D_L) of a drug is given to obtain a therapeutic plasma drug level as rapidly as possible. The D_L is calculated on the basis of a drug's apparent volume of distribution (V_D) and the desired plasma level of the drug.

27. The answer is E *[V E 2 a; VII B 2].*
Inulin is neither reabsorbed nor actively secreted and, thus, is excreted by glomerular filtration only. The inulin clearance rate is used as a standard measure of the glomerular filtration rate (GFR), a test that is useful both clinically and in the development of new drugs.

28. The answer is E *[V A 3 d; B 1 b (3)].*
Drugs that are highly bound to plasma proteins diffuse poorly into the tissues and, thus, have a small apparent volume of distribution (V_D).

29. The answer is B *[IV A 1 a].*
The onset time is the time from drug administration to the time when absorbed drug reaches the minimum effective concentration (MEC). The MEC is the drug concentration in the plasma that is proportional (not necessarily equal) to the minimum drug concentration at the receptor site that elicits a pharmacologic response.

30. The answer is A *[V A 3].*
The initial distribution of a drug is chiefly determined by blood flow, whereas drug affinity for the tissue determines whether the drug concentrates at that site. The glomerular filtration rate (GFR) affects the

renal clearance of a drug, not its initial distribution. The gastric emptying time and degree of plasma protein binding have an effect on drug distribution but are less important than the rate of blood flow to the tissues.

31. The answer is C *[V E 4 b (2)].*
The kidney, lung, skin, and intestine all have some capacity to biotransform (metabolize) drugs, whereas the brain has very little capacity for drug metabolism. The liver is the major organ with the highest capacity for drug metabolism activity.

32. The answer is D *[V B 4 c].*
The superposition principle, which underlies the design of multiple-dose regimens, assumes that the earlier drug doses do not affect subsequent doses. If any change in the elimination rate constant or total body clearance of the drug occurs during multiple dosing, then the superposition principle is no longer valid. Changes in the total body clearance (Cl_T) may be due to enzyme induction, enzyme inhibition, or saturation of an elimination pathway. Any of these would cause nonlinear pharmacokinetics.

33. The answer is D *[III B 2 a].*
A drug in solution is already dissolved and, thus, no dissolution is needed prior to absorption. Consequently, compared with other drug formulations, a drug in solution has a high rate of bioavailability. A drug in aqueous solution has the highest bioavailability rate and is often used as the reference preparation for other formulations. Drugs in hydroalcoholic solution (e.g., elixirs) also have good bioavailability. The rate of drug bioavailability from a hard gelatin capsule, compressed tablet, or suspension may be equal to that of a solution if an optimal formulation is manufactured and the drug inherently rapidly absorbed.

34–36. The answers are: 34-D, 35-E, 36-A *[V B 4 e, f].*
The oral maintenance dose (D_o) should maintain the patient's average drug concentration (C_{av}^{∞}) at the effective drug concentration. The drug's bioavailability (F), the apparent volume of distribution (V_D), the frequency of dosing (τ), and the excretion rate constant (k) must all be considered in calculating the dose. The equation used is:

$$C_{av}^{\infty} = \frac{FD_o}{kV_D\tau}$$

For the drug in question, $F = 0.75$, $k = 0.693/24$ hr, $V_D = 3$ L/kg $\times$ 65 kg, $\tau = 25$ hr, and $C_{av}^{\infty} = 1.5$ ng/ml, or 1.5 µg/L. Therefore, by substitution, $D_o = 270$ µg, or 0.270 mg. When the maintenance dose is given at a dosage frequency equal to the half-life, then the loading dose is equal to twice the maintenance dose; for the case in question, this would be 540 µg, or 0.540 mg. To determine the plasma drug concentration for a dosage regimen of 0.125 mg every 12 hours, one would again use the C_{av}^{∞} formula above. This time, $F = 0.75$, $D_o = 0.125$, $k = 0.693/24$ hr, $V_D = 3$ L/kg $\times$ 65 kg, and $\tau = 12$ hr. Therefore, $C_{av}^{\infty} = 1.39$ ng/ml. For cardiac glycosides, the peak (C_{max}) and trough (C_{min}) concentrations should be calculated, and plasma drug concentrations should be monitored after dosing. The loading dose (D_L) may be given in small increments over a period of time, according to the suggested dosage regimen by the manufacturer.

37. The answer is A (I) *[V A 1].*
The first equation in the question describes a zero-order reaction (dA/dt) in which the reaction rate increases or decreases at a constant rate (k). A zero-order reaction produces a graph of a straight line with the equation of $A = -kt + A_0$ when A is plotted against time (t). The other equations in the question represent first-order reactions.

Part II
Medicinal Chemistry and Pharmacology

David C. Kosegarten
Edward F. LaSala

7
Organic Chemistry and Biochemistry

Edward F. LaSala
John D. Leary

I. ORGANIC CHEMISTRY

A. Introduction. Medicinal chemistry is rooted in organic chemistry—the study of organic (carbon-based) compounds. These compounds are classified by **functional group**—a group of atoms that occurs in many molecules and confers on them a characteristic chemical reactivity, regardless of the carbon skeleton. Functional groups are part of the overall structure of the drug and determine such characteristics as water or lipid solubility, reactivity, chemical stability, and in vivo stability, which in turn determine drug properties.

1. Functional groups that impart **liposolubility** are likely to increase the drug's tendency to cross cellular membranes.
2. Functional group **reactivity** is most important for reactions occurring under **normal environmental conditions,** primarily air oxidation and hydrolysis. For example, benzene's characteristic reactions occur only with special reagents and in special laboratory conditions. Thus, benzene's shelf life is relatively long, and it requires no special storage conditions.
3. Functional groups affect drug reactivity and, hence, **drug shelf life** and **stability**.
4. Functional groups also affect **in vivo stability**—the susceptibility of the drug to biotransformation and determination of appropriate metabolic pathways.

B. Alkanes, which are also called **paraffins** or **saturated hydrocarbons,** have a general formula of $R—CH_2—CH_3$. (R = a radical, or a molecule fragment.)

1. Alkanes are **lipid soluble**.
2. The common reactions of alkanes are **halogenation** and **combustion**.
3. On the shelf, alkanes are **chemically inert** with regard to air, light, heat, acids, and bases.
4. In vivo, alkanes are **stable; side-chain hydroxylation may occur**.

C. Alkenes, also called **olefins** or **unsaturated hydrocarbons,** have a general formula of $R—CH{=}CH_2$.

1. Alkenes are **lipid soluble**.
2. The common reactions of alkenes are **addition of hydrogen or halogens, hydration** (to form glycols), and **oxidation** (to form peroxides).
3. On the shelf, **volatile alkenes and peroxides may explode** in the presence of oxygen and a spark.
4. In vivo, alkenes are **relatively stable**. **Hydration, epoxidation, peroxidation,** or **reduction** may occur.

D. Aromatic hydrocarbons are based on **benzene** (Figure 7-1). These molecules exhibit multicenter bonding, which confers unique chemical properties.

1. Aromatic hydrocarbons are **lipid soluble**.
2. The common reactions of aromatic hydrocarbons are **halogenation, nitration, sulfonation,** and **Friedel-Crafts alkylation**.

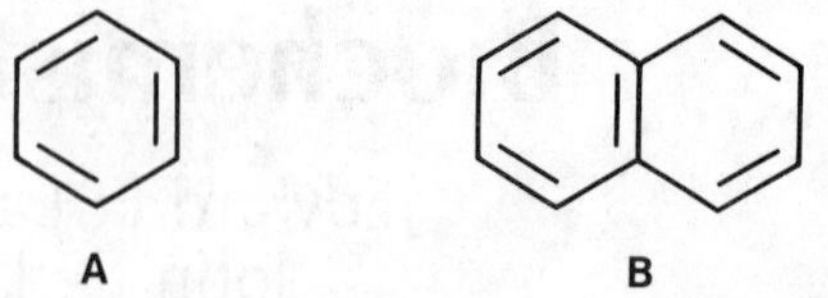

Figure 7-1. Chemical structures of (*A*) benzene and (*B*) naphthalene. Benzene and related compounds, such as naphthalene, are planar molecules in the form of a regular hexagon.

3. On the shelf, aromatic hydrocarbons are **quite stable.**
4. In vivo, aromatic hydrocarbons undergo **hydroxylation.**

E. Alkyl halides, also known as **halogenated hydrocarbons,** have a general formula of R—CH_2—X.

1. Alkyl halides are **lipid soluble**. Their **solubility increases with the extent of halogenation**.
2. The common reactions of alkyl halides are **nucleophilic substitution** and **dehydrohalogenation**.
3. On the shelf, alkyl halides are **stable.**
4. In vivo, alkyl halides **are not readily metabolized.**

F. Alcohols contain a **hydroxyl group** (—OH) and may be classified as primary, secondary, or tertiary. **Primary alcohols** have a general formula of R—CH_2—OH; **secondary alcohols** have a general formula of R—CH(CH_3)—OH; and **tertiary alcohols** have a general formula of R—C(CH_3)$_2$—OH.

1. Low molecular weight alcohols are **water soluble;** water solubility decreases as hydrocarbon chain length increases. Alcohols are also **lipid soluble.**
2. The common reactions of alcohols are **esterification** and **oxidation**.
   a. **Primary alcohols** are oxidized to **aldehydes** and then to **acids.**
   b. **Secondary alcohols** are oxidized to **ketones.**
   c. **Tertiary alcohols** ordinarily **are not oxidized.**
3. On the shelf, alcohols are **stable.**
4. In vivo, alcohols may undergo **oxidation, glucuronidation,** or **sulfation.**

G. Phenols are **aromatic compounds containing a hydroxyl group** (—OH). **Monophenols** have **one hydroxyl group,** and **catechols** have **two hydroxyl groups** (Figure 7-2).

1. Phenols are **lipid soluble;** phenol itself (carbolic acid) is **fairly water soluble**. Ring substitutions generally decrease water solubility.
2. The common reactions of phenols are **reactions with strong bases** (to form water-soluble salts), **esterification with acids,** and **oxidation** (to form quinones, usually colored).
3. On the shelf, phenols are **susceptible to air oxidation** and to **oxidation on contact with ferric ions.**
4. In vivo, phenols undergo **sulfation, glucuronidation, aromatic hydroxylation,** and ***O*-methylation.**

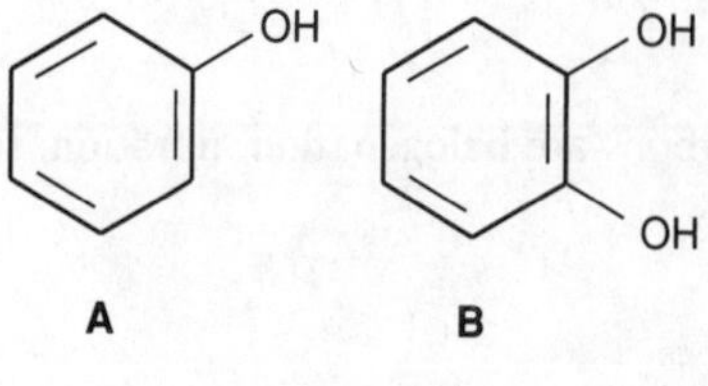

Figure 7-2. Structures of (*A*) monophenol and (*B*) catechol functional groups.

H. Ethers have a general formula of R—O—R, with an oxygen atom bonded to two carbon atoms.

1. Low molecular weight ethers are **partially water soluble;** water solubility decreases with an increase in the hydrocarbon portion of the molecule. Ethers are also **lipid soluble**.
2. The common reaction of ethers is **oxidation** (to form peroxides).
3. On the shelf, **peroxides may explode**.
4. In vivo, ethers undergo ***O*-dealkylation**. Stability increases with the size of the alkyl group.

I. Aldehydes have a general formula of R—CHO and contain a **carbonyl group** (C=O).

1. Aldehydes are **lipid soluble;** low molecular weight aldehydes are also **water soluble**.
2. The common reactions of aldehydes are **oxidation** and (for those of low molecular weight) **polymerization**.
3. On the shelf, aldehydes **oxidize to acids**.
4. In vivo, aldehydes may also undergo **oxidation to acids**.

J. Ketones have a general formula of R—CO—R and, like aldehydes, contain a **carbonyl group** (C=O).

1. Ketones are **lipid soluble**. Low molecular weight ketones are also **water soluble** with solubility decreasing as the hydrocarbon portion of the molecule increases.
2. Ketones are **relatively nonreactive,** although they may exist in equilibrium with their enol forms.
3. On the shelf, ketones are **very stable**.
4. In vivo, ketones may undergo **some oxidation** and **some reduction**.

K. Amines contain an **amine group** (—NH_2). **Primary amines** have a general formula of R—CH_2—NH_2; **secondary amines** have a general formula of R—CH_2—NH—R; **tertiary amines** have a general formula of R—CH_2—N—R_2; and **quaternary amines** have a general formula of R—CH_2—N^+—R_3.

1. Low molecular weight amines are **water soluble;** solubility decreases with increased branching (e.g., primary amines are more water soluble than secondary amines). However, quaternary amines, being ionic, are quite water soluble, as are most amine salts. Amines are also **lipid soluble**.
2. The common reactions of amines are **oxidation** and, for alkyl amines, **salt formation with acids**. Aromatic amines, which are less basic, have less tendency to react with acids.
3. On the shelf, phenolic amines are susceptible to **air oxidation**.
4. In vivo, amines may undergo minor **glucuronidation, sulfation,** and **methylation**. Primary amines also undergo **oxidative deamination**. Primary and secondary amines undergo **acetylation**. Secondary and tertiary amines undergo ***N*-dealkylation,** and tertiary amines undergo ***N*-oxidation**.

L. Carboxylic acids have a general formula of R—COOH and contain a **carboxyl group** (—COOH).

1. Low molecular weight carboxylic acids are **water soluble,** as are sodium and potassium salts. Carboxylic acids are also **lipid soluble**.
2. The common reactions of carboxylic acids are **salt formation with bases, esterification,** and **decarboxylation**.
3. On the shelf, carboxylic acids are **very stable**.
4. In vivo, carboxylic acids undergo **conjugation** (with glucuronic acid, glycine, and glutamine) and **β-oxidation**.

M. Esters have a general formula of R—COOR.

1. Esters are **lipid soluble;** low molecular weight esters are slightly **water soluble**.
2. The common reaction of esters is **hydrolysis**.

3. On the shelf, simple or low molecular weight esters are **susceptible to hydrolysis,** whereas complex, high molecular weight, or water-insoluble esters are resistant.

4. In vivo, esters undergo **enzymatic hydrolysis**.

N. **Amides** have a general formula of R—CONH$_2$ or R—CONH—R (lactam form).

1. Amides are **lipid soluble;** low molecular weight amides are **fairly water soluble**.

2. Amides have **no common reactions**.

3. On the shelf, amides are **very stable**.

4. In vivo, amides undergo **enzymatic hydrolysis,** primarily in the liver.

II. BIOCHEMISTRY

A. **Introduction.** Biochemistry is the study of molecular phenomena associated with life processes. It influences drug metabolism, therapeutic effectiveness, and biotransformation. Biochemically significant molecules include amino acids and proteins, carbohydrates, lipids, pyrimidines, and purines, and biopolymers—enzymes, which are built from amino acids, polysaccharides,which are built from carbohydrates, and nucleic acids, which are built from pyrimidines and purines.

B. **Amino acids and proteins**

1. **Amino acids** are the monomer units of proteins and have the following general formula:

$$R—\underset{\underset{NH_2}{|}}{CH}—COOH$$

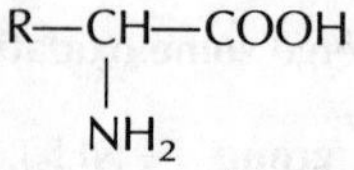

a. The amino acids that form proteins are **α-amino acids;** that is, the amino group (—NH$_2$) and the radical (R) are attached to the first (α) carbon removed from the carboxylic acid group. A protein can be hydrolyzed into its component α-amino acids by acids, bases, or enzymes.

b. Amino acids exist in two **enantiomorphs** (mirror-image forms), also known as **optical isomers**. Optical isomers are designated dextrorotatory (D) or levorotatory (L), depending on whether the molecule rotates polarized light in a clockwise direction (D) or a counterclockwise direction (L). The body synthesizes only **L-amino acids** into proteins.

c. Amino acids have a **zwitterion structure** (both positive and negative regions of charge), which accounts for their high melting point and low water solubility. Amino acids in solution have the following general formula:

$$R—\underset{\underset{NH_3{}^+}{|}}{CH}—COO^-$$

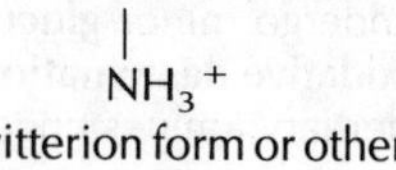

d. **Ionization** of amino acids to the zwitterion form or other forms depends on pH (Figure 7-3).

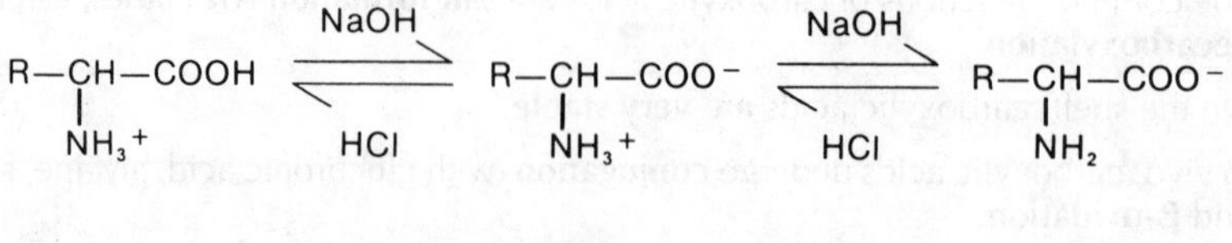

$$\underset{I}{R-\underset{\underset{NH_3{}^+}{|}}{CH}-COOH} \underset{HCl}{\overset{NaOH}{\rightleftharpoons}} \underset{II}{R-\underset{\underset{NH_3{}^+}{|}}{CH}-COO^-} \underset{HCl}{\overset{NaOH}{\rightleftharpoons}} \underset{III}{R-\underset{\underset{NH_2}{|}}{CH}-COO^-}$$

Figure 7-3. Amino acid ionization in solution. *Form I* is the dominant form in an acidic solution. *Form II* (the zwitterion form) dominates at the isoelectric point (the pH at which zwitterion formation occurs). *Form III* dominates in an alkaline solution.

e. Amino acids are linked to form proteins by the **peptide bond**—a link between the carbonyl carbon and the amino nitrogen (Figure 7-4).

2. Proteins, which result from amino acids linking by means of peptide bonds, have four levels of structure.

a. Primary structure refers to the sequence of amino acids in the protein.

b. Secondary structure refers to the spatial arrangement of sequenced amino acids; for example, α-conformation (helical coil) or β-conformation (pleated sheet).

c. Tertiary structure refers to the coiling and folding of protein chains into compact structures, such as globular shapes.

d. Quaternary structure refers to the arrangement of individual subunit chains into complex molecules.

C. Carbohydrates are **polyhydroxy aldehydes** or **ketones. Three major classes** of carbohydrates exist: monosaccharides, oligosaccharides, and polysaccharides.

1. Monosaccharides (simple sugars), such as glucose or fructose, consist of a single polyhydroxy aldehyde or ketone unit.

a. Aldehydic monosaccharides are reducing sugars.

b. Monosaccharides can be linked together by **glycosidic bonds,** which are hydrolyzed by acids but not by bases.

2. Oligosaccharides, such as sucrose, maltose, and lactose, consist of short chains of monosaccharides joined covalently.

a. Sucrose cannot be absorbed by the intestine until it is converted by sucrase into its components, glucose and fructose.

b. Maltose is hydrolyzed by maltase into two molecules of glucose.

c. Lactose (or milk sugar) cannot be absorbed by the intestine until it is converted by lactase into its components, galactose and glucose.

3. Polysaccharides, such as cellulose and glycogen, consist of long chains of monosaccharides.

D. Pyrimidines and purines are **bases** that, when bonded with ribose, form **nucleosides,** which when subsequently bonded to phosphoric acid form **nucleotides**—the structural building blocks of nucleic acids.

1. Pyrimidine bases include:

a. Cytosine (C), found in deoxyribonucleic acid (DNA) and ribonucleic acid (RNA)

b. Uracil (U), found in RNA only

c. Thymine (T), found in DNA only

2. Purine bases include:

a. Adenine (A), found in DNA and RNA

b. Guanine (G), found in DNA and RNA

3. Pyrimidines and purines exhibit **tautomerism** (a form of stereoisomerism) and can exist in either **keto** (lactam) or **enol** (lactim) forms (Figure 7-5).

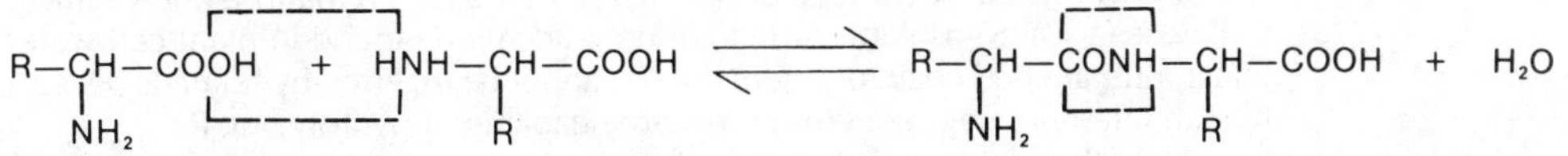

Figure 7-4. Peptide bond formation occurs as a result of the condensation of the carboxyl group of one amino acid with the amino group of another. Water is eliminated during this process.

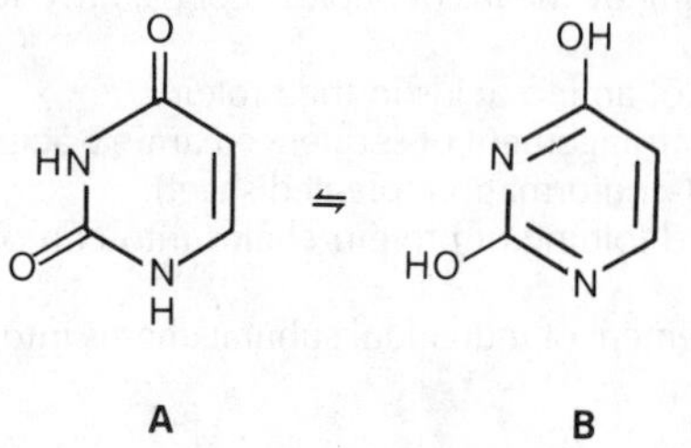

Figure 7-5. Uracil may exist in two tautomeric forms: (*A*) in a keto (or lactam) form and (*B*) in an enol (or lactim) form.

E. Biopolymers

1. **Enzymes**—linked chains of amino acids—are proteins capable of acting as catalysts for biologic reactions. They may be simple or complex and may require cofactors or coenzymes for biologic activity.
   a. An enzyme **enhances the rate of a specific chemical reaction** by lowering the activation energy of the reaction. It does not change the reaction's equilibrium point, and it is not used up or permanently changed by the reaction.
   b. A **cofactor** may be an inorganic component (usually a metal ion) or a nonprotein organic molecule. A cofactor may be biologically inactive without an **apoenzyme** (the protein portion of a complex enzyme). A cofactor firmly bound to the apoenzyme is called a **prosthetic group**. An organic cofactor that is not firmly bound but is actively involved during catalysis is called a **coenzyme**.
   c. A complete, catalytically active enzyme system is referred to as a **holoenzyme**.
   d. Enzymes fall into **six major classes**.
      (1) **Oxidoreductases** (e.g., dehydrogenases, oxidases, peroxidases) are important in the oxidative metabolism of drugs.
      (2) **Transferases** catalyze the transfer of groups, such as phosphate and amino groups.
      (3) **Hydrolases** (e.g., proteolytic enzymes, amylases, esterases) hydrolyze their substrates.
      (4) **Lyases** (e.g., decarboxylases, deaminases) catalyze the removal of functional groups by means other than hydrolysis.
      (5) **Ligases** (e.g., DNA ligase, which binds nucleotides together during DNA synthesis) catalyze the coupling of two molecules.
      (6) **Isomerases** catalyze various isomerizations, such as the change from D to L forms or the change from cis- to trans-isomers.
2. **Polysaccharides** (also called **glycans**) are long-chain polymers of carbohydrates and may be linear or branched. They are classified as homopolysaccharides or heteropolysaccharides.
   a. **Homopolysaccharides** (e.g., starch, glycogen, cellulose) contain only one type of monomeric unit.
      (1) **Starch** (a reserve food material of plants) is composed of two glucose polymers—amylose (linear and water soluble) and amylopectin (highly branched and water insoluble). It yields mainly maltose (a glucose disaccharide) after enzymatic hydrolysis with salivary or pancreatic amylase; only glucose after complete hydrolysis by strong acids.
      (2) **Glycogen,** like amylopectin, is a highly branched, compact chain of D-glucose. The main storage polysaccharide of animal cells, it is found mostly in liver and muscle and can be hydrolyzed by salivary or pancreatic amylase into maltose and D-glucose.
      (3) **Cellulose** (a water-insoluble structural polysaccharide found in plant cell walls) is a linear, unbranched chain of D-glucose. It cannot be digested by humans because the human intestinal tract secretes no enzyme capable of hydrolyzing it.
   b. **Heteropolysaccharides** (e.g., heparin, hyaluronic acid) contain two or more types of monomeric unit.
      (1) **Heparin** (an acid mucopolysaccharide) consists of sulfate derivatives of *N*-acetyl-D-glucosamine and D-iduronate. It can be isolated from lung tissue and is used medically to prevent blood clot formation.

(2) **Hyaluronic acid,** a component of bacterial cell walls as well as of the vitreous humor and synovial fluid, consists of alternating units of *N*-acetyl-D-glucosamine and *N*-acetylmuramic acid.

3. **Nucleic acids** are linear polymers of **nucleotides**—pyrimidine and purine bases linked to ribose or deoxyribose sugars (nucleosides) and bound to phosphate groups. The backbone of the nucleic acid consists of alternating phosphate and pentose units with a purine or pyrimidine base attached to each.
   a. Nucleic acids are **strong acids,** closely associated with cellular cations and such basic proteins as histones and protamines.
   b. The two main types of nucleic acids are **DNA** and **RNA**. RNA exists in three forms.
      (1) **Ribosomal RNA (rRNA)** is found in the ribosomes, but its functions are not fully understood yet.
      (2) **Messenger RNA (mRNA)** serves as the template for protein synthesis and specifies a polypeptide's amino acid sequence.
      (3) **Transfer RNA (tRNA)** carries activated amino acids to the ribosomes, where the amino acids are incorporated into the growing polypeptide chain.
   c. In both DNA and RNA, the successive nucleotides are joined by **phosphodiester bonds** between the 5′-hydroxy group of one nucleotide's pentose and the 3′-hydroxy group of the next nucleotide's pentose.
   d. **DNA differs from RNA** in that it lacks a hydroxyl group at the pentose's C_2' position, and it contains thymine rather than uracil.
   e. DNA structure consists of two α-helical DNA strands coiled around the same axis to form a double helix. The strands are antiparallel—the 5′, 3′-internucleotide phosphodiester links run in opposite directions.
      (1) **Hydrogen bonding** between specific base pairs—adenine and thymine (A—T) and cytosine and guanine (C—G)—holds the two DNA strands together. The strands are **complementary** (the base sequence of one strand determines the base sequence of the other).
      (2) The **hydrophobic bases** are on the inside of the helix; the **hydrophilic deoxyribose–phosphate backbone** is on the outside.

III. BIOCHEMICAL METABOLISM

A. Overview. Biochemical metabolism is the review of pathways that lead to the synthesis or breakdown of compounds important to the life of an organism.

1. **Control of metabolism.** Metabolism is controlled by substrate concentration, enzymes (constitutive or induced), allosteric (regulatory) enzymes, hormones, and compartmentation.

2. **Catabolism** is the sum of degradation reactions that usually release energy for useful work (e.g., mechanical, osmotic, biosynthetic).

3. **Anabolism** is the sum of biosynthetic (build-up) reactions that consume energy to form new biochemical compounds (**metabolites**).

4. **Amphibolic pathways** are those that may be used for both catabolic as well as anabolic purposes. The **Krebs cycle** breaks down metabolites primarily to release 90% of the total energy of an organism. It also draws off metabolites to form compounds such as amino acids (e.g., aspartic, glutamic, alanine). Hemoglobin has its heme moiety formed from succinyl coenzyme A (succinyl CoA) and glycine followed by a complex set of reactions.

B. Bioenergetics

1. **Substrate level phosphorylation** entails the formation of one unit of adenosine triphosphate (ATP) per unit of metabolite transformed (e.g., succinyl CoA to succinate, phosphoenolpyruvate to pyruvate). These reactions do not need oxygen.

2. **Oxidative phosphorylation** entails the formation of two or three units of ATP per unit of metabolite transformed by oxidoreductase enzymes (e.g., dehydrogenases); these enzymes use flavin adenine dinucleotide (FAD) formed from the vitamin riboflavin, or nicotinamide adenine dinucleotide (NAD^+) from the vitamin nicotinamide as cofactors. The reactions are coupled to the electron transport system, and the energy released is used to form ATP in the mitochondria.

C. Carbohydrate metabolism

1. **Catabolism.** This process releases stored energy from carbohydrates.
   a. **Glycogenolysis** is the breakdown of glycogen into glucose phosphate in the liver and skeletal muscle, controlled by the hormones glucagon and epinephrine.
   b. **Glycolysis** is the breakdown of sugar phosphates (e.g., glucose, fructose, glycerol) into pyruvate (aerobically) or lactate (anerobically).

2. **Anabolism.** This process consumes energy to build up complex molecules from simpler molecules.
   a. **Glycogenesis** is the formation of glycogen in the liver and muscles from glucose consumed in the diet; its synthesis is controlled by the pancreatic hormone insulin.
   b. **Gluconeogenesis** is the formation of glucose from noncarbohydrate sources, such as lactate, alanine, pyruvate, and Krebs cycle metabolites; fatty acids cannot form glucose.

D. Krebs cycle. This pathway serves both breakdown and synthetic purposes and occurs in the mitochondrial compartment.

1. **Catabolism.** This pathway converts pyruvate (glycolysis), acetyl CoA (fatty acid degradation), and amino acids to carbon dioxide and water with a release of energy. The cycle is strictly oxygen-dependent (aerobic). Mature red blood cells lack mitochondria; hence, there is no Krebs cycle activity.

2. **Anabolism.** This pathway forms amino acids such as aspartate and glutamate from cycle intermediates; also, the porphyrin ring of heme (e.g., hemoglobin, myoglobin, cytochromes) is formed from a cycle intermediate.

3. **Anaplerotic reactions.** Since metabolites were used to make amino acids or heme (e.g., succinyl CoA), the metabolite must be replaced by intermediates from other sources (e.g., glutamate from the breakdown of protein forms ketoglutarate).

4. **Electron transport system** accepts electrons and hydrogen from the oxidation of the Krebs cycle metabolites and couples the energy released to synthesize ATP in the mitochondria.

E. Lipid metabolism

1. **Catabolism.** Triglycerides (triacylglycerols) stored in fat cells (adipocytes) are hydrolyzed by hormone-sensitive lipases into three fatty acids and glycerol.
   a. **Fatty acids** are broken down by beta oxidation to acetyl CoA (two carbon units), which enter the Krebs cycle to complete the oxidation to carbon dioxide and water with release of considerable energy. Too rapid breakdown of fatty acids leads to ketone bodies (ketogenesis) as in diabetes mellitus.
   b. **Glycerol** enters glycolysis and is oxidized to pyruvate and, via the Krebs cycle, to carbon dioxide and water.
   c. **Steroids** may be converted to other compounds such as bile acids, vitamin D, or steroidal hormones (e.g., cortisone, estrogens, androgens); they are not broken down completely.

2. **Anabolism.** Biosynthesis forms fatty acids, steroids, and other terpene-related metabolites.
   a. **Fatty acids** are formed in the cytoplasm, and unsaturation occurs in the mitochondria or endoplasmic reticulum. Humans cannot make linoleic acid; thus, it is important that it be included in the diet (essential fatty acid).
   b. **Terpene compounds** are derived from acetyl CoA via mevalonate and include:
      (1) Cholesterol and other steroids
      (2) Fat-soluble vitamins (i.e., A, D, E, K)
      (3) Bile acids
   c. **Sphingolipids** contain sphingenine formed from palmitoyl CoA and serine. Sphingenine forms a ceramide backbone when joined to fatty acids. The addition of sugars, sialic acid, or choline phosphate form compounds such as cerebrosides, gangliosides, or sphingomyelin found in nerve tissues and membranes.
   d. **Phosphatidyl compounds,** such as phosphatidyl choline (lecithin), phosphatidyl serine, or ethanolamine, are also important parts of membranes.

F. Nitrogen metabolism involves amino acid metabolism and nucleic acid metabolism (see Chapter 9 for a discussion of the nucleic acid role in cell activity).

1. **Catabolism**
   a. **Amino acids.** The amino group is removed by a transaminase enzyme. The carbon skeleton is broken down to acetyl CoA (ketogenic amino acids) or to citric acid cycle intermediates (glycogenic amino acids) and oxidized to carbon dioxide and water for energy. Glycogenic amino acids form glucose as needed via gluconeogenesis; some amino acids are both ketogenic and glycogenic (e.g., tyrosine).
   b. **Purines** are salvaged (90%), and the remaining 10% are degraded in a sequence that includes xanthine oxidase forming uric acid in humans.
   c. **Pyrimidines** are catabolized to β-alanine, ammonia, and carbon dioxide.

2. **Anabolism**
   a. **Amino acids** are formed from the citric acid cycle intermediates (see III D 2); others must be eaten daily in dietary proteins. The latter are called essential amino acids [phenylalanine, valine, tryptophan, threonine, isoleucine, methionine (histidine, arginine in infants), lysine, leucine (PVT TIM HALL)].
   b. **Purines** are formed by complex reactions using carbamoyl phosphate, aspartate, glutamine, glycine, carbon dioxide, and formyl tetrahydrofolate.
   c. **Pyrimidines** are formed from aspartate and carbamoyl phosphate in a multistep process.

G. **Nitrogen excretion.** Excess nitrogen must be eliminated since it is toxic. Humans primarily excrete urea but also excrete uric acid.

1. **Urea synthesis.** The Krebs-Henseleit pathway is used to form urea principally in the liver. The ammonia is removed from amino acids by amino acid transferases (transaminases) that use pyridoxal phosphate (vitamin B_6) as a coenzyme. Glutamine is formed from glutamate (an intermediate) and ammonia; glutamine and carbon dioxide form carbamoyl phosphate, which enters the urea cycle and after several steps forms urea.

2. **Uric acid synthesis.** Though most purines are salvaged, humans excrete the remaining purines as uric acid.

STUDY QUESTIONS

Directions: Each of the numbered items or incomplete statements in this section is followed by answers or by completions of the statement. Select the **one** lettered answer or completion that is **best** in each case.

1. Which of the following classes of organic compounds reacts to form salts with hydrochloric acid?

(A) Tertiary amines
(B) Carboxylic acids
(C) Amides
(D) Ethers
(E) Secondary alcohols

2. Which of the following terms best describes the conversion of

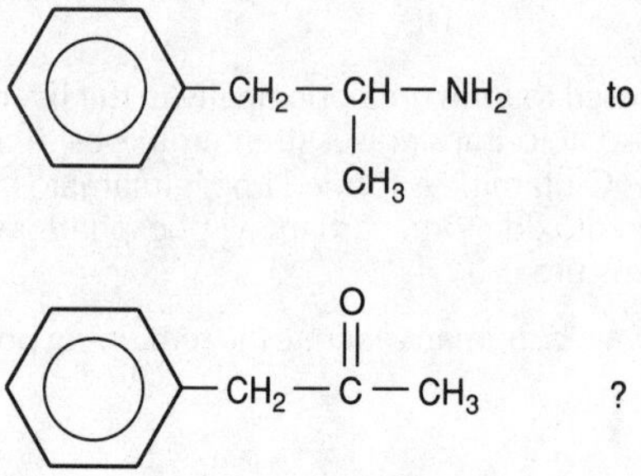

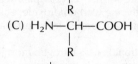

(A) *N*-dealkylation
(B) Oxidative deamination
(C) Acetylation
(D) Decarboxylation
(E) Reductive cleavage

3. Which of the following functional groups is most susceptible to hydrolysis?

(A) R—CO—R
(B) R—COOR
(C) R—O—R
(D) R—NH—CH_3
(E) R—COOH

4. Monomer units of proteins are known as

(A) monosaccharides
(B) prosthetic groups
(C) amino acids
(D) purines
(E) nucleosides

5. Which of the following formulas represents the zwitterion form of an amino acid?

(A) $H_2N—CH(R)—COO^-$
(B) $H_3\overset{+}{N}—CH(R)—COOH$
(C) $H_2N—CH(R)—COOH$
(D) $H_3\overset{+}{N}—CH(R)—COO^-$
(E) $H_2N—CH(R)—CONH—CH(R)—COOH$

6. Glucose is a carbohydrate that cannot be hydrolyzed into a simpler substance. It is best described as

(A) a sugar
(B) a monosaccharide
(C) a disaccharide
(D) a polysaccharide
(E) an oligosaccharide

7. All of the following carbohydrates are considered to be polysaccharides EXCEPT

(A) heparin
(B) starch
(C) glycogen
(D) maltose
(E) cellulose

8. Which of the following compounds are considered the building blocks of nucleic acids?

(A) Nucleotides
(B) Nucleosides
(C) Monosaccharides
(D) Purines
(E) Amino acids

1-A 4-C 7-D
2-B 5-D 8-A
3-B 6-B

9. Which of the following terms best describes a cofactor that is firmly bound to an apoenzyme?

(A) Holoenzyme
(B) Prosthetic group
(C) Coenzyme
(D) Transferase
(E) Heteropolysaccharide

10. Enzymes that uncouple peptide linkages are best classified as

(A) hydrolases
(B) ligases
(C) oxidoreductases
(D) transferases
(E) isomerases

11. The sugar that is inherent in the nucleic acids RNA and DNA is

(A) glucose
(B) sucrose
(C) ribose
(D) digitoxose
(E) maltose

Directions: Each question below contains three suggested answers, of which **one or more** is correct. Choose the answer

A if **I only** is correct
B if **III only** is correct
C if **I and II** are correct
D if **II and III** are correct
E if **I, II, and III** are correct

12. When certain functional groups are introduced into a benzene nucleus, they tend to decrease the liposolubility of benzene. These groups include

I. an ethyl group
II. a phenolic group
III. a carboxylic acid group

Questions 13–16

The following questions refer to the drug molecule

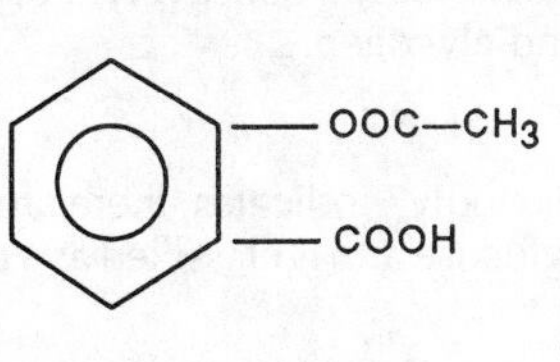

13. The drug molecule is soluble in

I. an aqueous base
II. water
III. an aqueous acid

14. Decomposition of the drug molecule at room temperature most likely would occur by

I. oxidation of the ester
II. reduction of the carboxylic acid
III. hydrolysis of the ester

15. Reactions that would be possible metabolic pathways for the drug molecule include

I. ring hydroxylation
II. enzymatic hydrolysis
III. glucuronide formation

16. Classes of organic compounds that have greater in vitro stability than in vivo stability include

I. carboxylic acids
II. alcohols
III. alkyl halides

9-B 12-D 15-E
10-A 13-A 16-C
11-C 14-B

ANSWERS AND EXPLANATIONS

1. The answer is A *[I K 2].*
Substances that react with acids to form salts must be bases. Only organic compounds that contain the nitrogen-containing amine group are bases. While amides contain nitrogen, the adjacent carbonyl group decreases the basicity; therefore, they are essentially neutral.

2. The answer is B *[I K 4].*
The reactant depicted contains a primary amine that is lost during the reaction; that is, the molecule is deaminated. The resultant product is a ketone formed from the oxidation of the carbon atom. Thus, this reaction would best be termed oxidative deamination.

3. The answer is B *[I M 2].*
Hydrolysis is a double decomposition reaction in which water is one of the reactants. Esters, particularly simple esters, commonly undergo hydrolysis. Certain types of ethers such as glycosides also undergo hydrolysis, but they usually require strongly alkaline conditions or a catalyst such as an enzyme. Ketones, amines, or carboxylic acids do not undergo hydrolysis.

4. The answer is C *[II B 1].*
Proteins are large molecules with molecular weights ranging from 5000 to over 1 million daltons. All proteins are composed of chains of amino acids and can be hydrolyzed to yield a mixture of their respective amino acids. There are 20 α-amino acids, which are commonly found in proteins. All the naturally occurring amino acids in proteins are L-enantiomers, with the exception of glycine. All have at least one amino group and one carboxyl group. The amino acids are linked together through the amino group of one amino acid and the carboxyl group of another amino acid with the splitting out of a water molecule to form an amide linkage, which in a protein is referred to as a peptide.

Monosaccharides are simple, nonhydrolyzable sugars. Purines and pyrimidines are organic bases, while a prosthetic group is a cofactor that is firmly bound to an apoenzyme.

5. The answer is D *[II B 1 c, d; Figures 7-3, 7-4].*
A zwitterion is a single species containing both negative and positive charges. It sometimes is referred to as an inner salt. Amino acids have an amino group and a carboxyl group in the same molecule. The amino group, which is basic, attracts the proton from the carboxyl group and becomes positively charged, while the carboxyl group becomes negatively charged when it donates its proton to the amino group. Amino acids exist as zwitterions at near neutral pH such as occurs within a cell or in the bloodstream.

6. The answer is B *[II C 1].*
While glucose is a sugar, it is more specifically a simple sugar that cannot be hydrolyzed into more simple sugars—thus, it is classified as a monosaccharide. Sugars may be simple, such as glucose, or complex, such as sucrose, and are classified as disaccharides or oligosaccharides, respectively. Polysaccharides consist of long chains of monosaccharides such as cellulose and glycogen.

7. The answer is D *[II C 2 b, 3, E 2 a, b].*
Polysaccharides are long-chain polymers of sugars. As the prefix "poly" indicates, there are many sugar units in the molecule. Maltose is composed of two molecules of glucose and is classified as a disaccharide or an oligosaccharide.

8. The answer is A *[II D, E 3].*
Nucleic acids are linear polymers of nucleotides that consist of three different molecules that are covalently linked to form one unit: (1) an organic base of either a purine or a pyrimidine; (2) a 5-carbon sugar (e.g., pentose); and (3) a phosphoric acid group. A nucleoside consists of the organic base and the pentose. A monosaccharide is a simple nonhydrolyzable carbohydrate, which may be considered a building block of polysaccharides. Purines are heterocyclic bases. Adenine and guanine are the two purines found in deoxyribonucleic acid (DNA) and ribonucleic acid (RNA). Amino acids are the building blocks of protein.

9. The answer is B *[II E 1 b].*
Complex, or conjugated, enzymes contain a nonprotein group called a cofactor, which is required for biologic activity. In many cases, the cofactor is quite firmly bound to the protein. In others, the binding occurs only during the reaction that the enzyme catalyzes. Cofactors that are firmly bound to the protein

are known as prosthetic groups, whereas those that are actively bound to the protein only during catalysis are referred to as coenzymes.

A holoenzyme is a complete, catalytically active enzyme system. A transferase is an enzyme that catalyzes the transfer of groups from one substance to another, such as catechol *O*-methyl transferase (COMT). A heteropolysaccharide is a polysaccharide that contains two or more different monomeric units, such as heparin.

10. The answer is A *[II E 1 d (3)].*
A peptide linkage is an amide functional group formed from the loss of a molecule of water from two amino acids. Uncoupling this linkage is the reverse of this reaction, a hydrolysis reaction. A hydrolase is an enzyme that catalyzes hydrolysis reactions. More specific terms for an enzyme that catalyzes the hydrolysis of proteins are amidase or peptidase. A ligase catalyzes the coupling of two molecules. An oxidoreductase catalyzes oxidation reactions. A transferase catalyzes the transfer of groups from one substance to another. An isomerase catalyzes the interconversion of one isomer to another.

11. The answer is C *[II D, E 3].*
Nucleic acids are biopolymers consisting of long chains of nucleotides. Nucleotides contain a pentose monosaccharide as one of their three constituents. Ribonucleic acid (RNA) contains, as the name suggests, the monosaccharide ribose, whereas deoxyribonucleic acid (DNA) contains deoxyribose. The only difference between these two sugars is the absence of oxygen in the 2 position of the ribose ring. Glucose, also known as dextrose, is a hexose. Digitoxose is a deoxyhexose present in the digitalis glycosides. Sucrose and maltose are disaccharides.

12. The answer is D (II, III) *[I A 1, G 1, L 1].*
The overall solubility of the various classes of organic compounds illustrates a tendency for functional groups containing oxygen or nitrogen to demonstrate a degree of water solubility, whereas functional groups containing only carbon and hydrogen have very little water solubility. The phenolic and carboxylic groups both contain oxygen. In addition, they are acidic groups capable of undergoing ionization. Thus, compared to the ethyl group, they are more likely to increase the water solubility of benzene.

13–16. The answers are: 13-A (I) *[I L 1],* **14-B (III)** *[I L 2, 3, M 2, 3],* **15-E (all)** *[I D 4, L 4, M 4],* **16-C (I, II)** *[I A, E, F, L].*
Organic substances generally are nonpolar; thus, they usually are insoluble in water. Since water is a polar solvent, only polar organics are water soluble. The most common type of polar organic compound is a salt. Since the molecule depicted is a carboxylic acid, it reacts with a base to form a water-soluble salt.

The molecule contains both a simple ester and a carboxylic acid. Simple esters are susceptible to hydrolysis from moisture in the air but are not susceptible to oxidation. Carboxylic acids are not reduced easily.

The molecule, acetylsalicylic acid, contains an aromatic hydrocarbon nucleus (which can undergo ring hydroxylation), a simple acetate ester (which can undergo hydrolysis), and a free carboxyl group (which can undergo glucuronide conjugation as well as glycine conjugation).

Molecules that have poor in vitro stability are usually those that are susceptible to air oxidation and hydrolysis, or they may be light sensitive. Alcohols undergo oxidation but not without the presence of oxidizing agents. Also, they do not hydrolyze; thus, they are stable in air and moisture. In the body, there are several common metabolic pathways available for their biotransformation. Acids do not hydrolyze, nor are they susceptible to oxidation, thus, are stable in the presence of air and moisture; whereas in vivo, acids easily undergo several common metabolic reactions, particularly conjugation reactions. Alkyl halides are not susceptible to either oxidation or hydrolysis and do not undergo common metabolic reactions in the body. Thus, alkyl halides are equally stable in vitro and in vivo.

8
Immunology

Vincent C. LoPresti

I. IMMUNE SYSTEM PHYSIOLOGY

A. Immunogens, antigens, and haptens

1. **Immunogens** are chemical compounds that provoke a specific immune response.
2. **Antigens** are chemical compounds that are recognized by and eliminated by a specific immune response.
3. **Immunogens/antigens.** Often, compounds associated with or secreted by parasitic bacteria, protozoa, fungi, and viruses, and of molecular weights (mol wt) greater than 5000 daltons normally act as both immunogens and antigens.
   - **a.** Molecular complexity is as important as molecular weight in determining the status of a compound as an immunogen; thus, proteins, glycoproteins, lipoproteins, and nucleoproteins are the most potent immunogens/antigens.
   - **b.** Drugs of sufficient molecular weight (e.g., insulin) can act as immunogens/antigens. The cells of another individual, and the cells of one's own body (see III) can act as immunogens/antigens. Immunogens/antigens can be contacted environmentally (e.g., pollens).
4. **Haptens** are low molecular weight compounds that cannot act as immunogens without first chemically complexing to a larger molecule or cell surface. Once they have stimulated the immune system in this complex, such compounds can then act as antigens in the uncomplexed state (with certain exceptions).
   - **a.** Haptens can be compounds present in the environment (e.g., pentadecyl catechol of poison ivy).
   - **b.** Drugs of several types may act as haptens (e.g., penicillin).
5. For the remainder of this chapter, the term "antigen" is used to represent compounds and cells that are both immunogens and antigens.

B. Cells of the immune system

1. **B lymphocytes and T lymphocytes** are the primary response cells of specific immune responses. All B and T lymphocytes are antigen specific by virtue of having specific antigen receptors as part of their plasma membranes. For the remainder of this chapter, the terms **B cell** and **T cell** are used instead of B lymphocyte and T lymphocyte.
2. **Antigen receptors of B cells** are antibody molecules.
   - **a.** B cells have thousands of identical antibodies in their membranes that allow them to bind chemically to a small group of chemically related antigens. This defines the antigen specificity of each B cell. Different B cells have different antigen specificities (Figure 8-1). The primary function of B cells in immune responses is to recognize specific antigens and divide to form many new B cells and **plasma cells (antibody-forming cells),** which secrete free, soluble ("humoral") antibody molecules into extracellular fluids.
   - **b. Virgin B cells** are those that have never responded to an antigen since their release into the circulation from bone marrow. Their membrane antibodies are of the immunoglobulin M and D (IgM, IgD) classes (see I D).
   - **c. Memory B cells** are derived by cell division from another B cell that has responded to an antigen. Their membrane antibodies are of immunoglobulin classes A, E, or G (IgA, IgE, IgG) [see I D].

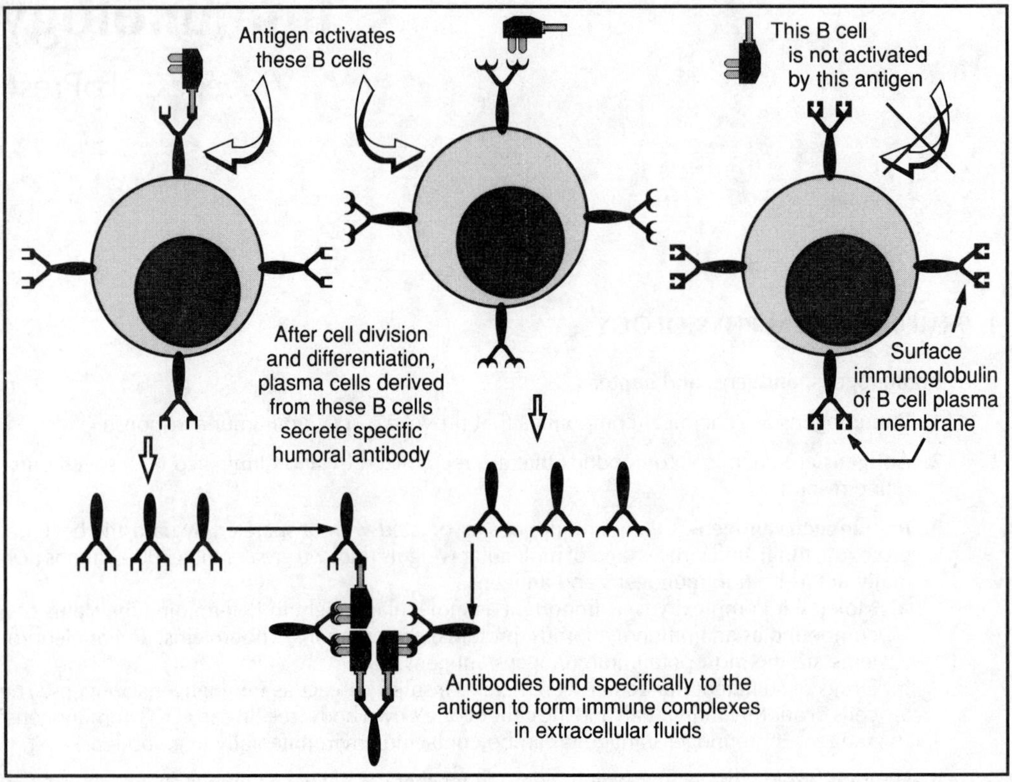
Antigen activates
these B cells
This B cell
is not activated
by this antigen
After cell division
and differentiation,
plasma cells derived
from these B cells
secrete specific
humoral antibody
Surface
immunoglobulin
of B cell plasma
membrane
Antibodies bind specifically to the
antigen to form immune complexes
in extracellular fluids

Figure 8-1. B cells: antigen specificity and activation.

3. Antigen receptors of T cells are composed of two membrane polypeptides (α and β) that define the antigen specificity of each T cell and several other polypeptides known as the **CD3 complex**. T cells are, thus, said to be **CD3$^+$**. Each T cell has thousands of identical antigen receptors in its membrane. Different T cells of different antigen specificities differ in the exact conformation of their antigen receptors.

a. Major histocompatibility complex (MHC) proteins. The antigen receptors of T cells do not chemically recognize antigens alone. Rather, they normally recognize **fragments of antigens (epitopes)** that are chemically combined with MHC proteins on the surface of other body cells (Figure 8-2). MHC proteins are divided into **two major classes**:

(1) Class I, which are present on the surfaces of almost all body cells

(2) Class II, which are present only on the surfaces of special **antigen presenting cells (APCs)**.

b. Thymus gland. T cells do not enter the circulation directly from bone marrow but rather must first enter the thymus gland to mature. Many T cells die in the thymus, particularly some of those that would respond against self-antigens.

(1) T cells that are released from the thymus into the circulation are **virgin T cells**.

(2) T cells that have originated by cell division from the responses of other T cells are **memory T cells**.

c. Glycoproteins. Most T cells can be classified by the presence of a membrane glycoprotein known as **CD4,** the **helper** or **T_H group,** or the presence of **CD8,** the **cytotoxic T lymphocyte (CTL) group**. There is also evidence for a group of **suppressor T cells** or **T_S,** also belonging to the CD8 group.

(1) T_H cells are primarily responsible for regulating the responses of B cells, CTL cells, macrophages, and other cells via the secretion of compounds known as **lymphokines**. CTL cells are primarily responsible for direct killing (cytotoxicity) of self-cells infected by viruses but also are lymphokine secretors. Lymphokines are small proteins that are usually secreted paracrinely.

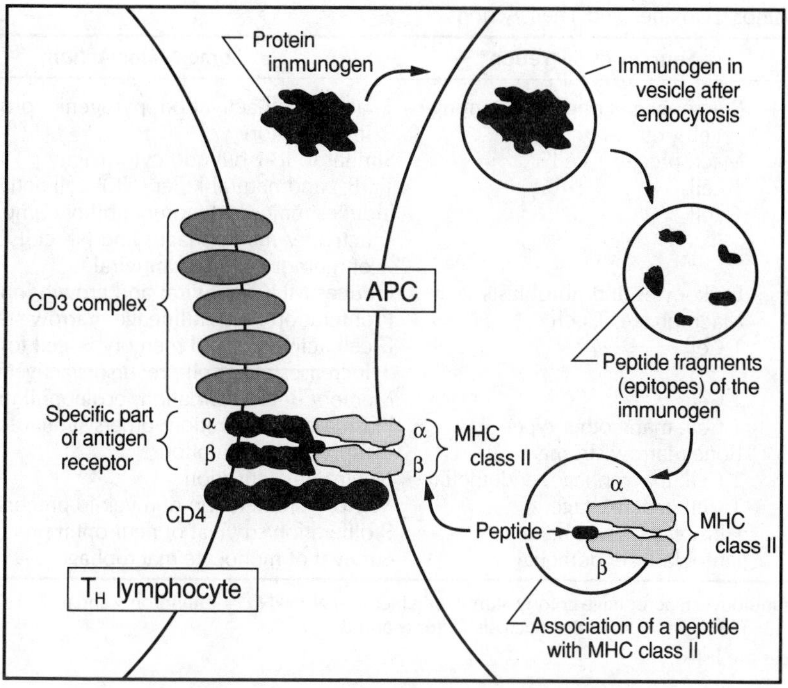

Figure 8-2. Helper T-cell antigen recognition.

(2) Lymphokines are part of a larger network of regulatory **cytokines,** which include secretions of other cell types in addition to those of lymphocytes. Table 8-1 summarizes the sources and actions of some important cytokines that regulate the immune system and inflammation.

4. Natural killer (NK) cells are large lymphocytes without a specific T- or B-cell antigen receptor but which possess cytotoxicity that appears to be similar to that of CTL.

5. Antigen presenting cells (APCs) are essential to most immune responses and define the sites at which immune responses usually originate.

a. The best understood APCs are the **fixed macrophages of lymph nodes, spleen,** and **other lymphoid tissue**. These cells begin most immune responses within these organs by presenting fragments of antigens (epitopes) bound to their surface MHC class II molecules to T_H (CD4) lymphocytes (see Figure 8-2) and by secreting cytokines as accessory signals.

b. Any body cell can serve as an APC for a subset of immune responses involving CTLs. Body cells can present fragments of antigens bound to their surface MHC class I molecules to CTL (CD8) lymphocytes.

c. Both T and B cells are continually circulated through the lymph nodes, spleen, and other lymphoid tissue, so that if their specific antigen is present, an immune response can begin.

6. Neutrophils, monocyte–macrophages, eosinophils, basophils, platelets, and **mast cells** serve a variety of functions that assist in eliminating antigens from the body. Their functions may be phagocytic, pro-inflammatory, cytotoxic, and regulatory.

C. Humoral immunity: primary and memory responses that produce antibodies

1. Overview. In most humoral immune responses, antigens are recognized by specific B cells and T_H cells. The T_H cells secrete cytokines, and B and T_H cells divide to increase their cell numbers. Non–antigen-specific B and T_H cells do not respond. Responding B cells produce both memory B cells and plasma cells (see Figure 8-1). In some humoral immune responses (e.g., to certain polysaccharide antigens), T_H cells are not involved (**T-independent responses**). B cells respond alone, producing only plasma cells that secrete IgM antibodies but no memory B cells.

Table 8-1. Major Cytokines and Their Actions

Cytokine	Sources of Secretion*	Some Major Actions
IL-1	Macrophage/antigen presenting cells, others	T- and B-cell activation, pyrogenic, pro-inflammatory
TNF α and β	Macrophage, T cell	Similar to IL-1 but add cytotoxicity
IL-2	T cell	T-, B-, and natural killer (NK)–cell activation
IFNγ	T cell	Induces major histocompatibility complex (MHC); activates macrophages and NK cells; formation of memory B cells; antiviral
IFN α and β	Leukocytes and fibroblasts	Induces MHC; antiviral and growth inhibition
IL-3	Macrophage, T cell	Proliferation of multilineage marrow stem cells
IL-4	T Cell	B-cell activation and memory B–cell formation; increases mast cell precursors/activates mast cells
IL-5	T Cell	Memory B–cell formation; eosinophil production
IL-6	T Cell, many other types	Plasma cell maturation; others similar to IL-1
IL-7	Bone marrow stroma	Lymphocyte maturation
IL-8	T Cell, macrophage, endothelial	Neutrophil activation
GM-CSF	T Cell, macrophage	Marrow proliferation of myeloid precursors
G-CSF	Fibroblasts, endothelial	Proliferation/survival of neutrophil precursors
M-CSF	Fibroblasts, endothelial	Survival of monocyte/macrophages

GM-CSF = granulocyte macrophage colony-stimulating factor; IFNγ, IFNα = interferon γ and α; IL-1 = interleukin-1, -2 through -8; TNFα, TNFβ = tumor necrosis factor α and β.

*Not all sources are listed.

2. **Primary immune response.** The first time a given antigen is encountered, only **virgin B cells** are present to respond to that antigen. These cells give rise to plasma cells that secrete IgM antibody, and memory cells that are committed to producing the other classes of antibody in later immune responses. Production of significant amounts of IgM antibodies does not occur until 7–10 days after the entry of antigen into the body. This is known as a primary immune response.

3. **Memory immune responses.** The second or subsequent encounter with the same or closely related antigen provokes responses by memory B cells and memory T_H cells. These responses are more rapid, since the numbers of antigen-specific B and T cells are greater in a memory immune response. Most antibody produced is IgG with smaller amounts of IgA and IgE. Production of significant amounts of antibodies occurs as rapidly as 2–3 days after the entry of antigen, and the absolute amount of antibody (measured in mg/dl of serum) is greater than in primary immune responses. The duration of memory varies for different antigens and probably for different individuals. Some, but not all, memory is lifelong.

4. **Major roles of antibodies**
   a. The first role is to **bind specifically to antigens to form antigen–antibody complexes (immune complexes)**.
   b. The second role is **to initiate other nonspecific mechanisms,** which eliminate antigens and antigen–antibody complexes from body fluids, prevent antigens from infecting or binding to cells, or provoke inflammation. These mechanisms depend upon the class of antibody involved.

D. Immunoglobulins: antigen binding and class-specific functions. The terms antibody and immunoglobulin can be used interchangeably.

1. **Structure.** The standard immunoglobulin unit is composed of four polypeptide chains: two identical light polypeptide chains, and two identical heavy polypeptide chains; thus, the structure is represented as H_2L_2. The two light chains and the two heavy chains can each be divided into a **C-terminal constant region** and an **N-terminal variable region** of amino acids.

2. **Class.** There are five general heavy-chain, constant region amino acid sequences. These determine the **five general classes of immunoglobulins: IgM, IgG, IgE, IgA,** and **IgD**. Within some classes, there are variants of the heavy-chain sequence that yield subclasses: IgM1, IgM2, IgG1 through 4, IgA1 and IgA2. The class of an immunoglobulin defines its nonspecific antigen elimination or inflammatory function. These functions are activated only after the formation of immune complexes, not in unbound antibodies.

a. **IgM** is the first immunoglobulin secreted during primary responses and plays a minor role during memory responses. It does not leave the blood in significant amounts due to its very large size (mol wt 900,000 daltons). It comprises about 20% of the adult serum immunoglobulin. Its class function is **to activate the complement system** (see I E). Its serum half-life is 9–11 days.

b. **IgG** is the predominant immunoglobulin secreted during memory responses and may also be secreted late during a primary response. It can diffuse from blood into other extracellular fluids, particularly in inflamed microvasculature, and crosses the placenta to enter the fetal circulation. It comprises about 70% of the adult serum immunoglobulin. Its class functions are **to opsonize antigens for phagocytosis** and **to activate the complement system**. Its serum half-life is 25–35 days.

c. **IgE** is secreted during memory responses and may also be secreted late during a primary response. It normally comprises less than 1% of serum immunoglobulin. Its class function is **to bind to IgE receptors located particularly on cell surfaces of blood basophils and connective tissue mast cells** to trigger the secretion of inflammatory mediators from these cells in the presence of specific antigens. Its serum half-life is 2–3 days, but its mast cell–bound half-life is several months.

d. **IgA** is secreted during memory responses and may also be secreted late during a primary response. It comprises 10% of serum immunoglobulin. Its class function is mainly **to be secreted across mucosal surfaces into gastrointestinal, respiratory, lacrimal, mammary, and genitourinary secretions, where it protects mucosal colonization** by bacteria and other microorganisms. Its serum half-life is about 5 days.

e. **IgD** comprises less than 1% of serum immunoglobulin and is not known to have a function as a secreted immunoglobulin.

3. **Specificity.** The specificity of each immunoglobulin for antigen-binding resides in the two identical antigen-binding sites, each formed by the combination of the variable regions of heavy and light chains. Secreted IgM antibodies have 10 identical antigen-binding sites via the combination of five H_2L_2 units with a "joining" polypeptide chain to form a pentamer. Likewise, IgA most commonly exists as a dimer with four binding sites.

4. **Quantitation of immunoglobulin—antigen-binding and cross-reactivity.** The immune system has the capacity to form between 10^8 and 10^{11} different specificities of immunoglobulin.

   a. Each immunoglobulin specificity can bind to several different, but structurally related, antigens. This illustrates the phenomenon of cross-reactivity of a single antibody for multiple antigens. Each immunoglobulin–antigen interaction is quantitated by its **association constant (K_a)**.

   b. Cross-reactivity may also derive from the sharing of some, but not all, antigens by two different strains of bacteria, virus, or other microorganism.

   c. Since each microorganism possesses several antigens, each elicits the production of multiple antibody specificities by the immune system. This combination of antibodies is known as a **polyclonal antiserum** and also defines the serotype of the immunizing organism.

5. **Fragments of immunoglobulin for clinical use.** Immunoglobulins can be enzymatically cleaved into fragments [e.g., **Fab** and **F(ab′)$_2$** (antigen-binding fragments), **Fc** (crystallizable fragment), **Fv** (variable region fragment)]. Fab and F(ab′)$_2$ fragments are clinically useful because they retain antigen specificity but not class-specific (e.g., inflammatory) functions and are more readily excreted renally. Conversely, this can also limit their effectiveness.

E. Antigen elimination and acute inflammatory mechanisms of humoral immunity

1. **Opsonization** is the preparation of any extracellular fluid antigen for phagocytosis via the formation of immune complexes. Neutrophils and monocyte–macrophages have a variety of receptors for the constant region of IgG antibodies, which bind immune complexes when the complexes are sufficiently large. This binding triggers phagocytosis of the immune complex and activates the phagocyte's metabolism, shifting it toward the production of bactericidal oxygen radicals (e.g., superoxide anion, hydrogen peroxide).

2. **Complement** is a group of about 20 serum proteins that, when activated, form a proteolytic cascade similar to the clotting and fibrinolytic sequences. Of these, certain proteins are activation inhibitors.

   a. In the **classic activation pathway,** immune complexes of IgM or IgG antibodies bind subunits of complement component 1 (C1) and trigger an initial series of proteolytic cleavages.

b. In the **alternative activation pathway,** the cell walls of certain microorganisms (e.g., gram-negative bacteria) trigger a similar sequence of cleavages that overcome normal inhibitory controls.
c. Certain complement proteins provide opsonization in addition to that provided by IgG in immune complexes.
d. Pro-inflammatory fragments of certain complement proteins act both by **direct activity on microvasculature,** promoting arteriole dilation and increased vascular permeability, and by triggering the release of histamine and other pro-inflammatory mediators from mast cells and basophils.
e. A complex of complement proteins known as the **membrane attack complex (MAC)** can insert into any lipid bilayer membrane, forming a large channel through which ions and water may diffuse. Many bacteria, enveloped viruses, and some human or mammalian cells are subject to this osmotic lysis.

3. Circulating basophils and connective tissue mast cells are mainly pro-inflammatory cells, which rapidly initiate acute inflammation. Triggers of secretion include mechanical and thermal trauma and the immunologic triggers, complement and IgE.
a. IgE antibodies, regardless of antigen specificity, equilibrate between serum and binding noncovalently to high affinity IgE receptors on mast cell and basophil surfaces. This "arms" the mast cells and basophils, but the triggering of secretion requires that antigen bind to and cross-link antigen-specific IgE molecules already affixed to their receptors.
b. Mast cells and basophils, when triggered, immediately secrete the contents of their storage granules, including histamine, proteases, and chemotactic proteins for neutrophils and eosinophils. In addition, activation of phospholipase A_2 releases arachidonic acid from membrane phospholipids and results in the synthesis of various leukotrienes, prostaglandins, and thromboxanes. The primary effects of these mediators are:
(1) Arteriole dilation
(2) Increased vascular permeability
(3) Contraction of respiratory and gastrointestinal smooth muscle
(4) Neutrophil and eosinophil chemotaxis

4. The purpose of acute inflammation is the increased ease of movement of crucial components of the blood into the tissues, including phagocytes, particularly neutrophils, IgG antibodies, complement, clotting proteins, and kinins. The adaptive result is the isolation and removal of invading microorganisms and necrotic tissues, followed by tissue repair and regeneration.

F. Cell-mediated immunity responses are considered to be those in which **antibody is not involved in the elimination of antigen.**

1. Nonviral intracellular parasites of monocyte–macrophages such as *Mycobacteria, Listeria,* and certain protozoa are primarily eliminated by T-cell–macrophage immunity. $CD4^+$ T cells recognize infected macrophages and secrete lymphokines, particularly interferon γ (IFNγ). These lymphokines activate macrophages to an even greater production of bactericidal oxygen radicals (e.g., superoxide anion, hydrogen peroxide) and enable them to kill intracellular parasites.

2. Viruses must be eliminated from both extracellular sites and from infected cells.
a. Antibodies opsonize virus particles in blood and tissue fluids for phagocytosis, but antibodies are generally ineffective against viral-infected cells.
b. CTL cells can recognize viral-infected cells and directly kill them in an antigen-specific manner, secreting lymphokines such as tumor necrosis factor α and β (TNFα, TNFβ). Often, the cells are killed before infectious virus particles can be assembled. When killed cells release infectious viral particles, these may be opsonized by antibody. Cell-mediated immunity and humoral immunity must, therefore, function in concert for optimal antiviral defenses.
c. NK cells are believed to kill viral-infected (and tumor) cells in a manner that is not antigen specific.
d. IFNγ, secreted by CTL, NK, and T_H cells, and **IFNα** and **IFNβ,** secreted by macrophages and other cells, provide additional antiviral immunity by binding to receptors on other cells and inducing synthesis of kinases and endonucleases (i.e., antiviral proteins) that inhibit viral and cellular growth. Interferons also up-regulate MHC proteins, which make viral-infected cells more "visible" to CTL cells.

II. HYPERSENSITIVITY REACTIONS describe **exaggerated, inappropriate,** or **overly prolonged immune responses, leading to tissue damage** (Figure 8-3). Five types of hypersensitivity reactions are recognized, primarily on the basis of mechanisms of pathogenesis. Note that a diverse array of etiologies may be included within each type. **Allergens** are broadly defined as antigens or haptens that induce hypersensitivity reactions.

A. IgE-mediated type I hypersensitivity reaction

1. **Pathogenesis** for a type I hypersensitivity reaction is due to **inappropriate hypersecretion of IgE** to specific allergens, plus auxiliary factors such as increased mucosal permeability to allergens (e.g., SO_2, NO_x, diesel fumes). The **propensity to hypersecrete IgE is inheritable;** a

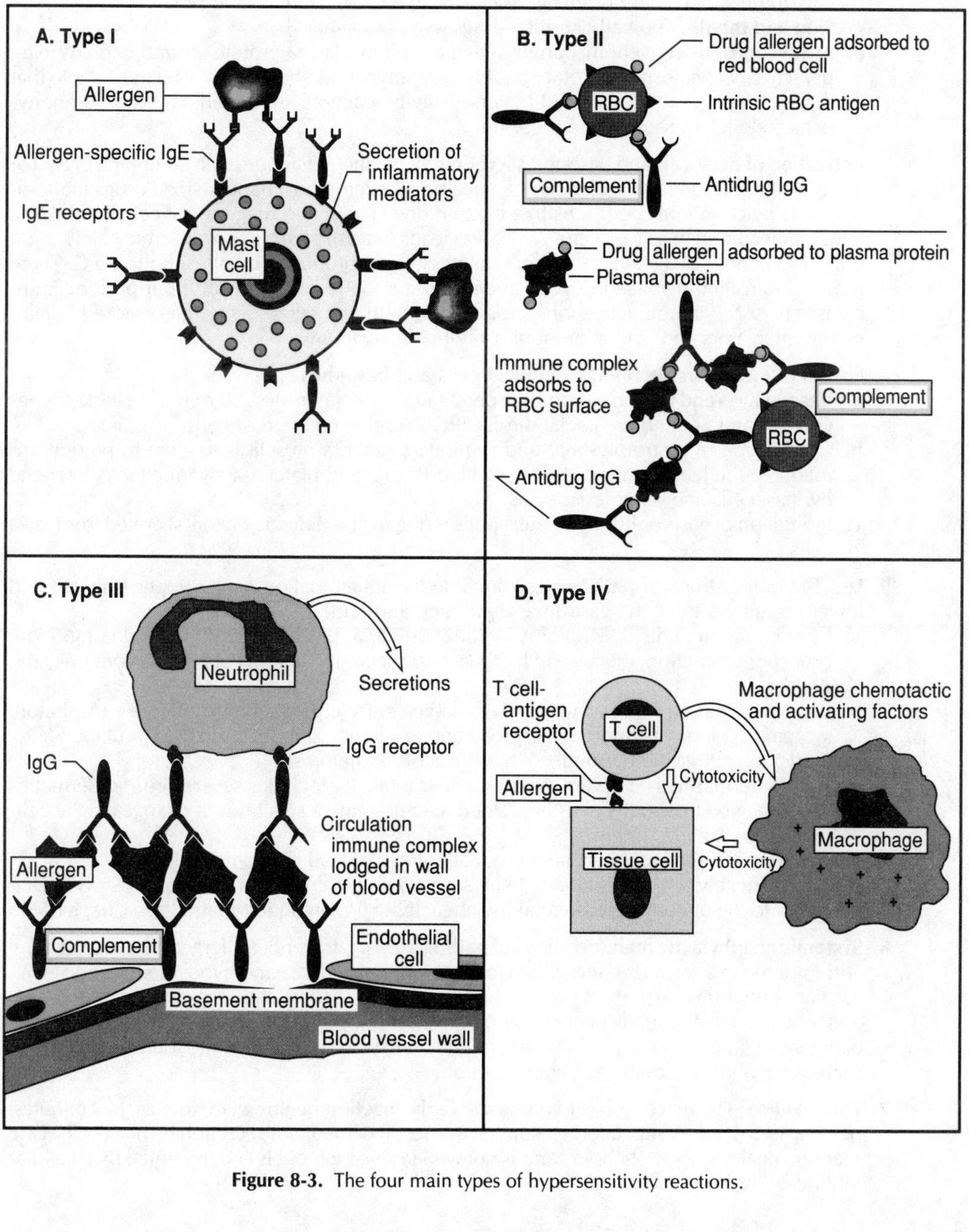

Figure 8-3. The four main types of hypersensitivity reactions.

child's probability of being a hypersecretor is 50% with one hypersecretor parent, and 75% with two such parents. Such individuals are said to be "atopic."

a. IgE is usually produced locally upon nonsystemic exposure to an antigen.
   (1) In **normosecretors** (1–10 μg/dl), arming of local mast cells occurs (see I).
   (2) In **hypersecretors** (typically 100 μg–1 mg/dl), there is a variable amount of IgE spillover, arming basophils and nonlocal mast cells, and causing a greater than normal occupancy of mast cell and basophil IgE receptors by IgE.
b. Because there is a lag period for IgE synthesis and cell arming, a type I reaction does not usually manifest upon first (or first seasonal) exposure to a given allergen.

2. **Common allergens**
   a. **Respiratory.** Pollens of various plants (e.g., ragweed, grasses, trees), fungi, animal fur, carpet mites, and other shed allergens
   b. **Gastrointestinal.** Dairy products, shellfish, soybeans, peanuts, and others
   c. **Skin and mouth.** Topically applied drugs (e.g., procaine)
   d. **Intravenous.** Insect venoms, drugs acting as cell or plasma protein–bound haptens (e.g., penicillin, cephalosporins, other antibiotics, polypeptide hormones, vaccines). Note that these may provoke type II or III hypersensitivity reactions in individuals who do not hypersecrete IgE in response to these drugs.

3. **Activation of mast cell and basophil secretion** by an allergen requires cross-linking of two or more receptor-bound IgE molecules by specific allergen. Thus, hapten-sized drugs that provoke this reaction must both sensitize the immune system and trigger mast cells bound to a larger molecule such as a protein. Activation leads to an increase in cytoplasmic calcium ion (Ca^{2+}), probably as a result of the second messengers produced by phospholipase C. There is also a transient increase in cyclic adenosine monophosphate (cAMP), but prolonged increases in cAMP inhibit activation of mast cells. Both immediate secretion of stored inflammatory mediators and activation of phospholipase A_2 follow.

4. **Effects of mediators secreted from mast cells and basophils**
   a. Vasodilation and increased capillary permeability occur due to histamine; the leukotrienes C4, D4, and E4; and prostaglandin D_2 (PGD_2) secreted by mast cells.
   b. Constriction of gastrointestinal and respiratory smooth muscle is thought to be due primarily to the leukotrienes C4, D4, and E4; PGD_2; and platelet-activating factor secreted by mast cells and other leukocytes.
   c. Infiltration of eosinophils and neutrophils is due to chemotactic factors secreted from mast cells.

5. **Local manifestations of pathogenesis** include the inflammation of the upper (rhinitis) and lower respiratory tract, the gastrointestinal tract, and skin.
   a. Most common clinical symptoms include, urticaria, pruritus (itching), nasal congestion, bronchoconstriction, mucus and lacrimal hypersecretion, laryngeal edema, vomiting, and diarrhea.
   b. Symptoms may be confined to portal of allergen entry (e.g., respiratory allergen: respiratory symptoms) or may be more widespread due to allergen spillover into the circulation (e.g., food allergen: gastrointestinal, skin, respiratory symptoms).
   c. **Atopic dermatitis** is a severe syndrome that typically includes severe pruritic dermatitis accompanied by rhinitis or asthma, food allergies, and a spectrum of changes in the cell-mediated immune system.
   d. In rare cases, the local introduction of allergen can lead to anaphylaxis.
   e. Approximately 50% of asthmatics hypersecrete IgE, and this is probably contributory but ancillary to the underlying bronchial hyperreactivity present in asthmatics (see Chapter 50).

6. **Systemic anaphylactic manifestations of pathogenesis.** Intravenous allergen (e.g., bee venom) administered to a sensitized individual leads to systemic edema and hypovolemic shock with cardiac arrhythmia, asphyxiation due to bronchoconstriction and mucous hypersecretion, and urticaria. Death usually occurs due to asphyxiation. In some individuals, intravenous drug allergens (e.g., penicillin) provoke only mild local symptoms, indicating a probable continuum of IgE normosecretion to hypersecretion.

7. **Time course.** The reaction has two phases: **Early reaction** begins as rapidly as 1–2 minutes, peaking in 1–2 hours after allergen contact as a result of mediator secretion by mast cells. **Late reaction** peaks at about 24 hours and is not well understood but is accompanied by a cellular infiltrate.

8. **Diagnosis.** Scratch tests inject a variety of allergens intradermally to screen for the presence of a wheal and flare (i.e., edema, erythema) response in the skin. The **radioallergosorbent (RAST)** and **radioimmunosorbent (RIST) assays** are radiolabeled tests that detect serum IgE concentrations. The results of these tests do not always agree nor do they always agree with the clinical manifestations.

9. **Prophylaxis**
   a. Identification and avoidance of allergens is the most important prophylactic measure.
   b. **Hyposensitization** is performed by administering increasing weekly doses of allergen injected subcutaneously and later by monthly maintenance injections. The best possible effects of the procedure are to elicit decreased allergen-specific IgE synthesis and increased allergen-specific IgG synthesis. IgG can bind entering allergen and prevent it from binding to basophil-bound IgE.
   c. Cromolyn sodium (cromoglycate) is a locally administered inhibitor of mast cell activation. Glucocorticoids block the late phase of the response but have less effect on the early phase.

10. **Therapy**
   a. **Competitive H_1 antagonists** of histamine are useful in local forms but do not completely reverse inflammation, since histamine is not the only inflammatory mediator. They have little effect in anaphylaxis. A variety of baths, creams, and corticosteroid ointments may be used in dermatitis.
   b. **Epinephrine** is the agent of choice to reverse anaphylaxis via its α- and β-agonist effects, and patients with systemic allergies are given the epinephrine self-administration kits. **β_2 agonists,** such as albuterol, are useful to promote bronchodilation, and **α_1 agonists,** such as phenylpropanolamine, diminish nasal congestion.

B. **Non–IgE-mediated type I hypersensitivity reactions.** These reactions are probably of several different types, mostly poorly understood and sometimes referred to as **anaphylactoid reactions**. The following factors may both contribute to non–IgE-mediated type I reactions and may exacerbate IgE-mediated type I reactions:

1. Respiratory β_2 receptor unresponsiveness, leading to a diminished bronchodilatory influence of the sympathetic nervous system.

2. Hyperreactivity of mast cells via H_2 receptor unresponsiveness, leading to a diminished negative feedback by histamine on the activation of mast cells

C. **Type II hypersensitivity reactions**

1. **Pathogenesis.** Antibody-mediated cytotoxicity occurs via production of IgM or IgG, which forms immune complexes that bind to their specific allergens located on cell surfaces.
   a. These allergens may be intrinsic cell surface components or extrinsic compounds adsorbed to the cell surface.
   b. Cytotoxicity may result from the activation of complement, phagocytosis of the IgG/IgM–opsonized cell, or both.
   c. A third cytotoxic mechanism involves direct killing of antibody-coated cells by macrophages, eosinophils, or NK cells and is known as antibody-dependent, cell-mediated cytotoxicity.
   d. Type II reactions can become anaphylactic if enough complement is activated, but usually they do not.

2. **Common allergens.** The etiologies of these subtypes of type II reactions are very diverse, and it is only the pathogenic mechanism that is common to all.
   a. Foreign blood cell surface antigens (allergens) in **transfusion mismatches** or in **Rh disease**
   b. **Drug allergens** (or drug metabolite allergens) acting as haptens, which are the **leading cause of hemolytic anemia**
      (1) These may directly adsorb to blood cell surfaces and be specifically bound by antibodies (e.g., penicillins, cephalosporins, quinidine, phenacetin).
      (2) Alternatively, they may form serum phase immune complexes, which adsorb nonspecifically to blood cell surfaces as "innocent bystanders" (e.g., rifampin, sulfonamides, chlorpromazine).
   c. **Certain autoimmunities,** where the allergens are self-antigens (e.g., Hashimoto's thyroiditis, myasthenia gravis, autoimmune thrombocytopenia purpura, autoimmune hemolytic anemia) [see III]. Autoimmune hemolytic anemia may sometimes be associated with the administration of α-methyldopa, resulting in autoantibodies against the red blood cell surface.
   d. **Hyperacute rejection** of renal cardiac grafts (see V)

3. **Chemical mediators.** Complement proteins produce cytotoxicity and inflammation and stimulate basophil secretions, which enhance inflammation.
4. **Clinical symptoms** depend upon the subtype (see II C 2). Hemolytic anemia and thrombocytopenia are predominant symptoms of pathologies involving blood cells. In autoimmune varieties, symptoms depend upon the cell type damaged by cytotoxicity. In hyperacute graft rejection, the transplanted tissue never successfully perfuses due to antibody-mediated cytotoxicity to its vasculature.
5. **Time course**
   a. If it is the first sensitization to a drug allergen, blood cell lysis and inflammation begin about 7–10 days after the initiation of drug therapy. Second exposure to the drug usually provokes symptoms within 3 days.
   b. **Transfusion mismatch.** Hemolysis begins in 1–2 hours after transfusion with peak effects at about 12 hours.
   c. **Rh disease** is not usually found in the first RhD^+ pregnancy of an RhD^- mother. In second and subsequent pregnancies, maternal IgG is produced usually upon sensitization of the mother to the RhD antigen by transplacental fetal red blood cells toward the end of the third trimester. Maternal anti-RhD IgG crosses the placenta, binds to fetal red blood cells, and activates the fetal complement system prenatally, leading to perinatal hemolytic anemia.
6. **Prophylaxis and therapy.** In drug-induced hypersensitivity reactions, withdrawing the drug usually reverses the pathology. Preventing recontact is clearly the best prophylaxis. In Rh disease, anti-RhD IgG is administered to the Rh^- mother within 72 hours postpartum for each Rh^+ delivery. The simplest mechanism of action is that this passive immunization (see VI B) binds fetal red blood cells in the maternal circulation and prevents sensitization of the maternal immune system.

D. **Type III hypersensitivity reactions** involve the persistence of immune complexes in the circulation or at local tissue sites as a result of a failure to be removed subsequent to the formation of specific antibodies. The etiologies of the subtypes of type III are very diverse, and it is only the pathogenic mechanism that is common to all.

1. **Pathogenesis.** Immune complexes activate complement, provoking inflammation, and induce positive chemotaxis in neutrophils. Persistence of immune complexes may be a result of:
   a. An extremely **high concentration of antigen,** leading to a disparity in the molar ratio of antigen to antibody. Hyposecretion of antibodies can also produce this type.
   b. **Chronic formation of immune complexes** in the circulation due to an underlying pathology, overloading the capacity of phagocytic cells to remove them rapidly
   c. Various other factors leading to the formation of insoluble immune complexes, which precipitate intravascularly or on basement membranes
2. **Common allergens**
   a. **Self-antigens in most nonorgan-specific** (rheumatologic) **autoimmune pathologies,** such as systemic lupus erythematosus or rheumatoid arthritis
   b. **Bacterial, protozoan, antigens in persistent or chronic infections** and transiently in the initial stages of viremia of certain viral infections [e.g., prodrome of hepatitis B virus (HBV) infection]
   c. **Drugs,** such as penicillin, sulfonamides, thiouracil, hydantoins, and streptomycin
   d. **Serum sickness.** Passive immunization with antisera from other species (e.g., horse)
   e. **Fungal and bacterial spores** in the local respiratory form of the pathology
3. **Chemical mediators. Complement proteins** produce inflammation and **stimulate mast cell and basophil secretions,** which enhance inflammation. The increased vascular permeability allows immune complexes both to leave the circulation and to affix to the basement membrane, underlying the endothelial lining of blood vessels. The kidney glomerulus and certain small arteries are particularly susceptible. Complement and mast cell proteins attract neutrophils, which in phagocytosing immune complexes release enzymes that damage local tissue and further intensify inflammation. Platelets aggregate, and microthrombi may form.
4. **Clinical symptoms** depend upon the severity and the systemic or local nature of immune complex persistence and deposition.
   a. The first symptoms of systemic pathology are lymphadenopathy, splenomegaly, fever, and skin rash, which are common in drug-induced and viremia-induced type III reactions.

b. More serious symptoms include vasculitis and glomerulonephritis, both of which may become necrotizing [common additional consequences of systemic lupus erythematosus (SLE)]. Arthralgia and arthritis may occur in both systemic and local varieties.
c. The most common local varieties are hypersensitivity pneumonitis to inhaled allergens of fungi and bacteria to which the patient may be occupationally exposed (e.g., mouldy hay in **farmer's lung**) or through exposure to spores borne in aerosol microdroplets from dirty ultrasonic humidifiers (e.g., **humidifier lung**). Symptoms include:
(1) Nasal congestion and bronchoconstriction
(2) Joint pain and inflammation of rheumatoid arthritis, which is due to joint-localized immune complexes involving rheumatoid factor and neutrophil phagocytosis (see Chapter 51).

5. **Time course**
a. **Systemic.** For patients with no prior exposure, symptoms may appear from 1–2 weeks (possibly longer) after exposure to allergen. For patients with preexisting antibodies, symptoms may appear within several hours to a day after exposure. Severe symptoms, such as glomerulonephritis, are usually delayed by about 2 weeks.
b. **Local.** In hypersensitivity pneumonitis, symptoms commonly appear 6–8 hours after exposure in a patient with preexisting antibodies.

6. **Prophylaxis and therapy.** In drug-induced varieties, **withdrawing the drug** usually reverses the pathology. Therapies may include antihistamines or corticosteroids. Transient infectious forms resolve spontaneously as complexes are removed by phagocytes.

E. Type IV hypersensitivity reactions

1. **Pathogenesis.** Among the situations classified as type IV reactions are prolonged inappropriate and appropriate immune responses. The common factor is the mediation of inflammation and tissue damage by antigen-specific T cells, usually in collaboration with activated macrophages. T cells may be of the helper (CD4) or cytotoxic (CD8) category, or both. These cells infiltrate tissues, producing cytotoxicity and tissue architecture disruption that is independent of antibody.
a. **Reactions to infections** entail a T-cell response against particular intracellular bacterial and protozoan parasites (e.g., *Mycobacteria*) and against the intracellular phases of viral infection. Significant tissue damage occurs when the response becomes ineffective and prolonged, ultimately leading to the formation of granulomas.
b. **Contact dermatitis** is an inappropriate skin inflammation against haptens, such as the pentadecyl catechols of poison ivy, which bind to epidermal cell surfaces, eliciting a T-cell response.
c. **Tuberculin reaction** is an appropriate dermal skin inflammation that is elicited by intradermal puncture with microorganismal allergens, indicating a state of either active T-cell immunity or T-cell memory to the organism in question. This form of type IV reaction is a convenient test for the status of an individual's T-cell immunity, the absence of an expected response indicating a state of anergy (unresponsiveness).
d. **Acute graft rejection** is an appropriate, albeit undesirable, T-cell response to a therapeutic graft of tissue from another individual.

2. **Common allergens**
a. **Infectious allergens.** *Mycobacterium tuberculosis, M. leprae, Listeria monocytogenes,* trypanosomes, and viruses
b. **Contact dermatitis.** Pentadecyl catechols from poison ivy, poison oak, chromates, nickel ions (leached from some jewelry clasps), acrylates, hair dyes containing *p*-phenylene diamine, and certain antibiotic ointments (e.g., topical neomycin)
c. **Tuberculin.** Skin testing with purified protein derivative (PPD) or tuberculin (Mantoux reaction), *Candida,* mumps, and other microorganismal antigens
d. **Grafted tissue.** Renal, cardiac, or other

3. **Chemical mediators** are thought to be most important in type IV pathogenesis: Cytokines of activated T cells attract and activate monocyte/macrophages to tissue sites where the pathogen is localized, such as the epidermis (in contact sensitivity), the dermis (in a tuberculin reaction), or to the site of a graft. Cytotoxicity can occur due to either CTL or macrophage secretions such as TNF. Macrophages also secrete inflammatory cytokines.

4. **Clinical symptoms** depend upon the subtype.
a. Skin rashes in measles infections and lesions of herpes simplex virus (HSV) infections are

due to CTL cytotoxicity to viral infected cells. Granulomas are local aggregations composed of T cells, monocyte/macrophages, and giant/epithelioid cells thought to derive from the fusion of activated macrophages. They occur around sites of chronic infectious organisms, such as the lungs in tuberculosis.

b. In contact sensitivity, cellular infiltration of the epidermis produces microvesicle formation with spongiosis.

c. Tuberculin tests are characterized by erythema and induration due to cellular infiltration of the dermis but no epidermal spongiosis.

d. Acute graft rejection shows perivascular infiltration by mononuclear cells with edema and necrosis of transplanted tissue.

5. Time course

a. Granulomas may form at various times after the onset of a chronic immune response but are generally delayed by 2 weeks.

b. Contact sensitivity may not manifest upon first transient exposure, but the onset of skin inflammation occurs within 12–24 hours and peaks within 24–48 hours of exposure. Susceptibility and severity varies widely. The same time course applies to tuberculin type reactions, often known as **delayed cutaneous hypersensitivity testing**.

c. Acute graft rejection usually commences 7–10 days after transplantation (see V).

6. Prophylaxis and therapy. Individual infectious pathologies are treated, depending upon the specific organism involved. Identification and avoidance of allergen is important in contact sensitivity dermatitis. This condition is often treated with topical corticosteroid ointments, which suppress T-cell and macrophage functions. Patients with widespread or unusually severe cases may require systemic corticosteroid treatment.

F. Type V hypersensitivity (antibody-mediated, hyperstimulatory) reactions represent situations in which **antireceptor antibodies act as agonists of normal ligands,** thereby activating receptor signaling. The best example is the antithyrotropin (anti-TSH) receptor antibody, which signals hypersecretion of thyroid hormone in **Graves' disease**.

III. AUTOIMMUNITY is a tissue-damaging immune response directed specifically and inappropriately against one or more self-antigens.

A. Etiology. The etiologies of "autoreactive" immune responses are not generally known and are likely to involve several different deregulations in the network of controls that normally prevent them. Aberration in normal regulation by CD4 T-helper and CD8 T-suppressor cells are most often cited as probable factors in etiology.

B. Epidemiology

1. Familial clustering is evident for many, if not most pathologies, representing a complex inherited predisposition toward development of autoimmunity. In some cases, this is associated with particular MHC types (e.g., the strong association of rheumatoid arthritis with the MHC class II type DR4).

2. For the most part, these pathologies are more common among women. The female:male incidence ratio is approximately 2:1 for myasthenia gravis and 10:1 for SLE. A few pathologies are more prevalent in males (e.g., Goodpasture syndrome).

C. Pathogenesis

1. Overview. In a given autoimmune pathology, the primary pathogenic mechanism may be mediated by antibodies (humoral) with or without a contribution by complement, may be primarily cell-mediated, or may involve both humoral and cell-mediated damage. Alternate exacerbation and remission of pathogenesis is a common feature of many of these pathologies.

2. Environmental factors are known to trigger pathogenesis, but specific factors have been identified in only a few types. These include associations between *Streptococcus* group A pharyngitis and rheumatic fever, exposure to organic solvents and Goodpasture syndrome, and ultraviolet radiation and SLE. In each case, environmental factors probably act against the background of genetic predisposition.

3. Organ-specific or non–organ-specific pathologies

a. Organ-specific pathologies (e.g., antithyroid autoimmunity). The immune response is limited to and directed specifically against self-antigens in one organ. Lesions and clinical symptoms are limited primarily to those arising from abnormal physiology of that organ. Cellular damage often arises via antibody and complement-mediated cytotoxicity (type II pathogenic mechanism) and sometimes via cell-mediated cytotoxicity (type IV pathogenic mechanism).

b. Non–organ-specific pathologies (e.g., SLE)

(1) These pathologies are also referred to as immunologic connective tissue, collagen vascular, or rheumatologic disorders. Autoantibodies are formed against self-antigens common to many or all tissues, particularly those located in the nuclei of cells and containing DNA or RNA (**antinuclear antibodies**). Pathologic changes occur systemically, primarily in connective tissues, and are at least partly due to the pathogenic mechanisms of type III hypersensitivity reactions (see II D). Clinical symptoms are observed in blood vessels, kidney glomerulus, skin, joints, serous membranes, and also may involve blood cells and plasma proteins.

(2) The non–organ-specific pathologies are sometimes difficult to distinguish from one another due to the similarities in autoantigens and pathogenesis. For example, virtually all SLE patients have circulating antinuclear antibodies, but these occur in about 50%–65% of patients with Sjögren syndrome and rheumatoid arthritis and a small percentage of clinically normal individuals as well. By contrast, rheumatoid factor (anti-IgG) is observed in 75%–90% of patients with Sjögren syndrome and rheumatoid arthritis but also in about 35% of patients with SLE. The synovitis of rheumatoid arthritis is often a clinical finding in SLE, and the vasculitis of SLE is found in some patients with rheumatoid arthritis (see Chapter 51).

D. Organ-specific autoimmunities

1. Rheumatic fever is not technically an autoimmune response, since antibodies are produced against group A streptococci and cross-react with cardiac muscle fibers that are damaged by complement. Increased risk is thought to be a function of strong immune responders to streptococcal M antigen.

2. Antithyroid autoimmunities (see Chapter 55). Aspects of several subtypes may occur in the same patient. Increased risk is associated with MHC class II types DR3 and DR5.

a. Primary autoimmune myxedema. Antibodies against the thyroid-stimulating hormone (TSH) receptor on thyroid follicle cells act as antagonists to the stimulation of growth of the follicle cells normally provoked by TSH. The result is thyroid atrophy with hypothyroidism.

b. Hashimoto's thyroiditis. Antibodies against thyroid peroxidase on follicle cells provoke cytotoxicity and inflammation via the activation of complement. Antibodies against thyroglobulin (colloid) itself also may be present. Cell-mediated immunity may account for some of the cytotoxic damage. The result is hypothyroidism that is treated with synthetic thyroid hormone.

c. Graves' disease. Antibodies act as agonists of TSH, binding to the TSH receptor and stimulating hypersecretion of thyroid hormone [thyroid-stimulating immunoglobulins (TSI)]. The result is hyperthyroidism treated by antithyroid drugs, such as propylthiouracil, or by thyroid ablation via surgery or radiation.

3. Myasthenia gravis

a. Pathogenesis. Antibodies against the nicotinic acetylcholine receptor on skeletal muscle plasma membrane at neuromuscular junctions act as competitive antagonists of **acetylcholine** binding. This provokes weakness and fatigue in skeletal muscles. In addition to this direct blockage of neuromuscular transmission, down-regulation of receptors and complement damage to muscle fibers also commonly occur. Much of the morbidity and mortality is a result of swallowing and respiratory muscle dysfunction. This may be provoked in some patients by penicillamine therapy. Increased risk is associated with MHC class I type B8.

b. Therapy. Anticholinesterase therapy (e.g., neostigmine) is used to increase acetylcholine synaptic concentrations (preservation of endogenous acetylcholine). Immunosuppression via corticosteroids is used in severe cases, and plasmapheresis to remove autoreactive antibodies from the blood also can be helpful. Thymectomy is beneficial in many patients.

4. Autoimmune pernicious anemia

a. Pathogenesis. Most commonly antibodies against intrinsic factor are secreted into the stomach lumen, where they inhibit the association of intrinsic factor with vitamin B_{12}. Absorption of vitamin B_{12} is diminished. It also can result from antibodies against gastrin receptors on parietal cells of stomach mucosa, which block stimulation of these cells by gastrin and diminish their secretion of intrinsic factor.

b. Therapy is via intramuscular injection of cyanocobalamin or orally administered concentrated intrinsic factor preparations.

5. Goodpasture syndrome

a. Pathogenesis. Antibodies against **glomerular capillary basement membrane (GBM)** activate complement and neutrophil-mediated damage. This leads to glomerulonephritis with rapid deterioration of renal function. These antibodies cross-react with pulmonary capillary basement membrane, producing pulmonary hemorrhage. Increased risk is associated with MHC class II type DR2.

b. Therapy. Immunosuppressive therapy generally consists of corticosteroids with plasmapheresis used to remove autoreactive antibodies.

6. Autoimmune hemolytic anemia (red blood cell), thrombocytopenia (platelet), neutropenia (neutrophil), and lymphopenia (lymphocyte)

a. Pathogenesis. Antibodies against membrane antigens of one or more of the indicated cell types may activate complement and opsonize the cells for rapid splenic phagocytosis. It may also occur as part of the spectrum of autoimmunity in non–organ-specific pathologies, particularly SLE. These autoimmune varieties should be distinguished from those precipitated by responses to external antigens (e.g., drugs), but the clinical consequences are similar.

b. Therapy. In adults, treatment begins with corticosteroids but often also requires splenectomy. Cyclophosphamide may be used in some patients.

7. Insulin-dependent diabetes mellitus (IDDM) (see Chapter 54). Progressive and ultimately complete destruction of pancreatic beta islet cells occurs in diabetes. Although predictively useful, antibodies against insulin and surface cytoplasmic antigens of the beta islet cell are present prior to clinical onset, the predominant cytotoxic mechansims appear to be mediated by T cells and perhaps macrophages. This view is supported by the beneficial effects of cyclosporine A therapy in early IDDM patients at levels that have little effect on antibody production. Increased risk is associated with MHC class II types DR3 and DR4.

8. Multiple sclerosis (MS)

a. Pathogenesis. T cells and macrophages, which are thought to be cytocidal for oligodendrocytes, infiltrate the central nervous system (CNS) and **attack the basic protein of myelin** as autoantigen. The immunologic component may be secondary to other unknown initiating agents. **CNS demyelination with sclerotic plaques** leads to symptoms of spasticity. Increased risk is associated with MHC class II type DR2. Guillain Barré syndrome is a related condition, involving peripheral nervous system (PNS) demyelination, which unlike MS, can be acute.

b. Therapy. Spasticity is treated with **baclofen** with variable effectiveness; the peripheral skeletal muscle relaxant **dantroline** is effective in some patients. Recently, **adrenocorticotropic hormone (ACTH)** rather than corticosteroids has become the favored immunosuppressive therapy.

E. Non–organ-specific autoimmunities. The similarities and differences in this class of pathologies is illustrated by comparison of Sjögren syndrome and SLE. For a discussion of rheumatoid arthritis, see Chapter 51.

1. Sjögren syndrome

a. Diagnosis is usually based upon lymphocytic infiltration and the presence of autoantibodies against salivary gland antigens and exocrine glands of the eyes, gastrointestinal and respiratory systems, and vagina. Hypergammaglobulinemia (50%) due to hyperactive B cells, antinuclear antibodies (50%–65%), and rheumatoid factors (anti-IgG) [75%–90%] are present in the indicated fractions.

b. Pathogenesis. Primary pathogenic events center around **inhibition of exocrine gland secretion** with dryness of eyes, mouth, and gastrointestinal, respiratory, and vaginal mucous membranes; and pain and edema in the salivary glands. However, patients with hypergammaglobulinemia are disposed to the pathogenesis of type III hypersensitivity reactions (see II D), such as vasculitis with CNS involvement and kidney disease.

c. **Therapy.** Treatment in milder cases is with **artificial tears** and frequent drinking of water. For more serious cases (e.g., vasculitis), treatment is similar to that for SLE, namely **systemic corticosteroids**.

2. **Systemic lupus erythematosus (SLE)**

a. **Diagnosis** is complicated and depends upon the presence of four or more of eleven criteria. Most useful among these are high concentrations of antinuclear antibodies directed against the following antigens: double-stranded DNA and the Smith (Sm) nuclear antigen, both of which are considered specific for a SLE diagnosis. Other diagnostic criteria include the presence of the lupus erythematosus cell (a neutrophil that has phagocytosed nuclei), a discoid erythematous facial rash, photosensitivity, oral ulcers, arthritis, renal dysfunction (persistent proteinuria), and anticardiolipin, antierythrocyte, or antileukocyte antibodies.

b. **Pathogenesis** is essentially that of **type III hypersensitivity**. There is always **hyperactivity of B cells** of unknown origin. This leads to hypergammaglobulinemia with circulating immune complexes of DNA and other nuclear antigens that precipitate onto vascular basement membranes, activating complement.

(1) Mild arthritis, fever, skin rash, and fatigue are common symptoms.

(2) Progressive necrotizing vasculitis with CNS involvement and glomerulonephritis are the most serious consequences, occurring in about 50% of patients.

(3) Hypertension may develop secondary to kidney disease.

(4) Hemolytic anemia and thrombocytopenia are common.

(5) A variety of behavioral changes occurs in approximately 25% of patients.

(6) Several drugs have been implicated in provoking a lupus-like syndrome, which usually resolves when the drug is withdrawn, and whose basis is not understood. These include **procainamide, hydralazine,** and **chlorpromazine**. There is no renal pathology in drug-induced forms.

c. **Therapy.** Patients with mild disease (low fever, arthritis) may be managed with nonsteroidal anti-inflammatory drugs (NSAIDs), but therapy for patients with more severe symptoms is usually oral methylprednisone. Cyclophosphamide may also be used, and plasmapheresis to remove circulating immune complexes may be helpful.

F. **Prospects for more specific immunologic therapies.** Current therapies comprise approaches that suppress all immune responses; however, current clinical trials seek to suppress only those lymphocytes that are activated; for example:

1. **Feeding autoantigens** to patients in an attempt to induce immunologic suppression

2. **Vaccination with autoreactive T cells** to induce immunologic suppression

3. **Anti-T_H monoclonal antibodies** (particularly anti-CD4) to attempt to eliminate autoreactive T cells

4. **Conjugates of interleukin-2 (IL-2) and toxins** from plants or bacteria to eliminate autoreactive T cells without generalized T-cell suppression

IV. IMMUNODEFICIENCY

IMMUNODEFICIENCY is either primary or secondary. **Primary immunodeficiencies** are those that are either **hereditary** or **congenital,** and in which one or more elements basic to the immune system fails to function properly or is absent. **Secondary immunodeficiencies** are the **consequence of some other systemic disorder** or are **iatrogenic in patients given immunosuppressive therapies**. They usually develop in patients who showed normal immune function prior to their onset. The expected clinical consequences of an immunodeficiency are governed by the specific portion of the immune system that is affected (e.g., B and T cells, complement).

A. **Primary immunodeficiencies** are with one exception rare pathologies. Some examples are:

1. **X-Linked agammaglobulinemia** (hypogammaglobulinemia) is an inherited deficiency in antibody production (humoral immunity) with relatively normal functioning of T cells but a failure of B cells to fully mature. Serum immunoglobulin levels are extremely low. As an X-chromosome–associated genetic disorder, it is found primarily in men.

a. **Pathogenesis** commences between 6 and 9 months postnatally and is representative of situations with antibody deficiency but intact T-cell function such as recurrent infections with extracellular pyogenic bacteria (e.g., streptococci, pneumococci, *Hemophilus*). Immunity to fungi and most viruses is generally functional.

b. **Clinical symptoms** include pneumonia, sinusitis, otitis, meningitis, and septicemia.

c. **Therapy.** Preferred treatment is via **passive immunization with intravenous human immune globulins (IGIV)** [see VI B 1 c].

2. **Common variable immunodeficiency** is believed to be an acquired deficiency of B cell maturation to plasma cells and can occur at any age in either sex. Pathogenesis, symptoms, and treatment are similar to X-linked agammaglobulinemia, although there is significant variation in the pathogenesis and etiology among individual patients.

3. **Selective IgA deficiency** is the most common primary immunodeficiency, affecting perhaps 0.5% of the U.S. population. It appears to be inherited. The low secretory IgA (sIgA) concentration predisposes to extracellular bacterial infections of mucosal surfaces, leading to respiratory, urogenital, and gastrointestinal infections. Some affected individuals are, however, asymptomatic for unknown reasons. Certain autoimmunities may be more prevalent. There is no specific immunologic therapy.

4. **DiGeorge syndrome** results from developmental failure of the thymus and parathyroid glands, accompanied by cardiovascular and other developmental anomalies. This leads to a decrease in total T-cell numbers but relatively normal immunoglobulin levels.

   a. **Pathogenesis** in severe cases (i.e., little functional thymic tissue) is representative of situations with T-cell deficiency, such as recurrent infections of skin, lung, genitourinary tract, and blood with opportunistic pathogens, particularly viruses (e.g., herpes viruses), fungi (e.g., *Candida*) and certain protozoa (e.g., *Pneumocystis carinii*), probable increased incidence of certain cancers, development of graft-versus-host disease (GVH) [see V C] after whole blood transfusion, and usually death in infancy or early childhood.

   b. **Therapy.** The only currently useful therapy for severe cases of T-cell deficiencies is bone marrow transplantation (see V C).

5. **Nezelof syndrome** is probably inherited and manifests as lymphopenia, thymic abnormalities, but normal or elevated serum immunoglobulin. Gram-negative sepsis may occur in addition to the opportunistic infections associated with T-cell deficiency.

6. **Severe combined immunodeficiency disorders (SCIDs)** are a heterogeneous group of inherited disorders with deficiencies in T cells, B cells (variable), and serum immunoglobulin. Infections with opportunistic organisms occur in the first few months postnatally, and survival past 1 year is rare without successful bone marrow transplantation. One form of SCIDs involves the inherited deficiency of the enzyme adenosine deaminase (ADA). Human trials for gene replacement therapy have begun.

7. **Chronic granulomatous disease (CGD)** has multiple modes of inheritance, all of which lead to the metabolic disorder where phagocytes are incapable of generating significant bactericidal oxygen-free radicals. Despite hypergammaglobulinemia and effective opsonization, chronic infections with catalase-positive bacteria (e.g., *Staphylococcus aureus*) occur due to the inability of phagocytes to kill these organisms subsequent to phagocytosis. Usually fatal early in life, some forms are probably candidates for gene replacement therapy.

B. **Secondary immunodeficiencies** include diminished immunologic responsiveness as a consequence of a variety of situations.

1. **Drug therapy with cytotoxic drugs** generally prevents division of responding lymphocytes, suppresses bone marrow production of blood cells, and may directly kill them. Corticosteroids have a broad suppressive action on immune system cells, including decreased division, cytokine secretion, and chemotaxis or emigration from the blood into tissues.

2. **Leukemias, lymphomas, and myelomas** are frequently associated with decreased immune responsiveness, at least some of which may result from destruction of the architecture of lymphoid organs (e.g., spleen, lymph nodes). There is evidence that suggests malignancy-related immunodeficiency in other cancers as well.

3. **Protein calorie malnutrition** can significantly decrease immune competence, particularly in children.

4. **Aging** is associated with decreased immunologic competence.

5. **Acute infections** can produce a transient immunodeficiency.

6. **Acquired immune deficiency syndrome (AIDS)** is a secondary immunodeficiency that is usually persistent and is very probably an indirect consequence of infection by **human immunodeficiency virus 1 (HIV-1)** and possibly **HIV-2**.
   a. **Pathogenesis.** The viral envelope glycoprotein 120 (gp120) has a strong affinity for CD4 (see I B 3 c), allowing the virus to directly infect T_H cells and certain monocyte/macrophages. As a retrovirus, viral entry and uncoating releases the viral RNA genome and the associated reverse transcriptase enzyme, which immediately synthesizes a double-stranded DNA copy of the genome (provirus). The proviral copy becomes integrated into the genome of the $CD4^+$ cell, and the virus enters a period of latency, essentially hidden from the immune system.
      (1) During **initial infection,** an acute illness, with an average duration of 3 weeks and resembling mononucleosis, occurs in an unknown percentage of individuals, while others are free of any symptoms.
      (2) **Seroconversion** (i.e., the appearance of antiviral antibodies) generally occurs within 3 weeks to 15 months after the initial exposure to HIV-1. A period of **asymptomatic infection** typically follows seroconversion.
      (3) Infected T_H cells are killed when **viral genes are reactivated from latency** and viruses bud from the cell. In addition, infected T cells may fuse to form "syncytia." This fusion may hasten the spread of virus to uninfected T cells and contribute to cell killing. A **progressive depletion of T_H cells** occurs (normal count about 800–1000/mm^3).
      (4) Monocyte/macrophages may produce new virus without being killed and may spread the virus to uninfected T cells as well as to other cell types. $CD4^-$ cell lines susceptible to HIV infection include neurons, liver, and fibroblasts. In direct cell-to-cell transfers of the virus, there may be minimal exposure to the extracellular immune system (e.g., antibody).
   b. **Clinical symptoms**
      (1) **Persistent generalized lymphadenopathy** (extrainguinal) is an indicator of impending progression to full disease. Unexplained fever, night sweats, diarrhea, and other conditions may also occur; these symptoms are often termed **AIDS-related complex (ARC)**.
      (2) Progression to full-blown AIDS may be delayed by 8 years or more from the time of initial infection. Depletion of T_H cells below 400/mm^3 and oral candidiasis are observations that suggest imminent disease. Since CD8 T cells are not greatly affected, the ratio of circulating CD4:CD8 cells becomes abnormal ("inverted").
      (3) Currently, a diagnosis of AIDS involves the occurrence of **opportunistic infections** or **neoplasms as a result of the progressive immunodeficiency** due to severe depletion of T_H-cell (CD4) function. Also included are the HIV-wasting syndrome and encephalopathy.
         (a) Opportunistic infections are the major consequence of AIDS, particularly by *P. carinii* (up to 80% of patients), *C. albicans, Mycobacterium avium-intracellulare,* HSV, cytomegalovirus (CMV), and others. Tuberculosis generally occurs as a reactivation of a latent infection in carriers. Cumulatively, **these opportunistic infections are the main cause of death**.
         (b) The otherwise rare cancer, **Kaposi's sarcoma,** occurs in less than half of patients, and the occurrence of non-Hodgkin's lymphoma is higher than in the general population.
      (4) **HIV-associated dementia complex (HADC)** may affect over half of AIDS patients. In HADC, macrophages infiltrate the brain and are the most productively infected cell by comparison to neurons or glia. Some patients show demyelination.
      (5) Other immune system abnormalities include polyclonal B-cell activation and hypergammaglobulinemia with a concomitant reduced ability to mount humoral immune responses to specific antigens. Chemotaxis, cytokine secretion, and cytotoxic ability of monocyte/macrophages are all diminished. These problems are believed to be consequences of impaired regulation by T cells.
   c. **Therapy**
      (1) Current therapies include antibiotics, azidothymidine (AZT), a viral reverse transcriptase inhibitor, dideoxyinosine (ddI), and interferon α (IFNα) (see VII D) for treatment of Kaposi's sarcoma. Many other drugs and immunomodulators are being tested.
      (2) Ultimately, an effective active vaccine is necessary to limit the spread of HIV infection. Viral antigenic variation, cell-to-cell transmission, and the uncertain role of antibodies

in protection make the process of vaccine development difficult. A live, attenuated vaccine (see VI C 2) is currently considered too great a risk. Trials of subunit vaccines are imminent.

V. GRAFT REJECTION

A. Overview. Individual differences in molecular structures in cells and tissues are to be expected (except in identical twins) because of the genetic variation inherent in humans. These molecular differences mean that transplanted tissues or organs (grafts) are likely to be antigenic to the recipient of the organs.

1. Although the MHC class I and II glycoproteins play an essential role in all immune responses of T cells (see I B 3 a), these molecules are both particularly variant in structure among different humans (polymorphic) and are also very antigenic.
2. An individual's particular set of MHC glycoproteins is called his or her **histocompatibility** or **human leukocyte antigen (HLA) type**. Class I glycoproteins are referred to as HLA-A, -B, and -C antigens; class II glycoproteins are referred to as HLA-DR, -DP, or -DQ antigens. Each individual receives one set of genes (a haplotype) encoding these protein antigens from each parent.
3. Other than identical twins, there is an approximately 25% (0.25) probability that two siblings with the same parents will be HLA identical or "matched" and approximately a 50% chance that they will be half HLA matched or haploidentical for this group of molecular structures. Parents and children are almost always haploidentical. The basis for rejection of transplanted tissues has, in some cases, resulted from HLA incompatibility but, in other cases, is unknown, since HLA matching does not always seem to be a factor in rejection.

B. Common solid organ transplants include kidney, heart, liver, heart/lung, and pancreas. Two sources of these organs are cadavers and living donors. The probability of an exact HLA match in cadaver grafts is approximately 1 in 10 million.

1. **HLA matching**
   a. Donation of an organ by an HLA-matched sibling is most desirable, but the primary problem in this type of transplantation is the rejection of the transplanted organ by the recipient's immune response, a host-versus-graft response.
   b. HLA-DR and HLA-B matching has been shown to be important in decreasing the rejection reaction in renal and cardiac grafts, but rejection still occurs in HLA-matched situations. HLA matching does not seem to be important in liver transplantation.
2. **Types of rejection of organ grafts**
   a. **Hyperacute rejection** is mediated by preexisting antibody in the recipient, usually against ABO mismatches. Complement is activated, clotting occurs, and the vasculature of the transplanted organ is occluded. Rejection is immediate (i.e., within the first 2 days after transplantation). An ABO mismatched graft is, therefore, attempted only in extremely rare instances. Once rejection has begun, it is essentially nontreatable.
   b. **Acute rejection** is most likely a T-cell–macrophage-mediated attack on the graft based on HLA and other tissue antigen mismatch. T cells and monocyte/macrophages infiltrate the graft, and by 10–14 days are provoking cellular necrosis and inflammation perivascularly. The entire graft begins to necrose if untreated.
   c. **Chronic rejection** occurs over several months to several years after transplantation. It is probably mediated by chronic immune complex formation and is manifested clinically as fibrosis and occlusion of small arteries and arterioles in the kidneys and by atherosclerosis in the heart. Despite the high success rate of MHC-matched, pharmacologically treated grafts in the first year post-transplantation (85%–90% kidney), the rejection rate after 5 years is still nearly 50%. This form of rejection is refractory to therapy.

C. Bone marrow transplantation is sometimes attempted in immunodeficiency diseases, aplastic anemias, some leukemias, and certain genetic diseases. In bone marrow transplantation, the graft contains a high proportion of donor lymphocytes that can respond against the host HLA and other antigens. This response causes graft-versus-host (GVH) disease.

1. Graft T-cell recognition of the host is important in GVH disease, as evidenced by the reductions of GVH disease after procedures that purge T cells from the donor marrow.

2. **Clinical manifestations** of GVH disease are most commonly seen in skin (e.g., rash, desquamation), gastrointestinal tract (e.g., pain, vomiting, intestinal bleeding), and liver (e.g., necrosis indicated by increased serum bilirubin). Death is frequent.

3. HLA matching is important in bone marrow transplantation, but the failure of even matched grafts due to GVH disease is high.

4. Since the recipient of the marrow (host) is immunosuppressed by drugs or radiation, the host-versus-graft response is less important.

D. Prophylaxis and therapy of graft rejection

1. **Immunosuppression of graft recipient**
   a. **Corticosteroids** (e.g., methylprednisolone, prednisone) are administered just prior to transplantation and then rapidly tapered thereafter due to their side effects. Corticosteroids may be used in combination with azathioprine, cyclosporine, or **antilymphocyte globulins/antithymocyte globulins (ALG/ATG)**.
   b. **Azathioprine** is given prior to transplantation with maintenance doses afterward.
   c. **Methotrexate** is mostly used for bone marrow transplantation in combination with ALG/ATG. It is administered either a few days before or at the time of transplantation.

2. **Specific suppression of T cells**
   a. **Cyclosporine** binds to an intracellular protein cyclophilin and somehow blocks transcription of cytokine genes in a T cell that has recognized antigens, thus inhibiting T-cell secretion of IL-2 and IFNγ and preventing complete T-cell activation. It is administered prophylactically, since it is more effective if present when rejection begins, and it is commonly combined with other agents. The major side effect of cyclosporine is nephrotoxicity.
   b. **ALG** and **ATG** are antisera derived from animals that contain a variety of antibody specificities against T-cell antigens. They are used both prophylactically and therapeutically in both bone marrow transplantation and organ transplantation.
   c. **Muromonab-CD3** (OKT3) is a mouse monoclonal antibody specific for the CD3 antigen, which is present on all peripheral T cells, and is used therapeutically to halt and reverse acute rejection upon its diagnosis.
      (1) Its main action is thought to be the opsonization of T cells for enhanced phagocytosis. It is administered daily for 10–14 days and is usually only usable once in a given patient since an immune response against the foreign mouse antibody occurs.
      (2) Acute side effects are common, probably due to nonspecific T-cell activation, leading to release of cytokines, and include high fever, chills, blood pressure changes, vomiting, diarrhea, and respiratory distress. Patients already in fluid overload have developed fatal pulmonary edema, and OKT3 is contraindicated in these patients.
      (3) Muromonab-CD3 may also be used in vitro as an agent to purge donor bone marrow of T cells to reduce the risk of GVH disease.

3. **Investigational agents** are being tested to prevent or reverse graft rejection. These include anti–T-cell immunotoxins (see VII C 1); conjugates of IL-2 and a toxin; and other monoclonals, which prevent T cells from adhering to foreign graft cells. These would be administered to the graft recipient. In addition, monoclonal antibodies are being used to mask HLA antigens on the graft tissue itself prior to its transplantation into the recipient.

VI. VACCINATION

A. Overview

1. **Passive vaccination** is the intramuscular or intravenous injection of antibody preparations for the purpose of immediately enhancing the immune competence of a patient. Protection depends upon the serum half-life of the injected antibody and is, thus, limited to several weeks to several months per administration (human sera).

2. **Active vaccination** is the intramuscular, subcutaneous, or oral introduction of one or more antigens designed to provoke the patient's immune system into a specific immune response, generating antibody, activated T cells, and specific memory. Protection via memory varies with the specific vaccine but, in some cases, can be for life.

B. Passive vaccination (Table 8-2)

1. **Preparations.** Doses of intramuscular preparations are sometimes given in units per kilogram, sometimes in milliliters per kilogram, and the dose varies with the individual vaccine and patient population. Intravenous preparations are commonly used in high doses.
   a. **Standard human serum immune globulin for intramuscular vaccination (IGIM)** is a polyclonal antiserum prepared from pooled plasma of donors and contains 165 mg of human immunoglobulin per milliliter, predominately the four subclasses of IgG. Side effects are rare and minimal, usually confined to minor inflammation and pain at the site of injection. This preparation is unsuitable for intravenous injection due to the formation of antibody aggregates that can activate complement and platelets.
   b. **Special IGIMs** are individual sera prepared from plasma lots of subjects actively immunized against or recovering from specific diseases. Each serum is, thus, enriched for antibodies of the desired specificity; for example, tetanus immune globulin (TIG) contains a higher proportion of antibodies against tetanus toxin than would be found in IGIM.
   c. **Intravenous human immune globulins (IGIV)** are preparations prepared from pooled human serum and modified to minimize antibody aggregation. Side effects of chills nausea and abdominal pain occur in about 10% of patients. Side effects may be diminished by reducing the rate of intravenous infusion. Premedication with corticosteroids is recommended, and epinephrine IV should be available in case of anaphylaxis.
   d. **Animal antisera.** Equine (horse) antisera is still used in certain applications (see Table 8-2). Mouse monoclonal antibody (muromonab-CD3) is approved for use in acute renal rejection (see V D 2 c). Half-lives of animal antibodies are generally much shorter in humans.

Table 8-2. Passive Vaccines

Illness	Vaccine	Rationale
Intramuscular		
Hepatitis B (HBV)	Hepatitis B immune globulin (HBIG)	Prophylaxis
Hepatitis A (HAV)	Immune globulin IM (IGIM)	Prophylaxis
Non-A, non-B hepatitis	IGIM	Prophylaxis and therapy
Measles	IGIM	Prophylaxis and therapy
Rabies	Rabies immune globulin (RIG)	Prophylaxis
Rubella	IGIM	Fetal prophylaxis in exposed mother
Varicella	Varicella zoster immune globulin (VZIG)	Prophylaxis and therapy in immunocompromised individual
Tetanus	Tetanus immune globulin (TIG)	Prophylaxis
Hypogammaglobulinemia	IGIM	Therapy of antibody deficiency
Rh disease	Rh_o(D) immune globulin (RhoGAM)	Prophylaxis after delivery of Rh^+ fetus by Rh^- mother
Diphtheria	Diphtheria antitoxin (Equine)	Prophylaxis and therapy
Botulism	Botulism antiserum (Equine)	Prophylaxis and therapy
Snakebite	Polyvalent antivenin (Equine)	Prophylaxis and therapy
Black widow bite	Black widow antivenin (Equine)	Prophylaxis and therapy
Intravenous*		
Hypogammaglobulinemia	Immune globulin IV (IGIV)	Therapy of antibody deficiency
Idiopathic thrombocytopenic purpura (ITP)	IGIV	Therapy
Chronic lymphocytic leukemia	IGIV	Therapy of antibody deficiency
Cytomegalovirus (CMV) infection	CMV IGIV	Therapy in renal transplant patients
Acute renal rejection	Muromonab-CD3 (murine)	Reversal of acute rejection

*Food and Drug Administration (FDA) approved uses; many others currently in trials.

2. Rationales for passive vaccination

a. Prophylaxis of infectious disease. Antibodies may be given prophylactically to prevent clinical symptoms of a viral or bacterial infectious process, particularly in an individual without prior exposure and, therefore, without memory. In this context, the vaccine often acts to protect during the incubation period for infection. For example:

(1) *Clostridium tetani* infection has an incubation period of about 5 days before significant quantities of tetanus toxin is produced. A primary immune response of 7–10 days would be too slow; passive vaccination with TIG binds the toxin and prevents pathology.

(2) Hepatitis B immune globulin (HBIG) should be administered to exposed individuals as soon as possible after exposure to prevent viral infection.

b. Prophylaxis or therapy aims to prevent or attenuate the pathologic consequences of an infectious pathology in special populations. Examples are the use of **varicella zoster immune globulin (VZIG)** in immunocompromised patients, and IGIM in pregnant mothers exposed to rubella who have not been actively vaccinated.

c. Therapy of antibody deficiency. Persons deficient in antibody production either due to primary immunodeficiency (see IV) or as a result of chronic lymphocytic leukemia receive periodic IGIV (preferred) or IGIM every 2–4 weeks to maintain humoral immunity.

d. Other situations. IGIV is used in therapy for idiopathic (autoimmune) thrombocytopenia purpura; intramuscular Rh_o(D) immune globulin (RhoGAM) in prophylaxis for Rh disease (see II C 5 c), and muromonab-CD3 (see V D 2 c) in acute renal graft rejection.

C. Active vaccination (Table 8-3) is always intended as a method of prophylaxis

1. Overview

a. Contents. Active vaccines always contain one or more antigens or whole pathogenic organisms but may in addition contain preservatives, low doses of antibiotics, and other compounds resulting from vaccine preparation in cells of nonhuman origin. The "valence" of a vaccine generally indicates the number of different strains of organism included (e.g., trivalent polio vaccine includes three strains of poliovirus).

b. Administration. Active vaccines are generally administered subcutaneously, intramuscularly, or intradermally. Some are introduced adsorbed to aluminum hydroxide or aluminum phosphate adjuvants. An adjuvant increases the antigenicity of the vaccine. A few vaccines are administered orally or intranasally.

c. Seroconversion. For most active vaccines, the success of the series of vaccinations is indicated by the seroconversion of the patient. This indicates that a person previously negative for specific serum antibodies (i.e., seronegative) is now positive for these antibodies (i.e., seropositive). This does not indicate established immunity for certain vaccines [e.g., bacille Calmette-Guérin (BCG) vaccine for tuberculosis].

d. A schedule of active vaccination is recommended for infants and young children (Table 8-3), but first vaccination is delayed until after 6 weeks of age due to the inadequate responses normally obtained from newborns, and the persistence of maternal antibodies in newborn circulation. Some vaccines are intended for use primarily in noninfant populations.

e. A series of vaccinations for effective immunity is required for certain vaccines. Others are effective with only a single vaccination. For those requiring a series, intervals between vaccinations greater than those recommended do not generally diminish protection. Duration of memory varies with the individual vaccine, and **booster vaccinations** may be necessary.

f. Side effects may include inflammation at the site of vaccination, malaise, mild febrile reactions, chills, headache, myalgia, and arthralgia. More severe side effects may include febrile illness, extreme somnolence, seizures, or anaphylactic hypersensitivity to vaccine antigens or accessory components (e.g., antibiotic, chicken protein). Severe reactions contraindicate continuation of a series. Individuals with severe febrile illness should not be actively vaccinated until the illness resolves.

2. Types of active vaccines

a. Live, attenuated vaccines consist of whole organisms (usually viruses), which multiply after vaccination but are attenuated to significantly reduce pathogenicity.

(1) A small dose provokes a strong immune response due to the increased antigen concentration achieved through multiplication of the organism. Some vaccines are, thus, capable of eliciting lifelong immunity in one or two doses [e.g., measles, mumps, rubella vaccine (MMR)]. The major problem with such vaccines is the relative genetic instability of viruses, which can produce reversion to virulence and, therefore, result in the very pathology against which the patient is being vaccinated [e.g., oral polio vaccine (OPV)].

Table 8-3. Commonly Administered Food and Drug Administration (FDA) Approved Active Vaccines

Vaccine	Target Population*	Number of Vaccinations	Schedule	Notes
Live, Attenuated				
Viral				
Oral polio (OPV) [trivalent]	Infants, children, health/day care workers	4	2, 4, 15–18 months; one at school entry	Approximately 1 in 2.6 million risk of vaccine-induced paralysis
Measles, mumps, rubella (MMR)	Infants, children	2	15 months (< 12 months if high risk); 1 at school entry	Generally affords lifelong immunity
Rubella	Adolescent females not previously vaccinated	1	Postpuberty	Protects future fetus from congenital rubella injury
Bacterial				
BCG tuberculosis	Persons exposed to sputum-positive tuberculosis patients	Varies	Depends upon success of initial vaccination	Unpredictable effectiveness; induces cell-mediated immunity
Killed, Inactivated				
Viral				
Influenza (tri- or polyvalent)	Geriatric, health care workers, those at risk for complications of flu	1 per year	Annually for maximal protection	Variant strains may appear each year; vaccine must be annually updated
Hepatitis B (HBV)	Homosexual males, prostitutes, health care workers, newborn of carrier mother	1 with boosters	Booster every 5 years for those with continuing risk	HBsAg from plasma of chronic carriers; routine infant vaccination now approved
Inactivated polio (IPV) [trivalent]	Immunodeficient children and families; as booster in health/day care workers	4	2, 4, 15–18 months; one at school entry	No sIgA, thus reduced protection; no paralysis risk
Rabies (HDCV)	Animal care worker	4 or 5† with boosters	7 days apart; boosters as required to maintain immunoglobulin (Ig)	Two doses to exposed, already immune individual
Bacterial				
Diphtheria, tetanus, pertussis (DTP)	Infants, children	4 with boosters	2, 4, 15–18 months, and one at school entry	Tetanus toxoid (Td) booster every 10 years or upon exposure via wound

Tetanus and diphtheria toxoids (Td)	Children ≥ 7 or adults with no prior vaccination	3 with boosters	Second dose in 4–8 weeks; third dose 6 months later	Td booster every 10 years or upon exposure via wound
Haemophilus b (Hib)	Infants, children; HIV-infected adults	Depends upon formulation	Depends upon formulation	Polysaccharide capsule is poor antigen; conjugate vaccines enhance potency
Pneumococcus (polyvalent)	At risk adults, children ≥ 2, (e.g., immunocompromised, geriatric)	1 or 1 per year	As necessary in at risk patients; not during active infection; 1 per year in geriatric patients	Poor response to polysaccharide antigen in children < 2
Subunit				
Recombinant HBV	See "hepatitis B" above	See above	See above	Generally interchangeable with plasma-derived vaccine

BCG = bacille Calmette-Guérin; HBsAg = hepatitis B surface antigen; HDCV = human diploid cell vaccine; HIV = human immunodeficiency virus; sIgA = secretory immunoglobulin A.
*Entire target population is not listed in all cases.
†5 Doses to already exposed individual.

(2) Live, attenuated viral vaccines are not recommended for pregnant women or for those intending to become pregnant within 3 months of vaccination. Live, attenuated viral or bacterial vaccines should, in general, not be given to immunocompromised individuals.

b. **Killed, inactivated vaccines** may contain whole killed cells (e.g., phenol killed *Bordetella pertussis*) or any antigenic fraction isolated from the organism. They are usually given adsorbed to adjuvant.

(1) Isolated antigens may require inactivation prior to use in a vaccine (e.g., formaldehyde modified toxin of *Clostridium tetani,* known as **tetanus toxoid (Td)** after modification). Such inactivation eliminates pathogenicity but preserves at least some antigenicity.

(2) Because no live organisms are present, reversion to pathogenicity is not a problem. However, doses of cells or antigens must be higher than in live, attenuated vaccines, and hypersensitivity reactions to vaccine components are more common. Minimum effective doses are usually measured in numbers of cells or micrograms of antigen.

(3) Vaccines where the antigenic fragment is a polysaccharide (e.g., *Haemophilus* b) are generally poor at eliciting immune responses and memory, probably due to their failure to evoke T-cell activation. Such vaccines have been improved by conjugating the polysaccharide to another antigenic compound such as Td. These are known as **conjugate vaccines**.

c. **Subunit vaccines.** Proteins and glycoproteins of an organism are produced by recombinant DNA technology in bacteria, yeast, or mammalian cells and are used as the antigens for vaccination. Currently, one such vaccine is approved by the Food and Drug Administration (FDA), that containing recombinant HBV surface antigen (rHBsAg).

d. **Experimental vaccines** include many other subunit vaccines, peptides produced by chemical, cell-free synthesis, recombinant DNA viruses containing genes for the antigens of multiple organisms, and anti-idiotype antibodies used for active vaccination.

3. **Specific vaccines** currently in common use and recommended schedules are listed in Table 8-3.

D. **Simultaneous administration of active and passive vaccines.** There are situations when it is desirable to administer simultaneously the active and passive vaccines against a pathogenic organism to maximize postexposure prophylaxis. The immune globulin offers immediate protection, while the active vaccine stimulates an immune response. These are given at separate sites to prevent antibody (passive) and antigen (active) from reacting and inactivating one another.

1. Infants with **HBV** born to mothers positive for the hepatitis B surface antigen (HBsAg) are significantly protected from becoming chronic carriers by this combined prophylaxis.

2. **Rabies.** Postexposure prophylaxis almost always includes combined use of active and passive vaccines due to the lethal nature of the unchecked infection. The exception is individuals with a history of an active vaccination who demonstrate sufficient existing serum antibody concentration.

3. **Tetanus.** The use of the combined prophylaxis is sometimes used but depends upon the type of wound and the previous history of tetanus active vaccination. A brief summary of recommended guidelines is as follows:

a. A **tetanus-prone wound** is one that produces anaerobic conditions (e.g., deep puncture) or in which exposure to *Clostridium* or its spores is probable (e.g., wound contaminated with animal feces). If a previous history of active vaccination is uncertain or includes less than three doses, both TIG and Td should be administered. The patient should then also be recalled to complete the toxoid series.

(1) If the wound is tetanus-prone but the individual has received a full series of active vaccination, no treatment is necessary if the interval since the last Td dose is 5 years or less.

(2) If the interval is more than 5 years, Td only (no TIG) should be given to boost memory immunity and antibody production.

b. For a **clean, minor wound,** if a previous history of active vaccination is uncertain or includes less than three doses, Td should be administered.

(1) If the wound is clean and minor, but the individual has received a full series of active vaccination, no treatment is necessary if the interval since the last Td dose is 10 years or less.

(2) If the interval is more than 10 years, Td only (no TIG) should be given to boost memory immunity and antibody production.

VII. PROSPECTS FOR IMMUNOMODULATION

A. **Fab antidigoxin antibody** preparations obtained from sheep are approved for the reversal of toxicity associated with toxic digoxin serum levels. The antibody binds digoxin, preventing its binding to its normal receptor site, and the Fab-digoxin complex is renally excreted.

B. **Monoclonal antibodies** are generally produced via the in vitro fusion of a cancerous plasma cell (myeloma) with an activated mouse B cell. The resulting **hybridoma** secretes murine (mouse) antibodies of a single defined specificity and has the immortality characteristic of the myeloma. Techniques for production of human monoclonal antibodies and a variety of hybrid mouse–human monoclonal antibodies are available but not as well refined as the hybridoma technology.

1. **Monoclonal antibodies** [e.g., whole antibodies or Fab or $F(ab')_2$ fragments] are routinely used for in vitro diagnostic tests such as blood group and tissue typing for HLAs, screening for cancer-related antigens such as carcinoembryonic antigen (CEA), urine testing for drugs and metabolites, and testing for HIV infection. In these and many other diagnostic applications, monoclonal antibodies are often conjugated to enzymes, radioisotopes, or fluorescent dyes.
2. The **murine muromonab-CD3** is used in therapy of acute graft rejection, and several other monoclonal antibodies are being tested (see V D 2 c).
3. **Monoclonal antibodies against T cells** are producing some improvement in clinical trials for certain autoimmune pathologies.
4. **Monoclonal antibodies against neoplastic cells** have had limited success but appear to be useful in certain leukemias and lymphomas.

C. **Monoclonal antibodies may be conjugated to enzymes, drugs, prodrugs, radioisotopes or plant and bacterial toxins** for the purpose of specific delivery of the conjugated agent to a focused in vivo site or sites of action. There are several types of problems with the use of these agents.

1. **Immunotoxins** are generally produced by conjugation of a monoclonal antibody to a biologic polypeptide toxin, such as diphtheria toxin, that is often modified to reduce nonspecific toxicity.
2. Although they are also being tested in aspects of graft rejection and autoimmunity, the principle effort has been directed toward the use of immunotoxins as antineoplastic agents. Clinical trials have produced moderate success in treating leukemia and lymphoma with lower success rates against tumors such as breast carcinoma.
3. **Monoclonal antibodies conjugated to radioisotopes** such as ^{90}Y have recently produced remissions in Hodgkin's and acute T-cell leukemia patients.
4. **Monoclonal antibodies conjugated to enzymes** that activate a prodrug to the active drug at some specific tissue site (e.g., neoplastic cell surface) are in early stages of human trials.

D. **Immunostimulation** has been attempted with a variety of compounds, ranging from cytokines (see Table 8-1) to bacterial products.

1. **IFNα** exists in multiple subtypes of which two are currently FDA approved. Its actions as an inhibitor of cell growth have led to its use in the treatment of hairy cell leukemia, Kaposi's sarcoma in AIDS patients, and genital warts. At lower doses, interferons may stimulate immune cellular functions (e.g., T cells, NK cells, macrophages), but at higher doses they can be immunosuppressive. The use of IFNα against other cancers has produced variable results.
2. **IFNγ** has greater activity in immunostimulation in the intact immune system, but its effects when administered also depend upon dose and timing. Combined use of both IFNα and IFNγ may yield better results. The most common side effects of interferon therapy are influenza-like symptoms. IFNγ is now approved for use as a macrophage-activating factor in patients with chronic granulomatous disease.
3. Several different protocols using **IL-2** have yielded promising results with some apparently complete remissions in melanoma patients. In this technique known as adoptive immunotherapy, a patient's peripheral blood lymphocytes, or tumor infiltrating lymphocytes, are removed,

cultured with IL-2, and later reinfused with additional IL-2. These IL-2 responsive cells are likely T cells and NK cells. Severe capillary leak syndrome with some patient mortality is a problematic side effect.

4. **Hormones of the thymus** that induce T-cell maturation and other functions have been used to increase certain cell-mediated immune functions with variable results.

5. Sulfur-containing compounds such as **levamisole** (a phenylimidothiazole anthelmintic) and **imuthiol** have been shown to have immunostimulatory activity with generally more effect on cell-mediated than humoral immunity. Levamisole has recently been approved as an oral agent for use in colon cancer in combination with fluorouracil.

6. **Inosine pranobex** is licensed for use in many other countries as an immunostimulant. It seems to induce T-cell differentiation and augment cell-mediated immune functions with minimal toxicity.

7. As a component of mycobacterial cell walls, **muramyl dipeptide (MDP)** is a stimulator of macrophage activation and may be used as an adjuvant given with antigen (see I), or as an immunostimulant given alone.

STUDY QUESTIONS

Directions: Each of the numbered items or incomplete statements in this section is followed by answers or by completions of the statement. Select the **one** lettered answer or completion that is **best** in each case.

1. A young child becomes infected by a serotype of *Streptococcus* to which his immune system has never before responded. What is the expected minimum latency between initial infection and the appearance of serum antibody specific to the organism?

(A) 2 days
(B) 4 days
(C) 7 days
(D) 14 days

2. Which of the following classes of antibody has the longest serum half-life and opsonizes antigens for phagocytosis through two different pathways?

(A) Immunoglobulin G (IgG)
(B) Immunoglobulin M (IgM)
(C) Immunoglobulin A (IgA)
(D) Immunoglobulin E (IgE)

3. Urticaria appearing rapidly after the ingestion of food is usually indicative of which type of hypersensitivity reaction?

(A) Type I
(B) Type II
(C) Type III
(D) Type IV

4. In which of the following autoimmune pathologies is the mechanism of pathogenesis classified as a type II hypersensitivity?

(A) Systemic lupus erythematosus (SLE)
(B) Insulin-dependent diabetes mellitus (IDDM)
(C) Graves' disease
(D) Hashimoto's thyroiditis

5. A patient presents with symptoms of nasal congestion and difficulty in breathing. The symptoms are not present during the day or prior to retiring, but the patient awakens with these symptoms. Which type of hypersensitivity would be most likely to account for these symptoms?

(A) Type I
(B) Type II
(C) Type III
(D) Type IV

6. Which of the following examples of type IV hypersensitivity reactions represents a situation where the tissue-damaging pathology could be considered as an "inappropriate" response by the immune system?

(A) Poison ivy dermatitis
(B) Chronic tuberculosis
(C) Acute graft rejection
(D) Tuberculin test

7. Which of the following agents is commonly used in the therapy of multiple sclerosis (MS)?

(A) Neostigmine
(B) Cyanocobalamin
(C) Adrenocorticotropic hormone (ACTH)
(D) Propylthiouracil

8. The therapeutic role of muromonab-CD3 in acute renal graft rejection is probably based upon which of the following effects?

(A) Activation of T-cell function and secretion of cytokines
(B) Destruction of T cells by complement
(C) Opsonization of T cells for phagocytosis
(D) Selective inhibition of the functioning of T_H cells

1-C 4-D 7-C
2-A 5-C 8-C
3-A 6-A

9. Which of the following is a current clinical application of intravenous human immune globulin (IGIV)?

(A) Prophylaxis after hepatitis B virus (HBV) exposure
(B) Therapy of humoral immunodeficiency
(C) Prophylactic infant immunization for polio
(D) Prophylaxis for Rh disease via infant immunization

10. Which of the following cytokines is currently approved for the therapy of certain forms of cancer?

(A) Interleukin-2 (IL-2)
(B) Interferon α (IFNα)
(C) Interferon γ (IFNγ)
(D) Imuthiol

Questions 11 and 12

A 6-year-old child presents with a deep puncture wound. The parent is unsure of the child's history of vaccination.

11. If no other information is available, the physician should recommend which of the following?

(A) No vaccinations
(B) Tetanus immune globulin (TIG)
(C) Tetanus toxoid (Td)
(D) Both TIG and Td at separate sites

12. If it were discovered that the child had received a full series of diphtheria, pertussis, tetanus (DPT) vaccinations, the last at entry into school, what should the physician recommend concerning immediate revaccination?

(A) None
(B) TIG
(C) Td
(D) Both TIG and Td at separate sites

13. Persistent infections by opportunistic pathogens such as *Candida albicans* and *Pneumocystis carinii* could be indicative of all of the following EXCEPT

(A) inherited T-cell immunodeficiency
(B) humoral immunodeficiency
(C) acquired immune deficiency syndrome (AIDS)
(D) combined immunodeficiency

14. Correct statements concerning human immunodeficiency virus (HIV) include all of the following EXCEPT

(A) individuals who become infected with the HIV-1 virus always demonstrate overt symptoms shortly after infection
(B) seroconversion to positive status for anti-HIV-1 antibodies is the primary criterion for diagnosis of a viral carrier
(C) the incubation period for the pathogenesis of acquired immune deficiency syndrome (AIDS) is currently believed to be 8 or more years after the initial infection with HIV
(D) $CD4^+$ T cells and macrophages may be able to spread the HIV virus to uninfected $CD4^+$ cells without the release of any extracellular virus particles

---

9-B	12-A
10-B	13-B
11-D	14-A

Directions: Each item below contains three suggested answers, of which **one or more** is correct. Choose the answer

A if **I only** is correct
B if **III only** is correct
C if **I and II** are correct
D if **II and III** are correct
E if **I, II, and III** are correct

15. Which of the following statements are true concerning the currently approved sheep Fab fragment used to counteract digoxin overdoses?

I. It is obtained by the immunization of sheep with a digoxin–protein conjugate and subsequent proteolytic cleavage of the collected antibody
II. It specifically binds digoxin, thereby preventing its activity
III. It has a serum half-life of about 3 weeks

16. $CD4^+$ T cells are capable of specifically recognizing antigens in which of the following forms?

I. Bound to major histocompatibility (MHC) class I molecules on the surface of any body cell
II. In free, soluble form in extracellular fluids
III. Bound to MHC class II molecules on the surface of special antigen presenting cells (APCs)

17. Which of the following describes a normal outcome of the activation of the complement system by either classical or alternative pathways?

I. Acute inflammation
II. Opsonization of immune complexes
III. Cytolytic action

18. In antiviral immunity, which of the following aspects of immunity is thought to provide the function of direct recognition and killing of viral-infected cells?

I. Cytotoxic T cells (CTL)
II. Antiviral antibodies
III. Interferons

19. Suppose that a patient has already been treated with penicillin and has produced antibodies against the drug that are still mostly present, when an emergency situation requires giving a dose of penicillin IV. If this patient is exhibiting a type I penicillin hypersensitivity reaction, which of the following pathologic consequences would be expected and within what time course of clinical onset?

I. Hemolytic anemia, onset of 1–2 hours after the intravenous dose
II. Anaphylaxis, onset of a few minutes after the intravenous dose
III. Cutaneous urticaria and pruritus, onset of a few minutes after the intravenous dose

20. Which of the following observations would be common to all instances of type IV hypersensitivity reactions?

I. Infiltration of the affected tissue by mononuclear cells
II. Twelve or more hour delay in clinical symptoms after allergen contact
III. Significant beneficial effect of the administration of H_1-antagonists

21. Which of the following immunologic findings is NOT unique to systemic lupus erythematosus (SLE)?

I. Hypergammaglobulinemia
II. Presence of circulating antinuclear antibodies
III. Presence of circulating rheumatoid factors

22. In seeking an organ donor who is human leukocyte antigen (HLA) matched with the recipient of the graft, which of the following individuals would be at least somewhat likely to provide an HLA match?

I. A sibling of the graft recipient
II. A parent of the graft recipient
III. A cadaver

15-C	18-A	21-E
16-B	19-D	22-A
17-E	20-C	

SUMMARY OF DIRECTIONS

A	B	C	D	E
I only	III only	I, II only	II, III only	All are correct

23. Graft-versus-host (GVH) disease is a problem associated primarily with which type of transplantation?

I. Kidney
II. Heart
III. Bone marrow

24. The prophylactic use of cyclosporine in graft rejection is probably based upon its ability to

I. inhibit the synthesis of antibodies, thereby preventing hyperacute rejection
II. inhibit the activation of T cells, thereby preventing acute rejection
III. block the transcription of interleukin-2 (IL-2) gene, and the synthesis/secretion of IL-2

25. Which of the following is a valid comparison of live, attenuated and killed, inactivated active vaccines?

I. Replication of the organisms in a live, attenuated vaccine increases the stimulation of the immune system, thereby often requiring a lower dose
II. Hypersensitivity reactions are more common with killed, inactivated vaccines
III. It is more likely that a killed, inactivated vaccine will produce lifelong immunity in one or two doses

26. Which of the following active vaccines is recommended for health care workers but is not routinely administered to infants?

I. Measles, mumps, rubella (MMR) vaccine
II. Influenza polyvalent
III. Tetanus toxoid (Td)

27. Which of the following is true about inactivated polio vaccine (IPV) as compared to oral polio vaccine (OPV)?

I. IPV is administered to immunocompromised children and families; otherwise, OPV is the vaccine of choice
II. OPV is thought to afford superior protection since the vaccine is introduced through the normal route of entry for poliovirus infection
III. The risks of severe side effects are greater for OPV than for IPV

23-B
24-D
25-C
26-D
27-E

ANSWERS AND EXPLANATIONS

1. The answer is C *[I C 2, 3].*
Assuming that the child has a normal primary immune response, significant production of serum antibody should occur during a 7–10 day period after exposure to the organism in question. The first antibody to appear will be IgM.

2. The answer is A *[I D 2 b, E].*
Immunoglobulin G (IgG) has a serum half-life of 25–35 days, longer than any other class [although mast cell-bound immunoglobulin E (IgE) has the longest half-life]. In general, immune complexes containing IgG are opsonized for phagocytosis through binding to the IgG receptors on neutrophils and macrophages, and additionally via the activation of complement. Although immunoglobulin M (IgM) also opsonizes, it only does so via the activation of complement.

3. The answer is A *[II A 5 a, b].*
Food allergies are usually type I pathologies. In an individual with preexisting hypersecreted immunoglobulin E (IgE) specific to a food allergen and bound to mast cells, the allergic response would be expected within a brief time after ingestion. Mast cell secretions would commonly lead to vomiting, and systemic spillover of allergen into the circulation could lead to milder effects in other tissues, such as urticaria.

4. The answer is D *[II C 2 c; III D 2 b].*
Anti-thyroid peroxidase antibodies can produce complement-mediated cytotoxicity to thyroid follicle cells, a type II pathogenic mechanism. In systemic lupus erythematosus (SLE), persistent circulating immune complexes are responsible for much of the pathogenesis (type III); in Graves' disease, an antibody acting as a thyroid-stimulating hormone (TSH) agonist hyperstimulates the thyroid (type V); in insulin-dependent diabetes mellitus (IDDM), T-cell cytotoxicity to beta islet cells is probably responsible for the major pathogenesis (type IV).

5. The answer is C *[II D 2, 4 b, 5 b].*
Local respiratory inflammation is a common possibility in types I and III due to inhaled allergens. In this case, the inflammatory response is not immediate, but requires several hours to develop, therefore arguing against type I pathogenesis. A common example of this local respiratory type III pathogenesis would be exposure to bacterial or fungal spores in the microdroplets produced by dirty ultrasonic room humidifiers.

6. The answer is A *[II E 1].*
Poison ivy contains a hapten, pentadecyl catechol, which in itself is not known to be toxic. Its capacity to elicit an immune response is, therefore, inappropriate since it serves no useful function. In chronic tuberculosis, the immune response is attempting (although unsuccessfully) to eliminate the mycobacterial pathogen. Acute graft rejection is also appropriate (even if unfortunate), since it is a response against foreign tissue. A tuberculin test is an appropriate manifestation of the existence of active immunity/memory to *Mycobacterium*.

7. The answer is C *[III D 8 b].*
Adrenocorticotropic hormone (ACTH) is the immunosuppressive agent of choice in multiple sclerosis (MS). Neostigmine is used as an anticholinergic in myasthenia gravis, cyanocobalamin is administered in autoimmune pernicious anemia to replace nonabsorbed vitamin B_{12}, and propylthiouracil is used as an antithyroid in Graves' disease.

8. The answer is C *[V D 2 c].*
Muromonab-CD3 is a mouse anti-CD3 monoclonal antibody that binds to all T cells, since CD3 is a constant part of each T cell's antigen receptor. The binding of muromonab-CD3 opsonizes the T cells for phagocytosis. Total T cell numbers are thereby reduced. Mouse antibodies are inefficient at activating human complement. Some T-cell activation with cytokine secretion does occur, but this is an undesirable side effect of muromonab-CD3 administration.

9. The answer is B *[VI B 1 c; Table 8-2].*
Intravenous human immune globulins (IGIV) are used to replace antibody in immunodeficient individuals. Hepatitis B immune globulin (HBIG) is administered intramuscularly. Anti-RhD antibody is also administered intramuscularly to the mother immediately postpartum (sometimes during pregnancy), but not to the infant. Prophylactic infant immunization for polio is via active, not passive vaccination.

10. The answer is B *[VII D].*
Interferon α (IFNα) is approved for use in patients with hairy cell leukemia and in acquired immune deficiency syndrome (AIDS) patients with Kaposi's sarcoma. At least some of its beneficial effects probably derive from its growth inhibitory activity. The other cytokines listed are in various stages of clinical trials as antineoplastic therapies, although interferon γ (IFNγ) is approved for use in patients with chronic granulomatous disease. Imuthiol is not a cytokine, but rather a synthetic drug.

11 and 12. The answers are: 11-D, 12-A *[VI D 3 a; Table 8-3].*
If the history of vaccination is uncertain, individuals with tetanus-prone wounds require both active and passive vaccination. The tetanus immune globulin (TIG) affords immediate protection in the event that the individual does not have memory. The tetanus toxoid (Td) begins the series leading to the establishment of memory. These recommendations should serve as general guidelines.

A tetanus-prone wound occurring in an individual with a full series of active vaccinations requires no treatment if the last vaccination in the series was administered less than 5 years before. Note that these are recommendations that should serve as general guidelines.

13. The answer is B *[IV A, B 6].*
Opportunistic infections by fungi, viruses, and parasites other than extracellular pyogenic bacteria would tend to suggest deficiency of T-cell functions. Choices A and C represent inherited and acquired T-cell deficiencies, respectively. Choice D includes both humoral and T-cell deficiency. Only choice B is a primarily humoral deficiency in which the expected signs would be recurrent infections by extracellular pyogenic bacteria.

14. The answer is A *[IV B 6].*
It is not known what percentage of individuals demonstrate overt symptoms subsequent to initial infections. Those individuals that do, generally show mononucleosis-like symptoms for an approximately 3-week period. However, it is believed that some individuals display no overt symptoms.

15. The answer is C (I, II) *[I A 4, D 2, 5; VII A].*
Digoxin is a hapten, a molecule that is too small to stimulate responses (be an immunogen) in its free form but which can be recognized by antibodies. Therefore, to obtain sheep antidigoxin antibodies, the sheep must be immunized with digoxin that has been coupled to a larger molecule (a protein in this case). The antibodies obtained from the sheep are then cleaved with proteolytic enzymes to yield the Fab fragment. This fragment is specific to and can bind digoxin, thereby blocking its biologic activity. Animal antibodies have a shorter serum half-life when injected into humans, and all Fab fragments (even human) have a short half-life by comparison to complete antibody molecules. Only complete human immunoglobulin G (IgG) has a half-life of approximately 1 month.

16. The answer is B (III) *[I B 3, 5].*
$CD4^+$ or helper T cells have receptors that recognize fragments (epitopes) of immunizing antigens (immunogens) only when these fragments are bound to an MHC class II molecule on the surface of antigen presenting cells (APCs). This prevents T cells from being inappropriately activated by soluble antigens. $CD8^+$ T cells recognize fragments bound to MHC class I molecules.

17. The answer is E (all) *[I E 2].*
When complement is activated, different proteins of the complement sequence have functions that lead to all three of the actions. Acute inflammation allows greater movement of plasma proteins and phagocytes from blood to tissues. Opsonization of immune complexes enhances their phagocytosis. Cytolysis of microorganisms often results in their killing.

18. The answer is A (I) *[I F 2].*
Antiviral antibodies are probably most important in extracellular immunity to viruses, binding virus particles for opsonization and preventing additional infection of cells. Interferons are secreted from viral-infected and other cells (e.g., macrophages, T cells) and after binding to receptors, induce the appearance of antiviral proteins in other cells. Cytotoxic T cells (CTLs) are capable of recognizing viral-infected cells and producing direct cytotoxicity.

19. The answer is D (II, III) *[II A 2 d, 6, 7, C 1 b, 5].*
If the patient has produced antibodies that are still present, and the hypersensitivity reaction is type I, these antibodies will be hypersecreted immunoglobulin E (IgE) mostly bound to mast cell and basophil IgE receptors (their half-life is several months). Intravenous introduction of penicillin results in rapid activation

of and secretion by blood basophils with rapid (within minutes) symptoms of type I hypersensitivity. These may be severe (anaphylaxis), or less severe (cutaneous, gastrointestinal, respiratory symptoms), depending upon the individual patient. Hemolytic anemia would be an expected result of a type II hypersensitivity to penicillin, based on the presence of immunoglobulin M (IgM) or immunoglobulin G (IgG) antibodies in serum, and the onset would be delayed by a few hours in a patient with preexisting antibodies.

20. The answer is C (I, II) *[II E 3–6].*
Type IV hypersensitivity reactions are always delayed after the introduction of allergen, as allergen-specific T cells become activated and attract other cells, such as macrophages, to the site of allergen introduction (e.g., the epidermis of the skin in contact sensitivity, the lungs in tuberculosis). These sites are, therefore, infiltrated by mononuclear cells. Inflammation is, however, mostly due to tissue disruption and necrosis and secretion of cytokines by the infiltrating cells. Although histamine secretion can also occur from local mast cells, H_1 antagonists of histamine should not be expected to have significant effects, since T-cell and macrophage activation, migration, and secretion will not be greatly affected by these drugs.

21. The answer is E (all) *[III C 3 b, E 1, 2].*
All three of the findings are common to more than one of the nonorgan specific autoimmune pathologies but are present in different percentages of patients with specific pathologies. For example antinuclear antibodies are probably present in all patients with systemic lupus erythematosus (SLE) but are found in only a fraction of rheumatoid arthritis and Sjögren syndrome patients. Rheumatoid factors are more common in rheumatoid arthritis than in SLE or Sjögren syndrome, and hypergammaglobulinemia is more prevalent in SLE than in Sjögren syndrome.

22. The answer is A (I) *[V A 3, B].*
Parents and children are almost never human leukocyte antigen (HLA) matched but are usually half-matched. The probability of an HLA match from a cadaver-derived organ is extremely low. The probability that two siblings will be HLA matched is 25% and 50% that they will be half-matched.

23. The answer is B (III) *[V B 2, C 1].*
In bone marrow transplantation, marrow containing competent lymphocytes is transplanted to a generally immunosuppressed host. Therefore, the greatest problem is an immune response by the graft against human leukocyte antigens (HLA) and other tissue antigens of the host. In renal and cardiac transplantation, the greatest problem is rejection of the foreign organ by the immune system of the host (host-versus-graft disease).

24. The answer is D (II, III) *[V B 2, D 2 a].*
Cell-mediated immune mechanisms are thought to be more important in acute graft rejection, and the inhibition of T-cell activation appears to be the key element in immunosuppression. Responding T cells require signalling from interleukin-2 (IL-2) to reach full activation and progress to cell division. IL-2 is produced by activated T cells and, therefore, can act autocrinely. Cyclosporine somehow blocks transcription of the IL-2 gene during T-cell activation, thereby inhibiting synthesis of IL-2 and preventing full T-cell activation and division. Its effects are, thus, limited to activated T cells. It has no direct effect on antibody synthesis and, therefore, is not useful in the hyperacute rejection phenomena that are based upon antibody-mediated mechanisms. Besides, hyperacute rejection is essentially nontreatable, since it depends upon the preexistence of antibodies in the graft recipient.

25. The answer is C (I, II) *[VI C 2 a, b].*
Live, attenuated vaccines introduce organisms competent to replicate, and this replication increases the amount of stimulation of the immune response. For this and probably other reasons, it is more likely that a live, attenuated, not a killed, inactivated, vaccine will provide lifelong immunity in one or two doses. Hypersensitivity reactions to vaccines are generally due to accessory components found in the vaccine as a result of its preparation. Such reactions are more common with killed, inactivated vaccines.

26. The answer is D (II, III) *[VI C 1 d; Table 8-3].*
The measles, mumps, rubella (MMR) vaccine is routinely administered to infants within or shortly after their first year, and a second dose is now recommended at school entry. Influenza active vaccine is generally targeted toward specific adult populations; health care workers are included in this target population, as are infants and children at risk, but the vaccine is not routinely administered to infants. Tetanus toxoid (Td) is not routinely administered to infants, who instead should receive diphtheria, tetanus, pertussis (DTP). Td is intended primarily for initial vaccinations in adults not previously vaccinated and for 10-year booster vaccinations in all individuals, including health care workers.

27. The answer is E (all) *[VI C 2; Table 8-3].*
Since oral polio vaccine (OPV) is a live, attenuated vaccine, it is not used in immunocompromised individuals who would have difficulty clearing the replicating virus; in general, live, attenuated vaccines are not given to immunocompromised individuals. Since individuals vaccinated with OPV become transient carriers of the attenuated virus, family members of such individuals are likewise not vaccinated, except with inactivated polio vaccine (IPV). OPV is the vaccine of choice for others and is given orally, the normal route of viral entry. This induces secretory immunoglobulin A (sIgA) in addition to immunoglobulin G (IgG), thereby providing increased protection. The risk of reversion to virulence (vaccine-induced polio) is small for OPV but probably nonexistent for IPV.

9
Biotechnology

John D. Leary

I. INTRODUCTION. Biotechnology is the application of the basic concepts of molecular biology to produce useful products for pharmaceutical, veterinary, clinical biochemistry, and agricultural uses. These products are proteins used for therapy (e.g., human insulin, erythropoietin) and immunotherapy, for diagnostic testing reagents, for the study of drug action, and as agricultural pesticides and chemicals.

II. BASIC BIOCHEMISTRY

A. Peptides and proteins

1. **Chemistry.** Peptides and proteins are formed from 20 L-amino acids via peptide (amide) covalent bonds. The peptide bond is the backbone of the protein molecule.
   a. **Dipeptides** contain two amino acids; **polypeptides** contain many amino acids.
   b. **Proteins** are polymers containing large numbers of amino acids (e.g., insulin, 51; chymotrypsin, 241).
      (1) **Globular proteins** are three-dimensional molecules with various sizes and shapes (see discussion of conformation in II A 2). Most proteins are of this type.
      (2) **Fibrous proteins** are most useful for structural purposes; these protein molecules hold things together. They include the proteins of skin and muscle tissue, and animal fibers such as hair, wool, and silk.
2. **Conformation**
   a. **Shape.** Native proteins fold into specific shapes, which affect biologic activity; for example, an extended linear molecule curls up into a spherical globular mass, which is needed for biologic activity.
   b. **Denaturation.** Loss of shape may be due to heat, pH, or urea, leading to loss of biologic action; for example, egg albumin, which is a liquid, is converted into a white solid on heating.
   c. **Storage.** Many proteins are stored at 4°C if in solution or suspension. Others are freeze-dried (lyophilized) powders, which are reconstituted when dispensed.
3. **Sequence** is the arrangement or succession of amino acids in a protein molecule.
   a. **Order.** The arrangement of amino acids starts with the free amino group (N-terminal) at one end and proceeds to the free carboxyl group (C-terminal) at the opposite end.
   b. **Control.** The orderly sequence of amino acids is under the control of genes and the genetic code (see II B 2 d).
   c. **Simple proteins** consist only of amino acids when they are completely hydrolyzed.
   d. **Conjugated proteins** require a nonprotein part joined to the protein part [e.g., sugar (glycoprotein), lipid (lipoprotein), and porphyrin (hemoglobin)] to be biologically useful. Hemoglobin can be separated in the laboratory into heme (the porphyrin unit containing iron) and the protein part called globin; however, this molecule cannot transport oxygen in the blood cells unless it is intact.
   e. **Levels of protein structure**
      (1) The **primary level of protein structure** consists of an orderly sequence of amino acids mentioned in II A 3 a.
      (2) The **secondary level of protein structure** consists of a helix that is formed by hydrogen bonding between a carboxyl group and a hydrogen atom. The hydrogen atom is attached to an amino group located several amino acids distant in the amino acid sequence.

(3) The **tertiary level of protein structure** consists of a folded protein molecule, which creates a biologically suitable shape that is stabilized by hydrogen bonds (R-groups), disulfide bonds, ionic attractions, hydrophobic attractions, or metals.
(4) The **quaternary level of protein structure** consists of two or more separate (identical or different) protein chains, which are needed to form a functional protein (e.g., hemoglobin has two α and two β protein chains in the globin portion of the molecule).

B. Nucleic acids

1. **Chemistry.** Nucleic acids are biopolymers composed of nucleotides with a sugar–phosphate backbone.
   a. **Nucleotides** consist of heterocyclic nitrogen bases (i.e., purines, pyrimidines) bonded to either deoxyribose-5′-phosphate or ribose-5′-phosphate.
   b. **Purines.** Adenine (A) and guanine (G) are the nitrogen bases found in both deoxyribonucleic acid (DNA) and ribonucleic acid (RNA).
   c. **Pyrimidines.** Cytosine (C) and either thymine (T) (DNA) or uracil (RNA) are the nitrogen bases found in nucleic acids.
2. **DNA** is a double-stranded polynucleotide molecule formed into a double helix to serve as an informational polymer.
   a. **Base pairing.** The nitrogen bases project into the center of the helix from the sugar–phosphate backbone.
   b. **Complementary base pairing.** Hydrogen bonds form between A and T or G and C.
   c. **Stability.** Base stacking and hydrogen bonds contribute to the stability of DNA.
   d. **Sequence.** The sequence of nucleotides on one strand of DNA form a unit called a **gene.** Genes contain information for the biosynthesis of peptides which then form proteins.
   e. **Location.** DNA is located in the nucleus of higher organisms (eukaryotes) or in the nucleoid of bacteria (prokaryotes). Some DNA is also located in plasmids (see IV B 3), mitochondria, and chloroplasts.
3. **RNA** is a polyribonucleotide, which is single-stranded and forms hydrogen bonds to other nucleic acids, such as DNA, or it forms hydrogen bonds within the same polynucleotide, as in tRNA.
   a. **Messenger RNA (mRNA).** Ribonucleotides of variable sizes take information from DNA genes and form polymers with codons (three adjacent nucleotides) used to determine the amino acid sequence in the proteins made by cells.
   b. **Transfer RNA (tRNA).** Polyribonucleotides of similar sizes are used to carry specific amino acids to the ribosomes to make the proteins. Anticodons on the second arm of the tRNAs form complementary base pairs with the mRNA codons to control the exact sequence of amino acids in proteins.
   c. **Ribosomal RNA (rRNA).** Several polyribonucleotides of differing sizes and shapes combine with peptides or proteins to form a supramolecular complex to serve as the site for protein synthesis in cells (i.e., the ribosome). For example, in prokaryotes, such as *Escherichia coli*, the ribosome is a 70S (S stands for Svedberg unit) molecule comprised of a 20S small subunit and a 50S large subunit.

C. DNA and RNA biosynthesis. An orderly progression of information from the DNA gene to the biosynthesis of the completed protein is divided into steps. The flow of information proceeds normally from DNA synthesis to the synthesis of the different RNA molecules to protein formation. These steps are described below.

1. **Replication** is the duplication of DNA by cells during **mitosis** (cell division).
   a. A semiconservative method of duplicating the DNA involves one strand from the original DNA, which serves as a **template,** or as a model, for adding deoxyribonucleotides by complementary base pairing to form the new strand. The other DNA strand from the original DNA serves as the template for the synthesis of the second new DNA strand and remains with it to eventually go to the new cell.
   b. Three kinds of DNA polymerases are involved in replication; of these, polymerase III is the major enzyme for synthesis, while the other polymerases serve to correct errors and perform related functions.
   c. Replication usually shows no mutations, so an exact copy of DNA is made; the term to indicate this is **fidelity.** Mutations may occur due to drugs, chemicals, or radiation.

2. **Transcription** entails the production of RNAs from ribonucleotides.
   a. Genes on DNA serve as templates to make RNAs.
   b. RNA polymerase is used in transcription.
3. **Translation** entails the production of specific proteins at the ribosome from information on DNA genes via the message on mRNA.
   a. Multiple copies of one strand of protein may be made from one mRNA, using several ribosomes (polyribosomes).
   b. Tailoring the final protein may remove unnecessary amino acids or may need the addition of nonprotein groups like heme.

III. PROTEIN ISOLATION

A. Physical and chemical properties

1. Generally, proteins are hydrophilic molecules. Proteins may have **hydrophobic regions** (inside of the folded protein) and **hydrophilic regions** (outside of the folded protein facing water); the polar and nonpolar character is based on the side chains of amino acids and their orientation.
2. The various levels of protein structure and the forces that hold the conformation together affect the biologic action.

B. Isolation

1. A dilute solution of salt (ammonium sulfate) or alcohol is used to extract most proteins at 4°C to reduce the risk of denaturation.
2. The protein mixture is precipitated by increasing the salt or alcohol concentration to decrease the water availability to the proteins.

C. **Purification.** The precipitated protein mixture is re-dissolved in buffer solutions and purified by the following methods:

1. Dialysis
2. Isoelectric precipitation (**pI** is the **point of minimum solubility,** which varies with each protein)
3. Gel filtration (molecular sieve)

D. Validation of purity

1. **Electrophoresis** separates proteins at a specific pH on buffered gel (based on the net charge of the protein molecule). A single band suggests purity.
2. **Comparison with reference protein.** The same electrophoretic behavior of two samples indicates purity of the isolated and purified protein.

E. Lyophilization

1. **Freeze-drying** of the protein removes water to increase stability for storage.
2. **Lability.** Many proteins are unstable in solution so they are packaged in the dried form.

IV. RECOMBINANT DNA TECHNOLOGY is the process by which DNA genes from a source organism are biochemically joined to DNA genes of a host cell to form a new hybrid DNA; for example, the human insulin gene is inserted into *E. coli,* and then the bacteria are grown to form human insulin.

A. **Human genome** is the **sum total** of all the genetic information contained in 23 pairs of chromosomes, containing thousands of genes composed of about four billion nucleotide pairs (base pairs). Basic research is underway to identify (map) the whole human genome to aid in understanding disease. Probes can locate many specific genes, both normal and mutated (defective).

1. **Desired genes,** capable of synthesizing the expected proteins, can be isolated.
2. **Defective genes,** causes of genetic disease, can be identified; data are then used by genetic counselors to assist patients and caregivers with the medical options available.

B. Biotechnology

1. **Gene removal.** Restriction enzymes selectively remove genes at specific points along DNA molecules.
2. **Gene synthesis.** If the amino acid sequence is known, small genes may be synthesized in the laboratory.
3. **Host organism.** *E. coli*, yeasts, or mammalian cells are selected to receive the new gene; plasmids are also often used to receive the new gene. **DNA ligase** is used to tie in the ends of the genes to the plasmid DNA.
4. **Protein synthesis.** New host cells are induced to form the desired protein from rRNA. Glycoproteins (e.g., erythropoietin), which require glycosylation of proteins, are usually carried out in mammalian cell culture.

V. BIOTECHNOLOGY POTENTIAL

A. New drug development. The development of new drugs is a promising prospect as evidenced by the burgeoning of both approved drug products (Table 9-1) and those currently in development or clinical trials.

B. Diagnostic agents. There are large numbers of drug products used as diagnostic agents for both animal and human subjects. These products are also useful as research tools (e.g., in drug-receptor studies).

C. Gene therapy. Isolated genes have been used to replace defective genes in a limited number of clinical trials of patients with blood disorders. The potential for gene therapy is limitless, but it is still in the early stages of development.

Table 9-1. Approved Biotechnology Drug Products

Class	Drug Product	Use	Year
Hormones	Human insulin	Diabetes	1982
	Somatotropin	Human growth hormone in children	1985
Interferons	Gamma-1b	Chronic granulomatous disease	1990
	Alfa-n3	Genital warts	1989
	Alfa-2b	Hairy cell leukemia	1986
		Genital warts	
		AIDS (Kaposi's sarcoma)	1988
		Hepatitis C (HCV)	1991
Blood	Erythropoietin	Anemia associated with chronic renal failure and anemia with zidovudine-treated HIV infection	1989
	Hemophilia factor VIII	Blood clotting factor	1992
Colony stimulating factors	GM-CSF	Autologous bone marrow transplantation	1991
	rG-CSF	Chemotherapy-induced neutropenia	1991
Vaccines	Hepatitis B (HBV) [recombinant]	HBV prevention	1986
Monoclonal antibody	Muromonab-CD3 (OKT3)	Acute kidney transplant rejection	1986
Tissue plasminogen activator	Alteplase	Acute myocardial infarction	1987
		Acute pulmonary embolism	1990
Enzyme	Glucocerebrosidase	Gaucher's disease (lipid storage disorder)	1992

AIDS = acquired immune deficiency syndrome; HIV = human immunodeficiency virus.

STUDY QUESTIONS

Directions: Each question below contains three suggested answers of which **one or more** is correct. Choose the answer

A if **I only** is correct
B if **III only** is correct
C if **I and II** are correct
D if **II and III** are correct
E if **I, II, and III** are correct

1. The conformation or shape of a globular protein is affected by

I. heat
II. pH
III. urea

2. What molecule controls the biosynthesis of proteins in living organisms?

I. DNA
II. RNA
III. Proteins

1-E
2-A

ANSWERS AND EXPLANATIONS

1. The answer is E (all) *[II A 2 b].*
The conformation of a protein is important to its intended activity and may be changed by pH, heat, or urea. Purified proteins are often buffered to control pH and stored at 4°C to minimize denaturation (altered conformation).

2. The answer is A (I) *[II B 2 d, e].*
The sequence of a DNA molecule forms a unit called a gene. It was proposed that each protein that is formed in a living organism has information that is contained in a gene. In some proteins, there may be two or more genes that code for the information; the original hypothesis has been modified to one gene–one peptide to account for proteins that are made up of two or more peptide chains. Most of the DNA that contains the genetic information is located on chromosomes that are found in the nucleus of eukaryotes; in prokaryotes, the information is in a region called the nucleoid.

10
Medicinal Chemistry

Edward F. LaSala

I. DRUG SOURCES AND MAJOR CLASSES

A. Natural products are drugs obtained from plant and animal sources.

1. **Alkaloids** are potent nitrogenous bases, obtained primarily from plants through extraction and purification (e.g., **morphine,** from the opium poppy; **atropine,** from the belladonna plant).
2. **Hormones** are potent organic substances (principally proteins and steroids) primarily obtained from animal sources (e.g., **insulin,** a protein obtained from the pancreas; **conjugated estrogens,** steroids obtained from the urine of pregnant mares).
3. **Glycosides** are organic substances consisting of a glucose (sugar) moiety bound to an aglycone (nonsugar) moiety by means of an ether bond (e.g., **digitoxin, amygdalin**).
4. **Antibiotics** are antimicrobial agents obtained from microorganisms (e.g., **penicillin, tetracycline**).

B. Synthetic products are drugs synthesized from organic compounds.

1. Synthetic products may have **chemical structures closely resembling those of active natural products** (e.g., **hydroxymorphone,** which resembles morphine; **ampicillin,** which resembles penicillin).
2. Synthetic products also may be **completely new products,** obtained by screening synthesized materials for drug activity (e.g., **barbiturates, antibacterial sulfonamides, thiazide diuretics, phenothiazine antipsychotics, benzodiazepine anxiolytics**).

II. DRUG ACTION AND PHYSICOCHEMICAL PROPERTIES

A. Drug action represents an artificial interference with an organism's natural (although not necessarily normal) function.

1. Systemically active drugs must **enter** and **be transported by body fluids**.
   a. The drug must **pass various membrane barriers, escape excessive distribution** into sites of loss, and **penetrate to the active site**.
   b. At the active site, the drug molecules must orient themselves and interact with the receptors to **alter function**.
   c. The drug must be removed from the active site and must be **metabolized** to a form that is easily **excreted by the body**.
2. Drug absorption, metabolism, utilization, and excretion all depend on the **drug's physicochemical properties** and the **host's physiologic and biochemical properties**. A drug's physicochemical properties can be altered; the host's properties cannot be altered.

B. Physicochemical properties of drugs include water solubility, liposolubility, ionization of acids or bases, ionization of salts, and hydrolysis of salts.

1. **Water solubility** depends on the drug's polarity. Polar substances are more water soluble than nonpolar substances; the degree of polarity depends on the extent of the drug's ionic character.
2. **Liposolubility** also depends on drug polarity.
   a. **Nonpolar substances** are more liposoluble than polar substances.

b. **Non–oxygen-containing functional groups,** such as alkyl and aryl groups, increase the drug's partition coefficient and impart liposolubility.
c. **Nonionized molecules** are nonpolar and, hence, liposoluble.

3. **Ionization of acids and bases** plays a role with substances that dissociate into ions.
a. The **ionization constant (K_a)** indicates the relative strength of the acid or base. An acid with a K_a of 1×10^{-3} is stronger (more ionized) than one with a K_a of 1×10^{-5}.
b. The **negative log of the ionization constant (pK_a)** also indicates the relative strength of the acid or base. An acid with a pK_a of 5 ($K_a = 1 \times 10^{-5}$) is weaker (less ionized) than one with a pK_a of 3 ($K_a = 1 \times 10^{-3}$).
c. **Strong acids** [e.g., hydrochloric acid (HCl), sulfuric acid (H_2SO_4), nitric acid (HNO_3), hydrobromic acid (HBr), iodic acid (HIO_3), perchloric acid ($HClO_4$)] are completely ionized. Almost all other acids, including organic acids, are weak. **Organic acids** contain one or more of these functional groups:
(1) Carboxyl group (—COOH)
(2) Phenolic group (Ar—OH)
(3) Sulfonic acid group (—SO_2H)
(4) Sulfonamide group (—SO_2NH—R)
(5) Imide group (—CO—NH—CO—)
d. **Strong bases** [e.g., sodium hydroxide (NaOH), potassium hydroxide (KOH), magnesium hydroxide [$Mg(OH)_2$], calcium hydroxide [$Ca(OH)_2$], barium hydroxide [$Ba(OH)_2$], and quaternary ammonium hydroxides] are also completely ionized. Almost all other bases including organic bases, are weak.
(1) **Organic bases** contain a primary, secondary, or tertiary aliphatic or alicyclic amino group (—NH_2, —NHR, or —NR_2).
(2) Most aromatic or unsaturated heterocyclic nitrogens are so weakly basic that they do not readily form salts with acids. Saturated heterocyclic nitrogens, in contrast, are similar to aliphatic amines.
e. **Weak acids.** Ionization of a weak acid (e.g., acetic acid, which has a pK_a of 4.76) takes place as follows:

$$CH_3COOH \rightleftharpoons CH_3COO^- + H^+$$

(1) When a weak acid (such as acetic acid) is placed in an **acid medium,** the equilibrium shifts to the left, suppressing ionization. This decrease in ionization conforms to **LeChatelier's principle,** which states that when a stress is placed on an equilibrium reaction, the reaction will move in the direction that tends to relieve the stress.
(2) When a weak acid is placed in an **alkaline medium,** ionization increases. The H^+ ions from the acid and the OH^- ions from the alkaline medium combine to form water, shifting the equilibrium to the right.
(3) **Weakly acid drugs** are less ionized in acid media than in alkaline media. When the pK_a of an acidic drug is greater than the pH of the medium in which it exists, it will be more than 50% in its nonionized (molecular) form and, thus, more likely to cross lipid cellular membranes.
f. **Weak bases.** Ionization of a weak base is the opposite of that for a weak acid.
(1) Weak bases are less ionized in a **basic (alkaline) medium** and more ionized in an **acid medium**.
(2) **Weakly basic drugs** are less ionized in alkaline media than in acid media. When the pK_a of a basic drug is less than the pH of the medium in which it exists, it will be more than 50% in its nonionized (molecular) form and, thus, more likely to cross lipid cellular membranes.

4. **Ionization of a salt** plays a role with salt forms that dissociate into ions.
a. **All salts** (with the exceptions of mercuric and cadmium halides and lead acetate) **are strong electrolytes**. Thus, they are very polar and not liposoluble.
b. Drug salts that do not undergo hydrolysis are ionized in both acid and alkaline media. Thus, they are transported across cell membranes with great difficulty. (**Amphoteric drugs,** containing both acid and basic functional groups, are also ionized in both acid and alkaline media and have the same transportation difficulties.)

5. **Hydrolysis of a salt** plays a role with salt forms that dissociate in aqueous media.
a. Salts of **strong acids** and **weak bases** hydrolyze in an aqueous medium to yield an **acidic solution**.
b. Salts of **weak acids** and **strong bases** hydrolyze in an aqueous medium to yield an **alkaline solution**.

c. Salts of **weak acids** and **weak bases** hydrolyze in an aqueous medium to yield an **acidic, basic,** or **neutral solution,** depending on the respective ionization constants involved.

d. Salts of **strong acids** and **strong bases** do not hydrolyze in an aqueous medium; thus, their **solutions are neutral.**

6. A **neutralization reaction** may occur when an acidic solution of an organic salt (a solution of a salt of a strong acid and a weak base) is mixed with a basic solution (a solution of a salt of a weak acid and a strong base). The nonionized organic acid or the nonionized organic base is likely to **precipitate** in this case. This reaction is the basis for many **drug incompatibilities,** particularly when intravenous solutions are mixed. Neutralization reactions may be avoided by knowing how to predict the approximate pH of the aqueous solutions of common drug salts.

a. Generally, a drug's **salt form** may be recognized when the generic or trade name consists of two separate words, indicating a **cation** and an **anion.**

b. Drugs with **nitrate, sulfate,** or **hydrochloride anions** (e.g., pilocarpine nitrate, morphine sulfate, meperidine hydrochloride) are salts of **strong acids.** Thus, their cation portions (e.g., pilocarpine, morphine, meperidine) must be **bases.**

(1) Because pilocarpine, morphine, and meperidine are neither metal nor quaternary ammonium hydroxides, they must be **weak bases.**

(2) Salts of weak bases and strong acids are water soluble and form **acidic aqueous solutions.**

c. Drugs with **sodium** or **potassium cations** (e.g., warfarin sodium, potassium penicillin G) are salts of **strong bases.**

(1) Because these drugs are organic, they must be **weak acids.**

(2) Salts of strong bases and weak acids are water soluble and form **basic aqueous solutions.**

d. Drugs whose **cation name ends with the suffix -onium** or **-inium** and whose anion is a chloride, bromide, iodide, nitrate, or sulfate (e.g., benzalkonium chloride, cetylpyridinium chloride) are salts of **strong bases** and **strong acids** and form **neutral aqueous solutions.**

III. STRUCTURAL FEATURES AND PHARMACOLOGIC ACTIVITY.

Drugs may be classified as structurally nonspecific and structurally specific.

A. Structurally nonspecific drugs are those for which the drug's interaction with the cell membrane depends more on the drug molecule's physical characteristics than on its chemical structure. Usually, the interaction is based on the **cell membrane's lipid nature** and the **drug's lipid attraction.** Most **general anesthetics,** as well as some **hypnotics** and some **bactericidal agents,** act through this mechanism.

B. Structurally specific drugs are those for which pharmacologic activity is determined by the drug's ability to bind to a **specific endogenous receptor.**

1. Receptor site theory describes the pharmacologic activity of such drugs.

a. The **lock-and-key theory** postulates a complementary relationship between the drug molecule and a specific area on the surface of the enzyme molecule (i.e., the **active,** or **catalytic, site**) to which the drug molecule is bound as it undergoes the catalytic reaction.

b. The **occupational theory of response** further postulates that, for a structurally specific drug, the intensity of the pharmacologic effect is directly proportional to the number of receptors occupied by the drug.

2. Receptor site binding. The **ability to bind to a specific receptor,** while not independent of the drug's physical characteristics, is primarily determined by the drug's **chemical structure.**

a. In such an interaction, the drug's **chemical reactivity** plays an important role, reflected in its **bonding ability** and in the **exactness of its fit** to the receptor.

b. Drug interaction with a specific receptor is analogous to the fitting together of jigsaw puzzle pieces. Only drugs of similar shape (i.e., similar chemical structure) can bind to a specific receptor and initiate a biologic response.

c. Often, only a **critical portion of the drug molecule** (rather than the whole molecule) is involved in receptor site binding.

(1) The functional group making up this critical portion is known as a **pharmacophore.**

(2) Drugs with **similar critical regions** but differences in other parts may have similar qualitative (although not necessarily quantitative) pharmacologic activity.

d. In general, the better a drug fits the receptor site, the higher the affinity between the drug and the receptor and the greater the observed biologic response. A drug that fits a receptor well is called an **agonist**.

e. Some drugs lacking the specific pharmacophore for a receptor may nonetheless bind to that receptor. Such a drug will have little or no pharmacologic effect and may also prevent a molecule having the specific pharmacophore from binding, blocking the expected biologic response. A drug that blocks a natural agonist and prevents it from binding to its receptor is called an **antagonist**.

3. Drug–receptor interaction. The stereochemistry of both the receptor site surface and the drug molecule helps determine the nature and efficiency of the drug–receptor interaction. **Stereoisomers**—compounds in which all the atoms are bonded in the same way but differ in their orientation in space—may differ in their biologic activities and are classified into two major groups.

a. Optical isomers have at least one asymmetric carbon atom, or **chiral center**—a carbon atom with four different groups attached to it.

(1) This asymmetric carbon atom gives rise to two possible isomers, or **enantiomorphs,** which differ in their spatial orientation (Figure 10-1). Enantiomorphs usually have identical properties, except that one rotates the plane of polarized light in a clockwise direction (**dextrorotatory,** designated D or +) and the other in a counterclockwise direction (**levorotatory,** designated L or −).

(2) An equal mixture of D and L enantiomorphs is called a **racemic mixture** and is optically inactive.

(3) Enantiomorphs may **differ in biologic activity** if their interaction with a receptor involves the asymmetric carbon and its attached groups. For example, **levorphanol** has narcotic, analgesic, and antitussive properties, whereas its mirror image, **dextrorphanol,** has only antitussive activity.

(4) A molecule with more than one asymmetric carbon gives rise to more than two isomers, only some of which are enantiomorphs. Those isomers that are not enantiomorphs are called **diastereomers**. They may differ in physicochemical and biologic properties.

b. Geometric isomers (cis–trans isomers) occur as a result of restricted rotation about a chemical bond, owing to double bonds or rigid ring systems in the molecule.

(1) Cis–trans isomers are not mirror images and have very different physicochemical properties and pharmacologic activity.

(2) Because the functional groups of these isomers are separated by different distances, they generally do not fit the same receptor equally well. If these functional groups are pharmacophores, the isomers will **differ in biologic activity**. For example, cis-diethylstilbestrol has only 7% of the estrogenic activity of trans-diethylstilbestrol (Figure 10-2).

c. Bioisosteres are molecules containing groups that are spatially and electronically equivalent and, thus, interchangeable without significantly altering the molecules' physicochemical properties. Replacement of a molecule with its isoteric analogue may produce selected biologic effects. For instance, the isostere may act as an antagonist to a normal metabolite (as in an antimetabolite drug).

(1) The **antibacterial sulfonamides,** for example, are isosteric with p-aminobenzoic acid and act as competitive antagonists to it (Figure 10-3).

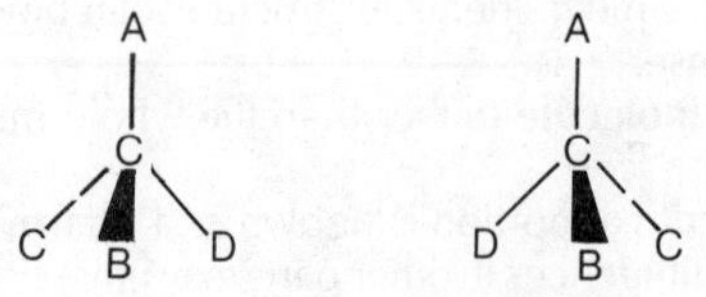

Figure 10-1. A tetrahedral carbon atom bonded to four different groups gives rise to two enantiomorphs, or optical isomers, which are mirror images of one another and cannot be superimposed.

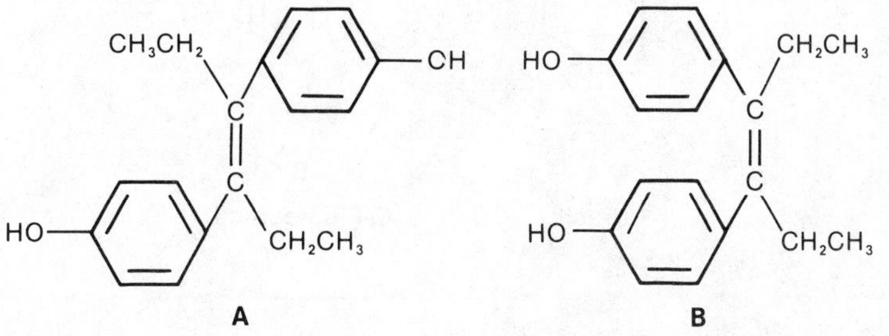

Trans-diethylstilbestrol Cis-diethylstilbestrol

Figure 10-2. These illustrations show (*A*) the trans-isomer of diethylstilbestrol and (*B*) the cis-isomer. The relationship of the functional groups changes relative to each other and to the carbon double bond.

(2) The anticancer agent **5-fluorouracil** is isosteric with uracil and interferes with the production of DNA (Figure 10-4).

IV. MECHANISMS OF DRUG ACTION

A. Action on enzymes

1. **Activation,** or **increased enzyme activity,** may result from induction of enzyme protein synthesis by such drugs as barbiturates, phenytoin and other antiepileptics, rifampin, antihistamines, griseofulvin, and oral contraceptives.
   a. **Allosteric binding.** A drug may enhance enzyme activity by allosteric binding, which triggers a conformational change in the enzyme system and, thus, alters its affinity for substrate binding. (This contrasts with the rigid lock-and-key theory of enzyme–substrate binding (see III B 1 a).
   b. **Coenzymes** play a role in optimizing enzyme activity. Coenzymes include **vitamins** (particularly the vitamin B complex) and **cofactors** [mainly metallic ions such as sodium (Na^+), potassium (K^+), magnesium (Mg^{2+}), calcium (Ca^{2+}), zinc (Zn^{2+}), and iron (Fe^{2+})]. Coenzymes activate enzymes by complexation and stereochemical interaction.

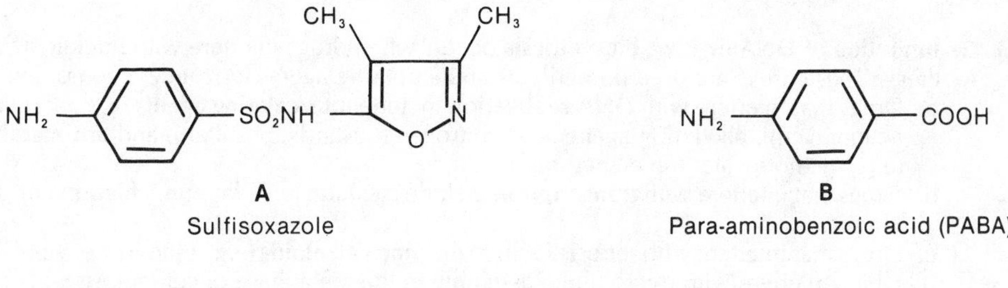

Sulfisoxazole Para-aminobenzoic acid (PABA)

Figure 10-3. The antibacterial sulfonamide sulfisoxazole (*A*) is isosteric with (*B*) p-aminobenzoic acid and acts as its competitive antagonist.

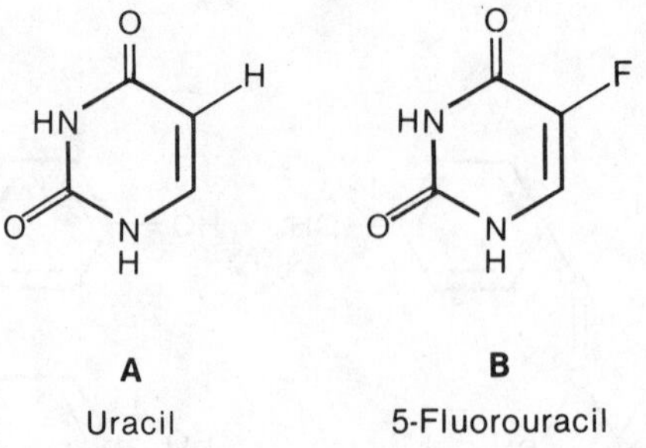

Figure 10-4. Substitution of a fluorine atom for a hydrogen atom of (*A*) uracil produces (*B*) 5-fluorouracil, which inhibits pyrimidine synthesis and interferes with DNA production.

2. **Inhibition,** or **decreased enzyme activity,** may result from drugs that interact with the apoenzyme, the coenzyme, or even the whole enzyme complex. The drug may modify or destroy the apoenzyme's protein conformation, react with the coenzyme (thus reducing the enzyme system's capacity to function), or bind with the enzyme complex (rendering it unable to bind with its substrate).
   a. **Reversible inhibition** is an equilibrium reaction between the enzyme and the drug. Maximum inhibition occurs when equilibrium is reached.
   b. **Irreversible inhibition** occurs when the drug binds with the enzyme to form a complex that does not dissociate. Inhibition increases with time if the drug is present in sufficient quantity.
   c. **Competitive inhibition.** The drug competes with the natural substrate for the same enzyme site, combining with the site reversibly. If the natural substrate's concentration is increased sufficiently, it will displace the drug from the binding site, reversing the inhibition.
   d. **Noncompetitive inhibition.** The drug combines with the enzyme or the enzyme–substrate complex at a site other than the catalytic site (where the substrate binds). An excess of natural substrate will not reverse the inhibition.

B. Suppression of gene formation

1. **Inhibition of nucleotide biosynthesis** occurs when folic acid antagonists or purine and pyrimidine analogues interfere with the biosynthesis of the purine and pyrimidine bases (the building blocks of nucleotides).
   a. **Antifolate drugs** (e.g., methotrexate) inhibit purine and thymidylic acid synthesis by inhibiting folate reductase.
   b. **Purine analogues** (e.g., 6-mercaptopurine, 6-thioguanine) act as antagonists in the synthesis of purine bases. These analogues do not act as active inhibitors until they are converted to their respective nucleotides.
   c. **Pyrimidine analogues** (e.g., 5-fluorouracil) inhibit the synthesis of thymidylic acid by inhibiting thymidine synthetase.

2. **Inhibition of DNA or RNA biosynthesis** occurs when drugs interfere with nucleic acid synthesis. These drugs are used primarily as antineoplastic agents for cancer chemotherapy.
   a. Drugs that interfere with **DNA replication** include **intercalating agents** (e.g., adriamycin, actinomycin), **alkylating agents** (e.g., nitrogen mustards, busulfan), and **antimetabolites** (e.g., methotrexate, 6-mercaptopurine).
   b. Drugs that interfere with **transcription** include **cisplatin** (cis-platinum), **bleomycin,** and **rifampicin.**
   c. Drugs that interfere with **mitosis** include the **vinca alkaloids** (e.g., vincristine, vinblastine), which interfere with microtubule assembly in the metaphase of cell mitosis.
   d. Drugs that **inhibit DNA polymerase** include **cytarabine** (ARA-C) and **vidarabine** (ARA-A), which act as antineoplastic agents as well as antiviral agents.

C. Inhibition of protein synthesis

1. **Tetracyclines** interfere with protein synthesis by inhibiting tRNA binding to the ribosome and blocking the release of completed peptides from the ribosome.
2. **Chloramphenicol** and **erythromycin** (which compete for the same binding site) bind to the ribosome and inhibit peptidyl transferase, blocking formation of the peptide bond and interrupting formation of the peptide chain.
3. **Aminoglycosides** decrease the fidelity of transcription by binding to the ribosome, which permits formation of an abnormal initiation complex and prohibits addition of amino acids to the peptide chain. Additionally, aminoglycosides cause misreading of the mRNA template, so that incorrect amino acids are incorporated into the growing polypeptide chain.

D. Inhibition of enzyme-catalyzed reactions. Antimetabolites that are structurally similar to normal cellular metabolites can replace these metabolites and react with enzymes to yield abnormal nonfunctional products. These agents are used to inhibit tumor growth, inhibit blood clotting, and inhibit bacterial growth.

1. Antimetabolites such as **6-mercaptopurine** and **methotrexate** inhibit tumor growth by interfering with nucleotide and nucleic acid biosynthesis.
2. Antimetabolites such as **warfarin** inhibit blood clotting by interfering with formation of clotting factors.
3. Antimetabolites such as **sulfonamides** inhibit bacterial growth by interfering with tetrahydrofolic acid formation.

E. Chelate formation

1. Chelate formation occurs when the ligand forms coordination bonds with a central metal ion at more than one site (usually, two sites are involved).
   a. **Biologic chelates** include the iron–hemoglobin chelate, the magnesium–chlorophyll chelate, and the iron–cytochrome chelate.
   b. Addition of a ligand with a greater affinity than the natural ligand for the essential metal causes formation of a more stable chelate, accounting for the ligand's medicinal properties. For example, both **isoniazid** and **8-hydroxyquinolone** can chelate with iron to exert antibacterial effects.
2. Chelating agents can also be used as **antidotes for metal poisoning**.
   a. **Ethylenediaminetetraacetic acid** (EDTA, edetate) chelates calcium and lead.
   b. **Penicillamine** (Cuprimine) chelates copper.
   c. **Dimercaprol** (BAL) chelates mercury, gold, antimony, and arsenic.

F. Action on cell membranes

1. **Digitalis glycosides** inhibit the cell membrane's sodium–potassium pump, inhibiting the influx of K^+ and the outflow of Na^+.
2. **Quinidine** affects the membrane potential of myocardial membranes by prolonging both the polarized and depolarized states.
3. **Local anesthetics** block impulse conduction in nerve cell membranes by interfering with membrane permeability to Na^+ and K^+.
4. **Antifungal drugs** (e.g., amphotericin B, nystatin) affect cell membrane permeability, causing leakage of cellular constituents.
5. **Certain antibiotics** (e.g., polymyxin B, colistin), affect cell membrane permeability through an unknown mechanism.
6. **Acetylcholine** increases membrane permeability to cations.

G. Nonspecific action

1. Structurally nonspecific drugs form a monomolecular layer over entire areas of certain cells. Because they involve such large surfaces, these drugs are usually given in relatively large doses.
2. Drugs that act by nonspecific action include the **volatile general anesthetic gases** (e.g., ether, nitrous oxide), some **depressants** (e.g., ethanol, chloral hydrate), and many **antiseptic compounds** (e.g., phenol, rubbing alcohol).

STUDY QUESTIONS

Directions: Each of the numbered items or incomplete statements in this section is followed by answers or by completions of the statement. Select the **one** lettered answer or completion that is **best** in each case.

1. Which of the following acids has the highest degree of ionization in an aqueous solution?

(A) Aspirin $pK_a = 3.5$
(B) Indomethacin $pK_a = 4.5$
(C) Warfarin $pK_a = 5.1$
(D) Ibuprofen $pK_a = 5.2$
(E) Phenobarbital $pK_a = 7.4$

2. Which of the following salts will most likely yield an aqueous solution with a pH below 7?

(A) Sodium salicylate
(B) Potassium chloride
(C) Magnesium sulfate
(D) Potassium penicillin
(E) Atropine sulfate

3. Which of the following salts forms an aqueous solution that is alkaline to litmus?

(A) Sodium chloride
(B) Benzalkonium chloride
(C) Meperidine hydrochloride
(D) Cefazolin sodium
(E) Chlordiazepoxide hydrochloride

4. All of the following medicinal agents are classified as natural products EXCEPT

(A) atropine
(B) diazepam
(C) digitoxin
(D) penicillin
(E) morphine

5. All of the following statements about a structurally specific agonist are true EXCEPT

(A) activity is determined more by its chemical structure than by its physical properties
(B) the entire molecule is involved in binding to a specific endogenous receptor
(C) the drug cannot act unless it is first bound to a receptor
(D) a minor structural change in a pharmacophore can produce a loss in activity
(E) the higher the affinity between the drug and its receptor, the greater the biologic response

6. The dextro (D) form of β-methacholine (see structure below) is approximately 500 times more active than its levo (L) enantiomer.

$$(CH_3)_3\overset{+}{N}{-}CH_2{-}\underset{\displaystyle CH_3}{\underset{|}{C}}HOOC{-}CH_3 \qquad C1^-$$

The observed difference in pharmacologic activity between the two isomers is most likely due to differences in the

(A) selectivity for a receptor
(B) rates of metabolism
(C) extent of distribution
(D) interatomic distance between pharmacophore groups
(E) penetrability to the site of action

1-A	4-B
2-E	5-B
3-D	6-A

Directions: Each question below contains three suggested answers, of which **one or more** is correct. Choose the answer

A if **I only** is correct
B if **III only** is correct
C if **I and II** are correct
D if **II and III** are correct
E if **I, II, and III** are correct

7. True statements concerning drugs that act systemically include

I. they must undergo biotransformation into an active form after reaching their active site
II. they must be in a form capable of passage through various membrane barriers
III. they must be in or be converted to a form that is readily excreted from the body

8. Examples of strong electrolytes (i.e., completely dissociated in an aqueous solution) include

I. acetic acid
II. pentobarbital sodium
III. diphenhydramine hydrochloride

9. Precipitation may occur upon mixing aqueous solutions of meperidine hydrochloride with which of the following solutions?

I. Sodium bicarbonate injection
II. Atropine sulfate injection
III. Sodium chloride injection

10. Drugs classified as antimetabolites include

I. 5-fluorouracil
II. sulfisoxazole
III. digoxin

11. The excretion of a weakly acidic drug generally is more rapid in alkaline urine than in acidic urine. This process occurs because

I. a weak acid in alkaline media will exist primarily in its ionized form, which cannot be reabsorbed easily
II. a weak acid in alkaline media will exist in its lipophilic form, which cannot be reabsorbed easily
III. all drugs are excreted more rapidly in an alkaline urine

Questions 12–15

All of the following questions refer to the drug meperidine (see structure below).

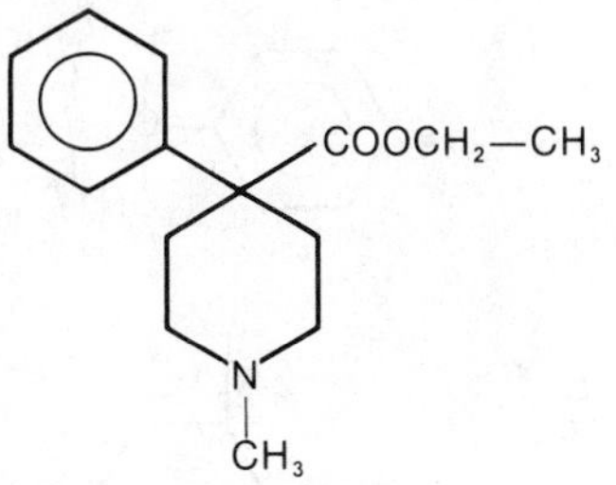

12. Functional groups present in the molecule shown include

I. an ester
II. a tertiary amine
III. a carboxylic acid

13. Meperidine is classified as a

I. weak acid
II. salt
III. weak base

14. Meperidine is soluble in which of the following substances?

I. Dilute hydrochloric acid
II. Dilute sodium hydroxide
III. Water

15. Assuming that meperidine is absorbed after oral administration and that a large percentage of the dose is excreted unchanged, the effect of alkalinization of the urine will increase its

I. duration of action
II. rate of excretion
III. ionization in the glomerular filtrate

7-D	10-C	13-B
8-D	11-A	14-A
9-A	12-C	15-A

Directions: The group of items in this section consists of lettered options followed by a set of numbered items. For each item, select the **one** lettered option that is most closely associated with it. Each lettered option may be selected once, more than once, or not at all.

Questions 16–19

For each pair of molecules, select the term that best fits the relationship.

(A) Geometric isomers
(B) Enantiomers
(C) Diastereomers
(D) Bioisosteres
(E) Same compound

16.

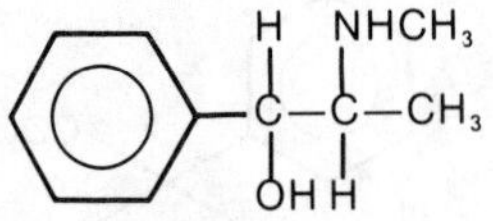

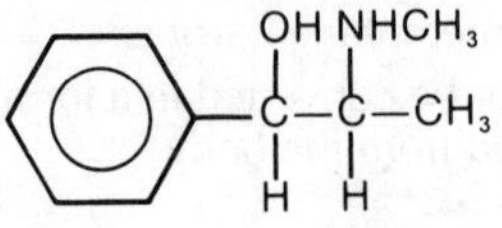

17.

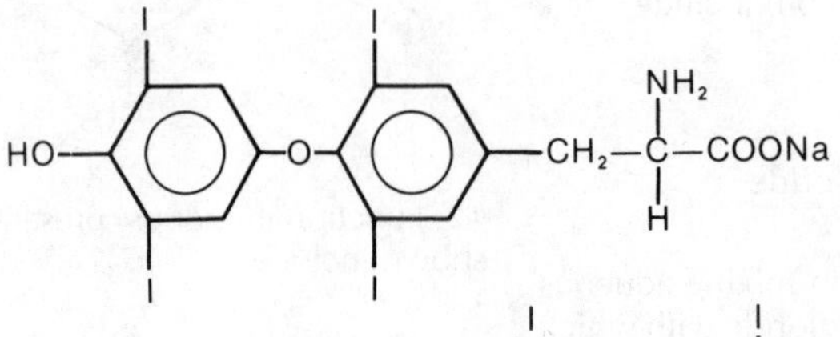

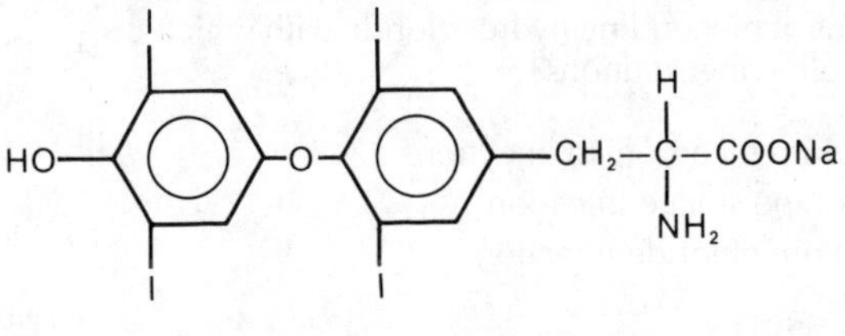

18.

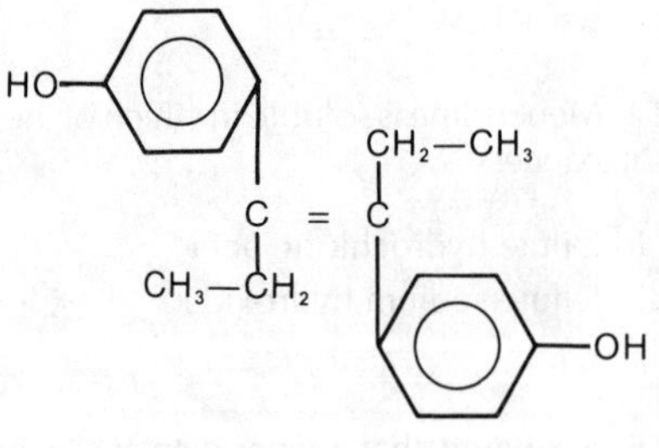

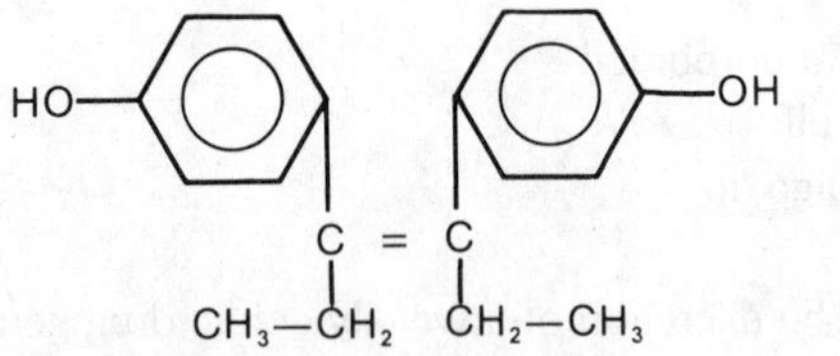

19.

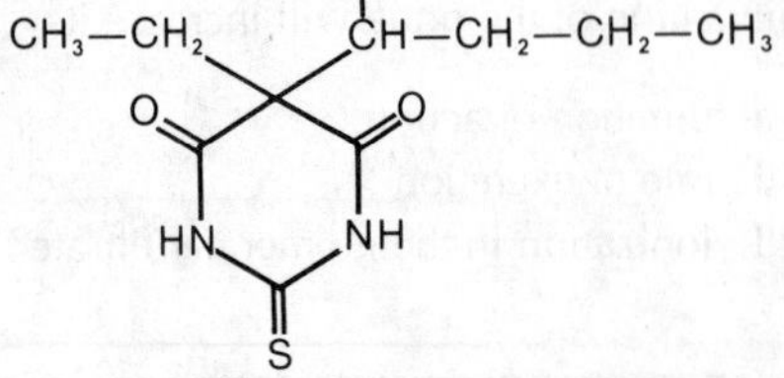

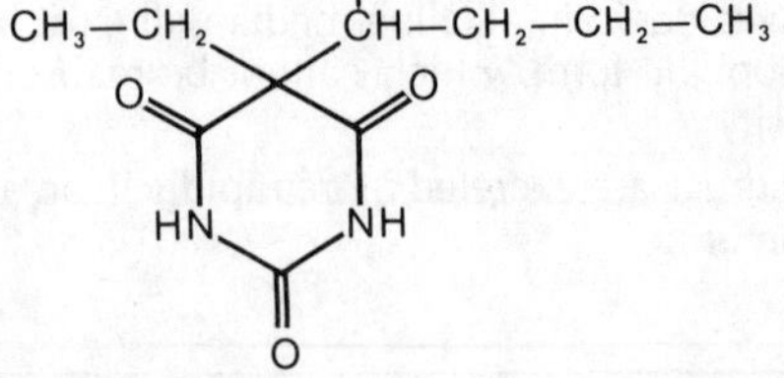

16-C
17-B
18-A
19-D

ANSWERS AND EXPLANATIONS

1. The answer is A *[II B 3 b].*
The pK_a (the negative log of the acid ionization constant) is indicative of the relative strength of an acidic drug. The lower the pK_a of an acidic drug, the stronger it is as an acid. A strong acid is defined as one that is completely ionized or dissociated in an aqueous solution; therefore, the stronger the acid, the greater the ionization.

2. The answer is E *[II B 5, 6].*
The solution must contain an acidic substance to have a pH below 7. Atropine sulfate is a salt of a weak base and a strong acid; therefore, its aqueous solution is acidic. Sodium salicylate and potassium penicillin are both salts of strong bases and weak acids; therefore, their aqueous solutions are alkaline. Magnesium sulfate and potassium chloride are salts of strong bases and strong acids; therefore, their aqueous solutions are neutral.

3. The answer is D *[II B 3 d, 5, 6].*
Only an aqueous solution of cefazolin sodium, which is a salt of a strong base and a weak acid, may be alkaline. Sodium chloride and benzalkonium chloride are both salts of strong bases and strong acids, and their aqueous solutions are neutral. Meperidine hydrochloride and chlordiazepoxide hydrochloride are salts of weak bases and strong acids, and their solutions are acidic.

4. The answer is B *[I A, B].*
Diazepam is a benzodiazepine anxiolytic, which, while it is a heterocyclic nitrogen-containing molecule, is not an alkaloid and is prepared synthetically. Natural products refer to those substances biosynthesized in plants or animals. The pure natural products are usually alkaloids, such as morphine or atropine; glycosides, such as digitoxin or digoxin; antibiotics, such as penicillin or streptomycin; or hormones, such as insulin or thyroxine.

5. The answer is B *[III B].*
While the whole molecule is attached (bound) to a specific endogenous receptor, the actual binding site may consist of only a specific functional group. For example, a drug containing a hydroxyl group may be attached by hydrogen bonding between the electropositive hydrogen of the hydroxyl group and an electronegative oxygen on the receptor. Binding of drugs to biologic constituents may involve chemical bonds such as covalent, ion–dipole, dipole–dipole, and Van der Waals forces, among others.

6. The answer is A *[III B 3 a; Figure 10-1].*
The term enantiomer and the D and L indicate that the β-methacholine has a chiral center and exhibits optical isomerism. Since the optical isomers have different orientations in space, one orientation will give a better fit than the other and will most likely have greater biologic activity than the other.

7. The answer is D (II, III) *[II A 1, 2].*
Generally, drugs must be lipophilic to pass through lipoprotein membranes and hydrophilic to be excreted by the kidney. Drugs do not have to be converted into an active form at their active site, although most drugs must be in their active form when they reach their active site. Many drugs are active in the form in which they are administered. Some drugs, usually referred to as prodrugs, are biotransformed into their active form after administration. Theoretically, drugs that reach their active site and then are metabolically activated should be more specific in their action and have fewer side effects. Currently, research efforts are underway to develop site-specific delivery systems and processes.

8. The answer is D (II, III) *[II B 3 c, 4 a, 6 a].*
Almost all salts (with very few exceptions) are strong electrolytes, and the terminology pentobarbital sodium and diphenhydramine hydrochloride indicate that both compounds are salts. Acetic acid is a weak acid; therefore, it is a weak electrolyte.

9. The answer is A (I) *[II B 5, 6].*
When meperidine hydrochloride solution is mixed with the alkaline solution of sodium bicarbonate, a neutralization reaction will occur with the possible precipitation of the water-insoluble free base meperidine. A neutralization reaction will occur when acidic solutions are mixed with basic solutions, or conversely. No reaction, in terms of acid–base, occurs when solutions are mixed with other acidic or neutral solutions or when basic solutions are mixed with other basic or neutral solutions. There should

be no reaction, then, when the meperidine hydrochloride solution, which is acidic, is mixed with the acidic solution of atropine sulfate or the neutral solution of sodium chloride.

10. The answer is C (I, II) *[III B 3 c; IV F 1].*
Both sulfisoxazole and 5-fluorouracil compete with and antagonize isosteric normal biologic molecules and, therefore, are antimetabolites. Digoxin is a drug that is thought to inhibit Na^+-K^+–ATPase or to affect intracellular influx or use of calcium ion (Ca^{2+}). Since digoxin is steroidal, it is not isosteric with either an enzyme, which is a protein, or an ion; therefore, it is not classified as an antimetabolite.

11. The answer is A (I) *[II B 2 c, 3 e (1)–(3)].*
A weakly acidic drug will be more ionized in an alkaline urine; therefore, it will be more polar and, thus, more soluble in the aqueous urine. It would also be less liposoluble, less likely to undergo tubular reabsorption, and thus be more likely to be excreted.

12–15. The answers are: 12-C (I, II), 13-B (III), 14-A (I), 15-A (I) *[II B 3, 4].*
The molecule contains a basic nitrogen, which is bonded to three carbon atoms (e.g., a tertiary amine), and an ethyl carboxylate, which is an ester group. An ester is the product of the reaction of an alcohol with a carboxylic acid that forms an alkyl carboxylate. There is no free carboxylic acid present. However, if this molecule is subjected to hydrolysis, it forms a carboxylic acid and ethyl alcohol.

Since meperidine contains a tertiary amine, it is classified as a base; because it is an organic base, it is considered weak. The nitrogen is not protonated. It is not ionic and, therefore, is not a salt.

A salt of meperidine is completely dissociated in water and, thus, is likely to be soluble. Since meperidine is a base, it can form a salt only with an acid. Meperidine is an organic base of relatively high molecular weight and, therefore, is most likely insoluble in water. Water-soluble organic compounds generally must be strongly ionic to dissolve in water since water is a highly polar solvent.

Alkalinization of the urine decreases the ionization of meperidine, making it more liposoluble and, thus, more likely to undergo reabsorption in the kidney tubule. This results in a decreased rate of excretion and an increased duration of action.

16–19. The answers are: 16-C, 17-B, 18-A, 19-D *[III B 3 a–c].*
The first pair of molecules are isomers that have two asymmetric carbon atoms. They are not superimposable and are not mirror images; therefore, they are known as diastereomers.

The second pair of molecules are isomers that have one asymmetric carbon atom.They are nonsuperimposable mirror images; therefore, they are enantiomers.

The third pair of molecules have different spatial arrangements and are isomers. The presence of the double bond, which restricts the rotation of the groups on each carbon atom involved in the double bond, characterizes this type of isomerism as geometric.

The last pair of molecules are neither isomers nor the same compound, since one contains three oxygens whereas the other contains two oxygens and a sulfur. Since oxygen and sulfur are in the same periodic family, they are isosteric, and the two compounds are known as bioisosteres.

11 Drug Metabolism

Edward F. LaSala

I. INTRODUCTION. Drug metabolism (also called **biotransformation**) refers to the biochemical changes drugs and other foreign chemicals (**xenobiotics**) undergo in the body, leading to the formation of different metabolites with different effects. Xenobiotics may undergo a variety of biotransformation pathways, resulting in the production of a mixture of intermediate metabolites and excreted products, including unchanged parent drug. Rarely is only one metabolite produced from a single drug.

A. Inactive metabolites. Some metabolites are inactive—their pharmacologically active parent compounds become inactivated or detoxicated.

1. The hydrolysis of **procaine** to p-aminobenzoic acid results in loss of anesthetic activity.
2. The oxidation of **6-mercaptopurine** to 6-mercaptouric acid results in loss of anticancer activity.

B. Metabolites that retain similar activity. Certain metabolites retain the pharmacologic activity of their parent compounds to a greater or lesser degree.

1. **Imipramine** is demethylated to the essentially equiactive antidepressant, **desipramine**.
2. **Acetohexamide** is reduced to the more active hypoglycemic, **L-hydroxyhexamide**.
3. **Codeine** is demethylated to the more active analgesic, **morphine**.

C. Metabolites with altered activity. Some metabolites develop activity different from that of their parent drugs.

1. The antidepressant **iproniazid** is dealkylated to the antitubercular, **isoniazid**.
2. The vitamin **retinoic acid** (vitamin A) is isomerized to the antiacne agent, **isoretinoic acid**.

D. Bioactivated metabolites. Some pharmacologically inactive parent compounds are converted to active species within the body. These parent compounds are known as **prodrugs**.

1. The prodrug **enalapril** is hydrolyzed to **enalaprilat,** a potent antihypertensive.
2. The prodrug **conjugated estrogen** is hydrolyzed to **active estrogen hormone**.
3. The antiparkinsonian **levodopa** is decarboxylated in the neuron to active **dopamine**.

II. BIOTRANSFORMATION PATHWAYS (Table 11-1)

A. Phase I reactions are those in which new functional groups are introduced into the molecule or unmasked by oxidation, reduction, or hydrolysis.

1. **Oxidation** is the most commonly encountered drug reaction.
   a. Many oxidative reactions take place in the **liver**.
   b. Oxidation is catalyzed by a complex of nonspecific enzymes called **NADPH-dependent mixed-function oxidases,** which are bound to the smooth endoplasmic reticulum within liver cells. (NADPH is the reduced form of nicotinamide-adenine dinucleotide phosphate.)

Table 11-1. Major Pathways of Drug Metabolism

Type of Reaction	Reaction Pathway	Examples
Oxidation		
Microsomal oxidations		
Aromatic hydroxylation	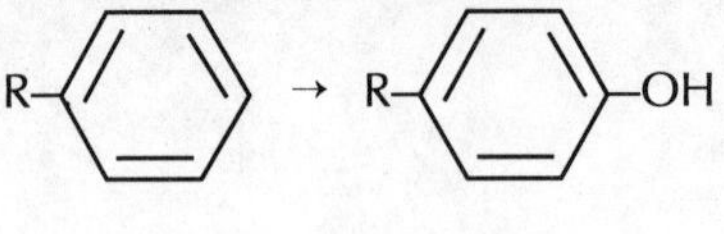	Phenylbutazone Phenytoin
Aliphatic hydroxylation	$R{-}CH_2{-}CH_3 \rightarrow R{-}CH(OH){-}CH_3$	Pentobarbital Meprobamate
Oxidative deamination	$R{-}CH(CH_3){-}NH_2 \rightarrow R{-}C(CH_3){=}O$	Amphetamine
N-dealkylation	$R{-}NH{-}CH_3 \rightarrow R{-}NH_2$	Ephedrine Morphine
O-dealkylation	$R{-}O{-}CH_3 \rightarrow R{-}OH$	Phenacetin Codeine
Sulfoxidation	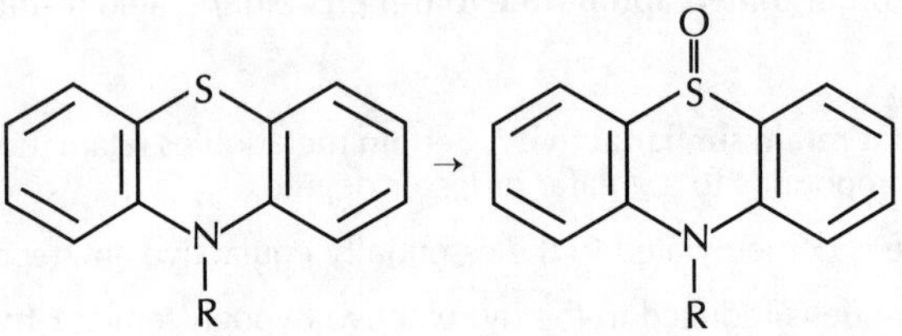	Chlorpromazine
Desulfuration	$R_2C{=}S \rightarrow R_2C{=}O$	Thiopental
Dehydrohalogenation	$R_2CH{-}CCl_3 \rightarrow R_2C{=}CCl_2$	Halothane
Nonmicrosomal oxidations		
Alcoholic oxidation	$R{-}CH_2OH \rightarrow R{-}CHO$	Ethanol
Aldehydic oxidation	$R{-}CHO \rightarrow R{-}COOH$	Acetaldehyde
Reduction		
Azoreduction	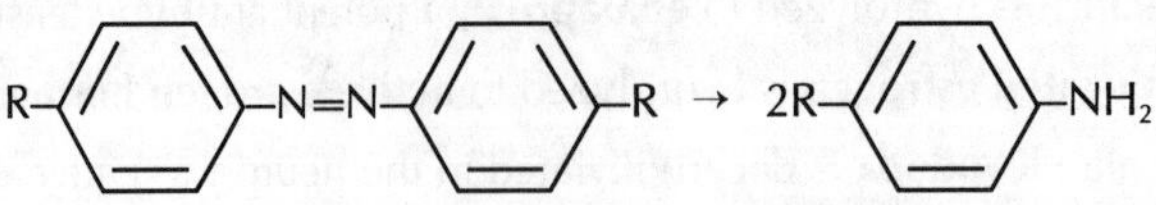	Sulfasalazine
Nitroreduction	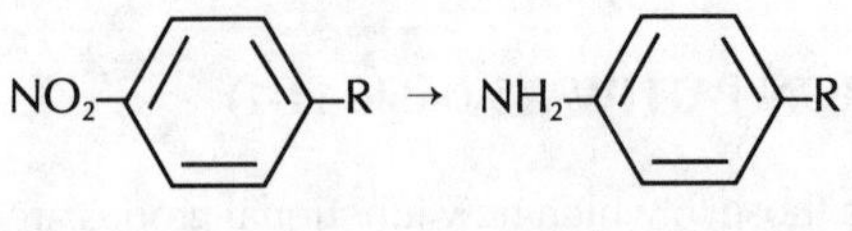	Chloramphenicol
Hydrolysis		
De-esterification	$R{-}COOR \rightarrow RCOOH + R{-}OH$	Procaine Meperidine
Deamidation	$R{-}CONH{-}R \rightarrow R{-}COOH + NH_2{-}R$	Lidocaine

(Continued on next page)

Table 11-1. Continued

Type of Reaction	Reaction Pathway	Examples
Conjugation		
Glucuronidation	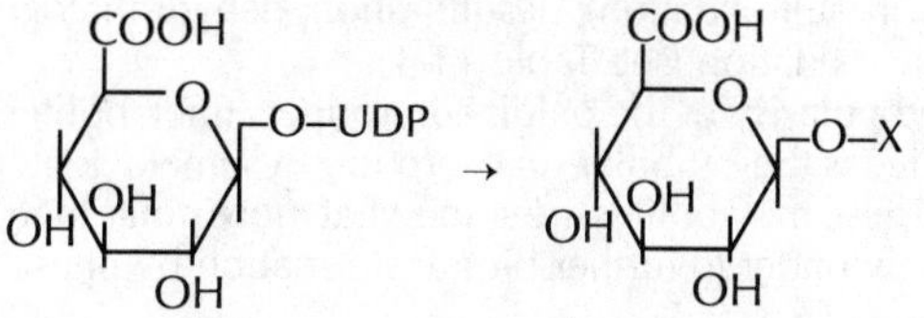	
Phenolic OH (X = –Ar)		Salicylates
Alcoholic OH (X = –R)		Oxazepam
Carboxyl (X = –OC–R)		Salicylates
Amine (X = –NH–R)		Sulfamethoxazole
Sulfhydryl (X = –SR)		Disulfiram
Glycine conjugation	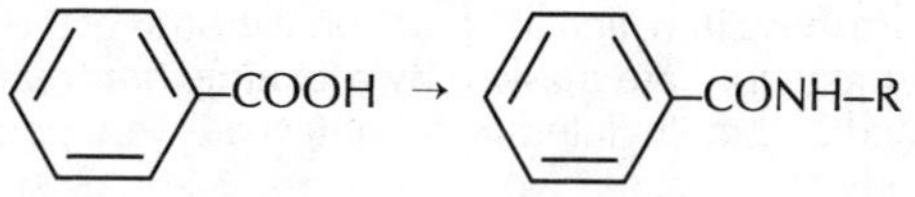	Salicylic acid Fenfluramine
Glutathione conjugation	HO–NH–Ar → NH_2–Ar–CH_2–S–CH(–NH–OC–CH_3)–COOH	Acetaminophen
Sulfate conjugation	R–OH → R–O–SO_2–OH	Steroids Terbutaline
Methylation		
Aromatic amines	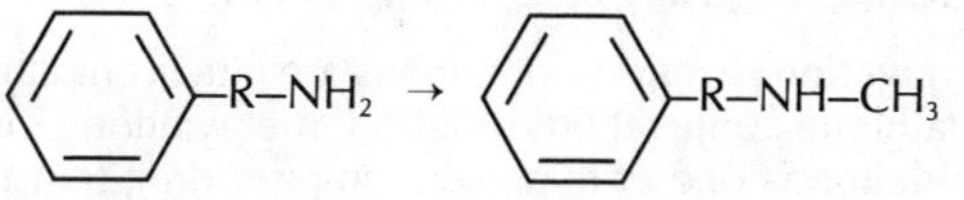	Oxprenolol
Catechols	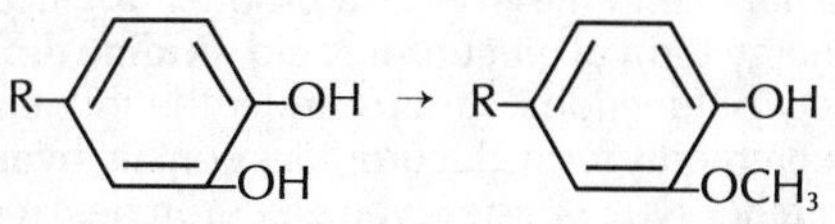	Levodopa
Acetylation		
Aromatic amines	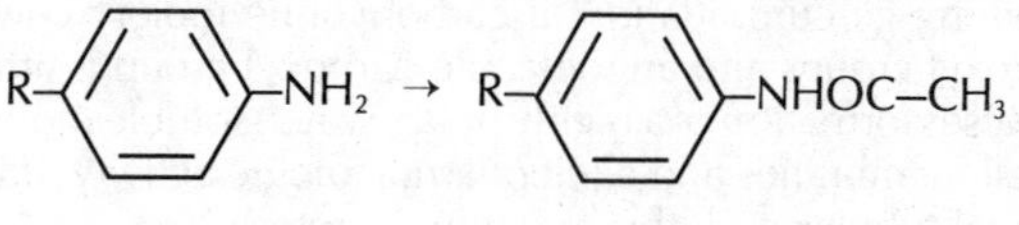	Sulfisoxazole Procainamide
Hydrazides	R–NH–NH_2 → R–NH–NHOC–CH_3	Isoniazid

c. NADPH-dependent mixed-function oxidases catalyze aliphatic hydroxylation; aromatic (or ring) hydroxylation; oxidative N-, O-, and S-dealkylation; oxidative deamination; N- and S-oxidation (sulfoxidation); desulfuration; dehydrohalogenation; alcoholic oxidation; and aldehydic oxidation (see Table 11-1).

d. The **increased polarity** of the oxidized products (metabolites) enhances their water solubility and reduces their tubular reabsorption to some extent, thus favoring their excretion in the urine. These metabolites are somewhat **more polar** than their parent compounds and very commonly undergo further biotransformation by phase II pathways (see II B).

2. **Reduction** is less commonly encountered than oxidation during drug metabolism. Different reductions, such as azoreduction or nitroreduction, lead to different types of polar functional groups (see Table 11-1).

3. **Hydrolysis** (an enzymatic process) results in more polar metabolites (see Table 11-1).
   a. **Esterase enzymes,** usually present in plasma and various tissues, are rather nonspecific and catalyze de-esterification, hydrolyzing relatively nonpolar esters into two polar, more water-soluble compounds—an alcohol and an acid.
   b. **Amidase enzymes** hydrolyze amides into amines and acids (deamidation). Deamidation occurs primarily in the liver.
   c. **Ester drugs** susceptible to plasma esterases (e.g., procaine) are usually shorter acting than structurally similar **amide drugs** (e.g., procainamide), which are not significantly hydrolyzed until they reach the liver.

B. **Phase II reactions** are those in which the functional groups of the original drug (or of a metabolite formed in a phase I reaction) are masked by a **conjugation reaction**. Most phase II conjugates (except for acetylated and methylated metabolites) are very polar, resulting in rapid drug elimination from the body.

1. **Conjugation reactions** combine the **parent drug** (or its metabolites) with certain **natural endogenous constituents,** such as glucuronic acid, glycine, glutamine, sulfate, glutathione, the two-carbon acetyl fragment, or the one-carbon methyl fragment. These reactions generally require both a **high-energy molecule** and an **enzyme**.
   a. The **high-energy molecule** consists of a **coenzyme** bound to the endogenous substrate, the parent drug, or the drug's phase I metabolite.
   b. The **enzymes** (usually called **transferases**) that catalyze conjugation reactions are found mainly in the liver and, to a lesser extent, in the intestines and other tissues.
   c. Most conjugates are **highly polar** and **unable to cross cell membranes,** making them almost always **pharmacologically inactive** and of little or no toxicity.

2. **Common conjugation reactions** in humans are glucuronidation, glycine and glutamine conjugation, glutathione conjugation, sulfation, methylation, and acetylation (see Table 11-1).
   a. **Glucuronidation** is one of the most common drug transformations, because glucuronic acid is readily available in the liver as a product of glucose metabolism.
      (1) The high-energy form of glucuronic acid, **uridine diphosphate glucuronic acid** reacts with a variety of functional groups under the influence of glucuronyl transferase.
      (2) Drugs that commonly form glucuronides contain **hydroxyl groups** or **carboxyl groups,** which form ether-type or ester-type glucuronides, respectively. (N-glucuronides and S-glucuronides are also possible.)
      (3) During glucuronidation, a carbohydrate moiety containing several hydrophilic hydroxyl groups and an ionizable carboxyl group is attached to a **lipophilic drug**. This causes formation of a highly polar, water-soluble molecule that is unlikely to penetrate cell membranes and elicit pharmacologic activity. It is also poorly reabsorbed by the renal tubules and, thus, readily excreted.
      (4) Glucuronides with **high molecular weight** (> 500) are often excreted into the bile and, eventually, into the intestines. The intestinal enzyme β-glucuronidase may then hydrolyze the conjugate, releasing the unaltered drug (or its primary metabolite) for reabsorption by the intestine.
   b. **Glycine and glutamine conjugation** occurs with aliphatic or aromatic acids to form amides. The high-energy molecule for this reaction is an **S-acyl-coenzyme A (CoA);** the reaction is catalyzed by a **transacylase**.
   c. **Glutathione conjugation** occurs when glutathione (present in the liver) acts as an endogenous nucleophile and, under the influence of **glutathione transferase,** reacts with electrophilic compounds such as halides or nitrates to form a mercapturic acid derivative.

d. **Sulfation** depends on the availability of endogenous sulfate, which is usually limited. Unlike glucuronidation, sulfate conjugation can become easily saturated. The high-energy form of sulfate (**3′-phosphoadenosine-5′-phosphosulfate**) reacts with phenols and alcohols under the influence of **sulfotransferase** (sulfokinase).

e. **Methylation** results primarily in O-, N-, and S-methylated products, which are usually less polar than the unaltered drugs. Thus, methylated metabolites may retain their pharmacologic activity, and the pathway is not significant in the elimination of foreign compounds from the body. The high-energy methyl form is **S-adenosylmethionine; methyltransferase** catalyzes the reaction.

f. **Acetylation** may occur with primary amines, hydrazides, sulfonamides, and, occasionally amides. It leads to the formation of N-acetylated products. These are usually less polar than the unaltered drug and, thus, may retain pharmacologic activity.

(1) N-acetylated metabolites may accumulate in tissues or in the kidneys, as in the case of certain **antibacterial sulfonamides**. Crystalluria and subsequent tissue damage may result.

(2) The high-energy molecule for acetylation is **acetyl-CoA**. **The reaction is catalyzed by N-acetyltransferase.**

III. FACTORS INFLUENCING DRUG METABOLISM

A. **Chemical structure** specifically influences a drug's metabolic pathway.

B. Species differences

1. **Qualitative differences** are differences in the actual metabolic pathway. Such a variation may result from a genetic deficiency of a particular enzyme or from a difference in a particular endogenous substrate. In general, qualitative differences occur primarily with **phase II reactions**.

2. **Quantitative differences** are differences in the extent to which the same type of metabolic reaction occurs. Such a variation may result from a difference in the enzyme level, a difference in the amount of endogenous inhibitor or inducer, or a difference in the extent of competing reactions. In general, quantitative differences occur primarily with **phase I reactions**.

C. Physiologic or disease state

1. Because the liver is the major organ involved in biotransformation, **pathologic factors that alter liver function** can affect a drug's hepatic clearance.

2. **Congestive heart failure** decreases hepatic blood flow by reducing cardiac output, which alters the extent of drug metabolism.

3. An **alteration in albumin production** (the plasma's major drug-binding protein) can alter the fraction of bound to unbound drug. Thus, a decrease in plasma albumin can increase the fraction of unbound (free) drug, which then becomes available to exert a more intense pharmacologic effect. The reverse is true when plasma albumin increases.

D. Genetic variations

1. The **acetylation rate** depends on the amount of N-acetyltransferase present, which is determined by genetic factors.

2. The general population can be divided into **fast acetylators** and **slow acetylators**. For example, fast acetylators are more prone to hepatotoxicity from the antitubercular agent isoniazid than slow acetylators, whereas slow acetylators are more prone to isoniazid's other toxic effects.

E. Drug dosage

1. As the **dosage is increased,** drug concentration in the body may saturate the metabolic enzymes. Because enzyme activity at high drug concentration is already at a maximum, any further increase in the drug level will not increase the rate of metabolism. Thus, the overall metabolism rate no longer follows first-order kinetics.

2. Once the metabolic pathway is **saturated** (either because of an exceedingly high drug level or because the supply of an endogenous conjugated agent is exhausted), an alternative pathway may be pursued. For example, at a low phenol level, phenol is conjugated to sulfate; at a high level, primarily to glucuronide.

F. Nutritional status

1. The levels of some **conjugating agents** (or endogenous substrates), such as sulfate, glutathione, and (rarely) glucuronic acid, are sensitive to body nutrient levels. For example, a **low-protein diet** may lead to a deficiency of certain amino acids, such as glycine. Low-protein diets also decrease oxidative drug metabolism capacity.
2. Diets **deficient in essential fatty acids** (particularly linoleic acid) reduce the metabolism of ethylmorphine and hexobarbital by decreasing synthesis of certain drug-metabolizing enzymes.
3. A **deficiency of certain dietary minerals** also affects drug metabolism. Calcium, magnesium, and zinc deficiencies decrease drug-metabolizing capacity, whereas iron deficiency appears to increase it. A copper deficiency leads to variable effects.
4. **Deficiencies of vitamins** (particularly vitamins A, C, E, and the B group) affect drug-metabolizing capacity. For example, a vitamin C deficiency can result in a decrease in oxidative pathways, whereas a vitamin E deficiency can retard dealkylation and hydroxylation.

G. Age

1. In **young children,** particularly **infants,** drugs may be more active than expected because the metabolizing enzyme systems are not fully developed at birth and develop variably. This is particularly significant with glucuronidation.
2. In **older children,** some drugs may be less active than in adults, particularly if the dosage is based on weight. The liver develops faster than the increase in general body weight and, thus, represents a greater fraction of total body weight.
3. In the **elderly,** metabolizing enzyme systems decline. The lowered level of enzyme activity slows the rate of drug elimination, causing higher plasma drug levels per dose than in young adults.

H. Gender.
In rats, males have a faster drug metabolism rate after puberty than females. In humans, the same pattern seems to exist with regard to antipyrine, diazepam, and some steroids.

I. Circadian rhythms.
The **nocturnal plasma levels** of drugs such as theophylline and diazepam are lower than the **diurnal plasma levels.**

J. Drug administration route

1. **Oral administration.** The drug is absorbed from the gastrointestinal tract and transported to the liver through the hepatic portal vein before entering the systemic circulation. Thus, the drug is subject to hepatic metabolism before it reaches its site of action—an effect known as the **first-pass effect,** or **presystemic elimination** (Table 11-2).
   a. The first-pass effect can cause **significant clinical problems**. Because drugs are metabolized in the liver from their active forms to inactive forms, this effect must be counteracted to achieve the desired plasma or tissue drug level.
   b. A common approach is to **increase the oral dose,** offsetting the loss of drug activity from the first-pass effect.
2. **Intravenous administration** bypasses the first-pass effect because the drug is delivered directly to the bloodstream without being metabolized in the liver. Thus, intravenous doses of drugs undergoing considerable first-pass effects are much smaller than oral doses.
3. **Sublingual administration** and **rectal administration** also bypass first-pass effects, although rectal administration may produce variable effects.

Table 11-2. Drugs Known or Suspected to Undergo First-Pass Metabolism

Alprenolol	Isoproterenol	Pentazocine
Cortisone	Meperidine	Progesterone
Desipramine	Metoprolol	Propoxyphene
Estradiol	Nitroglycerin	Propranolol
Fluorouracil	Nortriptyline	Salbutamol
Imipramine	Oxprenolol	Testosterone

K. Enzyme induction or inhibition can pose significant problems for the patient on a multiple-drug regimen, in which drug interactions are likely.

1. **Sequential or concurrent administration** of many structurally diverse drugs and environmental chemicals may increase the metabolism of some drugs—a phenomenon known as **enzyme induction**.
   a. Drugs such as phenobarbital, carbamazepine, and rifampin appear to act as enzyme inducers by increasing the synthesis or decreasing the degradation of drug-metabolizing enzymes (Table 11-3).
   b. Environmental chemicals such as the polycyclic aromatic hydrocarbons and the chlorinated insecticides also act as enzyme inducers. Cigarette smokers, for example, have lower plasma levels of drugs such as theophylline than do nonsmokers. The polycyclic aromatic hydrocarbon components of cigarette smoke appear to induce the N-demethylation pathway.

2. **Enzyme inhibition.** Some drugs and xenobiotics can decrease the metabolism of other drugs—a phenomenon known as enzyme inhibition. Inhibition may occur by destruction of drug-metabolizing enzymes, inhibition of enzyme synthesis, or complexation and inactivation of the drug-metabolizing enzymes (Table 11-4).

3. **Opposite effects** on drug activity occur when prodrugs are involved because these are inactive when administered and must be metabolized to their active forms.

4. **Tolerance** that develops with certain drugs, such as barbiturates, is related to enzyme induction. Induction results in increased metabolism and decreased activity compared to the effects of initial doses.

IV. EXTRAHEPATIC METABOLISM

A. Definition. Extrahepatic metabolism refers to drug biotransformation that takes place in **tissues other than the liver**. The most common sites include the **portals of entry** (e.g., skin, lungs, gut) and the **portals of excretion** (e.g., kidneys). However, metabolism may occur throughout the body.

B. Metabolism sites

1. **Plasma** contains esterases, which are primarily responsible for hydrolysis of esters. Simple esters (e.g., procaine, succinylcholine) are rapidly hydrolyzed in the blood.

2. **Intestinal mucosa** also contains drug-metabolizing enzymes.
   a. As a lipid-soluble drug passes through the intestinal mucosa during drug absorption, it may be metabolized into polar or inactive metabolites before entering the blood. The result is **comparable to a first-pass effect**.
   b. The intestinal mucosa's drug-metabolizing capacity compares to that of the liver. However, it shows much greater individual variation because of its greater exposure to the environment.

Table 11-3. Examples of Drug Interactions Involving Enzyme Induction

Activity of	Decreased by
Anticoagulants, oral	Phenobarbital
Anticoagulants, oral	Rifampin
Antidiabetics, oral	Rifampin
Carbamazepine	Phenobarbital
Contraceptives, oral	Carbamazepine
Contraceptives, oral	Phenobarbital
Contraceptives, oral	Rifampin
Digitoxin	Phenobarbital
Digitoxin	Rifampin
Theophylline	Phenobarbital
Theophylline	Rifampin

Table 11-4. Examples of Drug Interactions Involving Enzyme Inhibition

Activity of	Increased by
Acetaldehyde (from ethanol)	Disulfiram
Anticoagulants, oral	Chloramphenicol
Anticoagulants, oral	Cimetidine
Anticoagulants, oral	Disulfiram
Anticoagulants, oral	Metronidazole
Diazepam	Cimetidine
Phenytoin	Chloramphenicol
Phenytoin	Cimetidine
Phenytoin	Disulfiram
Phenytoin	Isoniazid
Theophylline	Cimetidine

3. **Intestinal bacterial flora** secrete a number of enzymes capable of metabolizing drugs and other xenobiotics.
   a. Any factor that **modifies the intestinal flora** may also **modify drug activity**. Age, diet, disease state, and exposure to environmental chemicals or drugs may all be important.
      (1) Certain **diseases,** particularly **intestinal disease,** affect intestinal flora. Ulcerative colitis, for example, promotes bacterial growth. Diarrhea reduces the number of bacteria.
      (2) Certain **environmental chemicals and drugs** also act on intestinal flora. Antibiotics, for example, decrease the number of bacteria.
   b. Bacterial flora secrete β-glucuronidase, which hydrolyzes the polar glucuronide conjugates of bile and allows the free, nonpolar bile acids to be reabsorbed. This **enterohepatic circulation** partially maintains the pool of bile acids. This same principle applies to certain glucuronide conjugates of drugs.
   c. Certain bacterial flora **convert vitamin precursors to their active forms,** as with vitamin K.
   d. Bacterial flora may also **convert certain substances to their toxic forms,** as with the conversion of the artificial sweetener cyclamate to cyclohexylamine, a suspected carcinogen.
   e. Intestinal bacteria produce **azoreductase,** which reduces the prodrug sulfasalazine to the active anti-inflammatory aminosalicylic acid and the active antibacterial sulfapyridine. Sulfasalazine is one of the few agents effective in the treatment of ulcerative colitis.

4. **Gastric acid** inactivates penicillin G. **Gastric acid** and **pepsin** inactivate insulin.

C. Placental and fetal metabolism

1. **Placenta.** In general, if a drug or other xenobiotic is lipid soluble enough to be absorbed into the circulation when administered to a pregnant woman, it will very likely also pass through the placenta.
   a. The placenta is not a physical nor a metabolic barrier to xenobiotics. Very little xenobiotic-metabolizing enzyme activity has been demonstrated in the placenta.
   b. Drugs present in their **active form** in the maternal circulation very likely pass **unchanged** into the fetal circulation.
   c. An exception to this lack of enzyme activity in the placenta is the presence of a small amount of **aryl aromatic hydroxylase,** which is **inducible in pregnant women who smoke cigarettes**. A potential consequence of this is an increase in the production of penultimate carcinogens from the action of this enzyme on the polycyclic aromatic hydrocarbons present in cigarette smoke and other environmental sources.

2. **Fetus.** In terms of fetal metabolism, there are varying degrees of drug-metabolizing activity dependent upon a number of factors including fetal age.
   a. A **major deficiency** is that of **glucuronic acid conjugating activity** both in the **fetus** and the **neonate**.
   b. Two consequences of this are the **gray baby syndrome,** resulting from decreased chloramphenicol glucuronidation, and **neonatal hyperbilirubinemia,** resulting from a decrease in bilirubin glucuronide formation.

V. PRINCIPLES OF DRUG METABOLISM are used to improve drug therapy to decrease the overall extent of metabolism, to overcome pharmaceutical problems, to overcome presystemic metabolism, to prolong the duration of action, to decrease toxicity, or to provide site-specific delivery of the parent drug molecules.

A. Dosage forms

1. **Nitroglycerin,** a rapidly acting antianginal agent, is essentially ineffective when administered orally because of its extremely high first-pass effect.
   a. Through the use of **sublingual tablets,** nitroglycerin enters the systemic circulation directly rather than the portal vein and, thus, is effective in small doses.
   b. Sublingual administration, however, is largely ineffective for prophylactic use because of its rapid inactivation; thus, **ointment** and **transdermal patch formulations** provide continuous absorption in selected cases.
2. **Methenamine** is a mild urinary antibacterial agent whose activity depends upon an acidic urine to be converted in situ to its active form (formaldehyde).
   a. Upon oral administration, it is subject to presystemic conversion to formaldehyde by gastric acid, thus potentially reducing its bioavailability.
   b. The use of **enteric-coated formulations** can protect methenamine during its passage through the acid environment.

B. Enzyme inhibitors

1. **Dopamine,** effective in the treatment of parkinsonism, is unable to penetrate the blood–brain barrier and, thus, cannot reach its site of action. Levodopa, the amino acid precursor of dopamine, does penetrate into the brain where it is decarboxylated to the active form. Thus, levodopa acts as a prodrug, providing site-specific delivery of the active drug, dopamine. The peripheral decarboxylation of levodopa can be inhibited by carbidopa [see Chapter 12 IX A 2 a].
2. **β-lactam antibiotics.** The antibacterial activity of a number of β-lactam antibiotics is reduced in infections caused by organisms capable of secreting the enzyme, **β-lactamase**.
   a. β-lactamase inactivates the susceptible antibiotic through its ability to hydrolytically cleave the β-lactam ring.
   b. Two agents, **clavulanic acid** and **sulbactam** are effective enhancers of such antibiotics. They inhibit the hydrolysis of the β-lactam ring by binding to and inactivating the β-lactamase enzyme. Since these agents are themselves destroyed in the process, they are termed **suicide inhibitors** [e.g., combinations of **clavulanic acid** with **amoxicillin** (Augmentin) and with **ticarcillin** (Timentin), **sulbactam** with **ampicillin** (Unasyn)].

C. Molecular modification

1. The high first-pass effect of certain drugs can be significantly reduced by modifying the molecule in such a way that the major metabolic pathway is **sterically hindered**.
   a. Estradiol has minimal oral activity because of a high first-pass effect. The introduction of an ethinyl group into its molecular structure produces a drug in which the position at which **conjugation** occurs is sterically hindered. The first-pass effect on **ethinyl estradiol** but not its estrogenic activity is markedly reduced and the drug is a potent, orally effective estrogenic substance.
   b. It and its methyl analog, **mestranol,** are extensively used as the estrogen components of the **combination type of oral contraceptive**.
   c. The same principle explains the fact that **methyltestosterone** is considerably more active when administered orally than is testosterone.
2. **Prodrugs** are used in a number of ways.
   a. **Esters** of estradiol, such as **benzoate, valerate,** and **cypionate,** are used to prolong estrogenic activity. Intramuscular injections of these esters in oil result in a depot of drug that is slowly hydrolyzed, thereby releasing free estradiol over a prolonged period of time. Other examples of this principle include **testosterone heptanoate** and **fluphenazine enanthate**.
   b. **Benzathine penicillin G** (Bicillin) is an early example of the prodrug concept. Inactive because of its insolubility, it is slowly broken down after injection as an aqueous suspension to release soluble penicillin G over a period of hours, resulting in an increase in the normal duration of action of penicillin G.

c. **Ampicillin,** although orally active, is not well absorbed due to its low liposolubility. Esterification of the carboxyl group markedly increases its liposolubility, affording more complete absorption. The modified ampicillin is rapidly hydrolyzed to its active form. **Bacampicillin** (Spectrobid) produces significantly higher serum levels of ampicillin.

d. **Chloramphenicol,** an antibiotic, is a neutral molecule; thus, it is not possible to prepare water-soluble salts that could be used in preparing parenteral dosage forms. Esterifying chloramphenicol with succinic acid produces a molecule that can form a water-soluble sodium salt. Although inactive, it is readily hydrolyzed to free chloramphenicol by plasma esterases.

e. **Stilbestrol,** the synthetic estrogen, may produce undesirable, feminizing side effects when used in the treatment of prostatic carcinoma. These side effects can be avoided by the use of the ester prodrug diethylstilbestrol diphosphate. Virtually inactive until dephosphorylated by acid phosphatase, which is highly active in prostatic carcinomatous tissue, it permits the largely localized release of free estrogen at its site of action with a reduction in systemic side effects.

f. **Epinephrine** is used locally in the eye for the treatment of glaucoma, although there is poor corneal penetrability due to its high polarity. The highly lipophilic, **dipivalyl ester** of epinephrine, **dipivefrine** (Propine) is able to penetrate unchanged into the cornea and is converted in situ to the active parent drug.

g. Both the anti-inflammatory activity and the gastrointestinal irritation of many nonsteroidal anti-inflammatory drugs (NSAIDs) appear to be related to their ability to inhibit prostaglandin synthesis. The NSAID **sulindac** (Clinoril) is the much less pharmacologically active sulfoxide derivative of sulindac sulfide. Absorbed as the inactive prodrug, it appears to cause less gastrointestinal irritation. Slow conversion to the active sulindac sulfide after absorption affords a relatively long duration of anti-inflammatory activity.

h. **Enalaprilat** is a potent angiotensin converting enzyme inhibitor that is active after parenteral administration, but, due to its high polarity, it is inactive orally. Its monomethyl ester prodrug **enalapril** (Vasotec) is considerably more lipophilic and, thus, provides good oral absorption. It is easily converted to the active form by serum esterases.

STUDY QUESTIONS

Directions: Each of the numbered items or incomplete statements in this section is followed by answers or by completions of the statement. Select the **one** lettered answer or completion that is **best** in each case.

1. Which of the following statements concerning drug metabolism is true?

(A) Generally a single metabolite is excreted for each drug administered
(B) Often a drug may undergo a phase II reaction followed by a phase I reaction
(C) Drug-metabolizing enzymes are found only in the liver
(D) All metabolites are less active pharmacologically than their parent drugs
(E) Phase I metabolites more likely are able to cross cellular membranes than phase II metabolites

2. Which of the following metabolites would be the least likely urinary excretion product of orally administered aspirin (see structure below)?

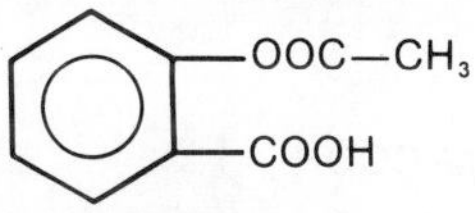

(A) Glycine conjugate
(B) Ester glucuronide
(C) Unchanged drug
(D) Ether glucuronide
(E) Hydroxylated metabolite

3. Sulfasalazine (see structure below) is a prodrug that is activated in the intestine by bacterial enzymes. The enzyme most likely responsible is

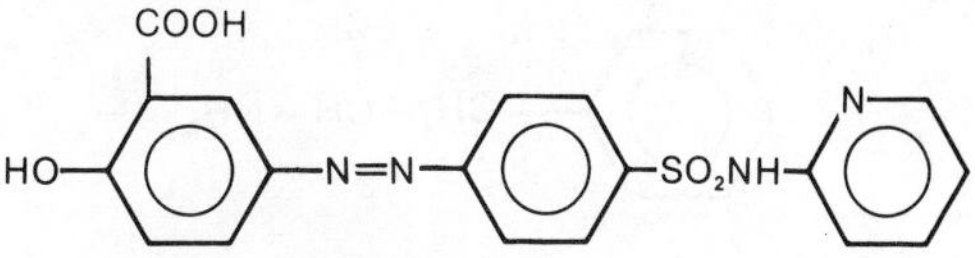

(A) azoreductase
(B) pseudocholinesterase
(C) N-acetyltransferase
(D) β-glucuronidase
(E) methyltransferase

4. Chloramphenicol (see structure below) is considered to be toxic in infants (gray baby syndrome). This is due to tissue accumulation of unchanged chloramphenicol, resulting from an immature metabolic pathway. Which of the following enzymes would most likely be deficient?

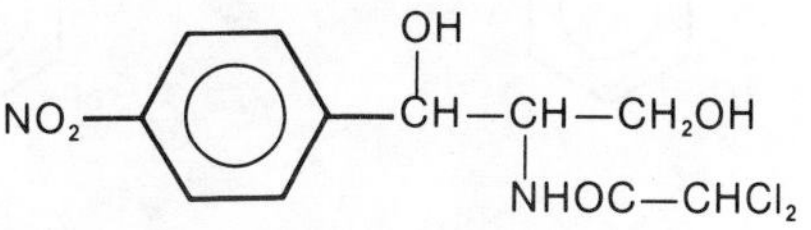

(A) Pseudocholinesterase
(B) Glucuronyl transferase
(C) N-acetyltransferase
(D) Azoreductase
(E) Methyltransferase

1-E
2-C
3-A
4-B

Directions: Each question below contains three suggested answers of which **one or more** is correct. Choose the answer

A if **I only** is correct
B if **III only** is correct
C if **I and II** are correct
D if **II and III** are correct
E if **I, II, and III** are correct

5. Terms that may be used to describe the following metabolic reaction include

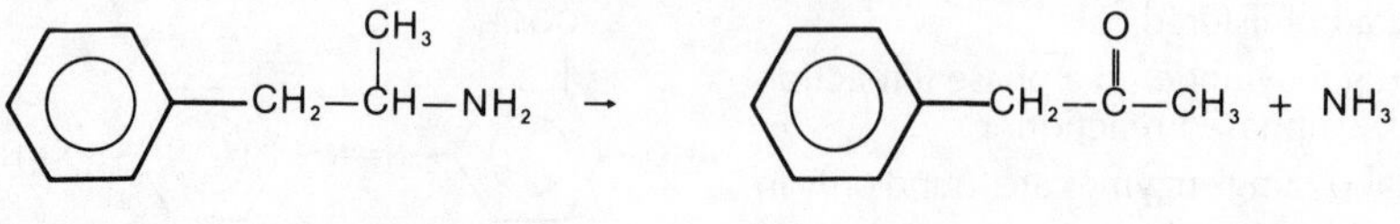

I. oxidative N-dealkylation
II. oxidative deamination
III. phase I reaction

6. Phase II metabolic reactions include which of the following?

I.

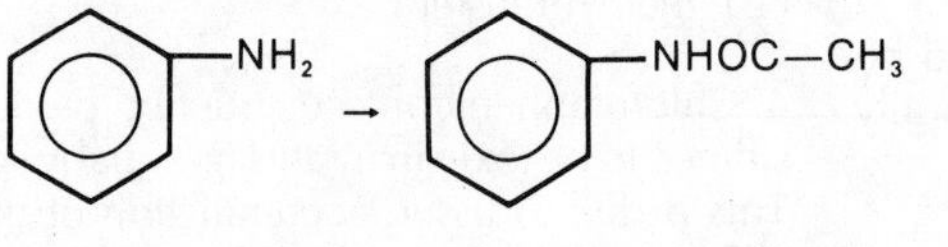

II.

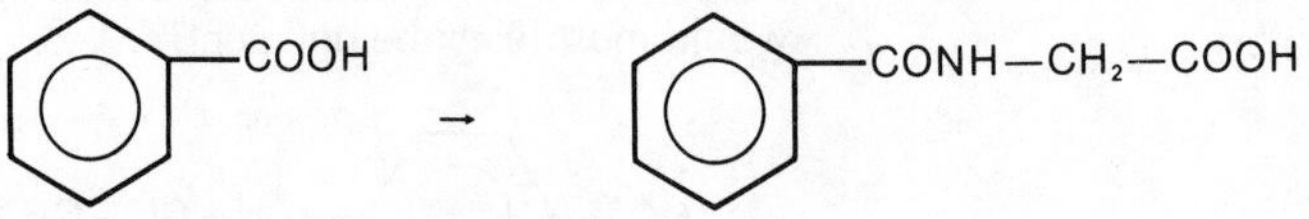

III.

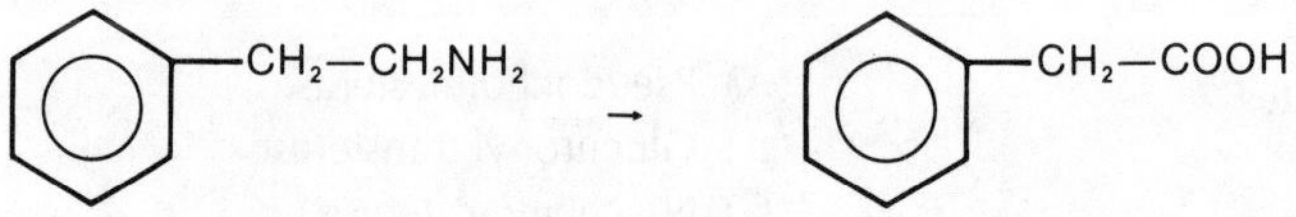

7. Conditions that tend to increase the action of an orally administered drug that undergoes phase II metabolism include

I. enterohepatic circulation
II. enzyme saturation
III. first-pass effect

8. Metabolic reactions likely to be affected by a protein-deficient diet include

I. glycine conjugation
II. hydrolysis
III. glucuronidation

5-D
6-C
7-C
8-A

Directions: The group of items in this section consists of lettered options followed by a set of numbered items. For each item, select the **one** lettered option that is most closely associated with it. Each lettered option may be selected once, more than once, or not at all.

Questions 9–12

For each drug, select the metabolic pathway that it would most likely follow.

(A) Ether glucuronidation
(B) Ester glucuronidation
(C) Azoreduction
(D) Oxidative deamination
(E) Hydrolysis

9. Benzoic acid

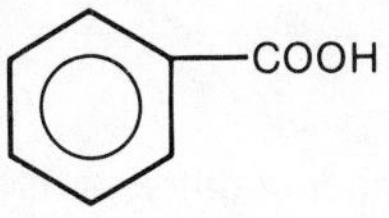

10. Procaine

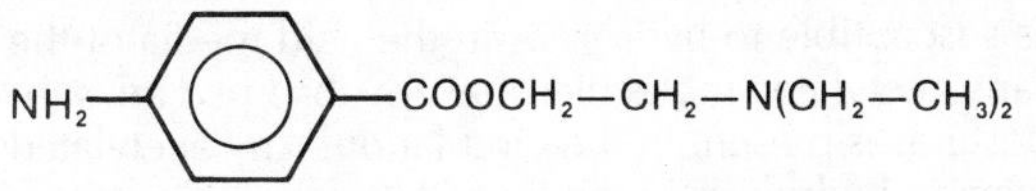

11. Acetaminophen

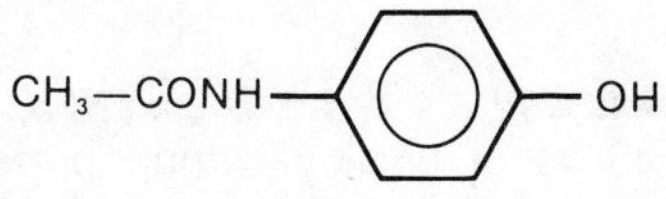

12. Amphetamine

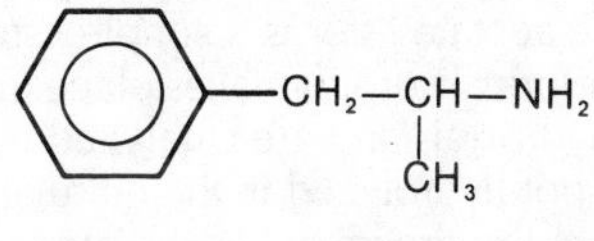

9-B
10-E
11-A
12-D

ANSWERS AND EXPLANATIONS

1. The answer is E *[I; II A 1 d, B].*
Phase I metabolites are often somewhat more polar than their parents. With the exception of acetylated and methylated metabolites, phase II metabolites are always much more polar than their parents. Thus, phase I metabolites are more likely to retain some liposolubility and are more likely to cross cellular membranes.

It is unusual for a single metabolite to be excreted for a given drug. Most drugs yield a mixture of metabolites. Because of the high polarity and subsequent high excretion of phase II metabolites, they are not likely to undergo further metabolism. Phase I metabolites, on the other hand, are less polar and are very likely to undergo further phase II metabolic reactions.

While the major site of metabolism is the liver, there are many extrahepatic sites that secrete drug-metabolizing enzymes. While many metabolites are less pharmacologically active than their parents, there are many drugs whose metabolites have equal or greater pharmacologic activity and sometimes greater toxicity as well. Prodrugs (i.e., drugs inactive in the form administered) always form at least one active metabolite.

2. The answer is C *[II A 1 c, 3 a, B 2 a (2), b; Table 11-1].*
Because of the types of functional groups present, aspirin may undergo a number of different metabolic reactions. These include hydroxylation of the aromatic nucleus, conjugation of the carboxyl group with glycine, conjugation of the carboxyl group with glucuronic acid with the formation of an ester glucuronide, hydrolysis of the acetate ester, and conjugation of the phenol group (resulting from hydrolysis of the acetate ester) with glucuronic acid to form an ether glucuronide.

Since the acetate ester is a simple ester, aspirin is susceptible to hydrolysis in the acid media of the stomach before absorption takes place. In addition, any acetylated molecules that are absorbed are subjected to hydrolysis and are catalyzed by the many esterases present in the circulation. Any acetylated molecules not hydrolyzed in the circulation are subject to hydrolysis in the liver. All of these processes occur before the drug reaches the glomerular filtrate; therefore, excretion of the unchanged acetylated drug is highly unlikely.

3. The answer is A *[II A 2; IV B 3 e; Table 11-1].*
Sulfasalazine has both anti-inflammatory and antibacterial activity when converted to aminosalicylic acid and sulfapyridine in the body. This reaction occurs by reductive cleavage of the "azo" linkage contained in the sulfasalazine molecule and is catalyzed in the intestine by bacterial azoreductase. This is a form of site-specific delivery since the intact drug is not absorbed from the stomach or upper intestine and reaches the colon, where it is metabolized. Sulfasalazine is one of a few drugs that is effective for the treatment of ulcerative colitis.

4. The answer is B *[II B 2 a (1); III G 1; IV C 2 b; Table 11-1].*
The chloramphenicol molecule contains an aromatic nucleus, which would be subject to hydroxylation, a nitro group that is subject to reduction, an amide group that is subject to liver hydrolysis, and alcohol groups that are subject to glucuronidation. Of all the enzyme systems responsible for these reactions, the system responsible for glucuronidation is developed poorly in premature infants and infants up to approximately 6–8 weeks of age.

5. The answer is D (II, III) *[II A; Table 11-1].*
The reaction shown in the question involves the conversion of one functional group to another (amine to carbonyl); thus, it is classified as a phase I reaction. The introduction of oxygen into the molecule indicates oxidation, and the loss of the amino group signifies deamination; thus, the reaction also can be classified as oxidative deamination. Oxidative N-dealkylation implies the removal of an alkyl group from a nitrogen. The nitrogen in the parent molecule does not have an alkyl group attached to it.

6. The answer is C (I, II) *[II A, B; Table 11-1].*
Phase II metabolic reactions involve masking of an existing functional group with a natural endogenous constituent. The formulas shown in choices I and II both represent this type of reaction, choice I being an acetylation reaction and choice II being a glycine conjugation reaction. Choice III represents a change in an existing functional group and, thus, represents a phase I reaction. It is an oxidative deamination reaction.

7. The answer is C (I, II) *[II B 2 a (4); III E 1, 2; IV B 3 b].*
Enterohepatic circulation refers to the process by which glucuronides, which are secreted into the intestine with the bile, are hydrolyzed by intestinal bacterial β-glucuronidase. The hydrolyzed free drug, which is no longer polar, becomes available for intestinal reabsorption into the system and subsequent penetration to its active site.

If an enzyme system becomes saturated, then the active drug cannot be inactivated by that pathway. If the drug cannot undergo an alternative pathway, the increased plasma levels of an unchanged active drug can result in increased activity or toxicity.

The first-pass effect results in metabolism of a drug by the liver before the drug reaches its site of action, resulting in an overall decrease in its activity. Drugs that undergo first-pass metabolism generally are effective in much smaller intravenous doses than oral doses.

8. The answer is A (I) *[III F 1].*
Phase II metabolic reactions require natural endogenous substrates, which normally are supplied in the diet. A deficiency of these substances would result in decreasing the biotransformation of drugs that use these pathways. Glycine conjugation is such a phase II reaction. Glycine is an amino acid that requires dietary protein. A diet deficient in protein, therefore, could lead to a deficiency of glycine and, thus, a decrease in glycine conjugation. Glucuronidation is also a phase II reaction that requires endogenous glucuronic acid, but this substance is supplied by dietary carbohydrates. Hydroxylation is a phase I metabolic reaction and does not require dietary protein.

9–12. The answers are: 9-B *[II B 2 a (2)],* **10-E** *[II A 3 a],* **11-A** *[II B 2 a (2)],* **12-D** *[II A 1 b].*
A common metabolic pathway of carboxylic acids is conjugation with the endogenous substrate, glucuronic acid, with the net equation involving the splitting out of a molecule of water by combining the hydrogen of the carboxyl group with the anomer OH of glucuronic acid. This essentially is a reaction of an acid and an alcohol, which results in the formation of an ester linkage. Carboxylic acids also undergo glycine or glutamine conjugation, which results in the formation of an amide linkage. Theoretically, it is also possible for benzoic acid to undergo ring hydroxylation, which is a common phase I pathway for aromatic nuclei.

Procaine is an ester-type local anesthetic. It is a simple ester and, therefore, very susceptible to hydrolysis in the body, due to the wide distribution of esterase enzymes and body water. This susceptibility to hydrolysis is the major reason why local anesthetics of this type have short durations of action when compared to other types of local anesthetics.

One of the principal functional groups in acetaminophen is the phenol, which commonly undergoes glucuronidation. The net result of the reaction is the splitting out of a molecule of water from the loss of the hydrogen atom of the phenol and the hydroxyl group of glucuronic acid, forming an ether linkage. Phenols also commonly undergo sulfate conjugation reactions and occasionally undergo O-methylation reactions. They may also undergo ring hydroxylation, due to the aromatic nucleus.

The principal functional group in amphetamine is a primary amine. Amines have a very low in vivo stability. Primary amines commonly undergo phase I oxidative deamination as well as phase II acetylation reactions.

12
Drugs Affecting the Autonomic Nervous System and the Neuromuscular Junction

David C. Kosegarten
Edward F. LaSala

I. INTRODUCTION. Drugs affecting the autonomic nervous system and the neuromuscular junction mimic or modify the actions of neurohumoral transmitters. They fall into five major categories: cholinergic agonists, cholinergic antagonists, adrenergic agonists, adrenergic antagonists, and neuromuscular blocking agents. Table 12-1 defines basic pharmacologic concepts.

Table 12-1. Basic Pharmacologic Concepts

Concept	Definition
Drug receptor	A specific cellular site that interacts with a drug molecule, mediating the drug's action. Drug receptors are located in or on the cell membrane or within the cell itself. They are affected by micromolar to nanomolar drug concentrations, demonstrate relative stereospecificity, and can be selectively blocked by drug antagonists.
Affinity	The ability of a drug to combine with a specific receptor.
Agonist	A drug that has both affinity for a receptor and intrinsic activity that produces a pharmacologic effect. A drug that has affinity but very little or low intrinsic activity is considered a partial agonist (or, alternatively, a partial antagonist).
Antagonist	A drug that has affinity for a receptor but lacks intrinsic activity.
Pharmacologic antagonism	The process that occurs when an antagonist combines with a receptor, preventing or limiting an agonist's ability to produce a pharmacologic effect.
Physiologic antagonism	The process that occurs when an agonist and an antagonist act independently on two different receptors for different cellular mechanisms or different physiologic systems. For example, a drug that mimics the activity of the parasympathetic nervous system may be antagonized by a drug that mimics the activity of the sympathetic nervous system.
Drug intrinsic activity	A measure of the drug's ability to produce a pharmacologic effect.
Drug efficacy	A drug's ability to produce a maximum drug effect.
Drug potency	The relative concentrations of two or more drugs that produce the same drug effect.
Drug potentiation	The process that occurs when administration of a second, active drug increases the effectiveness of a first drug that is ineffective when given alone.
Drug synergism	The process that occurs when co-administration of two drugs causes a greater therapeutic effect than administration of each drug individually.
Drug additive effect	The process that occurs when co-administration of two drugs causes a therapeutic effect equal to that obtained by administration of each drug individually.

(Continued on next page)

Table 12-1. Continued

Concept	Definition
Drug therapeutic index (margin of safety)	The relationship between the dosage that produces an undesirable effect (death) and the dosage that produces a desirable (therapeutic) effect. The greater the ratio of these dosages, the safer the drug and the higher its therapeutic index.
Tolerance	The phenomenon of decreased responsiveness to a drug following chronic administration.
Tachyphylaxis	The rapid development of tolerance.
Anaphylaxis	An acute systemic reaction (commonly characterized by urticaria, respiratory distress, and vascular collapse) that occurs in a previously sensitized individual after exposure to the sensitizing antigen.
Anaphylactoid reaction	A dose-dependent, idiosyncratic reaction, clinically similar to anaphylaxis, that can occur after the first administration of certain drugs.

II. CHOLINERGIC AGONISTS

A. Chemistry

1. **Acetylcholine,** the natural endogenous mediator and the most potent cholinergic agonist, is an ester of acetic acid and choline, a quaternary aminoalcohol (Figure 12-1). A hygroscopic simple ester, it is unstable and quickly hydrolyzed both in vitro and in vivo. Thus, it is extremely short-acting and usually is not a satisfactory therapeutic agent.

2. **Therapeutically useful cholinergic agonists** may be direct-acting or indirect-acting.
   a. **Direct-acting agonists** may be produced by replacing the acetyl group of acetylcholine with a carbamoyl group or by substituting a methyl group of the β-carbon. These actions decrease the drug's hydrolysis rate, providing such stable, useful agonists as methacholine chloride (Provocholine) and bethanechol chloride (Urecholine) [Figure 12-2].
   b. **Indirect-acting agonists** (e.g., acetylcholinesterase inhibitors) are divided into two major classes.
      (1) **Reversible (short-acting) agents** are principally carbamic esters, such as physostigmine (Eserine) and neostigmine (Prostigmin) [Figure 12-3].
      (2) **Irreversible (long-acting) agents** are principally organophosphate esters, such as isoflurophate and echothiophate (Phospholine) [Figure 12-4].

B. Pharmacology

1. **Cholinergic responses** are mediated by both muscarinic and nicotinic receptors.
   a. **Muscarinic receptors** are present at parasympathetic postganglionic neuroeffector cell sites (Table 12-2).
   b. **Nicotinic receptors** are present at the ganglia of both the parasympathetic and sympathetic nervous systems and also at the neuromuscular junctions of the somatic nervous system (see VI A 1).

2. Cholinergic agonists act by **mimicking the activity of endogenous acetylcholine** at muscarinic and nicotinic receptor sites.
   a. **Direct-acting agonists** interact directly with these receptors.
   b. **Indirect-acting agonists** inhibit or block the activity of cholinesterase enzymes (e.g., acetylcholinesterase, pseudocholinesterase), which block the action of endogenous acetylcholine. Thus, these agonists allow endogenous acetylcholine to accumulate at cholinergic receptors, producing cholinergic stimulation. Organophosphate cholinesterase inhibitors (e.g., certain agricultural insecticides and so-called nerve gases) bind to the enzyme to form a long-lasting enzyme inhibitor complex and are extremely toxic.

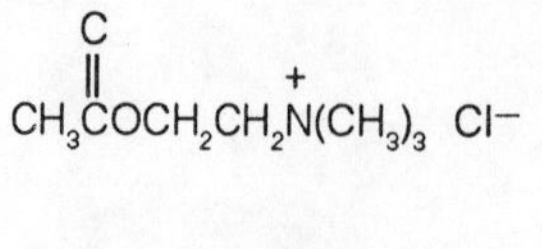

Figure 12-1. The structural formula of acetylcholine.

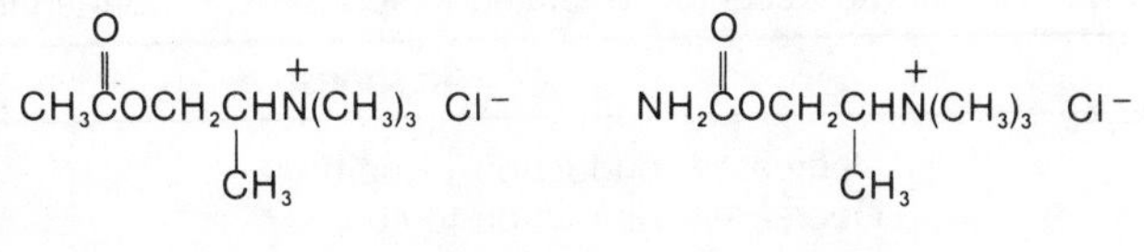

$$CH_3\overset{\overset{\displaystyle O}{\|}}{C}OCH_2\overset{\overset{\displaystyle CH_3}{|}}{C}H\overset{+}{N}(CH_3)_3 \quad Cl^-$$

$$NH_2\overset{\overset{\displaystyle O}{\|}}{C}OCH_2\overset{\overset{\displaystyle CH_3}{|}}{C}H\overset{+}{N}(CH_3)_3 \quad Cl^-$$

A   **B**

Figure 12-2. Clinically useful direct-acting cholinergic agonists include (*A*) methacholine chloride (Provocholine) and (*B*) bethanechol chloride (Urecholine).

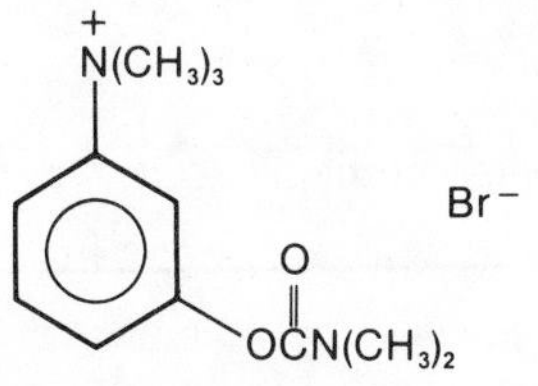

Figure 12-3. The structural formula of neostigmine bromide (Prostigmin), a reversible acetylcholinesterase inhibitor.

C. Therapeutic indications

1. **Direct-acting agonists** are indicated to:
   a. Initiate micturition in acute nonobstructive urinary retention (e.g., bethanechol)
   b. Produce miosis in the treatment of glaucoma (e.g., pilocarpine)

2. **Indirect-acting agonists** are indicated to:
   a. Produce miosis in the treatment of glaucoma (e.g., physostigmine, isoflurophate, echothiophate)
   b. Treat myasthenia gravis (e.g., ambenonium, neostigmine, pyridostigmine)
   c. Aid in the differential diagnosis of myasthenia gravis and cholinergic crisis (e.g., edrophonium)
   d. Counteract intoxication or adverse effects from compounds with anticholinergic activity (e.g., physostigmine)

D. Adverse effects

1. **Topical adverse effects** include congested conjunctivae, myopic accommodation, and transient lenticular opacity.

2. **Systemic adverse effects** include headache, syncope, nausea, vomiting, bradycardia, hypotension, bronchospasm, abdominal cramps, diarrhea, epigastric distress, salivation, sweating, lacrimation, flushing, and tremors.

III. CHOLINERGIC ANTAGONISTS

A. Chemistry

1. **Atropine,** an alkaloid obtained from the belladonna plant, is the prototypical cholinergic antagonist (anticholinergic agent). A portion of the atropine molecule is structurally similar to acetylcholine (Figure 12-5), permitting the molecule to bind to postganglionic receptors. However, the molecule has no intrinsic activity, and its bulky shape prevents acetylcholine from binding to the receptor.

2. **Synthetic anticholinergic agents** [e.g., dicyclomine (Bentyl), glycopyrrolate (Robinul), propantheline] are also available. These agents, like atropine, are bulky analogues of acetylcholine (Figure 12-6).

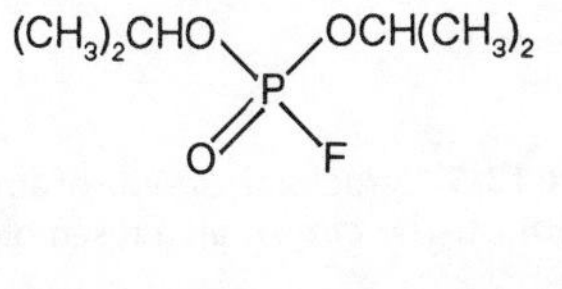

Figure 12-4. The structural formula of isoflurophate (Floropryl), an irreversible acetylcholinesterase inhibitor.

Table 12-2. Muscarinic Receptor-Mediated Responses to Cholinergic Agonists

Organ	Response
Heart	Decreases conduction velocity Decreases contraction force Decreases contraction rate
Eye	Contracts the iris sphincter muscle and the ciliary muscle, producing miosis
Lung	Contracts tracheal and bronchial muscles
Intestine	Increases peristalsis Increases secretions Relaxes sphincter
Urinary bladder	Relaxes trigone and sphincter muscles Contracts detrusor muscle

B. Pharmacology

1. Cholinergic antagonists **competitively inhibit the activity of endogenous acetylcholine.**
2. Antagonists that inhibit muscarinic receptor-mediated responses are called **antimuscarinic agents;** those that inhibit nicotinic receptor-mediated responses are called **ganglionic blocking agents.**

C. Therapeutic indications

1. **Antimuscarinic agents** are indicated to:
   a. Reduce glandular and bronchiolar secretions before anesthesia (e.g., atropine, scopolamine)
   b. Induce sedation (e.g., scopolamine)
   c. Alleviate motion sickness (e.g., scopolamine)
   d. Reduce vagal stimulation of the myocardium (e.g., atropine)
   e. Produce ophthalmic mydriasis and cycloplegia (e.g., homatropine)
   f. Reduce gastrointestinal smooth muscle spasms (e.g., propantheline)
   g. Treat bronchospasm associated with chronic obstructive pulmonary disease (e.g., ipratropium)
   h. Control Parkinson's disease and some neuroleptic-induced extrapyramidal disorders (e.g., benztropine, trihexyphenidyl)
   i. Treat intoxication by cholinergic agonists or by the rapid form of mushroom poisoning (e.g., atropine)
2. **Ganglionic blocking agents** are indicated to treat hypertensive crisis (e.g., trimethaphan).

D. Adverse effects

1. **Topical adverse effects** include hyperopic accommodation and increased intraocular pressure.
2. **Systemic adverse effects** include headache, nervousness, drowsiness, dizziness, palpitations, tachycardia, dry mouth, mydriasis, blurred vision, nausea, vomiting, constipation, urinary retention, and fever.

IV. ADRENERGIC AGONISTS

A. Chemistry

1. **Direct-acting adrenergic agonists** include norepinephrine and epinephrine (naturally occurring catecholamines) as well as their derivatives. Catecholamines are biosynthesized from tyrosine, an amino acid (Figure 12-7).
   a. The ethylamine chain common to these agonists is essential to their activity.

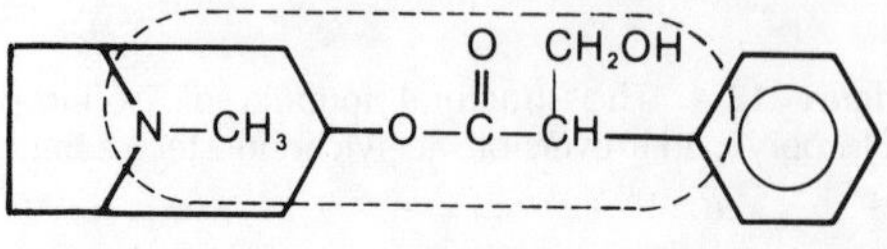

Figure 12-5. Structural formula of atropine, a cholinergic antagonist. The *circled area* resembles acetylcholine.

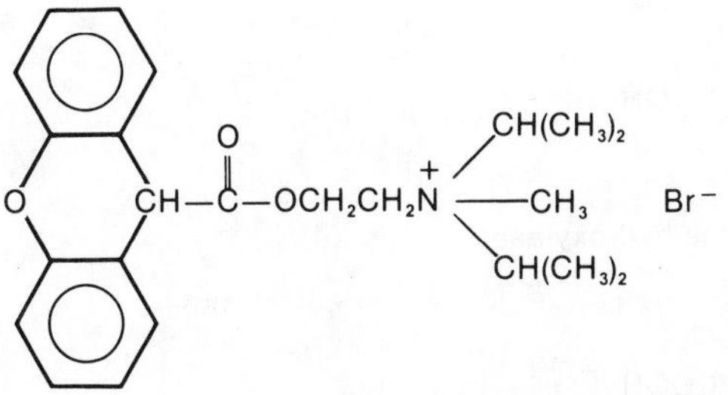

Figure 12-6. Structural formula of propantheline bromide (Probanthine), a synthetic cholinergic antagonist.

b. N-substituents alter drug activity. Small substituents (e.g., hydrogen, a methyl group) produce α-receptor activity, as with norepinephrine; larger substituents (e.g., an isopropyl group) produce β-receptor activity, as with isoproterenol.

c. Removal of the **para (4) hydroxyl group** leaves only α-receptor activity, as with phenylephrine.

d. The **meta (3) hydroxyl group** is essential for direct α- and β-activity. However, drugs in which the meta hydroxyl is replaced by a sulfonamide or a hydroxymethyl group retain activity.

e. The catecholamines are inactivated by methylation of the meta hydroxyl group (catalyzed by catechol O-methyltransferase) and by oxidation deamination [catalyzed by monoamine oxidase (MAO)].

2. **Indirect-acting agonists (sympathomimetic amines)** are compounds that are chemically related to the catecholamines and have similar effects. These are primarily synthetic compounds; examples include hydroxyamphetamine, ephedrine, tuaminoheptane, naphazoline, methamphetamine, protokylol, terbutaline, and dobutamine (Figure 12-8).
   a. Sympathomimetic amines may have one, two, or no hydroxyl groups. The fewer hydroxyl groups, the less intestinal destruction and the greater the drug's lipophilic character; thus, the greater the absorption and the duration of activity after oral administration.
   b. The benzene ring of these drugs may be replaced by cyclohexyl, naphthalene, or other rings or by aliphatic chains.
   c. Alkyl substitution at the α-carbon (adjacent to the amino group) retards destruction of phenol and phenyl compounds and increases lipophilic character, contributing to prolonged activity.
   d. N-substituents with bulky groups increase β-receptor activity, as with direct-acting agents.

B. Pharmacology

1. **Adrenergic peripheral responses** are mediated by both α- and β-receptors (Table 12-3).
   a. **α-Receptors** fall into two groups.
      (1) **Postjunctional α_1-adrenergic receptors** are found in the radial smooth muscle of the iris; in the arteries, arterioles, and veins; in the splenic capsule; and in the gastrointestinal tract. Drugs that are **α_1-selective agonists** include phenylephrine and methoxamine.
      (2) **Prejunctional α_2-adrenergic receptors** mediate the inhibition of release of adrenergic neurotransmitter. Drugs that are **α_2-selective agonists** include α-methylnorepinephrine and clonidine.
   b. **β-Receptors** also fall into two groups.
      (1) **Postjunctional β_1-adrenergic receptors** are found in the myocardium, the intestinal smooth muscle, and adipose tissue. Drugs that are **β_1-selective agonists** include dobutamine.
      (2) **Postjunctional β_2-adrenergic receptors** are found in bronchiolar and vascular smooth muscle. Drugs that are **β_2-selective agonists** include terbutaline.

2. **Direct-acting adrenergic agonists** (e.g., phenylephrine, clonidine, dobutamine, terbutaline) produce their effects primarily by direct stimulation of adrenergic receptors. They may be receptor-selective, as with the drugs listed above, or they may be nonselective. For example, the adrenergic neurotransmitter norepinephrine affects α_1-, α_2-, and β_1-receptors, whereas the adrenal medullary hormone epinephrine affects α_1-, α_2-, β_1-, and β_2-receptors. Isoproterenol affects both β_1- and β_2-receptors.

3. **Indirect-acting adrenergic agonists** work through other routes. For example, tyramine acts by releasing norepinephrine from storage sites in adrenergic neurons.

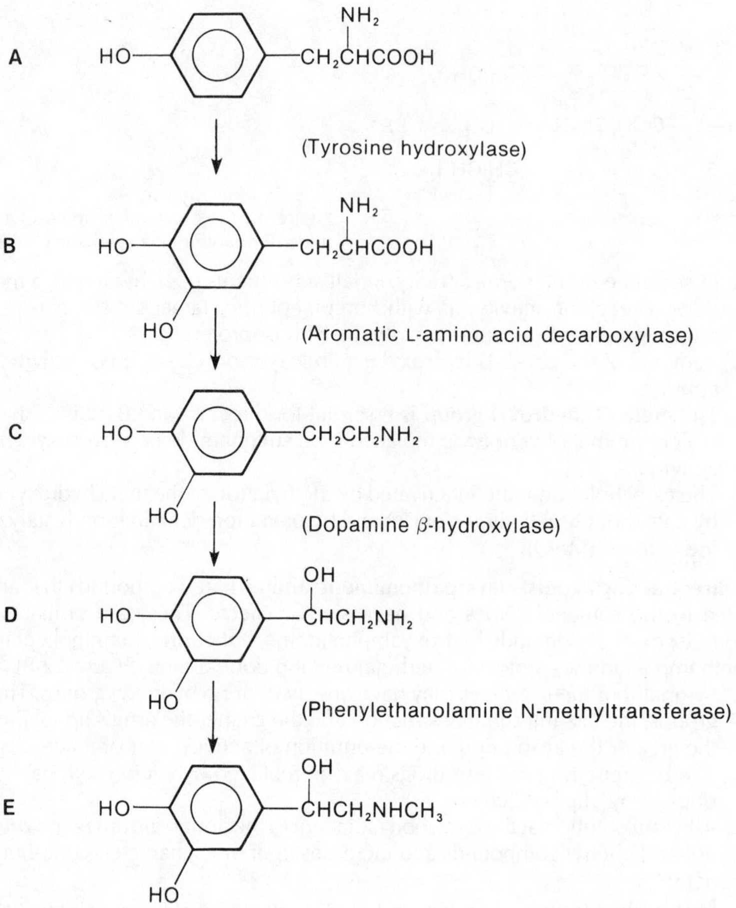

Figure 12-7. Synthesis of catecholamines from the amino acid tyrosine. In the presence of tyrosine hydroxylase, (*A*) tyrosine is converted to (*B*) dihydroxyphenylalanine (dopa). Further substitutions permit the synthesis of (*C*) dopamine, (*D*) norepinephrine, and (*E*) epinephrine.

4. Certain agonists (e.g., ephedrine, dopamine, metaraminol, mephentermine) produce their effects through both direct and indirect mechanisms.

C. Therapeutic indications

1. **Epinephrine** (an α- and β-adrenergic agonist) is indicated to treat bronchospasm and hypersensitivity reactions and is the agent of choice for anaphylactic reactions. It is also used to prolong the activity of local anesthetic solutions and to restore cardiac activity in cardiac arrest.
2. **Phenylephrine** (an α_1-selective agonist) is used to provide pressor activity, to prolong the activity of local anesthetic solutions, and to relieve paroxysmal atrial tachycardia.
3. **Clonidine** (an α_2-selective agonist) and the prodrug α-methyldopa (converts to methylnorepinephrine) are used as central-acting sympatholytic antihypertensives.
4. **Isoproterenol** (a β-adrenergic agonist) is used as a bronchodilator and as a cardiac stimulant in shock and cardiac arrest.
5. **Dobutamine** (a β_1-selective agonist) is used to improve myocardial function in congestive heart failure.
6. **Terbutaline** (a β_2-selective agonist) is used as a bronchodilator.

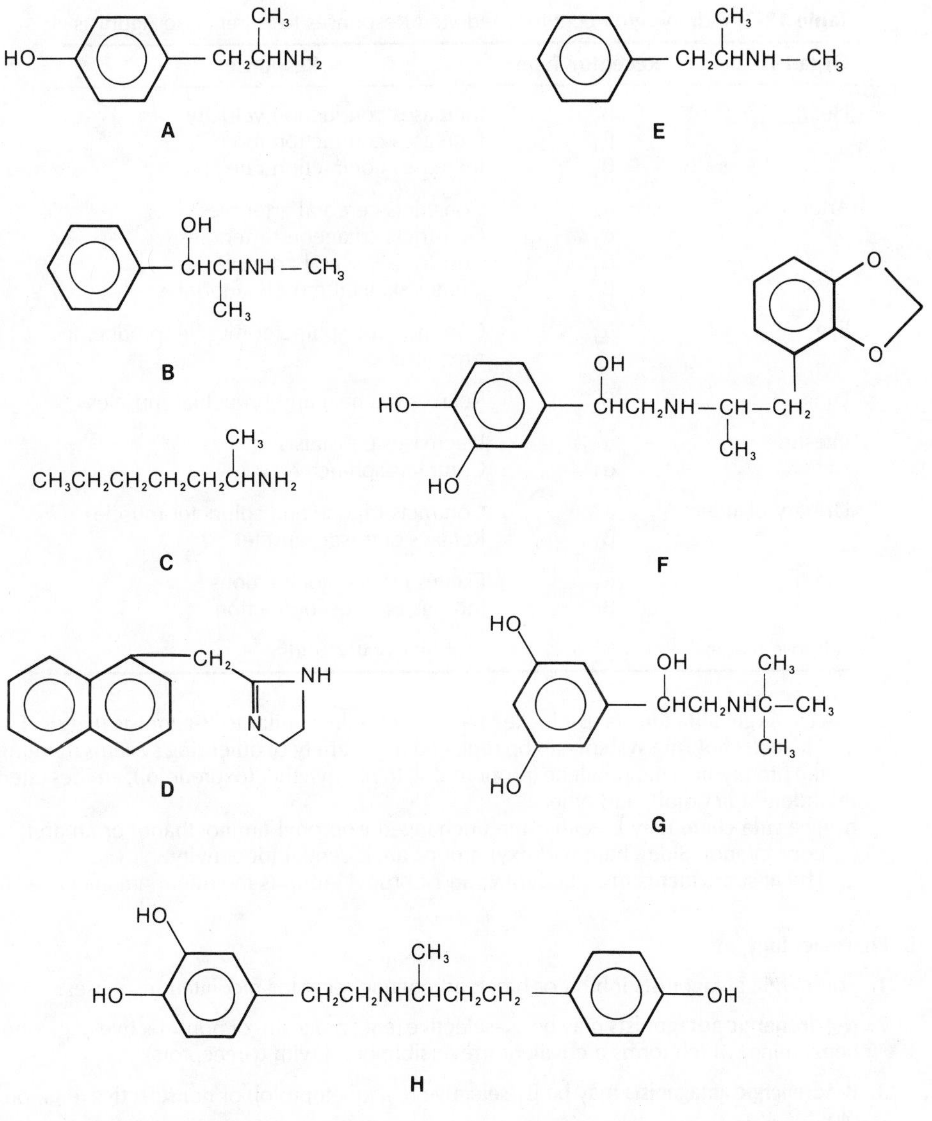

Figure 12-8. Structural formulas of representative sympathomimetic amines. (*A*) Hydroxyamphetamine (Paredrine); (*B*) ephedrine or pseudoephedrine (Sudafed); (*C*) tuaminoheptane (Tuamine); (*D*) naphazoline (Privine); (*E*) methamphetamine (Methedrine); (*F*) protokylol (Ventaire); (*G*) terbutaline (Brethine); (*H*) dobutamine (Dobutrex).

D. Adverse effects. Adrenergic agonists may cause cardiac dysrhythmias, cerebral hemorrhage, pulmonary hypertension and edema, anxiety, headache, and rebound nasal congestion.

V. ADRENERGIC ANTAGONISTS

A. Chemistry

1. **α-Adrenergic antagonists** (α-blockers) have varied structures and bear little resemblance to the adrenergic agonists. Antagonists include the ergot alkaloids (e.g., ergotamine), the dibenzamines (e.g., phenoxybenzamine), the benzolines (e.g., tolazoline), and the quinazolines (e.g., prazosin) [Figure 12-9].

Table 12-3. Adrenergic Receptor-Mediated Responses to Adrenergic Agonists

Organ/Tissue	Receptor Type	Response
Heart	β_1	Increases conduction velocity
	β_1	Increases contraction force
	β_1	Increases contraction rate
Arterioles	α_1	Constricts cerebral arterioles
	α_1	Constricts cutaneous arterioles
	α_1	Constricts visceral arterioles
	β_2	Dilates skeletal muscle arterioles
Eye	α_1	Contracts iris sphincter muscle, producing mydriasis
Lung	β_2	Relaxes tracheal and bronchial muscles
Intestine	α, β	Decreases peristalsis
	α_1	Contracts sphincter
Urinary bladder	α_1	Contracts trigone and sphincter muscles
	β_1	Relaxes detrusor muscle
Uterus	α_1	Excites uterine contractions
	β_2	Inhibits uterine contractions
Adipose tissue	β_1	Mobilizes fatty acids

2. **β-Adrenergic antagonists** (β-blockers) are structurally similar to β-agonists (Figure 12-10).
   a. The **catechol ring system** can be replaced by a variety of other ring systems, ranging from the prototypical naphthalene (propranolol) to phenylether (oxprenolol), amides (atenolol), indoles (pindolol), and others.
   b. The **side chain** may be either the unchanged isopropyl-aminoethanol or an aryloxyaminopropranol. Side-chain hydroxyl groups are essential for activity.
   c. The **N-substituents** must be bulky; an isopropyl group is the minimum effective size.

B. Pharmacology

1. Adrenergic antagonists inhibit or block adrenergic receptor-mediated responses.
2. **α-Adrenergic antagonists** may be α_1-selective (e.g., prazosin) or nonselective (e.g., phenoxybenzamine, which forms a covalent irreversible bond with α-receptors).
3. **β-Adrenergic antagonists** may be β_1-selective (e.g., metoprolol) or nonselective (e.g., propranolol).

C. Therapeutic indications

1. **Prazosin** (an α_1-selective antagonist) is used to produce vasodilation and is an important antihypertensive agent.

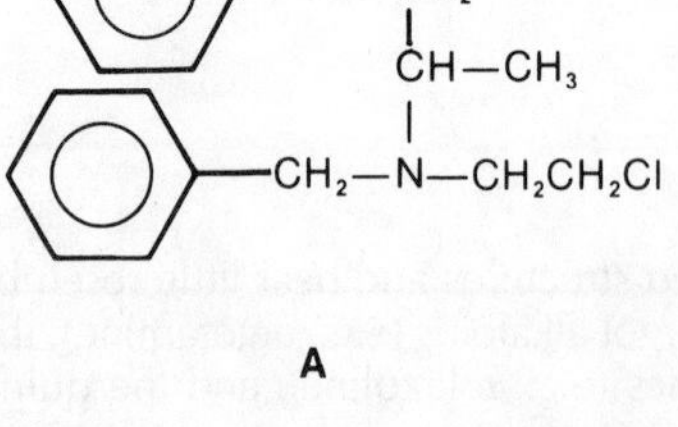

A

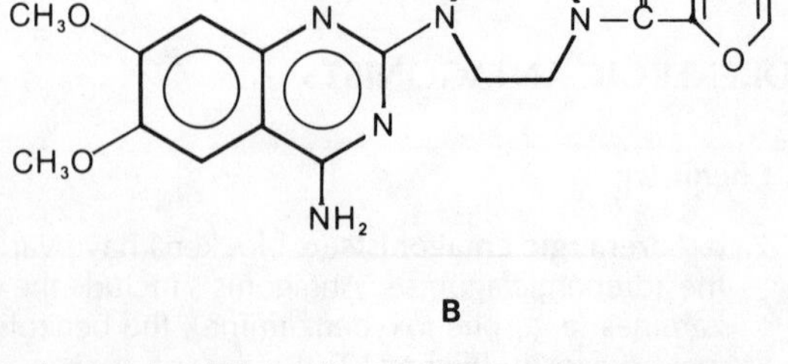

B

Figure 12-9. The structural formulas of (*A*) phenoxybenzamine (Dibenzyline) and (*B*) prazosin (Minipress), representative α-blockers.

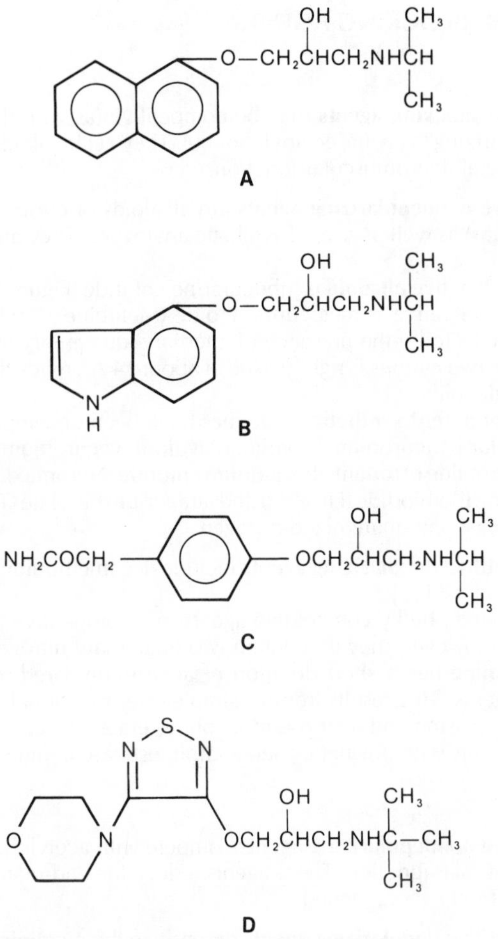

Figure 12-10. The structural formulas of (*A*) propranolol (Inderal); (*B*) pindolol (Visken); (*C*) atenolol (Tenormin); and (*D*) timolol (Blocadren), representative β-blockers.

2. **Phenoxybenzamine** (a nonselective α-antagonist) is used to relieve vasospasm in Raynaud's syndrome and for acute hypertensive emergencies resulting from MAO inhibitors, sympathomimetics, or pheochromocytoma.

3. **Propranolol** (a nonselective β-antagonist) is used for the prophylaxis of angina pectoris, supraventricular and ventricular dysrhythmias, and migraine headache. It is also used as an antihypertensive, as a negative inotropic agent in hypertrophic obstructive cardiomyopathies, and as a negative chronotropic agent in anxiety and hyperthyroidism.

4. **Metoprolol** (a β_1-selective antagonist) is used primarily as an antihypertensive agent.

D. Adverse effects

1. **Prazosin** may cause sudden syncope with the first dose, orthostatic hypotension, dizziness, headache, drowsiness, palpitations, fluid retention, and priapism.

2. **Phenoxybenzamine** may cause orthostatic hypotension, tachycardia, inhibition of ejaculation, miosis, and nasal congestion.

3. **Propranolol** may cause bradycardia and congestive heart failure, increased airway resistance, increased serum triglycerides, decreased high-density lipoprotein cholesterol, blood dyscrasias, psoriasis, depression, hallucinations, organic brain syndrome, and transient hearing loss. Sudden withdrawal may be cardiotoxic.

4. **Metoprolol** has adverse effects similar to those of propranolol, except that it is less likely to increase airway resistance because of its β_1-selectivity.

VI. NEUROMUSCULAR BLOCKING AGENTS

A. Chemistry

1. **Neuromuscular blocking agents** may be competitive (as with the prototypical curare alkaloids) or depolarizing (as with succinylcholine). They act by blocking the effects of acetylcholine at the skeletal neuromuscular junction.

2. The **competitive nondepolarizing agents** are alkaloids of **curare** (the arrow poison of South American Indians) as well as several synthetic analogues. They are primarily bulky, rigid molecules.
   a. The **principal active alkaloid** is tubocurarine chloride (Figure 12-11). A closely related trimethylated derivative is metocurine iodide (Metubine). Their most important structural feature appears to be the presence of a tertiary–quaternary amine in which the distance between the two cations is rigidly fixed at about 14 A°, twice the length of the critical moiety of acetylcholine.
   b. A number of **potent synthetic analogues** have been developed. They include the **structurally similar** pancuronium bromide (Pavulon), vecuronium bromide (Norcuron), pipecuronium bromide (Arduan), doxacurium chloride (Nuromax), and the **structurally dissimilar** gallamine triethiodide (Flaxedil) and atracurium besylate (Tracrium). All of these agents possess at least one quaternized nitrogen.

3. The **noncompetitive depolarizing agents** include decamethonium bromide and succinylcholine chloride (Figure 12-12).
   a. Unlike the large, bulky competitive agents, noncompetitive agents are slender aliphatic molecules. However, they do contain two quaternary nitrogens.
   b. **Succinylcholine** has a short duration of action compared to the other neuromuscular blocking agents. This results from its simple ester functional group, which is rapidly hydrolyzed by plasma and liver pseudocholinesterases. Its action may be prolonged, however, in patients with a genetic pseudocholinesterase deficiency.

B. Pharmacology

1. The **competitive nondepolarizing agents** compete with acetylcholine for nicotinic receptors at the neuromuscular junction. These agents reduce the end-plate potential so that the depolarization threshold is not reached.

2. The **noncompetitive depolarizing agents** desensitize the nicotinic receptors at the neuromuscular junction. These agents react with the nicotinic receptors, decreasing receptor sensitivity in a manner similar to that of excess released acetylcholine. They depolarize the excitable membrane for a prolonged period (2–3 minutes); the membrane then becomes unresponsive (desensitized).

C. Therapeutic indications. **Neuromuscular blocking agents,** which cause only skeletal muscle paralysis (the patient remains conscious and capable of feeling), are used to:

1. Promote skeletal muscle relaxation and facilitate endotracheal intubation, as an adjunct to surgical anesthesia

2. Limit trauma associated with skeletal muscle contraction during electroconvulsive shock therapy

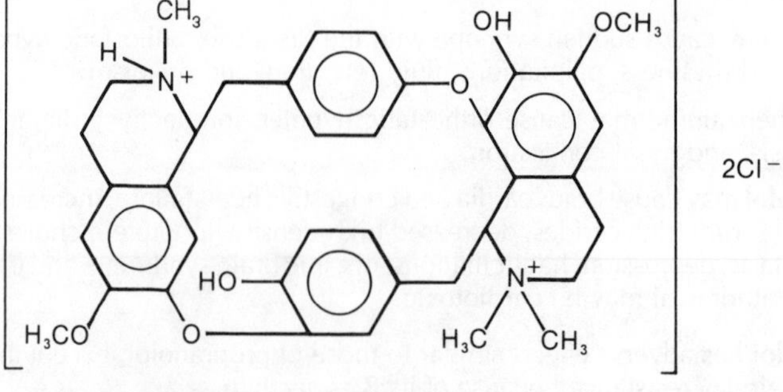

Figure 12-11. Structural formula of tubocurarine chloride (Tubarine), a competitive nondepolarizing agent.

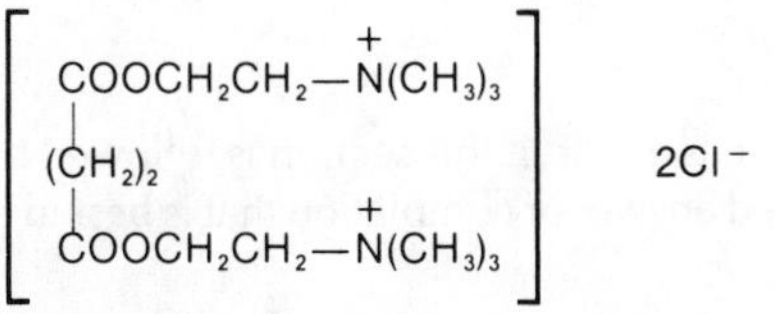

$$\left[\begin{array}{l} COOCH_2CH_2 \overset{+}{-} N(CH_3)_3 \\ (CH_2)_2 \\ COOCH_2CH_2 \overset{+}{-} N(CH_3)_3 \end{array} \right] \quad 2Cl^-$$

Figure 12-12. Structural formula of succinylcholine chloride (Anectine), a noncompetitive depolarizing agent.

D. Adverse effects

1. **Competitive nondepolarizing agents** may cause respiratory paralysis, histamine release, bronchospasm, and hypotension (e.g., tubocurarine) or respiratory paralysis, tachycardia, and hypertension (e.g., gallamine, pancuronium).

2. **Noncompetitive depolarizing agents** (e.g., succinylcholine, decamethonium) may cause respiratory paralysis, muscle fasciculation with pain, extraocular muscle contraction with increased intraocular pressure, and increased intragastric pressure. In addition, succinylcholine may cause muscarinic responses such as bradycardia, increased glandular secretions, and cardiac arrest. In combination with halothane, succinylcholine may cause malignant hyperthermia in genetically predisposed individuals.

STUDY QUESTIONS

Directions: Each of the numbered items or incomplete statements in this section is followed by answers or by completions of the statement. Select the **one** lettered answer or completion that is **best** in each case.

1. Which of the following drugs would most likely be used in the treatment of bronchospasm that is associated with chronic obstructive pulmonary disease?

(A) Edrophonium
(B) Ipratropium
(C) Ambenonium
(D) Propantheline
(E) Homatropine

2. All of the following adverse effects are manifestations of cholinergic agonists EXCEPT

(A) bradycardia
(B) bronchoconstriction
(C) xerostomia
(D) lacrimation
(E) myopic accommodation

3. Which of the following drugs is considered to be the agent of choice for anaphylactic reactions?

(A) Clonidine
(B) Isoproterenol
(C) Epinephrine
(D) Phenylephrine
(E) Terbutaline

4. Which of the following neuromuscular blocking agents may cause muscarinic responses such as bradycardia and increased glandular secretions?

(A) Tubocurarine
(B) Succinylcholine
(C) Pancuronium
(D) Decamethonium
(E) Gallamine

Directions: Each item below contains three suggested answers of which **one or more** is correct. Choose the answer

A if **I only** is correct
B if **III only** is correct
C if **I and II** are correct
D if **II and III** are correct
E if **I, II, and III** are correct

5. True statements concerning therapeutic indications of cholinesterase inhibitors include

I. they may be used as miotic agents in the treatment of glaucoma
II. they may be used to increase skeletal muscle tone in the treatment of myasthenia gravis
III. they decrease gastrointestinal and urinary bladder smooth muscle tone

6. Antimuscarinic agents are used in the treatment of Parkinson's disease and in the control of some neuroleptic-induced extrapyramidal disorders. These agents include

I. ipratropium
II. benztropine
III. trihexyphenidyl

7. Certain drugs are sometimes incorporated into local anesthetic solutions to prolong their activity and reduce their systemic toxicity. These drugs include

I. dobutamine
II. phenylephrine
III. epinephrine

1-B	4-B	7-D
2-C	5-C	
3-C	6-D	

Directions: Each group of items in this section consists of lettered options followed by a set of numbered items. For each item, select the **one** lettered option that is most closely associated with it. Each lettered option may be selected once, more than once, or not at all.

Questions 8–10

For each of the drug molecules below, select the most appropriate pharmacologic classification.

(A) Direct-acting cholinergic agent
(B) β-Adrenergic blocker
(C) Irreversible acetylcholinesterase inhibitor
(D) Anticholinergic agent
(E) Indirect sympathomimetic amine

8.

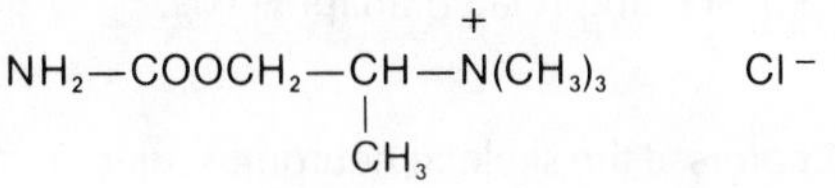

9.

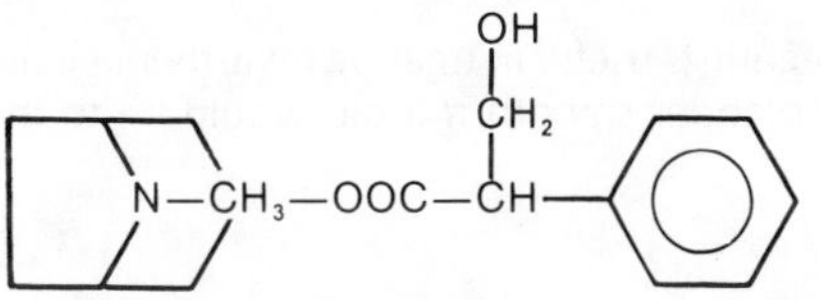

10.

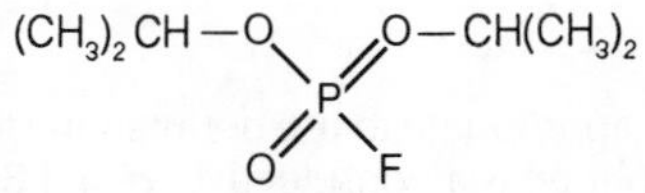

Questions 11–13

For each of the pharmacologic categories listed below, select the structure that it most likely represents.

(A)

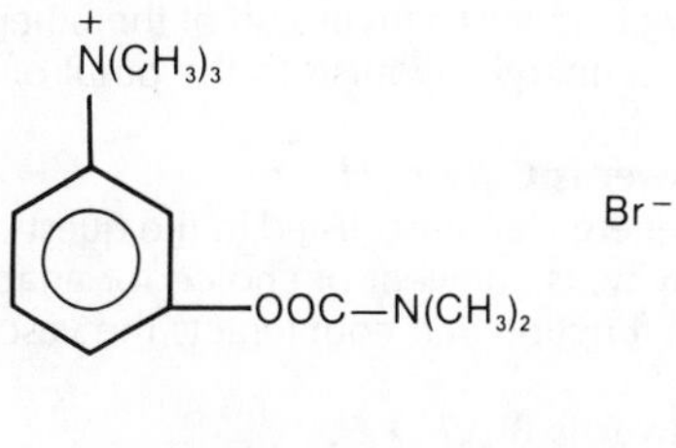

(B)

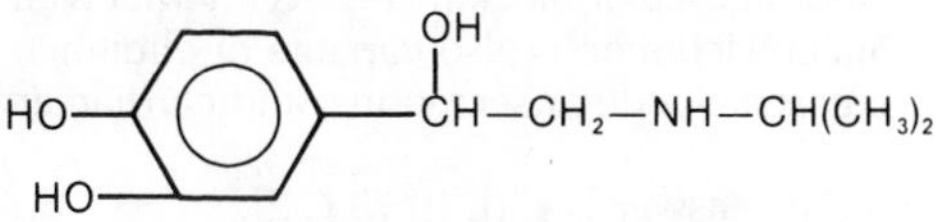

(C)

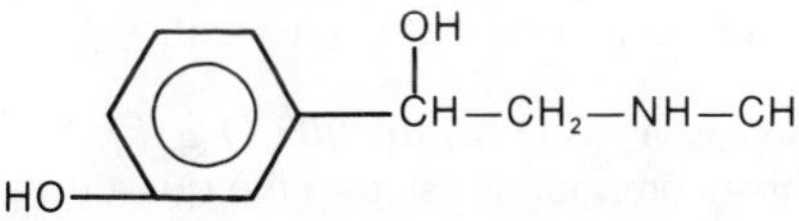

(D)

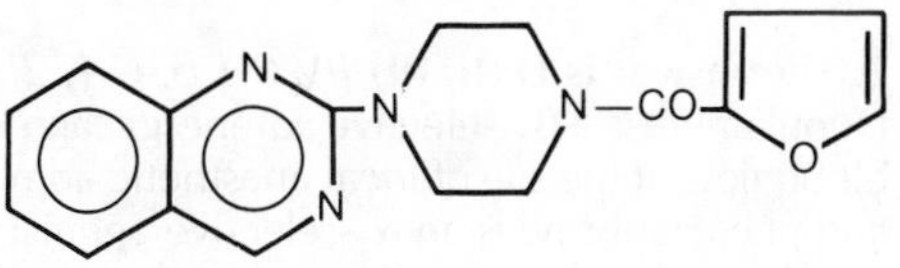

(E)

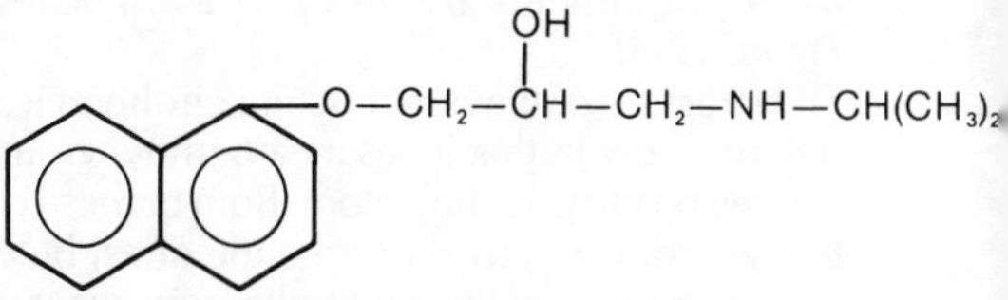

11. β-Adrenergic blocker
12. α-Adrenergic agonist
13. β-Adrenergic agonist

8-A	11-E
9-D	12-C
10-C	13-B

ANSWERS AND EXPLANATIONS

1. The answer is B *[II C 2 b, c; III C 1 e–g].*
Ipratropium is a newly approved antimuscarinic agent used to treat bronchospasm. Propantheline and homatropine are antimuscarinic agents used as a gastrointestinal antispasmodic and as a mydriatic, respectively. Edrophonium and ambenonium are indirect-acting cholinergic agonists and, as such, would be expected to induce bronchospasm.

2. The answer is C *[II D].*
Xerostomia, or dry mouth, results from reduced salivary secretions and, therefore, is not a manifestation of cholinergic agonist activity. All of the other effects listed in the question are extensions of therapeutic effects of cholinergic agonists to the point of being adverse effects.

3. The answer is C *[IV C 1].*
Of the adrenergic agonists listed in the question, only epinephrine, because of its broad, nonselective α- and β-activity, is an agent of choice for anaphylactic reactions. Epinephrine improves circulatory and respiratory function and counteracts the vascular effects of histamine-related anaphylaxis.

4. The answer is B *[VI D 2].*
Neuromuscular blocking agents interact with nicotinic receptors at the skeletal neuromuscular junction. Succinylcholine is also capable of eliciting autonomic muscarinic responses, such as bradycardia, increased glandular secretions, and cardiac arrest.

5. The answer is C (I, II) *[II C 2].*
Cholinesterase inhibitors are indirect-acting cholinergic agonists useful in treating myasthenia gravis and glaucoma. Their effects on gastrointestinal and urinary bladder smooth muscle would be to increase smooth muscle tone, not decrease it.

6. The answer is D (II, III) *[III C 1 g, h].*
All three compounds listed in the question are antimuscarinic agents; however, only benztropine and trihexyphenidyl are used to control parkinsonism and some neuroleptic-induced extrapyramidal disorders. Ipratropium is a newly approved agent for the treatment of bronchospasm.

7. The answer is D (II, III) *[IV B 1 b, C 1, 2].*
Dobutamine is a β_1-selective adrenergic agonist. It would be inappropriate to use dobutamine to reduce blood flow at the site of local anesthetic administration. Epinephrine is a nonselective α- and β-agonist, and phenylephrine is an α_1-selective agonist; both of these drugs can be used to limit the systemic absorption of local anesthetics and prolong their activity.

8–10. The answers are: 8-A *[II A 2 a; Figures 12-1, 12-2],* **9-D** *[III A 1; Figure 12-5],* **10-C** *[II A 2 b (2); Figure 12-4].*
The structure of the direct-acting cholinergic agent in question 8 is very similar to that of acetylcholine, differing only in that it has a carbamoyl group in place of the acetyl group and has a methyl group substituted on the β-carbon atom. Both of these changes decrease the rate of hydrolysis, resulting in an agent that acts directly, as acetylcholine does, but has a significantly longer duration of action.

The structure of the anticholinergic agent in question 9 also resembles that of acetylcholine, but with a significant difference in that the alcohol portion of the ester function is a large bulky group. This agent has no inherent cholinergic activity but can bind to the acetylcholine receptors in the postganglionic fibers, thus preventing acetylcholine molecules from interacting with these sites. This agent, which is atropine, is, therefore, an anticholinergic. Because it contains a fluorophosphate group, the structure in question 10 can be recognized as being an organophosphate ester. This agent can bind covalently to the acetylcholine receptor and acts as an irreversible indirect-acting cholinergic agonist.

11–13. The answers are: 11-E *[V A 2; Figure 12-10],* **12-C** *[IV A 1; Figure 12-7],* **13-B** *[IV A 1; Figure 12-8].*
Structure E resembles the prototype β-agonist isoproterenol. It differs by having isoproterenol's catechol ring replaced by a naphthyloxy group. This substitution destroys the agonist activity, resulting in the formation of a β-adrenergic blocking agent.

Structure C differs from the prototype α-adrenergic agent norepinephrine only in the removal of the parahydroxyl group. While this agent no longer has the catechol structure, it does have inherent α-adrenergic activity.

Structure B possesses the catecholamine moiety typical of adrenergic agonists. The presence of the bulky N-isopropyl group characterizes it as a β-agonist.

13 Drugs Affecting the Central Nervous System

David C. Kosegarten
Edward F. LaSala

I. INTRODUCTION. Drugs affecting the central nervous system (CNS) provide anesthesia, treat psychiatric disorders, relieve anxiety, provide sleep or sedation, prevent epileptic seizures, suppress movement disorders, and relieve pain. They include general and local anesthetics, antidepressants and antipsychotics, anxiolytics, sedative–hypnotics, antiepileptics, antiparkinsonian agents, and opioid analgesics and antagonists.

II. GENERAL ANESTHETICS

A. Chemistry

1. **Inhalation anesthetics** are drugs inhaled as gases or vapors. These diverse drugs are relatively simple lipophilic molecules, ranging from the inorganic agent nitrous oxide (N_2O) to the rarely used ethers, such as ethyl ether, and hydrocarbons, such as cyclopropane, both of which are extremely **flammable,** and to the frequently used, **nonflammable** halogenated hydrocarbons and ethers such as halothane (Fluothane) and enflurane (Ethrane).

2. **Nonvolatile anesthetics** are also lipophilic molecules. They range from the ultra–short-acting barbiturates such as thiopental, the cyclohexamines (e.g., ketamine), the benzodiazepines (e.g., midazolam), and the opioids (e.g., fentanyl), all of which are administered as **water-soluble salts** to the imidazole, etomidate, administered as an **aqueous propylene glycol solution** compatible with many preanesthetics and the dialkylphenol, propofol, administered as an **emulsion,** which should not be mixed with other therapeutic agents prior to administration (Figure 13-1).

B. Pharmacology

1. **General anesthetics** depress the CNS, producing a reversible loss of consciousness and loss of all forms of sensation.

2. **Inhalational anesthetics** are absorbed and primarily excreted through the lungs. Frequently, they are supplemented with analgesics, a skeletal muscle relaxant, and antimuscarinic agents.
   a. **Analgesics** permit a reduction in the required concentration of inhalational anesthetic.
   b. **Skeletal muscle relaxants** cause adequate muscle relaxation during surgery.
   c. **Antimuscarinic agents** decrease bronchiolar secretions.

3. **Nonvolatile anesthetics** are usually administered intravenously (e.g., thiobarbiturates, benzodiazepines).

C. Therapeutic indications

1. **Inhalation anesthetics** are indicated to provide general surgical anesthesia.

2. **Nonvolatile anesthetics** are indicated to induce drowsiness and provide relaxation prior to the induction of inhalational general anesthesia (e.g., thiopental, diazepam, midazolam).

D. Adverse effects. General anesthetics depress respiration and circulation as well as the CNS. They can also decrease hepatic and kidney function (e.g., methoxyflurane) and cause cardiac dysrhythmias as a result of increased myocardial sensitivity to catecholamines (e.g., halothane).

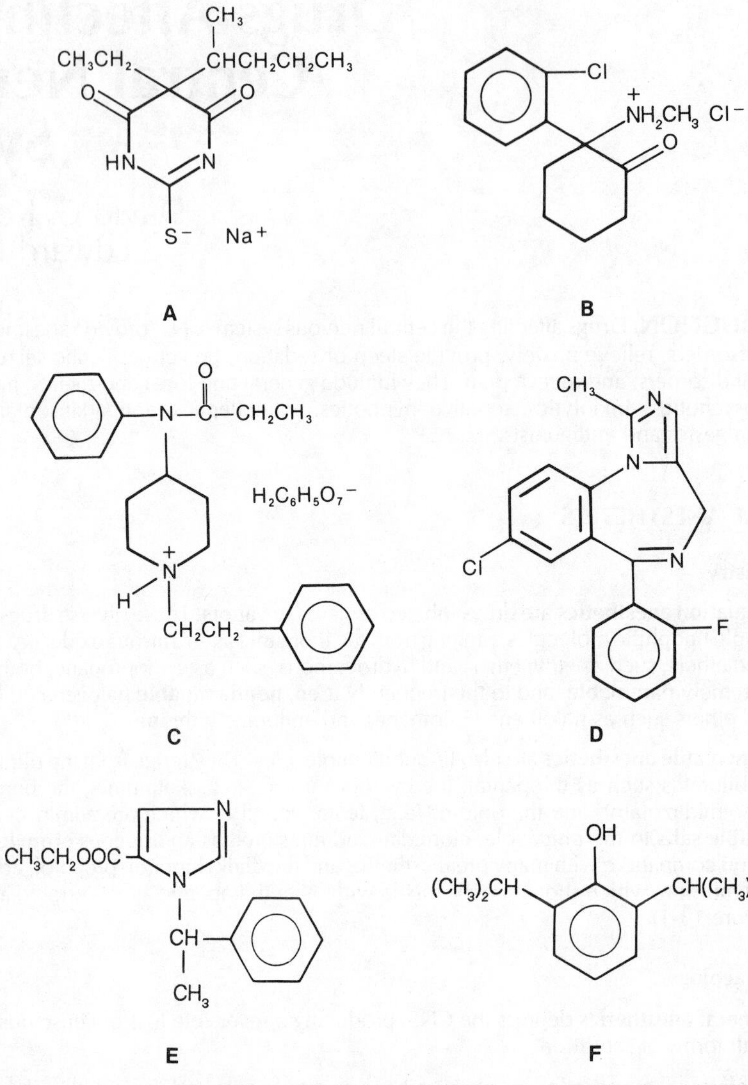

Figure 13-1. Structural formulas of nonvolatile general anesthetics: (*A*) thiopental sodium (Pentothal), (*B*) ketamine hydrochloride (Ketaject), (*C*) fentanyl citrate (Sublimaze), (*D*) midazolam (Versed), (*E*) etomidate (Amidate), and (*F*) propofol (Diprivan).

III. LOCAL ANESTHETICS

A. Chemistry. Most local anesthetics are structurally similar to the alkaloid cocaine (Figure 13-2). They consist of a hydrophilic amino group linked through an ester or amide connecting group to a lipophilic aromatic moiety. A few phenols and aromatic alcohols also have local anesthetic activity.

1. **Ester-type agents** are short-acting and are hydrolyzed by plasma esterases.

2. **Amide-type agents** are long-acting and are hydrolyzed in the liver.

3. The drug's pK_a (see Chapter 10 II B 3, 6) influences its state. At tissue pH, the drug can exist either as a lipophilic, uncharged, secondary or tertiary amine that crosses connective tissue and enters nerve cells or as a charged ammonium cation that appears to block the generation of action potentials by means of a membrane receptor complex.

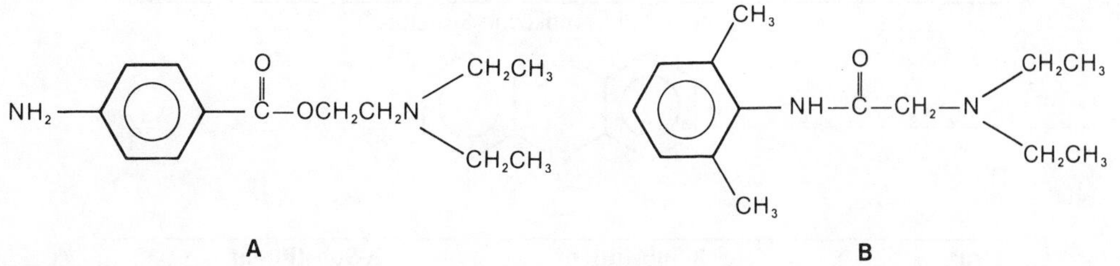

Figure 13-2. Structural formulas of local anesthetics structurally similar to cocaine: (*A*) procaine (Novocaine) and (*B*) lidocaine (Xylocaine).

B. Pharmacology

1. Local anesthetics **reversibly block nerve impulse conduction and produce reversible loss of sensation** at their administration site. They do not produce a loss of consciousness.
   - **a.** Small, nonmyelinated nerve fibers, which conduct pain and temperature sensations, are affected first.
   - **b.** Local anesthetics appear to become incorporated within the nerve membrane or to bind to specific membrane sodium ion (Na^+) channels, restricting Na^+ permeability in response to partial depolarization.
2. Local anesthetic solutions frequently contain the vasoconstrictor **epinephrine,** which reduces vascular blood flow at the administration site. This reduces systemic absorption, prolongs the duration of action, and reduces systemic toxicity.

C. Therapeutic indications.
Local anesthetics are indicated to:

1. Produce regional nerve block for the relief of pain, when injected close to the innervating nerve
2. Provide anesthesia for minor operations, when infiltrated around the tissue site
3. Provide anesthesia for surgery of the lower limbs and pelvis and for obstetric surgery, when injected into the epidural space or the subarachnoid space of the spinal cord
4. Provide anesthesia of the skin and mucous membranes, when applied topically

D. Adverse effects

1. Ester-type local anesthetics may cause hypersensitivity reactions in susceptible individuals.
2. Systemic absorption of toxic concentrations of local anesthetics may cause seizures; CNS, respiratory, and myocardial depression; and circulatory collapse.

IV. ANTIPSYCHOTICS.
The principal antipsychotics are phenothiazines, thioxanthenes, and butyrophenones. Other types of molecules having antipsychotic activity include the dihydroindolones such as molindone (Moban), the dibenzodiazepines such as clozapine (Clozaril), and the diphenylbutylpiperidines such as pimozide (Orap).

A. Chemistry

1. **Phenothiazines** (e.g., chlorpromazine, triflupromazine, thioridazine, prochlorperazine, trifluoperazine, fluphenazine) must have a **nitrogen-containing side-chain substituent** on the ring nitrogen for antipsychotic activity (Table 13-1). The ring and side-chain nitrogens must be separated by a three-carbon chain; phenothiazines, in which the ring and side-chain nitrogens are separated by a two-carbon chain, have antihistaminic or sedative activity only.
   - **a.** The side chains are either dimethylaminopropyl, piperazine, or piperidine derivatives. Piperazine side chains confer the greatest potency.
   - **b.** The ring substituent in position 2 must be electron-attractive for optimum activity. A trifluromethyl substituent confers the greatest activity.
   - **c.** Fluphenazine and long-chain alcohols form stable, **highly liposoluble esters** (e.g., enanthate, decanoate), which possess markedly prolonged activity.
2. **Thioxanthenes** (e.g., chlorprothixene, thiothixene) lack the ring nitrogen of phenothiazines and have a side chain attached by a double bond (Figure 13-3).

Table 13-1. Antipsychotic Phenothiazines

General Phenothiazine Structure*

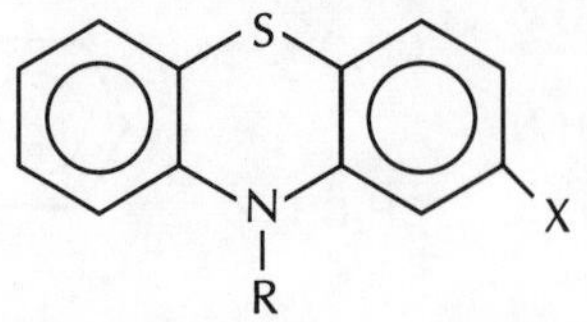

Drug	X-Substituent	R-Substituent
Chlorpromazine (Thorazine)	$-Cl$	$-(CH_2)_3-N(CH_3)_2$
Triflupromazine (Vesprin)	$-CF_3$	$-(CH_2)_3-N(CH_3)_2$
Thioridazine (Mellaril)	$-SCH_3$	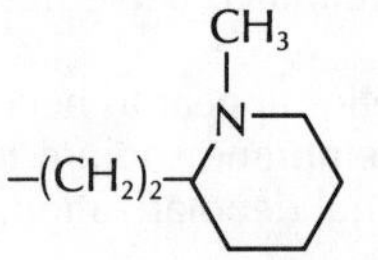
Prochlorperazine (Compazine)	$-Cl$	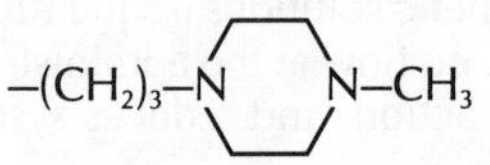
Trifluoperazine (Stelazine)	$-CF_3$	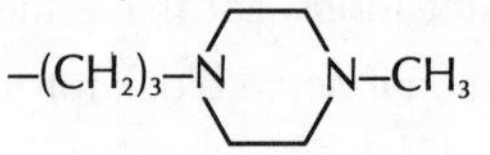
Fluphenazine (Prolixin)	$-CF_3$	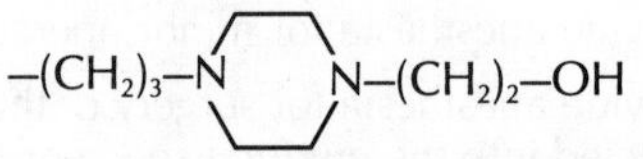

*Antipsychotic phenothiazines have the general structure illustrated in the table. Substituents at positions marked X and R result in different drugs.

3. **Butyrophenones** (e.g., haloperidol) are chemically unrelated to phenothiazines but have similar activity (Figure 13-4).

B. Pharmacology

1. Phenothiazines, thioxanthenes, and butyrophenones have similar pharmacologic effects. Their antipsychotic effects (i.e., improvement of mood and behavior) and their neuroleptic effects (i.e., emotional quieting, development of extrapyramidal symptoms) appear to result from their ability to antagonize central dopamine-mediated synaptic neurotransmission.
2. Other effects vary among the classes of antipsychotics. These include antiemetic activity and blockade of muscarinic, α_1-adrenergic, and H_1-histaminergic receptors.

C. Therapeutic indications.

C. Therapeutic indications. Antipsychotics are primarily indicated for the treatment of psychosis associated with schizophrenia, paranoia, and the manic symptoms of manic–depressive illness.

D. Adverse effects

1. **Centrally mediated adverse effects** include:
   a. Drowsiness

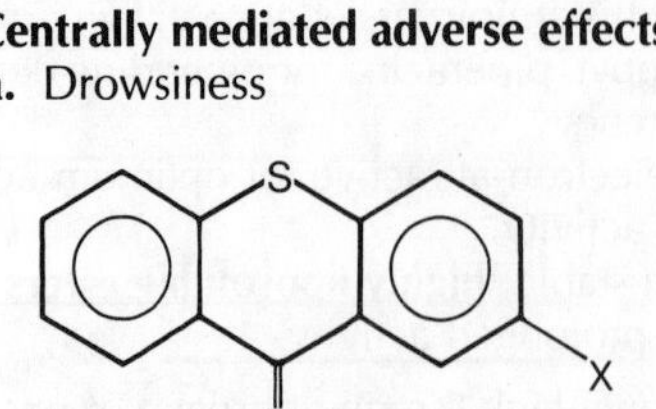

Figure 13-3. Thioxanthenes, similar to phenothiazines, have substituents at *X* and *R* positions that alter drug activity. Chlorprothixene (Taractan) has a $-Cl$ substituent at *X* and $CH-(CH_2)_2-N(CH_3)_2$ at *R*. Thiothixene (Navane) has a $-SO_2N(CH_3)_2$ substituent at *X* and the group:

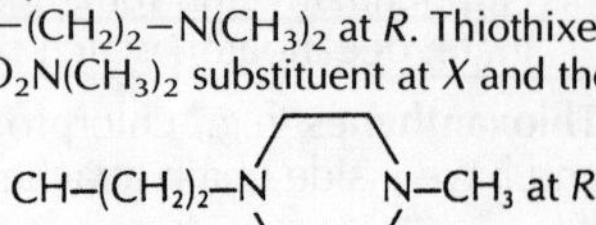

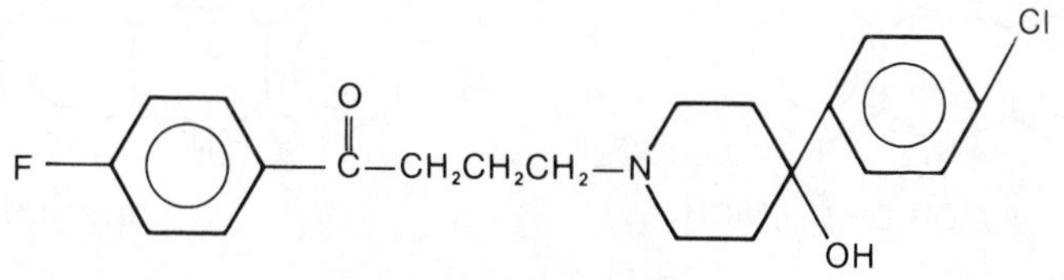

Figure 13-4. Structural formula of haloperidol (Haldol), a butyrophenone antipsychotic.

b. Extrapyramidal symptoms, such as akathisia, acute dystonia, akinesia, and tardive dyskinesia
c. Alteration of temperature-regulating mechanisms, including poikilothermy
d. Increased appetite and weight gain
e. Alterations in hypothalamic and endocrine function, such as increased release of corticotropin, gonadotropins, prolactin, growth hormone, and melanocyte-stimulating hormone

2. **Peripheral adverse effects** include:
   a. Postural hypotension and reflex tachycardia
   b. Hepatotoxicity and jaundice
   c. Failure of ejaculation
   d. Bone marrow depression
   e. Photosensitivity
   f. Xerostomia and blurred vision

V. ANTIDEPRESSANTS are classified into three structurally unrelated groups—the monoamine oxidase (MAO) inhibitors, the tricyclic antidepressants, and the atypical antidepressants.

A. Chemistry

1. **MAO inhibitors** may be weakly potent **hydralazines** [e.g., phenelzine isocarboxazid (Marplan)] or extremely potent **phenylcyclopropylamines** (i.e., ring-closed amphetamine derivatives, such as tranylcypromine) [Figure 13-5].
2. **Tricyclic antidepressants,** which are commonly used, are secondary or tertiary amine derivatives of molecules having a fused three-ring system.
   a. The principal tricyclic antidepressants are derivatives of **dibenzazepine** [e.g., imipramine, desipramine, clomipramine (Anafranil), trimipramine (Surmontil)] and **dibenzocycloheptadiene** (e.g., amitriptyline, nortriptyline) [Figures 13-6 and 13-7].
   b. Other closely related tricyclic antidepressants include doxepin (Sinequan), a **dibenzoxepine,** amoxapine (Asendin), a **dibenzoxazepine**, and protriptyline (Vivactil), a **dibenzocycloheptadiene.**
   c. A closely related **tetracyclic** agent is maprotiline (Ludiomil).
3. **Atypical antidepressants** have varied structures. They range from the complex **heterocycle,** trazodone, a **benzotriazole derivative** to the nonheterocycles, fluoxetine, a **phenyltolylpropylamine derivative** and bupropion (Wellbrutin), an **aminopropiophenone** [Figure 13-8].

B. Pharmacology

1. **MAO inhibitors** appear to produce their antidepressant effects by blocking the intraneuronal oxidative deamination of brain biogenic amines (i.e., norepinephrine, serotonin). This increases the availability of biogenic amines at central aminergic receptors. Other biochemical

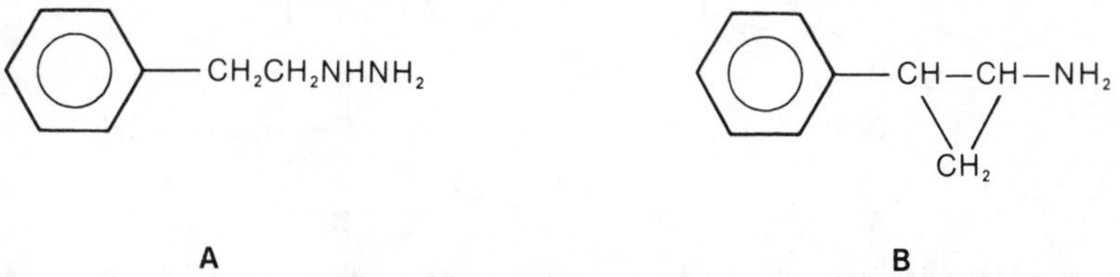

Figure 13-5. Structural formulas of (*A*) phenelzine (Nardil), a hydralazine derivative monoamine oxidase (MAO) inhibitor, and (*B*) tranylcypromine (Parnate), a cyclopropylamine derivative MAO inhibitor.

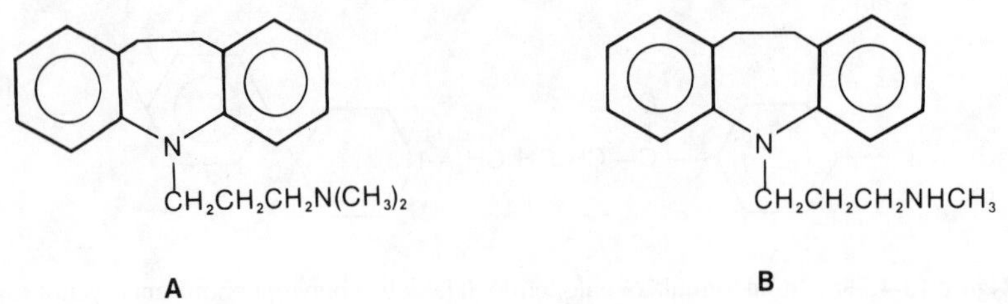

Figure 13-6. Structural formulas of tricyclic antidepressants derived from dibenzazepine: (*A*) imipramine (Tofranil) and (*B*) desipramine (Norpramin).

events (e.g., the down-regulation of central β-adrenergic and serotoninergic receptors) resulting from chronic inhibition of MAO and re-uptake blockade may also explain the therapeutic action of antidepressants. This explanation is suggested by the latency period of MAO inhibitors, which take 2–4 weeks to become effective.

2. **Tricyclic antidepressants** appear to act principally by reducing CNS neuronal re-uptake of biogenic amines (i.e., norepinephrine, serotonin). This prolongs the availability of biogenic amines at central aminergic receptors.

3. **Atypical antidepressants** have varying effects on re-uptake of biogenic amines. Trazodone and fluoxetine selectively inhibit serotonin re-uptake.

C. Therapeutic indications

1. **MAO inhibitors** are indicated to treat depression, phobic anxiety, and narcolepsy that has not responded to other treatments. However, their use is limited by their adverse effects (see V D).

2. **Tricyclic and atypical antidepressants** are the agents of choice for endogenous depression. The tricyclic imipramine is also used to treat enuresis.

D. Adverse effects

1. **MAO inhibitors** interact with sympathomimetic drugs and with foods that have a high tyramine concentration, such as cheese, wine, and sausage. Hypertensive crisis may result. In addition, MAO inhibitors can cause a wide range of adverse effects, including:
   a. CNS effects, such as CNS stimulation, tremors, agitation, overactivity, hyperreflexia, mania, and insomnia followed by weakness, fatigue, and drowsiness
   b. Cardiovascular effects, such as postural hypotension
   c. Gastrointestinal effects, such as nausea, abdominal pain, and constipation
   d. Antimuscarinic effects, such as dry mouth, urinary retention, and constipation

2. **Tricyclic antidepressants** can cause adverse effects that vary with the drug and may include:
   a. CNS effects, such as drowsiness, dizziness, weakness, fatigue, and confusion
   b. Cardiovascular effects, such as orthostatic hypotension, tachycardia, and interference with atrioventricular conduction
   c. Antimuscarinic effects, such as dry mouth, urinary retention, and constipation
   d. Gastrointestinal effects, such as nausea, vomiting, diarrhea, and anorexia
   e. Bone marrow depression
   f. Mania (in patients with manic–depressive illness)

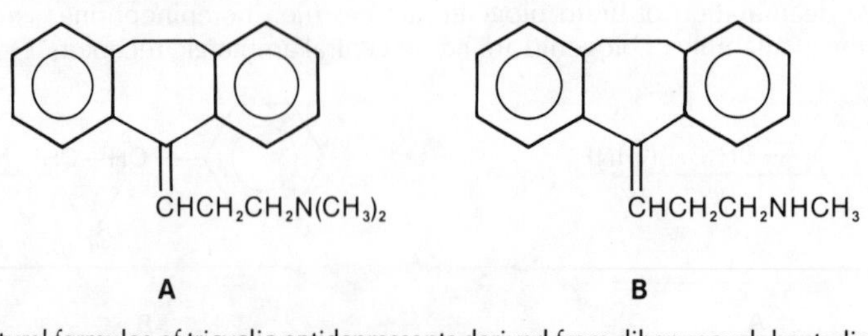

Figure 13-7. Structural formulas of tricyclic antidepressants derived from dibenzocycloheptadiene: (*A*) amitriptyline (Elavil), (*B*) nortriptyline (Aventyl).

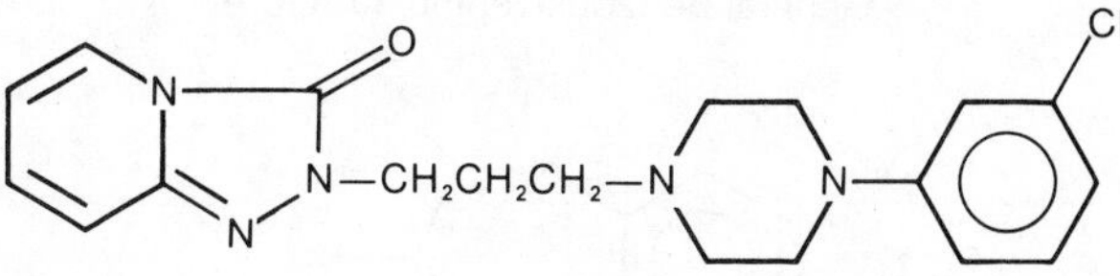

A

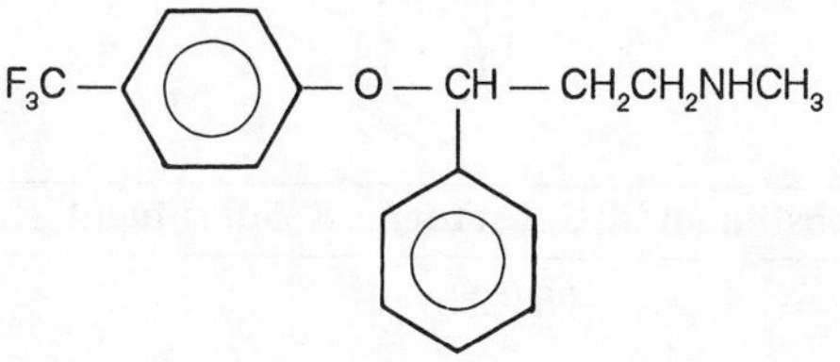

B

Figure 13-8. Structural formulas of (*A*) trazodone (Desyrel) and (*B*) fluoxetine (Prozac), atypical antidepressants.

3. **Atypical antidepressants** may cause adverse effects including:
   a. CNS effects, such as dizziness, nightmares, confusion, drowsiness, fatigue, headache, insomnia, impaired memory, akathisia, numbness, and tonic–clonic seizures
   b. Cardiovascular effects, such as hypertension, hypotension, tachycardia, chest pain, and syncope
   c. Gastrointestinal effects, such as nausea, vomiting, diarrhea, and constipation
   d. Blurred vision and tinnitus
   e. Antimuscarinic effects, such as urinary retention, dry mouth, and constipation
   f. Bone marrow depression
   g. Priapism and menstrual irregularities

VI. ANXIOLYTICS fall into four major classes—the highly effective benzodiazepines and azaspirodecanediones and the less effective propanediol carbamates and diphenylmethanes.

A. Chemistry

1. **Benzodiazepines** (e.g., chlordiazepoxide, diazepam, halazepam, clorazepate, prazepam, oxazepam, lorazepam, alprazolam) have varying durations of action, which can be correlated with their structures in some cases (Table 13-2).
   a. Agents with a 3-hydroxyl group are easily metabolized by phase II glucuronidation and are short-acting (see R_3-substituent column in Table 13-2).
   b. Agents lacking a 3-hydroxyl group must undergo considerable phase I metabolism, including 3-hydroxylation. These agents are long-acting. Most long-acting agents form the intermediate metabolite desmethyldiazepam, which has a very long half-life. Thus, these agents may have a cumulative action.
   c. Triazolobenzodiazepines (e.g., alprazolam) undergo a different pattern of metabolism and are intermediate in activity.
   d. Agents lacking an amino side chain are not basic enough to form water-soluble salts with acids. For example, intravenous solutions of diazepam contain propylene glycol as a solvent. Precipitation may occur if these solutions are mixed with aqueous solutions.

2. **Azaspirodecanediones** (e.g., buspirone) have anxiolytic activity resembling that of the benzodiazepines. However, these agents lack other CNS depressant activity (Figure 13-9).

3. **Propanediol carbamates** (e.g., meprobamate) **and diphenylmethanes** (e.g., hydroxyzine) are used much less commonly than the benzodiazepines for the treatment of anxiety (Figure 13-10).

Table 13-2. Benzodiazepine Anxiolytics

General Benzodiazepine Structure*

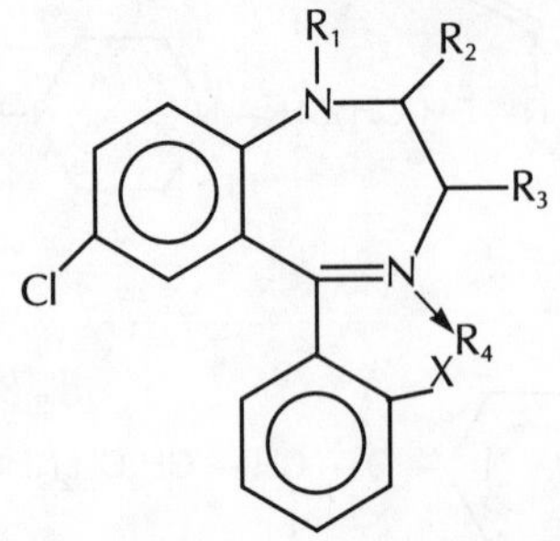

Drug	R_1-Substituent	R_2-Substituent	R_3-Substituent	R_4-Substituent	X-Substituent
Chlordiazepoxide (Librium)	=	$-NHCH_3$	. . .	O	. . .
Diazepam (Valium)	$-CH_3$	=O	. . .	. . .	. . .
Halazepam (Paxipam)	$-CH_2CF_3$	=O	. . .	. . .	. . .
Clorazepate dipotassium (Tranxene)	–H	–OH; –OK	–COOK	. . .	. . .
Prazepam (Centrax)	$-CH_2-CH(CH_2)_2$	=O	. . .	. . .	. . .
Oxazepam (Serax)	–H	=O	–OH	. . .	. . .
Lorazepam (Ativan)	–H	=O	–OH	. . .	–Cl
Alprazolam (Xanax)		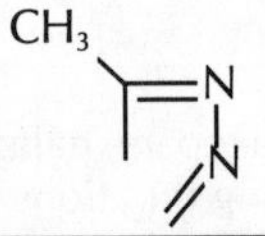	. . .	. . .	. . .

*Benzodiazepine anxiolytics have the general structure illustrated in the table. Substituents at the position marked R_1, R_2, R_3, R_4, and X result in different drugs.

B. Pharmacology

1. **Benzodiazepines** appear to produce their calming effects by depressing the limbic system and reticular formation through potentiation of the inhibitor neurotransmitter γ-aminobutyric acid (GABA).
   a. Anxiolytic activity correlates with the drug's binding affinity to a macromolecular GABA-chloride ionophore receptor complex.
   b. Hypnotic and anticonvulsant properties also exist (see VII and VIII).
   c. Benzodiazepines increase the depressant effects of alcohol and other CNS depressant drugs.
2. **Azaspirodecanediones.** Buspirone has an unknown mechanism of action.
   a. Buspirone binds to central dopamine and serotonic receptors rather than to GABA-chloride ionophore receptor complexes.
   b. It possesses no hypnotic or anticonvulsant properties and appears not to add to the depressant effects of alcohol or other CNS depressant drugs.

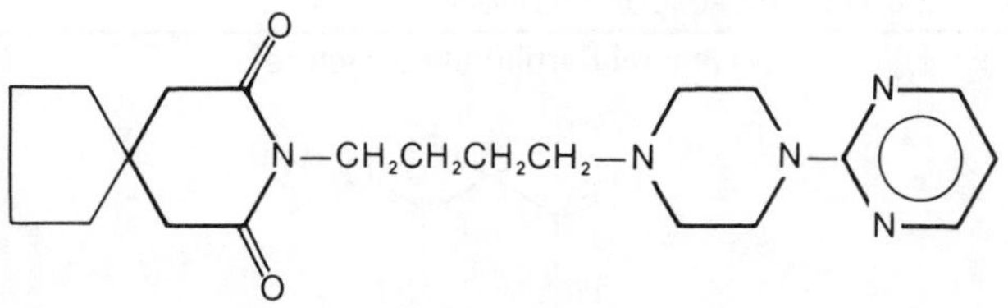

Figure 13-9. Structural formula of buspirone (Buspar), the prototypical azaspirodecanedione anxiolytic.

C. Therapeutic indications

1. Benzodiazepines and the azaspirodecanedione buspirone are indicated to treat anxiety.
2. Benzodiazepines are also indicated for use as a preanesthetic medication (see II A 2, C 2), as sedative–hypnotics (see VII), as anticonvulsants (see VIII), and during acute alcohol withdrawal.

D. Adverse effects

1. **Adverse effects associated with benzodiazepines** include:
   - a. CNS effects, such as CNS depression, drowsiness, sedation, ataxia, confusion, and dysarthria
   - b. Gastrointestinal effects, such as nausea, vomiting, and diarrhea
   - c. Psychiatric effects (rare), such as paradoxical excitement, insomnia, paranoia, and rage reactions
   - d. Abuse potential and possibly dependence
2. **Adverse effects of buspirone** are limited to restlessness, dizziness, headache, nausea, diarrhea, and paresthesias. However, tardive dyskinesia is possible with long-term therapy.

VII. SEDATIVE–HYPNOTICS.

Sedatives are principally long-acting or intermediate-acting barbiturates (e.g., phenobarbital, amobarbital), whereas **hypnotics** may be the widely used benzodiazepines (e.g., flurazepam, alprazolam), short-acting barbiturates (e.g., pentobarbital, secobarbital), piperidinediones (e.g., glutethimide), or aldehydes (e.g., chloral hydrate).

A. Chemistry

1. **Barbiturates** are 5,5-disubstituted derivatives of barbituric acid, a saturated triketopyramidine (Table 13-3).
   - a. Two side chains in position 5 are essential for sedative–hypnotic activity.
   - b. Long-acting agents have a phenyl and an ethyl group in position 5.
   - c. Branched side chains, unsaturated side chains, or side chains longer than an ethyl group tend to increase lipophilicity and metabolism rate. Increased lipophilicity leads to a shorter onset of action, a shorter duration of action, and increased potency.
   - d. Replacement of the position 2 oxygen with sulfur produces an extremely lipophilic molecule that distributes rapidly into lipid tissues outside the brain.

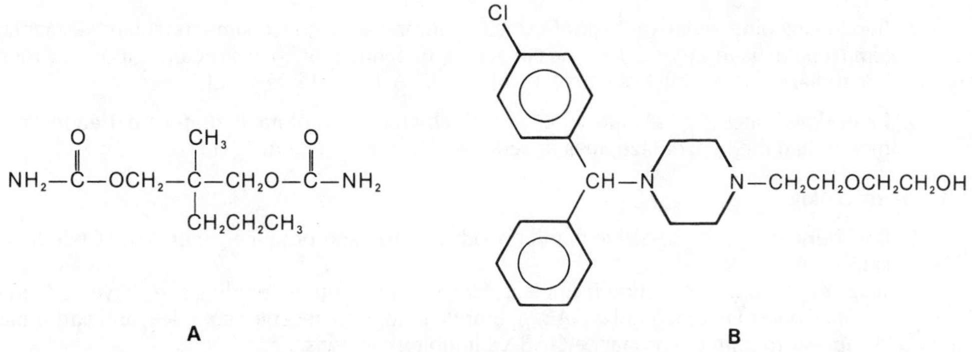

Figure 13-10. Structural formulas of (*A*) meprobamate (Miltown, Equanil), a propanediol carbamate anxiolytic, and (*B*) hydroxyzine (Atarax, Vistaril), a diphenylmethane anxiolytic.

Table 13-3. Barbiturate Sedative–Hypnotics

General Barbiturate Structure*

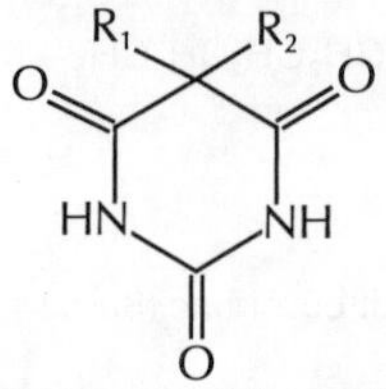

Drug	R_1-Substituent	R_2-Substituent	Duration of Action
Phenobarbital (Luminal)	$-CH_2CH_3$	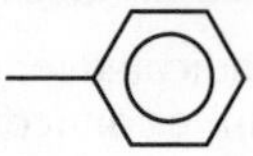	Long
Amobarbital (Amytal)	$-CH_2CH_3$	$-CH_2CH_2CH(CH_3)_2$	Intermediate
Butabarbital (Butisol)	$-CH_2CH_3$	$-CHCH_2CH_3$ (with CH_3 branch)	Intermediate
Pentobarbital (Nembutal)	$-CH_2CH_3$	$-CHCH_2CH_2CH_3$ (with CH_3 branch)	Short
Secobarbital (Seconal)	$-CH_2CH{=}CH_2$	$-CHCH_2CH_2CH_3$ (with CH_3 branch)	Short

*Barbiturate sedative–hypnotics have the general structure illustrated in the table. Substituents at R_1 and R_2 positions result in different drugs with different durations of action.

(1) These ultra–short-acting barbiturates are not useful as sedative–hypnotics but do act as effective induction anesthetics (see II A 2). The action of these drugs is terminated very quickly.

(2) The prototype ultra–short-acting barbiturate is thiopental (Pentothal), the 2-thio isostere of pentobarbital.

e. The barbiturates and many of their metabolites are weak acids, and changes in urinary pH greatly influence their excretion. This is particularly true with overdoses, when a relatively large amount of unchanged drug appears in the glomerular filtrate.

f. Phenobarbital is one of the most powerful and versatile enzyme-inducing agents known. Other barbiturates have less enzyme-inducing effect, except when they are used continuously in higher-than-normal doses.

2. **Benzodiazepine sedative–hypnotics** (e.g., flurazepam, quazepam, triazolam, estazolam, temazepam) have varying durations of action, depending on their structures, as is true for the benzodiazepine anxiolytics (Table 13-4) [see VI A 1 and Table 13-2].

3. **Piperidinediones** (e.g., glutethimide) **and aldehydes** (e.g., chloral hydrate) are used less commonly than the benzodiazepines as sedative–hypnotics (Figure 13-11).

B. Pharmacology

1. **Barbiturates** are less selective than benzodiazepines and produce generalized CNS depression.

a. The mechanism of action is unclear. However, barbiturate binding sites have been identified on a macromolecular GABA-chloride ionophore receptor complex, and barbiturates appear to mimic or enhance GABA's inhibitory actions.

b. Barbiturates have a wide range of dose-dependent pharmacologic actions related to CNS depression, including sedation, hypnosis, and anesthesia. They also act as potent respiratory depressants and as inducers of hepatic microsomal drug-metabolizing enzyme activity.

Table 13-4. Benzodiazepine Sedative–Hypnotics

General Benzodiazepine Structure*

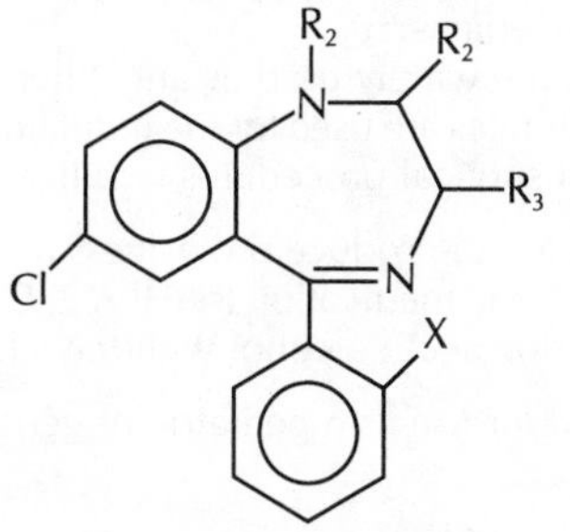

Drug	R_1-Substituent	R_2-Substituent	R_3-Substituent	X-Substituent	Duration of Action
Flurazepam (Dalmane)	$CH_2CH_2N(C_2H_5)_2$	=O	–H	–F	Long
Quazepam (Doral)	$-CH_2CF_3$	=S	–H	–F	Intermediate to long
Triazolam (Halcion)	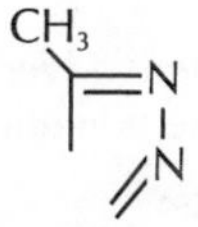		–H	–Cl	Intermediate
Estazolam (ProSom)	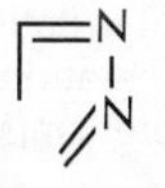		–H	–H	Intermediate
Temazepam (Restoril)	$-CH_3$	=O	–OH	–H	Short

*Benzodiazepine sedative–hypnotics have the general structure illustrated in the table. Substituents at the positions marked R_1, R_2, R_3, and X result in different drugs with different durations of action.

2. **Benzodiazepine sedative–hypnotics** act in the same way as benzodiazepine anxiolytics (see VI B 1). Unlike barbiturates, they do not significantly induce hepatic microsomal drug-metabolizing enzyme activity.

3. **Piperidinediones, aldehydes, and other nonbarbiturate sedative–hypnotics** have similar pharmacologic actions related to CNS depression.
   - **a.** Only chloral hydrate is a drug of choice to induce sleep in pediatric or geriatric patients.
   - **b.** Chloral hydrate's activity is mediated by the formation of the active metabolite trichloroethanol. Chloral hydrate induces hepatic microsomal drug-metabolizing enzyme activity.

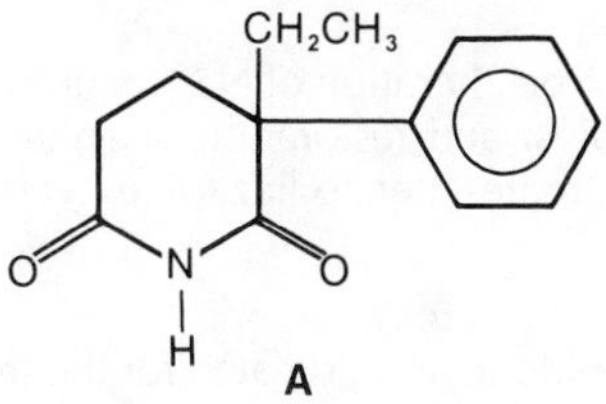

A

$Cl_3C{-}CH(OH)_2$

B

Figure 13-11. Structural formulas of (*A*) glutethimide (Doriden), a piperidinedione sedative–hypnotic, and (*B*) chloral hydrate (Noctec), an aldehyde sedative–hypnotic.

C. Therapeutic indications

1. **Barbiturates** are no longer considered appropriate as sedative–hypnotics in view of the availability of the safer benzodiazepines.
   a. Long-acting barbiturates are widely used as antiepileptics (see VIII).
   b. Ultra–short-acting barbiturates are used for the induction of general anesthesia and as general anesthetics for short surgical procedures (see II A 2, C 2).

2. **Benzodiazepines** are indicated to produce drowsiness and promote sleep. They are also indicated for use as a preanesthetic medication (see II A 2, C 2), as anticonvulsants (see VIII), as anxiolytics (see VI), and during acute alcohol withdrawal.

3. **Chloral hydrate** is indicated for use as a pediatric or geriatric hypnotic.

D. Adverse effects

1. **Barbiturates** may cause a variety of adverse effects, including:
   a. CNS effects, such as drowsiness, confusion, nystagmus, dysarthria, depressed sympathetic ganglionic transmission, hyperalgesia, impaired judgment, impaired fine motor skills, paradoxic excitement (in geriatric patients), and potentiation of other CNS depressant drugs
   b. Respiratory and cardiovascular effects, such as respiratory depression, bradycardia, and orthostatic hypotension
   c. Gastrointestinal effects, such as nausea, vomiting, constipation, diarrhea, and epigastric distress
   d. Exfoliative dermatitis and Stevens-Johnson syndrome
   e. Headache, fever, hepatotoxicity, and megaloblastic anemia (with the chronic use of phenobarbital)

2. **Benzodiazepine sedative–hypnotics** have the same adverse effects as benzodiazepine anxiolytics (see VI D 1). In addition, they have abuse potential and may cause dependence.

3. **Chloral hydrate** has the following adverse effects:
   a. Gastrointestinal effects, such as gastrointestinal irritation and upset, nausea, and vomiting
   b. CNS effects, such as CNS depression, disorientation, incoherence, drowsiness, ataxia, headache, and potentiation of other CNS depressants (particularly alcohol)
   c. Leukopenia

VIII. ANTIEPILEPTICS

A. Chemistry. Antiepileptics (anticonvulsants) vary widely in structure (Figure 13-12).

1. **Older agents,** which are still widely used, include derivatives of the long-acting barbiturates (e.g., phenobarbital, primidone), the hydantoins (e.g., phenytoin), the succinimides (e.g., ethosuximide), and the oxazolidinediones (e.g., trimethadione).

2. **Newer agents,** which are more structurally diverse, include derivatives of the dibenzazepines (e.g., carbamazepine), the benzodiazepines (e.g., clonazepam), the dialkylacetates (e.g., valproic acid), and others.

B. Pharmacology

1. Antiepileptics prevent or reduce excessive discharge and reduce the spread of excitation from CNS seizure foci.

2. The mechanisms of action of antiepileptics appear to be alteration of Na^+ neuronal concentrations by promotion of Na^+ efflux (e.g., hydantoins) and restoration or enhancement of GABA-ergic inhibitory neuronal function (e.g., barbiturates, benzodiazepines, valproic acid).

C. Therapeutic indications

1. Phenytoin, carbamazepine, phenobarbital, and primidone are indicated for the treatment of tonic–clonic (grand mal) seizures.

2. Ethosuximide, valproic acid, and clonazepam are indicated for the treatment of absence (petit mal) seizures.

3. Clonazepam is indicated for the treatment of myoclonic seizures.

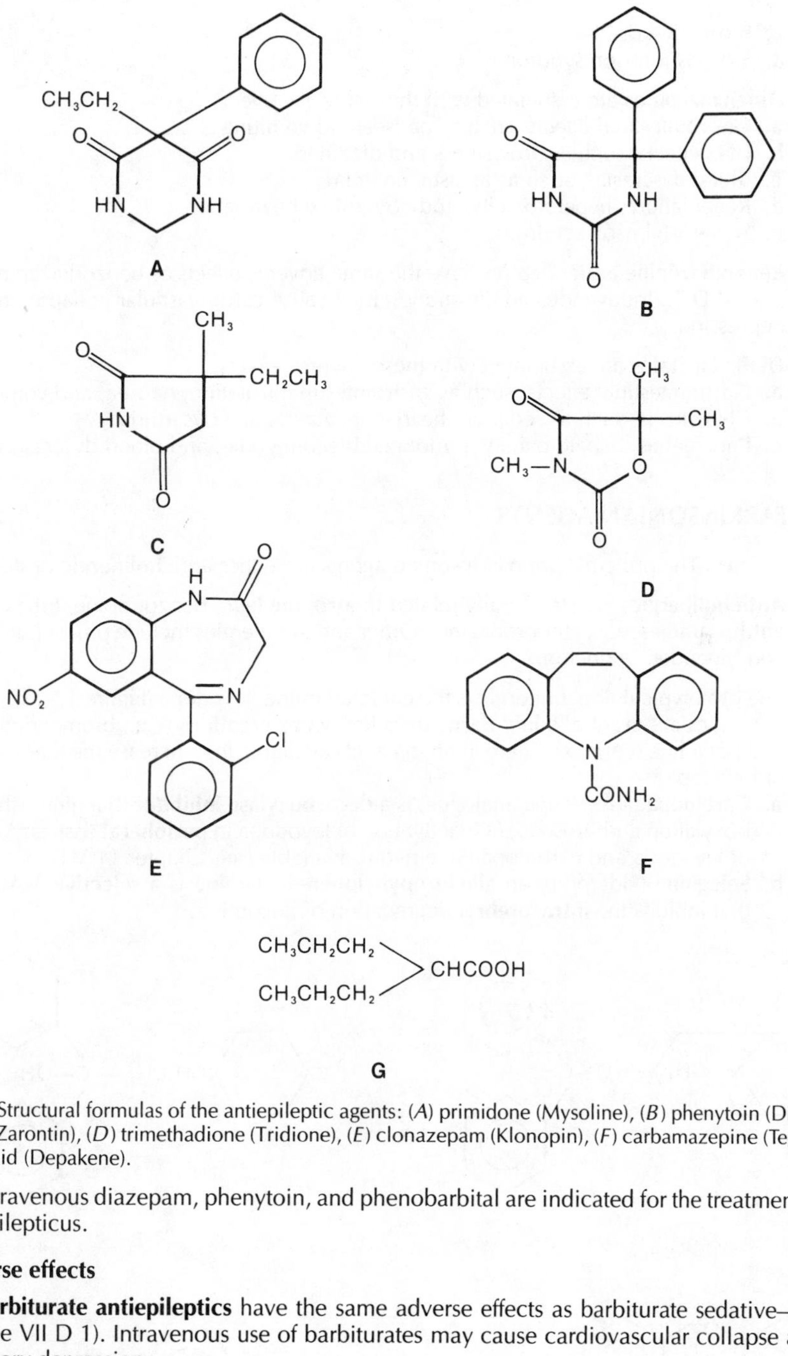

Figure 13-12. Structural formulas of the antiepileptic agents: (*A*) primidone (Mysoline), (*B*) phenytoin (Dilantin), (*C*) ethosuximide (Zarontin), (*D*) trimethadione (Tridione), (*E*) clonazepam (Klonopin), (*F*) carbamazepine (Tegretol), and (*G*) valproic acid (Depakene).

4. Intravenous diazepam, phenytoin, and phenobarbital are indicated for the treatment of status epilepticus.

D. Adverse effects

1. **Barbiturate antiepileptics** have the same adverse effects as barbiturate sedative–hypnotics (see VII D 1). Intravenous use of barbiturates may cause cardiovascular collapse and respiratory depression.
2. **Hydantoins** are associated with these adverse effects:
   a. Gastrointestinal effects, such as gastrointestinal irritation, nausea, and vomiting
   b. CNS effects, such as nystagmus, diplopia, and ataxia
   c. Blood dyscrasias, osteoporosis, and gingival hyperplasia
   d. Stevens-Johnson syndrome
   e. Cardiovascular collapse and respiratory depression (with intravenous administration)
3. **Succinimides** are associated with these adverse effects:
   a. Gastrointestinal effects, such as gastrointestinal irritation, nausea, and vomiting
   b. CNS effects, such as CNS depression, drowsiness, headache, and confusion

c. Blood dyscrasias
d. Stevens-Johnson syndrome

4. **Dibenzazepines** are associated with these adverse effects:
   a. Gastrointestinal effects, such as nausea and vomiting
   b. CNS effects, such as drowsiness and dizziness
   c. Blood dyscrasias, such as aplastic anemia
   d. Renal failure, hepatotoxicity, and congestive heart failure
   e. Stevens-Johnson syndrome

5. **Benzodiazepine antiepileptics** have the same adverse effects as benzodiazepine anxiolytics (see VI D 1). Intravenous administration may cause cardiovascular collapse and respiratory depression.

6. **Dialkylacetates** are associated with these adverse effects:
   a. Gastrointestinal effects, such as gastrointestinal irritation, nausea, and vomiting
   b. CNS effects, such as sedation, headache, ataxia, and dysarthria
   c. Pancreatitis, hepatotoxicity, prolonged bleeding time, and blood dyscrasias

IX. ANTIPARKINSONIAN AGENTS

A. Chemistry. The principal antiparkinsonian agents are either **anticholinergic** or **dopaminergic**.

1. **Anticholinergics** are structurally related to **atropine** (e.g., benzotropine, trihexyphenidyl) or **antihistamines** (e.g., ethopropazine). Other anticholinergics include procyclidine (Kemadrin) and biperiden (Akineton).

2. The prototypical **dopaminergic** is the **catecholamine,** levodopa (Figure 13-13). Newer dopaminergics are **ergot alkaloid derivatives** known as **ergolines** (e.g., bromocriptine (Parlodel) and pergolide (Permax). There are two agents available that increase the therapeutic efficacy of levodopa.
   a. **Carbidopa,** a levodopa analogue, is a **decarboxylase inhibitor** that diminishes the decarboxylation and subsequent inactivation of levodopa in **peripheral tissues**. A **combination** of levodopa and carbidopa (Sinemet) is available (see Chapter 11 V B 1).
   b. **Selegiline** (Elderpryl), an **alkylpropynylphenethylamine** is a **selective MAO-B inhibitor** that inhibits the **intracerebral** degradation of dopamine.

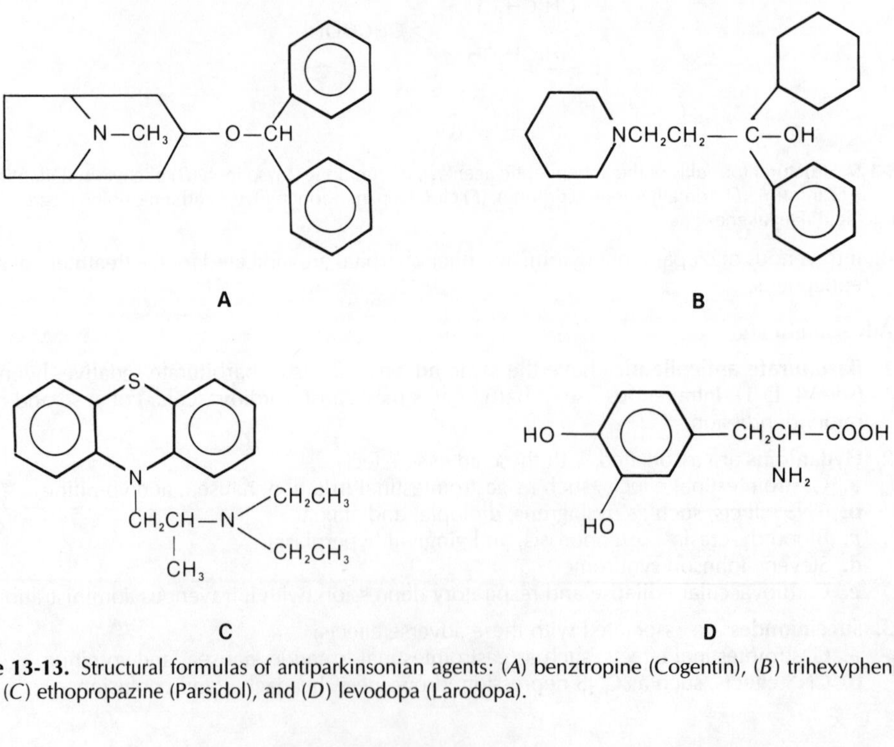

Figure 13-13. Structural formulas of antiparkinsonian agents: (*A*) benztropine (Cogentin), (*B*) trihexyphenidyl (Artane), (*C*) ethopropazine (Parsidol), and (*D*) levodopa (Larodopa).

B. Pharmacology. Antiparkinsonian agents act by restoring the striatal balance of dopaminergic and cholinergic neurotransmitters, which is disturbed in parkinsonism.

1. **Levodopa,** which can cross the blood–brain barrier, is the immediate precursor of the striatal inhibitory neurotransmitter dopamine and is converted to dopamine in the body.
2. **Amantadine,** an antiviral agent, appears to stimulate the release of dopamine from intact striatal dopaminergic terminals.
3. **Bromocriptine,** a dopaminergic receptor agonist, mimics the activity of striatal dopamine.
4. **Selegiline,** an inhibitor of the central MAO-B isoenzyme, blocks the central catabolism of dopamine, increasing its availability in the basal ganglia.
5. **Anticholinergics** such as trihexyphenidyl and benztropine block the excitatory cholinergic striatal system.
6. **Antihistamines** such as diphenhydramine possess anticholinergic properties.

C. Therapeutic indications

1. **Levodopa** is indicated to treat idiopathic, postencephalitic, or arteriosclerotic parkinsonism.
2. **Amantadine** is indicated to treat idiopathic, postencephalitic, or arteriosclerotic parkinsonism, as well as extrapyramidal symptoms induced by antipsychotic drugs (with the exception of tardive dyskinesia).
3. **Bromocriptine** is indicated to treat idiopathic or postencephalitic parkinsonism.
4. **Selegiline, anticholinergics,** and **antihistamines** are indicated for use as adjunctive therapy for all types of parkinsonism, including drug-induced extrapyramidal symptoms (with the exception of tardive dyskinesia).

D. Adverse effects

1. **Levodopa** is associated with these adverse effects:
   - **a.** Gastrointestinal effects, such as gastrointestinal upset, nausea, vomiting, anorexia, and excessive salivation
   - **b.** Cardiovascular effects, such as orthostatic hypotension, tachycardia, and dysrhythmias
   - **c.** CNS effects, such as headache, dizziness, and insomnia
   - **d.** Abnormal involuntary movements, such as dyskinesia and choreiform or dystonic movements
   - **e.** Psychiatric effects, such as delusions, hallucinations, confusion, psychoses, and depression
2. **Amantadine** is associated with these adverse effects:
   - **a.** CNS effects, such as drowsiness, insomnia, dizziness, slurred speech, and nightmares
   - **b.** Urinary retention and ankle edema
   - **c.** Livedo reticularis (mottling of skin on the extremities)
   - **d.** Psychiatric effects, such as hallucinations and confusion
3. **Bromocriptine** is associated with these adverse effects:
   - **a.** Nausea
   - **b.** Hypotension
   - **c.** Psychiatric effects, such as confusion and hallucinations
   - **d.** Livedo reticularis
   - **e.** Abnormal involuntary movements, such as dyskinesia and choreiform or dystonic movements
4. **Selegiline** is associated with adverse effects that are similar to those of bromocriptine, including dyskinesias and hallucinations.
5. Anticholinergic antiparkinsonian agents have the same adverse effects as other cholinergic antagonists (see Chapter 12, III D).
6. Antihistaminic antiparkinsonian agents have the same adverse effects as other antihistamines (see Chapter 14 II A).

X. OPIOID ANALGESICS consist of natural opiate alkaloids and their synthetic derivatives.

A. **Chemistry.** The opiate alkaloids are derived from opium, which is considered the oldest drug on record. Opium (the dried exudate of the poppy seed capsule) contains about 25 different alkaloids. Of these, morphine is the most important both quantitatively and pharmacologically (Figure 13-14).

1. The morphine molecule can be altered in a variety of ways; related compounds may also be synthesized from other starting materials.
2. Morphine's phenolic hydroxyl group is extremely important; however, analgesic activity appears to depend on a p-phenyl-N-alkylpiperidine moiety, in which the piperidine ring is in the chair form and is perpendicular to the aromatic ring. The alkyl group is usually methyl. Morphine's amphoteric character (phenolic hydroxyl and tertiary amine) contributes to its erratic absorption when administered orally.
3. The piperidine moiety of morphine is common to most opioid analgesics, including the morphine analogues (e.g., codeine, heroin, hydromorphone, oxycodone) and the piperidines (meperidine, diphenoxylate). The methadones (e.g., methadone, propoxyphene) appear to assume a pseudopiperidine ring configuration in the body (Figure 13-15).

B. **Pharmacology**

1. Opioid analgesics mimic endogenous enkephalins and endorphins at CNS opiate receptors, raising the pain threshold and increasing pain tolerance.
2. Opioid analgesics also cause chemoreceptor trigger zone stimulation and decrease α_1-adrenergic receptor responsiveness.

C. **Therapeutic indications.** Opioid analgesics are indicated to relieve moderate-to-severe pain, such as the pain associated with myocardial infarction. They are also used as preanesthetic medications, as analgesic adjuncts during anesthesia, as antitussives, and as antidiarrheals.

D. **Adverse effects.** Opioid analgesics are associated with these adverse effects:

1. CNS effects, including CNS depression, miosis, dizziness, sedation, confusion, disorientation, and coma
2. Gastrointestinal effects, including nausea, vomiting, constipation, biliary spasm, and increased biliary tract pressure
3. Cardiovascular effects, such as orthostatic hypotension, peripheral circulatory collapse, dysrhythmias, and cardiac arrest
4. Respiratory depression
5. Bronchoconstriction
6. Psychiatric effects, such as euphoria, dysphoria, and hallucinations
7. Abuse potential and dependence
8. Precipitation of withdrawal symptoms in opioid-dependent patients (when opioid agonist–antagonists, such as pentazocine or nalbuphine, are used as analgesics)

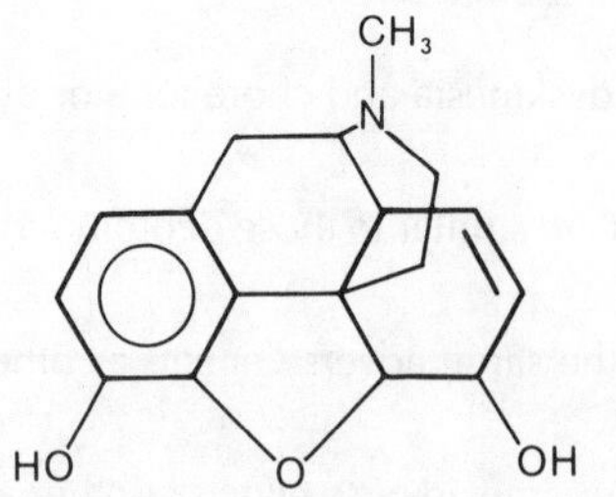

Figure 13-14. Structural formula of morphine.

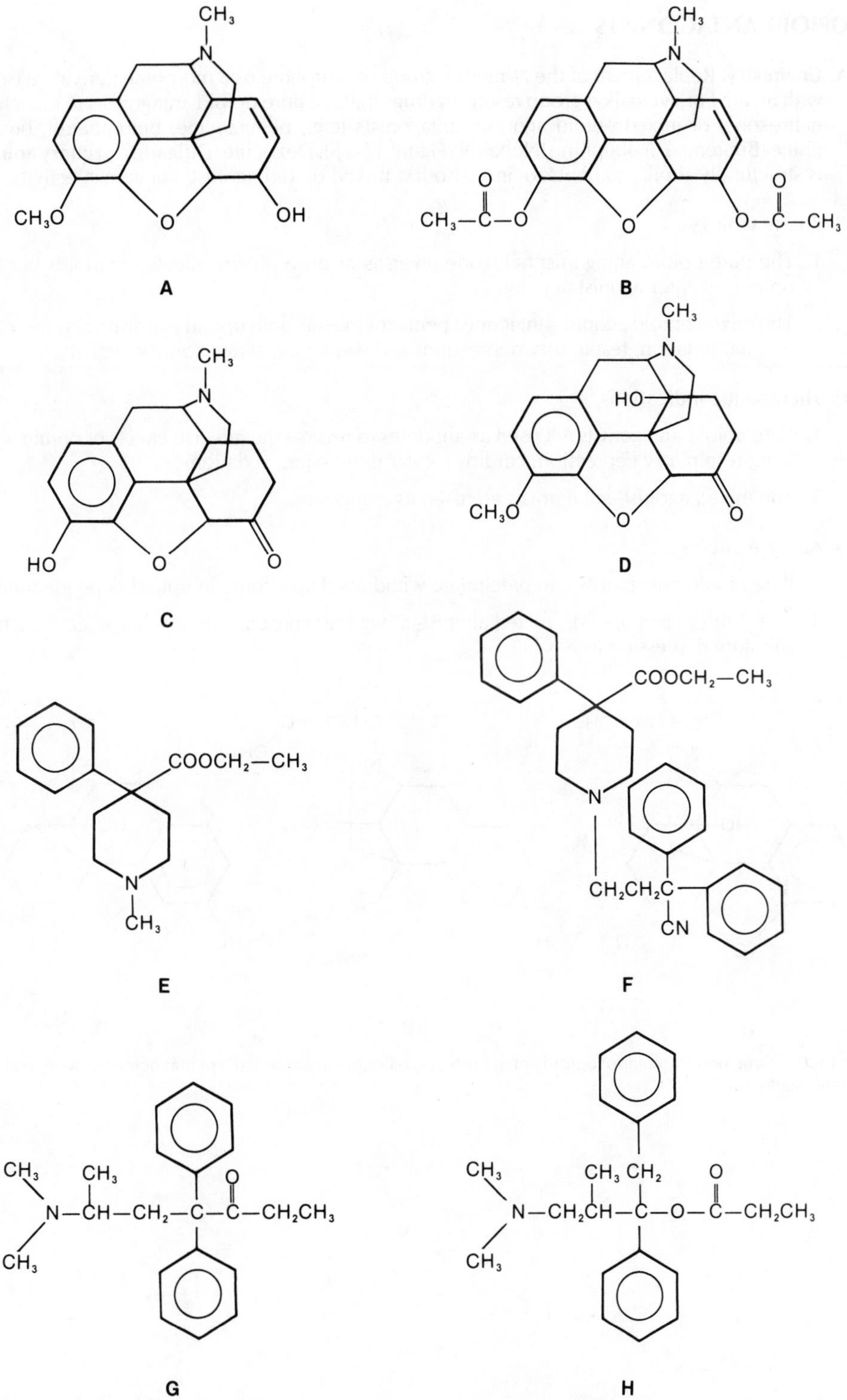

Figure 13-15. Structural formulas of selected opioid agonists, including (*A*) codeine, (*B*) heroin, (*C*) hydromorphone (Dilaudid), and (*D*) oxycodone (Percodan), morphine analogues; (*E*) meperidine (Demerol) and (*F*) diphenoxylate (Lomotil), piperidine analgesics; and (*G*) methadone (Dolophine) and (*H*) propoxyphene (Darvon), methadone analgesics.

XI. OPIOID ANTAGONISTS

A. Chemistry. Replacement of the N-methyl group of morphine or a morphine derivative (see X A) with an allyl or cycloalkyl group results in drugs that are pure opioid antagonists (e.g., naloxone, naltrexone) or mixed opioid agonists–antagonists [e.g., pentazocine, butorphanol, buprenorphine (Buprenex), nalbuphine (Nubain)] (Figure 13-16). **Dezocine** (Dulgan), a **primary amine** that is structurally similar to pentazocine, also has mixed opioid agonist–antagonist activity.

B. Pharmacology

1. The pure opioid antagonist naloxone reverses or prevents the effects of opioids but has no opioid-receptor agonist activity.
2. The mixed opioid agonist–antagonist pentazocine has both opioid agonistic actions (e.g., analgesia, sedation, respiratory depression) and weak opioid antagonistic activity.

C. Therapeutic indications

1. Pure opioid antagonists are used as antidotes to reverse the adverse effects of opioid agonists (e.g., respiratory depression, cardiovascular depression, sedation).
2. The mixed agonist–antagonists are used as analgesics.

D. Adverse effects

1. Pure opioid antagonists can precipitate withdrawal syndrome in opioid-dependent patients.
2. In the absence of opioids, mixed agonist–antagonists produce opioid-like effects, such as respiratory depression (see X D).

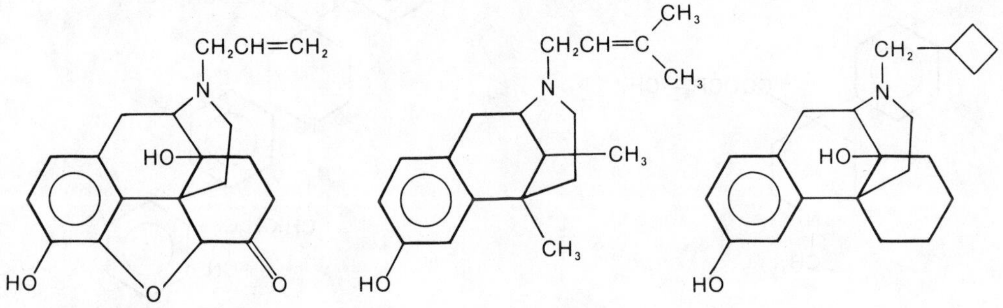

A B C

Figure 13-16. Structural formulas of opioid antagonists: (*A*) naloxone (Narcan), (*B*) pentazocine (Talwin), and (*C*) butorphanol (Stadol).

STUDY QUESTIONS

Directions: Each of the numbered items or incomplete statements in this section is followed by answers or by completions of the statement. Select the **one** lettered answer or completion that is **best** in each case.

1. Which of the following drugs is a volatile substance that is administered by inhalation?

(A) Thiopental
(B) Halothane
(C) Alprazolam
(D) Buspirone
(E) Phenytoin

2. The structure of prochlorperazine is shown below. Which of the following medications, because of its chemical relationship to prochlorperazine, would most likely cause similar side effects?

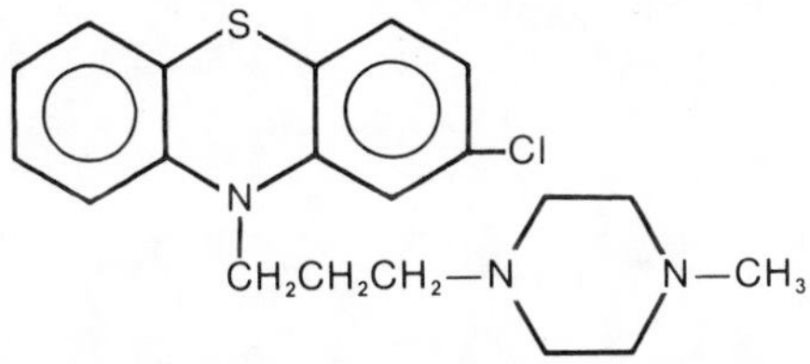

(A) Fluphenazine
(B) Thioridazine
(C) Alprazolam
(D) Buspirone
(E) Pentobarbital

3. The brief duration of action of an ultra–short-acting barbiturate is due to a

(A) slow rate of metabolism in the liver
(B) low lipid solubility, resulting in a minimal concentration in the brain
(C) high degree of binding to plasma proteins
(D) rapid rate of redistribution from the brain due to its high liposolubility
(E) slow rate of excretion by the kidneys

4. Which of the following mechanisms of action most likely contributes to the treatment of parkinsonism?

(A) The direct-acting dopaminergic agonist amantadine mimics the activity of striatal dopamine
(B) The antimuscarinic activity of diphenhydramine contributes to the restoration of striatal dopaminergic–cholinergic neurotransmitter balance
(C) Striatal H_1 receptors are blocked by the antihistaminic trihexyphenidyl
(D) The ergoline bromocriptine stimulates the release of striatal dopamine from intact terminals
(E) The ability of dopamine to cross the blood–brain barrier allows it to restore striatal dopaminergic–cholinergic neurotransmitter balance

5. All of the following adverse effects are associated with the use of levodopa EXCEPT

(A) sialorrhea
(B) orthostatic hypotension
(C) delusions, confusion, and depression
(D) dyskinesia and dystonia
(E) livedo reticularis

6. The activity of which of the following drugs is dependent upon a p-phenyl-N-alkylpiperidine moiety?

(A) Phenobarbital
(B) Chlorpromazine
(C) Diazepam
(D) Imipramine
(E) Meperidine

7. Opioids are used as all of the following agents EXCEPT

(A) antitussives
(B) analgesics
(C) anti-inflammatories
(D) antidiarrheals
(E) preanesthetic medications

1-B 4-B 7-C
2-A 5-E
3-D 6-E

Directions: Each question below contains three suggested answers of which **one or more** is correct. Choose the answer

A if **I only** is correct
B if **III only** is correct
C if **I and II** are correct
D if **II and III** are correct
E if **I, II, and III** are correct

8. Improper administration of local anesthetics can cause toxic plasma concentrations that may result in

I. seizures and central nervous system (CNS) depression
II. respiratory and myocardial depression
III. circulatory collapse

9. In addition to their anxiolytic properties, benzodiazepines are indicated for use

I. as preanesthetic medications
II. as anticonvulsants
III. during acute withdrawal from alcohol

Directions: Each group of items in this section consists of lettered options followed by a set of numbered items. For each item, select the **one** lettered option that is most closely associated with it. Each lettered option may be selected once, more than once, or not at all.

Questions 10–12

For each statement below, choose the drug that it most closely describes.

(A) Tranylcypromine
(B) Imipramine
(C) Buspirone
(D) Trazodone
(E) Phenelzine

10. An anxiolytic drug that does not possess either hypnotic or anticonvulsant properties

11. A prototype tricyclic antidepressant with antimuscarinic properties that make it useful in the treatment of enuresis

12. An antidepressant that inhibits serotonin reuptake and may cause adverse effects such as impaired memory, akathisia, and menstrual irregularities

---

8-E
9-E
10-C
11-B
12-D

Questions 13–15

For each of the following structures, select the most appropriate pharmacologic category.

(A) General anesthetic
(B) Local anesthetic
(C) Antidepressant
(D) Anxiolytic
(E) Opioid antagonist

13.

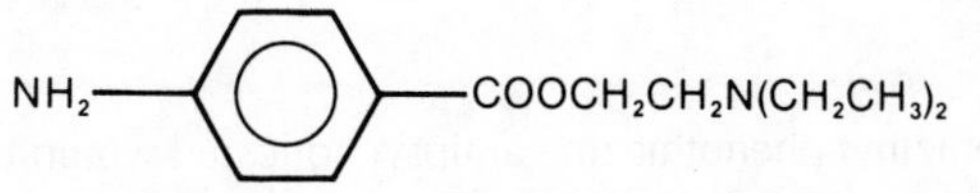

14.

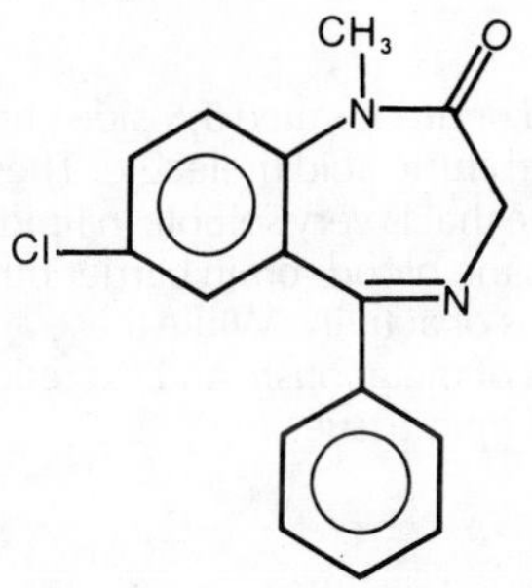

15.

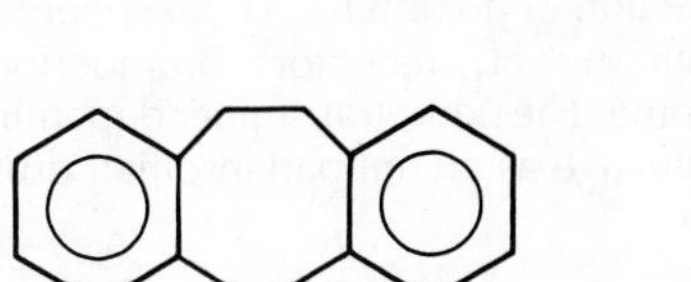

13-B
14-D
15-C

ANSWERS AND EXPLANATIONS

1. The answer is B *[II A 1].*
The general anesthetics are divided into two major classes of drugs: those that are gases or volatile liquids, which are administered by inhalation, and those that are nonvolatile salts, which are administered as intravenous solutions. Halothane is a halogenated hydrocarbon, which belongs to the former class. It has the advantage over older volatile anesthetics (e.g., ethyl ether, cyclopropane) of being nonflammable. Thiopental sodium, alprazolam, buspirone, and phenytoin are all nonvolatile substances that are administered orally or parenterally. Thiopental is a general anesthetic; it is sometimes referred to as a basal anesthetic since it does not produce significant third-stage surgical anesthesia. Alprazolam and buspirone are anxiolytics, whereas phenytoin is an anticonvulsant.

2. The answer is A *[IV A 1; Table 13-1].*
Fluphenazine, like prochlorperazine, is a piperazinyl phenothiazine antipsychotic and would be likely to cause similar side effects. While thioridazine is also a phenothiazine antipsychotic, it is a piperidyl derivative rather than a piperazinyl derivative. Alprazolam, phenytoin, and pentobarbital are not phenothiazines; therefore, structurally, they are not similar to prochlorperazine.

3. The answer is D *[VII A 1 c, d; Figure 13-1].*
Ultra–short-acting barbiturates are characterized by having branched or unsaturated 5,5-side chains and by having a sulfur atom in place of oxygen in the 2 position of the barbituric acid molecule. These modifications of barbituric acid result in an extremely liposoluble molecule that is very soluble in lipid tissues. After administration, an ultra–short-acting barbiturate readily crosses the blood–brain barrier but then is quickly redistributed into extra-cerebral tissue, resulting in a rapid loss of activity. While these agents do remain in the body for a long time and may appear to have slow rates of metabolism and excretion, their long retention time is due more to their slow rate of leaching out of lipid tissue.

4. The answer is B *[IX B].*
The H_1 antagonist diphenhydramine possesses antimuscarinic activity, which allows it to be of use in the restoration of striatal dopaminergic–cholinergic neurotransmitter balance. Amantadine appears to stimulate the release of striatal dopamine; it does not mimic the action of dopamine. Trihexyphenidyl is an antimuscarinic agent, not antihistaminic; it blocks cholinergic, not H_1, receptors. Bromocriptine is a dopaminergic agonist and mimics the activity of striatal dopamine. The neurotransmitter dopamine is not able to cross the blood–brain barrier and is, therefore, not effective as an antiparkinsonian drug.

5. The answer is E *[IX D 1].*
Livedo reticularis is a circulatory disorder characterized by large, bluish, discolored areas on the extremities. It is an adverse effect associated with the use of amantadine and bromocriptine but not with the use of levodopa.

6. The answer is E *[X A 2, 3; Figure 13-15, E].*
The p-phenyl-N-alkylpiperidine moiety is common to the structurally specific opioid analgesics. Meperidine is an opioid analgesic and is an N-methyl-p-phenylpiperidine derivative. Its chemical name is ethyl 1-methyl-4-phenylpiperidine-4-carboxylate. Phenobarbital is a barbiturate sedative. Chlorpromazine is a phenothiazine antipsychotic. Diazepam is a benzodiazepine anxiolytic. Imipramine is a tricyclic dibenzazepine antidepressant.

7. The answer is C *[X C].*
Unlike the salicylates, opioids do not possess anti-inflammatory activity. Opioids do suppress the cough reflex and are preeminent analgesics. Opioids cause constipation and are, thus, effective antidiarrheal agents. When used as preanesthetic medication, opioids permit a reduction in the amount of general anesthetic required for surgical anesthesia.

8. The answer is E (all) *[III D 2].*
Careful administration of a local anesthetic by a knowledgeable practitioner is essential to prevent systemic absorption and consequent toxicity. This is especially important when the patient has cardiovascular disease, poorly controlled diabetes, thyrotoxicosis, or peripheral vascular disease.

9. The answer is E (all) *[VII C 2].*
Benzodiazepines may serve as induction agents for general anesthesia; they also have anxiolytic properties. In addition, intravenous diazepam is used to treat status epilepticus, while clonazepam is used orally for myoclonic and absence (petit mal) seizures. Benzodiazepines also diminish alcohol withdrawal symptoms.

10–12. The answers are: 10-C *[VI B 2],* **11-B** *[V C 2],* **12-D** *[V B 3, D 3].*
Buspirone's mechanism of anxiolytic action is unknown. Unlike the benzodiazepines, buspirone lacks hypnotic and anticonvulsant properties. The tricyclic antidepressant imipramine is useful in the treatment of enuresis because the compound blocks muscarinic receptors mediating micturition. Trazodone is categorized as an atypical antidepressant that selectively blocks serotonin re-uptake.

13–15. The answers are: 13-B *[III A; Figure 13-2],* **14-D** *[VI A; Table 13-2],* **15-C** *[V A 2; Figure 13-6].*
The structure shown in question 13 is that of procaine, which is a diethylaminoethyl p-aminobenzoate ester. It contains a hydrophilic amino group in the alcohol portion of the molecule and a lipophilic aromatic acid connected by the ester linkage. The procaine molecule is typical of ester-type local anesthetics.

The structure in question 14 is that of diazepam, which has a benzo-1,4-diazepine as its base nucleus. The widely used benzo-1,4-diazepine derivatives have significant anxiolytic, hypnotic, and anticonvulsant activities.

The structure in question 15 is that of desipramine, which has a dibenzazepine as its base nucleus. Dibenzazepine derivatives that have a methyl- or dimethylaminopropyl group attached to the ring nitrogen have significant antidepressant activity. Similarly substituted dibenzocycloheptadienes also have antidepressant activity. Together these two chemical classes make up the majority of the tricyclic antidepressants.

14

Autacoids and Their Antagonists, Non-narcotic Analgesic–Antipyretics, and Nonsteroidal Anti-inflammatory Drugs

David C. Kosegarten
Edward F. LaSala

I. INTRODUCTION

A. Autacoids, which are also referred to as autopharmacologic agents or local hormones, have widely differing structures and pharmacologic actions. The two most important autacoids are histamine and the prostaglandins. Their antagonists also have important pharmacologic roles.

B. Non-narcotic analgesic–antipyretics have dissimilar structures but share certain therapeutic actions, including relief of pain, fever, and, sometimes, inflammation. They appear to work by inhibiting synthesis of prostaglandins and related autacoids.

C. Nonsteroidal anti-inflammatory drugs (NSAIDs) differ in structure and activity from the non-narcotic analgesic–antipyretics, but they all have anti-inflammatory properties and also appear to inhibit prostaglandin synthesis.

II. AUTACOIDS AND THEIR ANTAGONISTS

A. Histamine and antihistaminics

1. Chemistry

a. Histamine is a bioamine derived principally from dietary histidine, which is decarboxylated by L-histidine decarboxylase (Figure 14-1).

b. Antihistaminics (histamine antagonists) may be classified as **H_1-receptor antagonists** or **H_2-receptor antagonists**.

(1) **H_1-receptor antagonists,** the classic antihistaminic agents, are chemically classified as **ethylenediamines** (e.g., tripelennamine), **alkylamines** (e.g., chlorpheniramine), **ethanolamines** (e.g., diphenhydramine), **piperazines** (e.g., cyclizine), **phenothiazines** (e.g., promethazine), and **piperidines** (e.g., terfenadine) [Figure 14-2]. Astemizole (Hismanal), a piperidylamino benzimidazole, is also available.

(2) **H_2-receptor antagonists** are heterocyclic methylthioalkyl derivatives. These include cimetidine (Tagamet), ranitidine (Zantac), famotidine (Pepcid), and nizatidine (Axid) [Figure 14-3].

(3) An alternative to the H_2-antagonists is omeprazole (Prilosec), a **specific inhibitor of H^+,K^+-ATPase,** which is the ultimate mediator of gastric acid secretion. Its structure includes a sulfinyl bridge linking a substituted benzimidazole with a substituted pyridine ring.

2. Pharmacology

a. Histamine has powerful pharmacologic actions, mediated by two specific receptor types (Table 14-1).

(1) **H_1-receptors** mediate typical allergic and anaphylactic responses to histamine, such as bronchoconstriction, vasodilation, increased capillary permeability, and spasmodic contractions of gastrointestinal smooth muscle.

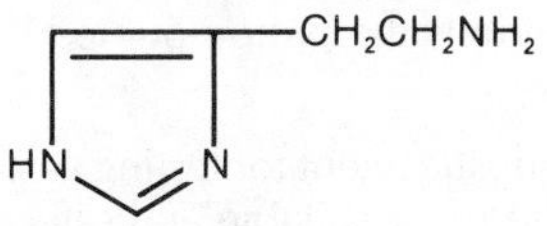

Figure 14-1. Structural formula of histamine, an autacoid.

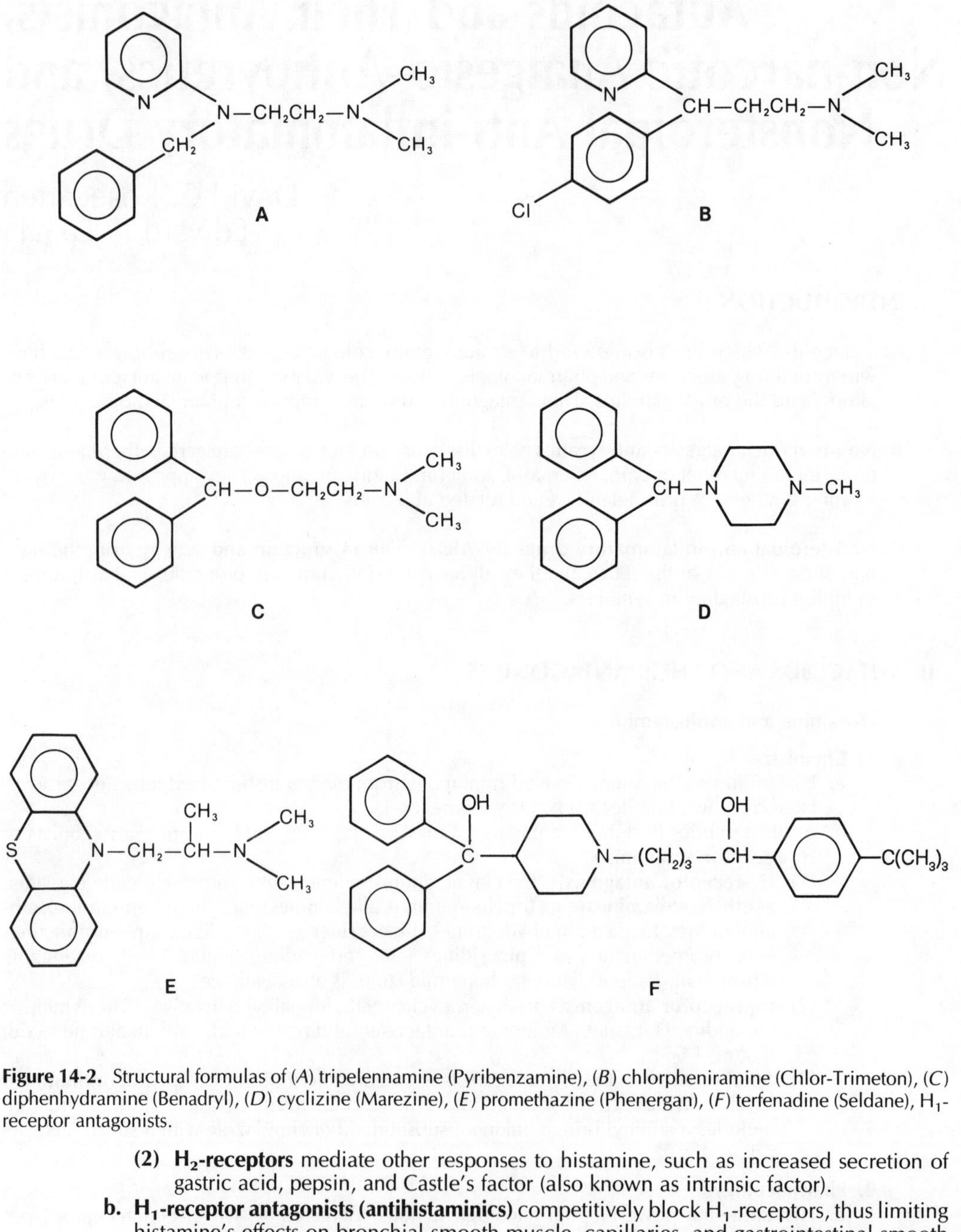

Figure 14-2. Structural formulas of (*A*) tripelennamine (Pyribenzamine), (*B*) chlorpheniramine (Chlor-Trimeton), (*C*) diphenhydramine (Benadryl), (*D*) cyclizine (Marezine), (*E*) promethazine (Phenergan), (*F*) terfenadine (Seldane), H_1-receptor antagonists.

(2) **H_2-receptors** mediate other responses to histamine, such as increased secretion of gastric acid, pepsin, and Castle's factor (also known as intrinsic factor).

b. H_1-receptor antagonists (antihistaminics) competitively block H_1-receptors, thus limiting histamine's effects on bronchial smooth muscle, capillaries, and gastrointestinal smooth muscle. They also prevent histamine-induced pain and itching of the skin and mucous membranes.

c. H_2-receptor antagonists competitively block H_2-receptors, thus limiting the effects of histamine on gastric secretions.

d. A new **antisecretory agent, omeprazole,** inhibits the proton pump H^+,K^+-ATPase.

3. Therapeutic indications

a. Exogenous histamine may be used as a diagnostic agent for testing gastric function. However, other stimulants of gastric secretion are more suitable and safer.

b. H_1-receptor antagonists are used to provide symptomatic relief of allergic symptoms, such

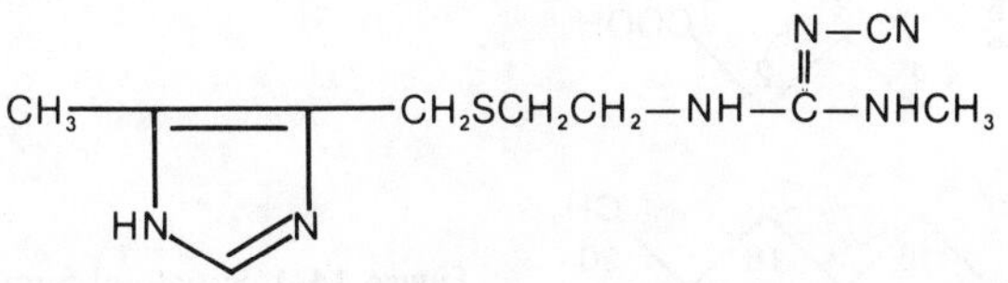

Figure 14-3. Structural formula of cimetidine, an H_2-receptor antagonist.

as seasonal rhinitis and conjunctivitis. Their anesthetic and antipruritic effects also make them useful for symptomatic relief of urticaria.

c. **H_2-receptor antagonists** are used to treat gastric hypersecretory conditions, such as duodenal ulcer and Zollinger-Ellison syndrome.

d. The **proton pump inhibitor,** omeprazole, is used to treat duodenal ulcers.

4. **Adverse effects**

a. **Histamine** may cause numerous adverse effects related to its basic pharmacology (see II A 2 a).

b. **H_1-receptor antagonists** are associated with the adverse effects listed below.

(1) Central nervous system (CNS) effects, such as CNS depression, sedation, fatigue, tinnitus, hallucinations, and ataxia

(2) Gastrointestinal effects, such as nausea and vomiting

(3) Antimuscarinic effects, such as dry mouth, urinary retention, and constipation

(4) Teratogenic effects (possible with piperazine compounds)

c. **Peripheral H_1-receptor antagonists,** terfenadine and astemizole, are devoid of significant sedative and antimuscarinic effects. However, elevated plasma levels of both astemizole and terfenadine have been associated with electrocardiographic QT prolongation, cardiac arrest, torsades de pointes, and other ventricular arrhythmias. Moreover, concomitant use of terfenadine with the antifungal ketoconazole or the macrolide antibiotics, erythromycin and troleandomycin, is contraindicated because such a combination results in significantly elevated terfenadine plasma levels.

d. **H_2-receptor antagonists** are associated with these adverse effects:

(1) CNS effects, such as confusion and dizziness

(2) Hepatic and renal dysfunction

(3) Inhibition of the hepatic microsomal drug-metabolizing enzyme system (with cimetidine)

Table 14-1. Selected Actions of Endogenous Histamine

Site	Action	Receptor Type
Cardiovascular		
Vascular	Arterial contraction	H_1
	Arteriolar relaxation	H_1 and H_2
	Venule contraction	H_1
	Venule relaxation	H_2
	Endothelial cells, release of EDRF	H_1
	Endothelial cells, contraction	H_1
Heart	Increased heart rate	H_2
	Increased force of contraction	H_2
	Slowed atrioventricular conduction	H_1
Respiratory	Bronchiolar smooth muscle contraction	H_1
Gastrointestinal		
Gastric mucosa	Increased secretion of acid and pepsin	H_2
Gastrointestinal smooth muscle	Contraction	H_1
Various		
Cutaneous nerve endings	Pain and itch	H_1

EDRF = Endothelium-derived relaxing factor.

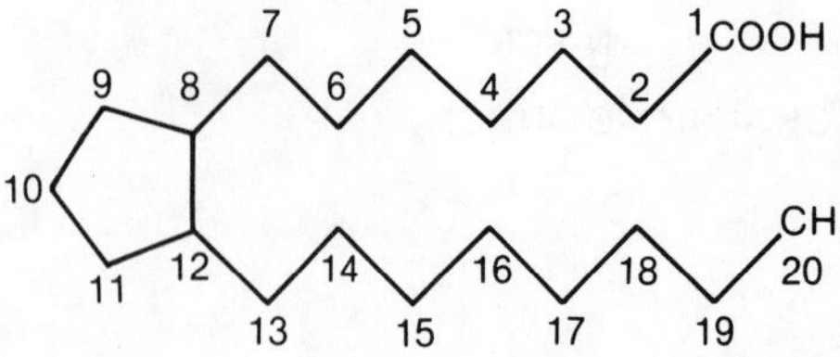

Figure 14-4. Structural formula of prostanoic acid from which the prostaglandins are derived.

(4) Androgenic effects (with high doses of cimetidine), such as impotence and gynecomastia in men and galactorrhea in women

e. **The H^+,K^+-ATPase inhibitor,** omeprazole, may cause painful nocturnal erection and gynecomastia, in addition to interfering with the metabolism of diazepam, warfarin, and phenytoin.

B. Prostaglandins

1. Chemistry

a. Prostaglandins are derivatives of prostanoic acid, a 20-carbon fatty acid containing a 5-carbon ring (Figure 14-4). In the body, prostaglandins are principally synthesized from arachidonic acid, a component of membrane phospholipids.

b. Classification of prostaglandins as prostaglandin A (PGA), prostaglandin B (PGB), prostaglandin E (PGE), and so forth relates to the presence or absence of keto or hydroxyl groups at positions 9 and 11 (see Figure 14-4). Subscripts relate to the number and position of double bonds in the aliphatic chains (Figure 14-5).

2. Pharmacology

a. Endogenous prostaglandins appear to affect virtually every body function. They are released in response to many chemical, bacterial, mechanical, and other insults, and they appear to contribute to the signs and symptoms of the inflammatory process, including pain and edema.

b. When given clinically, PGE inhibits platelet aggregation, stimulates intestinal and uterine smooth muscle, produces vasodilation, and relaxes the smooth muscle of the ductus arteriosus.

3. **Therapeutic indications.** PGE is used for temporary maintenance of a patent ductus arteriosus in infants awaiting corrective surgery for congenital heart defects.

4. **Adverse effects** associated with PGE include:

a. CNS effects, such as CNS irritability, fever, and seizures
b. Cardiovascular effects, such as hypotension, dysrhythmias, vasodilation, and cardiac arrest
c. Respiratory effects, such as respiratory depression and distress
d. Hematologic effects, such as anemia, thrombocytopenia, and disseminated intravascular coagulation (DIC)
e. Diarrhea
f. Decreased renal function

III. NON-NARCOTIC ANALGESIC–ANTIPYRETICS AND NSAIDS

A. Salicylates

1. Chemistry

a. Salicylates are derivatives of salicylic acid, which is found as the glycoside salicin in willow bark. The prototypical drug is aspirin, the acetyl ester of salicylic acid (Figure 14-6). A simple ester, aspirin hydrolyzes easily, is unstable in aqueous media, and is affected by moisture.

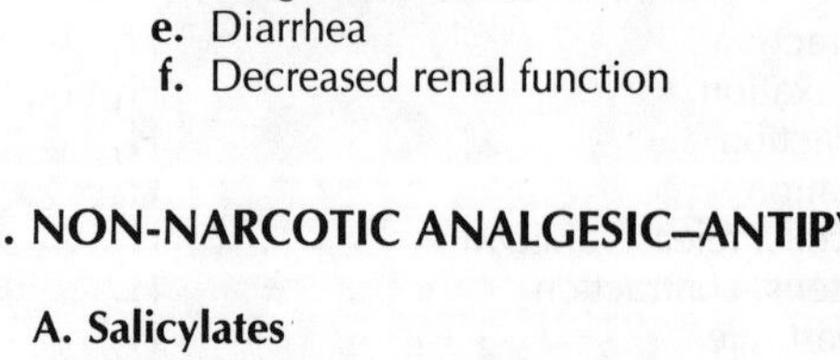

Figure 14-5. Structural formula of misoprostol (Cytotec), a derivative of prostaglandin E_1 (PGE_1).

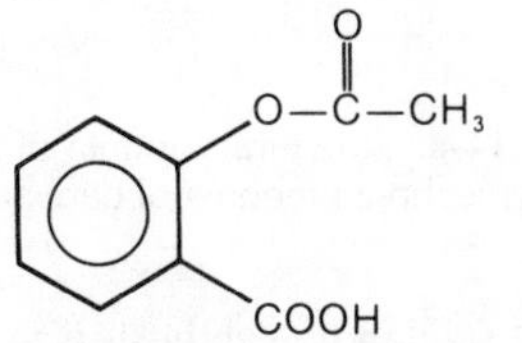

Figure 14-6. Structural formula of aspirin, the prototypical salicylate analgesic–antipyretic.

b. More stable salicylates include diflunisal and the topical agent methyl salicylate (wintergreen oil) [Figure 14-7].

c. Most salicylates are weak acids. Their excretion is influenced by changes in urinary pH.

2. Pharmacology

a. Salicylates inhibit the enzyme cyclooxygenase and, thus, inhibit local prostaglandin synthesis (see II B 2 a). As a result, they are analgesic for low-intensity integumental pain, antipyretic, and anti-inflammatory.

b. Salicylates also block platelet cyclooxygenase and subsequent formation of thromboxane A_2. As a result, they inhibit platelet aggregation and eventual thrombus formation.

3. Therapeutic indications

a. Salicylates are indicated for use as:

(1) Analgesics, for relief of skeletal muscle pain, headache, neuralgias, myalgias, and spasmodic dysmenorrhea

(2) Anti-inflammatory agents, for relief of rheumatoid arthritis symptoms and acute rheumatic fever

(3) Antipyretic agents, for relief of fever. (Children with varicella or influenza-type viral infections should not be given salicylates because of the observed association between salicylate use in these situations and Reye syndrome.)

b. Aspirin is also indicated for **prophylaxis of myocardial infarction.**

c. Methyl salicylate (wintergreen oil) is used topically as a **counter irritant.**

4. Adverse effects

a. Salicylates are associated with the following effects:

(1) Gastrointestinal effects, such as nausea, vomiting, and gastrointestinal irritation, discomfort, ulceration, and hemorrhage

(2) Increased depth of respirations

(3) Antagonism of vitamin K with associated hypoprothrombinemia

(4) Uncoupling of oxidative phosphorylation, hyperglycemia, glycosuria, and reduced lipogenesis

(5) Delayed onset of labor

(6) Salicylism (salicylate toxicity, usually marked by tinnitus, nausea, and vomiting)

b. Low daily doses of salicylates (2 g) decrease renal urate excretion and increase serum uric acid levels. **High daily doses** (5 g) have the opposite effect.

c. Ingestion of one teaspoon of the topical agent **methyl salicylate** (wintergreen oil) can cause fatal intoxication.

B. p-Aminophenol derivatives

1. Chemistry. The prototypical p-aminophenol derivative is **acetaminophen,** an active metabolite of phenacetin and acetanilid (Figure 14-8).

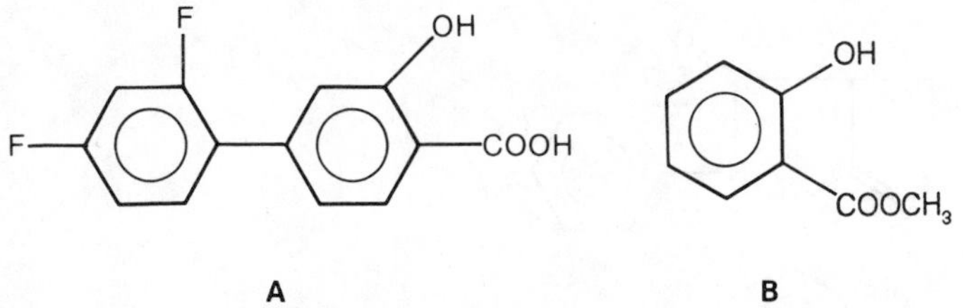

Figure 14-7. Structural formulas of (*A*) diflunisal (Dolobid) and (*B*) methyl salicylate (wintergreen oil), salicylate derivatives.

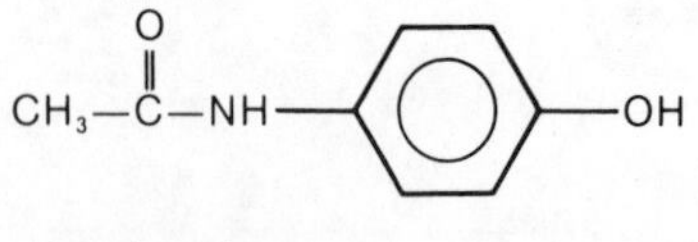

Figure 14-8. Structural formula of acetaminophen, the prototypical p-aminophenol derivative.

2. **Pharmacology**
   a. p-Aminophenol derivatives inhibit central prostaglandin synthesis (see II B 2 a). They are analgesic for low-intensity pain and are antipyretic.
   b. Because they are less effective than salicylates in blocking peripheral prostaglandin synthesis, they have no anti-inflammatory activity and do not affect platelet function.

3. **Therapeutic indications**
   a. **Acetaminophen** and **phenacetin** are indicated for use as **analgesics** and **antipyretics,** particularly in the patient unable to tolerate salicylates.
   b. Acetaminophen may be safely used as an alternative antipyretic in the child with varicella or an influenza-type viral infection [see III A 3 a (3)].

4. **Adverse effects**
   a. When given in therapeutic doses, adverse effects are limited to:
      (1) Skin rash
      (2) Hemolytic anemia (with long-term phenacetin use)
      (3) Methemoglobinemia
      (4) Renal dysfunction and tubular necrosis
   b. Acute acetaminophen overdose causes severe hepatotoxicity with necrosis and liver failure.

C. Pyrazolone derivatives

1. **Chemistry.** The most important pyrazolone derivatives are **phenylbutazone,** its metabolite **oxyphenbutazone,** and the uricosuric agent **sulfinpyrazone** (Anturane). Phenylbutazone is the prototypical agent (Figure 14-9).

2. **Pharmacology**
   a. **Phenylbutazone** and **oxyphenbutazone** inhibit prostaglandin synthesis (see II B 2 a) and stabilize lysosomal membranes. As a result, they have analgesic, antipyretic, and anti-inflammatory effects.
   b. **Sulfinpyrazone** inhibits proximal tubular absorption of urate and has a uricosuric effect. However, it is devoid of analgesic, antipyretic, or anti-inflammatory effects.

3. **Therapeutic indications**
   a. **Phenylbutazone** and **oxyphenbutazone** are used for short-term treatment of acute rheumatoid arthritic conditions and acute gout. However, they should be given only after other therapeutic measures have failed.
   b. **Sulfinpyrazone** is used to control hyperuricemia in the treatment of intermittent and chronic gout.

4. **Adverse effects**
   a. The adverse effects of **phenylbutazone** and **oxyphenbutazone** often limit their use and include:
      (1) Gastrointestinal effects, such as discomfort, nausea, vomiting, dyspepsia, and peptic ulceration
      (2) Blood dyscrasias, such as agranulocytosis, aplastic anemia, hemolytic anemia, thrombocytopenia, and petechiae

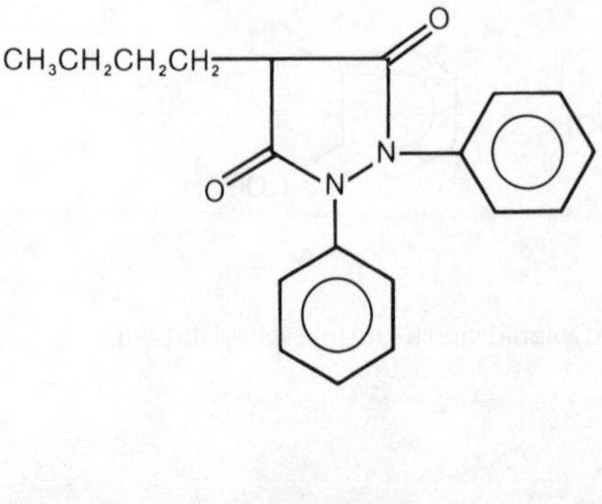

Figure 14-9. Structural formula of phenylbutazone (Butazolidin), a pyrazolone derivative.

(3) Cardiovascular effects, such as congestive heart failure with edema and dyspnea
(4) Renal effects, such as nephrotic lithiasis, renal necrosis, impaired renal function, and renal failure
(5) CNS effects, such as drowsiness, agitation, confusion, headache, lethargy, numbness, weakness, tinnitus, and hearing loss
(6) Hyperglycemia
(7) Skin rash

b. **Sulfinpyrazone** is associated with these adverse effects:
(1) Gastrointestinal effects, such as discomfort and upset
(2) Blood dyscrasias, as for phenylbutazone and oxyphenbutazone
(3) Renal failure

D. Agents used for the treatment of gout

1. Chemistry

a. Acute attacks of gout result from an inflammatory response to joint depositions of sodium urate crystals. Therapeutic agents counter this response by reducing plasma uric acid concentrations or inhibiting the inflammatory response.

b. Agents used for the treatment of gout have widely varying structures and include the pyrazolone derivative, sulfinpyrazone (see III C 2 b, 3 b, 4 b), the alkaloid colchicine, isopurines such as allopurinol, and benzoic acid derivatives such as probenecid (Figure 14-10).

2. Pharmacology

a. Although **colchicine's** exact mechanism of action is unknown, it appears to reduce the inflammatory response to deposited urate crystals by inhibiting leukocyte migration and phagocytosis. It also interferes with kinin formation and reduces leukocyte lactic acid production.

b. **Allopurinol** reduces serum urate levels by blocking uric acid production. It competitively inhibits the enzyme xanthine oxidase, which converts xanthine and hypoxanthine to uric acid.

c. **Probenecid,** a uricosuric agent, inhibits the proximal tubular reabsorption of uric acid, increasing uric acid excretion, thus reducing plasma uric acid concentrations.

3. Therapeutic indications

a. **Colchicine** is used principally for the treatment of acute gout attacks.

b. **Allopurinol,** which reduces uric acid synthesis and facilitates the dissolution of tophi (chalky urate deposits), is used to prevent the development or progression of chronic tophaceous gout.

c. **Probenecid** is used to treat chronic tophaceous gout. It is also used in smaller doses to prolong the effectiveness of penicillin-type antibiotics, by inhibiting their tubular secretion.

4. Adverse effects

a. Chronic use of **colchicine** is associated with these adverse effects:
(1) Agranulocytosis, aplastic anemia, myopathy, hair loss, and peripheral neuritis
(2) Nausea, vomiting, abdominal pain, and diarrhea (indications of impending toxicity)

b. **Allopurinol** is associated with these adverse effects:
(1) Gastrointestinal effects, such as gastrointestinal distress, nausea, vomiting, and diarrhea
(2) Skin rash, Stevens-Johnson syndrome, and hepatotoxicity
(3) Precipitation of an acute gout attack (with initial allopurinol therapy)

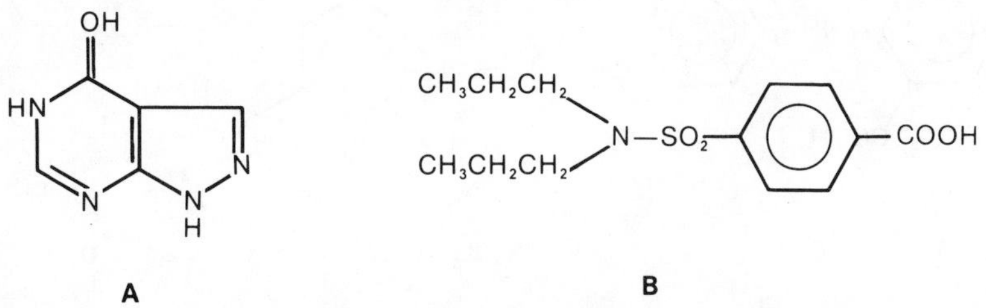

Figure 14-10. Structural formulas of (*A*) allopurinol (Zyloprim) and (*B*) probenecid (Benemid), agents used in the treatment of gout.

c. **Probenecid** is associated with these adverse effects:
   (1) Headache, nausea, vomiting, urinary frequency, sore gums, and dermatitis
   (2) Dizziness, anemia, hemolytic anemia, and renal lithiasis

E. Nonsteroidal anti-inflammatory drugs (NSAIDs)

1. **Chemistry.** The NSAIDs consist of a large number of structurally diverse acids. These include **arylacetic acids** (e.g., ibuprofen, naproxen), **indene derivatives** (e.g., indomethacin, sulindac), **fenamic acids** (e.g., mefenamic acid, diclofenac), and other structurally unrelated agents (e.g., piroxicam) [Figure 14-11].

2. **Pharmacology**
   a. NSAIDs have anti-inflammatory effects, resulting from their ability to inhibit the cyclooxygenase enzyme system and, thus, reduce local prostaglandin synthesis (see II B 2 a).
   b. NSAIDs also have analgesic and antipyretic effects.

3. **Therapeutic indications.** NSAIDs, like aspirin, are agents of choice for the treatment of rheumatoid arthritis, osteoarthritis, and ankylosing spondylitis.

4. **Adverse effects.** NSAIDs are associated with these adverse effects:
   a. Gastrointestinal effects, such as gastrointestinal distress and irritation, erosion of gastric mucosa, nausea, vomiting, and dyspepsia
   b. CNS effects, such as CNS depression, drowsiness, headache, dizziness, visual disturbances, ototoxicity, and confusion
   c. Hematologic effects, such as thrombocytopenia, altered platelet function, and prolonged bleeding time
   d. Skin rash

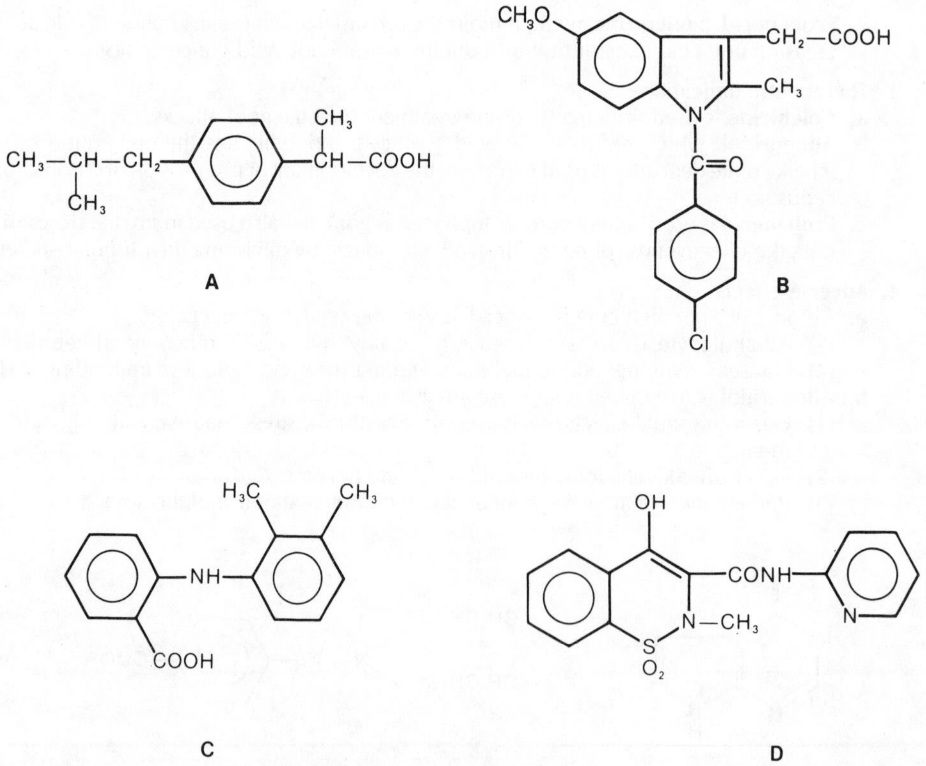

Figure 14-11. Structural formulas of (*A*) ibuprofen, (*B*) indomethacin, (*C*) mefenamic acid, and (*D*) piroxicam, representative nonsteroidal anti-inflammatory drugs (NSAIDs).

STUDY QUESTIONS

Directions: Each of the numbered items or incomplete statements in this section is followed by answers or by completions of the statement. Select the **one** lettered answer or completion that is **best** in each case.

1. All of the following are therapeutic indications for salicylates EXCEPT

(A) rheumatoid arthritis
(B) fever in children with influenza or varicella
(C) fever in adults with influenza
(D) spasmodic dysmenorrhea
(E) prophylaxis against myocardial infarction

2. All of the following statements describing acetaminophen are true EXCEPT

(A) it has anti-inflammatory activity similar to or greater than that of salicylates
(B) it acts as an analgesic and antipyretic
(C) it may cause skin rash
(D) it may be used in children with varicella or influenza-type viral infections
(E) acute overdose is characterized by severe hepatotoxicity

Directions: Each question below contains three suggested answers of which **one or more** is correct. Choose the answer

A if **I only** is correct
B if **III only** is correct
C if **I and II** are correct
D if **II and III** are correct
E if **I, II, and III** are correct

3. Correct statements regarding agents used in the treatment of gout include

I. allopurinol inhibits proximal tubular reabsorption of uric acid and may cause renal lithiasis and urinary frequency
II. probenecid blocks the conversion of xanthine and hypoxanthine to uric acid
III. impending colchicine toxicity is heralded by abdominal pain, nausea, vomiting, and diarrhea

4. Pharmacologic properties of histamine include

I. constriction of capillaries
II. elevated blood pressure
III. increased gastric secretions

5. True statements concerning cimetidine and ranitidine include

I. they are useful in the treatment of duodenal ulcers
II. they may cause dizziness, mental confusion, and hepatic dysfunction
III. they are useful in the treatment of allergic reactions

6. The antihistaminic drug famotidine is classified as a

I. classic antihistamine
II. H_1-receptor antagonist
III. H_2-receptor antagonist

1-B
2-A
3-B
4-B
5-C
6-B

Directions: The group of items in this section consists of lettered options followed by a set of numbered items. For each item, select the **one** lettered option that is most closely associated with it. Each lettered option may be selected once, more than once, or not at all.

Questions 7–11

For each characteristic given below, select the drug that most appropriately corresponds to it.

(A) Acetaminophen
(B) Indomethacin
(C) Aspirin
(D) Diphenhydramine
(E) Ibuprofen

7. Hydrolyzed in the bloodstream
8. An active metabolite of another drug
9. Classified as a salicylate
10. Excretion somewhat increased in an acidified urine
11. Classified as an arylacetic acid

7-C
8-A
9-C
10-D
11-E

ANSWERS AND EXPLANATIONS

1. The answer is B *[III A 3].*
The association of Reye syndrome with the use of salicylates in febrile children with varicella or influenza-type viral infections warrants that a nonsalicylate antipyretic be used if needed in such circumstances.

2. The answer is A *[III B 2 b, 3, 4].*
Acetaminophen has a limited peripheral effect on prostaglandin synthesis and, therefore, lacks anti-inflammatory capability. Acetaminophen is a nonsalicylate alternative antipyretic, which may be used in children with varicella or influenza-type viral infections. Adverse effects include skin rash or other allergic reactions, and acute overdose is accompanied by severe liver damage.

3. The answer is B (III) *[III D 2 b, c, 4 a (2), b, c].*
Gastrointestinal upset, with adverse effects such as nausea, vomiting, and diarrhea, is associated with the early stages of colchicine toxicity. Probenecid inhibits the proximal tubular reabsorption of uric acid, while allopurinol inhibits the formation of uric acid from xanthine and hypoxanthine. Probenecid, not allopurinol, may cause renal lithiasis and urinary frequency.

4. The answer is B (III) *[II A 2 a].*
While gastric secretions are stimulated by histamine, the autacoid causes increased capillary permeability, capillary dilation, vasodilation, and hypotension.

5. The answer is C (I, II) *[II A 3, 4 d].*
Cimetidine and ranitidine are examples of H_2-receptor antagonists. They restrict H_2-mediated gastric secretions. They are ineffective in the treatment of allergic reactions since they are not H_1-receptor antagonists. Adverse effects that limit their duration of use include altered hepatic and renal function, as well as dizziness and confusion.

6. The answer is B (III) *[II A 1 b].*
The generic name famotidine more closely resembles those of the widely used H_2-receptor antagonists, cimetidine and ranitidine—all three have the common suffix -tidine. The generic names of most of the H_1-receptor antagonists end in the suffix -amine, such as diphenhydramine and chlorpheniramine. The H_1-receptor antagonists, which are much older drugs, now often are referred to as the classic antihistamines.

7–11. The answers are: 7-C *[III A 1 a],* **8-A** *[III B 1; Figure 14-8],* **9-C** *[III A 1 a; Figure 14-6],* **10-D** *[II A 1 c; Figure 14-2],* **11-E** *[III E 1; Figure 14-11].*
Esters, particularly simple esters, readily undergo in vivo hydrolysis both with and without the aid of catalytic enzymes. Amides also undergo hydrolysis but require the aid of catalytic enzymes. There are a number of specific and nonspecific esterases circulating in the bloodstream but few, if any, amidases. Aspirin (acetylsalicylic acid) is the phenolic acetyl ester of p-hydroxybenzoic acid (i.e., salicylic acid) and, thus, is classified as a salicylate. Aspirin is readily hydrolyzed in the bloodstream and is the only drug listed that contains an ester linkage.

Acetaminophen is a metabolite of phenacetin. Phenacetin (N-acetyl-p-ethoxyaniline) undergoes oxidative O-dealkylation in the body, forming N-acetyl-p-aminophenol (acetaminophen).

In order for its excretion to be increased in an acidic urine, a drug must be a weak base. Aspirin, indomethacin, and ibuprofen are all weak acids, as are the other nonsteroidal anti-inflammatory agents (NSAIDs). Acetaminophen is a neutral molecule. Diphenhydramine, as the generic name implies, has an amino group present in its molecule. As can be seen in its structure (see Figure 14-2*C*), it contains a tertiary amine. Amines are weak bases; thus, diphenhydramine would be more ionized in acidic media and less likely to undergo tubular reabsorption from the glomerular filtrate. It would, therefore, be more easily excreted in acidic urine.

The NSAIDs are all acids, which contributes to their ability to penetrate synovial fluids. The NSAIDs are often classified as arylacetic acids or heteroarylacetic acids. Ibuprofen does not contain any hetero atoms and, thus, is classified as an arylacetic acid. Indomethacin, an indene derivative, contains a nitrogen in the pyrrole ring and, thus, is a heteroarylacetic acid. Aspirin, although an acid, is a salicylic acid derivative. Diphenhydramine is a base, and acetaminophen is neutral.

15
Drugs Affecting the Cardiovascular System

David C. Kosegarten
Edward F. LaSala

I. INTRODUCTION.

Numerous categories of drugs affect the cardiovascular system. Certain drugs can treat heart failure (e.g., cardiac glycosides), relieve angina pectoris (e.g., antianginal agents), and control dysrhythmias (e.g., antiarrhythmic agents). Others can reduce hypertension (e.g., antihypertensives, including a variety of diuretics, β-blocking agents, arteriolar smooth muscle dilators), treat the hyperlipidemias (e.g., antihyperlipidemic agents), reduce clotting and treat such conditions as venous thrombosis and pulmonary embolism (e.g., anticoagulants), and treat anemias (e.g., antianemic agents).

II. CARDIAC GLYCOSIDES

A. Chemistry

1. Almost all the cardiac glycosides (also called **cardiotonics**) are naturally occurring steroidal glycosides obtained from plant sources. **Digitoxin** is obtained from *Digitalis purpurea*, **digoxin** from *Digitalis lanata*, and **ouabain** from *Strophanthus gratus*.
2. The digitalis-like agents are closely related structurally, consisting of one or more sugars (i.e, **glycone portion**) and a steroidal nucleus (i.e., **aglycone or genin portion**) bonded through an **ether (glycosidic) linkage.** These agents also have an **unsaturated lactone substituent (cyclic ester)** on the genin portion. The prototypical agent is **digitoxin** (Figure 15-1).
   - a. **Digoxin** (Lanoxin) has an additional hydroxyl group at position 12 (see Figure 15-1).
   - b. **Ouabain** has a rhamnose glycone portion and additional hydroxyl groups at positions 1, 5, 11, and 19 (see Figure 15-1).
3. Removal of the glycone portion causes decreased activity and increased toxicity from changes in polarity that cause erratic absorption from the gastrointestinal tract.
4. The **duration of action** of a cardiac glycoside is **indirectly proportional to the number of hydroxyl groups,** which increase polarity. Increased polarity results in decreased protein binding, liver biotransformation, and tubular reabsorption.
   - a. **Digitoxin** has a long duration of action and may act cumulatively.
   - b. **Ouabain,** in contrast, has an extremely short duration of action and is effective only when given intravenously.
5. The one non-naturally occurring glycoside is **amrinone,** a bipyridine derivative (Figure 15-2).

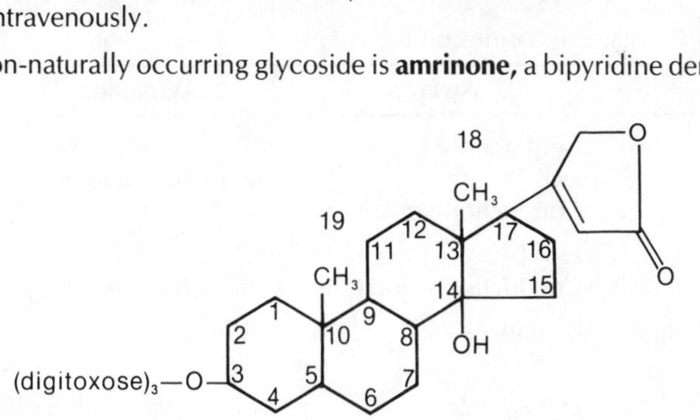

Figure 15-1. Structural formula of digitoxin (Crystodigin), the prototypical digitalis-like cardiac glycoside.

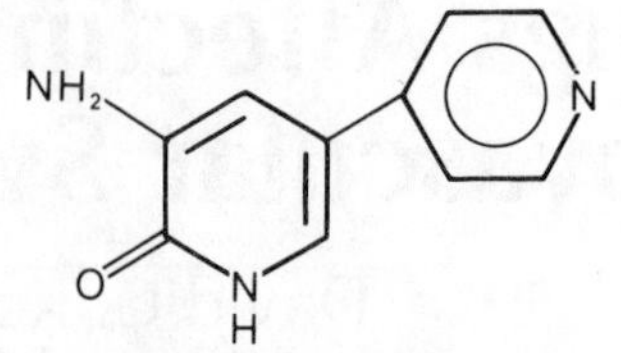

Figure 15-2. Structural formula of amrinone (Inocor), the bipyridine derivative cardiac glycoside.

B. Pharmacology. Cardiac glycosides increase myocardial contractility and efficiency, improve systemic circulation, improve renal perfusion, and reduce edema. They act through a variety of mechanisms (Table 15-1).

1. When given in therapeutic doses, cardiac glycosides have the following actions on the heart and its conduction system:
   - **a.** A positive inotropic effect (thought to involve either enhanced calcium entry into myocardial cells during depolarization or enhanced calcium release from intracellular sarcoplasmic reticulum binding sites)
   - **b.** An increase in systolic contraction velocity [probably initiated by inhibition of membrane-bound sodium (Na^+), potassium (K^+)–activated adenosinetriphosphatase]
   - **c.** An increase in the refractory period of the atrioventricular (AV) node
2. Therapeutic doses of cardiac glycosides also cause:
   - **a.** A negative chronotropic effect from increased vagal tone of the sinoatrial (SA) node
   - **b.** Diminished central nervous system (CNS) sympathetic outflow from increased carotid sinus baroreceptor sensitivity
   - **c.** Systemic arteriolar and venous constriction, which increases venous return and, thus, increases cardiac output

C. Therapeutic indications

1. Congestive heart failure
2. Atrial fibrillation
3. Atrial flutter
4. Paroxysmal atrial tachycardia

D. Adverse effects

1. **Early adverse effects** of cardiac glycosides represent the early stages of toxicity, including:
   - **a.** Gastrointestinal effects, such as anorexia, nausea, vomiting, and diarrhea
   - **b.** CNS effects, such as headache, visual disturbances (green or yellow vision), confusion, delirium, neuralgias, and muscle weakness
2. **Later adverse effects** represent intoxication and include such serious cardiac disturbances as premature ventricular contractions, paroxysmal and nonparoxysmal atrial tachycardia, AV dissociation or block, ventricular tachycardia, and ventricular fibrillation.

Table 15-1. Effects of Cardiac Glycosides on the Heart

	Atria	AV Node	Ventricles
Direct effects	Contractility ↑ ERP ↑ Conduction velocity ↓	ERP ↑ Conduction velocity ↓	Contractility ↑ ERP ↓ Automaticity ↑
Indirect effects	ERP ↓ Conduction velocity ↑	ERP ↑ Conduction velocity ↓	No effect
Effects on electrocardiogram	P changes	P-R interval ↑	Q-T ↓ ; T and ST depressed
Adverse effects	Extrasystole Tachycardia	AV depression or block	Fibrillation Extrasystole Tachycardia

AV = atrioventricular; ERP = Effective refractory period. Arrows indicate changes: ↑ = increased; ↓ = decreased.
Reprinted with permission from Jacob LS: *Pharmacology,* 3rd ed. Malvern, PA, Harwal, 1992, p 96.

III. ANTIANGINAL AGENTS AND PERIPHERAL VASODILATORS

A. Chemistry

1. **Antianginal agents** include **nitrites** (i.e., organic esters of nitrous acid), such as amyl nitrite; **nitrates** (i.e., organic esters of nitric acid), such as nitroglycerin and isosorbide; **β-blockers,** such as propranolol; and **calcium antagonists,** such as verapamil and nifedipine (Figure 15-3).
   a. **Amyl nitrite** is a very volatile and flammable liquid, administered by inhalation. It requires special precautions (especially restriction of smoking) during administration.
   b. **Nitroglycerin** is also a very volatile and flammable liquid and requires great care during storage. It must be dispensed from its original glass containers and protected from body heat.
      (1) When given intravenously, nitroglycerin requires the use of special plastic administration sets to avoid absorption and loss of potency.
      (2) Nitroglycerin is metabolically unstable and undergoes extensive first-pass metabolism.

2. **Peripheral vasodilators** include the dipiperidino-dipyrimidine dipyridamole (see Figure 15-3).

B. Pharmacology

1. **Nitrites and nitrates** are fast-acting antianginal agents that directly relax vascular smooth muscle. This causes peripheral pooling of the blood, diminished venous return (reduced preload), decreased systemic vascular resistance, and decreased arterial pressure (reduced afterload). These vascular effects:
   a. Reduce myocardial oxygen demand
   b. Cause redistribution of coronary blood flow along the collateral coronary arteries, improving perfusion of the ischemic myocardium

2. **β-Adrenergic blockers** decrease sympathetic-mediated myocardial stimulation (see Chapter 12 V A 2, C 3). The resulting negative inotropic and negative chronotropic effects reduce myocardial oxygen requirements.

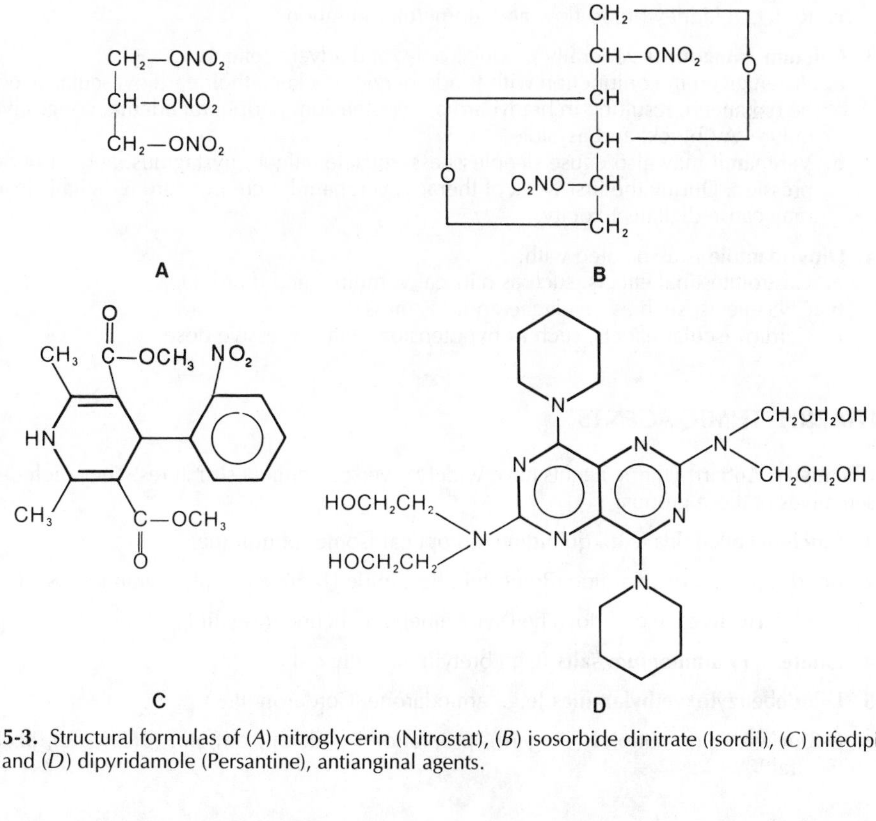

Figure 15-3. Structural formulas of (*A*) nitroglycerin (Nitrostat), (*B*) isosorbide dinitrate (Isordil), (*C*) nifedipine (Procardia), and (*D*) dipyridamole (Persantine), antianginal agents.

3. **Calcium antagonists** (also known as **calcium channel blockers**) block calcium entry through the membranous calcium ion (Ca^{2+}) channels of cardiac and vascular smooth muscle.
   a. Peripheral arterioles dilate and total peripheral resistance decreases, reducing afterload and reducing myocardial oxygen requirements.
   b. Calcium antagonists also increase oxygen delivery to the myocardium by dilating coronary arteries and arterioles.

4. **Dipyridamole** relaxes smooth muscles, decreasing coronary vascular resistance and increasing coronary blood flow.

C. Therapeutic indications

1. **Nitrites and nitrates** are used to relieve acute anginal attacks, as prophylaxis during anticipation of an acute anginal attack, and for long-term management of recurrent angina pectoris.

2. **β-Adrenergic blockers** are used for adjunctive prophylaxis of chronic stable angina pectoris in combination with nitrites or nitrates.

3. **Calcium antagonists** are used to treat chronic stable angina pectoris and variant (Prinzmetal's) angina.

4. **Dipyridamole** is used primarily for prophylaxis of angina pectoris, although its beneficial effects are not well understood.

D. Adverse effects

1. **Nitrites and nitrates** are associated with:
   a. CNS effects, such as headache, apprehension, dizziness, and weakness
   b. Cardiovascular effects, such as hypotension, tachycardia, palpitations, and syncope
   c. Skin effects, such as rash and dermatitis
   d. Methemoglobinemia

2. **β-Adrenergic blockers** are associated with:
   a. Worsening of congestive heart failure
   b. Bradycardia and hypotension
   c. Reduced kidney blood flow and glomerular filtration

3. **Calcium antagonists** generally produce only mild adverse effects.
   a. When given in conjunction with β-adrenergic blockers, their cardiovascular effects may be enhanced, resulting in bradycardia, hypotension, peripheral edema, congestive heart failure, AV block, and asystole.
   b. **Verapamil** may also cause sleeplessness, muscle fatigue, nystagmus, and emotional depression. During the first week of therapy, verapamil increases serum digitalis levels and may cause digitalis toxicity.

4. **Dipyridamole** is associated with:
   a. Gastrointestinal effects, such as nausea, vomiting, and diarrhea
   b. CNS effects, such as headache and dizziness
   c. Cardiovascular effects, such as hypotension (with excessive doses)

IV. ANTIARRHYTHMIC AGENTS

A. Chemistry. Antiarrhythmic agents have widely diverse chemical structures. They include representatives of these groups:

1. **Cinchona alkaloids** (e.g., quinidine, an optical isomer of quinine)

2. **Amides** [e.g., procainamide (Pronestyl), flecainide (Tambocor), disopyramide (Norpace)]

3. **Xylyl derivatives** [e.g., lidocaine (Xylocaine), mexiletine (Mexitil)]

4. **Quaternary ammonium salts** [e.g., bretylium (Bretylol)]

5. **Diiodobenzyloxyethylamines** [e.g., amiodarone (Cordarone)]

6. **β-Blockers** [e.g., nadolol (Corgard), propranolol (Inderal), esmolol (Brevibloc), acebutolol (Sectral)]

7. **Calcium antagonists** [e.g., diltiazem (Cardizem), verapamil (Calan)]
8. **Hydantoins** [e.g., phenytoin (Dilantin)]

B. Pharmacology. Antiarrhythmic agents are classified according to their ability to alter the action potential of cardiac cells (Tables 15-2 and 15-3).

1. **Class IA compounds** (e.g., quinidine, procainamide, disopyramide) slow the rate of rise of phase 0 (the phase of rapid depolarization and reversal of transmembrane voltage) and prolong repolarization.
2. **Class IB compounds** (e.g., lidocaine, tocainide, mexiletine, phenytoin) have a minimal effect on the rate of rise of phase 0 and shorten repolarization.
3. **Class IC compounds** (e.g., encainide, flecainide) have a marked effect in slowing the rate of rise of phase 0 and in slowing conduction. They have little effect on repolarization.
4. **Class II compounds** (e.g., propranolol, nadolol, esmolol, acebutolol) are β-adrenergic antagonists that competitively block catecholamine-induced stimulation of cardiac β-receptors and depress depolarization of phase 4.
5. **Class III compounds** (e.g., bretylium) prolong repolarization.
6. **Class IV compounds** (e.g., verapamil) are calcium antagonists that block the slow inward current carried by calcium during phase 2 (i.e., long-sustained depolarization or the plateau of the action potential) and increase the effective refractory period.

C. Therapeutic indications. Antiarrhythmic agents are used to reduce abnormalities of impulse generation (ectopic pacemaker automaticity) and to modify the disturbances of impulse conduction within cardiac tissue. (For indications for specific agents, see Table 15-4.)

D. Adverse effects

1. **Class IA compounds** are associated with cardiovascular effects, such as myocardial depression, AV block, ventricular dysrhythmias, asystole, and hypotension; and gastrointestinal effects, such as gastrointestinal upset, nausea, vomiting, and diarrhea. In addition:
   a. **Quinidine** may cause cinchonism, with tinnitus, confusion, photophobia, headache, and psychosis.
   b. **Procainamide** may cause systemic lupus erythematosus–like syndrome.
   c. **Disopyramide** may cause congestive heart failure and antimuscarinic effects.
2. **Class IB compounds** are associated with CNS effects, including CNS depression, drowsiness, disorientation, and paresthesias; cardiovascular effects, including hypotension and circulatory collapse; and hepatitis. In addition:
   a. **Lidocaine** may cause seizures and respiratory arrest.
   b. **Tocainide** may cause pneumonitis and blood dyscrasias.

Table 15-2. Major Effects of Antiarrhythmic Drugs on Electrocardiogram

Drug	QRS	Q-T	P-R*
Quinidine Procainamide Amiodarone	↑	↑	→↑
Disopyramide	↑	↑	→
Lidocaine Phenytoin Tocainide Mexiletine	→	↓	→↑↓
Propranolol	→	↓	→↑

Arrows indicate changes: ↑ = increased; ↓ = decreased; → = no change.

*P-R intervals: All antiarrhythmic drugs have a variable response, usually with little observable effect. However, lidocaine hardly ever affects the P-R interval, while phenytoin and propranolol usually increase the P-R interval.

Reprinted with permission from Jacob LS: *Pharmacology,* 3rd ed. Malvern, PA, Harwal, 1992, p 102.

Table 15-3. Effects of Antiarrhythmic Drugs on Electrophysiologic Properties of the Heart

	Automaticity		Effective Refractory Period		Membrane Responsiveness (Purkinje Fibers)
Drug	**Sinus Node**	**Purkinje Fibers**	**AV Node**	**Purkinje Fibers**	
Quinidine Procainamide Amiodarone Disopyramide	→	↓	↑→↓	↓	↓
Lidocaine Phenytoin Tocainide Mexiletine	→	↓	↑→↓	↓	↓
Propranolol	↓	↓	↑	↑	↓
Esmolol	↓	↓	↑	↑	↓
Acebutolol	↓	↓	↑	↑	↓
Bretylium	↑↓	↑↓	↓→↑	↑	→
Verapamil	↓	→↓	↑	→	→

AV = atrioventricular, arrows indicate changes: ↑ = increased; ↓ = decreased; → = no change.
Reprinted with permission from Jacob LS: *Pharmacology*, 3rd ed. Malvern, PA, Harwal, 1992, p. 101.

c. **Mexiletine** may cause hepatic injury and blood dyscrasias.
d. **Phenytoin** may cause nystagmus, decreased mental function, and blood dyscrasias.

3. **Class IC compounds** are associated with:
   a. Cardiovascular effects, including potentiation of arrhythmias in patients with ventricular arrhythmias, particularly patients with a history of myocardial infarction. They can potentiate sinus node dysfunction and aggravate heart failure.
   b. Visual disturbances, such as blurred or double vision

4. **Class II compounds** are associated with:
   a. Cardiovascular effects, such as hypotension, AV block, and asystole
   b. Respiratory effects, such as bronchospasm

5. **Class III compounds** are associated with:
   a. Cardiovascular effects, such as hypotension and initially increased dysrhythmias
   b. Gastrointestinal effects, such as nausea and vomiting

Table 15-4. Use of Antiarrhythmic Drugs in Common Cardiac Arrhythmias

Arrhythmia	Treatment of Choice	Alternatives
I. Supraventricular		
Atrial fibrillation or flutter	Digitalis to control ventricular rate, direct current (DC) shock for conversion	Quinidine to suppress recurrences after DC shock
Paroxysmal atrial or nodal tachycardia	Vagotonic maneuver; digitalis	Verapamil (quinidine, procainamide, disopyramide, and β-adrenergic antagonists may all be useful, especially prophylactically)
II. Ventricular		
Ventricular premature depolarization	Lidocaine	Procainamide, quinidine, or disopyramide for prolonged suppression
Ventricular tachycardia	DC shock	Lidocaine, procainamide, or mexiletine
III. Digitalis-induced	Lidocaine or phenytoin	Procainamide is somewhat useful; β-adrenergic antagonists are useful but have a high incidence of adverse effects

Reprinted with permission from Jacob LS: *Pharmacology*, 3rd ed. Malvern, PA, Harwal, 1992, p 102.

6. **Class IV compound verapamil** is associated with cardiovascular adverse effects, such as hypotension, bradycardia, AV block, congestive heart failure, and asystole.

V. ANTIHYPERTENSIVE AGENTS

A. Chemistry. Antihypertensive agents vary so widely in chemical structure that they are usually classified by mechanism of action rather than chemical class (Table 15-5).

B. Pharmacology. Antihypertensive agents lower blood pressure by reducing total peripheral resistance or cardiac output through a variety of mechanisms (see Table 15-5).

1. **Diuretics** (thiazides) create a negative sodium balance, reduce blood volume, and decrease vascular smooth muscle responsiveness to vasoconstrictors (see Chapter 16 IV).
2. **Vasodilators** (e.g., hydralazine) relax arteriolar smooth muscle, decreasing arterial resistance.
3. **Peripheral sympatholytics** interfere with adrenergic function by blocking postganglionic adrenergic receptors (e.g., propranolol, prazosin), limiting the release of neurotransmitters from adrenergic neurons (e.g., guanethidine) or depleting intraneuronal catecholamine storage sites (e.g., reserpine).
4. **Central α_2-sympathomimetics** (e.g., clonidine, methyldopa) appear to mediate their effects by stimulation of presynaptic α_2-inhibitory receptors, resulting in a negative sympathetic outflow and lowered peripheral resistance.
5. **Angiotensin-converting enzyme (ACE) inhibitors** (e.g., captopril) block the conversion of inactive angiotensin I to the potent vasoconstrictor angiotensin II. The reduced angiotensin II level also lowers aldosterone levels, which limits sodium retention.

C. Therapeutic indications

1. Antihypertensive agents are used separately or in combination to **treat high blood pressure.**

Table 15-5. Classification of Antihypertensive Agents by Their Mechanism of Action

Mechanism of Action	Drug	Chemical Class
Diuretic	Hydrochlorothiazide (Hydrodiuril)	Benzothiadiazide
Vasodilators		
Arteriolar	Diazoxide (Hyperstat IV)	Benzothiadiazide
	Hydralazine (Apresoline)	Phthalazine
	Minoxidil (Loniten)	Guanidine (cyclic)
Arteriolar and venous	Sodium nitroprusside (Nipride)	Nitroprusside
Peripheral sympatholytics	Atenolol (Tenormin)	β-blocker (selective)
	Guanadrel (Hylorel)	Guanidine (open-chain)
	Guanethidine (Ismelin)	Guanidine (open-chain)
	Labetalol (Trandate)	β-blocker (nonselective)
	Metoprolol (Lopressor)	β-blocker (selective)
	Nadolol (Corgard)	β-blocker (nonselective)
	Pindolol (Visken)	β-blocker (nonselective)
	Prazosin (Minipress)	Guanidine (cyclic)
	Propranolol (Inderal)	β-blocker (nonselective)
	Reserpine (Serpasil)	Rauwolfia alkaloid
Central α_2-sympathomimetics	Clonidine (Catapres)	Guanidine (cyclic)
	Guanabenz (Wytensin)	Guanidine (open-chain)
	Guanfacine (Tenex)	Guanidine (open-chain)
	Methyldopa (Aldomet)	Catecholaminoacid
Angiotensin-converting enzyme inhibitors	Captopril (Capoten)	Pyrrolidine
	Enalapril (Vasotec)	Pyrrolidine
	Lisinopril (Prinivil)	Pyrrolidine
	Ramipril (Altace)	Cyclopenta [b] pyrrole

2. These agents may also be administered parenterally to **treat hypertensive emergencies,** such as malignant hypertension, eclampsia, or the severe hypertension associated with excess catecholamines. Parenteral therapy may include some combination of these agents:
   a. **Arteriolar and venous vasodilator,** such as nitroprusside
   b. **Arteriolar vasodilator,** such as diazoxide or hydralazine
   c. **α-Adrenergic blocking agent** and **β-adrenergic blocking agent,** such as labetalol
   d. **β-Blocking agent,** such as propranolol
   e. **Ganglionic blocking agent,** such as trimethaphan

D. Adverse effects

1. **Diuretics (thiazides)** may cause:
   a. Fluid and electrolyte imbalances, such as hypokalemia, hypercalcemia, hyperuricemia, hypomagnesemia, hyponatremia, and hyperglycemia
   b. Increased serum low-density lipoprotein cholesterol and triglyceride levels
   c. Other effects (see Chapter 16 IV D)

2. **Vasodilators** are associated with:
   a. Gastrointestinal effects, such as gastrointestinal upset
   b. CNS effects, such as headache and dizziness
   c. Cardiovascular effects, such as tachycardia, fluid retention, and aggravation of angina
   d. Other effects, such as nasal congestion, hepatitis, glomerulonephritis, and systemic lupus erythematosus–like syndrome

3. **Peripheral sympatholytics** are associated with a variety of adverse effects, depending on the specific agent.
   a. **β-Blockers** (e.g., propranolol) are associated with:
      (1) Cardiovascular effects, such as bradycardia, congestive heart failure, and Raynaud's phenomenon
      (2) Gastrointestinal effects, such as gastrointestinal upset
      (3) Blood dyscrasias
      (4) CNS effects, such as depression, hallucinations, organic brain syndrome, and transient hearing loss.
      (5) Other effects, such as increased airway resistance, increased serum triglyceride levels, decreased high-density lipoprotein cholesterol levels, and psoriasis
      (6) Withdrawal syndrome if withdrawal is abrupt
   b. **Prazosin** is associated with:
      (1) Cardiovascular effects, such as sudden syncope with the first dose, palpitations, and fluid retention
      (2) CNS effects, such as headache, drowsiness, weakness, dizziness, and vertigo
      (3) Antimuscarinic effects and priapism
   c. **Guanethidine** is associated with:
      (1) Cardiovascular effects, such as bradycardia, orthostatic hypotension, and sodium and water retention
      (2) Diarrhea
      (3) Aggravation of bronchial asthma
   d. **Reserpine** is associated with:
      (1) CNS effects, such as nightmares, depression, and drowsiness
      (2) Cardiovascular effects, such as bradycardia
      (3) Gastrointestinal effects, such as gastrointestinal upset
      (4) Nasal stuffiness

4. **Central α_2-sympathomimetics** also have adverse effects that vary with the specific agent.
   a. **Clonidine** is associated with:
      (1) CNS effects, such as sedation and drowsiness
      (2) Dry mouth and severe rebound hypertension
      (3) Insomnia, headache, and cardiac dysrhythmias (with sudden withdrawal)
   b. **Methyldopa** is associated with:
      (1) Cardiovascular effects, such as orthostatic hypotension and bradycardia
      (2) CNS effects, such as sedation and fever
      (3) Gastrointestinal effects, such as colitis
      (4) Other effects, such as hepatitis, cirrhosis, Coombs-positive hemolytic anemia, and systemic lupus erythematosus–like syndrome

5. **Angiotensin converting enzyme inhibitors** are associated with:
   a. Cardiovascular effects, such as hypotension
   b. Hematologic effects, such as neutropenia and agranulocytosis
   c. Other effects, such as anorexia, polyuria, oliguria, acute renal failure, and cholestatic jaundice

VI. ANTIHYPERLIPIDEMIC AGENTS

A. Chemistry. Antihyperlipidemic agents vary in chemical structure and are usually classified by their site of action—locally in the intestine (nonabsorbable agents) or systemically (absorbable agents).

1. **Nonabsorbable agents** are **bile acid sequestrants**. These agents are hydrophilic, water-insoluble resins that bind to bile acids in the intestine. Examples include **cholestyramine chloride,** a basic anion-exchange resin consisting of trimethylbenzylammonium groups in a large copolymer of styrene and divinylbenzene, and **colestipol hydrochloride,** a copolymer of diethylpentamine and epichlorohydrin (Figure 15-4).

2. **Absorbable agents** include **nicotinic acid** (but not the structurally similar nicotinamide), the aryloxyisobutyric acid derivatives **clofibrate** (a prodrug ester) and **gemfibrozil,** the sulfur-containing bis-phenol **probucol,** the 3-hydroxy-3-methylglutaryl-coenzyme A (HMG-CoA) reductase inhibitor **lovastatin,** and the fatty fish oils containing large amounts of **eicosapentaenoic acid (EPA)** and **docosahexaenoic acid (DHA)** [Figure 15-5].

B. Pharmacology. Antihyperlipidemic agents help **reduce lipoprotein production** (e.g., lovastatin, clofibrate, gemfibrozil) or **increase the efficiency of lipoprotein removal** (e.g., cholestyramine, colestipol).

C. Therapeutic indications. These agents are used (in conjunction with appropriate diet and exercise) to reduce plasma lipoprotein levels.

D. Adverse effects

1. **Nonabsorbable agents** (e.g., cholestyramine, colestipol) are associated with gastrointestinal distress, including abdominal bloating, nausea, dyspepsia, steatorrhea, and constipation or diarrhea.

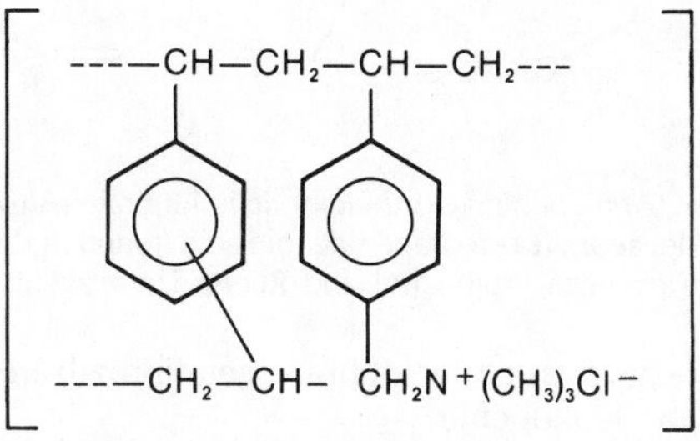

A

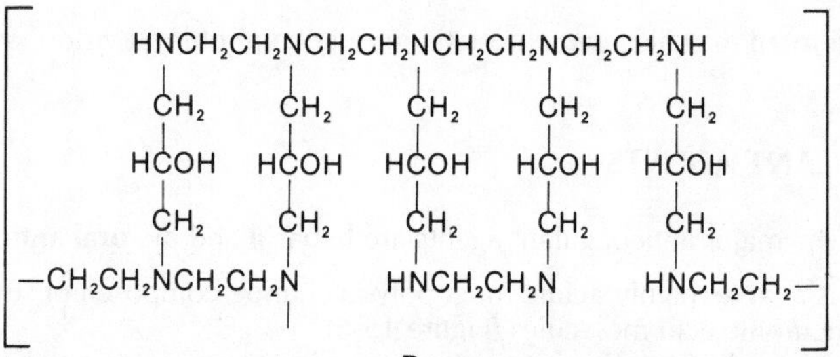

B

Figure 15-4. Structural formulas of (*A*) cholestyramine chloride (Questran) and (*B*) colestipol hydrochloride (Colestid), nonabsorbable antihyperlipidemic agents.

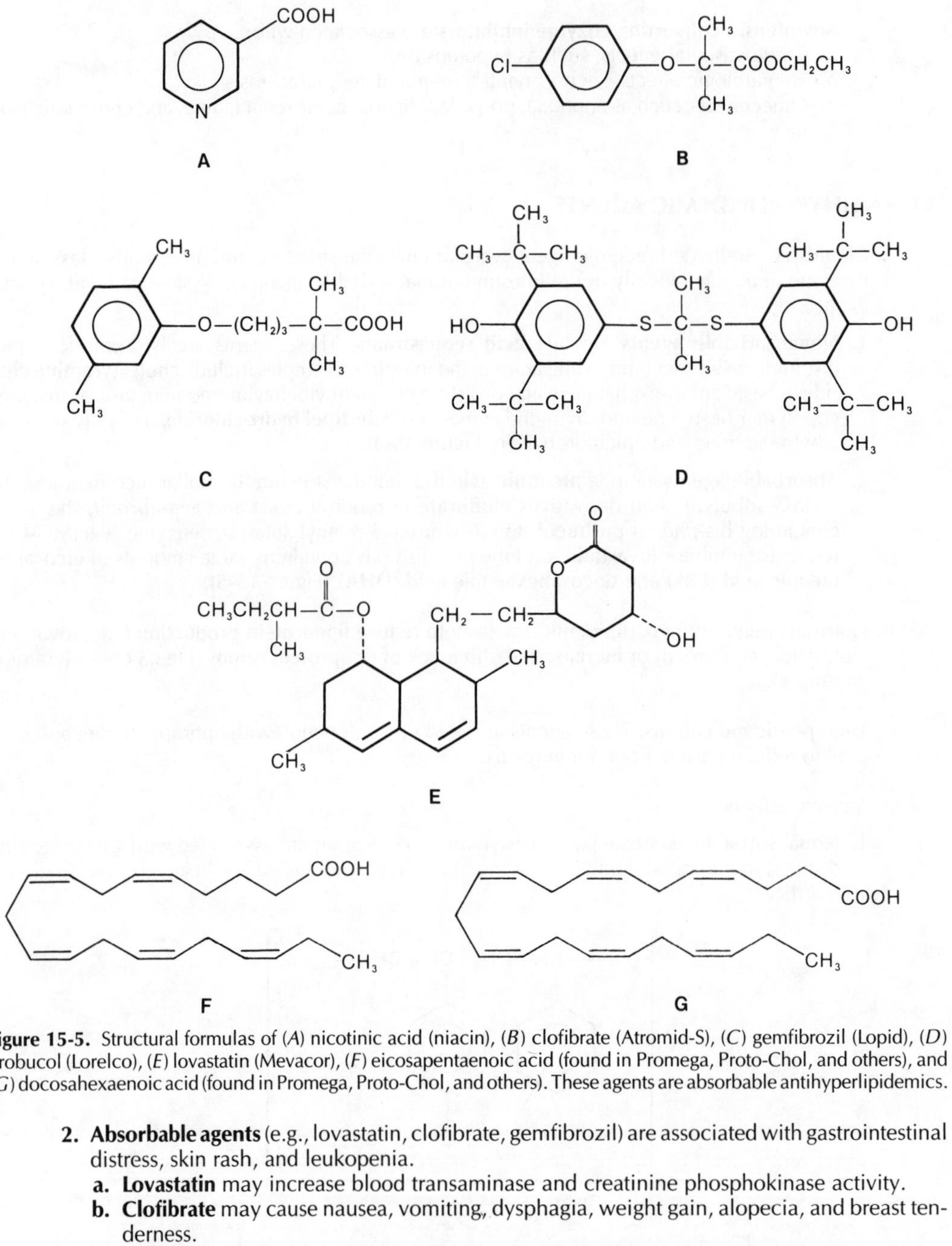

Figure 15-5. Structural formulas of (*A*) nicotinic acid (niacin), (*B*) clofibrate (Atromid-S), (*C*) gemfibrozil (Lopid), (*D*) probucol (Lorelco), (*E*) lovastatin (Mevacor), (*F*) eicosapentaenoic acid (found in Promega, Proto-Chol, and others), and (*G*) docosahexaenoic acid (found in Promega, Proto-Chol, and others). These agents are absorbable antihyperlipidemics.

2. **Absorbable agents** (e.g., lovastatin, clofibrate, gemfibrozil) are associated with gastrointestinal distress, skin rash, and leukopenia.
   a. **Lovastatin** may increase blood transaminase and creatinine phosphokinase activity.
   b. **Clofibrate** may cause nausea, vomiting, dysphagia, weight gain, alopecia, and breast tenderness.
   c. **Gemfibrozil** may also cause skeletal muscle pain, blurred vision, and anemia.

VII. ANTICOAGULANT AGENTS

A. Chemistry. The major anticoagulant agents are **heparin** and the **oral anticoagulants**.

1. **Heparin** is a large, highly acidic mucopolysaccharide composed of sulfated D-glucosamine and D-glucuronic acid molecules (Figure 15-6).
   a. Because it is highly acidic, it exists as an anion at physiologic pH and is very poorly absorbed from the gastrointestinal tract. Thus, it is usually administered parenterally as the sodium salt.

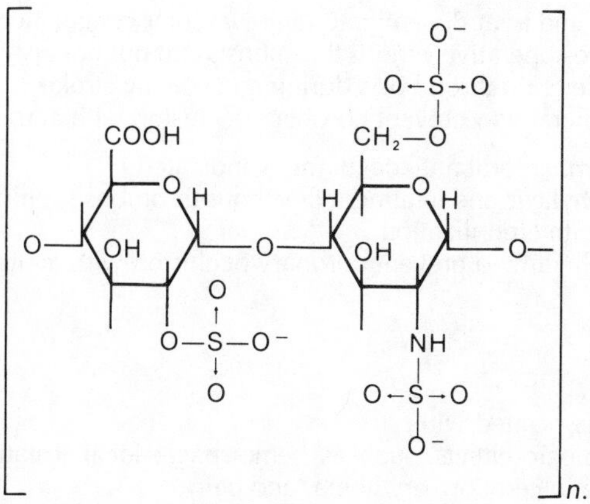

Figure 15-6. Structural formula of heparin, a mucopolysaccharide anticoagulant agent.

b. The action of heparin is quickly terminated by **protamine sulfate,** a highly basic protein that combines chemically with heparin in approximately equal amounts (mg:mg).

2. **Oral anticoagulants** consist of the highly effective **coumarin derivatives** and the relatively unimportant **indanedione derivatives.**

   a. The **coumarin derivatives** (e.g., **warfarin, dicumarol**) are water insoluble, weakly acidic 4-hydroxycoumarin lactones (Figure 15-7).

   (1) These agents are **chemically related to vitamin K,** and their mechanism of action is directly related to their antagonism of this vitamin.

   (2) These agents are also highly protein bound and extensively metabolized in the liver. These characteristics, in addition to their relatively narrow therapeutic index, make them very susceptible to significant drug interactions.

   b. Phenindione represents a typical **indanedione derivative** (Figure 15-8).

B. Pharmacology

1. **Heparin activates antithrombin III** (heparin cofactor), which, in turn, **inhibits the conversion of prothrombin to thrombin**. In combination with antithrombin III, heparin also **inactivates thrombin, inhibiting the conversion of fibrinogen to fibrin**. It **prolongs blood clotting time** both in vivo and in vitro.

2. **Oral anticoagulants interfere with the vitamin K–dependent hepatic synthesis of the active clotting factors** II (prothrombin), VII, IX, and X. These agents prolong blood clotting time in vivo only.

C. Therapeutic indications

1. **Heparin** is indicated:

   a. For the prophylaxis and treatment of venous thrombosis, pulmonary embolism, peripheral arterial embolism, and atrial fibrillation with embolization

   b. To prevent clotting during arterial surgery and cardiac surgery

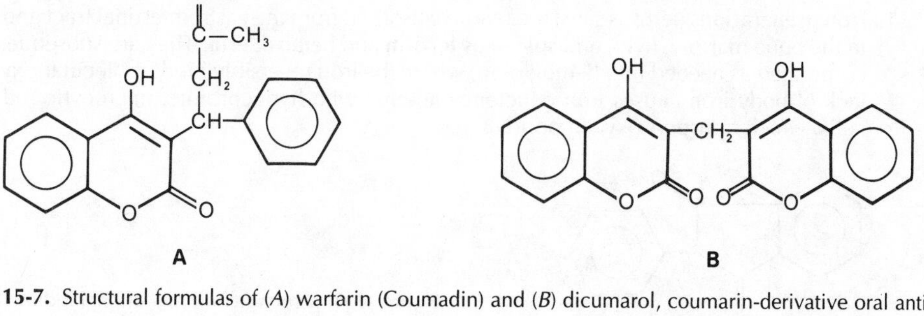

Figure 15-7. Structural formulas of (*A*) warfarin (Coumadin) and (*B*) dicumarol, coumarin-derivative oral anticoagulants.

c. To diagnose and treat disseminated intravascular coagulation (DIC)
d. To prevent postoperative venous thrombosis and pulmonary embolism (in low-dose form)
e. To prevent cerebral thrombosis during an evolving stroke
f. As adjunct therapy to prevent coronary occlusion with acute myocardial infarction

2. **Warfarin sodium,** an oral anticoagulant, is indicated:
a. For the prophylaxis and treatment of venous thrombosis, pulmonary embolism, and atrial fibrillation with embolization
b. As adjunct therapy to prevent coronary occlusion with acute myocardial infarction

D. Adverse effects

1. **Heparin**
a. Heparin is associated with:
(1) Hematologic effects, such as hemorrhage, local irritation, thrombocytopenia, hematoma, ulceration, erythema, and pain
(2) Other effects, such as hypersensitivity reactions, fever, chills, and urticaria
b. Severe adverse effects may be treated by administration of protamine sulfate, the specific antidote for heparin.

2. **Warfarin**
a. The oral anticoagulant warfarin sodium is associated with these adverse effects:
(1) Hemorrhage
(2) Anorexia, urticaria, purpura, and alopecia
b. Severe adverse effects may be treated by the administration of vitamin K (phytonadione), the specific antidote for warfarin sodium.

VIII. ANTIANEMIC AGENTS

A. Chemistry. The major antianemic agents are iron preparations, cyanocobalamin (vitamin B_{12}), and folic acid.

1. Most **iron preparations consist of ferrous salts,** which are absorbed from the gastrointestinal tract better than ferric salts or elemental iron.
a. Typical oral preparations include **ferrous sulfate** (e.g., Feosol), **ferrous gluconate** (e.g., Fergon), and **ferrous fumarate** (e.g., Feostat).
b. When parenteral administration is indicated, **iron dextran** (e.g., Imferon) may be used. This preparation consists of a complex of ferric hydroxide and low molecular weight dextrans, forming a colloidal solution.

2. **Cyanocobalamin** (vitamin B_{12}) is a nucleotide-like macromolecule with a modified porphyrin unit (a corrin ring) containing a trivalent cobalt atom. A cyanide ion is also coordinated to the cobalt atom, as is a benzimidazole group. The benzimidazole group is bonded to an α-ribosyl phosphate.

3. **Folic acid** consists of three major components: a pteridine nucleus bonded to the nitrogen of p-aminobenzoic acid, which is bonded through an amide linkage to glutamic acid (Figure 15-9).

B. Pharmacology

1. **Iron preparations** (ferrous salts) are readily absorbed from the gastrointestinal tract and stored in the bone marrow, liver, and spleen as **ferritin** and **hemosiderin**. They are subsequently incorporated as needed into hemoglobin, where the iron reversibly binds molecular oxygen. A lack of body iron causes iron deficiency anemia with hypochromic, microcytic red blood cells, which transport oxygen poorly.

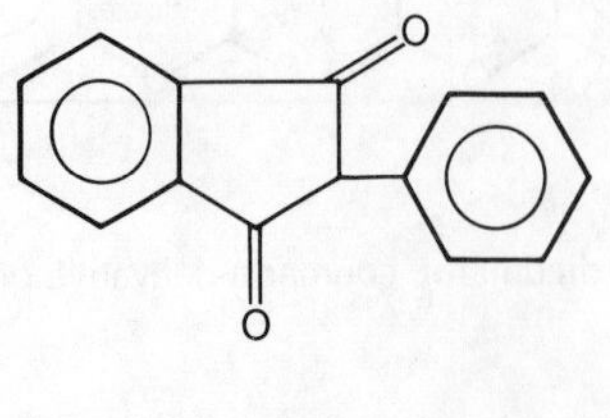

Figure 15-8. Structural formula of phenindione (Hedulin), an indanedione-derivative oral anticoagulant.

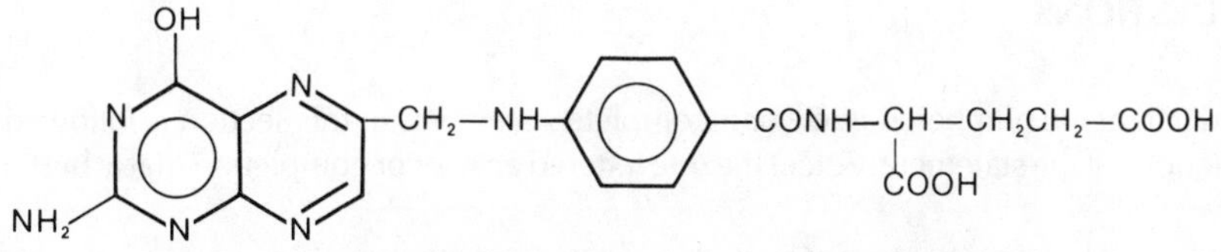

Figure 15-9. Structural formula of folic acid, an antianemic agent.

2. **Cyanocobalamin** is readily absorbed from the gastrointestinal tract in the presence of intrinsic factor (Castle's factor), a glycoprotein produced by gastric parietal cells, which is necessary for gastrointestinal absorption of cyanocobalamin.
   - **a.** Cyanocobalamin is transported to tissue by transcobalamin II. It is essential for cell growth, for maintenance of normal nerve cell myelin, and for the metabolic functions of folate.
   - **b.** Lack of dietary cyanocobalamin (or lack of intrinsic factor) causes a vitamin B_{12} deficiency and megaloblastic anemia with hyperchromic, macrocytic, immature red blood cells. Demyelination of nerve cells also occurs, causing irreversible CNS damage.
3. Folic acid is readily absorbed from the gastrointestinal tract, transported to tissue, and stored intracellularly. It is a precursor of several coenzymes (derivatives of tetrahydrofolic acid) that are involved in single carbon atom transfers. A lack of dietary folic acid causes folic acid deficiency and megaloblastic anemia with hyperchromic, macrocytic, immature red blood cells. However, folic acid deficiency causes no neurologic impairment.

C. Therapeutic indications

1. **Iron preparations** (ferrous salts) are used to treat iron deficiency anemia.
2. **Cyanocobalamin** is used to treat megaloblastic anemia resulting from vitamin B_{12} deficiency.
3. **Folic acid** is used to treat megaloblastic anemia resulting from folic acid deficiency.

D. Adverse effects

1. **Iron preparations** are associated with gastrointestinal effects, such as gastrointestinal distress, nausea, heartburn, diarrhea, and constipation.
2. **Cyanocobalamin** has only rare adverse effects.
3. **Folic acid** is associated only with rare allergic reactions after parenteral administration.

STUDY QUESTIONS

Directions: Each of the numbered items or incomplete statements in this section is followed by answers or by completions of the statement. Select the **one** lettered answer or completion that is **best** in each case.

1. Calcium channel blockers have all of the following characteristics EXCEPT

(A) they block the slow inward current carried by calcium during phase 2 of the cardiac action potential
(B) they dilate peripheral arterioles and reduce total peripheral resistance
(C) they constrict coronary arteries and arterioles and decrease oxygen delivery to the myocardium
(D) they are useful in treating stable angina pectoris and Prinzmetal's angina
(E) their adverse effects include aggravation of congestive heart failure

2. The termination of heparin activity by protamine sulfate is due to

(A) a chelating action
(B) the inhibition of gastrointestinal absorption of heparin
(C) the displacement of heparin–plasma protein binding
(D) an acid–base interaction
(E) the prothrombin-like activity of protamine

3. Which of the following cardiovascular agents is classified chemically as a glycoside?

(A) Nifedipine
(B) Digoxin
(C) Flecainide
(D) Cholestyramine
(E) Warfarin

4. Cardiac glycosides may be useful in treating all of the following conditions EXCEPT

(A) atrial flutter
(B) paroxysmal atrial tachycardia
(C) congestive heart failure
(D) ventricular tachycardia
(E) atrial fibrillation

5. Ingestion of which of the following vitamins should be avoided by a patient taking the oral anticoagulant?

(A) Vitamin A
(B) Vitamin B
(C) Vitamin D
(D) Vitamin E
(E) Vitamin K

1-C
2-D
3-B
4-D
5-E

Directions: Each item below contains three suggested answers of which **one or more** is correct. Choose the answer

A if **I only** is correct
B if **III only** is correct
C if **I and II** are correct
D if **II and III** are correct
E if **I, II, and III** are correct

6. In the oral treatment of iron deficiency anemias, iron is preferably administered as

I. ferrous iron
II. ferric salts
III. elemental iron

7. Parenterally administered antihypertensive agents used in the treatment of hypertensive emergencies include the

I. centrally acting antiadrenergic clonidine
II. arteriolar and venous vasodilator nitroprusside
III. ganglionic-blocking agent trimethaphan

8. Certain factors contribute to the longer duration of action of digitoxin when compared to that of digoxin. These include

I. greater protein binding
II. reduced polarity
III. greater tubular reabsorption

9. Correct statements concerning the properties of oral anticoagulants include

I. oral anticoagulants interfere with vitamin K–dependent synthesis of active clotting factors II, VII, IX, and X
II. adverse effects associated with oral anticoagulants are hemorrhage, urticaria, purpura, and alopecia
III. oral anticoagulants prolong the clotting time of blood both in vivo and in vitro

Directions: The group of items in this section consists of lettered options followed by a set of numbered items. For each item, select the **one** lettered option that is most closely associated with it. Each lettered option may be selected once, more than once, or not at all.

Questions 10–12

For each group of adverse effects, select the class of drug that most closely relates to it.

(A) Cardiac glycosides
(B) Calcium channel blockers
(C) Angiotensin-converting enzyme inhibitors
(D) β-Adrenergic blockers
(E) Nitrites and nitrates

10. Bradycardia, hypotension, increased airway resistance, and congestive heart failure

11. Visual disturbances (yellow or green vision), confusion, anorexia, vomiting, atrioventricular block, and ventricular tachycardia

12. Hypotension, acute renal failure, cholestatic jaundice, and agranulocytosis

---

6-A	9-C	12-C
7-D	10-D	
8-E	11-A	

ANSWERS AND EXPLANATIONS

1. The answer is C *[III B 3, C 3, D 3].*
Calcium channel blockers are used in the treatment of angina because they dilate coronary arteries and arterioles, thus decreasing coronary vascular resistance and increasing coronary blood flow.

2. The answer is D *[VII A 1, D 1 b; Figure 15-6].*
Heparin is a highly acidic mucopolysaccharide, whereas protamine is a highly basic protein. When administered subsequently to heparin, protamine chemically combines with it (presumably by an acid–base interaction) and inactivates its anticoagulant effect. Hence, it is an effective antidote for heparin. Caution must be employed in the use of protamine since an excess of protamine can cause an anticoagulant effect itself.

3. The answer is B *[II A 1].*
Most glycosides are natural products obtained from plant material. While there are very few medicinal agents that are glycosides, the group known as the cardiac glycosides are extremely important and are widely used in the treatment of congestive heart failure. Digoxin is a cardiac glycoside obtained from *Digitalis lanata*. Other cardiac glycosides include digitoxin, which is obtained from *Digitalis purpurea,* and ouabain, which is obtained from *Strophanthus gratus*.

4. The answer is D *[II C; Table 15-4].*
Ventricular tachycardia is produced by toxic cardiac glycoside dosage and would not be a therapeutic indication for the agents. Cardiac glycosides increase systolic contraction velocity and increase the refractory period of the atrioventricular (AV) node. They also have a positive inotropic effect.

5. The answer is E *[VII A 2 a (1), D 2].*
The oral anticoagulants such as warfarin act by inhibiting the liver biosynthesis of prothrombin, which is the precursor of the enzyme thrombin that catalyzes the conversion of soluble fibrinogen to the insoluble polymer fibrin, which results in clot formation. One of the principal factors in the biosynthesis of prothrombin is vitamin K, with which warfarin competes to inhibit this process. Since this is a reversible competition, vitamin K acts as an antagonist to the oral anticoagulants.

6. The answer is A (I) *[VIII A 1].*
Absorption of orally administered iron is significantly more complete with ferrous iron than with either ferric salts or elemental iron, presumably because of its better solubility characteristics. Iron preparations (ferrous salts) are more readily absorbed from the gastrointestinal tract and are stored in the bone marrow, liver, and spleen as ferritin and hemosiderin.

7. The answer is D (II, III) *[V B 4, C 2 a, e].*
Clonidine is not recognized as a drug of choice for hypertensive emergencies, possibly because of its central mechanism of action and the latent period required for its effect compared with other peripheral agents.

8. The answer is E (all) *[II A; Figure 15-1].*
Structurally, digitoxin has only one alcohol group on its steroidal nucleus, whereas digoxin has two. This slight difference in structure has a significant effect on the polarity of the molecule. Due to its greater liposolubility, digitoxin is more likely to undergo tubular reabsorption, to undergo enterohepatic cycling, to penetrate into the liver microsomes and undergo metabolism, and to be protein-bound, all of which contribute to its longer duration of action and potential cumulative effects.

9. The answer is C (I, II) *[VII A 2 a (1), D 2].*
Oral anticoagulants are only effective in vivo since they block hepatic synthesis of vitamin K–dependent coagulation factors (factors II, VII, IX, and X). This also explains the latency period associated with initiation of oral anticoagulant therapy.

10–12. The answers are: 10-D *[III D 2],* **11-A** *[II D],* **12-C** *[V D 5].*
Nonselective β-adrenergic blockers (e.g., propranolol) produce adverse effects associated with their mechanism of action on the autonomic nervous system. Thus, bronchospasm, lowering of blood pressure, and reduced heart rate result from blockade of autonomic β-adrenergic receptors. Visual disturbances (yellow or green vision) are peculiar to cardiac glycoside overdose. Atrioventricular (AV) dissociation and ventricular tachycardia are obviously more significant adverse effects. Angiotensin-converting enzyme inhibitors reportedly may cause blood dyscrasias in addition to cholestatic jaundice and acute renal failure.

16
Diuretics

David C. Kosegarten
Edward F. LaSala

I. INTRODUCTION. Diuretics increase the rate of urine formation, increasing urine volume and water and solute excretion. They fall into five major categories: osmotic diuretics, carbonic anhydrase inhibitors, benzothiadiazide diuretics, loop diuretics, and potassium-sparing diuretics.

II. OSMOTIC DIURETICS

A. Chemistry. Osmotic diuretics (e.g., mannitol, urea) are highly polar, water-soluble agents with a low renal threshold (Figure 16-1).

B. Pharmacology

1. Osmotic diuretics are relatively inert chemicals that are freely filtered at the glomerulus and poorly absorbed. By increasing the osmolarity of the glomerular filtrate, they **limit tubular reabsorption of water** and, thus, **promote diuresis**.
2. Because these agents increase water, sodium, chloride, and bicarbonate excretion, they cause an **increase in urinary pH**.

C. Therapeutic indications. Osmotic diuretics are used to:

1. Help prevent and treat oliguria and anuria
2. Reduce cerebral edema and decrease intracranial pressure
3. Reduce intraocular pressure

D. Adverse effects. Osmotic diuretics are associated with:

1. Headache and blurred vision
2. Increased blood volume (aggravates congestive heart failure)

III. CARBONIC ANHYDRASE INHIBITORS

A. Chemistry. Carbonic anhydrase inhibitors are aromatic or heterocyclic sulfonamides with a prominent thiadiazole nucleus. **Acetazolamide** is the prototypical agent (Figure 16-2).

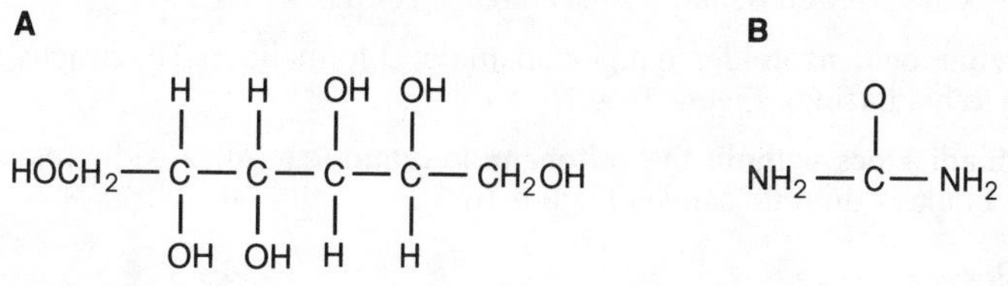

Figure 16-1. Structural formulas of (*A*) mannitol (Osmitrol) and (*B*) urea (Ureaphil), osmotic diuretics.

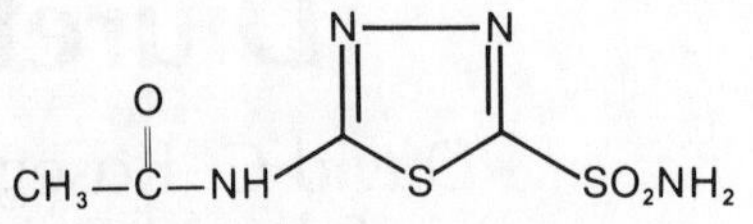

Figure 16-2. Structural formula of acetazolamide (Diamox), the prototypical carbonic anhydrase inhibitor.

B. Pharmacology

1. Carbonic anhydrase inhibitors **noncompetitively inhibit the enzyme carbonic anhydrase.** This prevents the enzyme from providing the tubular hydrogen ions needed for exchange with sodium, reducing sodium reabsorption in the proximal tubule and enhancing sodium's subsequent exchange with potassium in the distal tubule.

2. Because these agents increase water, sodium, potassium, and bicarbonate excretion, they cause an **alkaline urinary pH.**

C. Therapeutic indications. Carbonic anhydrase inhibitors are used:

1. To reduce edema (as adjunct diuretic therapy)
2. To reduce intraocular pressure (retard aqueous humor formation)
3. To alkalinize the urine, enhancing excretion of acidic drugs and their metabolites
4. As anticonvulsant agents in the treatment of petit mal epilepsy

D. Adverse effects. Carbonic anhydrase inhibitors are associated with:

1. Central nervous system (CNS) effects, such as CNS depression, drowsiness, sedation, fatigue, disorientation, and paresthesia
2. Gastrointestinal effects, such as gastrointestinal upset, nausea, vomiting, and constipation
3. Hematologic effects, such as bone marrow depression, thrombocytopenia, hemolytic anemia, leukopenia, and agranulocytosis
4. Hyperchloremic acidosis

IV. BENZOTHIADIAZIDE DIURETICS

A. Chemistry

1. The commonly used benzothiadiazide diuretics (**thiazides**) are primarily closely related **benzothiadiazines with variable substituents.** The prototypical agent is **chlorothiazide** (Figure 16-3; see Figure 16-3*A*).

2. Optimal diuretic activity depends on certain **structural features.**
   a. The benzene ring must have a **sulfonamide group** (preferably unsubstituted) in position 7 and a **halogen** (usually a chloro group) or a **trifluoromethyl group** in position 6 (see Figure 16-3).
   b. **Saturation of the 3,4-double bond** increases potency, as with hydrochlorothiazide (see Figure 16-3*B*).
   c. **Lipophilic substituents** at position 3 or **methyl groups** at position 2 enhance potency and prolong activity, as with cyclothiazide and bendroflumethiazide (see Figure 16-3*C*).
   d. **Replacement of the sulfonyl group** in position 1 by a **carbonyl group** results in prolonged activity, as with quinethazone (see Figure 16-3*D*).

3. A few **sulfamoylbenzamides** (e.g., indapamide, chlorthalidone) have activity similar to that of the benzothiadiazines (Figure 16-4).

4. **Benzothiadiazines without the sulfonamide group** (e.g., diazoxide) retain antihypertensive activity but lack diuretic activity (Figure 16-5).

B. Pharmacology

1. Benzothiadiazides **directly inhibit sodium and chloride reabsorption** at the proximal portion of the distal convoluted tubule.

2. These agents increase water, sodium, chloride, potassium, and bicarbonate excretion and decrease calcium excretion and uric acid secretion. They cause an **alkaline urinary pH.**

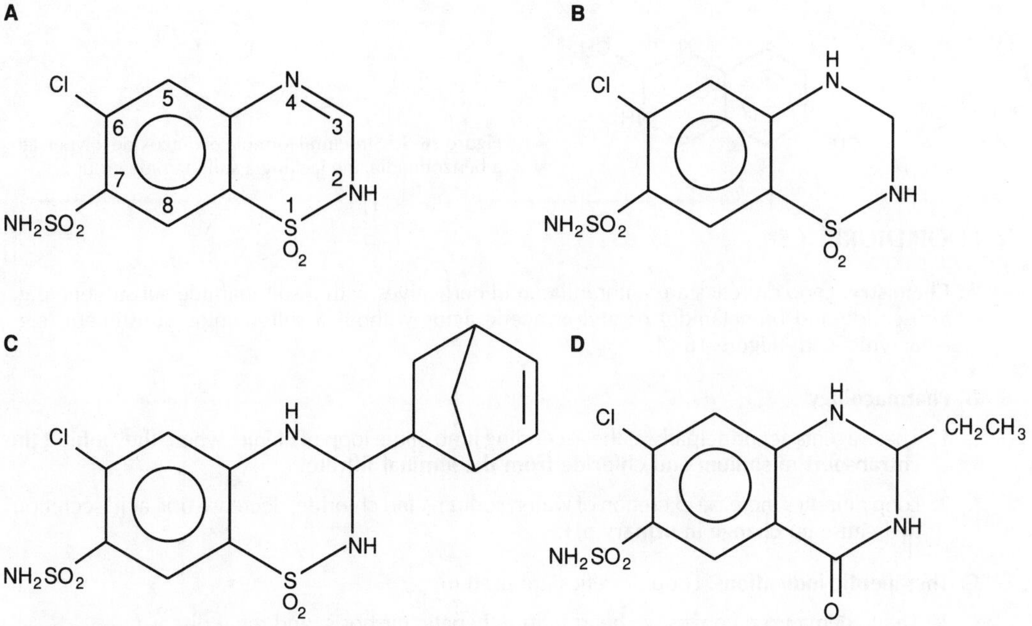

Figure 16-3. Structural formulas of (*A*) chlorothiazide (Diuril), the prototypical benzothiadiazide diuretic, and (*B*) hydrochlorothiazide (Hydrodiuril) as well as (*C*) cyclothiazide (Anhydron) and (*D*) quinethazone (Hydromox), related compounds with substituents that prolong activity and enhance potency.

C. Therapeutic indications. Benzothiadiazides are used to:

1. Treat chronic edema

2. Treat hypertension

3. Treat congestive heart failure (as adjunctive edema therapy)

D. Adverse effects. Benzothiadiazides are associated with:

1. CNS effects, such as headache, dizziness, paresthesias, drowsiness, and restlessness

2. Gastrointestinal effects, such as gastrointestinal irritation, nausea, vomiting, abdominal bloating, and constipation

3. Cardiovascular effects, such as orthostatic hypotension, palpitations, hemoconcentration, and venous thrombosis

4. Hematologic effects, such as blood dyscrasias, leukopenia, thrombocytopenia, agranulocytosis, aplastic anemia, hemolytic anemia, and rash

5. Fluid and electrolyte imbalances, such as hypokalemia, hypercalcemia, and hyperuricemia

6. Muscular cramps

7. Acute gout attacks

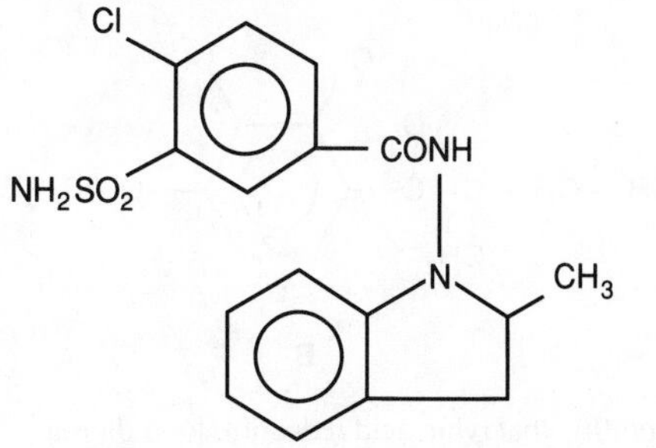

Figure 16-4. Structural formula of indapamide (Lozol), a sulfamoylbenzamide with pharmacologic activity similar to that of the benzothiadiazide diuretics.

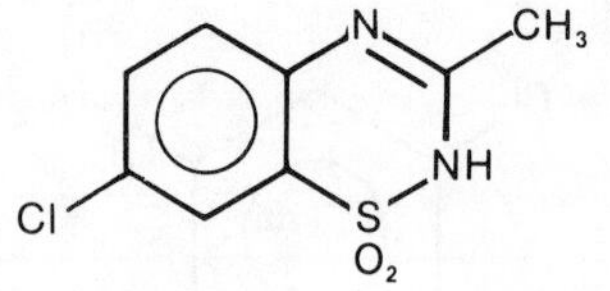

Figure 16-5. Structural formula of diazoxide (Hyperstat), a benzothiadiazine lacking a sulfonamide group.

V. LOOP DIURETICS

A. Chemistry. Loop diuretics are anthranilic acid derivatives with a sulfonamide substituent (e.g., furosemide and bumetanide) or aryloxyacetic acids without a sulfonamide substituent (e.g., ethacrynic acid) [Figure 16-6].

B. Pharmacology

1. These agents act principally at the ascending limb of the loop of Henle, where they **inhibit the cotransport of sodium and chloride from the luminal filtrate**.
2. Loop diuretics increase excretion of water, sodium, and chloride, decrease uric acid secretion, and cause **no change in urinary pH**.

C. Therapeutic indications. Loop diuretics are used to:

1. Treat edema from congestive heart failure, hepatic cirrhosis, and renal disease
2. Treat pulmonary edema and ascites

D. Adverse effects. Loop diuretics are associated with:

1. Fluid and electrolyte imbalances, such as hypokalemia, azotemia, dehydration, hyperuricemia, and hypercalciuria
2. CNS effects, such as headache, vertigo, blurred vision, tinnitus, and (rarely) irreversible hearing loss
3. Hematologic effects, such as thrombocytopenia and agranulocytosis
4. Cardiovascular effects, such as orthostatic hypotension
5. Gastrointestinal effects, such as nausea, vomiting, and diarrhea
6. Leg cramps

VI. POTASSIUM-SPARING DIURETICS

A. Chemistry. The potassium-sparing diuretics are pteridine or pyrazine derivatives (e.g., triamterene, amiloride) or steroid analogue antagonists of aldosterone (e.g., spironolactone) [Figure 16-7].

B. Pharmacology

1. **Spironolactone** acts as a **competitive inhibitor of aldosterone** at receptors in the distal tubule. It interferes with aldosterone-mediated sodium–potassium exchange, decreasing potassium secretion.

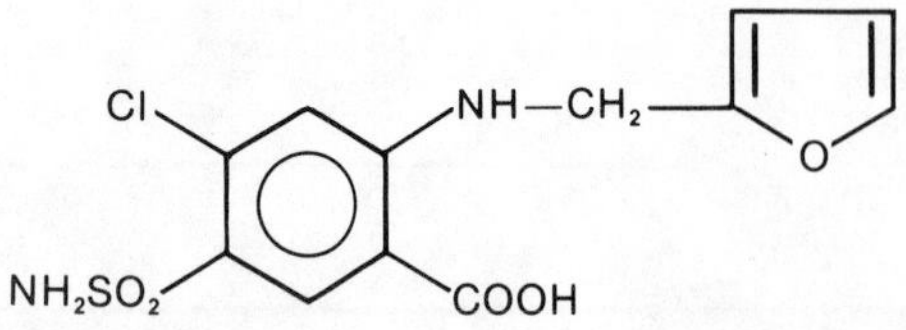

A

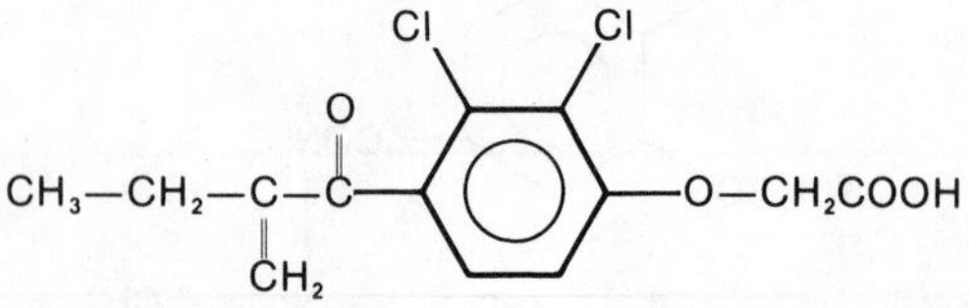

B

Figure 16-6. Structural formulas of (*A*) furosemide (Lasix) and (*B*) ethacrynic acid (Edecrin), loop diuretics.

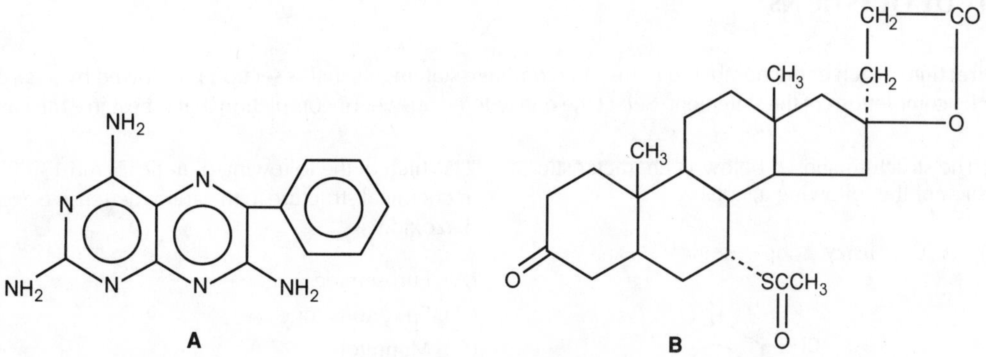

Figure 16-7. Structural formulas of (*A*) triamterene (Dyrenium) and (*B*) spironolactone (Aldactone), potassium-sparing diuretics.

2. **Triamterene,** which is not an aldosterone antagonist, **acts directly on the distal tubule** through an unknown mechanism. It interferes with sodium reabsorption and potassium transport, decreasing potassium secretion.

3. **Amiloride,** which also is not an aldosterone antagonist, appears to **inhibit sodium–potassium ATPase**. Thus, it inhibits active transport of sodium and potassium at the distal tubule, decreasing potassium secretion.

4. The potassium-sparing diuretics increase bicarbonate excretion and cause an **alkaline urinary pH**.

C. Therapeutic indications. Potassium-sparing diuretics are used:

1. As adjunctive therapy, to treat edema from congestive heart failure, hepatic cirrhosis, nephrotic syndrome, and hyperaldosteronism
2. As adjunctive therapy (with thiazides and loop diuretics), to treat hypertension
3. To treat or prevent hypokalemia

D. Adverse effects

1. **Spironolactone** is associated with:
   - **a.** Hyperkalemia
   - **b.** Gastrointestinal effects, such as gastrointestinal upset, nausea, abdominal cramps, and diarrhea
   - **c.** Endocrine effects, such as gynecomastia, menstrual irregularities, and hirsutism
   - **d.** CNS effects, such as mental confusion and lethargy

2. **Triamterene** and **amiloride** are associated with:
   - **a.** Hyperkalemia
   - **b.** Gastrointestinal effects, such as gastrointestinal upset, nausea, and vomiting
   - **c.** CNS effects, such as headache and dizziness
   - **d.** Increased uric acid levels in patients with gouty arthritis (with triamterene)
   - **e.** Methemoglobinemia in patients with alcoholic cirrhosis (with triamterene, which inhibits dihydrofolate reductase)

STUDY QUESTIONS

Directions: Each of the numbered items or incomplete statements in this section is followed by answers or by completions of the statement. Select the **one** lettered answer or completion that is **best** in each case.

1. The structure shown below is characteristic of which of the following agents?

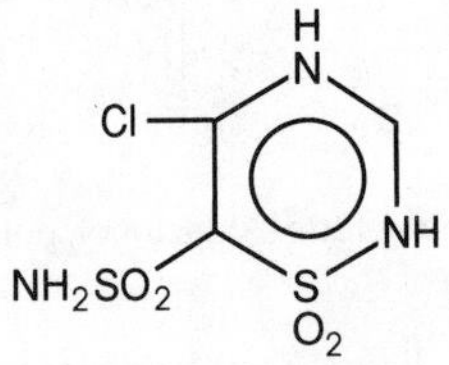

(A) Osmotic diuretics
(B) Carbonic anhydrase inhibitors
(C) Thiazides
(D) Loop diuretics
(E) Potassium-sparing diuretics

2. Which of the following diuretics is most similar in chemical structure to the antihypertensive agent diazoxide?

(A) Furosemide
(B) Spironolactone
(C) Mannitol
(D) Acetazolamide
(E) Chlorothiazide

Directions: The group of items in this section consists of lettered options followed by a set of numbered items. For each item, select the **one** lettered option that is most closely associated with it. Each lettered option may be selected once, more than once, or not at all.

Questions 3–5

For each statement listed below, select the drug that it most closely characterizes.

(A) Furosemide
(B) Hydrochlorothiazide
(C) Spironolactone
(D) Mannitol
(E) Acetazolamide

3. It interferes with distal tubular aldosterone-mediated sodium–potassium exchange, renders the urine alkaline, and may cause hyperkalemia, gynecomastia, and menstrual irregularities

4. Freely filtered, this drug limits tubular reabsorption of water and is useful in reducing cerebral edema and intracranial pressure

5. The principal site of action of this drug is on the thick ascending limb of Henle's loop; it is useful in treating pulmonary edema and ascites

---

1-C
2-E
3-C
4-D
5-A

ANSWERS AND EXPLANATIONS

1. The answer is C *[IV A; Figure 16-3].*
The structure can be recognized as a benzothiadiazine, which is known also as a thiazide. It represents the structure of hydrochlorothiazide, a sulfonamide diuretic. Other sulfonamide diuretics include the carbonic anhydrase inhibitors, such as acetazolamide, and the loop diuretics, such as furosemide. Neither of these subclasses contains drugs with a benzothiadiazine nucleus.

2. The answer is E *[IV A; Figures 16-3, 16-5].*
Diazoxide is a benzothiadiazine derivative; therefore, it would be most similar to chlorothiazide, which is also a benzothiadiazine. While both the thiazides and the diazoxides have antihypertensive activity, only the thiazides have significant diuretic activity. One of the structural requirements of the thiazide diuretics is an electron-withdrawing group, such as a halogen, ortho to the sulfonamide group on the benzene nucleus. The diazoxide molecule lacks such a group.

3–5. The answers are: 3-C *[VI B 1, D 1],* **4-D** *[II B 1, C 2],* **5-A** *[V B 1, C 1].*
Spironolactone interferes with aldosterone-mediated sodium–potassium exchange, reducing the amount of potassium excreted and is often used with other diuretics that promote the excretion of potassium, such as the benzothiadiazides. Mannitol increases the osmolarity of the glomerular filtrate since it is reabsorbed poorly. By increasing the osmolarity of the glomerular filtrate, mannitol limits tubular reabsorption of water, thus promoting diuresis. In this way, it reduces cerebral edema and decreases intracranial pressure. Furosemide is a diuretic of choice in the treatment of acute congestive heart failure because it promotes a significant rapid excretion of water and sodium.

17 Hormones and Related Drugs

David C. Kosegarten
Edward F. LaSala

I. INTRODUCTION. Hormones—substances secreted by specific tissues and transported to other specific tissues, where they exert their effects—may be classified pharmacologically as drugs. They may be obtained from **natural substances** (animal preparations), or they may be **synthetic or semi-synthetic compounds** resembling the natural products. They are often used for **replacement therapy** (e.g., exogenous insulin for treatment of diabetes mellitus). However, they can also be used for a variety of other therapeutic and diagnostic purposes. Certain drugs (e.g., thyroid hormone inhibitors and oral antidiabetic agents), while not hormones themselves, influence the synthesis or secretion of hormones. Therapeutically useful hormones and related drugs include the **pituitary hormones,** the **gonadal hormones,** the **adrenocorticosteroids,** the **thyroid hormones and inhibitors,** and the **antidiabetic agents**.

II. PITUITARY HORMONES

A. Chemistry. Pituitary hormones are divided into two groups by their site of secretion.

1. **Posterior pituitary hormones.** The two posterior pituitary hormones—**oxytocin** (Pitocin) and **vasopressin** (Pitressin)—are closely related octapeptides. They differ from each other in only two of their eight amino acids but have different biologic actions.

2. **Anterior pituitary hormones**
   a. **Protein molecules** are anterior pituitary hormones that are used therapeutically.
      (1) **Corticotropin** (Acthar)—commonly referred to as **adrenocorticotropic hormone,** or **ACTH**—is a single-chain polypeptide containing 39 amino acids. It has a molecular weight (mol wt) of 4600.
      (2) **Thyrotropin** (Thytropar)—commonly referred to as **thyroid-stimulating hormone (TSH)**—is a glycoprotein with a mol wt of 28,000.
      (3) **Thyrotropin-releasing hormone (TRH)** [Relefact]—commonly known as **protirelin**—is a tripeptide with a molecular weight of 363.
      (4) **Growth hormone** (Asellacrin)—commonly known as **somatotropin**—consists of 191 amino acids and has a mol wt of 21,500.
   b. **Pituitary gonadotropins** are anterior pituitary hormones that are not available for therapeutic use. These include **follicle-stimulating hormone (FSH), luteinizing hormone (LH),** and **prolactin** (commonly known as luteotropic hormone, or LTH). However, several related **nonpituitary gonadotropins** have FSH-like or LH-like actions and are used therapeutically, including:
      (1) **Menotropins** (Pergonal)—commonly known as **hMG** (human menopausal gonadotropin)—are high in FSH-like and LH-like activity and are obtained from the urine of postmenopausal women.
      (2) **Urofollitropin** (Metrodin) is high in FSH-like activity and is obtained from the urine of postmenopausal women.
      (3) **Human chorionic gonadotropin** (Follutein)—commonly known as **hCG**—has LH-like activity and is obtained from the urine of pregnant women.

B. Pharmacology. The therapeutically important pituitary hormones include the anterior pituitary agents **corticotropin, growth hormone** (somatotropin), and **menotropins** (gonadotropin), and the posterior pituitary agents **vasopressin** and **oxytocin**.

1. **Corticotropin** is secreted from the anterior pituitary, **stimulating the adrenal cortex to produce and secrete adrenocorticosteroids** (see IV).

2. **Growth hormone** stimulates protein, carbohydrate, and lipid metabolism to promote increased cell, organ, connective tissue, and skeletal growth, **causing a rapid increase in the overall rate of linear growth**.

3. **Menotropins produce ovarian follicular growth** and **induce ovulation** by means of FSH-like and LH-like actions.

4. **Vasopressin** has vasopressor and antidiuretic hormone (ADH) activity. It acts primarily on the distal renal tubular epithelium, where it **promotes the reabsorption of water**.

5. **Oxytocin stimulates uterine contraction** and plays an important role in the **induction of labor**.

C. Therapeutic indications

1. **Corticotropin** is used primarily for the diagnosis and differentiation of primary and secondary adrenal insufficiency.

2. **Growth hormone** is used for the long-term treatment of children whose growth failure is the result of lack of endogenous growth hormone secretion.

3. **Menotropins** are used to induce ovulation and pregnancy in anovulatory infertile women whose anovulation is not the result of primary ovarian failure. In men, menotropins are used to induce spermatogenesis.

4. **Vasopressin** is used to treat neurogenic diabetes insipidus and to treat postoperative abdominal distention.

5. **Oxytocin** is used to promote delivery by initiating and improving uterine contractions and to control postpartum bleeding or hemorrhage.

D. Adverse effects

1. **Corticotropin** is only rarely associated with adverse effects, which represent hypersensitivity reactions or corticosteroid excess.

2. **Growth hormone** is associated with adverse effects primarily related to the development of antibodies to growth hormone. The antibodies are nonbinding in most cases and do not interfere with continued growth hormone treatment.

3. **Menotropins** are associated with:
   - **a.** Hypersensitivity, arterial thromboembolism, febrile reactions, ovarian enlargement hyperstimulation syndrome, hemoperitoneum, and (rarely) birth defects in women
   - **b.** Gynecomastia in men

4. **Vasopressin** is associated with:
   - **a.** Gastrointestinal effects, such as abdominal cramps, flatulence, nausea, and vomiting
   - **b.** Central nervous system (CNS) effects, such as tremor, sweating, vertigo, and headache
   - **c.** Other effects, such as urticaria, bronchoconstriction, and anaphylaxis

5. **Oxytocin** is associated with:
   - **a.** Severe water intoxication with convulsions and coma, after slow (24-hour) infusion
   - **b.** Uterine hypertonicity, with spasm, tetanic contractions, or uterine rupture
   - **c.** Postpartum hemorrhage
   - **d.** Nausea, vomiting, and anaphylaxis
   - **e.** Fetal effects, such as bradycardia, neonatal jaundice, cardiac dysrhythmias, and premature ventricular contractions

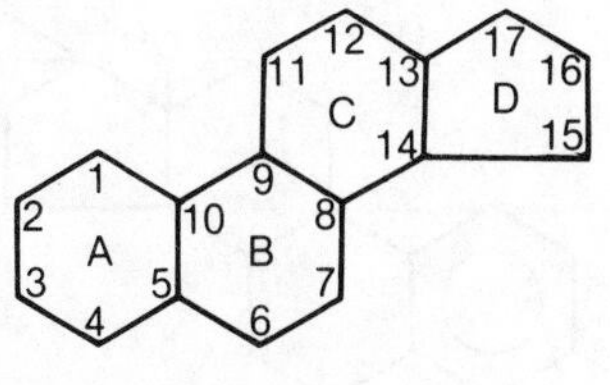

Figure 17-1. Structural formula of cyclopentanoperhydrophenanthrene, from which the gonadal hormones are derived. The letters *A* through *D* indicate the rings, which may be modified during subsequent conversions; the numbers *1* through *17* refer to carbon atom positions on the rings.

III. GONADAL HORMONES

A. Chemistry. Most natural and synthetic gonadal hormones are derivatives of **cyclopentanoperhydrophenanthrene** (Figure 17-1). All hormones having this fused reduced 17-carbon-atom ring system are classified as **steroids.**

1. **Natural estrogens.** The basic nucleus of the natural estrogens has a methyl group designated as C-18 on position C-13 of cyclopentanoperhydrophenanthrene. This basic nucleus is known as **estrane.**
   a. Unlike other steroid hormones, **all estrogens have an aromatic A ring** (see Figure 17-1).
   b. **Estradiol** (Estrace), the principal estrogenic hormone, exists in the body in equilibrium with **estrone**, which is converted to **estriol** prior to excretion (Figure 17-2).
      (1) Several **estradiol esters** [e.g., estradiol 17-cypionate (Depo-Estradiol) and estradiol 17-valerate (Delestrogen)] are prepared as intramuscular injections in oil, to prolong their action.
      (2) These estradiol esters are **slowly hydrolyzed in muscle tissues** before absorption and, thus, are considered to be prodrugs.
      (3) Addition of an α-ethynyl group (—C≡CH) at position C-17 of estradiol increases resistance to first-pass metabolism and enhances oral effectiveness. Two of these **estradiol derivatives, ethinyl estradiol** and its 3-methyl ether **mestranol,** are used principally as the estrogenic components of serial-type **oral contraceptives** (Figure 17-3). Another, **quinestrol** (Estrovis), is used principally for **estrogen replacement therapy.**
2. **Synthetic estrogens** (e.g., diethylstilbestrol, chlorotrianisene) are **nonsteroidal stilbene derivatives** that appear to assume an estradiol-like conformation in vivo (Figure 17-4). The **antiestrogens** clomiphene and tamoxifen citrate are **stilbene derivatives** that are structurally related to chlorotrianisene (Figure 17-5). However, these agents have different in vivo binding sites and activities.

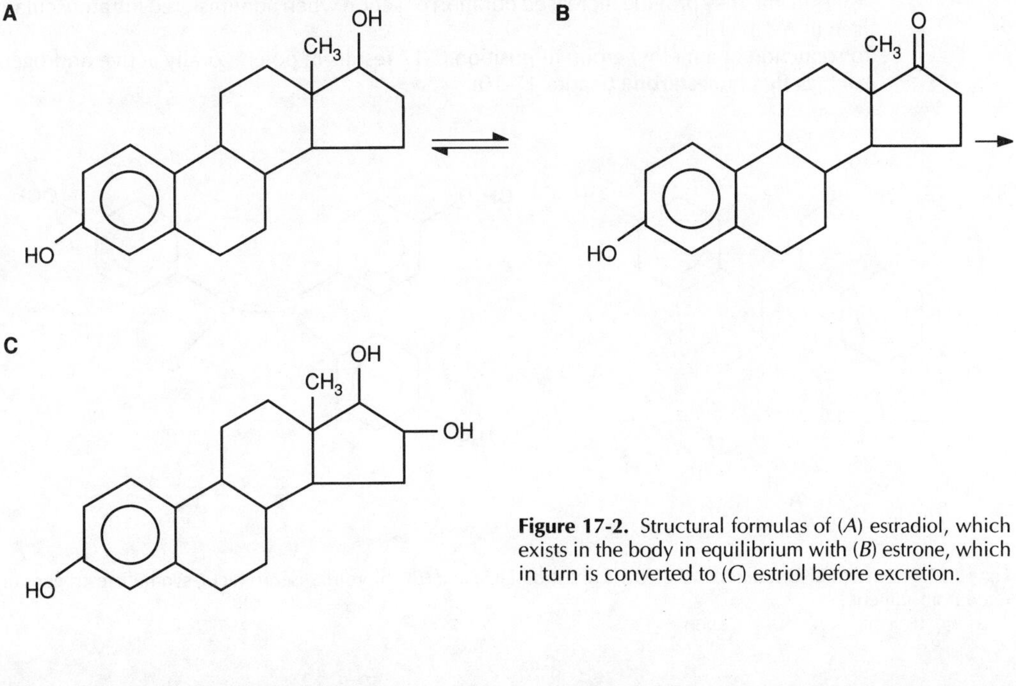

Figure 17-2. Structural formulas of (*A*) estradiol, which exists in the body in equilibrium with (*B*) estrone, which in turn is converted to (*C*) estriol before excretion.

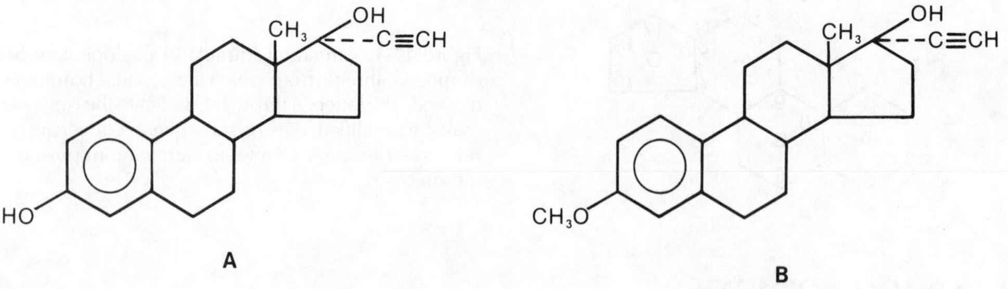

Figure 17-3. Structural formulas of (*A*) ethinyl estradiol and (*B*) mestranol, estradiol derivatives used principally as the estrogenic components of serial-type oral contraceptives.

3. **Progestins**
   a. The **naturally occurring progestin progesterone** is a C-21 steroid with a methyl group designated C-19 at position C-10 of estrane and a C-20–C-21 chain at position C-17 (see Figure 17-3). Its basic nucleus is known as **pregnane** (Figure 17-6).
   b. **Synthetic progestins,** which are also steroids, consist of two types.
      (1) The **progesterone derivatives** (e.g., medroxyprogesterone acetate, megestrol acetate) typically introduce a methyl group at position C-6 of progesterone and an acetoxy group at position C-17. These substitutions increase lipid solubility and decrease first-pass metabolism, **enhancing oral activity and the progestin effect** (Figure 17-7).
      (2) The **19-norprogestins** replace the C-19 methyl group of progesterone with a hydrogen; they also replace the C-17 acetyl group with a hydroxyl group and an ethynyl group. The prototypical agent of this type is **norethindrone** (Figure 17-8).
         (a) The 19-norprogestins are more liposoluble than progesterone and undergo less first-pass metabolism.
         (b) These agents have **potent oral activity** and are extensively used as **oral contraceptives.**
         (c) Other 19-norprogestins include the positional isomer of norethindrone, **norethynodrel,** its 18-methyl homologue **norgestrel,** and its 3,17-diacetate analogue **ethynodiol diacetate.**

4. The **primary natural androgen is testosterone,** a C-19 steroid structurally similar to progesterone (Figure 17-9). It differs from progesterone in having a hydroxyl group at position C-17, rather than a C-20–C-21 chain (see Figure 17-6).
   a. **Esters of testosterone,** such as testosterone 17-enanthate (Delatestryl), resemble estradiol esters in that they provide increased duration of action when administered intramuscularly [see III A 1 b (1)].
   b. Introduction of a methyl group at position C-17 results in potent, orally active androgens such as **fluoxymesterone** (Figure 17-10).

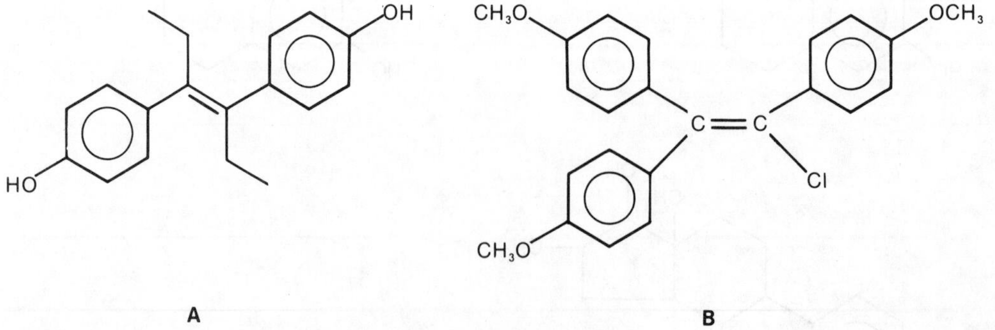

Figure 17-4. Structural formulas of (*A*) diethylstilbestrol (DES) and (*B*) chlorotrianisene (Tace), synthetic estrogens derived from stilbene.

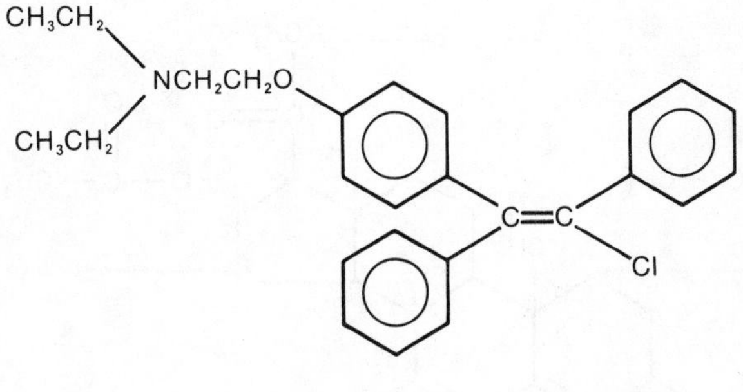

A

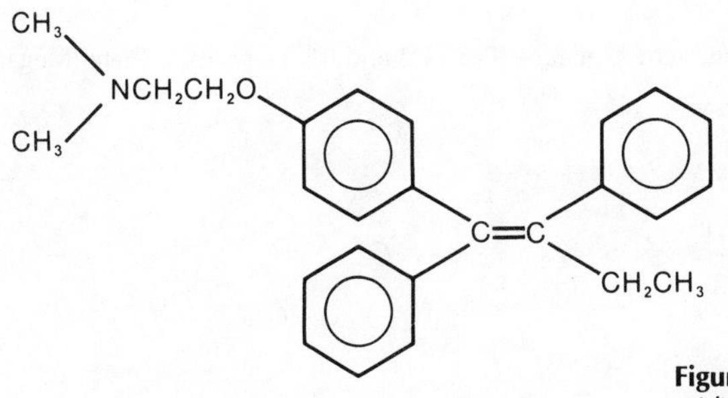

B

Figure 17-5. Structural formulas of (*A*) clomiphene (Clomid) and (*B*) tamoxifen (Nolvadex), antiestrogens that are structurally similar to chlorotrianisene.

c. Other structural modifications of testosterone result in drugs with a **much-enhanced anabolic-to-androgenic activity ratio** (e.g., oxandrolone, dromostanolone) [Figure 17-11]. Agents with 17-methyl groups are orally active.

B. Pharmacology. Gonadal hormones are steroids that require cytoplasmic receptors for transport to the nuclei of target-tissue cells, where they stimulate production of messenger and ribosomal ribonucleic acid (RNA). They also act in the feedback regulation of pituitary gonadotropins.

1. **Estrogens and progestins** mimic the activities of the female gonadal hormones (i.e., estradiol, progesterone), which initiate and control sexual development and maintain the integrity of the female reproductive system.
2. **Androgens** mimic the activity of the male gonadal hormone (testosterone), which initiates and controls sexual development and maintains the integrity of the male reproductive system.

C. Therapeutic indications

1. **Estrogens are used:**
   a. In oral contraceptives
   b. For replacement therapy, to treat menopause and female hypogonadism (Turner's syndrome)
   c. To treat prostatic carcinoma and breast carcinoma
2. **Progestins** are used:
   a. In oral contraceptives

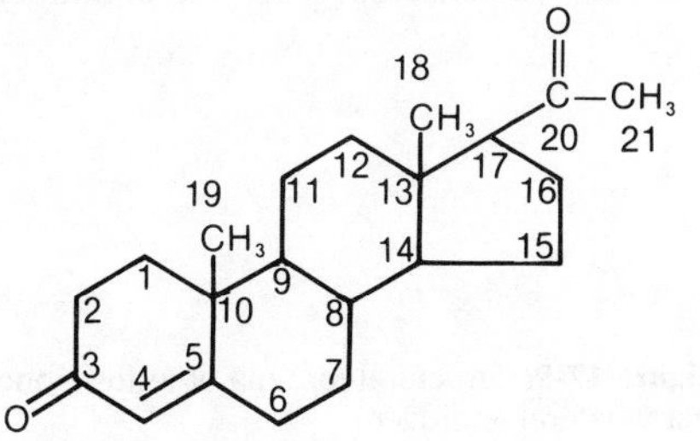

Figure 17-6. Structural formula of progesterone, which is a derivative of pregnane. The numbers *1* through *21* refer to carbon atom positions on the rings.

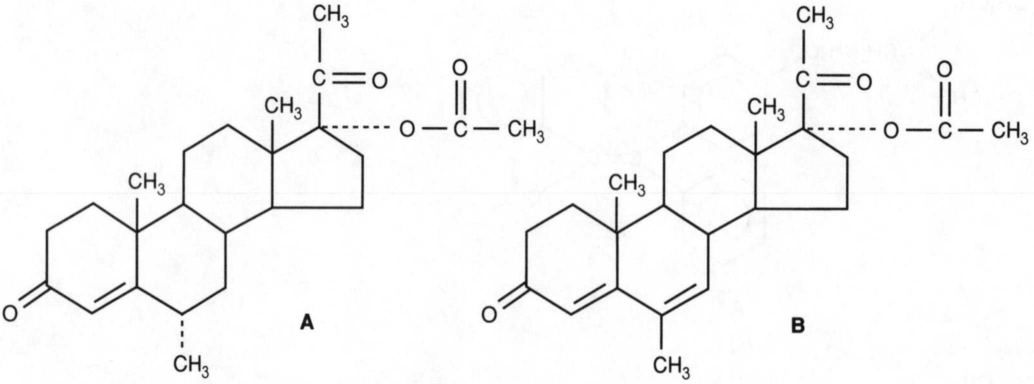

Figure 17-7. Structural formulas of (*A*) medroxyprogesterone acetate (Provera) and (*B*) megestrol acetate (Megace), synthetic progestins.

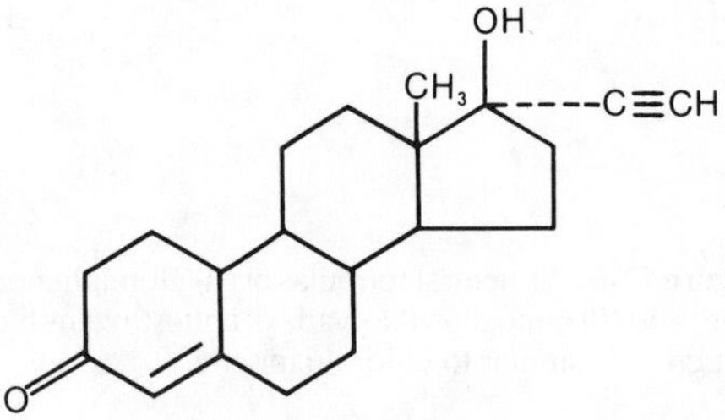

Figure 17-8. Structural formula of norethindrone, the prototypical 19-norprogestin.

b. To treat dysfunctional uterine bleeding
c. To treat endometriosis and dysmenorrhea
d. To treat endometrial carcinoma

3. **Androgens** are used to:
   a. Treat male hypogonadism
   b. Treat osteoporosis associated with hypogonadism
   c. Aid in the treatment of acute renal failure, by decreasing the rate of urea formation and, thus, decreasing the frequency of dialysis
   d. Stimulate erythropoiesis
   e. Treat hereditary angioneurotic edema

D. Adverse effects

1. **Estrogens** are associated with:
   a. Gastrointestinal effects, such as gastrointestinal distress, nausea, vomiting, anorexia, and diarrhea
   b. Cardiovascular effects, such as hypertension and an increased incidence of thromboembolic diseases, stroke, and myocardial infarction
   c. Fluid and electrolyte disturbances, such as increased fluid retention and increased triglyceride levels
   d. An increased incidence of endometrial cancer and hepatic adenomas (associated with long-term use)

2. **Progestins** are associated with:
   a. Gynecologic effects, such as irregular menses, breakthrough bleeding, and amenorrhea

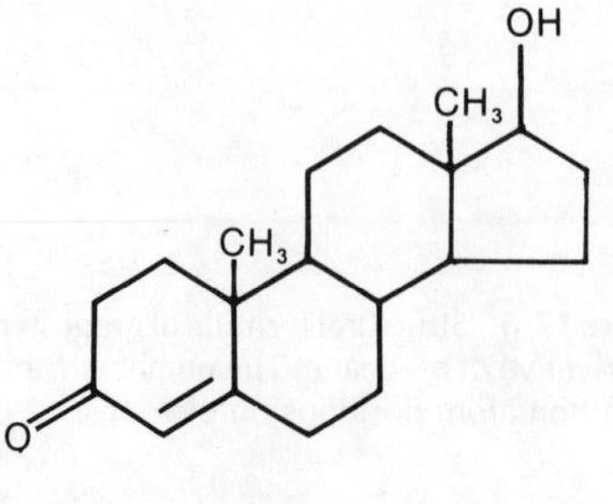

Figure 17-9. Structural formula of testosterone, the primary natural androgen.

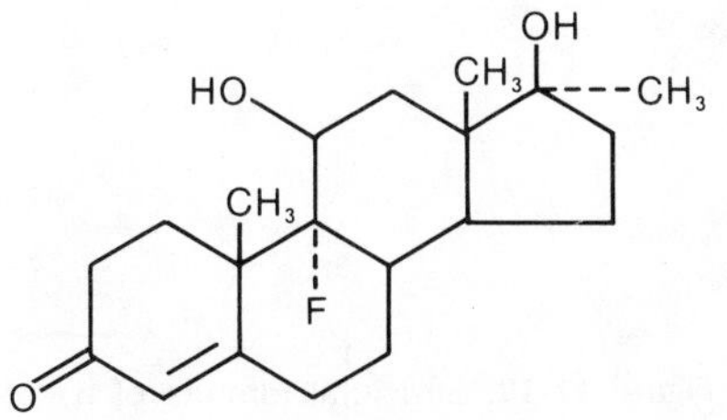

Figure 17-10. Structural formula of fluoxymesterone (Halotestin), a modified testosterone with potent androgenic activity.

b. Weight gain and edema
c. Exacerbation of breast carcinoma

3. **Androgens** are associated with:
   a. Hepatic effects, such as hepatic toxicity, jaundice, and hepatic adenocarcinoma
   b. Urogenital effects, such as prostatic enlargement, urinary retention, priapism, and azoospermia
   c. Edema
   d. Paradoxical gynecomastia

IV. ADRENOCORTICOSTEROIDS

A. **Chemistry.** The adrenal cortex synthesizes **nongonadal steroids** (adrenocorticosteroids), which may be classified as **mineralocorticoids,** possessing sodium-retaining and potassium-excreting effects, and **glucocorticoids,** possessing anti-inflammatory, protein-catabolic, and immunosuppressant effects. However, most naturally occurring adrenocorticosteroids have some degree of both mineralocorticoid and glucocorticoid activity. All adrenocorticosteroids are derived from the **C-21–pregnane steroidal nucleus.**

1. **Cortisone** and **hydrocortisone,** which are formed in the middle (fascicular) layer of the adrenal cortex (Figure 17-12), are the **prototypical glucocorticoids.**
   a. The 17 β-ketol side chain (—$COCH_2OH$), the 4-ene, and the 3-ketone structures are found in all clinically useful adrenocorticosteroids (see Figure 17-12).
   b. Many natural, semisynthetic, and synthetic glucocorticoids are available. **Modifications of the prototypes** cortisone and hydrocortisone **represent attempts to increase glucocorticoid activity while decreasing mineralocorticoid activity.**
      (1) The **oxygen atom** at position C-11 is essential for glucocorticoid activity.
      (2) A **double bond** between positions C-1 and C-2 increases glucocorticoid activity without increasing mineralocorticoid activity, as with **prednisolone** (Figure 17-13).
      (3) **Fluorination** at position C-9 greatly increases both mineralocorticoid and glucocorticoid activity, as with **fludrocortisone;** whereas fluorination at position C-6 increases glucocorticoid activity with less effect on mineralocorticoid activity, as with **fluprednisolone** (see Figure 17-13).
      (4) A **hydroxyl group** at position C-17 and a **hydroxyl group** (as with **triamcinolone**) or a **methyl group** (as with **dexamethasone**) at position C-16 enhance glucocorticoid activity and abolish mineralocorticoid activity (see Figure 17-13).
      (5) An **acetate ester** or a **16α, 17α-isopropylidenedioxy group** (also known as an **acetonide group**) at position C-21 enhances topical absorption, as with **fluocinonide** (see Figure 17-13).

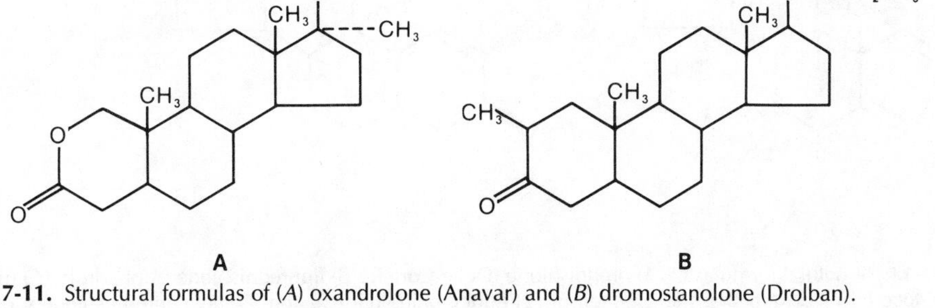

Figure 17-11. Structural formulas of (*A*) oxandrolone (Anavar) and (*B*) dromostanolone (Drolban).

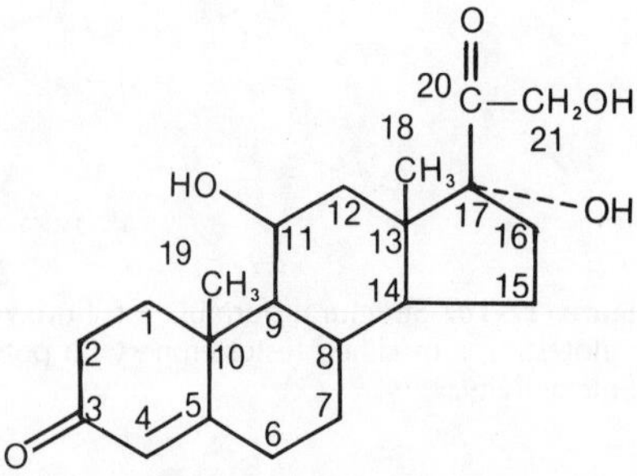

Figure 17-12. Structural formula of hydrocortisone, a prototypical glucocorticoid. The numbers *1* through *21* refer to carbon atom positions on the rings.

(6) **Sodium salts of 21-succinate or phosphate esters** result in water-soluble compounds, as with **methylprednisolone sodium succinate** and **betamethasone sodium phosphate** (see Figure 17-13).

2. **Aldosterone,** which is formed in the outer (glomerular) layer of the adrenal cortex, is the prototypical mineralocorticoid. The two clinically useful mineralocorticoids are **desoxycorticosterone acetate** and **fludrocortisone acetate** (Figure 17-14).

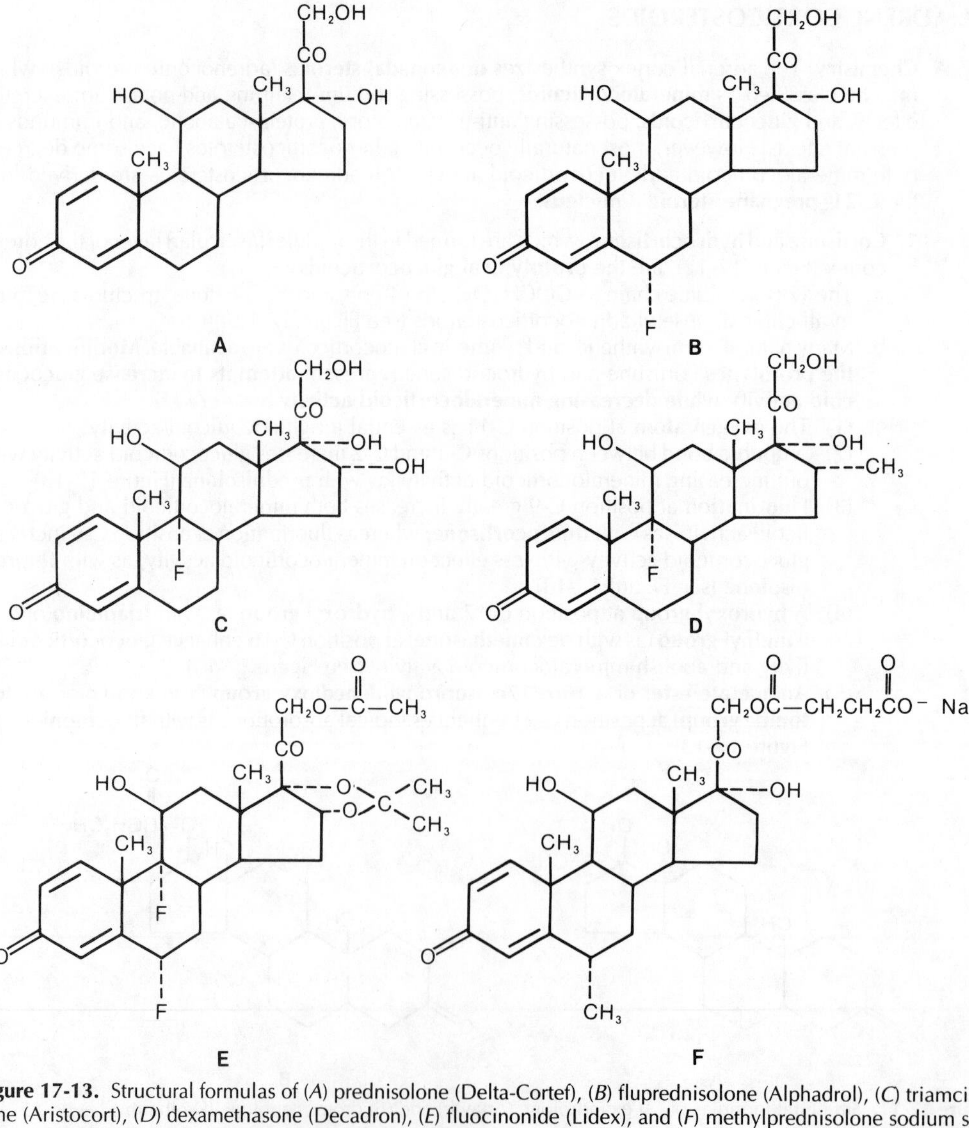

Figure 17-13. Structural formulas of (*A*) prednisolone (Delta-Cortef), (*B*) fluprednisolone (Alphadrol), (*C*) triamcinolone (Aristocort), (*D*) dexamethasone (Decadron), (*E*) fluocinonide (Lidex), and (*F*) methylprednisolone sodium succinate (Solu-Medrol), clinically important glucocorticoids.

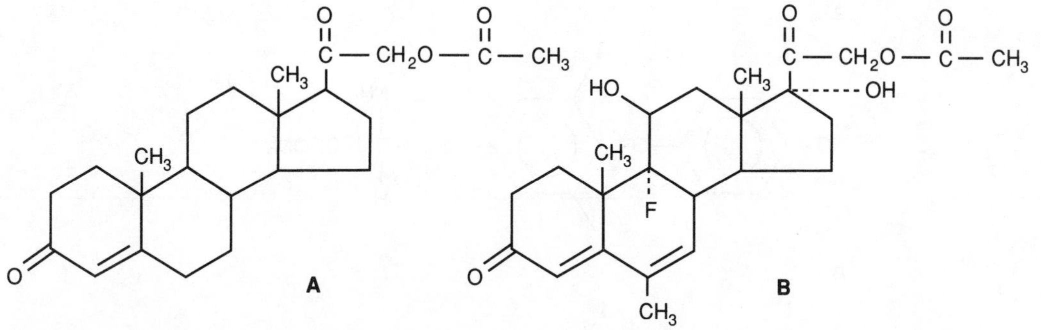

Figure 17-14. Structural formulas of (*A*) desoxycorticosterone acetate (Percorten Pivalate) and (*B*) fludrocortisone acetate (Florinef Acetate), the clinically useful mineralocorticoids.

B. Pharmacology

1. Therapeutically useful adrenocorticosteroids **mimic the activity of the natural glucocorticoids** and have **metabolic, anti-inflammatory,** and **immunosuppressive activity**.
2. Adrenocorticosteroids require cytoplasmic receptors for transportation to the nuclei of target tissue cells, where they **stimulate production of messenger and ribosomal RNA**. Adrenocorticosteroids also **act in the feedback regulation of pituitary corticotropin.**

C. Therapeutic indications. Adrenocorticosteroids are used:

1. As replacement therapy, to treat acute and chronic adrenal insufficiency
2. As the therapy of last resort, to treat severe, disabling arthritis
3. To treat severe allergic reactions
4. To treat chronic ulcerative colitis
5. To treat rheumatic carditis
6. To treat renal diseases, including nephrotic syndrome
7. To treat collagen vascular diseases
8. To treat cerebral edema
9. As topical agents, to treat skin disorders and inflammatory ocular disorders

D. Adverse effects. Adrenocorticosteroids are associated with:

1. Suppression of pituitary–adrenal integrity
2. Gastrointestinal effects, such as peptic ulcer, gastrointestinal hemorrhage, ulcerative esophagitis, and acute pancreatitis
3. CNS effects, such as headache, vertigo, increased intraocular and intracranial pressures, muscle weakness, and psychological disturbances (euphoria or dysphoria, depression, and suicidal tendencies)
4. Cardiovascular effects, such as edema and hypertension
5. Other effects, including weight gain, osteoporosis, hyperglycemia, flushed face and neck, acne, hirsutism, cushingoid "moon face" and "buffalo hump," and increased susceptibility to infection

V. THYROID HORMONES AND INHIBITORS

A. Chemistry

1. **Active thyroid hormones. Thyroxine (T_4)** and **triiodothyronine (T_3;** also known as **liothyronine**) are synthesized in the thyroid gland. Their precursor **thyroglobulin** (Proloid) is a large protein (mol wt about 650,000) obtained from partial purification of bovine or porcine thyroid gland extracts.
   a. The **sodium salts** of **T_3** and **T_4 are used therapeutically**. These agents contain aromatic rings and iodine, an essential component that must be obtained in the diet (Figure 17-15).
   b. A 4:1 mixture of T_4 and T_3, known as **liotrix** (Euthroid), is also employed therapeutically.

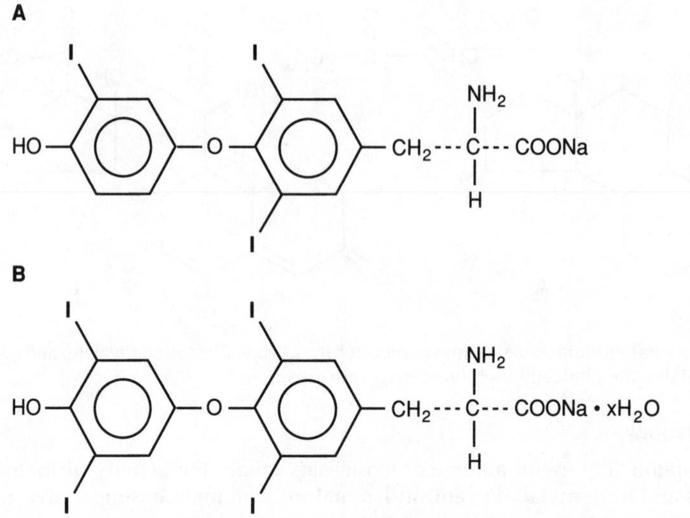

Figure 17-15. Structural formulas of (*A*) liothyronine (Cytomel) and (*B*) levothyroxine (Synthroid), clinically useful thyroid hormone preparations.

2. **Thyroid inhibitors** directly or indirectly interfere with the synthesis of thyroid hormones. These agents include the **iodides** (i.e., potassium salt, sodium salt), **radioactive iodine** (primarily sodium iodide 131(^{131}I)), and the **thioamides** (e.g., methimazole, propylthiouracil) [Figure 17-16].

B. Pharmacology

1. **Thyroid hormone preparations** mimic the activity of endogenous and thyroid hormones. These hormones regulate growth and development, have calorigenic and metabolic activity, and (through sensitization of β-adrenergic receptors) have positive inotropic and chronotropic effects on the myocardium. Thyroid hormones also act in the feedback regulation of pituitary thyrotropin.

2. **Thyroid inhibitors** act in various ways.
   a. **Iodides in high concentrations** acutely inhibit synthesis of iodotyrosine and iodothyronine. They also antagonize the effect of thyrotropin on endocytosis, proteolysis, and thyroid hormone secretion.
   b. **^{131}I** is rapidly trapped by the thyroid gland and incorporated into the colloid of the follicles. Its ionizing radiation, which is slowly released, is toxic to thyroid cells.
   c. **Thioamides** interrupt the synthesis of thyroid hormones by preventing iodine incorporation into the tyrosyl residues of thyroglobulin.

C. Therapeutic indications

1. **Thyroid hormone preparations** are used to treat myxedema, myxedema coma, hypothyroidism, simple goiter, and thyrotropin-dependent carcinoma.

2. **Thyroid inhibitors** are indicated for the treatment of hyperthyroidism.
   a. **High concentrations of iodide** (Lugol's solution) are used before thyroid surgery to make the thyroid gland firmer and reduce its size.

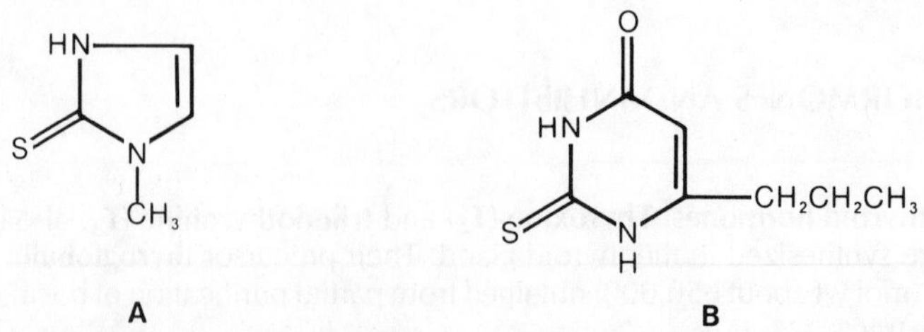

Figure 17-16. Structural formulas of (*A*) methimazole (Tapazole) and (*B*) propylthiouracil, thioamide thyroid hormone inhibitors.

b. **^{131}I** is especially useful to treat hyperthyroidism in older patients and in patients with heart disease.

c. **Thioamides** (e.g., methimazole, propylthiouracil) are used to treat hyperthyroidism—to control the disorder in mild cases, in conjunction with ^{131}I, or to prepare the patient before thyroid surgery.

D. Adverse effects

1. **Thyroid hormone preparations** are only rarely associated with adverse effects. Overdosage may cause palpitations, nervousness, insomnia, and weight loss.

2. **Thyroid inhibitors** are associated with adverse effects that depend on the agent used.

a. **Iodides** are associated with these adverse effects:

(1) Iodism, including increased salivation, brassy taste, sore teeth and gums, swollen eyelids, inflamed larynx and pharynx, frontal headache, skin lesions, and skin eruptions

(2) Hypersensitivity reactions, with fever, arthralgia, eosinophilia, and angioedema

b. **^{131}I** is associated with:

(1) Delayed hypothyroidism (relatively high incidence)

(2) Possible effects on the future offspring of young adults

c. **Thioamides** are associated with:

(1) CNS effects, such as drowsiness, headache, and paresthesias

(2) Gastrointestinal effects, such as gastrointestinal distress, nausea, and vomiting

(3) Hematologic effects, such as leukopenia, thrombocytopenia, and agranulocytosis

(4) Dermatologic effects, such as urticaria, rash, dermatitis, and alopecia

(5) Other effects, such as hepatitis, nephritis, jaundice, myalgia, arthralgia, edema, and systemic lupus erythematosus–like syndrome

VI. ANTIDIABETIC AGENTS

A. Chemistry. Antidiabetic agents include **insulin preparations** and **oral hypoglycemic agents.**

1. **Insulin** is an endocrine hormone secreted by the beta cells of the pancreas. It is composed of two polypeptide chains: an **A chain** of 21 amino acids and a **B chain** of 30 amino acids. Two **disulfide bonds** connect the A and B chains, and a third disulfide bond is found within the A chain.

a. **Source.** Insulin is available as **bovine insulin** (differs from human insulin by three amino acids), **porcine insulin** (differs from human insulin only in the terminal amino acid), and **human insulin.**

(1) **Single-species insulins** contain **only bovine** or **only porcine** insulin.

(2) **Mixed insulins** contain **both bovine and porcine** insulin.

(3) **Human insulins** are prepared either by enzymatic conversion of the terminal amino acid of porcine insulin (Novolin) or by means of recombinant DNA technology (Humulin).

(4) **Purified insulins** (also called single-peak insulins) are preparations containing less than 10 parts per million (ppm) of the insulin precursor proinsulin.

b. **Duration of action.** Insulins are classified by their duration of action as well as by their source and purity.

(1) **Short-acting insulins** include crystalline zinc insulin and semilente insulin.

(a) **Crystalline zinc insulin** (also called **regular insulin,** or **CZI**) is a soluble insulin prepared at neutral pH. It is the only type of insulin that can be mixed with all other insulins and also the only type forming a clear solution, which can be given intravenously.

(b) **Semilente insulin** is a finely divided, amorphous preparation also known as **prompt insulin zinc suspension**. The lente insulins [see VI A 1 b (2) (b), (3) (b)] contain no modifying protein and are prepared with an acetate buffer. **Lente insulins can be mixed with each other but cannot be mixed with either isophane insulin (NPH) or protamine zinc insulin (PZI).** Semilente insulin has a duration of action comparable to that of CZI.

(2) **Long-acting insulins** include PZI and ultralente insulin.

(a) **PZI** consists of insulin complexed with zinc and an excess of protamine in a phosphate buffer.

(b) **Ultralente insulin** is a large, crystalline form, also known as **extended insulin zinc suspension**. Its duration of action is comparable to that of PZI.

(3) **Intermediate-acting insulins** include NPH and lente insulin.

(a) **NPH** is similar to PZI but contains less protamine.

(b) **Lente insulin,** also known as **insulin zinc suspension,** is a mixture of 70% ultralente crystals and 30% semilente powder. Its duration of action is comparable to that of NPH.

2. **Oral hypoglycemic agents** are classified chemically as **sulfonylureas** and are derivatives of the phenylsulfonylurea nucleus. Therapeutically useful agents include **tolbutamide, chlorpropamide, tolazamide, acetohexamide, glyburide,** and **glipizide** (Table 17-1).

B. Pharmacology

1. **Insulin preparations** mimic the activity of endogenous insulin, which is required for the proper utilization of glucose in normal metabolism. Insulin interacts with a specific cell-surface receptor to facilitate the transport of glucose and amino acids.

2. **Oral hypoglycemic agents** stimulate insulin secretion from functioning pancreatic beta cells. These agents may also sensitize pancreatic beta cells to the insulin-releasing effects of glucose, and they may increase cell-surface receptors or increase the affinity of these receptors for insulin.

Table 17-1. General Structure of the Sulfonylurea Oral Hypoglycemic Agents

General Sulfonylurea Structure

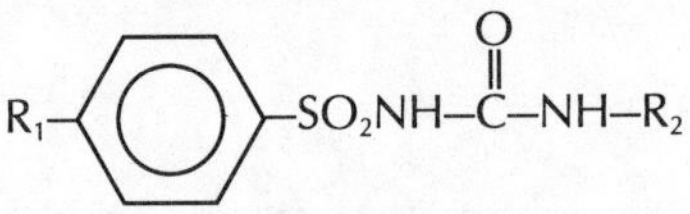

Drug	R_1-Substituent*	R_2-Substituent*
First-generation drugs		
Tolbutamide (Orinase)	CH_3–	$–CH_2CH_2CH_2CH_3$
Chlorpropamide (Diabinese)	Cl–	$–CH_2CH_2CH_3$
Tolazamide (Tolinase)	CH_3–	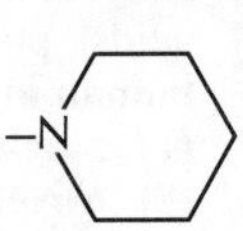
Acetohexamide (Dymelor)	CH_3CO–	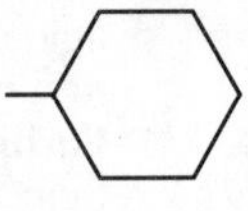
Second-generation drugs		
Glyburide (DiaBeta, Micronase)	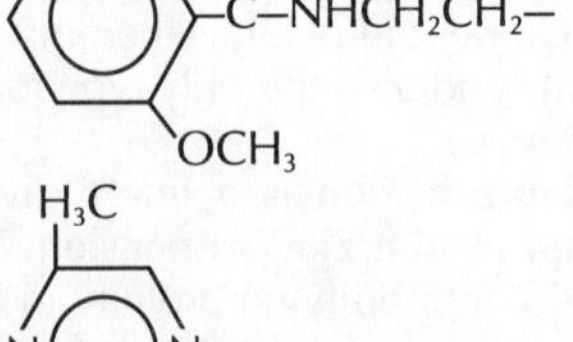	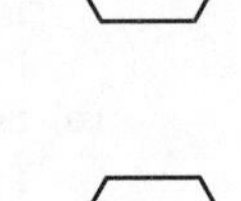
Glipizide (Glucotrol)	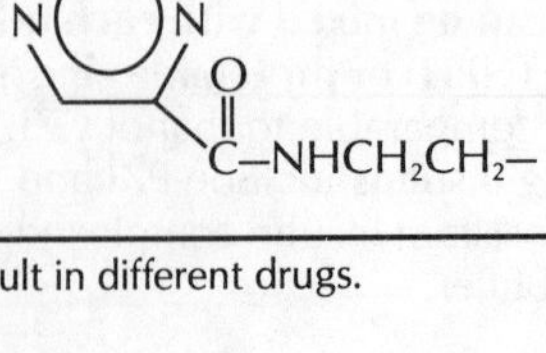	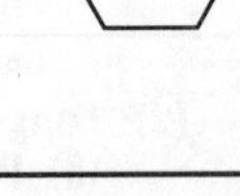

*Substituents at the positions marked R_1 and R_2 result in different drugs.

C. Therapeutic indications

1. **Insulin preparations** are used to treat diabetes mellitus that cannot be controlled by diet alone.

2. **Oral hypoglycemic agents** are used as an adjunct to diet—to **treat non-insulin–dependent diabetes mellitus** that cannot be controlled by diet alone.

D. Adverse effects

1. **Insulin preparations** are associated with these adverse effects:
   - **a.** Hypoglycemia, with sweating, tachycardia, and hunger; possibly progressing to insulin shock with hypoglycemic convulsions
   - **b.** Hypersensitivity reactions
   - **c.** Local irritation at the injection site

2. **Oral hypoglycemic agents** are associated with these adverse effects:
   - **a.** Hypoglycemia, particularly in patients with renal or hepatic insufficiency
   - **b.** Gastrointestinal effects, such as gastrointestinal disturbances, nausea, and vomiting
   - **c.** Blood dyscrasias, such as leukopenia, thrombocytopenia, agranulocytosis, and hemolytic anemia
   - **d.** Hypersensitivity reactions, with skin rash and photosensitivity
   - **e.** Cholestatic jaundice

STUDY QUESTIONS

Directions: Each of the numbered items or incomplete statements in this section is followed by answers or by completions of the statement. Select the **one** lettered answer or completion that is **best** in each case.

1. The following structure is a hormone. It would be classified best as

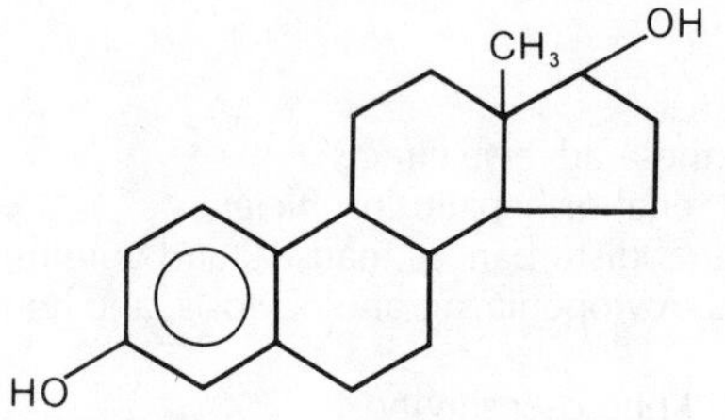

(A) an estrogen
(B) a progestin
(C) an androgen
(D) a gonadotropin
(E) an adrenocorticosteroid

2. All of the following substances are endogenous tropic hormones secreted by the pituitary gland EXCEPT

(A) somatotropin
(B) human chorionic gonadotropin (hCG)
(C) follicle-stimulating hormone (FSH)
(D) thyroid-stimulating hormone (TSH)
(E) corticotropin (ACTH)

3. Which of the following substances when present in urine is the most likely positive sign of pregnancy?

(A) Thyroid-stimulating hormone (TSH)
(B) Corticotropin (ACTH)
(C) Human chorionic gonadotropin (hCG)
(D) Interstitial cell-stimulating hormone (ICSH)
(E) Protamine zinc insulin (PZI)

4. All of the following hormonal drugs possess a steroidal nucleus EXCEPT

(A) ethinyl estradiol
(B) norethindrone
(C) liothyronine
(D) prednisolone
(E) fluoxymesterone

5. Which of the following glucocorticoids produces the least sodium retention?

(A) Cortisone
(B) Hydrocortisone
(C) Prednisolone
(D) Dexamethasone
(E) Fludrocortisone

6. Which of the following insulins can be administered intravenously?

(A) Regular insulin
(B) Isophane insulin (NPH)
(C) Protamine zinc insulin (PZI)
(D) Semilente insulin
(E) Ultralente insulin

1-A	4-C
2-B	5-D
3-C	6-A

Directions: Each question below contains three suggested answers of which **one or more** is correct. Choose the answer

A if **I only** is correct
B if **III only** is correct
C if **I and II** are correct
D if **II and III** are correct
E if **I, II, and III** are correct

7. Hormones that form lipophilic esters without prior structural modifications include

I. hydrocortisone
II. testosterone
III. progesterone

8. Water-soluble adrenocorticoid derivatives include

I. hydrocortisone acetate
II. fluocinonide
III. methylprednisolone sodium succinate

9. Insulin preparations that contain a modifying protein include

I. lente insulin
II. regular insulin
III. isophane insulin (NPH)

Directions: Each group of items in this section consists of lettered options followed by a set of numbered items. For each item, select the **one** lettered option that is most closely associated with it. Each lettered option may be selected once, more than once, or not at all.

Questions 10–12

For each pharmacologic property, select the hormone that most closely relates to it.

(A) Testosterone
(B) Insulin
(C) Corticotropin
(D) Estradiol
(E) Vasopressin

10. Secreted by pancreatic beta cells to facilitate glucose and amino acid transport for normal cellular metabolic processes

11. Initiates and controls male sexual development and maintains the integrity of the male reproductive system

12. Promotes the resorption of water at the renal distal convoluted tubule

Questions 13–15

For each adverse effect, select the class of drug that most closely relates to it.

(A) Antithyroid agents
(B) Sulfonylurea oral hypoglycemics
(C) Adrenocorticosteroids
(D) Progestins
(E) Androgens

13. Peptic ulceration and gastrointestinal hemorrhage; hyperglycemia, hypertension, and edema; "buffalo hump" and "moon face"; psychological disturbances; and increased susceptibility to infection

14. Agranulocytosis and other blood dyscrasias; cholestatic jaundice; nausea and vomiting; hypoglycemia; and photosensitivity

15. Hepatotoxicity and jaundice; urinary retention and azoospermia; prostatic hypertrophy and priapism; and paradoxical gynecomastia

7-C	10-B	13-C
8-B	11-A	14-B
9-B	12-E	15-E

ANSWERS AND EXPLANATIONS

1. The answer is A *[III A 1 a; Figure 17-2].*
Ring A is aromatic. Since the only type of steroidal hormone that has an aromatic A ring is an estrogen, this structure represents an estrogen. Other structural characteristics of estrogens include the fact that the structure contains 18 carbon atoms; thus, it is an estrane and contains a β-alcohol group in position 17.

2. The answer is B *[II A 2 a, b].*
Human chorionic gonadotropin (hCG) is produced by placental tissue and serves to stimulate the secretion of progesterone during pregnancy. Growth hormone (somatotropin), follicle-stimulating hormone (FSH), thyroid-stimulating hormone (TSH), and corticotropin (ACTH) are all secreted by the anterior pituitary gland.

3. The answer is C *[II A 2 b (3)].*
Human chorionic gonadotropin (hCG) is a proteinaceous tropic hormone that is secreted by chorionic (e.g., placental) tissue. Thus, hCG is present in the urine only after conception has occurred.

4. The answer is C *[V A 1; Figures 17-3, 17-8, 17-13, 17-15].*
Liothyronine is a thyroid hormone. Thyroid hormones consist of iodinated aromatic amino acids and are not steroidal in nature. Ethinyl estradiol is a steroidal estrogen, norethindrone is a steroidal 19-nor-progestin, prednisolone is an adrenocorticosteroid, and fluoxymesterone is a steroidal androgen.

5. The answer is D *[IV A 1 b (4); Figure 17-13].*
Glucocorticoids have varying degrees of mineralocorticoid activity. This mineralocorticoid activity, which can result in sodium and fluid retention, can be blocked by the introduction of a methyl or hydroxyl group in position 16 of the steroidal nucleus. Dexamethasone has a 16 α-methyl substituent.

6. The answer is A *[VI A 1 b].*
Most insulin preparations are suspensions; thus, they contain particulate matter. Only clear solutions may be administered intravenously. Regular insulin, which consists of water-soluble crystalline zinc insulin, is, therefore, suitable for intravenous administration. Insulin preparations normally are injected subcutaneously.

7. The answer is C (I, II) *[Figures 17-6, 17-12].*
Hydrocortisone has a 21-hydroxyl group, and testosterone has a 17-hydroxyl group; therefore, both of these agents can form esters (e.g., hydrocortisone acetate, testosterone propionate). Progesterone does not have any alcohol groups in its molecule; therefore, it cannot directly form any esters.

8. The answer is B (III) *[IV A 1 b (6); Figure 17-13].*
Methylprednisolone sodium succinate is the sodium salt of the succinate ester of methylprednisolone; thus, it is water-soluble. Hydrocortisone acetate is an ester, and fluocinonide is an acetonide; neither of which is water-soluble.

9. The answer is B (III) *[VI A 1 b].*
Regular insulin, which is a rapid-acting insulin preparation, contains only zinc insulin crystals. All lente insulins are free of modifying proteins, which contributes to their hypoallergenic properties. Isophane insulin is NPH insulin, which contains protamine, a strongly basic protein. The protamine reduces the water solubility of zinc insulin and lengthens its duration of action. Isophane insulin is classified as an intermediate-acting insulin preparation, having a duration of action of about 24 hours.

10–12. The answers are: 10-B *[VI B 1, 2],* **11-A** *[III B 2],* **12-E** *[II B 4].*
Insulin is required for the proper utilization of glucose and the transport of glucose and amino acids across cell membranes. Testosterone, which is produced principally from the Leydig cells of the testes, is responsible for male sexual characteristics. Vasopressin is secreted from the posterior pituitary and is sometimes referred to as an antidiuretic hormone.

13–15. The answers are: 13-C *[IV D],* **14-B** *[VI D 2],* **15-E** *[III D 3].*
Exogenously administered adrenocorticosteroids are effective anti-inflammatory agents but give rise to a wide range of metabolic and immunosuppressive effects that result in severe adverse effects. Oral antidiabetic agents of the sulfonylurea type may cause blood dyscrasias, impaired liver function, and photosensitivity. Exogenously administered androgens suppress sperm formation and cause paradoxical gynecomastia. Most significant is the hepatotoxicity produced by alkyl-substituted androgen compounds.

18
Antineoplastic Agents

Edward F. LaSala

I. INTRODUCTION.

I. INTRODUCTION. Chemotherapeutic agents used in the treatment of cancer are referred to by a number of terms, including antineoplastics, cytotoxic agents, carcinostatic agents, and anticancer agents.

A. Uses

1. As a group, these agents can, in certain cases, **relieve pain, prevent or delay metastasis after surgery, cause temporary remission,** and **significantly increase survival time**. However, they provide relatively few cures.
2. Common cancers that can be cured effectively by drugs include **Hodgkin's disease, acute lymphocytic and myelogenous leukemia, testicular cancer,** and **non-Hodgkin's lymphomas**. Other forms of human cancer, such as lung cancer and colon cancer, are more resistant to chemotherapy.

B. Mechanism of action

1. Antineoplastic agents work by **destroying cancer cells**. Many of the most potent agents act at specific phases of the cell cycle and are, thus, **effective only against dividing cells**.
2. Malignancies most susceptible to drugs are those that **grow rapidly** (those with a high percentage of cells in the process of division). Slow-growing tumors are often unresponsive to these drugs.
3. Antineoplastic agents are **selectively more toxic to cancer cells than to normal cells**. However, this selectivity is narrow, and these agents are **very toxic**.
   a. Toxicity is most evident in tissues with a high turnover rate, such as **bone marrow, hair follicles,** and **intestinal epithelium**.
   b. Common **adverse effects** of these drugs include bone marrow depression, alopecia, and severe nausea and vomiting.
   c. Such toxicity often **limits the use** of antineoplastic agents.
4. **Combination therapy**—the use of two or more drugs with differing fundamental actions, often results in greater effectiveness of action and reduced toxicity.
   a. In many cases, combination therapy permits **greater effect against a tumor** without a corresponding increase in toxicity.
   b. Combination therapy also **delays the development of resistance to a single agent** and **increases survival time**.

C. Classification. Antineoplastic agents are classified by their mechanism of action or physicochemical properties. Classes include alkylating agents, antimetabolites, hormones, antibiotics, plant products and derivatives, and miscellaneous agents.

II. ALKYLATING AGENTS.

II. ALKYLATING AGENTS. These highly reactive chemicals can alkylate, or bind covalently, with the cellular components of DNA.

A. Nitrogen mustards

1. **Chemistry.** These agents, which include mechlorethamine (Mustargen), cyclophosphamide (Cytoxan), ifosfamide (Ifex), melphalan (Alkeran), chlorambucil (Leukeran), and uracil mustard are mostly characterized by a *bis*-2-chloroethylamine substituent, R—$NH(CH_2CH_2Cl)_2$.

2. **Pharmacology.** In vivo, this substituent acts as a **bifunctional alkylating agent** on guanine bases in both DNA strands. This results in **cross-linking** (interstrand linking).
   a. Cross-linking **prevents division of the helical DNA strands** and, thus, subsequent reproduction of daughter cells.
   b. These agents act as **cell-growth inhibitors**.
3. **Therapeutic indications.** Nitrogen mustards are indicated for use with a variety of neoplastic diseases, including Hodgkin's disease, non-Hodgkin's lymphomas, acute and chronic lymphocytic leukemias, breast cancer, ovarian cancer, and others.
4. **Adverse effects.** Major adverse effects include leukopenia, anemia, thrombocytopenia, nausea, vomiting, hyperuricemia, dermatitis, and alopecia.

B. Ethylenimines

1. **Chemistry.** The prototypical agent is **triethylenethiophosphoramide** (Thiotepa) [Figure 18-1].
2. **Pharmacology.** This agent acts as a **bifunctional alkylating agent,** as a result of the in vivo opening of the ethylenimine rings. Ifosfamide produces serious urotoxic effects. Mesna (Mesenex) is ordinarily administered concurrently to reduce these effects.
3. **Therapeutic indications**
   a. Ethylenimines are seldom employed clinically today. Nitrogen mustards often are used instead.
   b. On occasion, triethylenethiophosphoramide may be indicated for treatment of Hodgkin's disease, non-Hodgkin's lymphomas, and breast, lung, and ovarian cancer.
4. **Adverse effects.** Major adverse effects include leukopenia, thrombocytopenia, neutropenia, nausea, vomiting, amenorrhea, decreased spermatogenesis, dermatitis, and hyperuricemia.

C. Alkyl sulfonates

1. **Chemistry. Busulfan** (Myleran) is the only clinically used agent in this group (Figure 18-2).
2. **Pharmacology.** In vivo, cleavage of busulfan's C—O bonds produces a bifunctional alkylating butyl carbonium ion, which **cross-links strands of DNA**.
3. **Therapeutic indications.** Busulfan has well-established beneficial effects when used to treat chronic granulocytic leukemia.
4. **Adverse effects**
   a. Major adverse effects include thrombocytopenia, anemia, nausea, vomiting, diarrhea, amenorrhea, impotence, sterility, and hyperuricemia.
   b. Less common effects include gynecomastia, alopecia, anhidrosis, generalized skin pigmentation, and pulmonary fibrosis.

D. Nitrosoureas

1. **Chemistry.** These agents, which include carmustine or BCNU (BICNU), lomustine or CCNU (CEENU), and streptozocin (Zanosar), have the general structure shown in Figure 18-3.
2. **Pharmacology.** These agents appear to act as **bifunctional alkylating agents,** cross-linking strands of DNA as monofunctional carbamoylating agents.
3. **Therapeutic indications**
   a. **Carmustine** and **lomustine** cross the blood–brain barrier, making them useful agents for the treatment of brain tumors. These agents are also indicated for use with Hodgkin's disease, non-Hodgkin's lymphomas, and renal cell, stomach, colon, and lung cancers.
   b. **Streptozocin** is used for metastatic pancreatic islet-cell cancer.

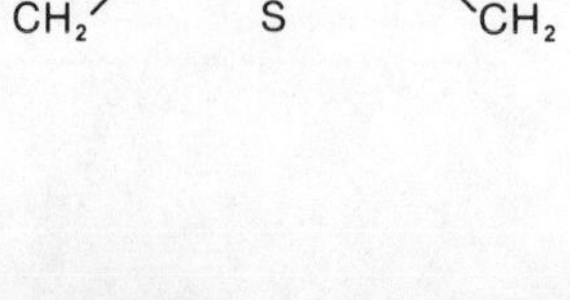

Figure 18-1. Structural formula of triethylenethiophosphoramide (Thiotepa), an ethylenimine alkylating agent.

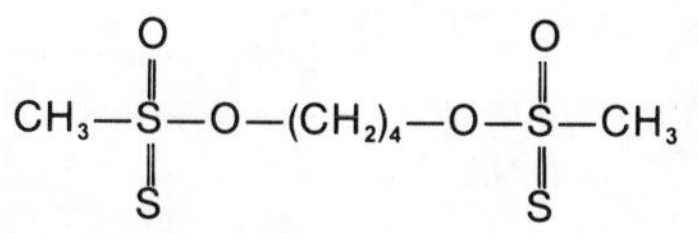

Figure 18-2. Structural formula of busulfan (Myleran), an alkyl sulfonate alkylating agent.

4. **Adverse effects**
   a. **Carmustine** and **lomustine** may cause leukopenia, thrombocytopenia, nausea, and vomiting. **Carmustine** may also cause hepatotoxicity, hyperuricemia, and pulmonary fibrosis. **Lomustine** may also cause nephrotoxicity and alopecia.
   b. **Streptozocin** may cause aplastic anemia, nausea, vomiting, diarrhea, nephrotoxicity, and hepatotoxicity.

E. Triazenes

1. **Chemistry. Dacarbazine** (DTIC) is the only agent used clinically in this group. It closely resembles the metabolite 5-aminoimidazole-4-carboxamide (AIC), which can be converted to inosinic acid.
2. **Pharmacology.** Dacarbazine appears to act as a **monofunctional alkylating agent**.
3. **Therapeutic indications.** Dacarbazine is used principally for the treatment of malignant melanoma. It also may be used in combination with other drugs to treat Hodgkin's disease and various sarcomas.
4. **Adverse effects.** Major adverse effects include severe nausea and vomiting, anorexia, leukopenia, thrombocytopenia, alopecia, fever, malaise, and myalgia.

F. Platinum coordination complexes

1. **Chemistry. Cisplatin** is the cis isomer of an inorganic platinum-containing complex. **Carboplatin** is an organic platinum-containing complex (Figure 18-4).
2. **Pharmacology.** These agents undergo hydrolysis, resulting in loss of chloride ion (cisplatin) and the bidentate dicarboxylato group (carboplatin), forming their respective activated species, which can form both **interstrand and intrastrand links** with DNA.
3. **Therapeutic indications.** Cisplatin is especially useful for advanced testicular cancer. It is also active against bladder and ovarian cancer. Carboplatin is approved for the treatment of ovarian cancers.
4. **Adverse effects.** Major adverse effects of cisplatin include nausea and vomiting, ototoxicity, leukopenia, thrombocytopenia, anemia, hyperuricemia, and nephrotoxicity. Carboplatin's dose-limiting toxic effect appears to be thrombocytopenia. Other effects are similar to cisplatin but to a lesser extent.

III. ANTIMETABOLITES.

These agents interfere with the biosynthesis of essential substances, either through enzyme inhibition or by incorporation into essential molecules to form false products. They ultimately block the synthesis or functioning of proteins, DNA precursors, or DNA itself, inhibiting cell growth.

A. Folic acid antagonists

1. **Chemistry. Methotrexate,** also known as **amethopterin** or MTX (Folex), the primary folic acid antagonist, is an analogue of folic acid that **combines irreversibly with** the enzyme **dihydrofolate reductase (DHF)**.
2. **Pharmacology**
   a. Inhibition of DHF by methotrexate reduces the production of **tetrahydrofolate (THF),** interfering with the metabolic conversion of deoxyuridine monophosphate (dUMP) to deoxythymidine monophosphate (dTMP).

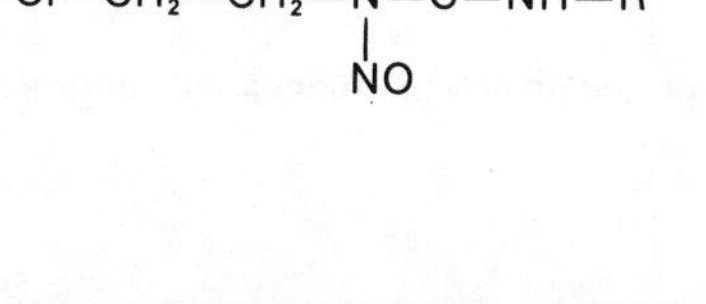

Figure 18-3. General structural formula of the nitrosourea alkylating agents.

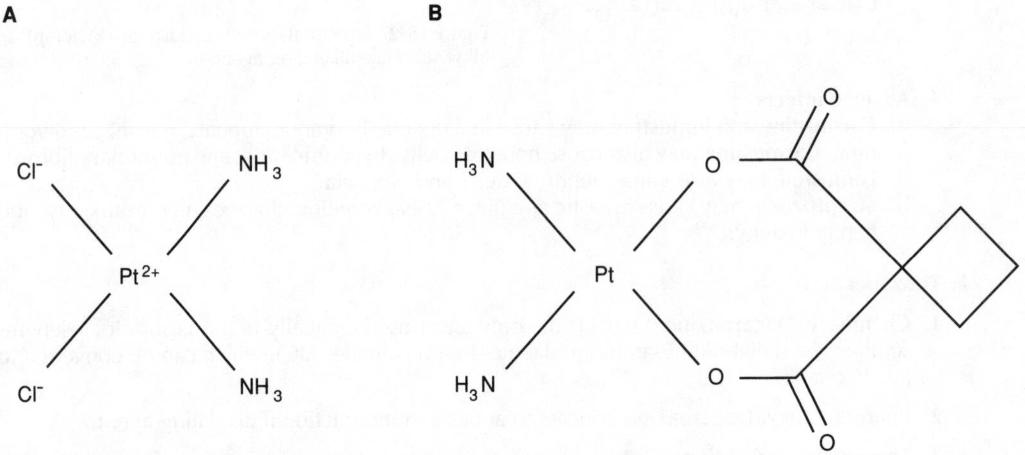

Figure 18-4. Structural formulas of (*A*) cisplatin (Platinol) and (*B*) carboplatin (Paraplatin), platinum coordination complexes.

b. This deficiency of dTMP results in **inhibited DNA synthesis**.

c. **Leucovorin** (a reduced form of folic acid) may be given after high-dose methotrexate therapy, to **reduce toxicity to normal cells**. Leucovorin provides intermediary THF, which reestablishes the conversion of dUMP to dTMP.

3. **Therapeutic indications.** Methotrexate may be used for treatment of acute lymphocytic leukemia, choriocarcinoma, mycosis fungoides, osteogenic sarcoma, and cancers of the breast, testis, lung, head, and neck.

4. **Adverse effects.** Toxic reactions to methotrexate are dose-related and may result in anemia, leukopenia, thrombocytopenia, stomatitis, diarrhea, nausea, vomiting, nephrotoxicity, hepatic dysfunction, alopecia, dermatitis, and hyperuricemia.

B. Purine antagonists

1. **Chemistry.** Purine antagonists include **mercaptopurine** or 6-MP (Purinethol) and **thioguanine** or 6-TG [Lanvis (Canada)] analogues of the natural purines hypoxanthine and guanine (Figure 18-5).

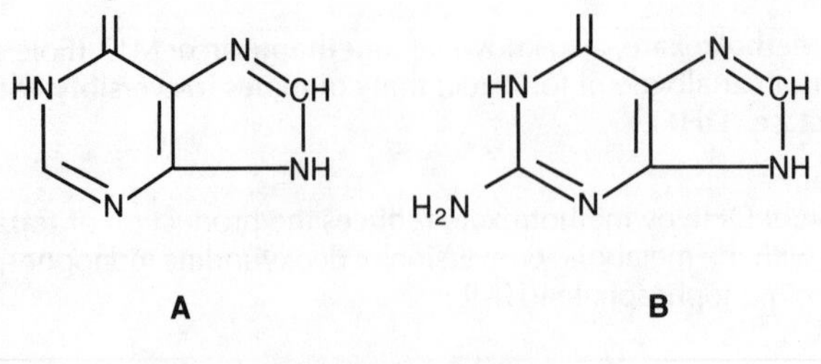

Figure 18-5. Structural formulas of (*A*) mercaptopurine and (*B*) thioguanine, purine analogue antimetabolites.

2. **Pharmacology**
   a. **Mercaptopurine** interferes with purine synthesis, ultimately interfering with adenine and guanine synthesis or with their incorporation into DNA.
   b. **Thioguanine** appears to be incorporated into DNA synthetic pathways, forming a false DNA code that interferes with the DNA template mechanism.
3. **Therapeutic indications.** Mercaptopurine and thioguanine may be used for treatment of acute lymphocytic, acute granulocytic, and chronic granulocytic leukemias.
4. **Adverse effects.** Major adverse effects of the purine antagonists include leukopenia, thrombocytopenia, anemia, nausea, vomiting, anorexia, jaundice, hepatotoxicity, and hyperuricemia.

C. Pyrimidine antagonists

1. **Chemistry.** Pyrimidine antagonists include **fluorouracil** or 5-FU (Adrucil) [Figure 18-6], **floxuridine** (FUdR), and **cytarabine** or araC (Cytosar-U).
2. **Pharmacology**
   a. **Fluorouracil** and **floxuridine** compete with deoxyuridine monophosphate (dUMP) for the enzyme thimidylate synthetase, thus inhibiting conversion of dUMP to deoxythymidine monophosphate (dTMP) and ultimately **inhibiting DNA synthesis**.
   b. **Cytarabine,** which differs from natural cytidine by having an arabinose sugar rather than a deoxyribose sugar, competes with cytidine nucleotide and **inhibits the action of DNA polymerase**.
3. **Therapeutic indications**
   a. **Fluorouracil** and **floxuridine** may be of palliative value when used to treat cancers of the breast, stomach, colon, pancreas, ovary, cervix, prostate, urinary bladder, head, and neck.
   b. **Fluorouracil** is also widely used topically for the treatment of premalignant skin keratoses and superficial basal cell cancers.
   c. **Cytarabine** is used for treatment of acute granulocytic and acute lymphocytic leukemias.
4. **Adverse effects**
   a. **Fluorouracil** and **floxuridine** may cause leukopenia, thrombocytopenia, anemia, anorexia, nausea, vomiting, diarrhea, stomatitis, dermatitis, hyperpigmentation, nail changes, alopecia, weakness, and malaise.
   b. **Cytarabine** may cause leukopenia, thrombocytopenia, anemia, megaloblastosis, nausea, vomiting, diarrhea, stomatitis, hepatic dysfunction, hyperuricemia, dermatitis, and fever.

IV. HORMONES.
For a complete discussion of the chemistry, pharmacology, major therapeutic uses, and adverse effects of hormones, see Chapter 17. Only the use of hormones for the treatment of neoplastic diseases is discussed here. For the most part, hormones are noncytotoxic.

A. Adrenocorticosteroids

1. Adrenocorticosteroids such as **prednisone** cause direct destruction of lymphocytes and provide **symptomatic relief of the complications of neoplastic disease**.
2. These agents are effective in the treatment of **certain lymphocytic leukemias** and are also widely used as adjuncts with other cytotoxic antineoplastic agents.

B. Estrogens

1. Estrogens such as **diethylstilbestrol phosphate** (Stilphostrol) sometimes are used to treat cancers of testosterone-dependent male reproductive tissue, such as **prostatic cancer**. These agents block the effects of androgens, producing chemical castration (see Chapter 11 V C 2 e).

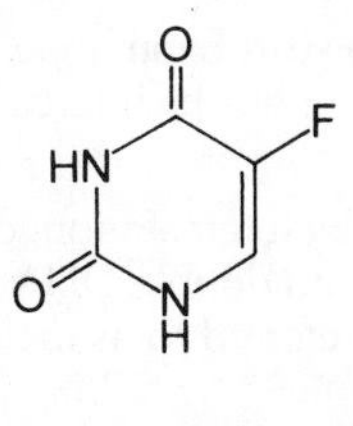

Figure 18-6. Structural formula of fluorouracil (Adrucil), a pyrimidine antagonist.

2. These agents also may be used for treatment of **breast cancer in postmenopausal women** for whom surgery and radiotherapy have not been effective.

3. A unique agent, **estramustine** (Emcyt) may be used for treatment of prostatic cancer. A *bis*-2-chloroethylamine derivative of estradiol, this agent is a prodrug that appears to act as a site-specific alkylating agent for estrogen-dependent tissues.

C. Androgens and anabolic steroids. Androgens, such as **fluoxymesterone** (Halotestin) and **testolactone** (Teslac), and anabolic steroids, such as **nandrolone phenpropionate** (Anabolin), are sometimes used to treat cancers of estrogen-dependent tissues, such as **breast cancer**.

D. Progestins. Megestrol acetate (Megace) is used for endometrial and breast carcinoma and medroxyprogesterone (Depo-Provera) is used for endometrial or renal carcinoma.

E. Antihormones

1. **Tamoxifen** (Nolvadex), a nonsteroidal triarylethylene derivative, acts as an **antiestrogen** by binding to cytoplasmic estrogen receptors and slowing the growth of estrogen-dependent tissues. It is used in the treatment of **breast cancer** in postmenopausal women.

2. **Aminoglutethimide** (Cytadren) acts as an **antiadrenal agent** by interfering with adrenocorticoid synthesis. It is used in the treatment of **adrenal cancer** and **metastatic breast cancer**.

3. **Flutamide** (Eulexin) is a nonsteroidal fluorinated *p*-nitroanilide that acts as a potent **antiandrogen** by inhibiting androgen uptake or by inhibiting nuclear binding of androgen in target tissues. **Ineffective alone,** it is used as an adjunct to the **gonadotropin-releasing hormone analogues** in the treatment of prostatic carcinoma to **suppress adrenal androgen production**.

4. **Gonadotropin-releasing hormone analogues**
   a. **Leuprolide acetate** (Lupron) is a synthetic nonapeptide analogue of **luteinizing hormone–releasing factor** (GnRH or LH–RH). It is a potent **LH–RH agonist** that binds to pituitary GnRH receptors and desensitizes them. When used continuously, it inhibits gonadotropin secretion, resulting in suppression of ovarian and testicular steroidogenesis. It is used in the treatment of **advanced prostatic cancer**.
   b. **Goserelin acetate** (Zoladex) is a synthetic decapeptide analogue of LH–RH or GnRH. Similarly to leuprolide, continuous administration leads to suppression of pituitary gonadotropins. It is used in the treatment of **advanced prostatic carcinoma.**

V. ANTIBIOTICS. The antibiotics used in cancer chemotherapy include dactinomycin, daunorubicin, doxorubicin, the bleomycins, plicamycin, and mitomycin.

A. Chemistry. These agents are produced by different species of the fungus *Streptomyces*.

1. **Doxorubicin** (Adriamycin, Rubrex), **daunorubicin** (Cerubidine), and **idarubicin** (Idamycin) are **anthracyclines** and similar in structure to the tetracyclines.

2. **Dactinomycin** also known as actinomycin D (Cosmegen) is a **phenoxazone chromopeptide**.

3. The **bleomycins,** which differ from each other only in their terminal amine moieties, are water-soluble, basic glycopeptides.

4. **Plicamycin** (Mithracin), which was formerly known as mithramycin, is a large structure somewhat similar to dactinomycin.

5. **Mitomycin** (Mutamycin) contains a urethane and a quinone group as well as an aziridine ring, which is essential to its antineoplastic activity.

6. **Mitoxantrone** (Novantrone) is an anthracenedione somewhat related to daunorubicin.

B. Pharmacology

1. All of the antibiotics used in cancer chemotherapy appear to act as **cell-growth inhibitors**.

2. **Dactinomycin, daunorubicin, idarubicin,** and **doxorubicin** appear to **bind noncovalently to guanine,** altering the character of the DNA double helix by intercalating with it. This interferes with the transcription of the DNA molecule.

3. **Bleomycin** (Blenoxane) binds to DNA, possibly by intercalation, causing hydrolysis of glycosidic linkages and reductive cleavage of single and double DNA strands. The resulting **fragmentation of the DNA molecule** is sometimes referred to as **nicking**.

4. **Plicamycin** appears to bind to DNA, resulting in an **inhibition of RNA synthesis**.
5. **Mitomycin** acts as a bifunctional alkylating agent, **inhibiting DNA synthesis**.
6. **Mitoxantrone** is a **DNA reactive agent** that stimulates the formation of **strand breaks** in DNA.

C. Therapeutic indications

1. **Dactinomycin** is used to treat Wilms' tumor, rhabdomyosarcoma, testicular cancer, and choriocarcinoma.
2. **Daunorubicin** is used to treat acute granulocytic and acute lymphocytic leukemias, and **idarubicin** is used to treat acute myeloid leukemias.
3. **Doxorubicin** is used to treat sarcomas, Hodgkin's disease, non-Hodgkin's lymphomas, acute leukemias, neuroblastomas, and cancers of the breast, thyroid, lung, stomach, and genitourinary tract.
4. **Bleomycin** is used to treat Hodgkin's disease, non-Hodgkin's lymphomas, and cancers of the head and neck, testis, skin, esophagus, and genitourinary tract.
5. **Plicamycin** is of limited value because of its severe toxicity. It may be used to treat malignant hypercalcemia and testicular cancer.
6. **Mitomycin** is used to treat cancers of the stomach, colon, pancreas, breast, bladder, and cervix.
7. **Mitoxantrone** is used to treat acute nonlymphocytic leukemias.

D. Adverse effects

1. **Dactinomycin** is associated with anemia, leukopenia, thrombocytopenia, anorexia, nausea, vomiting, diarrhea, stomatitis, erythema, desquamation, hyperpigmentation, alopecia, and soft-tissue damage.
2. **Daunorubicin** and **idarubicin** are associated with bone marrow depression, cardiac toxicity, nausea, vomiting, stomatitis, esophagitis, anorexia, diarrhea, nephrotoxicity, hepatotoxicity, dermatitis, and alopecia.
3. **Doxorubicin** is associated with leukopenia, thrombocytopenia, cardiac toxicity, nausea, vomiting, diarrhea, stomatitis, esophagitis, hyperpigmentation, and alopecia.
4. **Bleomycin** is associated with stomatitis, prolonged anorexia, nausea, vomiting, diarrhea, erythema, vesiculation, desquamation, ulceration, alopecia, pulmonary toxicity, and an acute allergic reaction with profound fever.
5. **Plicamycin** is associated with thrombocytopenia, nausea, vomiting, anorexia, diarrhea, stomatitis, and proteinuria. It is toxic to bone marrow, liver, and kidneys and also produces a severe bleeding syndrome, which may range from epistaxis to generalized hemorrhage.
6. **Mitomycin** is associated with thrombocytopenia, leukopenia, paresthesias, nausea, vomiting, anorexia, stomatitis, dermatitis, fever, malaise, and alopecia.
7. **Mitoxantrone** is associated with nausea and vomiting, alopecia, mucositis, stomatitis, and myelosuppression.

VI. PLANT PRODUCTS AND DERIVATIVES

A. Vinca alkaloids

1. **Chemistry. Vinblastine** (Velban) and **vincristine** (Oncovin) are alkaloids derived from the periwinkle plant (*Vinca rosea*). They are closely related dimeric compounds.
2. **Pharmacology.** The vinca alkaloids block mitosis by arresting cells in metaphase, thus **inhibiting cell growth**.
3. **Therapeutic indications**
   a. **Vinblastine** is used to treat Hodgkin's disease, non-Hodgkin's lymphomas, and cancers of the breast, testis, and renal cells.
   b. **Vincristine** is used to treat acute lymphoblastic leukemia, neuroblastoma, Wilms' tumor, rhabdomyosarcoma, Hodgkin's disease, and non-Hodgkin's lymphomas.

4. **Adverse effects**
   a. **Vinblastine** is associated with leukopenia, thrombocytopenia, depression, paresthesias, peripheral neuropathy, numbness, loss of deep tendon reflexes, muscle pain and weakness, nausea, vomiting, stomatitis, constipation, ileus, anorexia, abdominal pain, urinary retention, dermatitis, and alopecia.
   b. **Vincristine** is associated with mild anemia and leukopenia, peripheral neuropathy, loss of deep-tendon reflexes, paresthesias, muscle weakness and cramps, ataxia, hoarseness, headache, diplopia, ptosis, constipation, nausea, vomiting, anorexia, stomatitis, urinary retention, and alopecia.

B. Podophyllotoxin derivatives

1. **Chemistry. Etoposide** (VePesid) is a semisynthetic carbohydrate analogue of podophyllotoxin.
2. **Pharmacology.** Etoposide acts by **arresting cell mitosis**.
3. **Therapeutic indications.** This agent is used to treat acute nonlymphocytic leukemia, lymphosarcoma, Hodgkin's disease, testicular cancer, and small-cell lung cancer.
4. **Adverse effects.** Major adverse effects include myelosuppression, leukopenia, thrombocytopenia, nausea, vomiting, headache, fever, and alopecia. Anaphylaxis occurs rarely.

VII. MISCELLANEOUS AGENTS

A. Hydroxyurea (Hydrea) appears to inhibit ribonucleotide diphosphate reductase, causing inhibition of nucleotide synthesis. It is used to treat chronic granulocytic leukemia and malignant melanoma.

B. Procarbazine (Matulane) appears to cause depolymerization of the DNA molecule, interfering with DNA and RNA synthesis. It is used to treat Hodgkin's disease.

C. Asparaginase (Elspar) appears to hydrolyze asparagine, an amino acid commonly found in cancer cells that may be an essential nutrient for them. It is used to treat acute lymphocytic leukemia.

D. Interferons

1. **Chemistry.** Interferons, referred to as **biologic response modifiers,** are **human proteins** either natural, **interferon-alfa-N3** (Alferon N) or prepared by **recombinant DNA** technology, **interferon-alfa-2a** (Roferon A) and **interferon alfa-2b** (Intron A).
2. **Pharmacology.** They are **antiproliferative agents** that may have a direct effect on tumor cells and modify the host immune response.
3. **Therapeutic indications.**
   a. Interferon alfa-2a and interferon alfa-2b are indicated in the treatment of selected cases of **hairy cell leukemia** and **Kaposi's sarcoma** that is related to acquired immunodeficiency syndrome (AIDS).
   b. Interferon alfa-N3 is indicated for the treatment of selected cases of **condyloma acuminatum**.

STUDY QUESTIONS

Directions: Each of the numbered items or incomplete statements in this section is followed by answers or by completions of the statement. Select the **one** lettered answer or completion that is **best** in each case.

1. Assume that a type of cancer is susceptible to an individual drug. All of the following anticancer combinations are therapeutically rational EXCEPT

(A) triethylenethiophosphoramide–prednisone
(B) cyclophosphamide–6-mercaptopurine
(C) doxorubicin–methotrexate
(D) melphalan–chlorambucil
(E) floxuridine–vinblastine

2. Systemic antifolate therapy has been found to be useful in the treatment of psoriasis. Which of the following agents most likely would be dispensed for this purpose?

(A) Cyclophosphamide
(B) Vinblastine
(C) Bleomycin
(D) Methotrexate
(E) Carmustine

3. Most of the clinically available anticancer agents have an underlying mechanism of action that acts as

(A) cell-growth inhibitors
(B) stimulation of natural body defense mechanisms
(C) interference with cell wall production
(D) inhibition of cancer cell nutrient absorption
(E) receptor-site blockade of cancer cell secretions

Directions: Each item below contains three suggested answers, of which **one or more** is correct. Choose the answer

A if **I only** is correct
B if **III only** is correct
C if **I and II** are correct
D if **II and III** are correct
E if **I, II, and III** are correct

4. True statements concerning fluorouracil include

I. its chemical structure is a modified pyrimidine that is similar to uracil and thymine
II. bone marrow depression is a common side effect
III. it inhibits the methylation of deoxyuridine monophosphate to form deoxythymidine monophosphate

5. Anticancer agents that act as enzyme inhibitors include

I. doxorubicin
II. methotrexate
III. floxuridine

1-D
2-D
3-A
4-E
5-D

Directions: The group of items in this section consists of lettered options followed by a set of numbered items. For each item, select the **one** lettered option that is most closely associated with it. Each lettered option may be selected once, more than once, or not at all.

Questions 6–8

For each anticancer agent, select the mechanism of action that most appropriately describes it.

(A) Bifunctional alkylating agent
(B) Intercalating antibiotic
(C) Antimetabolite–antifolate
(D) Mitosis-blocking plant alkaloid
(E) Antimetabolite–pyrimidine antagonist

6. Cytarabine
7. Vinblastine
8. Doxorubicin

6-E
7-D
8-B

ANSWERS AND EXPLANATIONS

1. The answer is D *[I B 4; II A 1, 2].*
To be therapeutically rational, combinations of anticancer agents should consist of drugs that are individually effective in the type of cancer being treated and should belong to different antineoplastic classes, have different mechanisms of action, or both. Each of the pairs of drugs includes anticancer agents that belong to different classes and have different mechanisms of action except the melphalan–chlorambucil combination. Both of these agents are bifunctional alkylating agents that act by cross-linking guanine bases in both DNA strands, thus preventing their division and subsequent reproduction of daughter cells.

2. The answer is D *[I B 2; III A].*
An antifolate is an agent that antagonizes the action of folic acid. Methotrexate does this by inhibiting the action of dihydrofolate reductase, thus preventing the reduction of dihydrofolate to tetrahydrofolate. The deficiency of tetrahydrofolate interferes with conversion of deoxyuridine monophosphate (dUMP) to deoxythymidine monophosphate (dTMP) which, in turn, results in inhibited DNA synthesis. Thus, an antifolate acts as a cell-growth inhibitor. Psoriasis is a non-neoplastic disease of the skin but is similar to cancer in that it is characterized by abnormally rapid proliferation of epidermal cells. Methotrexate is indicated only for the treatment of severe, disabling psoriasis that is not adequately responsive to other forms of therapy.

3. The answer is A *[I B 1–3].*
Cancer cells, unlike most normal cells, continue to reproduce after maturation. Characteristically, this growth is described as uncontrollable. With the possible exception of the hormones (e.g., the adrenocorticoids when used as palliative adjuncts in the treatment of cancers other than certain lymphocytic leukemias), almost all of the approved anticancer drugs act to inhibit or slow down this uncontrollable growth. Another important characteristic of cancer cells is their ability to metastasize.

4. The answer is E (all) *[III C; Figure 18-6].*
Fluorouracil has a fluoro-group substituted on the 5 position of uracil. Thymine is 5-methyl uracil. Fluorouracil is a cell-growth inhibitor and as such is likely to cause bone marrow depression since it inhibits the growth of normal cells, particularly those that have a high turnover.

5. The answer is D (II, III) *[III A 1, C 2; V B 2].*
Methotrexate is an antifolate–antimetabolite that inhibits the action of dihydrofolate reductase. Floxuridine is a pyrimidine antagonist that inhibits the action of thymidylate synthetase. Doxorubicin is an antibiotic that acts by intercalation.

6–8. The answers are: 6-E *[III C]*, **7-D** *[VI A]*, **8-B** *[V B 2].*
Cytarabine is an analogue of the pyrimidine nucleoside, cytosine, in which the ribase sugar moiety has been replaced by arabinose. It is converted to the arabinonucleotide in the body, which then competitively inhibits DNA polymerase and, thus, blocks DNA synthesis.

Vinblastine is an alkaloid derived from the periwinkle plant (*Vinca rosea*). It and its structurally related homologue vincristine both act as mitotic antagonists by binding to contractile proteins in the mitotic spindle of dividing cells, which leads to inhibition of mitosis. Although the structures and mechanism of action of vinblastine and vincristine are quite similar, the two plant alkaloids are quite different in their therapeutic application and toxicities.

Doxorubicin is an antibiotic. Similar to dactinomycin and daunorubicin, it acts as an intercalating agent. Intercalating agents are substances that bind strongly to DNA by insertion into the space between adjacent base pairs of the double helix, thereby inhibiting DNA synthesis and DNA-directed RNA synthesis.

19
Nuclear Pharmacy

Stephen C. Dragotakes
Ronald J. Callahan

I. INTRODUCTION

A. Overview

1. **Nuclear pharmacy** is defined by the *American Pharmaceutical Association's Nuclear Pharmacy Practice Standards,* as "patient-oriented service that embodies the scientific knowledge and professional judgment required to improve and promote health through the safe, and efficacious use of radioactive drugs for diagnosis and therapy."*

2. **Radiopharmaceuticals** are chemical entities that contain radioactive elements. Most radiopharmaceuticals are used in diagnostic medical imaging; however, they are also used in therapeutic applications, such as in the treatment of hyperthyroidism, thyroid cancer, and polycythemia vera. This review primarily concerns diagnostic radiopharmaceuticals.

3. **Nuclear pharmacy practice** entails the:
   - **a.** Procurement of radiopharmaceuticals
   - **b.** Compounding of radiopharmaceuticals
   - **c.** Performance of routine quality control procedures
   - **d.** Dispensing of radiopharmaceuticals
   - **e.** Distribution of radiopharmaceuticals
   - **f.** Implementation of basic radiation protection procedures and practices
   - **g.** Consultation and education of the nuclear medicine community, patients, pharmacists, other health professionals, and the general public regarding:
     - **(1)** Physical and chemical properties of radiopharmaceuticals
     - **(2)** Pharmacokinetics and biodistribution of radiopharmaceuticals
     - **(3)** Drug interactions and other factors that alter patterns of distribution

B. Properties of radiopharmaceuticals

1. **Pharmacologic effects.** Radiopharmaceuticals do not produce pharmacologic effects since the quantities range from picogram (pg) to nanogram (ng) per kilogram (kg) of administered dose.

2. **Route of administration.** Most radiopharmaceuticals are prepared as sterile, pyrogen-free intravenous solutions to be administered directly to the patient. Other routes of administration include oral, interstitial, and inhalation (e.g., radioactive gases, aerosols).

3. **Radionuclides**
   - **a.** The radioactive component of a radiopharmaceutical is referred to as a radionuclide. Nuclides are identified as atoms having a specific number of protons and neutrons in the nucleus. A nuclide is typically identified by the chemical symbol of the element with a mass number to the upper left superscript, indicating the sum of protons and neutrons [e.g., iodide 131 (^{131}I)]. When the atom is radioactive, it is called a radionuclide.
   - **b.** Radionuclides undergo spontaneous radioactive decay accompanied by the release of energy. The distribution, metabolism, and elimination of the radiopharmaceutical can be determined by measuring this energy with imaging equipment. There are **four major types**

---

*Section on Nuclear Pharmacy: *American Pharmaceutical Association's Nuclear Pharmacy Practice Standards.* Academy of Pharmacy Practices, 1978.

of radiation emitted through this process: **alpha, beta, gamma,** and **x-rays**. Alpha and beta radiations are not useful in medical imaging. Most radiopharmaceuticals use penetrating gamma radiation, which can be easily detected and converted into imaging data.

4. **Half-lives of radiopharmaceuticals**
   a. **Physical half-life** of a radiopharmaceutical is the amount of time necessary for the radioactive atoms to decay to one-half their original number. Each nuclide is identified with a specific half-life.
   b. **Biologic half-life** of a radiopharmaceutical is the amount of time required for the body to eliminate one-half of the administered dose of any substance by the processes of biologic elimination.
   c. **Effective half-life** of a radiopharmaceutical is the time required for an administered radiopharmaceutical dose to be reduced by one-half due to both physical decay and biologic elimination. It is defined as:

$$t_e \text{ (effective half-life)} = (t_p \times t_b)/(t_p + t_b),$$

   where t_p = physical half-life and t_b = biologic half-life.

C. Criteria for optimal radiopharmaceuticals

1. They should have a half-life short enough to minimize radiation exposure to the patient yet long enough to allow for collection of imaging information.
2. They should incorporate a gamma-emitting radionuclide, which decays with the emission of a photon energy between 100–300 kilo electron volts (keV), which is efficiently detected with current instrumentation.
3. Radiopharmaceuticals should localize rapidly in the organ system of interest and be metabolized or excreted from the nontarget tissues to maximize contrast and minimize absorbed doses of radiation.
4. They should be readily available and cost-effective.

II. SODIUM PERTECHNETATE ^{99m}Tc GENERATOR

A. Overview

1. **Technetium 99m (^{99m}Tc).** The most commonly used radionuclide in diagnostic imaging today is ^{99m}Tc. This radionuclide is produced by the **radioactive decay of molybdenum 99 (^{99}Mo)**.
   a. ^{99m}Tc is obtained via commercially supplied sterile, pyrogen-free "generator" systems. A generator is a device used to separate a short half-life radionuclide from the longer-lived "parent" nuclide, while releasing the parent to produce more of the daughter nuclide. In this way, short half-life nuclides can be made available continuously at great distances from the sites of generator production.
   b. All of the commercially supplied generators currently use ^{99}Mo obtained from the fission of uranium 235 (^{235}U). This ^{99}Mo parent is absorbed on an alumina (Al_2O_3) ion exchange column, and the ^{99m}Tc formed from its decay is exchanged for the chloride ion (Cl^-) available in the 0.9% saline eluate solution washed through the column, as the sodium pertechnetate ^{99m}Tc ($Na^{+\,99m}Tc\,O_4^-$) form.
2. **The chemical valence state** of $Na^{+\,99m}TcO_4^-$ as it is eluted from the column is +7. Typically, it must be reduced to a valence state of +3, +4, or +5 before it is able to react with other compounds. Although ^{99m}Tc can be reduced by many processes, the **stannous ion (Sn^{2+}) reduction method** is most commonly used in ^{99m}Tc radiopharmaceutical kits.
   a. A radiopharmaceutical kit consists of sterile, pyrogen-free vials containing a reducing agent, the compound to be labeled, and any additional adjuvants to effect the reaction or stabilize the labeled product. In most cases they are lyophilized.
   b. The contents of radiopharmaceutical kits are stored under a nitrogen atmosphere so as to minimize oxidation of Sn^{2+}.

B. Sodium pertechnetate ^{99m}Tc USP ($Na^{+\,99m}TcO_4^-$) as eluted from a generator in 0.9% sodium chloride (NaCl) solution is an isotonic, sterile, nonpyrogenic, diagnostic radiopharmaceutical suitable for intravenous injection, oral administration, and direct instillation.

1. **Physical properties**
   a. The solution should be clear, colorless, and free of visible foreign material. The pH is 4.5–7.0.
   b. $Na^{+99m}TcO_4^-$ is used to radiolabel all other ^{99m}Tc radiopharmaceuticals.

2. **Biodistribution**
   a. $Na^{+99m}TcO_4^-$ is handled by the body in a fashion similar to ^{131}I; that is, it is taken up and released but not organified by the thyroid.
   b. After intravenous administration, $Na^{+99m}TcO_4^-$ concentrates in the choroid plexus, thyroid gland, salivary gland, and stomach, but remains in the circulation long enough for first-pass blood pool studies, organ perfusion, and major vessel studies.

3. **Decay data**
   a. $Na^{+99m}TcO_4^-$ decays by isomeric transition with a **physical half-life** of 6 hours.
   b. The primary **radiation emissions** are 140 keV gamma energy photons.

4. **Purity**
   a. **USP radionuclidic purity** requires a ^{99}Mo breakthrough limit of less than 0.15 μCi/mCi.
   b. **USP chemical purity** requires an aluminum ion (Al^{+3}) test result of less than 10 μg/ml.

5. **Administration and dosage.** All of the following imaging studies are administered intravenously except nasolacrimal imaging, which is instilled into the lacrimal canal.
   a. Brain imaging: 10–20 mCi [370–740 megabecquerels (MBq)]
   b. Thyroid imaging: 1–10 mCi (37–370 MBq)
   c. Salivary gland imaging: 1–5 mCi (37–185 MBq)
   d. Placenta localization: 1–3 mCi (37–111 MBq)
   e. Blood pool imaging: 10–30 mCi (370–740 MBq)
   f. Urinary bladder imaging: 0.5–1 mCi (18–37 MBq)
   g. Nasolacrimal imaging: $<$ 100 μCi ($<$ 3.7 MBq)

III. RADIOPHARMACEUTICALS FOR CARDIOVASCULAR IMAGING

A. **Perfusion agents for cardiac imaging.** Radiopharmaceuticals are useful in cardiac imaging as agents that provide information of regional myocardial blood perfusion. They typically are administered as part of a stress test so as to provide information at peak cardiac output. Pharmacologic augmentation of treadmill exercise stress test perfusion imaging includes the use of intravenous coronary vessel dilating agents, such as dipyridamole, adenosine, and dobutamine.

1. **Thallous chloride ^{201}Tl USP** (^{201}Tl) is a radionuclide that is produced by cyclotron. It is used for myocardial perfusion imaging in the diagnosis of coronary artery disease and localization of myocardial infarction.
   a. **Biodistribution**
      (1) ^{201}Tl is a monovalent cation with distribution analogous to potassium ion (K^+); myocardial uptake is by active transport via the Na^+–K^+-ATPase pump.
      (2) Biodistribution is generally proportional to organ blood flow at the time of injection with blood clearance by myocardium, kidneys, thyroid, liver, and stomach. The remainder is distributed uniformly throughout the rest of the body.
      (3) ^{201}Tl is excreted slowly and equally in both urine and feces.
   b. **Decay data**
      (1) The **physical half-life** is 73 hours.
      (2) The **effective half-life** is 2–4 days.
      (3) The **biologic half-life** is 11 days.
      (4) The **primary radiation emissions** are 68–80 keV x-rays and 167 keV and 135 keV gamma energy photons.
   c. **Administration and dosage.** Intravenous, 2–4 mCi (74–148 MBq)

2. **Technetium ^{99m}Tc sestamibi** (^{99m}Tc sestamibi) exists as a sterile, pyrogen-free intravenous injection after kit reconstitution with $Na^{+99m}TcO_4^-$ and heating at 100°C for 10 minutes.
   a. **Biodistribution**
      (1) ^{99m}Tc sestamibi is a cation complex that has been found to accumulate in viable myocardial tissue similar to ^{201}Tl.
      (2) The major pathway for clearance of ^{99m}Tc sestamibi is the hepatobiliary system. This agent is excreted without any evidence of metabolism via urine and feces.

b. Decay data

(1) **The effective half-life** is 3 hours.

(2) **The biologic half-life** is 6 hours.

c. Administration and dosage. Intravenous, 10–30 mCi (370–1110 MBq)

3. **Technetium ^{99m}Tc teboroxime** (^{99m}Tc teboroxime) is a myocardial perfusion kit that is useful in distinguishing normal from abnormal myocardium.

a. Biodistribution

(1) After kit reconstitution with $Na^{+\,99m}TcO_4^-$ and heating at 100°C for 15 minutes, ^{99m}Tc teboroxime is formed as a boronic acid ^{99m}Tc dioxime (BATO) derivative that exists as a sterile, pyrogen-free intravenous injection.

(2) ^{99m}Tc teboroxime is a neutral, lipophilic complex with high myocardial uptake and clearance rates.

(3) Peak myocardial uptake occurs within 2 minutes. Myocardial extraction efficiency is between 83%–95%.

(4) The major pathway for clearance of ^{99m}Tc teboroxime is the hepatobiliary system. This agent is excreted via urine and feces.

b. Decay data. Bi-exponential myocardial **biologic half-life** is 6 minutes and 13 hours.

c. Administration and dosage

(1) **Single dose:** Intravenous, 15–30 mCi (600–1110 MBq)

(2) **Combined rest/stress:** Intravenous, 35–50 mCi (1300–1850 MBq)

4. **Rubidium chloride** ($^{82}Rb^+$) is a generator-produced radiopharmaceutical obtained by the decay of its accelerator-produced parent (half-life is 25 days) adsorbed on a stannous oxide column.

a. Biodistribution

(1) When eluted with 0.9% NaCl at a rate of 50 ml/min, a solution of the short-lived daughter $^{82}Rb^+$ is eluted from the generator for direct intravenous administration.

(2) Following intravenous administration, $^{82}Rb^+$ rapidly clears from the blood and is extracted by the myocardial tissue in a manner analogous to K^+.

(3) Myocardial activity is visualized within 1 minute following administration.

b. Decay data

(1) The **physical half-life** is 75 seconds.

(2) The **decay mode** is by positron emission.

(3) The **primary radiation emissions** are annihilation 511 keV gamma energy photons.

(4) Parent strontium (^{32}Sr) and contaminant ^{85}Sr breakthrough must be closely monitored. Acceptable levels of strontium breakthrough are:

$$< 0.02\ \mu Ci\ ^{82}Sr/mCi\ ^{82}Rb^+$$
$$< 0.2\ \mu Ci\ ^{85}Sr/mCi\ ^{82}Rb^+$$

c. Administration and dosage. Intravenous, 30–60 mCi (1110–2220 MBq)

B. Agents used to measure cardiac function (regional myocardial wall motion)

1. **^{99m}Tc labeled red blood cells** are used for blood pool imaging, including cardiac first-pass and gated equilibrium imaging (regional cardiac wall motion).

a. Physical properties. Autologous red blood cells can be labeled by a number of techniques that use the Sn^{2+} radiolabeling method with three general steps.

(1) First, the cells are treated with Sn^{2+} (Sn^{2+}: 10–20 μg/kg) to provide an intercellular source of the reducing agent.

(2) Some procedures then allow for a removal of excess Sn^{2+} with scavenging agents.

(3) All of the methods include the addition of $Na^{+\,99m}TcO_4^-$. This ^{99m}Tc, while in the +7 valence state, crosses the intact erythrocyte membrane and binds to intercellular hemoglobin after being reduced by the available intercellular Sn^{2+}.

b. Biodistribution. Following intravenous injection, the labeling red blood cells distribute within the blood pool and are well maintained in the blood pool with a **bi-exponential whole body clearance** of 2.5–2.7 hours and 75–176 hours (e.g., major route of excretion is via the urine).

c. Administration and dosage. Intravenous, 10–20 mCi (370–740 MBq)

2. **Pyrophosphate injection USP and phosphates USP.** The major use for these agents in nuclear medicine is as convenient and stable sources of Sn^{2+} for the labeling of autologous red blood cells. In this application, the kits are reconstituted with sodium chloride injection USP and injected intravenously.

3. **Technetium ^{99m}Tc albumin (^{99m}Tc albumin) injection**
   a. **Biodistribution**
      (1) ^{99m}Tc albumin distributes initially within the intravascular space and leaves this space at a rate slow enough to permit imaging of the blood pool.
      (2) **Plasma clearance** is bi-exponential; a fast component clearing with a half-life of 2 hours and a slow component clearing with a half-life of 10–16 hours.
      (3) The major route of elimination is via the urine.
   b. **Administration and dosage.** Intravenous, 20 mCi (740 MBq)

C. **Agents for imaging myocardial infarction** include **pyrophosphate injection USP** and **phosphates USP**.

1. **Mechanism of localization.** The skeletal localizing radiopharmaceutical pyrophosphate has been shown to accumulate also in zones of myocardial infarction. This localization is thought to be due to binding of the pyrophosphate to microcalcification with hydroxyapatite crystals found in infarcted tissue.

2. **Biodistribution** of labeled pyrophosphate depends on the ability of phosphates to become involved with calcium ion (Ca^{2+}) metabolism in necrotic cardiac tissue.

IV. SKELETAL IMAGING

A. Skeletal imaging agents

1. **Overview.** ^{99m}Tc-labeled bone agents are useful in the detection of bone lesions that are associated with metastatic neoplasms, metabolic disorders, and infections of the bone. The imaging advantages of ^{99m}Tc, coupled with the sensitivity of bone agent localization in skeletal bone hydroxyapatite, allows for detection of bone pathology before evidence is shown by conventional x-rays.

2. **^{99m}Tc bone agents.** There are many different forms of ^{99m}Tc bone agents with minor differences in their individual chemical structure. Currently used bone imaging agents are based on the P — C — P diphosphonate structure, including ^{99m}Tc medronate disodium, ^{99m}Tc oxidronate, and ^{99m}Tc pyrophosphate. These bone agents are Sn^{2+} reduction method kits, which exist as sterile, pyrogen-free intravenous radiopharmaceuticals after reconstitution with $Na^{+\,99m}TcO_4^-$.
   a. **Physical properties**
      (1) All of the ^{99m}Tc bone agents are susceptible to radiologic decomposition with reoxidation of the ^{99m}Tc to a higher valence state. These agents sometimes include antioxidants (e.g., ascorbic or gentisic acid) in their formulation.
      (2) Most agents should be used within 6 hours after formulation.
      (3) They should be stored at room temperature before and after reconstitution.
   b. **Biodistribution**
      (1) It is believed that the localization of the diphosphonates occurs on the hydroxyapatite mineral matrix of skeletal bone with uptake related to bone metabolic activity and bone blood flow.
      (2) For ^{99m}Tc medronate disodium and ^{99m}Tc oxidronate, approximately 50% of the administered dose localizes in the skeleton, and 50% is excreted by the kidneys within the first 4–6 hours following intravenous injection.
   c. **Administration and dosage.** Intravenous, 10–20 mCi (370–740 MBq)

B. Bone marrow imaging (see VI B)

V. LUNG IMAGING.
Radiopharmaceuticals are used to evaluate both pulmonary perfusion and pulmonary ventilation, to detect pulmonary embolism, and to assess pulmonary function prior to pneumonectomy.

A. Pulmonary perfusion imaging

1. **Technetium ^{99m}Tc albumin aggregated USP (^{99m}Tc albumin aggregated)**
   a. **Physical properties**
      (1) The ^{99m}Tc albumin aggregated kit contains human serum albumin that has been aggregated by heat denaturization.

(2) This Sn^{2+} reduction method kit exists as a sterile, pyrogen-free suspension of radiolabeled aggregated particles after reconstitution with $Na^{+99m}TcO_4^-$.
(3) It should be stored at 2°–8°C after reconstitution.

b. Biodistribution

(1) After intravenous administration of ^{99m}Tc albumin aggregated, 80% of the radiolabeled albumin particles become trapped by capillary blockade in the pulmonary circulation.
(2) Following trapping, the particles are cleared from the lungs mainly by mechanical breakup. These smaller particles are ultimately cleared from the circulation by the reticuloendothelial system.
(3) Particle size should be controlled; that is, 90% of the particles should be between 10–90 μ, and none should be more than 150 μ to ensure adequate trapping by the lung capillary bed but no occlusion of the large bore vessels.
(4) Particle number should be between 200,000–700,000 particles per adult dose to obtain uniform imaging data without compromising capillary blood flow.

c. Decay data. Biologic half-life in the lung is 2–3 hours.

d. Administration and dosage. Intravenous, 1–4 mCi (37–148 MBq)

B. Pulmonary ventilation imaging with radioactive gases is a routine nuclear medicine procedure that can provide valuable information about regional lung ventilation. Radiopharmaceuticals that are used are either radioactive gases or radioaerosols.

1. Xenon ^{133}Xe USP (^{133}Xe) is supplied as a radioactive gas contained in glass septum vials to be administered by inhalation through a closed respiratory system or a spirometer. It is a byproduct of ^{235}U fission.

a. Biodistribution

(1) ^{133}Xe is a readily diffusible gas, which is neither used nor produced by the body. It passes through membranes and freely exchanges between blood and tissue, tending to concentrate more in body fat.
(2) Inhaled ^{133}Xe distributes within the alveoli and enters the pulmonary venous circulation via the capillaries with most of the absorbed ^{133}Xe returned and exhaled from the lungs after a single pass through the peripheral circulation.
(3) In concentrations used for diagnosis, the gas is physiologically inactive.

b. Decay data

(1) The **effective half-life** in the lung is 2 minutes.
(2) The **physical half-life** is 5.2 days.
(3) The **decay mode** is beta minus decay.
(4) The **primary radiation emissions** are 100 keV beta energy and 81 keV gamma energy photons.

c. Administration and dosage. Inhalation, 2–30 mCi (74–1110 MBq)

2. Xenon ^{127}Xe USP (^{127} Xe) is supplied as a radioactive gas contained in glass septum vials to be administered by inhalation through a closed respiratory system or a spirometer. It is produced by cyclotron.

a. Biodistribution. Localization is the same as ^{133}Xe.

b. Decay data

(1) The **physical half-life** is 36.4 days.
(2) The **decay mode** is by electron capture.
(3) The **primary radiation emissions** are 203 keV, 190 keV, 172 keV, and 375 keV gamma energy photons.

c. Administration and dosage. Inhalation, 5–10 mCi (185–370 MBq)

3. Krypton ^{81m}Kr USP (^{81m}Kr) is generator-produced by the decay of its parent radionuclide ^{81}Rb. It is supplied as a radioactive gas in the form of humidified oxygen eluted continuously through the generator and inhaled by the patient.

a. Decay data

(1) The **physical half-life** is 13 seconds.
(2) The **parent ^{81}Rb half-life** is 4.6 hours.
(3) The **primary radiation emissions** are 190 keV gamma energy photons.

b. Administration and dosage. Inhalation, 1–10 mCi (37–370 MBq)

4. Radioaerosols have become increasingly used with the advent of nebulizers that produce particles of a consistent size necessary for uniform lung distribution.

a. **Biodistribution**

(1) ^{99m}Tc pentetate radioaerosols of approximately 0.25 μ mass median aerodynamic diameter are useful in determining lung ventilation.

(2) After deposition of the nebulized droplets within the airways, the ^{99m}Tc pentetate is absorbed into the pulmonary circulation.

(3) The material is subsequently excreted by the kidneys. Clearance from the lungs is sufficiently slow to allow for imaging of the lungs in multiple projections from a single administration.

b. **Administration and dosage.** Inhalation, 8 mCi (296 MBq)

VI. HEPATIC IMAGING

A. **Overview.** Hepatic imaging requires the use of two different classes of radiopharmaceuticals to evaluate the two cell types responsible for hepatic function.

1. **Reticuloendothelial system imaging.** The liver, spleen, and bone marrow are evaluated with radiolabeled colloidal material, ranging in size from 0.1–3.0 μ. These particles are rapidly cleared from the blood by the Küpffer cells.

2. **Liver–spleen imaging.** Radiopharmaceuticals are useful in imaging space-occupying primary tumors and metastatic neoplasms, as well as hepatic defects caused by abscesses, cysts, and trauma.

3. **Radiopharmaceuticals** that localize in the bone marrow are useful in the evaluation of pathologies that affect bone marrow.

4. **Hepatobiliary imaging.** Hepatocyte function can be evaluated by substances meeting requirements of molecular weight, lipophilicity, and chemical structure, to be excreted by the polygonal cells into the hepatobiliary system. Hepatobiliary imaging radiopharmaceuticals are useful in the diagnosis of cystic duct obstruction in acute cholecystitis as well as defining post-cholecystectomy anatomy and physiology.

B. **Reticuloendothelial imaging agents**

1. **Technetium ^{99m}Tc sulfur colloid (^{99m}Tc sulfur colloid)** is a sterile, pyrogen-free intravenous radiopharmaceutical formed via a chemical reaction between $Na^{+99m}TcO_4^-$ and an acidified solution of sodium thiosulfate at 100°C.

a. **Physical properties**

(1) ^{99m}Tc sulfur colloid is thought to remain in the +7 valence state as the heptasulfide co-precipitate of elemental sulfur occurs during the reaction.

(2) The use of $Na^{+99m}TcO_4^-$ with Al^{+3} levels over 10 μg/ml can lead to the formation of particles more than 5 μm, which can result in lung uptake.

(3) Heating times should be controlled to preclude large particle formation.

b. **Biodistribution.** Following administration, approximately 80%–90% of the dose is phagocytized by the Küpffer cells of the liver, 5%–10% by the spleen, and the balance by the bone marrow. The blood clearance half-life is approximately 2.5 minutes. Particles are not metabolized and reside in the reticuloendothelial system for a prolonged period of time.

c. **Administration and dosage.** Intravenous, liver/spleen: 1–8 mCi (37–296 MBq); bone marrow: 3–12 mCi (111–444 MBq)

2. **^{99m}Tc albumin colloid** labeled with $Na^{+99m}TcO_4^-$ has been proposed as an alternative to ^{99m}Tc sulfur colloid. Possible advantages of this product include metabolism and clearance of the particle from the reticuloendothelial system and a single-step preparation, which does not require heating.

a. **Biodistribution.** Following administration, approximately 80%–90% of the dose is phagocytized by the liver, 5%–10% by the spleen, and the balance by the bone marrow.

b. **Administration and dosage.** Intravenous, 5–8 mCi (185–296 MBq)

C. **Hepatobiliary imaging agents**

1. **Overview**

a. **Iminodiacetic acid (IDA) derivatives** are useful as hepatobiliary imaging agents due to their ability to be selectively cleared by a carrier-mediated hepatocyte pathway. Since these agents share the same excretion pathway as bilirubin, patients with elevated bilirubin levels exhibit decreased hepatic clearance and an increased renal clearance. Lack of gallbladder visualization is an abnormal finding suggestive of acute cholecystitis.

b. **Cholecystokinetic agents,** such as sincalide, may be used to empty the contents of the gallbladder in fasting patients in an attempt to promote gallbladder filling and visualization.

c. **Narcotic analgesics,** such as morphine, have been used to constrict the sphincter of Oddi to produce elevated intraductal pressures to promote gallbladder filling.

2. **Technetium ^{99m}Tc disofenin (^{99m}Tc disofenin)**
   a. **Physical properties** (see II A 2 a, b)
   b. **Biodistribution**
      (1) ^{99m}Tc disofenin is rapidly cleared from the blood with 8% remaining in the blood after 30 minutes.
      (2) Approximately, 9% of the administered activity is excreted in the urine over the first 2 hours. The remainder of the activity is cleared through the hepatobiliary system.
      (3) Peak liver uptake is within 10 minutes with peak gallbladder uptake by 30–40 minutes.
      (4) Gallbladder and intestinal visualization occurs within 60 minutes postadministration.
   c. **Administration and dosage.** Intravenous, nonjaundiced patient: 1–5 mCi (37–185 MBq); jaundiced patient: 3–8 mCi (111–296 MBq)

3. **Technetium ^{99m}Tc lidofenin (^{99m}Tc lidofenin)**
   a. **Physical properties** (see II A 2 a, b)
   b. **Biodistribution**
      (1) After administration, ^{99m}Tc lidofenin is rapidly cleared from the blood circulation with 7% remaining after 26 minutes.
      (2) Approximately 14%–22% of the administered activity can be excreted in the urine within the first 90 minutes with the remainder of the activity clearing through the hepatobiliary system.
      (3) Peak liver uptake occurs within 10–15 minutes with visualization of the hepatic duct and gallbladder within 20–30 minutes.
      (4) Intestinal activity can be visualized within 30 minutes.
   c. **Administration and dosage.** Intravenous, nonjaundiced patient: 2–5 mCi (74–185 MBq); jaundiced patient: 3–10 mCi (111–370 MBq)

4. **Technetium ^{99m}Tc mebrofenin (^{99m}Tc mebrofenin)**
   a. **Physical properties** (see II A 2 a, b)
   b. **Biodistribution**
      (1) ^{99m}Tc mebrofenin is rapidly cleared from the blood with 17% remaining after 10 minutes. Only 1% of the administered activity is excreted in the urine within the first 3 hours, with the remainder of the activity clearing through the hepatobiliary system.
      (2) Peak liver uptake occurs within 10 minutes with visualizaion of the hepatic duct and gallbladder within 10–15 minutes, then intestinal activity within 30–60 minutes.
   c. **Administration and dosage.** Intravenous, nonjaundiced patient: 2–5 mCi (74–185 MBq); jaundiced patient: 3–10 mCi (111–370 MBq)

VII. RENAL IMAGING

A. Overview

1. Radiopharmaceuticals are used in renal imaging to determine renal function, renal vascular flow, and renal morphology. They are also useful for the evaluation of renal transplant patients for complications such as obstruction, infarction, leakage, tubular necrosis, and rejection.

2. The use of radiopharmaceuticals to determine renal function or renal morphology is based on the two physiologic mechanisms responsible for excretion: glomerular filtration and tubular secretion.

B. Agents cleared by glomerular filtration are useful in determining the glomerular filtration rate (GFR), renal artery perfusion, and the visualization of the collecting system.

1. **Technetium ^{99m}Tc pentetate USP (^{99m}Tc pentetate)**
   a. **Physical properties** (see II A 2 a, b)
   b. **Biodistribution**
      (1) After administration, ^{99m}Tc pentetate rapidly distributes throughout extracellular fluid space from which it is rapidly cleared by glomerular filtration.

(2) Up to 10% may be protein bound, leading to a decrease in measured GFR.
(3) After administration, 50% of the dose is cleared by the kidneys within 2 hours, and up to 95% is cleared by 24 hours.

c. **Administration and dosage.** Intravenous 10–20 mCi (370–740) MBq)

2. **Sodium iothalamate ^{125}I injection** is a commercially supplied sterile, pyrogen-free injection containing 1 mg sodium iothalamate per milliliter.

a. **Biodistribution**
(1) Sodium iothalamate ^{125}I is used for determination of the GFR but not for imaging due to poor imaging emissions of ^{125}I.
(2) Thyroid blockade with oral potassium iodide (KI) is suggested.

b. **Decay data**
(1) The **physical half-life** is 59 days.
(2) The **decay mode** is by electron capture.
(3) The **primary radiation emissions** are 35 keV gamma energy photons and x-rays.

c. **Administration and dosage.** Intravenous, 10–50 μCi (3.7–18.5 MBq)

C. **Tubular secretion agents** are used to evaluate renal tubular function and measure effective renal plasma flow.

1. **Iodohippurate ^{123}I hippuran and iodohippurate ^{131}I hippuran** are commercially supplied sterile, pyrogen-free, intravenous solutions. ^{123}I is produced by cyclotron and ^{131}I, by reactor.

a. **Biodistribution**
(1) Iodohippurate ^{123}I hippuran and ^{131}I hippuran are excreted 80% by tubular secretion and 20% by glomerular filtration.
(2) Whole body biologic half-life, excluding the bladder, is less than 1 hour.
(3) Approximately 50% of an administered dose is excreted within 30 minutes, with 90% excreted within 8 hours.
(4) Thyroid blockade with KI is suggested.

b. **Decay data and dosage**
(1) **Iodohippurate ^{123}I**
(a) The **physical half-life** is 13 hours.
(b) The **decay mode** is by electron capture.
(c) The **primary radiation emissions** are 159 keV gamma energy photons.
(d) **Administration and dosage.** Intravenous, 100–400 μCi (3.7–14.8 MBq)
(2) **Iodohippurate ^{131}I**
(a) The **physical half-life** is 8 days.
(b) The **decay mode** is by beta minus decay.
(c) The **primary radiation emissions** are 197 keV beta energy and 364 keV gamma energy photons.
(d) **Administration and dosage.** Intravenous, 10–100 μCi (0.4–3.7 MBq)

2. **Technetium ^{99m}Tc mertiatide (^{99m}Tc mertiatide)**

a. **Physical properties** (see II A 2 a, b)

b. **Biodistribution**
(1) ^{99m}Tc mertiatide is rapidly excreted via tubular secretion and glomerular filtration with 90% excreted in the urine within 3 hours.
(2) Renal clearance correlates with that of iodohippurate ^{131}I.

c. **Administration and dosage.** Intravenous, 10 mCi (185–370 MBq)

D. **Renal cortical imaging agents** are used to evaluate renal anatomy because of their ability to accumulate in the kidney and provide anatomic imaging data.

1. **Technetium ^{99m}Tc gluceptate (^{99m}Tc gluceptate)**

a. **Physical properties** (see II A 2 a, b)

b. **Biodistribution**
(1) ^{99m}Tc gluceptate rapidly distributes throughout the body with rapid blood clearance via glomerular filtration and tubular secretion.
(2) Approximately 25% of the administered dose is excreted within the first hour, 65% within 6 hours, and 70% within 24 hours.
(3) After 3–6 hours, a maximum of 5%–15% of the dose administered is concentrated in the proximal renal tubular cells of the renal cortex.

c. **Administration and dosage.** Intravenous, 10–20 mCi (370–740 MBq)

2. **Technetium ^{99m}Tc succimer USP (^{99m}Tc succimer)**
   a. **Physical properties** (see II A 2 a, b) ^{99m}Tc succimer complex must be allowed to incubate for 10 minutes postreconstitution and must be used within 30 minutes postincubation.
   b. **Biodistribution**
      (1) Within 3–6 hours postadministration, 40%–50% of the dose localizes in the renal cortex where it is taken up by the tubular cells.
      (2) Excretion into the urine is slow with 5%–20% being excreted within the first 2 hours, 10%–30% by 6 hours, and less than 40% by 24 hours.
   c. **Administration and dosage.** Intravenous, 2–6 mCi (74–222 MBq)

VIII. THYROID IMAGING

A. Overview

1. The basic function of the thyroid gland is the production of thyroid hormone for the regulation of metabolism. The thyroid hormones are produced within the gland with the organification of iodine obtained from the oxidation of available iodide circulating in the blood. The inability of the body to distinguish between the isotopes of iodine provides a perfect metabolic tracer for the thyroid biochemical system.

2. The function of the thyroid gland can be evaluated by the uptake of ^{131}I, allowing the detection of hypothyroidism with decreased uptake and hyperthyroidism with increased uptake.

3. $Na^{+\,99m}TcO_4^-$ is a monovalent ion with an ionic radius similar to iodide. As a result the pertechnetate ion is trapped by the thyroid gland in a fashion similar to iodide. The two species are sufficiently different that organification of the $Na^{+\,99m}TcO_4^-$ does not occur, and it is subsequently released.

B. Thyroid imaging agents

1. **Sodium iodide ^{123}I** is a radiopharmaceutical available in either solution or capsule form for oral administration. It is produced by cyclotron.
   a. **Biodistribution**
      (1) Orally administered iodine is rapidly absorbed from the gastrointestinal tract with thyroid gland uptake evident within minutes.
      (2) Sodium iodide ^{123}I is considered an ideal radiopharmaceutical for iodine uptake and imaging studies due to its short half-life and useful 159 keV primary gamma emissions.
   b. **Decay data**
      (1) The **physical half-life** is 13 hours.
      (2) The **biologic half-life** is 3.5 days.
      (3) The **decay mode** is by electron capture.
      (4) The **primary radiation emissions** are 159 keV, 27 keV, and 529 keV gamma energy photons.
   c. **Administration and dosage.** Oral thyroid uptake: 10–20 μCi (0.37–0.74 MBq); thyroid image: 100–500 μCi (3.7–18.5 MBq)

2. **Sodium iodide ^{131}I** is a classic radioiodine used for thyroid uptake and imaging studies; however, it is now used less often due to the high radiation dose absorbed.
   a. **Biodistribution**
      (1) Orally administered iodine is rapidly absorbed from the gastrointestinal tract with thyroid gland uptake within minutes.
      (2) Sodium iodide ^{131}I is not considered an ideal radioiodine radiopharmaceutical for iodine uptake and imaging studies because of its long half-life and the high radiation dose to the thyroid from its beta decay component.
      (3) The radiation dose from the high energy beta particle with the imaging potential of its gamma emissions make this radionuclide the agent of choice for therapeutic treatment of hyperthyroidism and thyroid cancer.
   b. **Decay data**
      (1) The **physical half-life** is 8.08 days.
      (2) The **decay mode** is by beta decay.
      (3) The **primary radiation emissions** are 606 keV and 333 keV beta energy and 364 keV, 637 keV, and 284 keV gamma energy photons.

c. **Administration and dosage.** Sodium iodide ^{131}I is available as either a capsule or in solution for oral administration.
(1) **Diagnostics**
(a) **Thyroid uptake:** 2–15 μCi (0.074—0.555 MBq)
(b) **Thyroid image:** 30–50 μCi (1.11—1.85 MBq)
(c) **Whole body image:** 1–5 mCi (37–185 MBq)
(2) **Therapeutics**
(a) **Thyroid ablation:** 5–15 mCi (185–550 MBq)
(b) **Thyroid carcinoma:** 50–200 mCi (1850–7400 MBq)

3. **$Na^{+99m}TcO_4^-$** (see II B)

4. **^{201}Tl (parathyroid imaging)**
a. **Biodistribution.** ^{201}Tl concentrates in the thyroid and also in parathyroid adenomas, which can be detected by a dual isotope subtraction technique of subtracting thyroid uptake counts from $Na^{+99m}TcO_4^-$ to unmask nonthyroid thallium uptake counts (see III A 1).
b. **Administration and dosage.** Intravenous, 2 mCi (74 MBq)

IX. BRAIN IMAGING

A. **Cerebral perfusion brain imaging agents.** Radiopharmaceuticals for evaluating brain perfusion must possess a lipophilic partition coefficient sufficient to diffuse passively across the blood–brain barrier almost completely within one pass of the cerebral circulation, as well as being sufficiently retained to permit data collection. The regional uptake of these agents is proportional to cerebral blood flow. This class of radiopharmaceuticals is useful in the diagnosis of altered regional blood perfusion in stroke.

1. **Technetium ^{99m}Tc exametazine (^{99m}Tc exametazine)** exists as a sterile, pyrogen-free, intravenous injection after reconstitution with $Na^{+99m}TcO_4^-$.
a. **Physical properties**
(1) ^{99m}Tc exametazime is a neutral, lipid-soluble complex, which freely crosses the blood–brain barrier. This is a relatively unstable complex, which converts to a water-soluble secondary complex incapable of penetrating into the brain. For this reason, the in vitro shelf life is 30 minutes, following radiolabeling.
(2) Additional limitations on kit preparation parameters require the use of high mole fraction $Na^{+99m}TcO_4^-$ generator eluates of less than 2 hours postelution from a generator previously eluted within 24 hours.
b. **Biodistribution**
(1) ^{99m}Tc exametazine rapidly clears from the blood with a maximum brain uptake of 3.5%–7%, with up to 2.5% remaining after 24 hours.
(2) The activity is widely distributed throughout the body with 30% distributing to the gastrointestinal tract.
(3) Within 48 hours, 50% of the dose is excreted via the urine and 40% via fecal elimination.
c. **Administration and dosage.** Intravenous, 10–20 mCi (370–740 MBq)

2. **Iofetamine hydrochloride ^{123}I** is not commercially available.
a. **Biodistribution**
(1) Iofetamine hydrochloride ^{123}I rapidly distributes throughout the body with rapid uptake in the brain; 5%–7% of the dose localizes in 20–60 minutes after administration due to its high lipophilicity.
(2) Following injection, iofetamine hydrochloride ^{123}I is rapidly metabolized with two major metabolites: p-iodoamphetamine and p-iodobenzoic acid.
(3) The primary route of elimination is via the urine with 20% excreted after 24 hours and 30% after 48 hours.
(4) Thyroid blockade wth oral KI is suggested.
b. **Decay data**
(1) The **physical half-life** is 13 hours.
(2) The **decay mode** is by electron capture.
(3) The **primary radiation emissions data** are 159 keV and 27 keV gamma energy photons.
c. **Administration and dosage:** Intravenous 3–6 mCi (111–222 MBq)

B. Carrier-mediated transport (cerebral metabolism) mechanisms are responsible for transporting glucose across the blood–brain barrier. Agents such as ^{18}F flurodeoxyglucose aid in the evaluation of cerebral function by mapping the distribution of glucose metabolism. ^{18}F flurodeoxyglucose is produced by cyclotron.

1. **Biodistribution.** Currently, there is a USP monograph for on-site–produced ^{18}F flurodeoxyglucose, which is a glucose analogue. ^{18}F flurodeoxyglucose concentrates in the brain where it is phosphorylated but does not undergo subsequent metabolism due to the replacement of the hydroxyl group in the 2 position with a fluorine atom. It is then metabolically trapped for a sufficient time to allow imaging.

2. **Decay data**
   a. The **physical half-life** is 109 minutes.
   b. The **decay mode** is by positron emission.
   c. The **primary radiation emissions** are 633 keV energy positrons and 511 keV gamma energy photons.

3. **Administration and dosage.** Intravenous 5–10 mCi (185–370 MBq)

C. Cerebrospinal fluid (CSF) dynamics. Radionuclide cisternography is useful in the evaluation of hydrocephalus and in detecting CSF leaks. In CSF imaging, the radiopharmaceutical **indium ^{111}In pentetate** (^{111}In pentetate) is introduced intrathecally into the spinal subarachnoid space, ascends through the basal cisterns, proceeds over the cerebral hemispheres, and drains eventually into the superior sagittal sinus. ^{111}In pentetate is commercially supplied as a sterile, pyrogen-free, unit dose injection. It is produced by cyclotron.

1. **Biodistribution**
   a. After intrathecal injection, this radiopharmaceutical normally ascends to the parasagittal region within 24 hours.
   b. After absorption into the bloodstream via the arachnoid villi, the major route of elimination is by kidney with 65% of the dose excreted within 48 hours and 85% within 72 hours.

2. **Decay data**
   a. The **physical half-life** is 67 hours.
   b. The **CSF biologic half-life** is 12 hours.
   c. The **effective half-life** is 10 hours.
   d. The **mode of decay** is by electron capture.
   e. The **primary radiation emissions** are 245 keV and 171 keV gamma energy photons.

3. **Administration and dosage.** Intrathecal, 500 μCi (18.5 MBq)

X. TUMORS, INFECTIONS, AND INFLAMMATION

A. Tumors

1. **Overview.** The usefulness of radiopharmaceuticals in the detection of tumors varies in sensitivity and specificity with differences in tumor location and type. **Gallium citrate ^{67}Ga USP (^{67}Ga)** may detect the presence of Hodgkin's disease, lymphoma, and bronchogenic carcinoma.

2. **Tumor detection agent ^{67}Ga** is commercially supplied as a sterile, pyrogen-free radiopharmaceutical. It is produced by a cyclotron.
   a. **Physical properties**
      (1) ^{67}GA accumulates in primary metastatic tumors as well as focal sites of infection.
      (2) It accumulates intercellularly bound to protein. Although the mechanism is unknown, it is thought that accumulation is dependent on the formation of a gallium transferrin complex in the serum or binding to transferrin receptors on tumor cells.
   b. **Biodistribution**
      (1) Following administration, the highest concentration of ^{67}Ga is in the renal cortex, other than sites of tumor or infection. After 24 hours, the maximum concentration shifts to bone and lymph nodes, but after 1 week, it is mainly concentrated in the liver and spleen.
      (2) ^{67}Ga is excreted relatively slowly from the body with 26% in the urine and 9% in the stools and with a whole body retention of 65% after 7 days.

c. **Decay data**
   (1) The **physical half-life** is 78 hours.
   (2) The **mode of decay** is by electron capture.
   (3) The **primary radiation emissions** are 93 keV, 185 keV, 300 keV, and 393 keV gamma energy photons.
d. **Administration and dosage.**
   (1) Intravenous, patients with infection: 3–8 mCi (111–300 MBq)
   (2) Intravenous, patients with tumor: 10 mCi (370 MBq)

B. Infection and inflammation

1. **Overview.** Evaluation of sites of infection include the use of radiolabeled white blood cells to image areas in which the cellular components of the natural defense mechanisms localize.
2. **Infection detection agents. Indium ^{111}In oxyquinoline USP (^{111}In oxyquinoline)** is a commercially supplied sterile, pyrogen-free radiopharmaceutical for the radiolabeling of autologous leukocytes. ^{111}In is produced by cyclotron.
   a. **Physical properties.** ^{111}In forms a saturated (1:3) neutral lipophilic complex with oxyquinoline, which enables it to penetrate a cell membrane. ^{111}In is then thought to become firmly bound to cytoplasmic components, thereby allowing the free oxine to be released by the cell.
   b. **Biodistribution**
      (1) After labeling, autologous leukocytes are reinjected, with 30% taken up by spleen and 30% by the liver, reaching a peak at 2–48 hours postinjection.
      (2) Pulmonary uptake is immediately evident postinjection but clears with minimal activity visible after 4 hours.
      (3) There is a bi-exponential blood clearance with 9%–24% clearing with a biologic half-life of 2–5 hours, and the remainder of 13%–18% clearing with a biologic half-life of 64–116 hours.
      (4) Elimination is mainly through radioactive decay with less than 1% excreted in feces and urine during the first 24 hours.
   c. **Decay data**
      (1) The **physical half-life** is 67 hours.
      (2) The **mode of decay** is by electron capture.
      (3) The **primary radiation emissions** are 245 keV and 171 keV gamma energy photons.
   d. **Administration and dosage.** Intravenous, 200–500 μCi (7.4–18.5 MBq)

STUDY QUESTIONS

Directions: Each of the numbered items or incomplete statements in this section is followed by answers or by completions of the statement. Select the **one** lettered answer or completion that is **best** in each case.

1. Which of the following emissions from the decay of radionuclides is most commonly used in nuclear medicine imaging?

(A) X-ray
(B) Beta
(C) Alpha
(D) Gamma
(E) Positron

2. Which of the following radionuclides is most commonly used in nuclear pharmacy practice?

(A) ^{67}Ga
(B) ^{201}Tl
(C) ^{99m}Tc
(D) ^{123}I
(E) ^{133}Xe

3. Which of the following radionuclides is generator-produced?

(A) ^{99m}Tc
(B) ^{201}Tl
(C) ^{67}Ga
(D) ^{133}Xe
(E) ^{123}I

4. Which of the following radiopharmaceuticals can be used in skeletal imaging?

(A) Technetium ^{99m}Tc albumin aggregated
(B) Technetium ^{99m}Tc medronate disodium
(C) Xenon ^{133}Xe USP
(D) Thallous chloride ^{201}Tl USP
(E) Technetium ^{99m}Tc disofenin

5. Which of the following radiopharmaceuticals is used in the diagnosis of acute cholecystitis?

(A) Technetium ^{99m}Tc sulfur colloid
(B) Technetium ^{99m}Tc medronate disodium
(C) Technetium ^{99m}Tc albumin
(D) Technetium ^{99m}Tc exametazime
(E) Technetium ^{99m}Tc disofenin

6. Which of the following cyclotron-produced radiopharmaceuticals is used for assessing regional myocardial perfusion as part of an exercise stress test?

(A) Thallous chloride ^{201}Tl USP
(B) Sodium iodide ^{123}I
(C) Gallium citrate ^{67}Ga USP
(D) Indium ^{111}In pentetate
(E) Cobalt ^{57}Co cyanocobalamin

7. Glomerular filtration and the urinary collection system can best be evaluated, using which of the following agents?

(A) Technetium ^{99m}Tc sulfur colloid
(B) Technetium ^{99m}Tc albumin
(C) Technetium ^{99m}Tc sestamibi
(D) Technetium ^{99m}Tc disofenin
(E) Technetium ^{99m}Tc pentetate

1-D
2-C
3-A
4-B
5-E
6-A
7-E

Directions: Each item below contains three suggested answers of which **one or more** is correct. Choose the answer

- **A** if **I only** is correct
- **B** if **III only** is correct
- **C** if **I and II** are correct
- **D** if **II and III** are correct
- **E** if **I, II, and III** are correct

8. The definition of the optimal radiopharmaceutical includes which of the following attributes?

   I. Short half-life
   II. Gamma photon with a 100–300 keV energy
   III. Rapid localization in target tissue and quick clearance from nontarget tissue

9. Which of the following statements are true for sodium pertechnetate ^{99m}Tc USP?

   I. It is used to radiolabel all other ^{99m}Tc radiopharmaceuticals
   II. The molybdenum 99 (^{99}Mo) breakthrough limit is less than 0.15 μCi ^{99}Mo/mCi ^{99m}Tc (< 0.15 kBq/37 MBq)
   III. It has a physical half-life of 16 hours

10. Which of the following organs can be imaged with technetium ^{99m}Tc sulfur colloid?

   I. Liver
   II. Spleen
   III. Bone marrow

11. Which of the following radiopharmaceuticals may be used to image the thyroid gland?

   I. Sodium iodide ^{131}I
   II. Sodium pertechnetate ^{99m}Tc USP
   III. Sodium iodide ^{123}I

Directions: The group of items in this section consists of lettered options followed by a set of numbered items. For each item, select the **one** lettered option that is most closely associated with it. Each lettered option may be selected once, more than once, or not at all.

Questions 12–16

Match each radiopharmaceutical with its mechanism of localization.

(A) Metabolic trapping
(B) Phagocytosis
(C) Capillary blockade
(D) Active transport
(E) Passive diffusion

12. Thallous chloride ^{201}Tl USP
13. Technetium ^{99m}Tc albumin aggregated USP
14. Technetium ^{99m}Tc sulfur colloid
15. Technetium ^{99m}Tc exametazime
16. ^{18}F flurodeoxyglucose

8-E	11-E	14-B
9-C	12-D	15-E
10-E	13-C	16-A

ANSWERS AND EXPLANATIONS

1. The answer is D *[I B 3 b].*
Current camera technology most efficiently detects gamma radiation. Alpha and beta emissions are not useful in nuclear medicine imaging due to their harmful particulate emissions and low tissue penetration. Although x-ray emissions can be used as in the case of the mercury daughter of the thallous chloride ^{201}Tl parent, they are not efficiently detected. Annihilation radiation associated with positron decay can be imaged, but this technology is currently limited to a few specialized centers.

2. The answer is C *[I C; II A 1].*
Technetium 99m (^{99m}Tc) has become the radionuclide of choice in current nuclear pharmacy practice since its introduction in the mid-1960s. ^{99m}Tc fulfills all of the requirements of the optimal radiopharmaceutical with its physical half-life of 6 hours, 140 keV gamma energy emission, ready availability, cost, and ability to be radiolabeled to a wide variety of biologically active compounds.

3. The answer is A *[II A 1 a].*
Technetium 99m (^{99m}Tc) is obtained via commercially supplied sterile, pyrogen-free "generator" systems. A generator is a device used to separate a short half-life radionuclide from the longer-lived "parent" nuclide, while retaining the parent to produce more of the daughter nuclide. In this way, short half-life nuclides can be made available on a continuous basis at great distances from the sites of generator production.

4. The answer is B *[IV A 2].*
The technetium 99m (^{99m}Tc) diphosphonate compounds are the most popular bone imaging agents currently used in nuclear medicine imaging. They are rapidly taken up by skeletal bone with 50% of the administered dose adsorbed onto bone hydroxyapatite and with the remainder excreted by the kidneys. The imaging advantages of the ^{99m}Tc, coupled with the sensitivity of bone agent localization in skeletal bone hydroxyapatite, allows for detection of bone pathology before evidence of pathology can be shown by conventional x-ray.

5. The answer is E *[VI C 1, 2].*
Technetium ^{99m}Tc disofenin is an iminodiacetic acid derivative, which is useful for hepatobiliary imaging due to its ability to be selectively cleared by a carrier-mediated hepatocyte pathway. Lack of gallbladder visualization is an abnormal finding suggestive of acute cholecystitis.

6. The answer is A *[III A 1].*
Regional uptake of thallous chloride ^{201}Tl USP (^{201}Tl) is proportional to myocardial blood supply. The injection of ^{201}Tl in concert with a treadmill exercise stress test determines myocardial perfusion at maximum cardiac output when cardiac demand outstrips supply and the distribution of ^{201}Tl is less affected by collateral blood supply within the myocardium. Regions that do not take up ^{201}Tl are interpreted as areas of infarct or ischemia. If these focal areas of decreased uptake subsequently fill in with redistributed ^{201}Tl, they are interpreted to be areas of ischemia in contrast to areas of infarct, which remain as diminished areas of activity.

7. The answer is E *[VII B 1].*
Technetium ^{99m}Tc pentetate is cleared through glomerular filtration in the same manner as inulin and can be used to determine the glomerular filtration rate (GFR) as well as in the evaluation of obstruction, vascular supply, and renal morphology.

8. The answer is E (all) *[I C].*
The optimal radiopharmaceutical has a half-life short enough to minimize radiation exposure to the patient yet long enough to allow for collection of imaging information. It should incorporate a gamma emitting radionuclide, which decays with the emission of a photon energy between 100–300 keV, which is efficiently detected with current instrumentation. The radiopharmaceutical should localize rapidly in the organ system of interest and be metabolized, excreted, or both from the nontarget tissues to maximize contrast and minimize radiation absorbed dose.

9. The answer is C (I, II) *[II A, B].*
Sodium pertechnetate ^{99m}Tc USP decays by isomeric transition with a physical half-life of 6 hours. The emission of a gamma photon has the energy of 140 keV.

10. The answer is E (all) *[VI B 1].*
Technetium ^{99m}Tc sulfur colloid localizes within the reticuloendothelial system with approximately 80%–90% of the dose of phagocytized by the Küpffer cells of the liver, 5%–10% by the spleen, and the balance by the bone marrow.

11. The answer is E (all) *[VIII B].*
Although all of the listed agents accumulate in the thyroid gland, only sodium iodide ^{123}I possesses ideal imaging characteristics and organification into thyroid hormone. While the imaging properties of sodium pertechnetate ^{99m}Tc USP are good, the pertechnetate ion is only trapped by the thyroid and not organified, thus limiting the information provided by the image.

12–16. The answers are: 12-D *[III A 1],* **13-C** *[V A 1],* **14-B** *[VI B 1],* **15-E** *[IX A 1],* **16-A** *[IX B 1].*
Thallous chloride ^{201}Tl USP is a monovalent cation with distribution analogous to potassium ion (K^+). Myocardial uptake is by active transport via the Na^+–K^+-ATPase pump.

After intravenous administration of technetium ^{99m}Tc albumin aggregated USP, 80% of the radiolabeled albumin particles become trapped by capillary blockade in the pulmonary circulation.

Following the administration of technetium ^{99m}Tc sulfur colloid, approximately 80%–90% of the dose is phagocytized by the Küpffer cells of the liver, 5%–10% by the spleen, and the balance by the bone marrow.

Technetium ^{99m}Tc exametazime is used for evaluating brain perfusion. It possesses a lipophilic partition coefficient sufficient to diffuse passively across the blood–brain barrier almost completely within one pass of the cerebral circulation, as well as being sufficiently retained to permit data collection.

^{18}F flurodeoxyglucose is used in evaluating cerebral function by mapping the distribution of cerebral glucose metabolism. As an analogue of glucose, ^{18}F flurodeoxyglucose is transported into the brain by carrier-mediated transport mechanisms responsible for transporting glucose across the blood–brain barrier. Because the presence of the F atom in the 2 position prevents metabolism beyond the phosphorylation step, ^{18}F flurodeoxyglucose becomes metabolically trapped within the brain.

Part III
Pharmacy Practice

Larry N. Swanson
Douglas J. Pisano

20
Reviewing and Dispensing Prescriptions and Medication Orders

Todd A. Brown

I. DEFINITIONS

A. **Prescriptions** are orders for drug or nondrug products that are written by a licensed practitioner who is authorized by statute to prescribe. Prescriptions are intended for use by patients on an ambulatory basis (see Appendix A). The following information should be included on a prescription:

1. **Patient information** (e.g., name, age, and home address)

2. **Date** on which the prescription was written

3. **Name and strength of the product.** The strength of the product is not required if only one strength is commercially available or if the product contains a combination of active ingredients. It is advisable to always include the strength to reduce the chance of misinterpretation of the prescription. The name may be any of the following:
   a. Proprietary (brand)
   b. Nonproprietary (generic)
   c. Chemical

4. **Quantity to be dispensed.** This should include the amount and the units of measure (e.g., grams, ounces, or tablets).

5. **Directions for the pharmacist.** Directions may be required for:
   a. Preparation (e.g., compounding)
   b. Labeling (information to be put on the prescription label)

6. **Directions for the patient.** This should include explicit instructions on the quantity and the schedule for proper use. "As Directed" should be avoided whenever possible.

7. **Refill information.** If refill information is not supplied, it is assumed that no refills are authorized.

8. **Prescriber information.** This should include the name, signature, office address, telephone number, and Drug Enforcement Administration number and/or state controlled substances number.

B. **Medication orders** are orders for drug or nondrug products that are intended for use by patients on an institutional rather than ambulatory basis. The medication order generally includes:

1. **Patient information** (e.g., name, age, and home address)

2. The **patient's identification number and known allergies**

3. **Date and time** the order was written

4. **Prescriber information** (e.g., name and signature)

5. **Name of the product.** This may include any of the following names:
   a. Proprietary (brand)
   b. Nonproprietary (generic)
   c. Chemical

6. **Product strength, dose, and route of administration.** The strength is not required if only one strength is commercially available or if the product contains a combination of active ingredients. It is advisable to include the strength to reduce the chance of misinterpreting the medication order.

7. **Directions for the pharmacist.** This may be used for:
   a. Preparation (e.g., compounding)
   b. Labeling (i.e., information to be put on the prescription label)

8. **Instructions for administration** including schedule and duration of use

9. Any **other relevant practitioner instructions** regarding patient care (e.g., radiologic procedures, laboratory tests, and diet)

II. UNDERSTANDING THE PRESCRIPTION OR MEDICATION ORDER AND EVALUATING ITS APPROPRIATENESS

A. Understanding the order

A complete understanding of all information contained in a prescription or medication order is required to ensure accurate dispensing. The pharmacist should read the entire prescription or medication order carefully to determine the prescriber's intent by interpreting the following information:

1. The patient's disease or condition requiring treatment
2. The reason the order is indicated, relative to the diagnosis or the patient's clinical condition (e.g., an antibacterial for an infection)
3. All terminology including units of measure (apothecary, metric, or English) and Latin abbreviations (see Tables 2-2, 2-3)
4. The name of the product, the quantity prescribed, and instructions for use
5. The name and address of both the patient and the physician

B. Evaluating the appropriateness of a prescription or medication order

Complete information is required on the prescription or medication order to ensure that the pharmacist could evaluate the appropriateness. When it is incomplete, the pharmacist should obtain the required information from the patient or the prescriber. The following should be considered during an evaluation:

1. The patient's disease or condition
2. The patient's allergies or hypersensitivities
3. The pharmacologic or biologic action of the prescribed product
4. The prescribed route of administration
5. Whether the prescribed product might result in a drug–drug, drug–disease, or drug–food interaction
6. Whether the dose, dosage form, and dosage regimen are safe and effective for the patient for whom the product is prescribed
7. Whether the patient will have any difficulties complying with the regimen and the potential impact on the patient's outcome
8. Whether the total quantity of medication prescribed is sufficient to allow proper completion of a course of therapy
9. Whether a physical or chemical incompatibility might result (i.e., if the product requires extemporaneous compounding)
10. Whether the prescription was issued in good faith, for a legitimate medical purpose, by a licensed practitioner, acting in the course and scope of practice

C. Discovering inappropriate prescriptions or medication orders

The pharmacist should not fill a prescription or medication order that is considered inappropriate, but should contact the prescriber. The process of calling a prescriber to discuss concerns is called **therapeutic intervention.**

1. When contacting the prescriber, the following information should be provided:
   a. A brief description of the problem
   b. A reference source which documents the problem
   c. A description of the clinical significance of the problem
   d. A suggestion or solution to the problem
2. The following resolutions are possible to solve the problem or concern:
   a. The prescription or medication order will be dispensed as written
   b. The prescription or medication order will not be dispensed
   c. The prescription or medication order will be altered and dispensed
3. If the pharmacist feels that, in his professional judgement, a prescription is inappropriate and could harm the patient, the pharmacist should not dispense the prescription. The pharmacist may also be required to explain the situation to the patient. If after a therapeutic intervention, the pharmacist feels that a medication order is still inappropriate, he should follow the guidelines of the institution.

III. PROCESSING AND DISPENSING MEDICATIONS requires that the pharmacist should follow appropriate guidelines.

A. On the prescription, the **pharmacist should record:**

1. The prescription number (for initial filling)
2. The date of filling or refilling
3. The quantity dispensed (if different from the quantity prescribed)
4. The pharmacist's initials
5. Any other information required by federal or state statutes

B. **The pharmacist must choose the correct product, dose, and dosage form** as indicated on the prescription or medication order.

C. **The pharmacist should prepare the prescription or medication order** for use by the patient. The following may be necessary for preparation:

1. Obtain the proper amount of medication to be dispensed
2. Reconstitution (addition of water or other liquid to make a solution or suspension)
3. Extemporaneous compounding (see Chapter 5)
4. Assembly of medication delivery unit
5. Performing necessary pharmaceutical calculations (see Chapter 2)

D. **The pharmacist must select the proper packaging and container** to ensure product stability, promote patient compliance, and comply with the legal requirements of packaging (see Chapter 25).

E. **Labeling the prescribed product**

1. **Prescription labels** (see Appendix A)
   The pharmacist must include the following information on the prescription label:
   a. Name and address of the pharmacy
   b. Patient's name
   c. Original date of filling
   d. Prescription number
   e. Directions for use
   f. Product's generic and/or trade name
   g. Product strength
   h. Quantity of medication dispensed
   i. Prescriber's name
   j. Lot number and expiration date
   k. Pharmacist's initials
   l. Any other information required by federal or state statutes

2. **Unit-dose packages** contain one dose or one unit of medication. For a medication order that is dispensed in **unit-dose packages,** the label should clearly identify the product's generic or trade name, product strength, lot number, and expiration date.
3. **Auxiliary and cautionary labels.** To ensure proper medication use, storage, and compliance with applicable statutes and to reinforce information provided during counseling, the pharmacist should affix **auxiliary and/or cautionary labels** as appropriate (see Appendix A).
4. For medication in Schedules II through IV (see Chapter 22), a federal transfer warning is required.

F. Record keeping

The pharmacist should maintain **prescription files and records** in accordance with standards of sound practice and statutory requirements (see Chapter 25). These records should include a **patient profile system** containing patient demographic information and a complete chronologic record of all medication use. The patient profile system may be automated (computerized) or manual (see also V A–L).

1. The patient profile should contain the following **patient information:**
   - **a.** Patient's name
   - **b.** Patient's address or room number (i.e., to identify patients that have identical names)
   - **c.** Allergies (i.e., to prevent drug allergy problems)
   - **d.** Birthdate (i.e., to assess the appropriateness of the prescribed dose)
   - **e.** Clinical condition(s) (i.e., to assist in ascertaining the appropriateness of drug/doses and to prevent drug–disease interactions)
   - **f.** Weight (i.e., to assess the appropriateness of the dose)
   - **g.** Occupation (i.e., to detect conditions associated with a particular occupation)
   - **h.** Nonprescription medication use (i.e., to prevent drug–drug interactions, drug–disease interactions, and other problems)
2. In addition, the patient profile should contain the following information from each prescription or medication order:
   - **a.** The name of the product
   - **b.** The strength of the product
   - **c.** The dosage form
   - **d.** The quantity dispensed
   - **e.** Complete directions for use
   - **f.** The prescription number
   - **g.** The dispensing date
   - **h.** The number of refills authorized or remaining
   - **i.** The prescriber's name
   - **j.** The initials of the dispensing pharmacist

IV. COUNSELING PATIENTS AND HEALTH PROFESSIONALS

The pharmacist's responsibilities include counseling patients and health professionals on the safe and effective use of medication.

A. Counseling patients

The pharmacist should evaluate the patient's understanding of each medication and supply additional information when the patient's information is incorrect or insufficient. The pharmacist may need to advise patients regarding the proper dosage, appearance, and name of the medication. Information about the route of administration, instructions for use, the duration of use, and the reason the products were prescribed may also be needed. In addition, the following topics may also be appropriate during the counseling session:

1. **Special procedures.** As appropriate, the pharmacist may advise patients on how to take the medication (e.g., on an empty stomach or with plenty of water) or may warn patients on what to avoid while taking the medication (e.g., alcoholic beverages or dairy products).
2. **Potential adverse effects.** The pharmacist may warn patients about possible adverse effects associated with the medication, may offer advice on ways to manage or minimize them, and may inform patients what action(s) should be taken if adverse effects occur.
3. **Proper storage.** The pharmacist should tell patients how to store products properly to ensure stability and potency.

4. **Over-the-counter (OTC) products.** The pharmacist should caution patients about the use of OTC products that may not be appropriate when taken with a prescribed product.

B. **Counseling nursing personnel.** The pharmacist should advise nurses regarding the indications, contraindications, adverse effects, monitoring parameters, and usual dosage for medication orders written for patients under their care.

C. **Counseling physicians and allied health professionals.** To ensure the safe and effective use of prescribed medications, the pharmacist may counsel health professionals on the following topics:

1. The choice of prescription product
2. The proper dosage, dosage regimen, and route of administration
3. The cost of the prescribed product and the costs associated with its use (i.e., administration costs and costs of treating possible adverse reactions)
4. Commercially available products and their strengths
5. Potential adverse drug effects
6. Drug interactions
7. Physical incompatibilities
8. Safe handling of chemotherapeutic agents
9. Nutritional support
10. Drug interference with laboratory tests

V. PATIENT MONITORING.

The pharmacist should establish effective monitoring practices to determine the therapeutic success or failure of a particular medication. Monitoring should be performed on a regular basis. A comprehensive **patient profile system** is required for good patient monitoring. It permits the pharmacist to detect the following:

A. **Late refills of maintenance products.** If this problem occurs, the pharmacist should discuss with the patient the importance of compliance.

B. **Acute medical conditions for which completion of therapy is essential** (i.e., completing the last 5 days of a 10-day course of antibiotic therapy). The pharmacist should monitor available refills to ensure completion of therapy.

C. **Adverse effects or iatrogenic disease.** The pharmacist should monitor situations in which the condition may have resulted from a prescribed product.

D. **OTC (nonlegend) interactions.** The pharmacist should attempt to monitor the patient's selection of OTC products to avoid interactions with prescribed products.

E. **Therapeutic parameters.** To ensure that the prescribed product has safe and effective results, the pharmacist should monitor parameters such as the patient's drug sensitivities, serum drug concentrations, and nutritional status when available.

F. **Duplicate prescribing of medication.** The pharmacist should monitor situations in which two medications that are exactly the same or similar are prescribed without the knowledge of the prescriber(s).

G. **Potential drug misuse or abuse.** With some medication (especially those used in chronic conditions) the focus is on patient compliance, however, with other medication (i.e., narcotics and other controlled substances) the pharmacist should check for the possibility of abuse.

H. **Potential allergies.** All allergies should be verified by the patient or by medical notes if possible as adverse effects are often misclassified as allergies.

I. **Unintended changes in therapy** that may result from mistakes in writing a prescription or medication order should be monitored.

J. Additive effects, which can result when unrelated medications contain similar pharmacologic effects, should be monitored.

K. Changes in patient's drug regimen. To prevent potential drug interactions or contraindications, the pharmacist must carefully consult the patient profile when new legend products are added to a patient's regimen.

L. Therapeutic failure. The pharmacist should monitor the patient's clinical condition for evidence of therapeutic failure (i.e., drug failure). Signs include:

1. The presence of symptoms of a condition that is currently being treated
2. A desire by the patient for a nonprescription medication that has similar effects to a prescribed medication

STUDY QUESTIONS

Directions: Each of the numbered items or incomplete statements in this section is followed by answers or by completions of the statement. Select the **one** lettered answer or completion that is **best** in each case.

1. Medication orders differ from prescriptions in which of the following ways?

(A) They are intended for ambulatory use
(B) They contain only the generic name of the drug
(C) They may contain nonmedication instructions from the practitioner
(D) They may be written by an unlicensed practitioner
(E) They contain the quantity of medication to be dispensed

2. A prescription label should contain all of the following EXCEPT

(A) the quantity dispensed
(B) the lot number
(C) the patient's diagnosis
(D) the expiration date
(E) the physician's name

3. Auxiliary/cautionary labels should be utilized for all of the following purposes EXCEPT

(A) to substitute for verbal consultation
(B) to ensure proper usage
(C) to inform the patient of storage requirements
(D) to comply with statutory requirements
(E) to warn against the concomitant use of certain drugs or foods

4. A pharmacist must monitor patients receiving medications to detect each of the following problems EXCEPT

(A) therapeutic failure
(B) adverse reactions
(C) drug interactions
(D) progression of the disease state
(E) noncompliance

5. The following items are essential for a patient profile system EXCEPT

(A) the patient's name
(B) the prescriber's Drug Enforcement Administration registration number
(C) the patient's allergies
(D) the patient's birthdate
(E) instructions for medication use

6. If therapeutic intervention is necessary, the following information should be communicated to the prescriber EXCEPT

(A) a declaration that a "mistake" was made
(B) a brief description of the problem
(C) a reference source that documents the problem
(D) an alternative or suggestion to the problem
(E) a description of the clinical significance of the problem

---

1-C
2-C
3-A

4-D
5-B
6-A

ANSWERS AND EXPLANATIONS

1. The answer is C *[I B]*.
Medication orders, because they are written for the care of inpatients, often contain laboratory, radiologic, and other nonmedication orders. Both medication orders and prescriptions may contain the trade or generic name of the drug. Only prescriptions contain the quantity of medication to be dispensed. Neither prescriptions nor medication orders are written by unlicensed practitioners.

2. The answer is C *[III E 1]*.
The quantity of medication dispensed, the lot number, the expiration date of the product, and the physician's name should appear on prescription labels. The patient's diagnosis, although listed on the patient's medication profile, is not included on the prescription label.

3. The answer is A *[III E 3; IV A 1]*.
Auxiliary/cautionary labels are an adjunct to verbal consultation, not a replacement. Appropriate uses for such labels include assuring the patient of proper use, citing storage requirements, complying with statutory requirements, and warning against food and drug interactions.

4. The answer is D *[V A, C, J, L]*.
Pharmacists have the clinical responsibility of monitoring patients for the therapeutic success or failure of drug therapy and for adverse reactions, drug interactions, and noncompliance. Monitoring patients for progression of their disease state is generally the responsibility of the patient's physician.

5. The answer is B *[III F 1, 2; V A–L]*.
The patient's name is required to identify each patient. Often the address or room number is required to identify patients with similar names. The patient's allergies, birthdate, and instructions for medication use are required to prevent drug allergy problems and assess the appropriateness of the medication and dose. The prescriber's Drug Enforcement Administration registration number is not necessary for a patient profile system.

6. The answer is A *[II C 1]*.
Information provided to the prescriber during a therapeutic intervention should include a description of the problem, a reference source, a description of the clinical significance, and an alternative. Informing the prescriber that a mistake was made does not encourage cooperation and resolution of the problem.

21 Drug Information Resources

Paul F. Souney
Brian F. Shea

I. DEFINITION. Drug information is current, critically examined, relevant data about drugs and drug use in a given patient or situation.

A. Current information uses the most recent, up-to-date sources possible.

B. Critically examined information should meet the following criteria.

1. More than one source should be used when appropriate.
2. The extent of agreement of sources should be determined; if sources do not agree, good judgment should be used.
3. The plausibility of information, based on clinical circumstances, should be determined.

C. Relevant information must be presented in a manner that applies directly to the circumstances under consideration (e.g., patient parameters, therapeutic objectives, alternative approaches).

II. DRUG INFORMATION RESOURCES. There are three sources of drug information: journals (primary sources), indexing and abstracting services (secondary sources), and textbooks (tertiary sources).

A. Primary sources

1. **Benefits.** Journal articles provide the most current information about drugs and, ideally, should be the source for answering therapeutic questions. Journals enable pharmacists to:
   a. Keep abreast of professional news
   b. Learn how a second clinician handles a particular problem
   c. Keep up with new developments in pathophysiology, diagnostic agents, and therapeutic regimens
   d. Distinguish useful from useless or even harmful therapy
   e. Enhance communication with other health care professionals and consumers
   f. Obtain continuing education credits
   g. Share opinions with other health care professionals through letters-to-the-editor columns
   h. Prepare for the Board certification examination in pharmacotherapy
2. **Limitations.** Although publication of an article in a well-known, respected journal enhances the credibility of information contained in an article, this does not guarantee that the article is accurate. Many articles possess inadequacies that become apparent as the ability to evaluate drug information improves.

B. Secondary sources

1. **Benefits.** Indexing and abstracting services (Table 21-1) are valuable tools for quick and selective screening of the primary literature for specific information, data, citation, and articles. In some cases, the sources provide sufficient information to serve as references for answering drug information requests.

Table 21-1. Examples of Abstracting/Indexing Services

Secondary References	Journals Indexed	Lag Time
ClinAlert	150	1–6 weeks
Current Contents	1200	1–6 weeks
Drugs in Use	1000	6–24 months
Drugdex		3–6 months
Index Medicus	2700	3–12 months
Inpharma	1700	3 weeks – 6 months
International Pharmaceutical Abstracts	500–1000	6–14 months
Iowa Drug Information System	160	3–12 months
Pharmaceutical News Index		2–8 weeks
Reactions	1700	3 weeks – 6 months
Science Citation Index	2000	3–12 months

2. **Limitations.** Each indexing or abstracting service **reviews a finite number of journals**. Therefore, relying on only one service can greatly hinder the thoroughness of a literature search. Another important fact to remember is the substantial difference in lag time (i.e., the interval between publication of an article and citation of the article in an index) among various services. Several examples are given in Table 21-1.
   a. Secondary sources **usually describe only articles and clinical studies** from journals. Frequently, readers respond to, criticize, and add new information to published articles and studies through letters. Services such as Index Medicus, Drugs in Use, or the Iowa Drug Information System generally do include pertinent letters to the editor within the scope of coverage.
   b. Indexing and abstracting services are primarily used to locate journal articles. In general, abstracts should not be used as primary sources of information, since they are generally interpretations of a study and may be a misinterpretation of important information. Pharmacists should obtain and evaluate the original article, since abstracts may not tell the whole story.

C. Tertiary sources

1. **Benefits.** General reference textbooks can provide easy and convenient access to a broad spectrum of related topics. Background information on drugs and diseases is often available. However, while a textbook may answer many drug-related questions, the limitations of these sources should not be overlooked.
   a. It may take several years to publish a text, so information available in textbooks may not include the most recent developments in the field. Other resources should be used to update or supplement information obtained from textbooks.
   b. The author of a textbook may not have done a thorough search of the literature, so pertinent data may have been omitted. An author may also have misinterpreted the primary or secondary literature. Reference citations should be available to verify the validity and accuracy of the data.
2. **General considerations** when examining and utilizing textbooks as sources of drug information include:
   a. The author, publisher, or both: What are the author's and publisher's track records?
   b. The year of publication (copyright date)
   c. The edition of the text: Is it the most current edition?
   d. The presence or absence of a bibliography: If a bibliography is included, are important statements accurately referenced? When were the references published?
   e. The scope of the textbook: How accessible is the information?
   f. Alternative resources that are available (e.g., primary and secondary sources, other relevant texts)

III. ELECTRONIC BULLETIN BOARDS (EBB)

A. Benefits. An EBB expands the ability to monitor therapies recently published or discussed in the media. The use of EBBs may prevent duplication of drug information searches by users.

B. Limitations

1. Unlike information published in journals or textbooks, information obtained from an EBB is generally not peer reviewed or edited prior to release.
2. Information from the EBB is only as reliable as the person who posted it and the users who read and comment on its contents.

C. Use. EBBs can be reached using a computer with a modem and communication software to access telephone communication lines. Specifics regarding modem settings required to access the EBB may be obtained via the EBB's system operator. Information obtained from the EBB should be used in the same way information obtained from a consultation with a colleague is handled. See Table 21-2 for a list of EBBs specific for pharmacists.

IV. STRATEGIES FOR EVALUATING INFORMATION REQUESTS.

It is important to obtain as many clues as possible about drug information requests before beginning a literature search. Both time and money can be wasted on doing a vast search. Below are important questions to ask the inquirer or evaluate prior to a manual or computerized search.

A. Talk with the inquirer. Before spending time searching for information, talk to the person who is requesting the information and acquire any necessary additional information.

1. **Determine the reason for the inquiry.** Find out where the inquirer heard or read about the drug. Is he or she taking the medication? If so, why? Determine if the inquirer has a medical condition, since the search may be able to be done by drug name or disease name. Ascertaining the reason for the inquiry helps in determining what additional information should be provided. For example, if the inquiry concerns a foreign drug, the inquirer may ask for a domestic equivalent.
2. **Clarify the drug's identification and availability.** Make sure that the drug in question is available and double check information about the drug, such as:
   - a. The **correct spelling** of the drug's name
   - b. Whether it is a **generic or brand-name drug**
   - c. What **pharmaceutical company** manufactures the drug and in what **country** the drug is manufactured
   - d. Whether the drug is **prescription or nonprescription**
   - e. Whether the drug is still **under investigation** and, if it is on the market, **the length of time on the market**
   - f. The **dosage form** of the drug
   - g. The **purpose of the drug** (i.e., what medical condition or symptom is the drug intended to alleviate; this information helps narrow the search if products with similar names are found)

Table 21-2. Selected Pharmacy-Oriented Electronic Bulletin Boards (EBBs)

EBB	Sponsor	Availability	Baud rate*	Phone number
ClinNet	American College of Clinical Pharmacy (ACCP)	For ACCP members only	1200 or 2400	412-648-7893
F.I.X.	The Formulary	Annual subscription fee	1200 or 2400	800-262-8664
PharmLine	American Association of Colleges of Pharmacy (AACP)	For AACP members only	1200 or 2400	800-247-4276
PharmNet	American Society of Hospital Pharmacists (ASHP)	For ASHP members only	1200 or 2400	800-848-8980 (call for local number)
FDA	Food and Drug Administration (FDA)	Anyone can access; no fee	1200 or 2400	800-222-0185

*Baud rate signifies the type of modem that can be used to connect with the EBB.

B. To identify or assess product availability, consider using noncomputerized resources (see also Appendix D).

1. For drugs manufactured in the **United States,** the following resources are available:
   a. *Martindale: The Extra Pharmacopoeia,* which is updated every 5 years
   b. The *American Drug Index,* which is updated annually
   c. *Drug Facts and Comparisons,* which is updated monthly and bound annually
   d. *Drug Topics Red Book* or *Blue Book,* which releases supplements and is updated annually
   e. The *Physician's Desk Reference,* which is updated annually
   f. The *American Hospital Formulary Service (AHFS) Drug Information,* which is supplemented quarterly and updated annually

2. For drugs manufactured in **foreign countries,** the following resources are available:
   a. *Martindale: The Extra Pharmacopoeia*
   b. *Index Nominum*
   c. *United States Adopted Names (USAN)* and the *United States Pharmacopeia (USP) Dictionary of Drug Names*

3. For **investigational drugs,** the following resources are available:
   a. *Martindale: The Extra Pharmacopoeia*
   b. *Drug Facts and Comparisons*

4. For **orphan drugs** [i.e., drugs that are used to prevent or treat a rare disease (affect < 200,000 people in the United States, so the cost of development is not likely to be offset by sales) and for which the FDA offers assistance and financial incentives to sponsors undertaking the development of the drugs], the following resources are available:
   a. *Drug Facts and Comparisons*
   b. The *National Information Center for Orphan Drugs and Rare Diseases* (NICODARD)

5. For **an unknown drug** (i.e., one that is in hand but not identified) chemical analysis can be performed or the drug can be identified by physical characteristics, such as color, special markings, and shape. Consult the following sources for help:
   a. The *Physician's Desk Reference*
   b. Identidex
   c. The manufacturer
   d. A laboratory

V. SEARCH STRATEGIES. To develop an effective search strategy for locating drug information literature, the following tactics should be followed after determining whether primary or secondary sources are desired.

A. Determine whether the question at hand is clinical or research-related. **Define the question as specifically as possible.** Also, identify appropriate index terms (also called keywords or descriptors) with which to search for the information.

B. Determine the type of information that is needed and how much is needed (i.e., only one fact, the most recent journal articles, review articles, or a comprehensive database search).

C. Ascertain as much information as possible about the drug being questioned and the inquirer's association with it. Remember that data on adverse drug effects or drug interactions is often fragmented and inadequately documented. See IV A 2 for the specific drug information that should be acquired, and also determine answers to the following questions.

1. What is the indication for the prescribed drug?

2. Is the drug's use approved or unapproved? This information can be found in the following resources (remember to check how often these resources are updated to ensure having the latest information):
   a. **Approved uses** of drugs can be checked in:
      (1) *AHFS Drug Information* for the current year and in the year's supplements
      (2) *Drug Facts and Comparisons*
      (3) *Physician's Desk Reference*
   b. **Unapproved uses** of drugs can be found in:
      (1) *AHFS Drug Information*
      (2) *Drug Facts and Comparisons*

(3) *Martindale: The Extra Pharmacopoeia*
(4) Index Medicus or other computer programs (e.g., Medline, Paperchase)
(5) Drugdex
(6) *Inpharma*

3. What is the age, sex, and weight of the patient in question?

4. Does the patient have any other medical conditions or renal or hepatic disease?

5. Is the patient taking any other medications?

6. What drugs has the patient taken over the past 6 months and what were the dosages?

7. Did the patient experience any signs or symptoms of a possible adverse drug reaction? If so:
a. How severe was the reaction?
b. When did the reaction appear?
c. Has the patient (or any member of the patient's family) experienced any allergic or adverse reactions to medications in the past?
d. Consult the following resources for more information:
(1) Meyler's *Side Effects of Drugs* (SEDBASE online)
(2) A general drug reference
(3) *Reactions* (ADIS)
(4) Index Medicus

8. Did the patient experience any signs or symptoms of an adverse drug interaction? If so:
a. What were the specific drugs in question?
b. What were the respective dosages of the drugs?
c. What was the duration of therapy?
d. What was the length of the course of administration?
e. What are the details of the events secondary to the suspected reaction?
f. Consult the following resources for more information:
(1) A drug interactions reference [e.g., *Drug Interaction Facts,* Hansten's *Evaluations of Drug Interactions* (*EDI*)]
(2) A general drug reference (e.g., *Martindale: The Extra Pharmacopoeia)*
(3) *Reactions*
(4) Index Medicus

9. What is the patient's current medication status?

10. Does the patient have any underlying diseases?

11. How has the patient been managed so far?

12. What is the stability of the drug and how is compatibility of the drug with other drugs, the administration technique, and the equipment that holds it? Resources to check for this information include:
a. Trissel's *Handbook on Injectable Drugs*
b. King's *Guide to Parenteral Admixtures*

D. Explore other possible information resources if necessary. For example, it may be useful to find background material in textbooks (tertiary references) then go to the journal literature (primary references) for more current information. Also, the manufacturer of the drug may be a useful source for missing information. In exchange for information, most companies expect to receive an adverse drug reaction form.

VI. EVALUATING A CLINICAL STUDY. Resource identification is followed by a critical assessment of the available information. This step is critical in developing an appropriate response for the inquirer.

A. Evaluate the objective of the study. Determine the aim of the research that was performed. What did the researchers intend to examine? Is this goal stated clearly (i.e., is the objective specific)? Was the research limited to a single objective, or were there multiple drugs or effects being tested?

B. Evaluate the subjects of the study. Determine the profile of the study population by looking for the following information.

1. Were healthy subjects or affected patients used in the study?

2. Were the subjects volunteers?
3. What were the criteria for selecting the subjects?
4. How many subjects were included and what is the breakdown of age, sex, and race?
5. If a disease was being treated, did any of the subjects have diseases other than that being initially treated? Were any additional treatments given? Were there any contraindications to the therapy?
6. What was the patient selection method and who was excluded from the study?

C. **Evaluate the administration of the drug treatment.** For each drug being investigated, determine the following information:

1. **Details of treatment with the agent being studied:**
   a. Daily dose
   b. Frequency of administration
   c. Hours of day when administered
   d. Route of administration
   e. Source of drug (i.e., the supplier)
   f. Dosage form
   g. Timing of drug administration in relation to factors affecting drug absorption
   h. Methods of ensuring compliance
   i. Total duration of treatment
2. **Other therapeutic measures in addition to the agent being studied**

D. **Evaluate the setting of the study.** Try to determine the environment of the study as well as the dates on which the trial began and ended. Look for the following information:

1. People who made the observations (Various professionals offer different and unique perspectives based on their backgrounds and interests. Were the same people making observations throughout the study?)
2. Whether the study was done on an inpatient or outpatient basis
3. Description of physical setting (i.e., hospital, clinic, ward)
4. Length of the study (dates on which the trial began and ended)

E. **Evaluate the methods and design of the study.** The study design (e.g., retrospective, prospective, blind, crossover) and the methods used to complete the study are very important in judging whether the study and the results are valid. From the study, try to determine answers to the following questions:

1. Are the methods of assessing the therapeutic effects clearly described?
2. Were the methods standardized?
3. Were control measures used to reduce variation that might influence the results? Examples of such control methods include:
   a. Concurrent controls
   b. Stratification or matched subgroups
   c. A run-in period
   d. The patient as his or her own control (i.e., crossover design)
   e. Identical ancillary treatment
4. Were controls used to reduce bias? Examples of such controls include:
   a. **Blind assessment,** which means that the people observing the patients do not know who is a subject and who is a control
   b. **Blind patients,** which means that the patients do not know whether they received the substance being studied or a placebo
   c. **Random allocation,** which means that patients involved in the study have an even chance of being assigned to either the group of subjects receiving the active drug or the group receiving controls

   d. **Matching dummies,** which are placebos that are physically identical to the active agent being studied
   e. **Comparison** of a placebo or a therapy to a recognized standard practice

F. Evaluate the analysis of the study. After looking at specific areas of the study separately, pull all of the information together to determine whether the trial is acceptable and the conclusions are justified by determining answers to the following questions.

1. Were the subjects suitably selected in relation to the aim(s) of the study?
2. Were the methods of measurement valid in relation to the aim(s) of the study?
3. Were the methods adequately standardized?
4. Were the methods sufficiently sensitive?
5. Was the design appropriate?
6. Were there enough subjects?
7. Was the dosage appropriate?
8. Was the duration of treatment adequate?
9. Were carryover effects avoided or were compensations made for them?
10. If no controls were used, were they unnecessary or overlooked?
11. If controls were used, were they adequate?
12. Was the comparability of treatment groups examined?
13. Are the data adequate for assessment?
14. If statistical tests were not done, were they unnecessary or overlooked?
15. If statistical tests are reported, assess the following:
    a. Is it clear how the statistical tests were done?
    b. Were the tests appropriately used?
    c. If results show no significant difference between test groups, were there enough patients (i.e., statistical power)?

VII. GENERAL GUIDELINES FOR RESPONSES TO DRUG INFORMATION REQUESTS

A. Do not guess!

B. Responses to a member of the public must take several ethical issues into account.

1. Patient privacy must be protected.
2. Professional ethics must be maintained.
3. The patient/physician relationship cannot be breached.
4. Response is not necessary if the inquirer intends to misuse or abuse information that is provided. The inquirer often admits intent or offers clues to potential abuse, such as in the following examples.
    a. A patient asks how a certain drug is dosed (i.e., how much the drug can be increased, when it can be increased, and what the maximum daily dose is). This kind of inquiry signals that the patient may be adjusting his or her own therapy.
    b. A patient asks a pharmacist to identify a tablet that is a prescription product known for a high rate of abuse.

C. Organize information before attempting to communicate the response to the inquirer. Anticipate additional questions.

D. Tailor the response to the inquirer's background. Also, consider the environment of the practice, institutional policy and procedure, and formulary.

E. Inform the inquirer where the information was found. Exercise caution with statements such as, "There are no reports in the literature."

F. Use **extreme** caution with statements such as, "I recommend . . ." Do not hesitate to refer consumers to their physicians.

G. Use more than abstracts to answer drug information questions, since abstracts may be taken out of context and do not include all of the data that is available in the original article.

H. Alert the inquirer of a possible delay when it takes longer than anticipated to answer the question.

I. Ask if the information that is provided answers the inquirer's questions.

J. Ask if the inquirer wishes to have reprints of articles or a written response.

22
Federal Pharmacy Law

Douglas J. Pisano
F. Randy Vogenberg

I. HISTORICAL PERSPECTIVE: 1900 TO 1970. Prior to 1900, pharmacy depended on compendia such as the *United States Pharmacopeia (USP)–National Formulary (NF)* to regulate or standardize pharmacy practice. Between 1900 and 1970, the following acts were put into effect.

A. 1906: The Pure Food and Drug Act (PFDA) required all foods and drugs to meet a standard of strength and purity.

B. 1911: The Sherley Amendment to the PFDA prohibited any company from making false therapeutic claims when labeling medicines for the purpose of defrauding the purchaser and put the responsibility of proving fraud on the government.

C. 1914: The Harrison Narcotic Act regulated the importation, sale, manufacture, and use of opium, cocaine, marijuana, many synthetic analgesics, and derivatives that produce or sustain physical or psychologic dependence.

D. 1931: The Food and Drug Administration (FDA) was renamed in order to enforce existing drug laws.

E. 1938: The Federal Food, Drug, and Cosmetic Act (FFDCA) resulted from the "Elixir of sulfanilamide" tragedies, in which 107 people died from taking elixir of sulfanilamide that contained the toxic solvent ethylene glycol.

1. This act required that the following criteria be met.
   a. Manufacturers of drugs and cosmetics must prove that their products are safe.
   b. Medical devices must be proven effective.
2. This act gave the FDA limited authority to remove products from the marketplace if they are found to be ineffective or unsafe.

F. 1952: The Durham–Humphrey Amendments to the FFDCA further clarified the distinction between prescription and over-the-counter (OTC) drugs based on whether or not the drugs were habit-forming, narcotic, hypnotic, or potentially harmful. These amendments required a physician's consent in order to dispense refills, giving rise to the legend, "Caution: Federal law prohibits dispensing without a prescription."

G. 1962: The Kefauver-Harris Amendments to the FFDCA required drug manufacturers to prove the safety and efficacy of their products before approval was given by the FDA for marketing. These amendments resulted from the thalidomide tragedies in which the sedative thalidomide was used in Europe as an antinauseant for pregnant women, and it caused severe deformities in their offspring. Thalidomide was never approved for use in the United States.

H. 1966: The Drug Efficacy Study Implementation (DESI) review took place when the FDA contracted an outside agency (the National Academy of Sciences/National Research Council) to establish panels of scientists in order to examine the efficacy of all drugs that were manufactured between 1938 and 1962. Approximately 4000 of these drugs were then rated as effective, probably effective, possibly effective, or ineffective.

II. SIGNIFICANT FEDERAL DRUG LAWS: 1970 TO 1991. Many of the laws and regulations that pharmacists must follow are partly due to amendments of the FFDCA of 1938.

A. 1970: Controlled Substances Act (CSA). The CSA is Title II of a much larger piece of legislation, the Comprehensive Drug Abuse Prevention and Control Act of 1970, which was enacted to improve the administration and regulation of all parties involved with the manufacturing, distribution, and dispensing of controlled substances.

1. Scheduling. The CSA places medicinal substances in schedules (or classes) in descending order, based on their potential for abuse, psychologic or physiologic dependence, and medical use.

a. Schedule I drugs include heroin, hallucinogenic substances, marijuana, opiates, and opium derivatives.

(1) These drugs have high abuse potential and no accepted medical use in the United States.

(2) Prescriptions may not be written for drugs of this class.

b. Schedule II drugs include morphine, short-acting barbiturates and amphetamines, and glutethimide.

(1) These drugs have high abuse potential, accepted medical use, and severe psychological and physiologic dependence.

(2) Prescriptions are not refillable and require a new, original prescription order.

(3) Dispensing part of the written amount requires pharmacists to record the number of units dispensed and to dispense the remainder within 72 hours. If the remaining units cannot be dispensed to the patient within this time frame, further quantities cannot be dispensed, and the physician must be notified.

(4) Partial dispensing of prescriptions in Schedule II for patients in a long-term care facility (LTCF) or who are medically diagnosed as terminally ill is valid for 60 days from the date of issuance.

(a) The pharmacist must record that the patient is in a LTCF or is terminally ill.

(b) The pharmacist must record the date, quantity dispensed, and quantity remaining.

(c) The pharmacist's initials or signature must appear on the back of the prescription.

(5) In an emergency situation, prescriptions involving Schedule II drugs may be called into a pharmacy via telephone provided that certain criteria are met:

(a) Immediate administration is necessary for proper treatment.

(b) No appropriate alternative is available, including a non–Schedule II controlled substance.

(c) The prescribing physician cannot reasonably provide a written prescription.

c. Schedule III drugs include tablet combinations with codeine, any suppository containing a barbiturate, and anabolic steroids.

(1) These drugs have less potential for abuse and dependence than Schedule II drugs.

(2) Prescriptions may be refilled up to five times within 6 months of the date that the prescription was first issued.

(3) Dispensing part of prescriptions requires pharmacists to record the quantity dispensed and the initials of the dispensing pharmacist either on the face of the original order or on the back of a refill.

(4) All partial dispensing must be done within 6 months of the issuance of the original prescription.

d. Schedule IV drugs include benzodiazepines, meprobamate, and propoxyphene. These drugs have less potential for abuse than Schedule III drugs. The rules for dispensing are the same as for Schedule III drugs.

e. Schedule V drugs include preparations containing opium derivatives for the control of coughs and diarrhea.

(1) These drugs have a low potential for abuse or dependence as compared to Schedule III or IV drugs.

(2) There are no refill limitations on prescriptions except that all refills must be dispensed in good faith based on the professional judgment of the pharmacist and the physician.

(3) Schedule V drugs include controlled substances that may be legally sold over the counter without a prescription (i.e., historically referred to as exempt narcotics) provided the following criteria are met.

(a) The substance must be sold by a pharmacist.

(b) Not more than 240 ml (or 48 solid dosage units) of opium-containing substances or 120 ml (or 24 solid dosage units) of non–opium-containing controlled substances may be dispensed within a 48-hour period.

(c) The purchaser must be at least 18 years of age and, if requested, submit identification to the pharmacist.

(d) The pharmacy must maintain a bound book to record the dispensing of Schedule V substances for a period of 2 years. The following information must be included:

(i) Name and address of purchaser

(ii) Name and quantity of controlled substance

(iii) Date of sale

(iv) Initials or name of dispensing pharmacist

2. **Order forms.** Schedule II controlled substances must be ordered by using a **DEA-222 order form.**
   - **a.** Upon receipt of ordered Schedule II controlled substances, the registrant must record on the retained store copy the number and date of each item received.
   - **b.** Persons with proper power of attorney may sign the DEA-222 order form as well.
   - **c.** Significant **loss or theft** of controlled substances must be reported to the Drug Enforcement Administration (DEA) using **form 106.**

3. **Recordkeeping and inventory**
   - **a.** The DEA requires that a registrant take an inventory every 2 years (biennially) within 4 days of the anniversary of the initial inventory date.
   - **b.** A registrant may change the date of the biennial inventory as long as the nearest DEA office is notified in advance and the date does not vary more than 6 months from the date of anniversary of the initial inventory date.
   - **c.** All records of receipt and distribution of controlled substances must be kept for 2 years.

4. **Controlled substance warning label.** Labels of any drug listed in Schedules II–IV must contain the following warning statement: "CAUTION: Federal law prohibits the transfer of this drug to any person other than the patient for whom it was prescribed."

5. **Corresponding responsibility.** A prescription for a controlled substance must be issued in good faith for a legitimate medical purpose by a practitioner in the usual course of his or her professional practice. Likewise, **pharmacists** have the corresponding responsibility to ensure that the prescription is issued and dispensed in good faith for a legitimate medical purpose by a practitioner acting in the usual course of his or her practice.

6. **United States postal regulations.** Pharmacists may not mail narcotic drugs in any schedule or quantity through the United States mail unless they are carrying out the duties of the Veterans Administration, the DEA, the military, law enforcement, or civil defense.
   - **a.** Opiates, semisynthetic narcotics, and their derivatives (e.g., meperidine, propoxyphene, diphenoxylate) may not be mailed.
   - **b.** Cocaine may not be mailed.
   - **c.** Schedule II controlled substances that are not in the above categories may be mailed to the patient.

B. 1970: Poison Prevention Packaging Act was passed in response to accidental poisonings in children. With certain qualifications, the act generally requires a child-resistant closure on aspirin, acetaminophen, methylsalicylate, controlled substances, iron-containing drugs, diphenhydramine, and most oral prescription drugs.

1. **Exemptions.** Some examples of drug products that are exempt from this act and do not require child-resistant closures include sublingual nitroglycerine, cholestyramine powder, and effervescent potassium supplements.

2. **Request for non–child-resistant containers.** Physicians and patients may request that prescriptions be dispensed in containers with non–child-resistant closures. Only the patient may give a blanket authorization requesting that all of his or her prescriptions be dispensed in non–child-resistant containers.

3. **Reusing containers.** Plastic child-resistant containers may not be reused. Glass containers may be reused as long as the safety closure is replaced.

C. 1972: OTC drug review. The FDA appointed advisory panels to evaluate approximately 80 therapeutic classes of drugs in order to assure that they are safe and effective for use by the public for self treatment. Ingredients for OTC use were classified in one of three categories:

1. **Category I.** Drugs are safe and effective and not misbranded (i.e., do not include false, misleading, or incomplete labeling).

2. **Category II.** Drugs are not safe and effective, or they are misbranded.

3. **Category III.** The data available are insufficient for classification of these drugs.

D. **1982: The Federal Anti-Tampering Act** was enacted in response to the 1982 deliberate contamination of Tylenol R capsules. This act requires the following.

1. Tamper-resistant packaging must be used for certain OTC products, cosmetics, and medical devices.

2. Packages "must have an indicator or barrier to entry that, when breached or missing, can reasonably be expected to provide visible evidence to consumers that tampering has occurred."

E. **1983: The Orphan Drug Act** allows manufacturers to gain incentives for the research, development, and marketing of drug products that are used to treat rare diseases or conditions that would otherwise be unprofitable.

F. **1984: The Drug Price Competition and Patent Term Restoration Act (Waxmann-Hatch Amendments to the FFDCA)** was enacted to create a fair environment between the pioneer drug manufacturer and the emerging generic drug industry.

1. **Title I** of this act allows generic drug firms to use Abbreviated New Drug Applications (ANDA) to gain quicker FDA approval for their products.

2. **Title II** provides pioneer drug companies with patent extensions for those products that lose marketing time while in the regulatory review process.

G. **1987: The Prescription Drug Marketing Act** was enacted to address the problems associated with the diversion of prescription drugs from legitimate commercial channels. This act:

1. Requires states to license wholesalers

2. Bans the sale, trade, or purchase of drug samples

3. Requires that all requests for drug samples by practitioners be made in writing and that records be maintained concerning the receipt and storage of drug samples

III. DRUG RECALLS.

Manufacturers usually recall products when requested by the FDA, which has no authority to recall a drug but may remove a drug from the marketplace through its seizure powers.

A. **Class I recalls** exist when there is a reasonable possibility that the use of a product will cause either serious adverse effects on health or will cause death.

B. **Class II recalls** exist when the use of a product may cause temporary or medically reversible adverse effects on health or when the probability of serious adverse effects on health is remote.

C. **Class III recalls** exist when the use of a product is not likely to cause adverse health consequences.

IV. PATIENT PACKAGE INSERTS (PPIs)

are required by FDA regulation to be provided to the patient when dispensing certain drugs. All of the following are drugs that must be dispensed with a PPI:

A. Isoproterenol inhalation products

B. Oral contraceptives

C. Estrogenic drug products

D. Intrauterine devices

E. Progestational drug products

F. Isotretinoin

STUDY QUESTIONS

Directions: Each of the numbered items or incomplete statements in this section is followed by answers or by completions of the statement. Select the **one** lettered answer or completion that is **best** in each case.

1. The Federal Food, Drug, and Cosmetic Act (FFDCA) of 1938 was enacted due to which one of the following situations?

(A) Thalidomide deaths
(B) Elixir of sulfanilamide deaths
(C) Necessary restriction for the dispensing of controlled substances
(D) Necessary allowance for granting generic drugs access to the market

2. An example of a drug product that cannot be sent through the United States mail is

(A) diazepam
(B) ranitidine
(C) pentazocine
(D) meprobamate

3. If a nonprescription medication is classified as Category I, per the ongoing over-the-counter (OTC) drug review, it is

(A) safe and effective and not misbranded
(B) effective but unsafe or misbranded
(C) safe but ineffective and not misbranded
(D) none of the above

4. An exempt narcotic is subject to which of the following restrictions?

(A) It may be sold in a quantity of not more than 360 ml in a 24-hour period
(B) It may be sold to persons under 18 years of age with parental permission
(C) It may be sold without keeping record of the transaction
(D) It may be sold with 240 ml or less of opium-containing substances

5. In the 1970 Poison Prevention Packaging Act, certain substances were allowed to be dispensed or sold to consumers without a child-resistant closure. An example of a substance exempt from child-resistant closure requirements is

(A) acetaminophen in a dosage form for children
(B) antihistamines
(C) cholestyramine powder preparations
(D) potassium chloride liquid

6. The major piece of legislation that further clarified the distinction between drug products that require a prescription and drug products that do not require a prescription was which one of the following?

(A) The Federal Food, Drug, and Cosmetic Act of 1938 (FFDCA)
(B) The Pure Food and Drug Act of 1906
(C) The Durham-Humphrey amendments to the FFDCA
(D) The Kefauver-Harris amendments to the FFDCA

7. The label that states "CAUTION: Federal law prohibits the transfer of this drug to any person other than the patient for whom it was prescribed" must be affixed to prescriptions that have been dispensed for drugs in all of the following schedules EXCEPT

(A) Schedule II
(B) Schedule III
(C) Schedule IV
(D) Schedule V

1-B
2-C
3-A
4-D
5-C
6-C
7-D

ANSWERS AND EXPLANATIONS

1. The answer is B *[I E]*.
Prior to 1938, manufacturers were only required to provide drug products that were pure and labels that accurately reflected the ingredients. When the Federal Food, Drug, and Cosmetic Act (FFDCA) was passed, proof of safety became the responsibility of the manufacturer.

2. The answer is C *[II A 6]*.
According to United States postal regulations, substances containing a narcotic, an opiate, or any of their derivatives may not be mailed. Pentazocine is an opioid, and therefore falls into this category of restricted drugs. Diazepam is a benzodiazepine, ranitidine is an histamine$_2$ (H_2)-receptor antagonist, and meprobamate is a sedative–hypnotic that is similar to the benzodiazepines.

3. The answer is A *[II C 1–3]*.
The Federal Drug Administration (FDA) assigns one of three categories to chemicals that are destined for over-the-counter (OTC) use. A rating of Category I allows a substance to be used in OTC products, since it has been found to be safe, effective, and not misbranded.

4. The answer is D *[II A 1 e (3)]*.
Exempt narcotics are those controlled substances that may be sold over the counter without a prescription, provided that they contain less than 100 mg per 100 g or 100 ml of mixture. Opium-containing products may not be sold in quantities greater than 240 ml in any 48-hour period.

5. The answer is C *[II B 1]*.
There are several prescription drugs that are exempt from child-resistant closure requirements issued by the Poison Prevention Packaging Act of 1970. These include cholestyramine powder, nitroglycerin, and effervescent potassium supplements. The exemptions were made due to either the packaging of the drug, as in the case of unit–dose potassium supplements, or the drug's likelihood of safety.

6. The answer is C *[I F]*.
The Durham-Humphrey amendments to the Federal Food, Drug, and Cosmetic Act (FFDCA) imposed many actions that tightened controls on prescription drug products. Included in this was determining what drug products required a physician's authorization for refill.

7. The answer is D *[II A 4]*.
According to federal regulations, all prescriptions in Schedules II, III, and IV must have the transfer warning label affixed to the container. Schedule V drugs include ingredients found in over-the-counter (OTC) compounds.

23
Hospital Pharmacy Practice

Joseph Sceppa
Jerome Janousek

I. HISTORICAL PERSPECTIVE. Institutional pharmacy practice has undergone dramatic changes in the last 20 years.

A. **During the 1960s,** the responsibilities of the hospital pharmacist generally involved supplying medication in bulk to ward stocks and extemporaneously compounding topical ointments, creams, and an occasional sterile ophthalmic preparation.

B. **Two major changes** in recent decades significantly affected hospital pharmacists and thrust them into leadership positions in the new era of pharmacy practice.

1. The unit-dose drug distribution system and pharmacy preparation of intravenous admixtures greatly enhanced the hospital pharmacist's role.
2. The clinical pharmacist emerged as an integral member of the patient care team.

C. Pharmacist involvement as a part of the patient care team and the development of doctor of pharmacy (Pharm D) and residency programs further enhanced the stature of the hospital pharmacist.

D. The **American Society of Hospital Pharmacists (ASHP)** has become a leading pharmacy organization in the United States, with a membership and range of activities extending beyond institutional walls.

E. Today, hospital pharmacists are vital players on the health care team, acting in such important capacities as therapeutic experts, drug information specialists, nutritional service members, and pharmacokinetic consultants.

F. Pharmacists share the responsibility for providing pharmaceutical care that results in achieving definite outcomes that improve the quality of life of patients.

II. ADMINISTRATIVE STRUCTURE OF THE HOSPITAL PHARMACY

A. **Director of Pharmacy.** Sometimes known as the chief pharmacist or pharmacy manager, the pharmacy director has varied leadership responsibilities.

1. Like all hospital departmental managers, the pharmacy director oversees both personnel and budgetary (fiscal) matters.
2. The director also serves on various hospital committees, typically acting as secretary of the pharmacy and therapeutics committee.
3. As a member of the hospital team, the pharmacy director may be involved in community outreach programs (see III C 4).
4. The pharmacy director sets quality standards for the department, evaluating policies and procedures and implementing changes and innovations as necessary.
5. The director is responsible for developing management strategies to assure cost effective pharmaceutical services and for implementing total quality management (TQM) concepts.
6. Compliance with accrediting and regulating agencies (e.g., the Joint Commission on Accreditation of Healthcare Organizations, the Department of Public Health, the Board of Registration in Pharmacy).

B. Associate or assistant director of pharmacy. Depending on department size, the pharmacy may have one or more associate or assistant directors.

1. The associate or assistant director aids the pharmacy director in the operation of the pharmacy.
2. Specific tasks may include overseeing day-to-day pharmacy operations, supervising the sterile products room, and directing pharmacy purchasing.
3. When the pharmacy director is absent, the associate or assistant director assumes administrative responsibility.

C. Staff pharmacists. These employees have daily responsibility for the pharmacy's distributive and clinical duties.

1. **Distributive duties** include:
   - **a.** Physician order review and filling
   - **b.** Unit-dose cart checking
   - **c.** Extemporaneous compounding of parenteral admixtures, oral solutions, and topical preparations
   - **d.** Specific assigned tasks, such as purchasing, inventory control, and narcotic distribution and control
2. **Clinical duties** of staff pharmacists are varied.
   - **a. Therapeutic assessment.** In addition to evaluating the appropriateness of prescribed drugs and dosages, staff pharmacists monitor for drug–drug interactions and adverse drug effects.
   - **b.** Staff pharmacists also advise physicians, participate in physician rounds, and may serve on the nutritional support team.
   - **c.** Other clinical duties of staff pharmacists include pharmacokinetic monitoring, patient discharge counseling, and in-service education.

D. Clinical pharmacists. Because of their specialized education and training, these pharmacists are responsible for providing clinical activities for the hospital pharmacy.

1. Most clinical pharmacists have an advanced degree, such as a master of science (MS) in clinical pharmacy or a Doctor of Pharmacy degree (PharmD). Some also may have completed a residency or fellowship in a clinical specialty.
2. The clinical pharmacist plays a major role in monitoring and evaluating drug therapy and intervening when appropriate.
3. Depending on departmental organization and hospital size, the clinical pharmacist also may have drug distribution duties.
4. Some clinical pharmacists hold appointments at colleges or schools of pharmacy, serving as preceptors to graduate and undergraduate students.

E. Hospital pharmacy residents. As graduates of pharmacy programs, these staff members have a special interest in hospital practice.

1. Generally, pharmacy residencies are 1-year or 2-year programs offered by hospitals alone or in conjunction with a college or school of pharmacy.
2. Hospital pharmacy residents gain intensive experience in the distributive, clinical, and administrative aspects of institutional practice.
3. Many pharmacy residents go on to graduate school, clinical fellowships, or entry-level hospital pharmacy management positions.
4. The ASHP matches potential pharmacy residents with ASHP residency programs to facilitate the selection process for both residency candidates and hospitals.

F. Technicians and other support personnel play an important part in hospital pharmacy operation.

1. Technicians may be pharmacy students fulfilling their internship requirements, or they may be high school graduates.

2. Technicians work under the direct supervision of a pharmacist. In fulfilling their primary duty (i.e, helping to carry out the pharmacist's responsibilities) technicians perform the following tasks:
   a. Fill unit-dose carts
   b. Fill floor stock pharmacy supplies
   c. Extemporaneously compound and prepare intravenous admixtures for approval by a pharmacist
3. Many hospitals and several schools of pharmacy and community colleges have established 1-year and 2-year technician training programs.
4. The Association of Pharmacy Technicians, a national organization, includes support personnel working in community pharmacies, hospitals, and other settings. Training programs, competency-based examinations and certification have been initiated in several states.

G. **Clerical and secretarial support staff.** These employees may be involved in pharmacy purchasing and patient billing as well as standard clerical and secretarial duties.

III. RESPONSIBILITIES OF THE HOSPITAL PHARMACY

A. **Drug distribution** is the primary responsibility of the hospital pharmacy.

1. **Drug distribution methods** continue to undergo major changes. For instance, to place pharmacy services closer to patient care areas, many large hospitals have decentralized drug distribution by creating satellite pharmacies using mobile cart systems. Automated dispensing machines are also starting to be used more in institutional practice.
2. **Drug distribution systems** fall into two major categories: floor stock and unit-dose systems.
   a. **Floor stock drug distribution**
      (1) The traditional drug distribution system, the floor stock system, involves a separate pharmacy area in a secured area on each patient care floor.
         (a) Generally, each **nursing area** has 10 to 100 dosage forms on hand for use by the nursing staff.
         (b) **Floor stock** may include many bulk supplies of the medications carried in the hospital pharmacy. In many cases, floor stock consists of a predetermined list of medications, with others sent on request to the nursing staff if physicians' orders are received for nonstock items.
      (2) **Drawbacks** of the floor stock system include an increased potential for medication errors.
         (a) **The floor stock system does not give pharmacists the opportunity to review physicians' orders** for accuracy of dosage and scheduling or potential drug interactions. The choice of medication is made by the medication nurse from floor stock, without the involvement of a dispensing pharmacist.
         (b) **Pharmacists have no chance to review the patient's medication profile** to monitor drug therapy. They must guess, based on nurses' requests for a resupply, when a particular drug is being used. Modified floor stock systems were developed in an attempt to address the issue of pharmacist review of medication profiles; however, these systems do not deal with the issue of nurses dispensing drugs.
   b. **Unit-dose drug distribution system.** Developed to reduce medication errors, this system guarantees pharmacist medication review and individual patient dispensing. It has largely replaced the floor stock system.
      (1) The unit-dose system has **two main components**.
         (a) **All physician medication orders are reviewed by a pharmacist** before they are dispensed. The pharmacist may review orders directly in the patient care area or may review copies of orders sent to the pharmacy.
         (b) **Medications are dispensed as unit-doses or units-of-use,** in an individually labeled box or drawer for each patient. Typically, a 24-hour medication supply is sent. For instance, for a patient who is to receive 250 mg of amoxicillin orally three times daily, the pharmacy sends three individually packaged, 250-mg capsules of amoxicillin.

(2) **Advantages.** Besides allowing pharmacists to review and dispense all medications, the unit-dose system reduces medication errors and helps cut pharmacy costs (by eliminating floor stock medication supplies and reusing certain doses).

(3) **Drawbacks.** Although the unit-dose system generally is superior to the floor stock system, it has certain flaws.

(a) Delays may occur in initiating new medication orders.

(b) Pharmacy labor costs are higher.

3. **Intravenous admixture programs**

a. Pharmacy personnel, after specialized training, prepare patient-specific doses of parenteral medications for the unit-dose system.

b. Pharmacy personnel allow for standardized dosing, labeling, and packaging.

c. Centralized manufacturing allows bulk preparation and minimizes waste.

d. Typical admixture areas minimize environmental contamination by using laminar airflow hoods, which also protect manufacturing personnel from exposure to potentially toxic products (e.g., antineoplastics).

B. Clinical functions of the hospital pharmacy

1. **Therapeutic consultation** may be the most important service provided by the hospital pharmacy staff.

a. Acute-care patients typically receive multiple drug therapy: such complex regimens necessitate the involvement of a pharmacist.

b. The hospital pharmacist also performs other clinical activities, such as:

(1) Selecting an antimicrobial therapy regimen or parenteral nutrition formula

(2) Monitoring the pharmacokinetic aspects of any therapy (e.g., aminoglycoside therapy)

(3) Assessing for drug interactions and monitoring for adverse effects

2. **Drug information centers,** which are operated by the pharmacies of many large teaching hospitals, field drug-related questions.

a. Textbooks, journals, and on-line computer information sources serve as the data base.

b. Health care professionals, both within and outside the hospital, may have access to the drug information center.

c. Some drug information centers act as poison control centers for their geographic region, which requires that the pharmacist interact with the public.

3. **Other clinical functions.** Hospital pharmacists participate in in-service and patient education programs. For example, they may give formal lectures to physicians, nurses, and other allied health personnel, and they may instruct patients about medications upon discharge.

C. Miscellaneous functions of the hospital pharmacy

1. **Purchasing.** This important administrative function has been simplified by advanced technology, such as computer-generated purchase orders and the use of bar codes when ordering.

a. Generally, a pharmacist or pharmacy technician coordinates pharmacy purchasing.

b. Pharmaceuticals may be purchased from the manufacturer or a drug wholesaler. To reduce drug acquisition costs, the pharmacies of several hospitals may unite to negotiate group contracts with manufacturers.

(1) A **prime-vendor contract,** in which the pharmacy guarantees that it will purchase a specific dollar amount from the wholesaler, also helps reduce pharmacy costs. In return for the guarantee, the wholesaler reduces the standard mark-up, which is a practice known as "cost plus."

(2) Under a **cost plus prime-vendor contract,** the wholesaler may use a cost plus formula, charging only the manufacturer's price plus a significantly lower handling fee.

(3) Prime vendor arrangements increase purchases from the wholesaler (rather than from the manufacturer), thereby reducing inventory and increasing inventory turns.

2. **Inventory control**

a. Hospital pharmacies usually take periodic (e.g., annual, semi-annual, or quarterly) physical inventories to determine the asset value of undispensed medications.

b. To maintain the proper inventory, the pharmacy's turnover rate can be determined.

(1) The **turnover rate** is calculated as follows:

$$\text{Turnover rate} = \frac{\text{Annual purchases (in dollars)}}{\text{Annual inventory (in dollars)}}$$

(2) A low turnover rate may indicate that inventory is too high, often associated with multiple stock locations (e.g., satellite).

3. Committee work

a. As mentioned in II A 2, the pharmacy director typically serves on the **pharmacy and therapeutics committee,** which oversees the use of medications in the hospital.

(1) Working with the committee chairperson (usually a physician), the pharmacy director sets the committee agenda. (Other pharmacy staff—for instance, a clinical pharmacist—also may hold committee membership).

(2) The committee determines which drugs should be carried on the hospital's formulary; it also oversees the use of investigational drugs and the handling of hazardous waste.

(3) The committee oversees quality assurance and quality improvement activities, and reports on medication incident reports as well as adverse drug events.

b. Other hospital committees that may include pharmacy personnel are the pharmacy–nursing committee, infection control committee, human studies committee, and quality assurance committee.

4. Community relations. A hospital pharmacist may coordinate community outreach programs such as hypertension and cholesterol screening, poison prevention awareness, and substance abuse prevention programs.

STUDY QUESTIONS

Directions: Each of the numbered items or incomplete statements in this section is followed by answers or by completions of the statement. Select the **one** lettered answer or completion that is **best** in each case.

1. Hospital pharmacy residency programs are governed by the

(A) ASCP
(B) ASHP
(C) APhA
(D) ACA
(E) NARD

2. Clinical pharmacists often possess which of the following advanced degrees?

(A) PD
(B) PhD
(C) MBA
(D) PharmD
(E) JD

3. Responsibilities often delegated to hospital pharmacy technicians include

(A) counseling of patients being discharged
(B) review of physicians' medication orders
(C) preparation of intravenous admixtures
(D) pharmacokinetic monitoring
(E) administration of intravenous admixtures

4. A patient's medication order states that she is to receive "ampicillin 500 mg po q6h." How many doses of ampicillin 250-mg capsules should be placed in the patient's unit-dose drawer daily?

(A) 2
(B) 4
(C) 6
(D) 8
(E) 10

5. In inventory control, the turnover rate is calculated by which of the following formulas (in dollar amounts)?

(A) Annual purchases + annual inventory
(B) Annual purchases × annual inventory
(C) Annual inventory ÷ annual purchases
(D) Annual purchases ÷ annual inventory
(E) Annual purchases − annual inventory

6. All of the following are considered desirable functions of a contemporary hospital pharmacy EXCEPT

(A) clinical consultation services
(B) intravenous admixture programs
(C) floor stock distribution systems
(D) selecting antimicrobial therapy regimens
(E) purchasing and inventory control

7. All of the following are advantages of unit-dose drug distribution systems EXCEPT

(A) prompt delivery of new medication orders
(B) pharmacist review of medication orders
(C) a decrease in medication errors
(D) reduced pharmacy costs
(E) pharmacist dispensing of medications

8. The clinical functions of a hospital pharmacist may include all of the following EXCEPT

(A) monitoring drug interactions
(B) administration of medications
(C) pharmacokinetic consultation
(D) participation on a nutritional support team
(E) making rounds with physicians

9. Information sources used by drug information centers may include all of the following EXCEPT

(A) popular literature
(B) medical journals
(C) textbooks
(D) on-line computer information sources
(E) pharmacy journals

1-B	4-D	7-A
2-D	5-D	8-B
3-C	6-C	9-A

ANSWERS AND EXPLANATIONS

1. The answer is B *[II E 4]*.
The American Society of Hospital Pharmacists (ASHP) matches potential pharmacy residents with residency programs. The ASHP also acts as the accrediting body for hospital pharmacy residencies.

2. The answer is D [*II D 1*].
The Doctor of Pharmacy degree (PharmD), a clinically oriented doctorate, is held by many clinical pharmacists in both institutional and academic settings.

3. The answer is C [*II F 2*].
Counseling patients about medication upon discharge, reviewing physicians' medication orders, and pharmacokinetic monitoring are all functions that must be performed by a pharmacist. The preparation of intravenous admixtures, under the direct supervision of a pharmacist, is an activity often delegated to technicians. The administration of intravenous admixtures is, in most cases, the responsibility of the nursing staff. Very few hospitals use pharmacy personnel to administer medications.

4. The answer is D [*III A 2 b (1) (b)*].
Typically, with the unit-dose distribution system, the pharmacy provides a 24-hour medication supply for each patient in an individually labeled unit-dose box or drawer. The patient in the question is to receive 500 mg of ampicillin orally every 6 hours—that is, four times each day. With only 250-mg capsules available, a daily unit-dose supply of eight capsules is necessary.

5. The answer is D [*III C 2*].
The annual purchases of a pharmacy (in dollars) divided by the pharmacy's annual inventory (in dollars) will yield the turnover rate. A low turnover rate may indicate that inventory is relatively high.

6. The answer is C [*III A 2 a (2), b, B 1 b (1)*].
Floor stock drug distribution systems have numerous drawbacks. Therefore, these systems have been replaced largely by unit-dose drug distribution systems in most hospital pharmacies. Clinical consultation services, intravenous admixture programs, providing drug information to hospital staff and to patients, community outreach services, and drug purchasing and inventory control are all important functions of the contemporary hospital pharmacy.

7. The answer is A [*III A 2 a, b*].
Although unit-dose systems offer numerous advantages, the prompt delivery of new medication orders is not one of them. Traditional floor stock systems, which kept "mini pharmacy" supplies of medications in the patient care area, provided much faster access to medications for the initiation of new therapy—at the cost, however, of numerous medication errors and other serious problems.

8. The answer is B [*II C 2; III B*].
Despite the pharmacist's assumption of numerous clinical functions in recent years, the administration of medications to patients has remained a nursing function.

9. The answer is A [*III B 2*].
While many different information sources are used for drug information centers, popular literature (e.g., *Time, Newsweek, People*) is not considered appropriate.

24
Community Pharmacy Practice

Stephen L. DePietro
Douglas J. Pisano

I. EVOLUTION OF PHARMACY PRACTICE. Pharmacy practice has changed as rapidly as any other profession in recent decades. In the not-so-distant past, a pharmacist's responsibilities were heavily concentrated in compounding and preparing a variety of dosage forms. A pharmacist would routinely prepare tablets, capsules, suppositories, and elixirs. As the pharmaceutical industry expanded, compounded prescriptions became commercially available. Neighborhood pharmacists were generally seen as extensions to physicians and an important provider of medical services. Pharmacists are now becoming increasingly more involved with therapeutic selection, monitoring drug regimens, and emphasizing patient compliance through education.

A. Professional changes. The pharmacist's role has changed from one who primarily compounded and dispensed prescription drugs to one who:

1. Is a more active source of prescription and over-the-counter (OTC) drug information
2. Has a greater focus on improving patient compliance
3. Recognizes drug interactions and counsels patients
4. Develops other professional cognitive services (i.e., hypertension screening, cholesterol screening)

B. Pharmacy practice

1. In the past 20 years, **technologic changes** have been dramatic.
   a. New therapeutic drug entities have been developed (e.g., calcium channel blockers).
   b. New diagnostic and treatment modalities have been expanded (e.g., radiopharmacy).
   c. Medical specialties have become more complex (e.g., immunology).
2. **Pharmacy education** has been changing to meet the challenging new roles of today's pharmacist through:
   a. Clinical clerkship/externship rotations
   b. Hospital/community residencies
3. **Continuing education** requirements have become mandatory to assure competence of existing practitioners. In addition to a required number of continuing education credits per year, many states have begun mandating a specific number of credits on a particular subject (e.g., pharmacy law, AIDS).

C. Socio/demographic influences on pharmacy practice

1. Society as a whole has become busier and more complex, which has changed the emphasis in marketing pharmacy services. Accessibility, convenience, home health care services, and the concept of pharmaceutical care are of increased importance. These changes are due to a variety of factors, including:
   a. Increases in two-income households
   b. Increases in women in the workplace
   c. Increases in the elderly population with an increase in average life expectancy
2. Consumers' desire for convenience has heightened (e.g., the expansion of chain pharmacy practice offers consumers multiple locations, well-merchandised nonprescription departments, and 24-hour pharmacy services).
3. Third-party insurance carriers began offering extended coverage for prescription drugs.

II. TYPES OF PHARMACY SETTINGS. Pharmacy has many types of practice settings. Each one is dynamic and subject to the same influences as other health care settings.

A. Independent community pharmacies. Local, independent pharmacies have long been considered by many to be among the pillars of a community, in that they were typically open long hours with pharmacists available at all times to address a variety of public health concerns.

B. Chain pharmacies are small to large corporations that operate numerous facilities under a single, corporate banner. They include large health and beauty aid departments along with prescription services. Chain pharmacy settings are typically characterized by:

1. Greater product selection due to larger facilities and buying power
2. Perception of lower prices
3. Major prescription and health and beauty aid marketing strategies
4. High prescription volume

C. Supermarket/combination store pharmacies have been successful by including prescription departments in a supermarket or grocery-type store. These are similar to chain pharmacy operations because many supermarkets are also part of a larger chain organization. The main advantage offered by supermarket/combination type pharmacy settings is the convenience of one-stop shopping for the majority of a consumer's needs.

D. Mail-service pharmacies have primarily a dispensing/supervisory role. In most cases, there is a contract with associations and third-party payers to provide prescription services.

1. **Advantages** of these types of pharmacies include potentially lower out-of-pocket expenses and the convenience of having prescriptions delivered by mail. Mail-service pharmacies are considered high-volume prescription operations, and pharmacists generally participate more routinely in checking prescriptions filled by technicians rather than filling prescriptions themselves.

2. **Disadvantages** include the absence of a pharmacist to answer any questions concerning medication, regimen, or ancillary medical concerns that patients may have when they are having their prescriptions filled.

E. Nursing home pharmacies. In addition to routine dispensing functions, nursing home pharmacies also stock durable medical equipment and intravenous and enteral feeding supplies. Services that are routinely provided include medication inspections, in-service education to nursing and staff members, and drug utilization reviews.

III. ACTIVITIES OF THE COMMUNITY PHARMACIST. A community pharmacist conducts and is involved in many activities that impact and affect health care delivery. A partial list of these services include the following:

A. Dispensing prescription medications and medical devices. A principle function of the community pharmacist is the preparation and dispensing of prescription medications and medical devices.

1. Pharmacists must be certain of the correct medication, dosage form, and directions for use prior to filling the prescription (see Chapter 20).

2. A pharmacist's intervention into a patient's drug therapy is crucial to assure that the intended medication with appropriate instructions is used correctly.

B. Information source. The dispensing of health care information is a rapidly growing function of the pharmacist due to their specialized training. The general public, members of the health care profession, and local civic groups depend on pharmacists for information regarding illnesses, over-the-counter (OTC) medications, prescription drugs, medical devices, and home health care concerns (see Chapter 21).

C. Home health care services. Home health care is rapidly becoming an important addition to a pharmacy's circle of services. Many pharmacists have invested a great deal of time and resources to specialize in this area so that they can provide a "full-service pharmacy" to encompass all health care needs. These needs may include:

1. The selection, fitting, training, and delivery of durable medical equipment
2. Nutritional supplies and services
3. Home parenteral drug or feeding devices and support

D. Monitoring drug therapy. The increased use of computers makes it easier for pharmacists to promote patient profile screening and prescription drug monitoring and follow-up as a new service. Pharmacists can conveniently monitor for:

1. Potential allergies
2. Drug interactions
3. Drug utilization review, which is useful to detect inappropriate drug use or abuse

E. Health care screening. Health care screening programs have become increasingly popular as a way for community pharmacies to promote their services. These programs may include screening for:

1. Cholesterol
2. Hypertension
3. Diabetes
4. Occult fecal blood
5. Hearing loss

F. Consulting services. Pharmacists may contract with nursing homes or other extended-care facilities as consultants to provide health care consulting services to both patients and staff. These services may include:

1. Patient profile monitoring
2. Staff education and in-services
3. Regulation compliance
4. General supply of house stock items

IV. ADMINISTRATIVE/PROFESSIONAL FUNCTIONS

A. Supervisory functions. Although their function may be less professional in orientation and more administrative (i.e., sales review and monitoring, inventory control, loss prevention, and personnel), pharmacists are often in a position to manage a department and personnel in the following settings:

1. An independent pharmacy
2. A multiple unit chain pharmacy operation
3. A nursing home pharmacy
4. A home health care pharmacy
5. A mail-service pharmacy
6. A community health center

B. Managerial functions include the day-to-day responsibility for efficiently running the business and developing the prescription department of an individual store.

C. Preceptor functions include training and supervising interns and externs during their required work experiences.

D. Community service functions include the types of specialized functions that require a pharmacist's expertise in order to benefit the community at large, such as:

1. Senior citizen activities and seminars
2. Brown bag projects (i.e., lunch-time seminars or lectures at business centers, clinics, schools, or other community centers)
3. Drug awareness programs for schools
4. Participation in civic organizations

STUDY QUESTIONS

Directions: Each of the numbered items or incomplete statements in this section is followed by answers or by completions of the statement. Select the **one** lettered answer or completion that is **best** in each case.

1. Which of the following statements regarding changes in pharmacy practice is correct?

(A) Commercial availability of prescription drugs resulted in an increase in pharmacist compounding
(B) Continuing education is intended to expand and maintain competence in the profession
(C) Recent technologic advances in medicine include limited diagnostic and treatment modalities, resulting in a decrease in third-party payments
(D) Pharmacists are now becoming less involved with patient education

2. Advantages that an independent pharmacy business may have over a chain pharmacy business include which one of the following?

(A) Greater product selection
(B) Home health care services
(C) Lower pricing
(D) Higher prescription volumes
(E) Greater advertising power

3. Staff education and in-services are regarded as functions of which one of the following aspects of community pharmacy practice?

(A) Drug therapy monitoring
(B) Health care screening
(C) Counseling services
(D) Home health care services
(E) None of the above

4. Pharmacists monitoring drug therapy would typically be checking all of the following EXCEPT

(A) proper utilization of medicine
(B) drug–drug interactions
(C) allergy contraindications
(D) appropriate diagnosis

5. Chain pharmacies have addressed the need for convenience shopping by offering all of the following EXCEPT

(A) well-stocked stores with a wide product selection
(B) centrally located 24-hour stores
(C) ample free parking
(D) multiple stores
(E) mail order service

6. Community health service functions involve every level of pharmacy practice and include all of the following EXCEPT

(A) senior citizen activities
(B) lunch-time seminars
(C) drug awareness programs
(D) participation in civic organizations
(E) in-service education to nursing home pharmacy staff

7. Community service activities allow a pharmacist to perform all of the following functions EXCEPT

(A) present drug awareness programs in schools
(B) give lectures to business people
(C) develop drug abuse/prevention programs
(D) offer extended coverage for prescription drugs
(E) offer presentations at area clinics

1-B 4-D 7-D
2-B 5-E
3-E 6-E

Directions: The question below contains three suggested answers of which **one or more** is correct. Choose the answer

A if **I only** is correct
B if **III only** is correct
C if **I and II** are correct
D if **II and III** are correct
E if **I, II, and III** are correct

8. Changes within the pharmacy profession include which of the following?

I. Deemphasizing cognitive services such as blood pressure screening
II. Routinely preparing suppositories and elixirs
III. Taking a more active role in patient counseling

8-B

ANSWERS AND EXPLANATIONS

1. The answer is B *[I A, B 1 a–b, 3, C 3].*
Technologic advances in medicine necessitate that all health care professionals continue their education in order to stay abreast of current theories and products. The scope of pharmacy practice has changed to include a modified emphasis on prescription compounding and a more advanced approach to therapeutics, diagnostics, and treatment.

2. The answer is B *[II A–B; III C].*
Independent pharmacies often carry home health care items, even though a great deal of time and effort must be expended before profits can be realized. Chain pharmacy operations may consider these items to be unprofitable or unimportant to their inventory.

3. The answer is E *[III F].*
Staff education and in-services are considered a function of the pharmacy consultant. Pharmacy consultants have the responsibility to educate nursing home and long-term care workers about pharmaceutical products and services.

4. The answer is D *[III D].*
Diagnoses are the responsibility of the physician. Prescription drug monitoring for drug interactions and allergic reactions is, however, a part of the increase in cognitive services offered by pharmacists. These services also include drug utilization review.

5. The answer is E *[I C 2; II B, D].*
Mail-service pharmacies exist, but are a separate entity. The chain pharmacy industry has attempted to draw clientele to their outlets by utilizing the one-stop shopping concept, which offers consumers a wide variety of products in stores with convenient location, hours, and parking.

6. The answer is E *[II E; IV A–D].*
In-service education is a routine facet of the operation of a pharmacy. Community health service functions, however, are specialized functions that benefit the community at large.

7. The answer is D *[IV D].*
Third-party insurance carriers offer extended coverage for prescription drugs. Since pharmacy as a profession is becoming more interactive, pharmacists are expected to do more for patients than the traditional dispensing duties. Many community pharmacists give a variety of presentations to all demographic groups in the community.

8. The answer is B (III) *[I A 3, 4, III E].*
Recent professional initiatives and legislative changes have led to a greater emphasis on cognitive services, in addition to product dispensing that is traditionally done by pharmacists. However, with expansion of the pharmaceutical industry, pharmacists are preparing far fewer compounds like suppositories and elixirs.

25
Long-Term Care Pharmacy Practice

Louise Mallet

I. DEMOGRAPHICS

A. Nursing facilities

1. There are approximately 19,000 nursing facilities representing 1.8 million nursing home beds.
2. The majority of nursing homes are for-profit facilities, with the cost for nursing home care averaging $2500 per month per resident.
3. The average occupancy rate in nursing care facilities is 96%.

B. Nursing home residents

1. **Percentage.** Approximately 5% of older Americans live in a nursing home. The percentage of patients who live in nursing homes increases with age, from 2% for those who are 65 to 74 to 22% for those who are age 85 and older.
2. **Age.** The average age for nursing home residents is 78 years, with women representing the majority of this population.
3. **Length of stay.** The mean length of stay in a nursing facility is 19 months. Fifty percent of the residents admitted to a nursing home die in that setting.

C. Chance of being placed in a nursing home

1. It is estimated that 25% to 50% of Americans over the age of 65 require nursing home services during their lifetimes.
2. **Risk factors** increase the chance of nursing home placement. Such risk factors include age (i.e., 70 years or older), sex (i.e., female), living alone, suffering from dementia, being recently discharged from the hospital, being immobilized, having numerous medical problems, suffering from depression or incontinence, being socially isolated, and not having supportive relatives.

II. DEFINITIONS

A. **Long-term care (LTC)** is care that is provided over an extended period of time.

B. **Skilled nursing facilities (SNFs)** provide medical and nursing care in addition to physical therapy, speech therapy, and occupational therapy.

C. **Intermediate-care facilities (ICFs)** provide medical, nursing, and social services for individuals who are unable to live independently. The level of care provided for individuals in ICFs is less than that provided for individuals in hospitals or SNFs.

D. **Intermediate-care mental retardation facilities (ICF-MRs)** provide care for mentally retarded individuals.

E. **Assisted living homes** (also called rest homes, domiciliary care homes, or board and care homes) provide care for individuals who need some assistance with daily activities.

F. The **Health Care Financing Administration (HCFA)** is the agency responsible for developing the requirements for meeting the needs of LTC residents.

G. **Consultant pharmacy practice** is a type of practice in which the pharmacist solves problems and serves as an advocate for health care professionals and patients.

H. **Drug regimen review (DRR)** is an active process whereby a licensed pharmacist reviews a patient's drug regimen at least once every month. Information collected from a variety of sources, such as the physician's orders, nurses' notes, laboratory reports, and medication administration records, is evaluated to determine whether there are any potential problems with the patient's drug therapy. The consultant pharmacist then communicates these findings and recommendations of the evaluation to the health care professionals.

III. EVOLUTION OF CONSULTANT PHARMACY PRACTICE.

Consultant pharmacy practice is less than 25 years old in the United States. Currently, more than 10,000 pharmacists are practicing in this area. The American Society of Consultant Pharmacists (ASCP) is the national professional association representing the interest of pharmacists practicing in this area.

A. **Before 1965,** standards for pharmaceutical services in nursing homes were regulated at the state level, and requirements for pharmacy services were limited.

B. **In 1965,** with the enactment of Medicare and Medicaid programs, federal regulations governing LTC facilities were developed and implemented through the HCFA.

C. **In 1974,** pharmacists, who are now referred to as consultant pharmacists, were mandated to perform monthly DRR for each resident's drug therapy in SNFs, to report findings to the facility's medical director and administrator, and to serve on the pharmaceutical services and infection control committees.

1. **In ICFs,** DRR can be performed by a nurse.
2. **In ICF-MRs,** DRR can be performed by a pharmacist or a nurse on a quarterly basis.

D. **In 1982,** a set of guidelines known as Indicators for Surveyor Assessment of the Performance of DRR were developed by the HCFA to help surveyors evaluate the quality of DRR. These indicators are not regulations; they are used by surveyors to determine patterns of performance by the consultant pharmacist in conducting DRR. The **indicators for assessing DRRs** include:

1. Reviews performed versus average census
2. Reviews performed in the facility
3. Average prescription utilization
4. Excessive reviews on the same day
5. Potential drug therapy problems

E. **In 1987,** pharmacists were mandated to conduct DRR in both SNFs and ICFs. Also in 1987, as part of the Omnibus Budget Reconciliation Act (OBRA), Congress enacted legislation to improve the quality of care in nursing homes (see VI).

F. **In 1988,** new regulations required that consultant pharmacists review the medication regimen of each ICF-MR resident on a quarterly basis, to report any irregularities to the prescribing physician and interdisciplinary team, and to participate as needed in the development, implementation, and review of each resident's individual care plan.

IV. WORK ENVIRONMENTS FOR CONSULTANT PHARMACISTS

A. Types of practices

1. Approximately 41% of consultant pharmacists have a **community-based practice** that provides consultant and provider services to nursing facilities and other LTC environments. Of these, 60% of consultant pharmacists provide services to five or fewer nursing facilities, 10% of consultant pharmacists serve six to ten facilities, and 20% of consultant pharmacists serve more than twenty facilities.

2. Approximately 23% of consultant pharmacists have a **closed-door pharmacy practice**.

B. Services

1. Nearly 47% of consultant pharmacists provide **dispensing and consulting** services.
2. About 16% of consultant pharmacists provide only **consultant** services.
3. Approximately 10% of consultant pharmacists provide **only dispensing** services.
4. An estimated 22% of consultant pharmacists provide **only administrative** services.

C. Practice sites. Consultant pharmacists provide services in a variety of practice sites, such as nursing homes, residential care facilities, adult day-care operations, home health care organizations, senior centers, hospices, retirement communities, prisons, community mental health centers, rehabilitation centers, and ICF-MRs.

V. PHARMACEUTICAL SERVICES.

Federal regulations require nursing facilities to provide pharmaceutical services to meet the needs of each resident, including procedures that ensure the accurate acquiring, receiving, dispensing, and administering of all drugs and biologicals, such as vaccines.

A. The facility must obtain the services of a **licensed pharmacist** to provide consultation on all aspects of the provision of pharmacy services in the facility and to establish a system of records of receipt and disposition of all controlled drugs.

B. DRRs for each resident must be conducted every month in nursing facilities by a licensed pharmacist, who must report any irregularities to the attending physician, the director of nursing, or both. These reports must be followed up with action.

C. Pharmaceutical services in nursing homes are usually divided into provider services and consultant services.

1. **Provider services** include the drug distribution system, record keeping, emergency drug supply, and audit systems for controlled substances.
2. **Consultant services** include activities such as the monthly DRR and the following:
   - **a.** Reporting recommendations to the physician, director of nursing, or administrator
   - **b.** Participation in quality assessment and the assurance committee or other committees
   - **c.** Development of a policy and procedure manual
   - **d.** Implementation of formulary
   - **e.** Therapeutic drug monitoring
   - **f.** In-service education programs
   - **g.** Publication of newsletter
   - **h.** Participation in planning resident care
   - **i.** Medication review
   - **j.** Implementation of research activities
   - **k.** Family and patient conferences

VI. OBRA REGULATIONS

went into effect on October 1, 1990. With these new regulations, consultant pharmacists must now focus on the quality of care. Pharmacists are now required to report any irregularities to the attending physician, the director of nursing, or both. The OBRA regulations mandate the following:

A. Comprehensive resident assessment, including ensuring that patients are not given unnecessary drugs. Each resident must be free from unnecessary drugs, which are defined by the following:

1. Drugs given in an excessive dose
2. Drugs given for excessive periods of time
3. Drugs given without adequate monitoring
4. Drugs given in the absence of a diagnosis

5. Drugs given in the presence of adverse effects that indicate that the dose should be reduced or discontinued

B. Monitoring of psychoactive medications. Based on a comprehensive assessment of a resident, the facility must ensure the following.

1. Residents who have not used antipsychotic drugs are not given these drugs unless therapy is necessary to treat a specific condition as diagnosed and documented in the patient's clinical record.

2. Residents who use antipsychotic drugs receive gradual dose reductions and behavioral interventions, unless clinically contraindicated, in an effort to discontinue these drugs.

C. Assuring the proper use of physical restraints

D. Ensuring the rights of each resident

E. Training nursing aides

F. Providing competency evaluation programs and regular in-service education

G. Providing 24-hour licensed nursing service

STUDY QUESTIONS

Directions: Each of the numbered items or incomplete statements in this section is followed by answers or by completions of the statement. Select the **one** lettered answer or completion that is **best** in each case.

1. What percent of older Americans reside in nursing homes?

(A) 2%
(B) 5%
(C) 10%
(D) 50%

2. The indicators for assessing drug regimen reviews (DRRs) can best be described as

(A) regulations
(B) guidelines
(C) laws
(D) standards of practice

3. The practice of consultant pharmacy in this country is

(A) less than 10 years old
(B) less than 25 years old
(C) more than 50 years old
(D) more than 100 years old

4. Drug regimen review (DRR) for each resident in nursing facilities must be conducted how often?

(A) Monthly
(B) Bimonthly
(C) Quarterly
(D) Annually

5. Omnibus Budget Reconciliation Act (OBRA) regulations mandate all of the following EXCEPT

(A) comprehensive resident assessment
(B) monitoring psychoactive medications
(C) monitoring research in nursing homes
(D) proper use of physical restraints

6. An unnecessary drug may include all of the following EXCEPT

(A) a drug given in excessive dose
(B) a drug given for an excessive period of time
(C) an antipsychotic drug for a symptomatic patient
(D) a drug given in the absence of a diagnosis

Directions: The question below contains three suggested answers of which **one or more** is correct. Choose the answer

A if **I only** is correct
B if **III only** is correct
C if **I and II** are correct
D if **II and III** are correct
E if **I, II, and III** are correct

7. An 85-year-old woman living alone with a history of congestive heart failure, urinary incontinence, osteoarthritis, constipation, and glaucoma was recently discharged from the hospital with a right hip fracture. She does not have any relatives living nearby. Which of the following risk factors predispose this patient for nursing home placement?

I. Having multiple medical problems
II. Being recently discharged from hospital
III. Being an 85-year-old woman

1-B 4-C 7-E
2-B 5-C
3-B 6-C

ANSWERS AND EXPLANATIONS

1. The answer is B *[I B 1].*
Approximately 5% of older Americans age 65 and older are living in nursing homes.

2. The answer is B *[III D].*
The indicators for assessing drug regimen reviews (DRRs) are not regulations; they are guidelines used by surveyors to determine patterns of performance by the consultant pharmacists.

3. The answer is B *[III C].*
In 1974, pharmacists referred to as consultant pharmacists were mandated to perform drug regimen reviews (DRRs) for each resident's drug therapy in skilled nursing facilities (SNFs).

4. The answer is C *[II H; V B].*
In nursing facilities, a drug regimen review must be conducted for each resident on a monthly basis by a licensed pharmacist.

5. The answer is C *[III E; VI].*
Omnibus Budget Reconciliation Act (OBRA) regulations do not encompass monitoring research in nursing homes. Implementation of research activities is an activity of a consultant pharmacist, however. Mostly, OBRA regulations mandate proper and adequate care and treatment of long-term care patients.

6. The answer is C *[VI A].*
An unnecessary drug is defined as a drug given in an excessive dose for excessive periods of time without adequate monitoring, a drug given in the absence of a diagnosis or in the presence of adverse effects that indicate that the dose should be reduced or discontinued.

7. The answer is E (all) *[I C 2].*
Risk factors for nursing home placement include being age 70 or older; being a woman; living alone; having multiple medical problems; being incontinent, depressed, immobilized, or demented; and having no supportive relatives nearby.

26
Managed Care

F. Randy Vogenberg

I. HISTORICAL PERSPECTIVE. Managed care organizations (MCOs) evaluate the need for a patient to use or undergo particular physician services or other health care services. The goal of MCOs is to eliminate excessive and unnecessary services, thereby keeping health care costs down and manageable. MCOs are now a significant factor in the delivery of pharmaceutical care in the United States, with more than 36 million people enrolled among 575 MCOs.

A. Health maintenance organizations (HMOs) began in the late 1800s and became a major method for health care delivery when Henry Kaiser, inspired by a prepaid health care program for Grand Coulee Dam workers, developed a comprehensive HMO (Kaiser-Permanente) for industrial workers and the public at the end of World War II.

1. Types of HMOs

a. The **Independent Practice Association (IPA)** was formed in 1954, and served as a model for the most common type of HMO currently available. Approximately 60% of HMOs are of the IPA prototype, which contract physicians either in solo or group practice to provide services to HMO members.

(1) The physicians can have a private practice that is not limited to patients on HMO plans.

(2) Physicians in an IPA-type HMO have more input into utilization review criteria and quality assurance than do physicians in the staff, group, or network models.

b. Staff-model HMOs. This type of HMO hires physicians and pays them a salary. The physicians work at the HMO office and their practice is limited to HMO subscribers.

c. Group-model HMOs. This type of HMO contracts with a private group practice that has physicians from a variety of specialties. The HMO pays the group, and the group divides the money among themselves.

d. Network-model HMOs. In this type, the HMO contracts more than one group practice to serve its members.

2. Legislation

a. In 1971, Congress passed legislation for **MCO grants and loans,** which made it financially feasible for these organizations to prosper.

b. In 1973, the **Health Maintenance Organization Act** was passed requiring businesses with more than 25 employees to offer MCOs to their employees, if MCOs were available in their area.

c. In the late 1970s and early 1980s, additional legislation fueled the growth of MCOs. The philosophy of MCOs changed as private and corporate investors saw profit-making opportunities in this method of delivering health care.

B. Preferred Provider Organizations (PPOs) differ from HMOs in that PPOs do not employ only physicians. Rather, in PPOs, a group consisting of physicians, hospitals, therapists, and others, such as pharmacists, work as a team to provide care and service to a specific group of people at a lower than normal rate.

1. Advantages. Traditional PPOs were community based with an independent physician and hospital for the purpose of decreasing cost. All services are attained through a contract.

2. Disadvantages of PPOs include variability in the network and a potential decrease in cost-effectiveness as compared with an HMO.

C. Pharmacy service in MCOs. Initially an afterthought, pharmacy services have become a major additional benefit for an MCO to offer its enrollees.

1. Pharmacy service is the most visible and most often used option from an MCO or employee marketing perspective.
2. Pharmacy service is among the most frequently used benefits in an MCO.
3. In recent times, the pharmacy benefit has come under more scrutiny as costs of pharmaceuticals have risen from less than 6% to nearly 15% of the health care dollar.
4. Sixty percent of pharmacists say their pharmacy is affiliated with an MCO.
5. Fifty percent of pharmacists believe that affiliation with an MCO positively affects their business (Schering Report XIII, 1986).
6. Overall trends in health care show that more services are shifting from inpatient to ambulatory care settings, including pharmaceutical care.

II. BASIC ELEMENTS OF A MANAGED CARE PRESCRIPTION BENEFIT.

The managed care prescription benefit (MCPB) is designed to manage both the cost of drugs and quality of care.

A. Common elements in an MCPB include:

1. Benefit limitations
2. Provider networks
3. Communication programming
4. Benefit cost-calculations
5. Drug utilization review
6. Formularies
7. Member cost-sharing
8. Claims processing and administration

B. Most **statistics and cost calculations** in an MCO are done on a **per member per month (PMPM) basis**. For example, an MCO with total pharmacy program costs of $250,000, an average number of members per month of 10,000, and a total number of member months [members times 12 months] of 120,000 would have a PMPM program cost of $2.08 [i.e., $\$250,000 \div (10,000 \times 12)$].

C. Managed care plan members share in the **cost of care** either through a deductible, co-payment, or a combination of both.

1. **Co-payment cost** ranges between $1 and $12 or can be expressed as a percentage of retail cost.
2. **Co-payment differentials** for generic and brand-name medications may be used where the brand-name drug would have a higher co-payment fee.
3. **Nonprescription [i.e., over-the-counter (OTC)] drugs** are not covered in MCO pharmacy programs.

D. Pharmacy reimbursement may be either the usual and customary charges paid or a formula [i.e., the average drug price plus dispensing fee] or a variation of both, depending on the plan design.

E. Payment and processing of claims may be handled in the following ways:

1. **Direct claim basis.** These are fee-for-service payments made by the patient.
2. **Card system.** A co-payment is collected and any claims are filed by the pharmacy.
3. **Point of sale (POS) system.** This requires on-line claims adjudication, which eliminates paper documentation while utilizing state-of-the-art computer systems to replace the prescription card. On-line systems are fast becoming the standard for processing pharmaceutical claims by pharmacists.

F. Drug use review, or drug utilization review (DUR) systems are utilized to some degree by most MCOs.

1. The **purpose of a good DUR system is to:**
   a. Reduce mistakes in pharmaceutical care
   b. Help contain costs

2. The **major steps in a DUR system** include:
   a. Collection of data from all sources
   b. Analysis of information to determine any variations in care
   c. Communication or intervention with providers and patients when there is a problem
   d. Continuing reassessment to determine success of the DUR program

III. ADMINISTRATIVE STRUCTURE IN A MANAGED CARE PHARMACY.

The common practice settings in an MCO for pharmacy include staff-model HMOs that may have an in-house clinic pharmacy or administrative positions in IPAs or PPOs, which primarily involve managing the pharmaceutical benefits.

A. Staff model HMOs

1. **The pharmacy director,** sometimes known as the chief pharmacist or pharmacy manager, has several responsibilities within the HMO, including:
   a. Overseeing both personnel and budgetary matters, including drug purchasing decisions
   b. Serving on various HMO committees and typically acting as secretary of the pharmacy committee
   c. Setting quality standards for the department
   d. Establishing policy and procedures for pharmacy operations
   e. Implementing changes or innovations as necessary

2. **Associate or assistant director.** Depending on the size and complexity of the HMO pharmacy department, the pharmacy may have one or more of these positions to aid the director. Specific tasks may include:
   a. Overseeing day-to-day operations
   b. Supervising discrete areas of operation
   c. Directing pharmacy purchasing
   d. Assuming managerial responsibility when the pharmacy director is absent

3. **Clinical pharmacists.** Depending on the size and location of the HMO, a pharmacist with a masters or doctor of pharmacy degree may be responsible for providing clinical services. The clinical pharmacist plays a major role in:
   a. DUR programs
   b. Formulary development
   c. Educational programs
   d. Distribution or patient counseling responsibilities

4. **Staff pharmacists.** These professional employees have daily responsibility for the pharmacy distributive and clinical duties, which can include:
   a. Supervision of support personnel
   b. Physician order review and filling
   c. Extemporaneous compounding
   d. Narcotic drug dispensing
   e. Purchasing
   f. Patient counseling
   g. Medical and nursing staff drug information and in-service education

5. **Technicians or support personnel.** These technical employees work under the direct supervision of a pharmacist and may be pharmacy students fulfilling their internship requirements, or they may be high school graduates.
   a. Many hospitals, colleges, and large MCOs have established technician training programs.
   b. The Association of Pharmacy Technicians, a national organization, includes support personnel working in all pharmacy settings, including HMOs.

6. **Clerical and secretarial support staff** may be involved in:
   a. Pharmacy purchasing

b. Billing
c. Communications
d. Standard clerical or secretarial duties

B. IPAs and PPOs differ from HMOs primarily in the management of drug distribution through a network of pharmacies rather than an in-house type operation. The administrative structure has the following positions.

1. **Director of pharmacy.** This person is primarily responsible for assuring the appropriate delivery of pharmaceutical care through the contracted pharmacy network of community retail pharmacies.

2. **Pharmacy department.** People in this department do not dispense drugs. They act to manage and supervise the participating pharmacies to assure consistency as well as quality of pharmaceutical care being provided to the IPA or PPO members.

3. **Clinical duties** include:
   a. Ensuring appropriate patient counseling to the ambulatory population in the pharmacy network
   b. Providing in-service education to the participating medical staff
   c. Assisting in managing the drug formulary including DUR
   d. Providing or developing selected drug monitoring programs for the IPA or PPO

4. **Purchasing or formulary duties.** Generally, a pharmacist coordinates the negotiated group purchasing activities with the assistance of a clerical or secretarial staff. Unlike pharmacists in most pharmacy settings, an IPA pharmacist is not responsible for **inventory control**. To reduce drug acquisition costs, most IPAs and PPOs will work with their pharmacy network to:
   a. Maximize purchasing discounts
   b. Establish prime-vendor contracts
   c. Negotiate rebates to the IPA and PPO as a means of reducing pharmacy program costs

5. **Committee work.** The pharmacy director typically serves on the pharmacy committee, which oversees the use of medications in the IPA. Working with the committee chairperson (who is usually a physician), the pharmacy director sets the committee's agenda.
   a. The agenda may include:
      (1) Drug formulary additions or deletions
      (2) Reports from DUR
      (3) Policies for handling of therapeutic issues
      (4) Policies for the use of investigational drugs in the IPA or PPO
   b. Other IPA committees may include:
      (1) Quality assurance
      (2) Professional practice (nursing–pharmacy) committees

6. **Community relations.** An IPA or PPO pharmacist may be involved in helping to coordinate IPA or PPO community-wide educational outreach programs on such topics as:
   a. Hypertension
   b. Diabetes
   c. Poison prevention
   d. Substance abuse prevention

IV. RESPONSIBILITIES OF THE MANAGED CARE PHARMACY

A. Drug distribution. Managed care pharmacies distribute drugs to patients from typical retail-type pharmacies, emergency (or night) drug cabinets, and internal supplies of medications for use in the HMO facility, such as vaccines or stock vials of injectables.

B. Clinical duties of pharmacists in a managed care pharmacy include:

1. Providing patient counseling to the ambulatory population

2. Providing in-service education to the medical and nursing staff

3. Assisting in managing the drug formulary including DUR

4. Providing or developing selected drug monitoring programs for the HMO

C. Purchasing and inventory control. This administrative function has been simplified by use of the computer and has become more critical to the overall financial success of the HMO. Generally, a pharmacist coordinates the purchasing with the assistance of clerical or secretarial staff. Drug acquisition costs are reduced by the following.

1. **A group purchasing organization and a prime-vendor contract.** The combined purchasing volume and guarantee of that volume provides the HMO with a discount, which helps reduce pharmacy costs.

2. **Responsible pharmacists.** Inventory control is a part of every pharmacists responsibility. HMO pharmacies usually take an annual physical inventory in addition to monthly inventory that is tracked by computer.

D. Committee work. The pharmacy director typically serves on the pharmacy committee that oversees the use of medications in the HMO. Working with the committee chairperson (usually a physician), the pharmacy director sets the committee's agenda.

1. The agenda may include:
   - **a.** Drug formulary additions or deletions
   - **b.** Reports from DUR
   - **c.** Guidelines for handling hazardous waste
   - **d.** Policy statements on the use of investigational drugs in the HMO
2. Other HMO committees may include:
   - **a.** Infection control
   - **b.** Human studies
   - **c.** Quality assurance
   - **d.** Professional practice (nursing–pharmacy) committees

E. Community relations. An HMO pharmacist may be involved in helping to coordinate HMO and community-wide educational outreach programs on such topics as:

1. Hypertension

2. Diabetes

3. Poison prevention

4. Substance abuse prevention

REFERENCE

Schering Laboratories: *Schering Report XIII.* Schering Report Series, Schering Pharmaceuticals, Kenilworth, New Jersey, 1986.

STUDY QUESTIONS

Directions: Each of the numbered items or incomplete statements in this section is followed by answers or by completions of the statement. Select the **one** lettered answer or completion that is **best** in each case.

1. An independent practice association (IPA) is one example of a

(A) managed care organization (MCO)
(B) pharmacy services administration organization (PSAO)
(C) hospital
(D) clinic
(E) insurance company

2. Responsibilities often delegated to managed care organization (MCO) pharmacy technicians include which one of the following?

(A) Billing and drug purchasing
(B) Patient counseling
(C) Drug dispensing to patients
(D) Review of physicians' prescriptions
(E) Drug monitoring

3. Most statistical revenue or expense reports in a managed care organization (MCO) are expressed in which one of the following terms?

(A) Per member per month (PMPM)
(B) Annual
(C) Monthly
(D) Daily
(E) Weekly

4. The sustained, rapid growth and expansion of managed care organizations (MCO) occurred in the United States after

(A) World War II
(B) legislative changes in the 1970s
(C) the completion of the Grand Coulee Dam
(D) the initiation of Henry Kaiser's health maintenance organization (HMO)
(E) Franklin D. Roosevelt's "New Deal"

5. Payment for pharmaceutical care, including processing of prescription drug claims, typically involve managed care organization (MCO) patients by having them use an identification card and which one of the following?

(A) A computer
(B) An on-line drug utilization review
(C) A claims processor
(D) A co-payment
(E) Communication with the physician

6. Unlike the health maintenance organization's (HMO's) pharmacy director or pharmacist, an independent practice association/preferred provider organization pharmacy director is not responsible for which of the following?

(A) Education
(B) Purchasing and contracts
(C) Dispensing drugs
(D) Quality assurance
(E) Supervising pharmacy personnel

7. In a managed care organization (MCO) plan with a differential deductible or co-payment, the patient pays a higher cash payment when receiving their medication when it is which of the following?

(A) A brand-name drug
(B) A generic drug
(C) A therapeutically interchangeable drug
(D) An over-the-counter (OTC) drug
(E) A multisource drug

1-A 4-B 7-A
2-C 5-D
3-A 6-C

ANSWERS AND EXPLANATIONS

1. The answer is A *[III B].*
A managed care organization (MCO) is an open network, which can allow for the management of drug distribution through a network of pharmacies as in an independent practice association (IPA).

2. The answer is C *[III A 5].*
Managed care organization (MCO) pharmacy technicians may be pharmacy students or well-trained lay people. Their duties may include the technical functions of pharmacy, such as dispensing drugs and entering information into a computer.

3. The answer is A *[II B].*
The real cost analysis in a managed care organization (MCO) is determined by the members. Group premiums are determined by how much a member utilizes a service.

4. The answer is B *[I A 2].*
The 1970s ushered in a period of loans and grants for the specific purpose of nurturing managed care. The federal government appropriated sizable funds to managed care organizations (MCOs) in order to upgrade and expand services.

5. The answer is D *[II C].*
Managed care organization patients are issued an identification card and are required to pay a predetermined co-payment for services, such as prescriptions.

6. The answer is C *[III B 1].*
Independent practice association (IPA)/preferred provider organization (PPO) pharmacy directors are not responsible for dispensing drugs. IPA/PPO directors coordinate pharmacy benefits from a central office where no pharmacy establishment is present.

7. The answer is A *[II C 2].*
Higher cash co-payments are required on single source or brand-name medications as an incentive to use less expensive generic drug products, which have a lower overall cost and therefore a lower co-payment.

27
Home Health Care

William W. McCloskey

I. INTRODUCTION. Home health care, which provides equipment and services that restore or maintain the maximal level of comfort, function, and health of patients in their homes, has become an acceptable and cost-effective alternative to hospitalization. **Respiratory therapy, physical therapy,** and **occupational therapy** can be provided to patients in their homes. However, this chapter focuses on the type of home health care in which pharmacists are involved—**home infusion therapy**.

II. HOME INFUSION THERAPY

A. Growth of home infusion therapy. Home infusion therapy enables patients to receive parenteral medications in their homes that otherwise require inpatient administration. The growth of this area of home health care is projected to grow more than 25% annually through 1994, which can be attributed to the following factors.

1. The **increasing cost of health care,** especially hospital care, makes it more cost-effective to treat patients at home.
2. **Advances in drug delivery technology.** An example is the development of ambulatory infusion devices, such as the **elastomeric infusion pump,** which enables patients to safely and conveniently administer medications at home.
   a. The elastomeric infusion pump is a **disposable** infusion device that delivers parenteral medication with the aid of pressure that is generated by deflation of a balloon-like reservoir.
   b. The pump is designed for **ambulatory delivery of drugs** such as antimicrobials.
3. There is an **increased acceptance** by both physicians and third-party payers regarding the suitability of administering parenteral medications at home.

B. Patient selection for home infusion therapy. Not every patient is a candidate for home infusion therapy. Each provider of home infusion therapy generally develops his or her own criteria for patient selection with a primary concern for patient safety. Most providers consider the following basic criteria when evaluating a patient for treatment.

1. The **patient's medical condition** must be stable or predictable.
2. The **patient or caregiver** must be willing and able to participate in the patient's care.
3. The **home environment** must be suitable for the safe storage and administration of medication and supplies. This includes the presence of electricity, running water, and a telephone.
4. There must be **adequate venous access**. This may include either peripheral access for short courses of therapy (i.e., a few weeks or less) or central venous access for therapy that may last months or longer. Central access usually is established via a minor surgical procedure prior to the patient leaving the hospital or clinic.
5. The patient or caregiver must be able to comprehend and demonstrate **proficiency and competency** in maintaining the access device, medication storage, and admixture when necessary.

C. Home infusion therapies. A number of parenteral therapies are now commonly administered in the home. The following outlines therapies that are more commonly administered.

1. **Total parenteral nutrition (TPN)** is indicated when patients have severe gastrointestinal disease or other conditions that preclude adequate oral ingestion or absorption of sufficient nutrition to maintain normal weight, strength, and fluid and electrolyte balance (see Chapter 29 V A, B).
   a. **Base TPN solution.** The typical parenteral solution contains dextrose, amino acids, electrolytes, vitamins, and trace elements. Since glucose concentrations are usually greater than 10%, these solutions are administered via a central vein.
   b. **Total nutrient admixture (TNA) contains intravenous fat emulsion,** which is administered as a source of calories and is mixed directly with the base TPN solution in the same container.
   c. **Administration.** Most home patients administer their solutions over a period of 8–16 hours, tapering the rate up and down at the beginning and end of their infusion. Some infusion pumps may be programmed to taper the rate automatically.

2. **Antimicrobial therapy.** Antimicrobials, including antibiotic, antifungal and antiviral medications are administered for a variety of infections such as osteomyelitis, bacterial endocarditis, cellulitis, and AIDS-related opportunistic infections (e.g., *Pneumocystis carinii* pneumonia, cryptococcal meningitis, cytomegalovirus).
   a. **Pharmacokinetics.** If given several options for selecting a parenteral antimicrobial to treat an infection, the pharmacokinetics of the drug should be considered. Those agents that can be administered once or twice a day, such as a long-acting cephalosporin, are more convenient for the patient in the home setting than those that require more frequent administration.
   b. **Administration.** Antimicrobials may be administered either through peripheral or central venous access, depending on the anticipated duration of therapy.
   c. **Types of infusion devices** that may be used to administer antimicrobials at home include:
      (1) Disposable ambulatory devices such as the elastomeric pump (see II A 2)
      (2) Syringe pumps for administering prefilled syringes
      (3) Programmable infusion pumps that allow intermittent infusion of doses at preset intervals and keep a vein open between intervals
   d. **Aerosols.** Aerosolized antimicrobials may also be supplied by home infusion therapy providers. Aerosolized pentamidine is commonly given for prophylaxis of *Pneumocystis carinii* pneumonia.

3. **Parenteral analgesic therapy** is appropriate for patients with advanced stages of neoplastic disease who experience chronic, severe pain that is not relieved by more conventional means of pain control. Medication can be delivered by an infusion pump that can be programmed to allow the patient to self-administer small bolus doses as needed. This concept is referred to as **patient-controlled analgesia (PCA).**
   a. The most accepted **method of dosing patients** at home is to continuously administer a short-acting narcotic analgesic, such as morphine, over 24 hours and allow the patient to administer additional bolus doses as needed via PCA.
   b. **Continuous infusion** may be either intravenous, intraspinal, or subcutaneous, if the volume of solution delivered does not exceed 2 ml/hr (the recommended maximum for subcutaneous absorption).

4. **Home chemotherapy.** Chemotherapy may be provided in the home for ambulatory patients who wish to avoid hospitalization or office visits, homebound patients who require chemotherapy, and patients receiving adjuvant therapy or prophylactic chemotherapy for extended periods of time (e.g., many sessions over a 6-month period).
   a. **Administration.** Depending on the chemotherapeutic agent and protocol, home chemotherapy may be administered intravenously, intraarterially, or subcutaneously.
      (1) Patients should have a central venous access established for administration of a drug that is either a **vesicant** or **irritant.**
      (2) If patients have available sites, peripheral administration may be used for administration of a **nonvesicant** agent.
   b. **Waste disposal.** Patients and caregivers should be instructed as to the proper handling and disposal of cytotoxic waste.

5. **Other infusion therapies**
   a. **Common therapies.** Blood products and derivatives, intravenous hydration, iron overload therapy, human growth hormone, and heparin are other common therapies administered in the home.

b. **Inotropic agents** such as dobutamine, dopamine, and amrinone are now being administered at the homes of selected patients who have heart failure refractory to conventional treatment.

c. **Hematopoietic growth factors** [e.g., epoetin alfa, granulocyte–colony-stimulating factor (G-CSF), granulocyte-macrophage–colony-stimulating factor (GM-CSF)], interferon, and other medications developed via biotechnologic advances (e.g., recombinant DNA technology) are gaining wider acceptance for home administration.

D. Role of the pharmacist in home infusion therapy

1. **Initial patient assessment.** A critical step in the provision of home infusion therapy is determining whether or not the patient is a suitable candidate (see II B).
   a. The pharmacist works in conjunction with other caregivers to determine whether or not it would be **safe and effective** to administer a particular therapy based on the patient's medical history and home environment.
   b. As part of this **initial assessment,** the pharmacist takes a comprehensive **drug history** and documents it on a **medication profile**.
      (1) The history should include both **prescription and nonprescription medications**.
      (2) In addition, a **pharmaceutical care plan** is developed to establish what the desired goal of therapy should be.

2. **Pump selection and programming.** One skill that is required of the home infusion pharmacist is an understanding of the variety of devices that may be used to administer parenteral medication. The pharmacist is actively involved in selecting the appropriate infusion device for the therapy based on the type of drug, safety, patient comfort level, reliability, and cost. If necessary, pharmacists program pumps prior to delivery to the patient's home.

3. **Therapeutic drug monitoring.** Since many intravenous medications are associated with toxicities if the dose is not individualized for the patient, routine monitoring of serum drug levels is conducted when appropriate. Serum levels of standard indicators of a patient's health [e.g., blood urea nitrogen (BUN), aspartate aminotransferase (AST), alanine aminotransferase (ALT)] are monitored and the drug regimen is adjusted as necessary.

4. **Patient education.** Patients and their significant others need to learn the skills required to administer parenteral medications including catheter care, aseptic technique, and infusion device troubleshooting. It is also important that they understand what the untoward effects of the medication may be and what to do should they occur.

5. **Parenteral product preparation.** Pharmacists employ principles of sterile product preparation and clean room technology in home infusion therapy, as well as develop quality control procedures for assessing both the final product and the integrity of the environment in which it was prepared (see Chapter 29 IX A–C).

E. Providers of home infusion therapy can be community pharmacy-based, hospital pharmacy-based, or independent commercial vendors. Those providing home care, including home infusion therapy, comprise a team of individuals who work together with patients and their physicians to help assure optimal care of the individual at home.

1. In addition to pharmacists and nurses, this team may include but is not limited to dietitians, social workers, supply coordinators/representatives, and insurance coordinators.

2. There may also be individuals who coordinate the patient's durable medical equipment (e.g., air compressors, wheelchairs).

STUDY QUESTIONS

Directions: Each of the numbered items or incomplete statements in this section is followed by answers or by completions of the statement. Select the **one** lettered answer or completion that is **best** in each case.

1. Which of the following intravenous antibiotics would be most suitable for home infusion therapy if all are equally effective in treating the infection?

(A) Ampicillin
(B) Ceftriaxone
(C) Penicillin G
(D) Cephapirin
(E) Ampicillin/sulbactam

2. Which of the following administration rates is most suitable for continuous subcutaneous administration of morphine sulfate?

(A) 10 ml/hr
(B) 5 ml/hr
(C) 1 ml/hr
(D) 1 ml/min
(E) 0.5 ml/min

3. All of the following factors have attributed to the rapid growth of home infusion therapy EXCEPT

(A) increased cost of hospitalization
(B) development of drug administration devices that enable patients to safely and conveniently administer medications in their home
(C) increased clinical acceptance on the part of physicians and other health care providers
(D) increased acceptance on the part of third-party payers
(E) home infusion therapy is for all patients who receive parenteral medications

4. Home infusion pharmacists may participate directly in all of the following areas of the patient's care EXCEPT

(A) development of a pharmaceutical care plan
(B) programming infusion devices
(C) monitoring serum drug levels
(D) educating patients on their medication
(E) establishing central venous access

1-B
2-C
3-E
4-E

ANSWERS AND EXPLANATIONS

1. The answer is B *[II C 2 a].*
A long-acting cephalosporin, such as ceftriaxone, may be conveniently dosed once or twice a day, making it more suitable for home care than the other agents listed.

2. The answer is C *[II C 3 b].*
Infusion rate should not exceed 2 ml/hr—the recommended maximum for subcutaneous absorption.

3. The answer is E *[II A, B].*
Not every patient is a candidate for home infusion therapy. There are generally specific criteria developed by providers to determine which patients are suitable.

4. The answer is E *[II B 4, D].*
Central venous access is usually established via a minor surgical procedure in a hospital or clinic.

28 Third Party Reimbursement

F. Randy Vogenberg
Dennis G. Lyons

I. INTRODUCTION. For pharmacists, the third party in third party reimbursement is an organization (e.g., an insurance company) or government program (e.g., Medicaid) that reimburses a pharmacy for products or services given to a patient. Third party administrators (TPAs) manage, on behalf of their clients, benefit plans that vary in size and scope of health care services coverage. Prescription drug programs for consumers represented less than 12% of all prescriptions in 1970; however, they are estimated to grow to at least 70% by the year 2000.

A. **Insurance carriers.** Employers or government agencies provide eligible patients, called subscribers, coverage for prescription drugs by one of the following methods.

1. **Full or partial payment.** The agency pays in full or in part for prescription drugs provided by participating pharmacies, who are called **providers**. These pharmacies usually agree to a method of payment or reimbursement based upon the following:
   - **a.** Fee for service (cost of the drug plus a fee)
   - **b.** Capitated payment (a fixed amount per patient per month)
   - **c.** Usual charges (based on retail prices charged to cash-paying patients)

2. **Limited coverage.** Insurers generally limit the coverage for services to specific drugs or classes of drugs, which are defined as the **covered drugs**. Limits may exist for:
   - **a.** The amount of drug (units dispensed)
   - **b.** The duration of therapy (days supply)
   - **c.** The number of prescription refills
   - **d.** The maximum number of days for which a prescription is valid

B. **Pharmacy formats**

1. **Preferred provider organizations (PPOs)** agree contractually to provide services to insured patients at a discounted rate.

2. **Pharmacy services administrative organizations (PSAOs)** provide prescription services on the basis of a contracted rate and may also include claims processing or drug purchasing on a group basis.

3. **Managed care** (see Chapter 26) is a new method of providing pharmaceutical services under a fixed budgeted amount that contains prescreening or utilization controls. Some requirements of managed care include:
   - **a.** Prior authorization of prescriptions, whereby the plan pays for particular drugs or services on the basis of a defined medical necessity
   - **b.** Review of claims that require prior authorization of drugs or service before the claim is paid

II. PRESCRIPTION PAYMENTS. Payment for covered pharmaceutical services is generally defined contractually between participating pharmacies and plan sponsors. The method of payment usually is one of the following.

A. A **fixed fee for service reimbursement** includes payment for the "drug ingredient cost," which is defined as:

1. **Actual acquisition cost (AAC),** which is the pharmacist's net payment made to purchase a drug product, after taking into account such items as purchasing allowances, discounts, and rebates

2. **Average wholesale price (AWP),** which is the composite wholesale price charged on a specific commodity set by the manufacturer and published in the Red Book or Blue Book.
3. **Estimated acquisition cost (EAC),** which is an estimate of the pharmacist's cost based on an analysis of purchasing by various groups classified by dollar volume of drug sales
4. **Maximum allowable cost (MAC),** which is a maximum cost assigned to a particular generic class of drugs usually calculated by a plan administrator or federally funded program (e.g., Medicaid's MACs are usually 150% of the lowest listed AWP of a particular generic drug product)

B. A **dispensing fee** is usually a fixed dollar amount added to the ingredient cost that includes any applicable state or federal tax.

C. Partial payment by patient. Most plans require a portion of the prescription to be paid by the patient while at the pharmacy. This payment may be one of the following:

1. **Copayment.** A copayment is a fixed dollar amount for each dispensed prescription that may vary for brand and generic drugs. The co-payment for generic drugs is set substantially lower than that for brand name drugs to encourage patients to request generic drugs. This is an incentive to urge patients to help keep the cost of health care down.
2. **Deductible.** Some plans require the patient to pay a set dollar amount for a predetermined period of coverage, usually quarterly or annually. The patient assumes the full liability for any prescription until the deductible amount has been expended, then the insurer covers subsequent prescription claims.
3. **Coinsurance.** With coinsurance, patients pay a portion of the prescription cost based on a percentage of the total prescription price, and the insurer covers the balance.

D. Risk sharing (capitation). Under this arrangement, the insurer pays the pharmacy or PSAO a fixed dollar amount per eligible member per month in advance of the service delivery. In this type of program:

1. The pharmacy makes a profit if the actual cost of services utilized by members is less than the amount paid by the plan.
2. The pharmacy loses profit if the cost of services exceeds the amount paid by the plan.

E. Usual and customary charges. Under this system, the pharmacy provides services to eligible members and charges the normal retail price for the prescription. The patient submits a claim to the insurer to be reimbursed by the plan less any coinsurance or deductible. This type of plan is referred to as a **subscriber submit** program.

III. CLAIMS PROCESSING.

Most prescription claims are submitted to a processor referred to as a fiscal intermediary.

A. Fiscal intermediaries perform the following functions.

1. They apply computer verification to submitted claims to ensure that:
   - **a.** Claims are accurate
   - **b.** Patients are eligible for the benefit
2. They provide professional consulting to the plan.
3. They audit participating pharmacies for verification of services.

B. Claims processing procedure. Claims filing varies according to whether the submission is by mail or electronic filing (e.g., via modem, on-line).

1. **Universal claim forms (UCFs),** which were developed in 1977, are the most common format and the national standard for all insurers to pay pharmacies. The National Council of Prescription Drug Programs (NCPDP) is the organization responsible for developing and maintaining UCFs.

2. **On-line claims processing.** The newest and most popular method of submitting pharmacy transactions is via computer.
   a. Claims that are sent by **modem** are sent on computerized forms. These may be sent one of two ways:
      (1) Directly to the TPA
      (2) Through a clearinghouse that verifies the basic elements of the claim
   b. **When the prescription is filled,** on-line claims processing performs the following functions:
      (1) Allows claims to be submitted from the point of sale directly to the fiscal intermediary
      (2) Verifies the eligibility of the patient
      (3) Verifies drug and proper reimbursed amount
      (4) Reduces the number of rejected claims
      (5) Significantly speeds the processing of claims for the pharmacy
   c. On-line drug utilization review. Many plan sponsors are adding drug utilization review capabilities to on-line systems, which can:
      (1) Screen for fraud or abuse
      (2) Target selected higher cost therapies
      (3) Change prescribing practices and patterns of prescribers
      (4) Screen for underuse of drug therapy

IV. ADMINISTRATIVE STRUCTURE AND RESPONSIBILITIES OF THIRD PARTY PRESCRIPTION DRUG PROGRAMS

A. Management

1. Generally, a nonpharmacist is responsible for the overall management of the TPA or prescription program.

2. Lower level management typically may include physicians, nurses, and pharmacists who assist in managing more of the routine daily operations of the benefit program.

B. Sales

1. Sales representatives for third party prescription drug programs are generally not pharmacists. These people are responsible for calling on potential clients in:
   a. Industry
   b. Small or large businesses
   c. Government
   d. Associations

2. The third party prescription drug programs may compete with traditional insurance programs (e.g., Blue Cross)

C. Claims administration handles the computer and claims aspects of the business. This department is staffed primarily with computer engineers and programmers.

D. Drug utilization review (DUR; also called drug use review or drug regimen review) is a relatively new area of focus for TPA firms. Historically, part of the general utilization review program was managed by physicians or nurses. Recent increases in costs for prescription drug benefit programs have resulted in the hiring of specially trained pharmacists to oversee this area of operation. There are **three types of DURs:**

1. **Retrospective,** which is based upon a past claims history by a single patient, a group of patients, or a drug

2. **Concurrent,** which is done during processing of prescriptions for dispensing and compares new prescriptions with what the patient had previously been taking

3. **Prospective** (overlap with concurrent DURs), which are intended to be done before filling a prescription or, in the case of active intervention, before a physician writes a prescription so that any potential harmful interactions can be avoided and the best medication can be given to a patient

STUDY QUESTIONS

Directions: Each of the numbered items or incomplete statements in this section is followed by answers or by completions of the statement. Select the **one** lettered answer or completion that is **best** in each case.

1. Of the following organizations, which one is responsible for establishing and maintaining standards for prescription drug claims?

(A) NCPDP
(B) APhA
(C) AACP
(D) NABP
(E) PSAO

2. When pharmacies organize into a group to provide prescription services on the basis of a contracted rate, this group is called a

(A) TPA
(B) PRO
(C) PPO
(D) RxNET
(E) PSAO

3. An example of a payment method to a pharmacy for providing the drug component of prescription services includes all of the following EXCEPT

(A) average wholesale price (AWP)
(B) actual acquisition cost (AAC)
(C) maximum allowable cost (MAC)
(D) estimated manufacturer's cost

4. A dispensing fee paid to the pharmacy in addition to reimbursement for the drug cost may be paid at the time of service if the patient has to make which one of the following?

(A) Deposit
(B) Co-payment
(C) Deductible
(D) Co-insurance
(E) Down payment

5. The newer and rapidly expanding on-line drug programs offer advantages to the pharmacy and processor in being able not only to facilitate payment of claims, but also to verify patient

(A) eligibility
(B) clinical problems
(C) drug refills
(D) poor credit
(E) transactions

6. Due to the rapid growth and acceptance of prescription drug programs, it is estimated that by the year 2000 these programs will result in which of the following estimated percentages of prescription business?

(A) 50%
(B) 65%
(C) 70%
(D) 85%
(E) 90%

7. When pharmacies agree to contractually provide services to an insured group of patients at a discounted rate, this type of organization or arrangement is called a

(A) health maintenance organization (HMO)
(B) pharmacy services administrative organization (PSAO)
(C) preferred provider organization (PPO)
(D) preferred vendor arrangement
(E) prime-vendor contract

1-A
2-E
3-D
4-B
5-A
6-C
7-C

ANSWERS AND EXPLANATIONS

1. The answer is A *[III B 1].*
Since the development of the first universal claim form (UCF) in 1977, the National Council of Prescription Drug Programs (NCPDP) has been the organization responsible for establishing and maintaining standards for prescription drug claim processing in the United States.

2. The answer is E *[I B 1–2].*
Unlike other pharmacy organizations, groups or associations, a Pharmacy Services Administrative Organization (PSAO) allows pharmacies to organize in a single group on the basis of a negotiated, contracted reimbursement rate. PSAOs do not violate provisions of the federal antitrust laws. They are different from preferred provider organizations (PPOs), which are organizations of providers preferred by a company or insurance group, which requires each of its members to sign an agreement.

3. The answer is D *[II A 1–4].*
The three major examples of payment for the drug cost component in a fixed fee for service pharmacy reimbursement model are the average wholesale price (AWP), the actual acquisition cost (AAC), and the maximum allowable cost (MAC). Manufacturers costs are not factored into the pharmacy-based reimbursement formula.

4. The answer is B *[II B].*
Generally, the dispensing or professional fee component in pharmacy reimbursement formulae has been the target for cost-shifting by all third party payers by way of requiring the patient to make a payment (i.e., a co-payment) to the pharmacy at the time of dispensing. Typically, these fees range from $2 to $15, depending on the plan design. Since the average pharmacy fee is $3.50, many feel that the patient is incurring the cost of service rather than the third party payer.

5. The answer is A *[III A 1 b, B 2 a (2), b (2)].*
A cornerstone to claims processing is being able to assure the eligibility of the individual receiving the pharmacy benefit. This is designed to reduce fraud or improper payment in prescription drug programs.

6. The answer is C *[I].*
Data from the 1980s showed that approximately 12% of all prescriptions in the United States took place via a prescription drug program. Although current estimates place drug programs at nearly 50%, that number is projected to increase to 70% by the year 2000.

7. The answer is C *[I B 1].*
A preferred provider organization (PPO) is a group of pharmacies who contractually agree to provide services as a network to an insured group, usually at some discount, arranged by or through a third party insurer. This is different from a pharmacy services administrative organization (PSAO) in that the pharmacies are a network who sign one contract with the insurer to provide pharmacy services. Preferred vendor arrangements are merely a list of vendors who may be preferred by an insurer for any number of reasons, and a prime vendor refers to a selected wholesaler.

29
Sterile Products

Ernest R. Anderson, Jr.

I. INTRODUCTION

A. Sterility, an absolute term, means the absence of living microorganisms.

1. **Sterile products** are pharmaceutical dosage forms that are sterile. Such products include parenteral preparations, irrigating solutions, and ophthalmic preparations. (For information on ophthalmic preparations, see Chapter 33.)
2. **Aseptic technique** refers to the procedures used to maintain the sterility of pharmaceutical dosage forms.
3. **Parenteral preparations** are pharmaceutical dosage forms that are injected through one or more layers of skin. Because the parenteral route bypasses the protective barriers of the body, parenteral preparations must be sterile. The pH of a solution may markedly influence the stability and compatibility of parenteral preparations (see V B).
4. **Pyrogens** are metabolic by-products of live or dead microorganisms that cause a pyretic response (i.e., a fever) upon injection.
5. **Tonicity** refers to the tone of a solution and is directly related to the osmotic pressure exerted by the solute.
   a. **Hypotonic solutions** have a lower osmotic pressure than blood or 0.9% sodium chloride solution. Because these solutions cause cells to expand, administration may lead to pain and hemolysis.
   b. **Isotonic solutions** exert the same osmotic pressure as blood or 0.9% sodium chloride solution.
   c. **Hypertonic solutions** have a greater osmotic pressure than blood or 0.9% sodium chloride solution. These solutions are administered through a central vein to avoid the pain caused by red blood cell shrinkage (resulting from water loss).

B. Design and function of sterile product areas

1. **Clean rooms.** These areas are specially constructed, filtered, and maintained to prevent environmental contamination of sterile products during the manufacturing process. Clean rooms must meet several **requirements**:
   a. **High-efficiency particulate air (HEPA) filters** are used to cleanse the air entering the room. These filters remove all airborne particles size 0.3 mm or larger with an efficiency of 99.97%. In addition, HEPA-filtered rooms generally are classified as Federal Class 10,000, which means that they contain no more than 10,000 particles size 0.5 mm or larger per cubic foot of air.
   b. **Positive-pressure air flow** is used to prevent contaminated air from flowing into the clean room. In order to achieve this, the air pressure inside the clean room is greater than the pressure outside the room, so that when a door to the clean room is opened, the air flow is outward.
   c. **Counters** in the clean room are made of stainless steel or other nonporous, easily cleaned material.
   d. **Walls and floors** are free from cracks or crevices and have rounded corners. If walls or floors are painted, epoxy paint is used.
   e. **Air flow.** As with the HEPA filters used in clean rooms, the air flow moves with a uniform velocity along parallel lines. The velocity of the air flow is 90 (+/− 20) feet per minute.

2. **Laminar flow hoods.** These clean-air work benches are specially designed, like clean rooms, to ensure the aseptic preparation of sterile products. Laminar flow hoods are generally used in conjunction with clean rooms. However, not all pharmacies involved in preparing sterile products have clean rooms; in these instances, laminar flow hoods are vital to ensure aseptic preparation.
   a. **HEPA filter requirement.** Like clean rooms, laminar flow hoods use HEPA filters, but the hoods use a higher efficiency air filter than do clean rooms. Laminar flow hoods are classified as Federal Class 100, meaning that they contain no more than 100 particles size 0.3 μm or larger per cubic foot of air with an **efficiency of 99.99%**.
   b. **Types of laminar flow hoods**
      (1) **Horizontal** laminar flow hoods were the first hoods used in pharmacies for the preparation of sterile products. Air flow in horizontal hoods moves across the surface of the work area, flowing first through a prefilter and then through the HEPA filter. The major **disadvantage** of the horizontal hood is that it offers no protection to the operator, which is especially significant when antineoplastic agents are being prepared (see V D).
      (2) **Vertical** laminar flow hoods provide **two major advantages** over horizontal flow hoods.
         (a) The air flow is vertical, flowing down on the work space. This air flow pattern protects the operator against potential hazards from the products being prepared.
         (b) A portion of the HEPA-filtered air is recirculated a second time through the HEPA filter. The remainder of the filtered air is removed through an exhaust filter, which may be vented to the outside to protect the operator from chronic, concentrated exposure to hazardous materials.
3. **Inspection and certification.** Clean rooms and laminar flow hoods are inspected and certified when they are first installed, at least every 6 to 12 months thereafter, and, in the case of hoods, when moved to a new location.
   a. **Inspections** are conducted by companies with the sensitive equipment needed for testing procedures and with personnel who are specially trained in these procedures.
   b. The **dioctyl phthalate (DOP) smoke test** ensures that no particle larger than 0.3 mm passes through the HEPA filter. In addition, an anemometer is used to determine air flow velocity, and a particle counter is used to determine the particle count.

II. STERILIZATION METHODS AND EQUIPMENT.

Sterilization is performed to destroy or remove all microorganisms in or on a product. Sterilization may be achieved through thermal, chemical, radioactive, or mechanical methods.

A. Thermal sterilization

A. Thermal sterilization involves the use of either moist or dry heat.

1. **Moist heat sterilization** is the most widely used and reliable sterilization method.
   a. Microorganisms are destroyed by **cellular protein coagulation**.
   b. The objects to be sterilized are exposed to saturated steam under pressure at a minimum temperature of **121°C** for at least **15 minutes**.
   c. An **autoclave** commonly is used for moist heat sterilization.
   d. Because it does not require as high a temperature, moist heat sterilization causes **less product damage** compared to dry heat sterilization.
2. **Dry heat sterilization** is appropriate for materials that cannot withstand moist heat sterilization. Objects are subjected to a temperature of at least **160°C** for **120 minutes** (if higher temperatures can be used, less exposure time is required).

B. Chemical (gas) sterilization is used to sterilize surfaces and porous materials (e.g., surgical dressings) that other sterilization methods may damage.

1. In this method, **ethylene oxide** is generally used in combination with heat and moisture.
2. **Residual gas** must be allowed to dissipate after sterilization and before use of the sterile product.

C. Radioactive sterilization is suitable for the industrial sterilization of contents in sealed packages that cannot be exposed to heat (e.g., prepackaged surgical components and some ophthalmic ointments).

1. This technique involves either **electromagnetic or particulate radiation**.
2. Accelerated drug decomposition sometimes results.

D. Mechanical sterilization (filtration) removes but does not destroy microorganisms and clarifies solutions by eliminating particulate matter. For solutions rendered unstable by thermal, chemical, or radiation sterilization, filtration is the preferred method. A depth filter or screen filter may be used.

1. **Depth filters** usually consist of fritted glass or unglazed porcelain—substances that trap particles in channels.
2. **Screen (membrane) filters** are films measuring 1–200 mm thick made of cellulose esters, microfilaments, polycarbonate, synthetic polymers, silver, or stainless steel.
   a. A **mesh** of millions of microcapillary pores of identical size filter the solution by a process of physical sieving.
   b. **Flow rate.** Because pores make up 70%–85% of the surface, screen filters have a higher flow rate than depth filters.
   c. **Types of screen filters**
      (1) **Particulate filters** remove particles of glass, plastic, rubber, and other contaminants.
         (a) **Other uses.** These filters also are used to reduce the risk of phlebitis associated with administration of reconstituted powders. Filtration removes any undissolved powder particles that may cause venous inflammation.
         (b) The **pore size** of standard particulate filters ranges from 0.45 mm–5 mm. Consequently, particulate filters cannot be used to filter blood, emulsions (e.g., fat emulsions), or suspensions because these preparations have a larger particle size. Special filters are available for blood filtration.
      (2) **Microbial filters,** with a pore size of 0.22 μm or smaller, ensure complete microbial removal or sterilization that is referred to as **cold sterilization**.
      (3) **Final filters,** which may be either particulate or microbial, are in-line filters used to remove particulates or microorganisms from an intravenous solution before infusion.

III. PACKAGING OF PARENTERAL PRODUCTS.

Parenteral preparations and other sterile products must be packaged in a way that maintains product sterility until the time of use and prevents contamination of contents during opening.

A. Types of containers

1. **Ampules,** the oldest type of parenteral product containers, are made entirely of **glass**.
   a. Intended for **single use only,** ampules are opened by breaking the glass at a score line on the neck.
   b. **Disadvantages.** Because glass particles may become dislodged during ampule opening, the product must be filtered before it is administered. Their unsuitability for multiple-dose use, the need to filter solutions before use, and other safety considerations have markedly reduced ampule use.
2. **Vials** are glass or plastic containers closed with a rubber stopper and sealed with an aluminum crimp.
   a. Vials have several **advantages** over ampules.
      (1) Vials can be designed to hold multiple doses (if prepared with a bacteriostatic agent).
      (2) It is easier to remove the product from vials than from ampules.
      (3) Vials eliminate the risk of glass particle contamination during opening.
   b. However, vials also have certain **disadvantages**.
      (1) The rubber stopper may become cored causing a small bit of rubber to enter the solution.
      (2) Multiple withdrawals (as with multiple-dose vials) may result in microbial contamination.
   c. Some drugs that are unstable in solution are packaged in vials unreconstituted and must be reconstituted with sterile water or sterile sodium chloride for injection before use.
      (1) To accelerate the dissolution rate and permit rapid reconstitution, many powders are lyophilized (freeze-dried).
      (2) Some of these drugs come in vials that contain a double chamber.
         (a) The top chamber, containing sterile water for injection, is separated from the unreconstituted drug by a rubber closure.
         (b) To dislodge the inner closure and mix the contents of the compartments, external pressure is applied to the outer rubber closure. This system eliminates the need to enter the vial twice, thereby reducing the risk of microbial contamination.

3. Some drugs come in vials that may be attached to an intravenous bag for reconstitution and administration (Add-Vantage by Abbott).
   a. The Add-Vantage vial is screwed into the top of an Add-Vantage intravenous bag, and the rubber diaphragm is dislodged from the vial allowing the intravenous solution to dissolve the drug.
   b. The reconstituted Add-Vantage vial and intravenous bag are ready for administration when hung.

4. **Prefilled syringes and cartridges** are designed for maximum convenience.
   a. **Prefilled syringes.** Drugs administered in an emergency (e.g., atropine, epinephrine) are available for immediate injection when packaged in prefilled syringes.
   b. **Prefilled cartridges** are ready-to-use parenteral packages that offer improved sterility and accuracy. They consist of a plastic cartridge holder and a prefilled medication cartridge with a needle attached. The medication is premixed and premeasured.

5. **Infusion solutions** are divided into two categories: small volume parenterals (SVP), those having a volume less than 100 ml; and large volume parenterals (LVP), those having a volume of 100 ml or greater. Infusion solutions are used for the intermittent or continuous infusion of fluids or drugs (see VIII B).

B. Packaging materials. Materials used to package parenteral products include glass and plastic polymers.

1. **Glass,** the original parenteral packaging material, has superior clarity, facilitating inspection for particulate matter. Compared to plastic, glass less frequently interacts with the preparation it contains.

2. **Plastic polymers** used for parenteral packaging include polyvinylchloride (PVC) and polyolefin.
   a. **PVC** is flexible and nonrigid.
   b. **Polyolefin** is semi-rigid; unlike PVC, it can be stored upright.
   c. Both types of plastic offer several **advantages** over glass including durability, easier storage, reduced weight, and improved safety.

IV. PARENTERAL ADMINISTRATION ROUTES.

Parenteral preparations may be given by a variety of administration routes.

A. Subcutaneous administration refers to injection into the subcutaneous tissue beneath the skin layers—usually of the arm or thigh. Insulin is an example of a subcutaneously administered drug.

B. Intramuscular administration means injection into a muscle mass. The mid-deltoid area and gluteus medius are common injection sites.

1. No more than 5 ml of a solution should be injected by this route.
2. Drugs intended for prolonged or delayed absorption (e.g., methylprednisolone) commonly are administered intramuscularly.

C. Intravenous administration is the most important and most common parenteral administration route. It allows an immediate therapeutic effect by delivering the drug directly into the circulation. However, this route precludes recall of an inadvertent drug overdose. Antibiotics, cardiac medications, and many other drugs are given intravenously.

D. Intradermal administration involves injection into the most superficial skin layer. Because this route can deliver only a limited drug volume, its use generally is restricted to skin tests and certain vaccines.

E. Intra-arterial administration is injection directly into an artery. It delivers a high drug concentration to the target site with little dilution by the circulation. Generally, this route is used only for radiopaque materials and some antineoplastic agents.

F. Intracardiac administration is injection of a drug directly into the heart.

G. Hypodermoclysis refers to injection of large volumes of a solution into subcutaneous tissue to provide a continuous, abundant drug supply. This route occasionally is used for antibiotic administration in children.

H. Intraspinal administration refers to injection into the spinal column.

I. Intra-articular administration means injection into a joint space.

J. Intrasynovial administration refers to injection into the joint fluid.

K. Intrathecal administration is injection into the spinal fluid; it sometimes is used for antibiotics.

V. PARENTERAL PREPARATIONS

A. Intravenous admixtures. These preparations consist of one or more sterile drug products added to an intravenous fluid—generally dextrose or sodium chloride solution alone or in combination. Intravenous admixtures are used for drugs intended for continuous infusion and for drugs that may cause irritation or toxicity when given via direct intravenous injection.

B. Intravenous fluids and electrolytes

1. **Fluids** used in the preparation and administration of parenteral products include sterile water and sodium chloride, dextrose, and Ringer's solutions, all of which have multiple uses. For example, these fluids serve as vehicles in intravenous admixtures, they provide a means for reconstituting sterile powders, and they serve as the basis for correcting body fluid and electrolyte disturbances and for administering parenteral nutrition.
   a. **Dextrose (D-glucose) solutions** are the most frequently used glucose solutions in parenteral preparations.
      (1) **Uses.** Generally, a solution of 5% dextrose in water (D5W) is used as a vehicle in intravenous admixtures. D5W may also serve as a hydrating solution. In higher concentrations (e.g., a 10% solution in water), dextrose provides a source of carbohydrates in parenteral nutrition solutions.
      (2) **Considerations.** Because the pH of D5W ranges from 3.5 to 6.5, instability may result if it is combined with an acid-sensitive drug.
         (a) Dextrose concentrations greater than 15% must be administered through a central vein.
         (b) Dextrose solutions should be used cautiously in patients with diabetes mellitus.
   b. **Sodium chloride** usually is given as a 0.9% solution. Because it is isotonic with blood, this solution is called normal saline solution (NSS). A solution of 0.45% sodium chloride is termed half-normal saline.
      (1) **Sodium chloride for injection,** which is a solution of 0.9% sodium chloride, is used as a vehicle in intravenous admixtures and for fluid and electrolyte replacement. In smaller volumes, it is suitable for the reconstitution of various medications.
      (2) **Bacteriostatic sodium chloride for injection,** which is also a 0.9% solution, is intended solely for multiple reconstitutions. It contains an agent that inhibits bacterial growth (e.g., benzyl alcohol, propylparaben, methylparaben), which allows for its use in multiple-dose preparations.
   c. **Waters** are used for reconstitution and for dilution of such intravenous solutions as dextrose and sodium chloride. Waters suitable for parenteral preparations include sterile water for injection and bacteriostatic water for injection.
   d. **Ringer's solutions,** which are appropriate for fluid and electrolyte replacement, commonly are administered to postsurgical patients.
      (1) **Lactated Ringer's injection** (i.e., Hartmann's solution, Ringer's lactate solution) contains sodium lactate, sodium chloride, potassium chloride, and calcium chloride. Frequently, it is combined with dextrose (e.g., as 5% dextrose in lactated Ringer's injection).
      (2) **Ringer's injection** differs from lactated Ringer's injection in that it does not contain sodium lactate and has slightly different concentrations of sodium chloride and calcium chloride. Like lactated Ringer's injection, it may be combined in solution with dextrose.

2. **Electrolyte preparations.** Ions present in both intracellular and extracellular fluid, electrolytes are crucial for various biologic processes. Surgical and medical patients who cannot take food by mouth or who need nutritional supplementation require the addition of electrolytes in hydrating solutions or parenteral nutrition solutions.
   a. **Cations** are positively charged electrolytes.
      (1) **Sodium** is the chief extracellular cation.
         (a) **Importance.** Sodium plays a key role in interstitial osmotic pressure, tissue hydration, acid–base balance, nerve impulse transmission, and muscle contraction.

(b) **Parenteral sodium preparations** include sodium chloride, sodium acetate, and sodium phosphate.

(2) **Potassium** is the chief intracellular cation.

(a) **Importance.** Potassium participates in carbohydrate metabolism, protein synthesis, muscle contraction (especially of cardiac muscle), and neuromuscular excitability.

(b) **Parenteral potassium preparations** include potassium acetate, potassium chloride, and potassium phosphate.

(3) **Calcium**

(a) **Importance.** Calcium is essential to nerve impulse transmission, muscle contraction, cardiac function, and capillary and cell membrane permeability.

(b) **Parenteral calcium preparations** include calcium chloride, calcium gluconate, and calcium gluceptate.

(4) **Magnesium**

(a) **Importance.** Magnesium plays a vital part in enzyme activities, neuromuscular transmission, and muscle excitability.

(b) **Parenteral preparation.** Magnesium is given parenterally as magnesium sulfate.

b. Anions are negatively charged electrolytes.

(1) **Chloride** is the major extracellular anion.

(a) **Importance.** Along with sodium, it regulates interstitial osmotic pressure and helps to control blood pH.

(b) **Parenteral chloride preparations** include calcium chloride, potassium chloride, and sodium chloride.

(2) **Phosphate** is the major intracellular anion.

(a) **Importance.** Phosphate is critical to various enzyme activities. It also influences calcium levels and acts as a buffer to prevent marked changes in acid–base balance.

(b) **Parenteral phosphate preparations** include potassium phosphate and sodium phosphate.

(3) **Acetate**

(a) **Importance.** Acetate is a bicarbonate precursor that may be used to provide alkali to assist in the preservation of plasma pH.

(b) **Parenteral acetate preparations** include potassium acetate and sodium acetate.

C. Parenteral antibiotic preparations are available as sterile unreconstituted powders, which must be reconstituted with sterile water, normal saline, or D5W, or as a sterile liquid parenteral.

1. **Administration methods.** Parenteral antibiotics may be given intermittently by direct intravenous injection, short term infusion, intramuscular injection, or intrathecal injection.

2. **Uses.** Parenteral antibiotics are used to treat infections that are serious and require high blood levels or when the gastrointestinal tract is contraindicated, such as in ileus.

3. **Dosing frequencies** of parenteral antibiotics vary from once daily to as often as every 2 hours depending on the kinetics of the drug, the seriousness of the infection, and the patient's disease or organ status (e.g., renal disease).

D. Parenteral antineoplastic agents. These medications may be toxic to the personnel who prepare and administer them, necessitating special precautions to ensure safety. In addition, patients receiving antineoplastics may experience various problems associated with drug delivery.

1. **Administration methods.** Parenteral antineoplastics may be given by direct intravenous injection, short-term infusion, or long-term infusion. Some are administered by a nonintravenous route, such as the subcutaneous, intramuscular, intra-arterial, or intrathecal route.

2. **Safe antineoplastic handling guidelines.** All pharmacy and nursing personnel who prepare or administer antineoplastics should receive special training in the following guidelines to reduce the risk of injury from exposure to these drugs.

a. A **vertical laminar flow hood** should be used during drug preparation, with exhaust directed to the outside.

b. All syringes and intravenous tubing should have **Luer-Lok fittings** (see VII B 1, 4).

c. **Clothing.** Personnel should wear closed-front cuffed surgical gowns and double-layered latex surgeon's gloves.
d. **Negative-pressure technique** should be used during withdrawal of medication from vials.
e. **Final dosage adjustment** should be made into the vial or ampule, or directly into an absorbent gauze pad.
f. **Priming equipment.** Special care should be taken when intravenous administration sets are primed.
g. Proper procedures should be followed for **disposal** of materials used in the preparation and administration of antineoplastics.
(1) **Needles** should not be clipped or recapped.
(2) **Preparations** should be discarded in containers that are puncture-proof, leak-proof, and properly labeled.
(3) **Hazardous waste** should be incinerated at a temperature sufficient to destroy organic compounds (1000°C).
h. After removal of gloves, personnel should **wash hands** thoroughly.
i. Personnel and equipment involved in the preparation and administration of antineoplastic agents should be **monitored** routinely.

3. **Patient problems.** Infusion phlebitis and extravasation are the most serious problems that may occur during the administration of parenteral antineoplastics.
a. **Infusion phlebitis**—inflammation of a vein—is characterized by pain, swelling, heat sensation, and redness at the infusion site. Drug dilution and filtration may eliminate or minimize the risk of phlebitis.
b. **Extravasation**—infiltration of a drug into subcutaneous tissues surrounding the vein—is especially harmful when antineoplastics with vesicant properties are administered. Measures must be taken immediately if extravasation occurs.
(1) Depending on the drug involved, emergency measures may include stopping the infusion, injecting hydrocortisone or another anti-inflammatory agent directly into the affected area, injecting an antidote (if available), and applying a cold compress (to facilitate a drug–antidote reaction).
(2) A warm compress may then be applied to increase the flow of blood, and thus the vesicant, away from damaged tissue.

E. **Parenteral biotechnology products** are created by the application of biologic processes to the generation of therapeutic agents such as monoclonal antibodies, various vaccines, and colony-stimulating factors.

1. **Potential uses** of these agents include cancer therapy, septic shock, infections, transplant rejection and vaccines against cancer, HIV infection, hepatitis B, herpes, and malaria.

2. **Characteristics.** Protein and peptide biotechnology drugs have a shorter half-life, often require special storage such as refrigeration or freezing, and must not be shaken vigorously lest the protein molecules be destroyed.

3. **Administration.** Many biotechnology products require reconstitution with sterile water or normal saline and may be parenterally administered by direct intravenous injection or infusion, or by intramuscular or subcutaneous injection.

VI. IRRIGATING SOLUTIONS.

Although these sterile products are manufactured by the same standards used to process intravenous preparations, they are **not intended for infusion into the venous system**.

A. **Topical administration.** Irrigating solutions for topical use are packaged in pour bottles so that they can be poured directly onto the desired area. These solutions are intended for such purposes as irrigating wounds, moistening dressings, and cleaning surgical instruments.

B. **Infusion of irrigating solutions.** This procedure, using an administration set attached to a Foley catheter, is commonly used for many surgical patients. Surgeons performing urologic procedures often use irrigating solutions to perfuse tissues in order to maintain the integrity of the surgical field, to remove blood, and to provide a clear field of view. To decrease the risk of infection, 1 ml of Neosporin G.U. Irrigant, an antibiotic preparation, is often added to these solutions.

C. Dialysis. Dialysates are irrigating solutions used in the dialysis of patients with such disorders as renal failure, poisoning, and electrolyte disturbances. These products remove waste materials, serum electrolytes, and toxic products from the body.

1. In **peritoneal dialysis,** a hypertonic dialysate is infused directly into the peritoneal cavity via a surgically implanted catheter. The dialysate, which contains dextrose and electrolytes, removes harmful substances by osmosis and diffusion. After a specified period of time, the solution is drained. Antibiotics and heparin may be added to the dialysate.

2. In **hemodialysis,** the patient's blood is transfused through a dialyzing membrane unit that removes the harmful substances from the patient's vascular system. After passing through the dialyzer, the blood reenters the body through a vein.

VII. NEEDLES AND SYRINGES

A. Hypodermic needles are stainless steel or aluminum devices that penetrate the skin for the purpose of administering or transferring a parenteral product.

1. **Needle gauge** refers to the outside diameter of the needle shaft; the larger the number, the smaller the diameter. Gauges in common use range from 13 (largest diameter) to 27. Subcutaneous injections usually require a 24-gauge or 25-gauge needle. Intramuscular injections require a needle with a gauge between 19 and 22. Needles between 18-gauge and 20-gauge are commonly used for compounding parenterals.

2. **Bevels** are slanting edges cut into needle tips to facilitate injection through tissue or rubber vial closures.
   a. **Regular-bevel needles** are the most commonly used type, and they are suitable for subcutaneous and intramuscular injections and hypodermoclysis.
   b. **Short-bevel needles** are used when only shallow penetration is required (as in intravenous injections).
   c. **Intradermal-bevel needles** are designed for intradermal injections and have the most bevelled edges.

3. **Needle lengths** range from 1/4 inch to 6 inches. Choice of needle length depends on the desired penetration.
   a. For **compounding parenteral preparations,** 1½ inch-long needles are commonly used.
   b. **Intradermal injection** necessitates a needle length of 1/4 inch to 5/8 inch.
   c. **Intracardiac injection** requires a needle length of 3½ inches.
   d. **Intravenous infusion** requires needles that range in length from 1¼ inches to 2½ inches.

B. Syringes are devices for injecting, withdrawing, or instilling fluids. Syringes consist of a glass or plastic barrel with a tight-fitting plunger at one end; a small opening at the other end accommodates the head of a needle.

1. The **Luer syringe,** the first syringe developed, has a universal needle attachment accommodating all needle sizes.

2. **Syringe volumes** range from 0.3–60 ml. Insulin syringes have unit gradations (100 units/ml) rather than volume gradations.

3. **Calibrations,** which may be in the metric or English system, vary in specificity depending on syringe size; the smaller the syringe, the more specific the scale.

4. **Syringe tips** come in several types.
   a. **Luer-Lok tips** are threaded to ensure that the needle fits tightly in the syringe. Antineoplastic agents should be administered with syringes of this type (see V D 2).
   b. **Luer-Slip tips** are unthreaded so that the syringe and needle do not lock into place. Because of this, the needle may become dislodged.
   c. **Eccentric tips,** which are set off center, allow the needle to remain parallel to the injection site and minimize venous irritation.
   d. **Catheter tips** are used for wound irrigation and administration of enteral feedings. They are not intended for injections.

VIII. INTRAVENOUS DRUG DELIVERY

A. Injection sites

1. **Peripheral vein injection** is preferred for drugs that do not irritate the veins, for administration of isotonic solutions, and for patients who require only short-term intravenous therapy. Generally, the dorsal forearm surface is chosen for venipuncture.
2. **Central vein injection** is preferred for administration of irritating drugs or hypertonic solutions, for patients requiring long-term intravenous therapy, and for situations in which a peripheral line cannot be maintained. Large veins in the thoracic cavity, such as the subclavian, are used.

B. Infusion methods

1. **Continuous-drip infusion** is the slow, primary-line infusion of an intravenous preparation to maintain a therapeutic drug level or provide fluid and electrolyte replacement.
   a. **Flow rates** must be carefully monitored. Generally, these rates are expressed as volume per unit of time (e.g., ml/hr or drops/min) and sometimes as μg/min for certain drugs.
   b. **Administration.** Such drugs as aminophylline, heparin and pressor agents typically are administered by this method.
2. **Intermittent infusion** allows drug administration at specific intervals (e.g., every 4 hours) and is most often used for antibiotics.
   a. **Three different techniques** may be used.
      (1) **Direct (bolus) injection** rapidly delivers small volumes of an undiluted drug. This method is used to:
         (a) Achieve an immediate effect (as in an emergency)
         (b) Administer drugs that cannot be diluted
         (c) Achieve a therapeutic serum drug level quickly
      (2) **Additive set infusion,** using a volume-control device, is appropriate for the intermittent delivery of small amounts of intravenous solutions or diluted medications. The fluid chamber is attached to an independent fluid supply or placed directly under the established primary intravenous line.
      (3) The **piggyback method** is used when a drug cannot be mixed with the primary solution. A special coupling for the primary intravenous tubing permits infusion of a supplementary secondary solution through the primary system.
         (a) This method eliminates the need for a second venipuncture or further dilution of the supplementary preparation.
         (b) **Admixtures** in which the vehicle is added to the drug are known as manufacturers' piggybacks. Admixtures in which a special drug vial is attached to a special intravenous bag are known as the Add-Vantage system.
   b. In some cases, **intermittent infusion injection devices** are used. Also called scalp-vein, heparin-lock, or butterfly infusion sets, these devices permit intermittent delivery while eliminating the need for multiple venipunctures or prolonged venous access with a continuous infusion. To prevent clotting in the cannula, dilute heparin solution or normal saline solution may be added. Benefits of intermittent infusion injection devices include the following.
      (1) This method is especially suitable for patients who do not require, or would be jeopardized by, administration of large amounts of intravenous fluids (e.g., those with congestive heart failure).
      (2) Because intermittent infusion injection devices do not require continuous attachment to an intravenous bottle or bag and pole, they permit greater patient ambulation.

C. Pumps and controllers

C. Pumps and controllers are the electronic devices used to administer parenteral infusions when the use of gravity flow alone might lead to inaccurate dosing or risk patient safety. Pumps and controllers are used to administer parenteral nutrition, chemotherapy, cardiac medications, and blood and blood products.

1. **Pumps** are used to deliver intravenous infusions with accuracy and safety.
   a. Two **types of mechanisms** are used in infusion pumps.
      (1) **Piston-cylinder mechanisms** use a piston in a cylinder or a syringe-like apparatus to pump the desired volume of fluid.
      (2) **Linear peristaltic mechanisms** use external pressure to expel the fluid out of the pumping chamber.

b. Types of pumps

(1) **Volumetric pumps** are used for intermittent infusion of medications such as antibiotics. They are also used for continuous infusion of intravenous fluid, parenteral nutrition, anticoagulants, and anti-asthma medications.

(2) **Syringe pumps** are used to administer intermittent or continuous infusions of medications (e.g., antibiotics and opiates) in concentrated form.

(3) **Mobile infusion pumps** are small infusion devices designed for ambulatory and home patients, and are used for administering chemotherapy and opiate medications.

(4) **Implantable pumps** are infusion devices surgically placed under the skin to provide a continuous release of medication, typically an opiate. The reservoir in the pump is refilled by injecting the medication through a latex diaphragm in the pump. This type of pump allegedly has a lower incidence of infection.

(5) **Patient-controlled analgesia pumps** are used to administer narcotics intermittently or on demand by the patient within the patient-specific parameters, which are ordered by the physician and programmed into the pump.

c. Benefits. Pumps, despite their extra costs and the training required by personnel, provide a number of important benefits. They maintain a constant, accurate flow rate; they detect infiltrations, occlusions, and air; and they may save nursing time.

2. Controllers, unlike pumps, exert no pumping pressure on the intravenous fluid. Rather, they rely on gravity and control the infusion by counting drops electronically, or they infuse the fluid mechanically and electronically (e.g., volumetric controllers). In **comparison to pumps,** the following are characteristics of controllers.

a. Controllers are less complex and generally are less expensive.

b. They achieve reasonable accuracy.

c. Controllers are very useful for uncomplicated infusion therapy but cannot be used for arterial drug infusion or for infusion into small veins.

D. Intravenous incompatibilities. When two or more drugs must be administered through a single intravenous line or given in a single solution, an undesirable reaction may occur. Although such incompatibilities are relatively rare, their consequences may be significant. A patient who receives a preparation in which an incompatibility has occurred may experience toxicity or an incomplete therapeutic effect.

1. Types of incompatibilities

a. A **physical incompatibility** occurs when a drug combination produces a visible change in the appearance of a solution.

(1) An **example** of physical incompatibility is the evolution of carbon dioxide when sodium bicarbonate and hydrochloric acid are admixed.

(2) Various **types** of physical incompatibilities may occur:

(a) Visible color change or darkening

(b) Formation of precipitate, which may result from the combination of phosphate and calcium

b. A **chemical incompatibility** reflects the chemical degradation of one or more of the admixed drugs, resulting in toxicity or therapeutic inactivity.

(1) The degradation is not always visible. **Nonvisible chemical incompatibility** may be detected only by analytical methods.

(2) Chemical incompatibility occurs in several **varieties**.

(a) **Complexation** is a reaction between products that inactivates them. For example, the combination of calcium and tetracycline leads to formation of a complex that inactivates tetracycline.

(b) **Oxidation** occurs when one drug loses electrons to the other, resulting in a color change and therapeutic inactivity.

(c) **Reduction** takes place when one drug gains electrons from the other.

(d) **Photolysis**—chemical decomposition caused by light—may lead to hydrolysis or oxidation, with resulting discoloration.

c. A **therapeutic incompatibility** occurs when two or more drugs, intravenous fluids, or both are combined and the result is a response other than that intended. An example of a therapeutic incompatibility is the reduced bactericidal activity of penicillin G when given after tetracycline. Since tetracycline is a bacteriostatic agent, it slows bacterial growth; penicillin, on the other hand, is most effective against rapidly proliferating bacteria. To prevent therapeutic incompatibility in this case, penicillin G should be given before tetracycline.

2. **Factors affecting intravenous compatibility**
   a. **pH.** Incompatibility is more likely to occur when the components of an intravenous solution differ significantly in pH. This increased risk is explained by the chemical reaction between an acid and a base, which yields a salt and water; the salt may be an insoluble precipitate.
   b. **Temperature.** Generally, increased storage temperature speeds drug degradation. To preserve drug stability, drugs should be stored in a refrigerator or freezer, as appropriate.
   c. **Degree of dilution.** Generally, the more diluted the drugs are in a solution, the less chance there is for an ion interaction leading to incompatibility.
   d. **Length of time in solution.** The chance for a reaction resulting in incompatibility increases with the length of time that drugs are in contact with each other.
   e. **Order of mixing.** Drugs that are incompatible in combination, such as calcium and phosphate, should not be added consecutively when an intravenous admixture is being prepared. This keeps these substances from pooling, or forming a layer on the top of the intravenous fluid, and, therefore, decreases the chance of an incompatibility. Thorough mixing after each addition is also essential.
3. **Preventing or minimizing incompatibilities.** To reduce the chance for an incompatibility, the following steps should be taken.
   a. Solutions should be administered promptly after they are mixed to minimize the time available for a potential reaction to occur.
   b. Each drug should be mixed thoroughly after it is added to the preparation.
   c. The number of drugs mixed together in an intravenous solution should be kept to a minimum.
   d. If a prescription calls for unfamiliar drugs or IV fluids, compatibility references should be consulted.

E. **Hazards of parenteral drug therapy.** A wide range of problems can occur with parenteral drug administration.

1. **Physical hazards**
   a. **Phlebitis,** which is generally a minor complication, may result from vein injury or irritation. Phlebitis can be minimized or prevented through proper intravenous insertion technique, dilution of irritating drugs, and a decreased infusion rate.
   b. **Extravasation** may occur with administration of drugs with vesicant properties (see V D 3 b).
   c. **Irritation** at the injection site can be reduced by varying the injection site and applying a moisturizing lotion to the area.
   d. **Pain** of infusate is most common with peripheral intravenous administration of a highly concentrated preparation. Switching to central vein infusion and diluting the drug may alleviate the problem.
   e. **Air embolism,** potentially fatal, can result from entry of air into the intravenous tubing.
   f. **Infection,** a particular danger with central intravenous lines, may stem from contamination during intravenous line insertion or tubing changes. Infection may be local or generalized (septicemia). The infection risk can be minimized by following established protocols for the care of central lines.
   g. **Allergic reactions** may result from hypersensitivity to an intravenous solution or additive.
   h. **Central catheter misplacement** may lead to air embolism or pneumothorax. To prevent this problem, catheter placement should always be verified radiologically.
   i. **Hypothermia,** possibly resulting in shock and cardiac arrest, may stem from administration of a cold intravenous solution. This problem can be prevented by allowing parenteral products to reach room temperature.
   j. **Neurotoxicity** may be a serious complication of intrathecal or intraspinal administration of drugs containing preservatives. Preservative free drugs should be used in these circumstances.
2. **Mechanical hazards**
   a. **Infusion pump or controller failure** may lead to runaway infusion, fluid overload, or incorrect dosages.
   b. **Intravenous tubing** may become kinked, split, or cracked. It also may produce particulates, allow contamination, or interfere with the infusion.
   c. **Particulate matter** may be present in a parenteral product.
   d. **Glass containers** may break, causing injury.
   e. **Rubber vial closures** may interact with the enclosed product.

3. **Therapeutic hazards**
   a. **Drug instability** may lead to therapeutic ineffectiveness.
   b. **Incompatibility** may result in toxicity or reduced therapeutic effectiveness.
   c. **Labeling errors** may cause administration of an incorrect drug or improper dosage.
   d. **Drug overdose** may be caused by runaway intravenous infusion, failure of an infusion pump or controller, or nursing or pharmacy errors.
   e. **Preservative toxicity** may be a serious complication, especially in children. For example, premature infants receiving parenteral products containing benzyl alcohol may develop a fatal acidotic toxic syndrome, which is referred to as the gasping syndrome.

IX. QUALITY CONTROL AND QUALITY ASSURANCE

A. Definitions

1. **Quality control** is the day-to-day assessment of all operations from the receipt of raw material to the distribution of the finished product, including analytic testing of the finished product.

2. **Quality assurance,** an oversight function, involves the auditing of quality control procedures and systems, with suggestions for changes as needed.

B. Testing procedures. Various types of tests are used to ensure that all sterile products are free of microbial contamination, pyrogens, and particulate matter. In addition, ampules are subjected to a leaker test to ensure that the container is completely sealed.

1. **Sterility testing** ensures that the process used to sterilize the product was successful.
   a. The **official *United States Pharmacopeia (USP)* standard** for sterility testing calls for the following:
      (1) A 10-test sample for batches of 20 to 200 units
      (2) A minimum of two test samples for batches of less than 20 units
   b. The **membrane sterilization method** is often used to conduct sterility testing. Test samples are passed through membrane filters and a nutrient medium is then added to promote microbial growth. After an incubation period, microbial growth is determined.

2. **Pyrogen testing** by means of qualitative fever response test in rabbits and an in vitro limulus lysate test is often difficult to conduct because of lack of facilities. Therefore, people handling sterile products should attempt to avoid problems with pyrogens by purchasing pyrogen-free water and sodium chloride for injection from reputable manufacturers and by using proper handling and storage procedures. Commercial laboratories are available to perform these tests.

3. **Clarity testing** is used to check sterile products for particulate matter. Before dispensing a parenteral solution, pharmacy personnel should check it for particulates by swirling the solution and looking at it against both light and dark backgrounds, using a clarity testing lamp or other standard light source.

C. Practical quality assurance programs for noncommercial sterile products include training, monitoring the manufacturing process, quality control check, and documentation.

1. **Training of pharmacists and technicians** in proper aseptic techniques and practices is the single most important aspect of an effective quality assurance program. Training should impart a thorough understanding of departmental policies and procedures.

2. By **monitoring the manufacturing process,** a supervisor can check adherence to established policies and procedures and take corrective action as necessary.

3. **Quality control** checking includes monitoring the sterility of a sample of manufactured products. The membrane sterilization method is practically employed using a commercially available filter and trypticase soy broth media.

4. **Documentation** of training procedures, quality control results, laminar flow hood certification, and production records are required by various agencies and organizations.

STUDY QUESTIONS

Directions: Each of the numbered items or incomplete statements in this section is followed by answers or by completions of the statement. Select the **one** lettered answer or completion that is **best** in each case.

1. Parenteral products with an osmotic pressure greater than that of blood or 0.9% sodium chloride are referred to as

(A) isotonic solutions
(B) hypertonic solutions
(C) hypotonic solutions
(D) iso-osmotic solutions
(E) neutral solutions

2. Sterilization of an ophthalmic solution could be achieved in a community pharmacy by

(A) using a 0.45-μm filter
(B) using a 0.22-μm filter
(C) incorporating the drug into an already sterile vehicle
(D) radiation sterilization
(E) heat sterilization

3. Which needle has the largest diameter?

(A) 25-gauge × 3/4 ″
(B) 24-gauge × 1/2″
(C) 22-gauge × 1″
(D) 20-gauge × 3/8″
(E) 26-gauge × 5/8″

4. Intradermal injection refers to injection into the

(A) muscle mass
(B) subcutaneous tissue
(C) spinal fluid
(D) superficial skin layer
(E) joint fluid

5. Advantages of the intravenous route include

(A) ease of removal of the dose
(B) a depo effect
(C) low incidence of phlebitis
(D) rapid onset of action
(E) a localized effect

6. The central vein may be considered a suitable route for intravenous administration in which of the following situations?

(A) When a nonirritating drug is given
(B) When isotonic drugs are given
(C) For short-term therapy
(D) When venous access is poor
(E) For postoperative hydration

7. The formation of an insoluble precipitate as a result of admixing calcium and phosphate is an example of what type of incompatibility?

(A) Chemical
(B) Physical
(C) Pharmacologic
(D) Medicinal
(E) Therapeutic

8. Parenteral drug products undergo what type of testing to ensure that all microorganisms have been destroyed or removed?

(A) Clarity testing
(B) Leaker testing
(C) Pyrogen testing
(D) Sterility testing
(E) Solubility testing

9. Which of the following drugs should NOT be prepared in a horizontal laminar flow hood?

(A) Aminophylline
(B) Dopamine
(C) Doxorubicin
(D) Nitroglycerin
(E) Bretylium tosylate

10. True statements about D5W include all of the following EXCEPT

(A) its pH range is 8 to 10
(B) it is isotonic
(C) it is a 5% solution of D-glucose
(D) it should be used with caution in diabetic patients
(E) it is often used in intravenous admixtures

1-B	4-D	7-B	10-A
2-B	5-D	8-D	
3-D	6-D	9-C	

11. As a packaging material for parenteral products, plastic offers all of the following advantages over glass EXCEPT

(A) unbreakability
(B) improved clarity for visual inspection
(C) ease of storage
(D) decreased weight
(E) safety

12. Procedures for the safe handling of antineoplastic agents include all of the following EXCEPT

(A) use of Luer-Lok syringe fittings
(B) wearing double-layered latex gloves
(C) use of positive-pressure technique when medication is being withdrawn from vials
(D) wearing closed-front, surgical-type gowns with cuffs
(E) not recapping or clipping used needles

11-B
12-C

ANSWERS AND EXPLANATIONS

1. The answer is B *[I A 5 c].*
Hypertonic solutions have an osmotic pressure greater than that of blood (or 0.9% saline), whereas hypotonic solutions have an osmotic pressure less than that of blood, and isotonic or iso-osmotic solutions have an osmotic pressure equal to that of blood.

2. The answer is B *[II D 2 c (2)].*
The use of a microbial 0.22 μm or smaller filter is necessary to achieve sterilization. The addition of a nonsterile drug to a sterile vehicle will not accomplish this. Radiation sterilization is an industrial technique and is not suitable for use in a community pharmacy. Heat sterilization might degrade the ophthalmic drug, making it unsafe to use.

3. The answer is D *[VII A 1].*
The gauge size refers to the outer diameter of the needle. The lower the gauge size number, the larger the needle.

4. The answer is D *[IV D].*
Intradermal injection refers to parenteral administration into the most superficial layer of skin. This administration route generally is used for certain types of vaccines and skin tests.

5. The answer is D *[IV C].*
The intravenous route of drug administration allows for rapid onset of action and, therefore, immediate therapeutic effect. There can be no recall of the administered dose, and phlebitis, or inflammation of a vein, may occur. In addition, a depo effect (i.e., accumulation and storage of the drug for distribution) cannot be achieved by administering a drug intravenously. Delivering a drug intravenously results in a systemic rather than a localized effect.

6. The answer is D *[VIII A 1].*
Nonirritating drugs, isotonic drugs, short-term therapy, and postoperative hydration are best given by peripheral intravenous administration. Central vein injection is used when access to a peripheral vein is poor, for administration of irritating drugs or hypertonic solutions and for long-term intravenous therapy.

7. The answer is B *[VIII D 1 a].*
Physical incompatibilities occur when two or more products are combined and produce a change in the appearance of the solution, such as the formation of a precipitate.

8. The answer is D *[IX B].*
Sterility testing ensures that parenteral products are free from microbial contamination. Pyrogen testing checks products for the presence of pyrogens, clarity testing tests for the presence of particulates, and leaker testing ensures that ampules have been completely sealed during the manufacturing process. Solubility testing may be done to determine the maximum soluble concentration of a drug.

9. The answer is C *[I B 2].*
Doxorubicin is an antineoplastic agent and consequently should be prepared only in a vertical laminar flow hood due to the potential hazard of these toxic agents to the operator.

10. The answer is A *[V B 1 a].*
D5W [dextrose (D-glucose) 5% in water] is acidic, its pH ranges from 3.5 to 6.5, and it is isotonic. It is often used in intravenous admixtures and should be used with caution in diabetic patients.

11. The answer is B *[III B].*
As a packaging material for parenteral products, a major disadvantage of plastic is its relative opacity, since visual inspection of the solution for particulate matter or a change in color is an important safety measure.

12. The answer is C *[V D 2].*
In order to prevent drug aerosolization, a negative-pressure technique (not a positive-pressure technique) should be used when an antineoplastic agent is being withdrawn from a vial. The other precautions mentioned in the question are important safety measures for handling parenteral antineoplastics. All pharmacy and nursing personnel who handle these toxic substances should receive special training.

30
Parapharmaceuticals, Home Diagnostics, and Medical Devices

Todd A. Brown
Joseph F. Palumbo

I. AMBULATORY AIDS

A. Wheelchairs. Many different types of wheelchairs are available. The patient's disabilities, size, weight, and activities are the main considerations in wheelchair selection. The following options should be considered when selecting a wheelchair.

1. **Seat size.** The standard chair width is 16–18 inches, with seats available up to 24 inches. The chair should be 2 inches wider than the widest part of the patient's body (usually around the buttocks or thighs).
2. **Arms** can be fixed, detachable, tilt-back, half, or full. The armrests and padding must also be considered.
3. **Tires** can be hard rubber or pneumatic (i.e., air-filled).
4. **Wheels** can be reinforced with spokes or can be composite based.
5. **Leg rests** can be different sizes and are available with padding.
6. **Footrests** can be different sizes and are available with or without heel loops.
7. **Casters (i.e., front wheels)** can be hard rubber or pneumatic.
8. **Calf rests** can be different sizes and are available with padding.
9. **Seat drapery** can be made of mesh or vinyl.
10. **Back drapery** can be made of mesh or vinyl.
11. **Cross braces** add stability and durability to the chair.
12. **Weight.** Standard wheelchairs weigh 35–50 pounds. Lightweight chairs are available for those who are unable to manipulate a standard chair and for ease of transport.

B. Sports chairs are designed for very active people and are usually lightweight and durable.

C. Powered wheelchairs are designed for people who cannot wheel themselves. They contain a motor and battery that power the wheelchair.

D. Powered carts are designed for people that have some mobility and are active.

E. Walkers are lightweight devices that are made of metal tubing and have four widely placed legs.

1. **Use.** They are used by patients who need more support than a cane but have reasonably good arm, hand, and wrist function. The patient holds onto the walker and takes a step, then moves the walker and takes another step.
2. **Types of walkers** include:
   - **a.** Adult adjustable walker
   - **b.** Adult nonadjustable walker
   - **c.** Child adjustable walker
   - **d.** Folding walker
   - **e.** Reciprocating walker
   - **f.** Wheeled walker

g. Side-walker
h. Hemiwalker

F. Canes. These simple ambulatory aids provide balance and transfer weight off a weakened limb.

1. **Types.** Canes may be wooden or metal.
   a. **Wooden canes** made for males typically are heavier than those made for females. The highest-quality wooden canes are those that have been cut with a handsaw.
   b. **Metal canes** come in adjustable and nonadjustable models and may be monopod or multipod. Good metal canes are those that have been cut with a tubing cutter.
   c. **Folding canes** fold into four sections and can be made of wood, metal, or plastic.

2. **Fitting a cane.** Each cane must be adjusted or cut to fit the individual patient.
   a. To support the arm muscles, the cane should provide about 25° of elbow flexion.
   b. The crease on the inside of the patient's wrist should be level with the top of the hand grip.
   c. The tip of the cane should be 4 inches in front of the toes at approximately a 45° angle.
   d. The cane should be cut about ½ inch shorter than the required length to allow for the thickness of the tip.

3. **Using a cane.** In most cases, the patient should carry the cane on the strong side to provide a wide base of support and permit the center of gravity to move forward rather than from side to side.

G. Crutches. These devices generally are used by patients with temporary disabilities (e.g., sprains, fractures) or by those who require more support than a cane.

1. **Sizes of crutches** range from toddler to large adult.

2. **Crutch accessories** include arm pads, handgrip cushions, and crutch tips.

3. **Types of crutches.** Crutches can be made of wood or aluminum; either type can be fixed or adjustable. Types of crutches include the forearm crutch, the axillary crutch, the quad crutch, and the shepherd's crook crutch.
   a. The **forearm crutch** (also called a Canadian or Lofstrand crutch) supports the wrists and elbows, attaching to the forearm by a collar or cuff. It is used by patients who need crutches on a long-term basis.
   b. The **axillary crutch,** which is the most commonly used crutch, provides more support than the forearm crutch.
   c. The **quad crutch** is a forearm crutch with a quadrangular base that is attached to the main shaft with a flexible rubber mount. This design allows the quad feet to maintain constant contact with the ground.
   d. The **shepherd's crook crutch,** a type of axillary crutch, resembles a forearm crutch except that the handgrips point to the rear and axillary rather than forearm support is provided.

4. **Fitting a crutch.** A crutch must be properly measured to prevent "crutch paralysis" (i.e., injury to axillary nerves, blood vessels, and lymph nodes).
   a. The patient should stand erect, supported by the wall or a chair, for the fitting.
   b. The crutch tip should fall 2 inches away from and 6 inches in front of the toes.
   c. The top rest should fall 2 inches below the axilla.
   d. The handgrips should be set so that the arms form roughly a 30° angle.

II. ORTHOPEDIC BRACES AND SURGICAL FITTINGS.

By limiting patient movement, orthopedic braces and surgical fittings promote proper body alignment. Pharmacists must undergo special training before attempting to fit an orthopedic device.

A. Back supports

1. **Uses.** These devices are worn by patients with various **spinal disorders,** including the following.
   a. **Kyphosis** (known in lay terms as "hump back") refers to increased convexity of the curvature of the thoracic spine (as viewed from the side).
   b. **Lordosis** (sometimes called "swayback") is an abnormal increase in the curvature of any spinal region.
   c. **Scoliosis** is a lateral spinal curvature.

2. **Types**
   a. A **sacral belt,** also called a sacral cinch or sacroiliac belt, provides varying degrees of compression and support to the sacrum and sacroiliac region of the spine.
   b. A **lumbosacral support** provides support to the lumbar and sacral areas.
   c. A **thoracolumbar support** provides support to higher areas of the back.

B. Cervical collars

1. **Uses.** These devices are used to provide support or limit the range of motion of the neck.
2. **Types**
   a. A **soft, or foam, cervical collar** provides mild support and stability to the neck.
   b. A **hard, or rigid, cervical collar** provides semirigid support to the neck and is used for soft-tissue damage, osteoarthritis, and whiplash injuries.
   c. A **Philadelphia, or extrication, collar** is used to immobilize the neck and is commonly used in emergency situations.

C. Shoulder immobilizers keep the shoulder and arm still. They are used for separations, dislocations, and injuries to the shoulder area.

D. Clavicle supports are sometimes called figure eight straps because of their appearance. They are used as aids for the reduction and stabilization of clavicle (i.e., collarbone) fractures.

E. Tennis elbow supports apply pressure to inflamed forearm muscles to provide support and comfort to those with tennis elbow (i.e., epicondylitis).

F. Wrist braces are used to reduce motion and to protect and stabilize the wrist from sprains and strains. They are also often used after cast removal.

G. Arm slings are used to provide comfort and support during recuperation from fractures, sprains, and surgery.

H. Rib belts are used to stabilize rib fractures. Female rib belts are shaped to go under the breasts.

I. Abdominal supports are used to provide abdominal support and to hold surgical dressings in place after surgery.

J. Knee braces, also called knee cages, are used for stabilization and support of the knee. They may have spiral stays, hinges, and an open or closed patella horseshoe pad.

K. Knee immobilizers prevent any motion of the knee and are used for severe injuries or fractures.

III. HOSPITAL BEDS AND ACCESSORIES.

Hospital beds may be manually or electrically operated.

A. Use. Hospital beds are used by patients who are confined to the bed for long periods of time or who require elevation of the head or feet as part of their treatment.

B. Features. Most hospital beds have an adjustable height feature and adjustable head and foot sections.

1. **Electrically operated beds** can be positioned by the patient while he or she is in bed using hand-held controls.
2. **Bed rails** are safety devices that prevent the patient from falling out of bed.

IV. OSTOMY APPLIANCES AND ACCESSORIES

A. Definitions. An **ostomy** is a surgical procedure in which an artificial opening is created between a hollow organ and the abdominal wall, or between two hollow organs. The opening is called a **stoma,** and it is created to allow passage of feces or urine.

B. An **ostomy procedure** is named for its anatomic location.

1. In a **colostomy,** part of the colon is removed. This procedure is done mainly in patients with colon or rectal cancer, lower bowel obstruction, or diverticulitis.
   a. The stoma may be located on the ascending, transverse, descending, or sigmoid colon segment.
   b. A colostomy may be temporary (as with bowel resection) or permanent (as with removal of the rectum). Eventually, the patient can resume normal activities. However, if the lower rectum has been removed, the male patient may be impotent or sterile.
   c. Stomal discharge may range from liquid to semisolid (as with an ascending colostomy) to solid (as with a sigmoid or descending colostomy).
2. In an **ileostomy,** a portion of the ileum is removed. This procedure usually is reserved for patients with severe ulcerative colitis or Crohn's disease.
   a. A loop of the proximal ileum is brought to the abdominal wall to create the stoma.
   b. Stomal discharge is liquid or semisolid. Because it contains digestive enzymes, it is highly irritating to skin surrounding the stoma.
   c. As with a colostomy, the patient eventually can resume normal activities.
3. **Urinary diversion** with stoma creation may be performed in patients undergoing cystectomy.
   a. In an **ileal conduit** (the preferred method), urine is diverted through a loop in the ileum to a stoma on the abdominal surface at the umbilicus. After surgery, the patient wears an external pouch continuously.
   b. Other types of urinary diversion procedures include ureterostomy, nephrotomy, and ileal bladder.

C. Ostomy appliances. The selection of an ostomy appliance (the collecting device for stomal discharge) depends mainly on the type of discharge produced. Other considerations include size of the gasket openings that fit around the stoma, method of attachment to the stoma, and types of activities the patient engages in.

1. **Solid waste appliances** (used for most colostomy patients) are disposable, detachable pouches with a relatively large gasket size. Most are sealed at the bottom.
2. **Semisolid waste appliances** (used for most ileostomy patients) usually are permanent devices attached to the skin either with cement or karaya gum washers to maintain a watertight seal. Instead of being sealed at the bottom, most of these appliances must be folded, then secured with a rubber band or clip; for drainage, the patient removes the rubber band or clip and unfolds the bottom.
3. **Urinary diversion appliances** are similar to semisolid waste appliances in that they are permanent rubber pouches that are cemented to the skin. They must be close-fitting and have a leak-proof seal.

D. Ostomy accessories

1. **Karaya gum washers** may be used to ensure a leak-proof seal around the stoma.
2. **Karaya gum powder,** used to prepare the skin for ostomy fitting, absorbs moisture and protects the skin from irritation.
3. **Foam pads,** usually made of nonabsorbent foam rubber, are placed between the appliance faceplate and the skin.
4. **Elastic belts** are used to attach some ostomy appliances over the stoma.
5. **Cement or adhesive disks** may be used to affix the ostomy appliance to the skin.
6. **Skin barriers** (e.g., Stomahesive) help protect the skin around the stoma from the discharge.
7. Special **irrigating sets** may be used instead of pouches by some colostomy patients.
8. **Hypoallergenic tape** is used to attach or support the ostomy appliance.
9. **Deodorizers** help control fecal odor. For local control, either an aerosol or a liquid concentrate deodorant can be used in the pouch. For systemic odor control, the patient may ingest bismuth subgallate, chlorophyll tablets, or charcoal tablets.
10. **Solvents** are used to remove the ostomy adhesive.
11. **Protective skin dressings** protect the skin when the ostomy appliance is removed.

E. Fitting of an ostomy appliance is usually done by an enterostomal therapist.

F. Special considerations for ostomy patients. To establish regular, conveniently timed bowel evacuation, the patient may administer an enema to the colon via the stoma daily or every few days.

1. Many ostomates may stop wearing a pouch after adequate bowel control has been established.
2. To protect the stoma, the patient places a gauze sponge or stoma cap over it.
3. Ostomates may be required to crush tablets or to take oral drugs in liquid form to ensure adequate absorption, since coated or sustained-release products may not dissolve in the intestine after an ostomy. Antibiotics, sulfa drugs, laxatives, and diuretics may cause problems in ostomates.

V. URINARY CATHETERS. These devices allow for collection and removal of urine from the bladder. Types of urinary catheters include the following.

A. External catheters

1. **Use.** External catheters are used for heavy incontinence problems or complete loss of urine control. They are connected to a leg bag by tubing, which allows the user to walk freely.
2. **Types** of external catheters include the following.
   a. The **male external catheter** is also called a condom catheter because it is placed over the penis. Some male catheters contain adhesive that assists in keeping the catheter secure; these are known as Texas catheters.
   b. The **female external collection system** is a contoured device that fits snugly around the female urinary opening. It is connected to a leg bag that is similar to the male external catheter.

B. Internal catheters

1. **Use.** Internal catheters are used in healthcare institutions during surgery or when external catheters are inappropriate. Internal catheters can also be used at home, but the patient must be taught proper insertion techniques to prevent infection. The catheter is inserted through the urethra into the bladder and attached to a urinary leg bag or a bedside collection bag.
2. **Size.** Most urinary catheters are sized by the French scale: the larger the number, the larger the diameter of the catheter.
3. **Types** of internal catheters include the following.
   a. The **straight catheter** consists of a rubber or plastic tube. One end is flared and connects to tubing or a collection device. The other end is inserted and has an opening into which the urine flows.
   b. The **Foley catheter** is sometimes called an indwelling catheter. It can be used for up to 30 days before changing and must be inserted by a trained health professional. The end inserted into the bladder has a balloon that is inflated with sterile water or sterile saline, which holds the catheter in place.

VI. THERMOMETERS. These instruments, which measure body temperature, are essential to medical practice and should be kept in every home.

A. Types

1. The **standard fever thermometer** has a sealed glass constriction chamber that contains liquid mercury. Responding to temperature changes, the mercury rises or falls in a column as it expands or contracts. It will then remain at the maximal temperature registered until it is shaken back into the reservoir at the bottom. (The constriction chamber acts as a valve check, preventing the mercury from flowing back into the reservoir.) **Fever thermometers** come in three main types. Their range is from 94°F to 106°F. Graduations are in two-tenths of a degree.
   a. The **oral thermometer** has a slender reservoir and bulb. Usually, it is placed under the tongue and left there for 3 minutes.
   b. The **rectal thermometer** has a blunt, pear-shaped bulb for added safety and retention. It is inserted into the rectum and left there for 4 minutes. A lubricant (e.g., petroleum jelly) should be used to aid insertion. Rectal temperature is normally 1° higher than oral temperature.

c. The **security thermometer** (also called a stubby thermometer) has a short, stubby bulb. It is used to take the oral or rectal temperature of a child or noncompliant patient.
d. If oral or rectal temperature cannot be taken, **axillary temperature** may be taken with any standard fever thermometer. It usually takes 10 minutes to achieve an accurate measurement. (Axillary temperature is 1° lower than oral temperature.)

2. The **basal thermometer** records temperatures ranging from 96°F to 100°F. It is graduated in tenths of a degree and is used to estimate the time of ovulation. This thermometer can be placed in the mouth or rectum.

3. **Electronic thermometers** register body temperature quickly and precisely. Heat alters the amount of current running through the resistor, and a digital readout then displays body temperature.

4. **Liquid crystal strips,** which are placed directly on the skin, calculate core body temperature from surface temperature. These stick-on strips are valuable for continuous temperature monitoring.

5. **Disposable thermometers** are presterilized and intended for single-use only. Also available are disposable thermometer covers, which are thin, sterile plastic sheaths that can be placed over oral thermometers for each temperature measurement and then discarded.

VII. HEAT AND COLD THERAPY.

For musculoskeletal disorders (e.g., sprains, strains, arthritis), physicians may recommend application of heat or cold to specific body regions.

A. **Heat** may be applied in a dry or moist form.

1. **Dry heat** commonly is recommended to induce vasodilation and leukocytosis, to relax muscles and connective tissue, or to hasten suppuration. It may be delivered via a **hot-water bottle** or an **electric heating pad**.

2. **Moist heat** penetrates more deeply into muscle tissues than dry heat.
   a. A **moist-heat pack** (i.e., a hydrocollator) is a bag filled with tiny silica beads. When boiled, the beads form a gelatinous substance that holds its temperature for up to 40 minutes.
      (1) The moist-heat pack must be wrapped in several layers of towels before it is placed on the body.
      (2) Between uses, the pack should be wrapped in plastic and stored in the refrigerator (or, if a long storage period is anticipated, the freezer).
   b. **Other moist-heat devices** include electric heating pads with a wettable sponge or cover, chemical hot packs, paraffin baths, and poultices.

B. **Cold application** is indicated mainly as acute therapy to decrease circulation to a local area (e.g., sprains), thereby reducing swelling. Also, severe arthritis may respond better to cold than to heat.

1. Cold application may be delivered via an ice bag, gel pack, or chemical pack.

2. Cold application is **contraindicated** in patients with circulatory stasis or injured tissue.

VIII. INCONTINENCE AND INCONTINENCE PRODUCTS

A. **Urinary incontinence** is partial or complete loss of control of the bladder. It is a major health problem in the elderly (up to 50% of all people admitted to nursing homes have incontinence problems). Types of urinary incontinence include:

1. **Urge incontinence** is an uncontrolled contraction of the bladder.

2. **Stress incontinence** is characterized by a weakness in the internal sphincter that causes leakage of urine when intra-abdominal pressure suddenly increases as occurs in coughing, laughing, and sneezing.

3. **Overflow incontinence** is caused by an obstruction of the bladder, weakness of the bladder muscle, or impaired sensory input to the bladder.

4. **Functional incontinence** is related to physical or psychological problems that limit a patient's ability to get to the bathroom in time.

5. **Iatrogenic incontinence** is caused by drugs that the patient is taking.

B. Incontinence products

1. Intractable, heavy incontinence may require use of an **external catheter** (see V A).
2. **Shields** are pads that are placed in the underwear and held in place by an adhesive strip that is on the back of the shield. These are designed for light incontinence problems.
3. **Undergarments** are worn under underwear and are kept in place by elastic straps. These are designed for moderate incontinence problems.
4. **Briefs** look like adult diapers and are kept in place with adhesive strips. These are designed for heavy incontinence problems and for nonambulatory patients.
5. **Underpads** are placed on the bed underneath an incontinent person to protect the bedding.
6. **Waterproof sheets** are plastic or vinyl sheets that protect the mattress. They may be lined with flannel for comfort.
7. **Incontinence systems** are garments that look like underwear. A reusable or disposable pad is placed in a specially designed pouch or pocket that is sewn into the garment.

IX. BATHROOM SAFETY EQUIPMENT

A. Elevated toilet seats are used by people who cannot stand from a low sitting position, such as those with limited mobility or those undergoing therapy for a hip fracture.

B. Toilet safety rails are used by people who require additional support getting on and off the toilet.

C. Commodes are portable toilets used by people with limited mobility who are unable to walk to the bathroom. Commodes contain a frame (with or without a backrest), a seat, and a bucket. Some commodes are adjustable in height, and some have drop arms to facilitate transfer to and from the commode. To make storage easier, folding commodes are available.

D. Three-in-one commodes function as a commode or elevated toilet seat and have toilet safety rails.

E. Bath benches are seats that fit in the bathtub and allows the user to sit while taking a shower.

F. Transfer benches are placed over the outside edge of the bathtub to assist the user in getting in and out of the bathtub.

X. HOME DIAGNOSTIC AIDS

A. Self-care tests or kits, which are sold in pharmacies for home use, detect specific conditions or measure levels of certain substances for monitoring purposes. Some are used to screen patients that require additional medical attention or follow-up.

1. **Limitations.** These tests have limitations as they are generally not as accurate as laboratory tests and are intended for use by patients under a physician's care. Often, a laboratory test is performed once a positive result is obtained.
   - **a.** Many factors can affect the accuracy of home tests, usually the instructions included with the test cover this information in detail.
   - **b. Outdated tests** can give misleading or inaccurate results.
2. **Role of the pharmacist.** Pharmacists should familiarize themselves with the tests they sell and be prepared to counsel patients on their use. Assistance should be given in the following areas:
   - **a.** Proper use and interpretation
   - **b.** Referral for appropriate medical follow-up if necessary

B. Types of home diagnostic aids

1. **Pregnancy tests.** New brands of pregnancy tests appear on the market frequently, and consumers must follow all test instructions carefully. Pregnancy tests detect the presence of human chorionic gonadotropin (hCG) in the urine.

2. **Ovulation tests** help predict when ovulation occurs and are used to increase the chance of conception. These tests measure the surge of luteinizing hormone (LH) that occurs before ovulation. The period of time for testing is individualized and is dependent on the length and regularity of the menstrual cycle.

3. **Ketone tests** detect the presence of ketones in the urine. This test is used by patients with diabetes as an indication of glucose control.

4. **Glucose tests** assist diabetic patients in monitoring their glucose levels.
   a. **Blood glucose tests** contain test strips onto which patients place a drop of their blood. To measure blood glucose levels, these strips change color or are inserted into a blood glucose monitor, which gives a more accurate result.
   b. **Urine glucose tests** include such products as Benedict's solution, tablets, and test strips. These tests are not as accurate as blood glucose tests and are more appropriate for stable diabetics with a low renal threshold.

5. **Occult blood (stool guaiac) tests** detect the presence of blood in the feces and are used as screening tests for colorectal cancer.
   a. **Patient education** is essential to ensure successful testing. The patient must avoid certain foods for a prescribed period of time before these tests are performed.
   b. **Limitations of occult blood tests**
      (1) These tests cannot differentiate upper and lower gastrointestinal tract bleeding.
      (2) False-positive results may occur.

6. **Blood pressure monitors** (i.e., sphygmomanometers) are used by patients with histories of borderline or high blood pressure to monitor their condition. These readings may be used by a physician to assess the efficacy of a patient's therapy. Pharmacists can play an important role by giving instructions on proper technique and interpretation of results. The patient's ability to use the test correctly should be the main consideration when selecting a test. **Types of monitors** include:
   a. The **mercury model**. This model is the most accurate and does not require calibration. It is generally more expensive and requires the use of a stethoscope, which could be difficult for patients with impaired dexterity or hearing.
   b. The **aneroid model**. This model is the least expensive and is easily portable but must be calibrated yearly. It may be difficult for certain patients to use, since a stethoscope is required for proper readings.
   c. **Electronic or digital models.** These models are the easiest to operate, and they do not require a stethoscope. They are the most expensive to buy and repair.

XI. HOME THERAPY.

Home infusion therapies are discussed in detail in Chapter 27. Other types of home therapy include the following.

A. Home apnea monitoring may be established for pediatric patients whose apnea has been documented by pneumography or for adults with sleep apnea. Treatment may include continuous positive airway pressure (CPAP) to prevent the airway from becoming obstructed.

B. Home phototherapy may be administered to newborns with hyperbilirubinemia, which occurs because the glucuronyl transferase pathway may not be fully matured for several weeks after birth. Exposure to fluorescent light breaks down bilirubin into harmless metabolites.

C. Home respiratory therapy

1. **Oxygen** commonly is administered at home to patients with various respiratory or cardiovascular conditions.
   a. Usually, oxygen is supplied as a **compressed gas or liquid** or via an oxygen concentrator.
   b. A **registered respiratory therapist** should be consulted for information on the correct procedures, cautions, and laws regarding oxygen use.

2. **Mechanical ventilation** (e.g., intermittent positive-pressure breathing) is administered to patients who cannot be weaned from a ventilator. This may be required for patients with severe chronic obstructive pulmonary disease (COPD), muscular dystrophy, or spinal cord injuries.

3. **Nebulizers** are used to deliver medication to the respiratory tract by inhalation. It is used by patients with respiratory infections, asthma, or COPD.

4. **Vaporizers** are used to deliver moisture to room air by heating water with electricity to produce steam.
   a. Vaporizers need to be cleaned regularly to prevent accumulation of minerals or dirt.
   b. A pinch of baking soda may be added to soft water to help conduct the electric current.
   c. Some vaporizers contain a cup used to deliver medication to the steam. The effectiveness of using medication with a vaporizer has not been established.
   d. Vaporizers can cause severe burns and should be used with caution around children.
5. **Humidifiers** deliver moisture to the air by making water particles small enough to make them airborne. The humidity produced promotes expectoration in patients with tenacious mucus. Humidifiers require regular cleaning to prevent the distribution of bacteria and molds. There are two types of humidifiers.
   a. The **simple humidifier** contains a small motor that breaks water into small droplets. A fan then blows these droplets into the air where they evaporate.
   b. The **ultrasonic humidifier** contains a transducer, which produces an ultra-fine mist and much more moisture than a simple humidifier. This type of humidifier is quieter than a simple humidifier but is more expensive.

STUDY QUESTIONS

Directions: Each of the numbered items or incomplete statements in this section is followed by answers or by completions of the statement. Select the **one** lettered answer or completion that is **best** in each case.

1. How far should the top of crutches rest below the axilla?

(A) 0.5 inch
(B) 1 inch
(C) 2 inches
(D) 3 inches
(E) 4 inches

2. What angle should the arms form when the handgrips on crutches are set properly?

(A) 10°
(B) 30°
(C) 45°
(D) 60°
(E) 90°

3. A product that delivers moisture to the air by heating water to produce steam is called

(A) a nebulizer
(B) a simple humidifier
(C) a ventilator
(D) a vaporizer
(E) an ultrasonic humidifier

4. A product that is designed for an ambulatory patient with a light incontinence problem is

(A) a brief
(B) a shield
(C) an undergarment
(D) an underpad
(E) waterproof sheeting

5. Home phototherapy is used to treat newborns who have

(A) hyperbilirubinemia
(B) azotemia
(C) hyperglycemia
(D) hypercalcemia
(E) hypernatremia

6. The diameter of urinary catheters is measured by which of the following scales?

(A) Luer
(B) Spanish
(C) French
(D) Gauge
(E) Metric

7. A cervical collar that immobilizes the neck is called a

(A) soft cervical collar
(B) hard cervical collar
(C) foam cervical collar
(D) extrication collar
(E) rigid cervical collar

8. Incontinence that is caused by an obstruction of the bladder is called

(A) overflow incontinence
(B) urge incontinence
(C) stress incontinence
(D) functional incontinence
(E) iatrogenic incontinence

9. A colostomy or ileostomy could be performed for all of the following conditions EXCEPT

(A) lower bowel obstruction
(B) malignancy of the colon or rectum
(C) ulcerative colitis
(D) duodenal ulcer
(E) Crohn's disease

1-C	4-B	7-D
2-B	5-A	8-A
3-D	6-C	9-D

Directions: The group of items in this section consists of lettered options followed by a set of numbered items. For each item, select the **one** lettered option that is most closely associated with it. Each lettered option may be selected once, more than once, or not at all.

Questions 10–11

Match the following phrases about body temperature (in degrees Fahrenheit) to the correct degree.

(A) 2 degrees lower
(B) 1 degree lower
(C) the same
(D) 1 degree higher
(E) 2 degrees higher

10. Relative to oral temperature, rectal temperature is

11. Relative to oral temperature, axillary temperature is

10-D
11-B

ANSWERS AND EXPLANATIONS

1. The answer is C *[I G 4].*
When a patient is measured for crutches, the top rest should be 2 inches below the axilla.

2. The answer is B *[I G 4].*
When a patient is measured for crutches, the handgrips are set so that the arms form about a 30° angle.

3. The answer is D *[XI C 4].*
A vaporizer delivers moisture to room air by heating water with electricity to produce steam.

4. The answer is B *[VIII B 2].*
Shields are pads that are placed in the underwear. They are designed for light incontinence problems.

5. The answer is A *[XI B].*
Newborn infants who have hyperbilirubinemia may require an extended course of phototherapy until the enzymes in the liver have matured. Home phototherapy allows the infant to be cared for at home, rather than in the hospital for a prolonged period.

6. The answer is C *[V B 2].*
The French scale is used to measure the diameter of urinary catheters. The Luer scale is used to measure the syringe-tip size on Luer-Lok and Luer-Slip syringes. The gauge scale is used to measure the outer diameter of needles, and the metric scale is a general system of measurement.

7. The answer is D *[II B 2 c].*
An extrication collar (also known as a Philadelphia cervical collar) is used to immobilize the neck. It is commonly used in emergency situations. Soft and foam are synonymous for the type of cervical collar that provides mild support and stability to the neck. Hard and rigid are synonymous for the type of cervical collar that provides semirigid support.

8. The answer is A *[VIII A 3].*
Overflow incontinence is caused by an obstruction of the bladder, weakness of the bladder muscle, or impaired sensory input. Urge incontinence is caused by an uncontrolled contraction of the bladder. Stress incontinence is caused by a increase in the intra-abdominal pressure. Functional incontinence is related to physical or psychological problems, and iatrogenic incontinence is caused by medication.

9. The answer is D *[IV B].*
Lower bowel obstruction, malignancy of the colon or rectum, and diverticulitis may all require a colostomy. Severe ulcerative colitis and Crohn's disease may require an ileostomy. The treatment of a duodenal ulcer does not include a colostomy or an ileostomy.

10–11. The answers are 10-D, 11-B *[VI A 1 b, d].*
Relative to oral temperature, rectal temperature is 1 degree higher, while axillary temperature is 1 degree lower. For example, if a patient's oral temperature is 100°, the rectal temperature would be 101° and the axillary temperature would be 99°.

31 Drug Use in Special Patient Populations: Pediatrics, Pregnancy, Geriatrics

Alan H. Mutnick
Suellen O'Neill
H. William McGhee

I. DRUG THERAPY IN PEDIATRIC PATIENTS

A. General considerations

1. Pediatric drug therapy challenges the pharmacist, since children are uniquely different from adults. Many of the assumptions made in adult drug therapy do not apply to children. For example, in contrast to the relatively stable pharmacokinetic profile that characterizes most of the adult years, **pharmacokinetic parameters in children change as they mature from birth to adolescence**. Complex processes relating to drug absorption, distribution, metabolism, and elimination are not fully developed at birth and mature at varying rates throughout childhood.

2. Drug selection, doses, and dosage intervals change throughout childhood making **drug therapy monitoring** essential. The outline below describes pharmacokinetic differences in childhood that influence drug therapy. Following this is a discussion of problems inherent to pediatric drug monitoring as well as some brief comments on adverse drug reactions. At the end, some cautions are suggested concerning drug dosing in children.

B. Pharmacokinetic considerations

1. **Absorption.** Oral drug absorption is a complex and variable process. Many drug- and patient-related factors influence absorption, although drug-related factors are generally fixed and patient-related factors change. These include gastric pH, gastric emptying time, an underlying disease state, bile salt production, and pancreatic enzyme function.
   - a. **Gastric pH.** Neonates are relatively achlorhydric. Increases in acid production correlate with initiation of enteral feedings. Acid production rises steadily from age 7 days to 1 month but is variable. Relative achlorhydria (i.e., pH > 4) is present in approximately 20% of neonates at 1 week of age, 15% at 2 weeks, and 8% at 3 weeks. By 6 weeks of age, gastric acid production is comparable to that in older infants and reaches adult values at 2 years of age. Relative achlorhydria may explain the increased bioavailability of basic drugs and the unpredictable, slower absorption of acidic agents.
   - b. **Gastric emptying.** The rate of gastric emptying is an important determinant of the rate and extent of drug absorption. Gastric emptying is highly variable in neonates and is affected by gestational and postnatal ages and the type of feeding administered. Infants acquire the same rate of gastric emptying as adults at 6 to 8 months of age.
     - (1) Since most drugs are absorbed in the small intestine, a **reduced rate of emptying** slows the rate of absorption, which can reduce peak drug concentrations. **Prematurity** slows gastric emptying from an already reduced rate in term neonates [half-life ($t_{1/2}$) of gastric emptying is 90 minutes] in comparison to adults ($t_{1/2}$ gastric emptying is 65 minutes).
     - (2) An **increased rate of emptying** may reduce the extent of absorption, since contact time with absorptive surfaces in the small intestine is reduced.
     - (3) **Breast-fed infants** empty their stomachs twice as fast as formula-fed infants, in whom gastric emptying is slower when formula feedings of increasing caloric density are administered.
   - c. **Underlying disease state**
     - (1) Disease states that can significantly **prolong gastric emptying** include pyloric stenosis, gastroesophageal reflux, respiratory distress syndrome, and congenital heart disease.

(2) Short bowel syndrome greatly **reduces the total surface area available for drug absorption.**

(3) Cholestatic liver disease, biliary obstruction, and distal ileum resection can **interfere with bile acid excretion or reabsorption and reduce the absorption of lipid-soluble substances** including vitamins A, D, and E.

d. **Bile salt production.** The bile salt pool and the rate of bile salt synthesis are reduced approximately 50% in premature and young term infants in comparison to adults. Decreased fat absorption from enteral feedings, as well as decreased drug absorption, can occur. For example, when vitamin D (i.e., calcifediol, also called 25-hydroxycholecalciferol) is administered to neonates, absorption is only 30% as compared to 70% in adults.

e. **Pancreatic enzyme function.** The absorption of lipid-soluble drugs is also affected by gastrointestinal concentrations of pancreatic enzymes. Neonates have low levels of lipases, and, when combined with reduced bile acid production, lipid-soluble drugs may be left insoluble and thus unabsorbed in the intestine. Oral suspensions, such as chloramphenicol palmitate, which require intraluminal hydrolysis by pancreatic lipases prior to absorption, have been associated with unreliable absorption of the active moiety in premature and term infants.

2. **Distribution.** How a drug distributes in the body is important in both the selection and dosage of a drug. Volume of distribution is affected by many age-dependent factors including the degree of protein binding, the sizes of various body compartments, and the presence of various endogenous substances.

a. **Protein binding.** Acidic drugs bind to **albumin** while basic substances bind primarily to **alpha$_1$-acid glycoprotein**. Both of these proteins are reduced in neonates, which allows for greater amounts of free drug in the serum and tissues. This has been demonstrated for phenytoin, phenobarbital, chloramphenicol, penicillin, propranolol, lidocaine, and several other substances. The increase in the free fraction of certain drugs in neonates and infants challenges the reliability of serum concentration monitoring, which utilizes parameters derived from adult populations. Adult levels for albumin and alpha$_1$-acid glycoprotein occur at approximately 10 to 12 months of age.

b. **Size of body compartments.** At birth, extracellular fluid volume constitutes approximately 40% of total body weight, decreasing to 25% by 6 months and 20% by 12 years. For polar compounds, such as the aminoglycosides that distribute into extracellular spaces, **loading doses** (i.e., the approximate amount of drug contained in the body during steady state) are required in neonates to achieve therapeutic concentrations. Loading doses are not necessary in older infants and children.

c. **Endogenous substances.** In neonates, various endogenous substances can bind to plasma proteins and reduce the degree of drug–protein binding. The two most important substances are **free fatty acids** and **unconjugated bilirubin,** which, when present in high concentrations, can increase the unbound:bound drug ratio in the plasma.

(1) The serum concentration of these two substances normalizes in early infancy.

(2) Caution is urged, however, in evaluating bilirubin- or free fatty acid-induced drug displacement reactions, since significant increases in the plasma concentrations of free drug occur only when the displaced drug is more than 90% bound and its metabolism is rate-limited.

(3) Usually, increases in unbound concentrations are only transient, since hepatic metabolism for most drugs is not rate-limited.

d. Since **bilirubin** competes with certain drugs for albumin binding sites, it can be displaced, which presents a theoretical concern for the development of **drug-induced kernicterus**. In neonates, **hyperbilirubinemia** develops because heme catabolism is accelerated and the conjugating ability of the liver is reduced.

(1) Unconjugated bilirubin normally binds noncovalently to plasma albumin, but the binding affinity is reduced in neonates, not approaching **adult values** until 6 months of age. Thus, it potentially can be displaced when certain highly bound acidic compounds are administered.

(2) The concern for drug-induced bilirubin displacement is theoretical, since it is derived from in vitro studies. It may be that drug-induced displacement of bilirubin and the development of clinical kernicterus is unlikely, since the affinity of bilirubin for albumin greatly exceeds that of most drugs. This remains controversial, however, and requires further study.

3. **Metabolism.** Drug metabolism occurs primarily in the liver, with additional biotransformation occurring in the intestine, lung, adrenal gland, and skin. In the liver, metabolism involves a series of **phase I and phase II reactions,** both of which are susceptible to enzyme-inducing (e.g., phenytoin, phenobarbital, carbamazepine, rifampin) and enzyme-inhibiting (e.g., cimetidine, erythromycin) agents.
   a. **Phase I reactions** are nonsynthetic reactions (i.e., oxidation, reduction, hydrolysis, and hydroxylation) that result either in inactive compounds or in metabolites with equal, lesser, or, rarely, greater pharmacologic action.
      (1) The major **enzymes** responsible for phase I oxidation reactions are those in the cytochrome P_{450} monooxygenase system, which at birth are at levels approximately 50% those of adult values.
      (2) Consequently, the **metabolism of many drugs** (e.g., phenobarbital) **is reduced** and **drug serum half-lives are prolonged** correspondingly.
         (a) The **ability to oxidize** drugs increases with increasing postnatal age so that by several weeks of postnatal life, metabolic rates generally are equal to or greater than adult rates.
         (b) **Metabolic rates** remain high for 1 to 5 years and gradually decline to adult levels at puberty.
   b. **Phase II reactions** are synthetic reactions (i.e., conjugation with glycine, glucuronide, or sulfate) that result in polar, water-soluble, inactive compounds for renal and bile elimination.
      (1) The underlying **enzyme systems** are unevenly depressed at birth and mature at varying rates.
      (2) For example, the **ability to conjugate drugs with glucuronide** (e.g., chloramphenicol) is greatly reduced at birth and does not reach adult values until 3 to 4 years of age.
      (3) Also, the **acetylation of sulfonamides** is significantly reduced at birth.
      (4) However, the **ability to conjugate sulfate groups** (e.g., acetaminophen) is well-developed at birth.
      (5) The **ability to conjugate carboxyl groups with glycine** apparently is only slightly reduced at birth and adult levels are achieved by about 6 months of age.
4. **Elimination.** The kidney is the major route of drug elimination for both water-soluble drugs and water-soluble metabolites of lipid-soluble drugs. Three basic processes contribute to renal elimination: glomerular filtration, tubular secretion, and tubular reabsorption. Both glomerular filtration and secretion promote the renal elimination of drugs, whereas reabsorption reduces it. All three processes display age-dependent changes in maturity.
   a. At birth, **glomerular filtration** in **full-term neonates** is 30% to 50% of the adult value and matures quickly, approaching 85% of adult values by 3 to 5 months of age. **Premature infants** (i.e., < 34 weeks) at birth have glomerular filtration rates that are further reduced and do not obtain rates comparable to full-term infants until 4 to 6 weeks of age.
   b. **Tubular function.**
      (1) **Tubular secretion** is an active process, utilizing separate protein carriers for acids and bases. In contrast to glomerular filtration, secretion matures at a slower rate. At birth, **full-term infants** have secretory rates of approximately 20% of adult values and do not achieve adult rates until 6 to 7 months of age. Before secretion is fully mature, some drugs (e.g., penicillin) may stimulate their own secretion, leading to decreased efficacy unless the dosage is increased.
      (2) **Tubular reabsorption** can be an active or passive process. It increases with postconceptional age and is reduced in neonates. Unlike tubular secretion, its development remains poorly understood.
   c. **Two other considerations** in renal elimination include renal blood flow and drug–protein binding.
      (1) **Renal blood flow** is the driving force underlying glomerular filtration. As cardiac output increases and renal vascular resistance decreases, renal blood flow increases, and adult values are attained by 6 to 12 months.
      (2) **Protein binding** significantly affects glomerular filtration, since only unbound drug is filtered.

C. **Problems in pediatric drug monitoring.** Several problems are inherent to pediatric pharmacotherapy and lack of recognition or concern for them may lead to greater morbidity or drug-related toxicity.
   1. As previously discussed, children display unique **age-dependent changes** in pharmacokinetic parameters. The absorption, distribution, metabolism, and elimination of a drug can vary

greatly between different age groups. Lack of proper clinical monitoring can lead to underdosage, overdosage, therapeutic failure, or drug-related toxicity.

2. **Therapeutic drug monitoring** assumes a correlation exists between serum drug concentrations and therapeutic effects. Many of these correlations have been displayed in adult patients but not in children. Extrapolating target serum drug concentrations, which are derived from adults, to children may not always be justified. Drug–protein binding differences, different metabolite patterns, and other factors can change the amount of free drug availability at the receptor site and alter the therapeutic effects of a drug.
   a. A potential complication in interpreting serum drug levels is the **presence of endogenous substances,** which may cross-react with analytical drug assays. This has been demonstrated for digoxin in neonates and infants, and the potential exists that it may be applicable to other drugs.
   b. **Drug levels are not constant** (except when administered by continuous infusion) in the serum and may fluctuate greatly during dosage intervals. Correct timing of drawing blood is essential for interpreting drug concentrations correctly.

3. **Technical problems** may interfere with proper drug delivery. Pediatric drug doses often are in small fluid volumes, which may greatly prolong drug delivery when administered through certain intravenous administration sets. Microbore tubing and infusion pumps can help prevent this problem. Drugs administered by enteral feeding tubes present similar problems.

D. Adverse Drug Reactions. Adverse drug reactions are not uncommon in children. Antibiotics (especially vancomycin, cephalosporins, and penicillins), anticonvulsants, narcotics, antiemetics and contrast agents are leading causes of reactions in children. The majority of these are mild (e.g., red-man syndrome with intravenous vancomycin) and are treated relatively simply.

1. However, approximately **three out of every ten reactions prolong or require hospitalization** (e.g., syndrome of inappropriate antidiuretic hormone (SIADH) with carbamazepine) and approximately one out of ten is considered severe (i.e., the reaction is life-threatening, or fatal, requires a prolonged recovery time, or is permanently disabling).

2. Examples of severe reactions include anaphylaxis after administration of a cephalosporin or respiratory arrest, following the combined intravenous use of diazepam and phenobarbital.

E. Dosing considerations in pediatric patients. Paracelsus' (1493–1541) statement concerning drug dosages is applicable to children: "All substances are poisons, there is none which is not a poison. The right dose differentiates a poison from a remedy."

1. **Drug dosages** for adults cannot be extrapolated to children. This is especially true in neonates and infants and for drugs with a narrow therapeutic index. As previously reviewed, children differ considerably pharmacokinetically from adults, and various rules for dosing children based upon age or weight are unreliable and are not recommended. Pediatric dosages rarely need to be calculated. If a pediatric dosage needs to be calculated, the use of body surface area (BSA) is recommended, and it can be determined by using a BSA nomogram or the following equation:

$$\text{BSA (in m}^2\text{)} = \sqrt{\frac{\text{height (cm)} \times \text{weight (kg)}}{3600}}$$

2. Pediatric drug dosages for nearly all drugs can be obtained from standard **pediatric references,** such as the *Harriet Lane Handbook* or *The Pediatric Drug Handbook* or the *Manual of Pediatric Therapeutics*. Dosages are based primarily upon weight and occasionally upon body surface area.

3. **Dosing intervals** are often different for children. For example, because of reduced renal and hepatic function, neonates generally require a longer dosing interval compared to children and adults. Older infants and children may require a shorter interval because of their enhanced elimination of drugs.

4. **Underlying disease states** may also affect pediatric doses and dosage intervals. For example, cystic fibrosis and oncology patients often require larger doses and shorter dosing intervals for aminoglycoside antibiotics.

5. **Errors in dosage calculations or drug preparation** are more likely to occur in pediatric patients than in adults. Arithmetic errors are prone to occur during extemporaneous preparation of pediatric dosage forms or in the calculation of dosages.

II. DRUG USE IN PREGNANT PATIENTS.

Pregnant women may require drug therapy for preexisting medical conditions or for problems associated with their pregnancy. This patient population may be exposed to drugs or environmental agents that have adverse effects on the unborn. Clinical situations also exist where the fetus may be pharmacologically treated via maternal administration of medication. It is important to understand the principles of drug use in these patients, since any drug administered to a pregnant woman may directly harm the developing fetus or adversely influence her pregnancy. Furthermore, pharmacotherapy in such a patient population requires knowledge of drug clearance as well as latent effects that are unique in pregnancy.

A. **Fetal development.** The effects of drug therapy in pregnancy depend largely upon the **stage of fetal development** during which exposure occurs. Limited information exists regarding the effects of drugs in the period of conception and implantation. However, it is suggested that, women who are at risk of conceiving or who wish to become pregnant, should withdraw all unnecessary medication 3 to 6 months prior to conception.

   1. **Blastogenesis.** During this stage (the first 15–21 days after fertilization), cleavage and germ layer formation occur. The embryonic cells are in a relatively undifferentiated state.
   2. **Organogenesis** (14–56 days). All major organs start to develop during this period. Exposure of the embryo to certain drugs at this time may cause major congenital malformations. Organogenesis is the most critical period of development.
   3. **Fetal Period** (ninth week to birth). At the ninth week the embryo is referred to as a fetus. Development during this time is primarily maturation and growth. Exposure to a drug during this period is generally not associated with major congenital malformations. However, the developing fetus may be at risk from exposure to the pharmacologic effects of a variety of fetotoxic drugs and microorganisms.

B. **Placental transfer of drugs.** The placenta, a product of conception, is the functional unit between the fetal body and the maternal blood.

   1. The **functions** of the placenta include nutrition, respiration, metabolism, excretion, and endocrine activity to maintain the fetal and maternal well-being. In conjunction with the fetus, the placenta produces a number of pregnancy-related hormones that are mainly secreted into the maternal circulation. In order for a drug to cause a teratogenic or pharmacologic effect in the embryo or fetus, it must cross from the maternal circulation to the fetal circulation or tissues. Generally, this passage occurs via the placenta.
   2. **The placenta is not a protective barrier.** Previously, the placenta was considered to be a protective barrier that isolated the fetus from drugs and toxins present in the maternal circulation. However, the protective characteristics of the placenta are, in fact, limited. The concept that a placental barrier exists should be disregarded. The transfer of most nutrients, oxygen, waste products, drugs, and other substances occurs via **passive diffusion** primarily driven by the concentration gradient. A few compounds, however, are actively transported across the placental membranes.
   3. **Factors affecting placental drug transfer.** Generally, the principles that apply to drug transfer across any lipid membrane can be applied to placental transfer of a drug. Most substances administered for therapeutic purposes have, by design, the ability to cross the placenta to the fetus. The critical factor is whether the rate and extent of transfer are sufficient to cause significant drug concentrations in the fetus. There are many factors that affect the rate and extent of placental drug transfer.
      a. **Molecular weight.** Low molecular weight drugs [i.e., less than 500 daltons (d)] diffuse freely across the placenta. Drugs of a higher molecular weight (500–1000 d) cross less easily. Drugs comprised of very large molecules (e.g., heparin) do not cross the placental membranes.
      b. **pH.** The pH gradient between the maternal and fetal circulation and the pH of the drug itself affects the degree of placental transfer. Weakly acidic drugs and weakly basic drugs tend to rapidly diffuse across the placental membranes.

c. **Lipid solubility.** Moderately lipid-soluble drugs easily diffuse across the placental membranes. It is important to note that many drugs that have been formulated for oral administration, and hence gastrointestinal absorption, are designed for optimal lipid membrane transfer. Generally, these drugs have the ability to undergo placental transfer.

d. **Drug absorption.** During pregnancy, gastric tone and motility are decreased, which results in delayed gastrointestinal emptying time. This may affect oral drug absorption. Nausea and vomiting, which are common in the first trimester, may also affect oral drug administration and absorption.

e. **Drug distribution.** The volume of distribution increases significantly during pregnancy and increases with advancing gestational age. The alteration in volume of distribution is the result of a combination of changes associated with pregnancy, including increased plasma volume and increased cardiac output secondary to an increase in stroke volume and heart rate. Total body fluid (i.e., both intravascular and extravascular volume) increases as does fat content.

f. **Plasma protein binding.** Placental transfer of plasma protein–bound drug is unlikely, since only the free unbound drug crosses the placenta. During pregnancy, a reduction in the levels of two major drug-binding proteins is observed, namely albumin and alpha$_1$-acid glycoprotein.

(1) The reduction of these two important proteins potentially alters the free fraction of a drug.

(2) When these plasma protein concentrations are decreased there are fewer binding sites available for acidic drugs, and an increase in free drug concentration may result.

(3) However, concomitant increases in drug catabolism in the liver, renal clearance, increased tissue uptake, and altered receptor activity may counteract the effect of changes in plasma protein binding.

g. **Physical characteristics of the placenta.** As pregnancy progresses, the placental membranes become progressively thinner resulting in a decrease in diffusion distance.

h. **The pharmacologic activities of the drug.** Drugs with vasoactive properties may affect maternal and placental blood flow, and therefore influence the amount of drug reaching the fetus.

i. **Co-existent disease states.** Maternal hypertension or diabetes may reduce or enhance placental drug transfer, as a result of alterations in placenta permeability.

j. **Rate of maternal and placental blood flow.** Factors that influence maternal blood flow (e.g., exercise, meals, vasoactive medications) may affect drug absorption, maternal drug concentration deliverable to the placenta, and ultimately the fetus.

4. **Embryotoxic drugs** are drugs that harm the developing embryo, resulting in termination of pregnancy or shortening of gestational length.

a. Many drugs (e.g., hormones, antidepressants, angiotensin-converting enzyme (ACE) inhibitors, and certain antibiotics) administered in early pregnancy may be embryotoxic.

b. Because the placenta has not quite fully formed by organogenesis (see II A 2), the embryo risks damage from a wide variety of compounds.

c. The administration of some drugs may result in miscarriage by causing a severe chemical insult to the products of conception.

5. **Teratogenic drugs** cause physical defects in a developing fetus. This risk of teratogenesis is highest during the first trimester.

a. Teratogenesis may lead to physical malformation and/or mental abnormalties.

b. Because fetal organ systems develop at different times, specific teratogenic effects depend mainly on the point of gestation when the drug was ingested.

c. The Food and Drug Administration has developed a **classification system** that groups drugs according to the degree of their potential risk during pregnancy [*Federal Register* 44(124): 37434–37467, June 26, 1979].

(1) **Category A.** Controlled studies that were performed in women who took these drugs during pregnancy did not demonstrate a risk to the fetus.

(2) **Category B.** Either no well-controlled human studies exist, or animal reproduction studies with these drugs did not demonstrate any risk to the fetus. Or, the animal reproduction studies demonstrated an adverse effect on animal fetuses, but well-controlled human studies did not demonstrate similar results.

(3) **Category C.** The human fetal risk associated with drugs in this category is unknown. Either adverse effects in animal studies were demonstrated, and similar human studies were not performed, or studies in animals and humans are not available.

(4) **Category D.** Drugs in this category demonstrated evidence of human fetal risk. However, pregnant women may benefit from treatment of a serious disease or a life-threatening situation with these drugs, which may be acceptable despite the risk to the fetus.

(5) **Category X.** Drugs in this category caused fetal abnormalities in human or animal studies, or there is evidence of fetal risk based on human experience, or both. The risk to the fetus from using these drugs clearly outweighs any possible benefit to the pregnant woman. Also, drugs in this category should not be used in women who are planning to conceive.

d. Examples of teratogenic and potentially toxic drugs include the following.

(1) **Vitamin A derivatives.** The drugs in this group, which includes vitamin A, isotretinoin, and etretinate, are potent animal teratogens. Use of these agents shortly prior to or during pregnancy may result in severe human deformities.

(2) **ACE inhibitors.** It remains unclear if this class of antihypertensive drugs produces structural abnormalities in the developing human fetus. These drugs may, however, compromise the fetal renal system and result in severe renal failure and possibly fetal death.

(3) **Warfarin and warfarin derivatives.** The use of warfarin during the first trimester has been associated with a pattern of defects that commonly include nasal hypoplasia and a depressed nasal bridge. The characteristic defects are collectively referred to as fetal warfarin syndrome (FWS). Use of warfarin during the second and third trimesters is associated with increased risk of fetal central nervous system (CNS) malformations. Heparin, which is poorly transferred across the placenta, may be substituted for warfarin when anticoagulant therapy is necessary.

(4) **Estrogen and androgens.** These category X drugs may cause serious genital tract malformations.

(5) **Other hormonal agents.** Drugs such as thyroid preparations and cortisone may affect the development of fetal endocrine glands. Methimazole and carbimazole have been associated with malformations in newborns exposed in utero. Propylthiouracil (PTU) is the drug of choice in pregnancy and lactation for anti-thyroid therapy.

(6) **Ethanol.** Consumption of alcohol in large amounts or for prolonged periods of time during pregnancy has been associated with a pattern of defects collectively referred to as fetal alcohol syndrome (FAS). Features of FAS include abnormalities in growth and cardiac, skeletal, craniofacial, muscular, genitourinary, cutaneous, and CNS development.

(7) **Antibiotics**

(a) Mottling of the teeth may occur when **tetracycline** is taken by the mother after week 18 of pregnancy. This teratogenic effect does not become evident until later in childhood when tooth eruption occurs.

(b) **Metronidazole** is mutagenic in animals and is contraindicated for the treatment of trichomoniasis during the first trimester. Use for other indications must be carefully evaluated, especially in the first trimester.

(c) **Quinolone** antibiotics are not recommended for use during pregnancy because of arthropathies observed in immature animals.

(8) **Anticonvulsants** such as phenytoin, trimethadione, valproic acid, and sodium valproate have been associated with malformations following their use during the first trimester.

(9) **Lithium.** Congenital malformations, primarily in the cardiovascular system, have been associated with first trimester administration of lithium. Ebstein's anomaly (i.e., tricuspid valve malformation) has been reported in a significant number of fetuses exposed to the drug during this period. Exposure to the drug near term has resulted in neonatal lithium toxicity, which is generally reversible.

(10) **Antineoplastics.** Many agents belonging to this class of drugs have been associated with fetal malformations following first trimester exposures. Examples include busulfan, chlorambucil, cyclophosphamide, and methotrexate.

(11) **Finazteride** may cause abnormal development of the genitalia of male fetuses exposed to the drug in utero. Pregnant women should avoid handling crushed tablets of the drug and should avoid contact with the semen of men who are taking this medication.

6. **Fetotoxic drug effects** are the result of pharmacologic activity of a drug that may cause physiologic effects in the developing fetus.

a. During the **fetal period,** these effects are more likely to occur than are teratogenic effects.

b. **Clinically significant** fetotoxic effects include the following:

(1) **CNS depression** may occur with barbiturates, tranquilizers, antidepressants, and narcotics. Also, analgesics and anesthetics commonly given during labor may cause significant CNS and respiratory depression in newborns.

(2) **Neonatal bleeding.** Maternal ingestion of agents such as nonsteroidal anti-inflammatory drugs (NSAIDs) and anticoagulants at therapeutic doses near term may cause bleeding problems in the newborn. NSAIDs may prolong gestation and interfere with the progress of labor. Acetaminophen is a safe and effective analgesic for use in pregnancy.

(3) **Drug withdrawal.** Habitual maternal use of barbiturates, narcotics, benzodiazepines, alcohol and other substances of abuse may lead to withdrawal symptoms in newborns.

(4) **Reduced birth weight.** Pregnant women who smoke cigarettes, consume large amounts of alcohol, or abuse drugs have an increased risk of delivering a low birth weight infant.

(5) **Constriction of the ductus arteriosus.** Maternal use of NSAIDs in the third trimester may cause premature closure of the ductus arteriosus and may result in pulmonary hypertension in the newborn.

C. Drug excretion in breast milk. Recent appreciation of the benefits of breast-feeding for the infant and mother has become evident. Today more than 60% of women choose to breast-feed their infants. Of these women, 90%–95% receive a medication during the first postpartum week. It is important to understand the principles of drug excretion in breast milk and specific information on the various medications in order to minimize risks from drug effects in the nursing infant.

1. Transfer of drugs from plasma to breast milk is governed by many of the same principles influencing human membrane drug transfer.

a. Many drugs cross the mammary epithelium via **passive diffusion** along a concentration gradient formed by the un-ionized drug content on each side of the membrane.

b. This membrane is a **semi-permeable lipid barrier** like other human membranes.

c. The membrane also consists of **small pores** that allow for direct passage of low molecular weight substances (i.e., less than 200 d).

(1) **Larger drug molecules,** which are unable to pass through the pores, must dissolve in the lipid part of the membrane in order to pass through to the breast milk.

(2) **Active transport mechanisms** are decribed for some substances; however, there are no drugs known to utilize this process.

2. Physiochemical characteristics of the drug and its environment that **influence the rate and extent** of drug passage into the breast milk include:

a. Molecular weight of the drug (see II C 1 c)

b. The **pH gradient between the breast milk and plasma.** Human milk tends to be more acidic than plasma.

(1) Therefore, weak acids may diffuse across the membrane and remain un-ionized, allowing for passage back into the plasma.

(2) Weak bases may diffuse into the breast milk and ionize, which causes drug trapping (i.e., a clinically significant increase in the concentration of weak bases in the breast milk).

c. Degree of drug ionization. Only the ionized form of a drug is able to pass through the lipid membrane. Drugs that exist ionized in large concentrations in the plasma would not be available to diffuse across the lipid membrane.

d. Plasma protein binding. Only the unbound portion of a drug is available to pass into the breast milk. In general, drugs with high plasma protein binding properties tend to remain in the plasma and pass into the breast milk in low concentrations. While milk proteins exist and drug binding to these proteins may occur, the clinical relevance is limited.

e. Lipid solubility of the drug. Lipid solubility is necessary for drug passage into the breast milk. Highly lipid-soluble drugs (e.g., diazepam) may pass into the breast milk in relatively high amounts and therefore may present a significant dose of drug to the nursing infant.

3. Following administration of a drug to a nursing mother, the drug may be partially activated or inactivated in the maternal liver. The drug may be metabolized to active or inactive metabolites.

a. Maternal pharmacology plays a significant role in the rate and extent of drug passage into breast milk. The extent of plasma protein binding as well as changes in the mother's ability to metabolize or eliminate the drug influence the amount of drug in the plasma that is available to pass into the breast milk.

b. Equally important in affecting breast milk drug concentrations is the **maternal dose of the drug,** the **dosing schedule or frequency,** and the **route of administration.**

4. **Drugs affecting hormonal influence of breast milk production.** The primary hormone responsible for controlling breast milk production is **prolactin.**
   a. **Following delivery,** serum prolactin levels increase to promote the production and secretion of breast milk. Prolactin continues to be released in response to infant feeding.
   b. However, infant feeding is not the only influence of serum prolactin levels. There are frequently prescribed **medications that may alter serum prolactin levels** and, therefore, the amount of breast milk produced.
      (1) A decrease in milk production may result in diminished weight gain in the nursing infant, the need for supplementation, or premature cessation of breast-feeding.
      (2) **Drugs that decrease serum prolactin levels.** Drugs such as **bromocriptine** have been used to suppress lactation in women who choose not to breast feed. Other drugs include:
         (a) Ergot alkaloids
         (b) L-dopa
      (3) **Drugs that increase serum prolactin levels. Metoclopramide and sulpiride** have been useful therapeutically to enhance milk production. The following drugs are known to increase serum prolactin levels, but they have not been used therapeutically.
         (a) Methyldopa
         (b) Amphetamines
         (c) Haloperidol
         (d) Phenothiazines
         (e) Theophylline

5. **Factors to assess the risk of toxicity to the infant,** including:
   a. Inherent toxicity of the drug
   b. Amount of drug ingested
   c. Degree of prematurity
   d. Nursing pattern of the infant

6. **Factors to minimize drug exposure to the infant.** One of the goals in the use of medications in the breast-feeding mother is to maintain a natural, uninterrupted pattern of nursing. In many instances, it may be possible to withhold a drug when it is not essential or delay therapy until after weaning. Other factors include:
   a. **Product selection.** When a specific product is being selected from a class of drugs, it is important to choose the product that is distributed into the milk the least.
      (1) Other desirable characteristics include a short half-life, inactive metabolites, and no accumulation in breast milk.
      (2) Additionally, selection of a particular route of administration associated with less concentration of the drug in breast milk is desirable.
   b. **Maternal dose relative to infant feeding.** One of the goals of drug dosing in lactating women is minimal infant exposure to the drug. In drugs taken on a scheduled basis, it is desirable to adjust the dosing and nursing schedules so that a drug dose is administered immediately prior to the infant's feeding.

7. **Examples of drugs that readily enter breast milk** and should be used with caution in nursing mothers include the following.
   a. **Narcotics, barbiturates, and benzodiazepines,** such as diazepam, may have a hypnotic effect on the nursing infant. These effects are related to the maternal dose. Alcohol consumption may have a similar effect.
   b. **Antidepressants and antipsychotics.** These classes of drugs appear to pass into the breast milk, however, no serious adverse effects are reported. The long-term behavioral effects of chronic exposure to these drugs on developing newborns is unknown.
   c. **Metoclopramide.** This antiemetic passes readily into the breast milk and may accumulate as a result of ion trapping. There are no published reports involving serious effects associated with use of this drug in lactating women. The use of metoclopramide may be of concern because of its potential strong CNS effects.
   d. **Anticholinergic compounds.** These drugs may result in adverse CNS effects in the infant and may reduce lactation in the mother. Dicyclomine is contraindicated in nursing mothers since it may result in neonatal apnea.

III. DRUG USE IN GERIATRIC PATIENTS

A. General considerations

1. The elderly currently represent approximately 12% of the population, and they consume 25% of all prescription medications. If the amount of nonprescription medications are added to this number, estimates increase the drug usage of those over age 65 to 50% of all drugs used in the United States.

2. Drug response in elderly patients is affected by age-related changes in physiology and pharmacokinetics.

3. Numerous reasons help explain why the elderly are more susceptible than younger patients to adverse drug reactions.
   a. Many geriatric patients have multiple diseases that directly impact the body's ability to handle various medications.
   b. As the number of diseases increase in any given patient, the number of medications that the patient is likely to take also increases. Recent studies reveal that most people over age 65 take between five to six different medications per day.
   c. As the number of medications in any given patient increases, so does the likelihood of an adverse drug reaction.
   d. In many cases, more than one physician may be prescribing medications for a single patient without knowledge of other agents being prescribed by another physician.
   e. Studies reveal that on average, geriatric patients self-medicate more frequently than their younger counterparts, who self-medicate as much as 1.5 times every 2 weeks.
   f. Studies reveal that as many as 40% of elderly patients stop taking their medications prematurely.
   g. The methods of administration, frequency of dosing, and combinations of drug products add to noncompliance of dose regimens.
   h. Changes in body composition, renal elimination, metabolism, and distribution can make it difficult to predict geriatric responses to many medications.

B. Pharmacokinetics in geriatric patients

1. **Drug absorption**
   a. **Age-related changes** in the stomach and small intestine, such as increased gastric pH and delayed gastric emptying time, do not create significant variations in the parameters of absorption in the elderly.
   b. Drugs such as antacids, which increase gastric pH, and anticholinergics, which further delay gastric emptying, may lead to significant decreases in bioavailability of various products such as digoxin, chlorpromazine, cimetidine, and tetracycline.

2. **Volume of distribution**
   a. **Body composition.** As a group, the elderly tend to be smaller than the young, with a greater composition of fat (approximately 35%), less muscle, and less body water.
   b. **Lipophilic and hydrophilic drugs.** Drugs that are lipid soluble (i.e., lipophilic) show increased volumes of distribution in the elderly, while those that are water soluble (i.e., hydrophilic) show decreased volumes of distribution. This becomes significant due to the fact that many drugs are dosed based on lean body weight.
   c. **Serum albumin** tends to be reduced in the elderly, resulting in an increased amount of unbound (free) drug for those agents that are highly bound to albumin (e.g., warfarin).
   d. **Other factors** that affect the volume of distribution include obesity, drug interactions, malnutrition, and bed rest. Several of these factors are common in the geriatric population.

3. **Metabolism.** It is difficult to quantify metabolizing capabilities for numerous drugs in specific patient populations.
   a. The **size of the liver** and its capacity for metabolism result in a reduction in the rate of active drug metabolism in the elderly.
   b. **Reduced hepatic artery flow,** as well as a consistent reduction in various microsomal enzyme reactions, may lead to prolonged serum half-lives of drugs and potential toxicity.

4. **Renal elimination.** Unlike metabolism, the effect of aging on renal clearance can be quantified.

a. **Serum creatinine levels** may be considered to be normal, when, in reality, the elderly do have a reduction in creatinine clearance.
b. The **Cockcroft-Gault formula** has been used with several other nomograms to depict the relationship that exists between serum creatinine and creatinine clearance.
c. Drugs that are excreted unchanged in the urine (e.g., digoxin, aminoglycosides, and penicillins) may remain in the body for longer periods of time, and may result in a higher incidence of toxicity.

C. Pharmacologic considerations in the geriatric population

1. The **site of action** of a given drug plays a major role in the response elicited by an elderly patient.
2. **Reductions in the cell population of organs,** oxygen consumption, tissue blood flow, and overall organ efficiency create a significant degree of scatter in the physiologic responses of elderly patients receiving numerous drugs. This typically results in either a heightened or diminished response to a drug.
3. **Drugs that act on the CNS** occasionally result in bizarre responses in elderly patients (e.g., increased excitement, mania). Barbiturates, benzodiazepines, antidepressants, and antiparkinsonian agents must be monitored closely for the development of such effects.
4. **Cardiotonics,** such as digitalis, tend to accumulate in the elderly due to decreased excretion, and they pose a significant risk for toxicity. Additionally, hypokalemia, hypothyroidism, and hypercalcemia also increase such toxicity.
5. **Anticoagulants,** due to the numerous reported drug–drug interactions encountered clinically, pose a significant threat to the elderly and should be monitored closely.
6. The elderly seem to have a higher incidence of fluid and electrolyte disturbances as compared to younger people, and this may pose a potential problem in those patients receiving diuretics.
7. The elderly are predisposed to a higher-than-normal rate of falls as compared to the younger population. Consequently, medications with **hypotensive** properties (e.g., calcium channel blockers, beta-adrenergic blockers, angiotensin-converting enzyme inhibitors, centrally acting sympatholytics, and peripherally acting vasodilators) pose a major threat in causing falls among the elderly.
8. Frequently, the elderly suffer adverse side effects from drug substances due to the failure of health professionals to recognize many of the traditionally accepted complaints of aging. Nausea, vomiting, fatigue, and upset stomach are not insignificant and may need further investigation.
9. When it comes to initiating drug therapy in the elderly, start low, and go slow.

D. Principles of drug therapy in the elderly. Prior to the preparation of any pharmaceutical for the elderly, the following should help the practitioner decide on specific therapeutic options.

1. The practitioner must be convinced that the drug therapy is required and that the diagnosed illness is amenable to drug therapy.
2. Elderly patients present with various obstacles when taking medications. In many situations, it is the dosage form of a drug and the frequency of administration that best determine the chances for a successful outcome, based on the establishment of maximal patient compliance.
3. Elderly patients cannot be expected to respond to all drugs in the same way that younger patients do. Efficacy of a product in the young does not always translate to the same in the elderly.
4. Ensure that the appropriate medication instructions have been given to the patient and that the importance of taking the medication as directed is stressed to the patient.
5. Provide the elderly with an added amount of empathy and be prepared to discuss their concerns. Listen extra carefully for messages that others may ignore.

STUDY QUESTIONS

Directions: Each of the numbered items or incomplete statements in this section is followed by answers or by completions of the statement. Select the **one** lettered answer or completion that is **best** in each case.

1. All of the following medications should not be routinely used during the third trimester EXCEPT

(A) acetaminophen
(B) nonsteroidal anti-inflammatory drugs
(C) warfarin
(D) lithium
(E) aspirin

2. Factors that affect the absorption of drugs in the elderly include all of the following EXCEPT

(A) lengthened gastric emptying time
(B) decreased plasma albumin
(C) elevated gastric pH
(D) decreased intestinal blood flow
(E) decreased gastrointestinal motility

3. Placental transfer of a drug is affected by all of the following characteristics EXCEPT

(A) molecular weight
(B) fetal sex
(C) gestational age
(D) lipid solubility of the drug
(E) plasma protein binding

4. All of the following are taken into account when calculating dosage for children EXCEPT

(A) height
(B) weight
(C) hepatic and renal function
(D) age
(E) body surface area

5. When selecting a benzodiazepine product for a woman who has chronic panic disorder, all of the following drug properties are desirable for breast-feeding her 8-month-old infant who was born at term EXCEPT

(A) hepatic metabolism to inactive metabolites
(B) a short half-life
(C) a rapid onset of action
(D) a tendency to bind to milk proteins

6. All of the following drugs may enhance breast milk production by increasing prolactin levels EXCEPT

(A) haloperidol
(B) methyldopa
(C) metoclopramide
(D) bromocriptine
(E) theophylline

Directions: The question below contains three suggested answers of which **one or more** is correct. Choose the answer

A if **I only** is correct
B if **III only** is correct
C if **I and II** are correct
D if **II and III** are correct
E if **I, II, and III** are correct

7. According to the principles of drug excretion into the breast milk, which combination of the following properties would result in the *highest* drug concentration in breast milk?

I. Low molecular weight, moderately lipophilic
II. Low plasma protein bound, weakly basic
III. Highly plasma protein bound, weakly acidic

1-A 4-D 7-C
2-B 5-D
3-B 6-D

ANSWERS AND EXPLANATIONS

1. The answer is A *[II B 5 d (3), (9), 6 b (2)].*
Acetaminophen is a safe and effective analgesic that can be used in therapeutic doses during pregnancy. Nonsteroidal anti-inflammatory drugs (NSAIDs) may interfere with the onset or progress of labor when used in the third trimester. NSAIDs and warfarin, when used near delivery, may cause bleeding problems in the newborn infant. Additionally, warfarin use in the third trimester may be associated with fetal central nervous system (CNS) abnormalities. Lithium use in the third trimester may cause neonatal lithium toxicity.

2. The answer is B *[III B 1, 2].*
Lengthened gastric emptying time, elevated gastric pH, decreased intestinal blood flow, and decreased gastrointestinal motility all may affect drug absorption. Decreases in plasma albumin may alter a drug's distribution but would not affect its absorption.

3. The answer is B *[II B 3].*
Fetal sex does not affect placental transfer of a drug. The molecular weight and the lipid solubility of a drug greatly influence its ability to cross the placental membranes. Plasma protein binding affects the amount of free drug available to cross the placenta. Gestational age influences the volume of distribution of the drug as well as the thickness of the placental membranes.

4. The answer is D *[I E].*
When calculating dosage for children, the child's height, weight, body surface area, and renal and hepatic function must be taken into account. Age, although sometimes used, may result in improper dosing due to the variations in body size and level of development found in children of the same age.

5. The answer is D *[II C 6 a (1)].*
When any drug is used by a nursing mother, it is desirable to have the least amount of active drug available in the maternal circulation to diffuse into the breast milk. A rapidly acting (for maternal onset of action), rapidly eliminated (i.e., short half-life) drug with inactive metabolites is optimal. If the drug binds in high quantities to milk proteins, it may tend to remain or accumulate in the breast milk.

6. The answer is D *[II C 4 b (3)].*
Bromocriptine effectively decreases serum prolactin levels and has been used therapeutically to suppress lactation. Haloperidol, methyldopa, metoclopramide, and theophylline may increase serum prolactin levels. Of these drugs, only metoclopramide (as well as sulpiride) has been useful therapeutically to enhance milk production.

7. The answer is C (I, II) *[II C 1–3].*
High molecular weight substances are less likely to pass into breast milk because of their size. Drugs that are highly plasma protein bound may only reach the breast milk in small amounts, since a large portion of the drug is bound to the maternal plasma proteins, and, therefore, only a small amount is free to diffuse into breast milk. A low molecular weight, moderately lipophilic drug passes easily into breast milk. A drug that has a low degree of plasma protein binding has a significant amount of drug free to diffuse into breast milk. A weakly basic drug may ionize after reaching the breast milk and therefore remain trapped in the milk.

32
Nonprescription Medication: An Overview

Larry N. Swanson

I. OVER-THE-COUNTER (OTC) DRUGS

A. OTC criteria. According to the **Food and Drug Administration (FDA) regulations,** a drug must be safe and effective in order to be sold over the counter.

1. An OTC drug is **safe** if it has a low incidence of adverse reactions or significant side effects under adequate directions for use as well as low potential for harm, which may result from abuse under conditions of widespread availability.

2. An OTC drug is **effective** if there is a reasonable expectation that for a significant portion of the target population the drug, when used under adequate directions for use, with warnings against unsafe use, provides clinically significant relief of the type claimed.

B. OTC labels. Whereas prescription drug labels for the patient carry minimal information, the FDA requires that OTC labels be much more detailed so the consumers can properly use the products without the advice of a health professional. The **label** on each nonprescription medicine includes:

1. Product name and statement of identity
2. Active ingredients
3. Inactive ingredients
4. Name and location of the manufacturer, distributor, or packer
5. Net quantity of contents
6. Description of tamper resistant features
7. Indications for use
8. Directions and dosage instructions
9. Warnings, cautionary statements, and drug-interaction precautions (if any)
10. Expiration date and lot or batch code

C. The **OTC drug market** for 1991 was approximately $12 billion. With more medications being transferred from prescription to OTC status in years to come, it is estimated that by the year 2000 the OTC market may be as large as $20 billion per year.

1. The OTC drug market is a very important component in the nation's overall health care. One study estimated that if 2% of the OTC drug consumers chose to visit a physician rather than selecting an OTC drug for their particular health problems, physician office visits would increase by 62%.

2. **A significant portion of the OTC medication sales occur outside of the pharmacy,** which is due in part to a general complacency of pharmacists toward OTC medications.
   - **a.** Some pharmacists have not considered OTC medications to be as effective or important as prescription drugs.
     - **(1)** The **importance of OTC medications** is especially apparent with the increasing number of prescription **agents moving to nonprescription status**. There are many conditions in which an OTC medication can or should be the primary therapy. Head lice, acne, vaginal candidiasis, constipation and dysmenorrhea are a few examples.

(2) OTC agents have the potential for significant **interactions** with prescription medications (e.g., aspirin and warfarin, antihistamines and alcohol). Additionally, some OTC agents used by people affected by certain diseases may cause serious problems (e.g., oral decongestants should be avoided generally by patients with hypertension, arrhythmias, or ischemic heart disease).

b. Pharmacists might be complacent about OTC medications because they believe that OTC labels are complete enough and that there is no role for the pharmacist in providing drug information. Studies have indicated that patients often do not read the labels or that some patients may not understand what is written. Even with good labeling and counseling on the part of the pharmacist, patients still need better assistance and monitoring of their OTC medication use.

c. Some pharmacists may just simply consider themselves "drug vendors" as opposed to true sources of medication information. A study of the questions posed to pharmacists by patients indicated that a greater number of professional questions were related to nonprescription medications than to prescription items.

D. OTC drug therapy requires a very definite role for the pharmacist both professionally and economically.

1. Because of the abundance of nonprescription medications available, helping a person select an OTC medication for that patient's particular need is one of the most professionally rewarding activities of the community pharmacist.

2. The pharmacist is the most accessible health care practitioner, and a pharmacist's advice about OTC medications is very imporant. In one study, the following data were produced. Of those surveyed:

a. Ninety-five percent would purchase a pharmacist-recommended product.
b. Ninety-two percent were satisfied with previous pharmacist-recommended products.
c. Ninety percent would consult with a physician if a pharmacist said to do so.
d. Seventy-six percent would take a pharmacist's advice over the advice of a friend.
e. Seventy-eight percent would buy a product recommended by a pharmacist over one they had picked up on a display.

3. The **"self-care" movement** of recent years has also increased the role that pharmacists can play in nonprescription medication use. This movement has been stimulated by the following:

a. Rising educational levels of the general population
b. Greater dissemination of health care information via print (e.g., newspapers, magazines) and electronic (e.g., television, radio) media.
c. A lack of available medical services to some individuals
d. A greater awareness of the limitations of medicine
e. A general increase in consumerism

II. THE FDA OTC DRUG REVIEW

A. History

1. In 1938, Congress enacted the **Federal Food, Drug, and Cosmetic Act (FFDCA)** (see Chapter 22 I E), which required manufacturers to market safe products.

2. In 1951, the **Durham-Humphrey Amendment** to the FFDCA was passed (see Chapter 22 I F). For the first time, medications were separated into **two distinct classes: prescription (legend) products and nonprescription, or OTC products.**

3. In 1962, Congress passed the **Kefauver-Harris Amendment** to the FFDCA (see Chapter 22 I G). This act required manufacturers to prove that their products were not only safe but also truly effective.

a. Implementation of the amendment (see Chapter 22 I H). To implement the Kefauver-Harris Amendment, the FDA contracted the National Academy of Sciences/National Research Council to assess drug efficacy for agents marketed between 1938 and 1962. This was followed by the FDA's implementation procedure, which is called the Drug Efficacy Study Implementation (DESI).

b. Drugs reviewed for efficacy. Of the approximately 4000 drugs that were reviewed, about 500 were OTC medications. Of these, about 300 were considered to be ineffective, which made it clear to the FDA that a comprehensive OTC drug review was necessary.

c. **Official start of the FDA OTC drug review.** The FDA OTC drug review officially began in 1972 and was expected to be completed within approximately 5 years. To date, the review is still not complete, but the process should be essentially finished in 1997.

B. Focus of the FDA OTC drug review. The principal focus of the review is to establish the safety, effectiveness, and proper labeling of OTC medications. Originally, 17 advisory review panels were established to look at 70 product categories. Because of the large number of OTC products available (approximately 300,000), the OTC review focused on active ingredients, which ultimately totalled approximately 800.

1. **Original panels.** The original panels reviewed medications in various product categories and classified the ingredients into **three categories:**
   a. **Category I.** Ingredients are generally recognized as safe and effective for the claimed therapeutic indication.
   b. **Category II.** Ingredients are not generally recognized as safe and effective or have unacceptable indications.
   c. **Category III.** Because of insufficient data, the FDA cannot classify these ingredients into category I or II.

2. **Completed reports.** Once the advisory panels completed their reports, they submitted information to the FDA, which was published in the *Federal Register* as Advanced Notices of Proposed Rulemaking (ANPRs). After FDA evaluation of this material, the FDA published its findings as a tentative final monograph and gave manufacturers and others an opportunity to incorporate additional information into the final monograph.

3. **Final monographs.** Once final monographs are published, manufacturers must comply with the requirements for marketing only those agents that are considered to be category I (monograph condition; original categories II and III are nonmonograph conditions). Manufacturers may petition the FDA with new supportive data for their product to amend a monograph, or they may submit a new drug application (NDA) for OTC use for the desired agent.

C. Implications of the OTC drug review process on pharmacists

1. **Pharmacists are now able to recommend products that contain ingredients that have been reviewed by a panel of experts and the FDA.** There has been a trend away from multiple drug combination products. Because many OTC agents were found to be ineffective, many products in a particular therapeutic category now contain identical active ingredients. Most OTC products contain only one category I agent (with the rare exception of cough and cold products).

2. **Pharmacists need to stay current on product ingredients.** A trade name for a product may remain the same even though there is a change in the ingredients. For example, Kaopectate®, which previously contained kaolin and pectin, now contains attapulgite, based on the final recommendations of the FDA after review of the available OTC antidiarrheal agents.

3. **Pharmacists need to stay current on what prescription drugs are given OTC status.** During the FDA OTC review process, many of the panels recommended that certain prescription drugs be switched to OTC drug status.
   a. Examples of **OTC drugs that had been prescription drugs** include topical hydrocortisone, oxymetazoline, chlorpheniramine in higher strengths, diphenhydramine, miconazole, tolnaftate, and ibuprofen.
   b. **Prescription drugs that are possible candidates to become OTC drugs** include a long list of agents (e.g., terfenadine, cimetidine, naproxen, nitroglycerin, and tretinoin).

III. A "PHARMACIST-ONLY" CLASS OF DRUGS

III. A "PHARMACIST-ONLY" CLASS OF DRUGS (also referred to as the third class of drugs) has been advocated for many years, the principal impetus being to protect the public from improperly using some of the OTC medications. Countries that have a "pharmacist-only" drug class include Canada, France, Germany, and Switzerland.

A. Benefits

1. The public would have some measure of **protection against misdiagnosing and self-prescribing,** but those who need the drugs could still obtain them without prescription.
   a. According to the National Council on Patient Information and Education, 50% of all medications are taken incorrectly.

b. The patient counseling required for a third class of drugs could significantly improve drug use outcomes.

2. The pharmacist has patient profiles for prescription drugs, so possible **incompatibilities with prescription medication could be checked** and OTC sales could be entered onto the patient profile.

3. This class of drugs would provide consumers with **monitoring and follow-up,** which is not available when patients select certain drugs themselves.

4. The designation of an additional class of drugs could also help in **monitoring drugs that are switched from prescription to nonprescription status**. An estimated 50 prescription drugs will be switched to OTC status in the next 4 to 5 years.

5. The advocated change might **save money** for patients both by preventing inappropriate drug selections and reducing the need for some office visits.

B. **Opposition** to the creation of such a class of drugs focuses primarily on the restrictions to consumer access to these agents.

1. **Fewer hours and areas of availability.** OTC drugs are currently sold to consumers in more than 1 million retail outlets, while the proposed third class of drugs would be available only in an estimated 65,000 pharmacies. This may limit the access of consumers to these drugs, particularly at night and in rural areas.

2. **Increased prices due to decreased competition.** Another objection to moving to a third class of drugs focuses on the concern that prices would increase if competition from other retail outlets is eliminated.

IV. THE FDA OFFICE OF OTC DRUG EVALUATION was recently established because of an increase in the creation, categorizing, and use of OTC drugs.

A. **Purpose.** This office was established to insure the regulation of OTC medications and is on the same operational level as the office responsible for regulation of prescription drugs.

B. **Functions.** The office has nine functions:

1. Coordinating and/or reviewing and deciding on the appropriate action, including approval or disapproval of all applications for OTC drug products, prescription drug switches to OTC status, and applications for other related drug products with the exception of new molecular entities and generic drug applications

2. Overseeing the development and implementation of standards for the safety and effectiveness of OTC drugs

3. Formulating, implementing, and publishing OTC drug monographs

4. Developing policy and procedures for the development of OTC drug reviews

5. Coordinating research activities throughout the FDA on all OTC drug issues

6. Serving as the primary agency contact for OTC drug information, regulation, and status

7. Maintaining a document control system for OTC drug submissions and a management information system for the office

8. Initiating actions based on recommendations made by OTC advisory panels, public comments, and new data

9. Participating in agency-sponsored consumer and professional educational programs on OTC drugs

C. **The OTC Drugs Advisory Committee** was also recently created as part of the FDA's efforts to expand and reorganize the office of OTC Drug Evaluation in response to the increasing demand for OTC products. The OTC Drugs Advisory Committee is responsible for the following **functions:**

1. Reviewing and evaluating available data concerning the safety and effectiveness of OTC drugs for use and treatment of a broad spectrum of human symptoms and diseases

2. Advising the commissioner on the approval of new drug applications
3. Serving as a forum to discuss the potential for some drug products to be switched from prescription to nonprescription status
4. Advising the commissioner on the promulgation of monographs establishing conditions under which OTC drugs are generally recognized as safe and effective and not misbranded
5. Conducting peer review and extramural scientific biomedical programs in support of the FDA's mission and regulatory responsibilities.

STUDY QUESTIONS

Directions: Each of the numbered items or incomplete statements in this section is followed by answers or by completions of the statement. Select the **one** lettered answer or completion that is **best** in each case.

1. Which one of the following statements regarding the Food and Drug Administration's (FDA's) over-the-counter (OTC) Drug Review process is correct?

(A) In the FDA OTC Drug Review process, individual products on the market were reviewed rather than individual ingredients
(B) Patients were found to be reluctant to follow a pharmacist's advice regarding OTC products
(C) The FDA OTC Drug Review has been underway for the last 20 years
(D) Approximately 500 OTC drugs were found to be ineffective

2. All of the following statements concerning over-the-counter (OTC) drugs are correct EXCEPT

(A) category I OTC agents are now referred to as a monograph condition
(B) the 1938 Federal Food, Drug, and Cosmetic Act (FFDCA) required medications to be safe
(C) the Durham-Humphrey Amendment created prescription and nonprescription categories of medications
(D) the Kefauver-Harrris Amendment requires pharmacists to counsel patients on all OTC medications
(E) category III OTC agents do not have sufficient data to be classified as category I or II agents

3. All of the following are required on the label of an over-the-counter (OTC) medication EXCEPT

(A) the name and address of the store selling the product
(B) the directions and dosage instructions
(C) the expiration date
(D) a list of inactive ingredients
(E) the net quantity of the contents

4. All of the following results stem from the Food and Drug Administration's (FDA's) over-the-counter (OTC) Drug Review EXCEPT

(A) many products that required prescriptions were made available as OTC products
(B) a third class of drugs was created in addition to prescription and nonprescription
(C) many products in a particular therapeutic class have the same active ingredient(s)
(D) pharmacists can recommend products more confidently because of the rigorous review of the ingredients in each product
(E) trade names of many products have remained the same while the ingredients have changed

---

1-C
2-D
3-A
4-B

ANSWERS AND EXPLANATIONS

1. The answer is C *[II A 3 c, B].*
The Food and Drug Administration's (FDA's) review of over-the-counter (OTC) drugs began in 1972, was expected to take 5 years, and is now expected to be finished in 1997. Approximately 4000 drugs were reviewed as a result of implementing the Kefauver-Harris Amendment to the Federal Food, Drug, and Cosmetic Act (FFDCA). Of those 4000 drugs, 500 were OTC products and 300 of them were found to be ineffective. This finding reinforced the need for a comprehensive OTC drug review. The complete review focused on approximately 800 active ingredients, which are found in approximately 300,000 OTC products. The large number of OTC products rendered a complete review of all products infeasible.

2. The answer is D *[II A 3].*
The 1962 Kefauver-Harris Amendment to the 1938 Federal Food, Drug, and Cosmetic Act (FFDCA) required that manufacturers of pharmaceuticals prove the effectiveness, as well as safety, of their products.

3. The answer is A *[I B 1].*
There are 10 items that are required to be on the labels of OTC medications; however, there is no requirement to have the name and address of the store selling the product.

4. The answer is B *[III].*
The third class of drugs, which do not require a prescription but can only be sold by the pharmacist (not off the shelf), has been frequently discussed but does not presently exist in the United States.

33
OTC Products: Otic, Dental, and Ophthalmic

Larry N. Swanson
Connie Lee Barnes
Constance McKenzie Fleming

I. OTIC OVER-THE-COUNTER (OTC) PRODUCTS

A. The ear structure

1. The **external ear** consists of the auricle (pinna), which is the visible outer structure of the ear that serves to funnel sounds into the ear canal.

2. The **ear canal,** also known as the external auditory meatus, is a channel that is about 1 inch in length, points downward, and ends in a cul-de-sac at the tympanic membrane (ear drum).
   - **a.** The **skin lining the ear canal** is very thin and tightly stretched. The slightest degree of inflammation elicits a significant amount of pain. This canal is also lined with glands that secrete substances that form cerumen (ear wax), which lubricates the lining of the ear canal and aids the removal of organisms and other foreign debris.
   - **b.** The **tympanic membrane** vibrates when hit by sound waves and it transmits that sound into the middle ear.

3. The **middle ear** is a small chamber about the size of a pea and contains the three small bones known as the **ossicles,** which amplify and transmit the sound waves further into the inner ear.
   - **a.** The middle ear is normally filled with air. The **eustachian tubes,** which are about the size of a pencil lead, connect the middle ear with the nasopharynx and equilibrate air pressure between the middle ear and the outer atmosphere. The "popping" sensation that is heard upon swallowing is the sound of air bubbles passing through these tubes, which then open.
   - **b.** In the presence of a cold or allergy, these eustachian tube walls may swell, which in turn prevents air from passing through. A pressure drop in the middle ear may create a vacuum, which draws fluid into the middle ear. Bacteria may then grow in this fluid and produce a condition known as **otitis media** (middle ear infection).

4. The **inner ear** consists of the **cochlea** (the organ of hearing) and the **vestibular apparatus,** which is involved with maintaining balance and equilibrium.

B. Common ear disorders.
Table 33-1 differentiates the symptoms of the common otic disorders encountered by pharmacists. There are three ear-related conditions for which pharmacists may recommend over-the-counter medications: Ear wax softening, pressure due to altitude changes, and prevention of otitis externa (i.e., swimmer's ear).

Table 33-1. Symptoms of Otic Disorders

	Boil	Bacterial External Otitis	Impacted Cerumen	Suppurative Otitis Media
Pain*	Often	Often	Rarely	Usually
Hearing deficit	Rarely	Possibly	Often	Possibly
Purulent discharge	Rarely	Often	Rarely	Occasionally, when present, it indicates perforation
Bilateral symptoms	Rarely	Possibly	Rarely	Occasionally
Appropriateness of self-medication	Auricle only	Never	Never	Never

*Pain is increased with chewing, traction on the auricle, and medial pressure on the tragus, except in otitis media, where it is knife-like and steady.

1. **Excessive ear wax**
   a. Functions of cerumen include:
      (1) Lubrication of the lining of the ear canal
      (2) Aiding the removal of organisms and debris by its outward movement, which is caused by movement of the jaw during chewing and talking
      (3) Helping to protect the ear canal through its bacteriostatic and possibly fungistatic properties
   b. There are primarily **four reasons why cerumen may accumulate**:
      (1) Overactive ceruminous glands, which are rare
      (2) An anatomically narrowed ear canal
      (3) A large amount of hair in the canal, which occurs often in the elderly
      (4) Inefficient or insufficient chewing or talking, which may also occur in the elderly
   c. **Improper removal methods.** Attempts should not be made to remove ear wax by using cotton-tipped applicators, match sticks, or hairpins, as this usually pushes the ear wax down further in the canal and makes it more difficult to remove. **Ear wax-softening agents** include:
      (1) **Carbamide peroxide** (urea hydrogen peroxide) is the only approved monograph agent for ear wax removal (not impacted ear wax).
         (a) **Action.** Carbamide peroxide releases oxygen and, via a mechanical action of effervescence, loosens the wax debris and aids in its removal.
         (b) **To prevent vertigo** one should warm the vial of this medication in the hands and put 5 to 10 drops in the ear.
         (c) **Use.** Carbamide peroxide should be used twice a day for 4 days, and the ear canal may be irrigated with the use of an ear syringe.
      (2) **Cerumenolytics** such as triethanolamine polypeptide oleate may be used for **impacted ear wax**. This is available via prescription and must be administered under the supervision of a physician.

2. **Altitude and ear pressure.** During situations such as airplane descent, where there are rapid changes in air pressure, the eustachian tubes may not function properly. Going from low atmospheric pressure down closer to the earth, where the air pressure is higher, causes a vacuum to form in the middle ear. As a result, the ear drum retracts and cannot vibrate, which creates a muffled sound and some pain. Patients with a cold or allergy may be more susceptible to this problem.
   a. The act of **swallowing** (induced by chewing gum or letting hard candy dissolve in the mouth), activates the muscles that pull open the eustachian tubes and helps to unblock the ears.
   b. **Yawning** is also effective in opening the eustachian tubes.
   c. Another effective method of unblocking the ears is pinching the nostrils and, using the cheek and throat muscles, **forcing air into the back of the nose** as if trying to blow off the thumb and fingers from the nostrils.
   d. The use of **decongestant** medication may be recommended, either in the form of an oral agent such as pseudoephedrine, which should be taken about an hour before descent, or a topical decongestant such as oxymetazoline, which should be administered 10 to 15 minutes prior to descent.

3. **Otitis externa** (also called swimmer's ear or hot weather ear) usually occurs during the summer months.
   a. **Pathophysiology**
      (1) Typically, this condition develops when water accumulates in the external ear canal after swimming. The combination of heat and humidity results in softening and swelling of the ear wax, which interferes with the normal protective function of the ear wax. The pH in this area then increases and sets the stage for bacterial invasion.
      (2) The resulting itching makes affected patients scratch the area, which further interferes with the integrity of the ear canal.
      (3) In more than 50% of cases, the microorganism that is involved is *Pseudomonas aeruginosa*.
      (4) The infection is commonly unilateral.
   b. The **symptoms** are as follows:
      (1) Itching
      (2) Pain that is accentuated by moving the ear (i.e., pulling upward on the auricle or pressing on the tragus)
      (3) A fluid discharge from the canal (in severe cases)

(4) A decrease or loss of hearing (if the ear canal is completely blocked)

c. **Treatment**

(1) There is **no OTC treatment** for this condition.

(2) Prescription treatment usually includes an antibiotic/steroid combination, such as neomycin, polymyxin, hydrocortisone, or an acetic acid and hydrocortisone combination.

d. **Prevention**

(1) After swimming or showering, the head should be turned to the side to drain water out of the ear. If otitis externa is a frequent occurrence, wax stopples, which are placed in the ear before swimming, may be recommended.

(2) To dry the ear after swimming, several drops of a **50/50 solution of isopropyl alcohol and white vinegar,** which contains acetic acid and restores the acid pH to the external auditory canal, can be instilled in the ear.

(3) A **2% acetic acid prescription eardrop** or one of the **OTC boric acid products** can be recommended for prevention of otitis externa.

4. **Boils (i.e., furuncles)** are infected hair follicles in the ear canal that usually involve the organism *Staphylococcus aureus*. This condition is usually self-limiting and is best treated by the application of warm compresses, which brings the boil to a head.

5. **Otitis media** is an infection of the middle ear with *S. pneumoniae* and *Haemophilus influenzae* being the most frequent organisms encountered. Next to colds, this is the most common infection in young children.

a. The **symptoms** include pain in the ear, fever, and possibly decreased hearing.

b. The **treatment** involves the use of oral antibiotics, which are available on prescription.

c. Because of the relatively short eustachian tubes and their horizontal configuration in infants, **bottle feeding infants in a supine position should be avoided,** because this allows milk to drain down the eustachian tubes into the middle ear. Occasionally, when an infant is bothered by middle ear infections, a physician may choose to insert tympanostomy tubes into the ear drum for drainage and pressure equalization purposes.

II. DENTAL OTC PRODUCTS

A. Dental anatomy.

A. Dental anatomy. Anatomically, the teeth are divided into two parts: the **crown** (above the gingival line) and the **root** (below the gingival line).

1. **Enamel** is crystalline calcium salts (hydroxyapatite) that cover the crown of the tooth to protect the underlying tooth structure.

2. **Dentin** is the largest part of the tooth structure that is located beneath the enamel. It protects the dental pulp.

3. **Cementum** is a bonelike structure that covers the root and provides the attachment of the tooth with the periodontal ligaments.

4. **Pulp** consists of free nerve endings.

B. Common dental problems and OTC products

1. **Dental caries** (i.e., cavities) are formed by the growth and implantation of cariogenic microorganisms.

a. **Causes**

(1) **Bacteria** (primarily *Streptococcus mutans* and Lactobacillaceae) produce acids (e.g., lactic acid) that demineralize enamel. Initially, demineralized enamel appears as a white, chalky area and becomes bluish-white and eventually brown or yellow.

(2) Also, **diet** is another factor in the development of dental caries. Foods with a high concentration of refined sugar (i.e., sucrose) increase the risk of dental caries. Sucrose is converted by bacterial plaque into volatile acids that destroy the hydroxyapatite.

(a) **Fructose and lactose** are less cariogenic than sucrose.

(b) **Noncariogenic sugar substitutes** are xylitol, sorbitol, and aspartame.

b. **OTC products** for dental caries include products that can alleviate the pain and sensitivity until the patient can get to the dentist. Examples of ingredients that are beneficial in this regard include eugenol, benzocaine (e.g., Anbesol®, Orajel®), or an oral analgesic (e.g., aspirin, acetaminophen).

2. **Plaque and calculus**
   a. **Causes**
      (1) **Plaque** is a sticky substance formed by the attachment of bacteria to the pellicle, which is a thin, acellular, glycoprotein–mucoprotein coating that adheres to the enamel within minutes after cleaning a tooth.
      (2) **Calculus** (also known as **tartar**) is the substance formed when plaque is not removed within 24 hours. The plaque begins to calcify into calculus when calcium salt precipitates from the saliva. Calculus can be removed only by a professional dental cleaning.
   b. **OTC products**
      (1) **Toothbrushes.** Soft, rounded, nylon bristles are preferred by dentists, since hard bristles can irritate the gingival margins and cause the gums to recede. Electric toothbrushes may benefit patients who require someone to clean their teeth for them or patients who have orthodontic appliances.
      (2) **Irrigating devices** direct a high-pressure stream of water through a nozzle to the hard-to-clean areas by gently lifting the free gingiva to rinse out crevices. Two types are available: **pulsating** (i.e., intermittent low- and high-pressure water streams) and **steady** (i.e., constant and consistent water pressure), neither of which has shown superior irrigating ability.
         (a) Irrigating devices should serve as adjuncts in maintaining oral hygiene.
         (b) **Examples** include Dento-Spray®, Hydro Pik®, Propulse 7618®, and the Water Pik® Oral Irrigator.
   c. **Dental floss** is available waxed, unwaxed, thick, thin, flavored, or unflavored. There are no differences between dental flosses in terms of plaque removal and prevention of gingivitis. There is no evidence of a residual wax film with the use of waxed dental floss.
      (1) The selection of dental wax depends upon characteristics of the patient, such as tooth roughness or tightness of tooth contacts (e.g., waxed floss is recommended for tight-fitting teeth because it can pass easily between the teeth without shredding).
      (2) The American Dental Association (ADA) recognizes the following brands as safe and effective: Butler®, Johnson & Johnson®, Dr. Flosser®, and Oral-B®.
   d. **Dentifrices** are products that enhance the removal of stains and dental plaque by the toothbrush. These include toothpastes, antiplaque and anticalculus mouthwashes, cosmetic whiteners, desensitizing agents, and disclosing agents.
      (1) **Toothpastes** are beneficial in decreasing the incidence of dental caries, reducing mouth odors, and enhancing personal appearance. **Ingredients** include the following.
         (a) **Abrasives** are responsible for physically removing plaque and debris. Examples include silicates, sodium bicarbonate, dicalcium phosphate, sodium metaphosphate, calcium pyrophosphate, calcium carbonate, magnesium carbonate, and aluminum oxides.
         (b) **Humectants** prevent the preparation from drying. Examples include sorbitol, glycerin, and propylene glycol.
         (c) **Suspending agents** add thickness to the product. Examples include methylcellulose, tragacanth, and karaya gum.
         (d) **Flavoring agents** include sorbitol or saccharin.
         (e) **Pyrophosphates** are found in tartar-control toothpastes. These products retard tartar formation; however, they form an alkaline solution that may irritate the skin. Some patients may experience a rash around the outside of the mouth. These patients should use only regular toothpaste or use regular toothpaste with occasional uses of tartar-control toothpaste.
         (f) **Fluoride** is anticariogenic because it replaces the hydroxyl ion in hydroxyapatite with the fluoride ion to form fluorapatite on the outer surface of the enamel. Fluorapatite hardens the enamel and makes it more acid-resistant. Fluoride has also demonstrated antibacterial activity.
            (i) Fluoride is **most beneficial if used from birth through age 12 or 13,** since unerrupted permanent teeth are mineralizing during that time. Whether or not a patient receives fluoride depends upon the concentration in their drinking water (Table 33-2).
            (ii) **Common fluoride compounds** in toothpaste include 0.24% sodium fluoride and 0.76% or 0.80% sodium monofluorophosphate (e.g., Aim®, Crest®, Aqua-Fresh®, Colgate®).

Table 33-2. Daily Fluoride Supplement Requirements for Children Based on Concentration of Fluoride in Drinking Water

Water Concentration	Age	Fluoride Supplement Required
> 0.7 ppm of fluoride	—	None
0.3–0.7 ppm of fluoride	Newborn–2 years	None
	2–3 years	0.25 mg/day
	3–13 years	0.50 mg/day
< 0.3 ppm of fluoride	Newborn–2 years	0.25 mg/day
	2–3 years	0.50 mg/day
	3–13 years	1.0 mg/day

ppm = parts per million.

(2) **Antiplaque dentifrices** include micronized silica abrasives and sodium bicarbonate as ingredients. To date, no antiplaque dentifrices have been accepted by the ADA as efficacious.

(3) **Anticalculus dentifrices** include zinc chloride, zinc citrate, and 3.3% pyrophosphate as ingredients to prevent calculus formation. To date, anticalculus products have not been evaluated by the ADA, therefore they do not carry the seal of acceptance.

(4) **Cosmetic whitening agents.** The most common ingredient in these products that is responsible for whitening the teeth is 10% carbamide peroxide (e.g., in Rembrandt®). This ingredient is a white crystal that reacts with water to release hydrogen peroxide, which in turn liberates free oxides. Some cosmetic whiteners may contain calcium peroxide (e.g., EpiSmile®).
   - (a) **Possible risks** associated with using whitening products include alteration of normal flora, tissue irritation, teeth sensitivity, and gingivitis.
   - (b) **Antiseptics** have been used as whiteners (e.g., Gly-Oxide®, Proxigel®).

(5) **Desensitizing agents** reduce the pain in sensitive teeth caused by cold, heat, or touch. These products should be nonabrasive and should not be used on a permanent basis unless directed by a dentist.
   - (a) **Examples of 5% potassium nitrate compounds** include Denquel®, Promise®, and Fresh Mint Sensodyne®.
   - (b) An **example of 10% strontium chloride hexahydrate product** is Original Formula Sensodyne®.
   - (c) An **example of a dibasic sodium citrate product** is Protect®.

(6) **Disclosing agents** aid in visualizing where dental plaque has formed. These products are for occasional use only and should not be swallowed. The Food and Drug Administration (FDA)-approved products are D&C Red No. 28 and FD&C Green No. 3. Following use, the consumer should rinse the mouth with water and expectorate.

(7) **Mouthwashes** may contain astringents, demulcents, detergents, flavors, germicidal agents, and fluoride. They can be used for cosmetic purposes, for reducing plaque, or for supplementing fluoride consumption.
   - (a) **Cosmetic mouthwashes** freshen the breath. They are nontherapeutic and are not effective as an antiseptic agent. These mouthwashes are classified by their active ingredients, alcohol content, and appearance. The most popular products are those that contain medicinal phenol and mint. The higher the percent of alcohol, the higher the impact of flavor within the mouth.
   - (b) **Antiplaque mouthrinses.** Products that have received the ADA seal are Kmart® Antiseptic Mouthrinse, Listerine® Antiseptic, and Peridex® Oral Rinse.
   - (c) **Fluoridated mouthwashes** are used after cleaning the teeth and should be expectorated. Nothing should be put into the mouth for 30 minutes after using these mouthwashes. The ADA has approved the following products: ACT® Anti-Cavity Dental Rinse, ACT® for Kids, Fluorigard® Anti-Cavity Dental Rinse, and Reach® Fluoride Dental Rinse.

3. **Gingivitis** is inflammation of the gingiva. The gingiva may appear larger in size with a bluish hue due to engorged gingival capillaries and a slow venous return.

a. **Cause.** Gingivitis is caused by microorganisms that eventually damage cellular and intercellular tissues. **Chronic gingivitis** may be localized or generalized. The gums readily bleed when probed or brushed, and the patient should seek dental assistance.
b. **OTC products** that a person with gingivitis may use include anesthetics containing eugenol or benzocaine (e.g., Orajel®) to relieve the pain. Mouthwashes may freshen the breath; however, it is important to consider the potential of these products to disguise and delay treatment of pathologic conditions (e.g., gingivitis) prior to use. Also, acetaminophen (Tylenol®) may be recommended. The patient should seek the advice of his or her dentist.

4. **Periodontal disease** is the result of chronic gingivitis left untreated. The periodontal ligament attachment and alveolar bone support of the tooth deteriorate.

5. **Acute necrotizing ulcerative gingivitis (ANUG)** is also called **trench mouth** and is characterized by necrosis and ulceration of the gingival surface with underlying inflammation. This condition is usually seen in teens and young adults.
a. **Signs and symptoms** of ANUG include severe pain, halitosis, bleeding, foul taste, and increased salivation.
b. The **cause** of ANUG is unknown. It is postulated that it may be associated with the overgrowth of spirochete and fusiform organisms.
c. **Risk factors** include anxiety, stress, smoking, malnutrition, and poor oral hygiene.
d. **Treatment** consists of local debridement. Also, penicillin VK (penicillin V is a derivative of penicillin G, however it is more stable in an acidic medium and, therefore, is better absorbed from the gastrointestinal tract; K stands for potassium) or metronidazole may be used in certain cases (e.g., widespread lesions).
e. **OTC products** that can alleviate some of the symptoms include acetaminophen and products with benzocaine (not eugenol because it may cause soft tissue damage). The patient should be advised to see his or her dentist. The use of salicylates is not recommended if the patient is predisposed to bleeding. Also, adequate nutrition, high fluid intake, and rest are essential. Rinsing the mouth with warm normal saline or 1.5% peroxide solution may be helpful for the first few days.

6. **Temporomandibular joint (TMJ) syndrome** is caused by an improper working relationship between the chewing muscles and the TMJ.
a. **Signs and symptoms** include a dull, aching pain around the ear; headaches; neck aches; limited opening of the mouth; and a clicking or popping noise upon opening the mouth.
b. **Risk factors** include bruxism (i.e., grinding the teeth) and occlusal (i.e., bite) abnormalities.
c. **Treatment** consists of moist heat applied to the jaw, muscle relaxants, bite plates or occlusal splints, a diet of soft foods, correcting the occlusion, or surgery.
d. **OTC products** that can help relieve the pain include oral analgesics (e.g., acetaminophen, ibuprofen).

7. **Teething pain.** The ADA has not accepted any product for teething pain. A **frozen teething ring** may provide symptomatic relief. Persisting pain may be treated with a local anesthetic such as benzocaine (found in Baby Anbesol® and Baby Orajel®). If a teething child presents with a fever, a physician should be contacted.

8. **Xerostomia** (i.e., dry mouth) is caused by improper functioning of the salivary glands (as in Sjögren's syndrome). **Artificial saliva** is available as an OTC product. The ADA has approved the following artificial salivas: Moi-Stir®, Salivart®, Xero-Lube®, and Saliva Substitute®.

C. Common oral lesions and OTC products

1. **Canker sores** (also referred to as **recurrent aphthous ulcers** or **recurrent aphthous stomatitis**)
a. The **cause** of canker sores is unknown. Recent studies suggest that the cause may be due to dysfunction of the immune system initiated by minor trauma.
b. **Lesions** can occur on any nonkeratinized mucosal surface in the mouth (i.e., tongue, lips) and usually appear gray-to-yellow with an erythematous halo of inflamed tissue surrounding the ulcer. Most lesions persist for 10 to 14 days and heal without scarring.
c. **OTC products** can control the pain of canker sores, shorten the duration of current lesions, and prevent new lesions. Products include **protectants** and **local anesthetics**.
(1) **Protectants** include Orabase®, denture adhesives (see II E 2), and benzoin tincture. Denture adhesives are not approved for this use by the FDA.
(2) **Local anesthetics** such as benzocaine or butacaine are the the most common anesthetics found in these OTC products.

(a) The FDA has approved the following ingredients:
(i) Benzocaine (5% to 20%)
(ii) Benzyl alcohol (0.05% to 0.1%)
(iii) Dyclonine (0.05% to 0.1%)
(iv) Hexylresorcinol (0.05% to 0.1%)
(v) Menthol (0.04% to 2%)
(vi) Phenol (0.5% to 1.5%)
(vii) Phenolate sodium (0.5% to 1.5%)
(viii) Salicyl alcohol (1% to 6%)

(b) Examples of OTC local anesthetics for oral use include Anbesol®, Blistex®, Campho-Phenique®, Orajel®, and Benzodent®.

(c) The use of products containing substantial amounts of menthol, phenol, camphor, and eugenol should be discouraged due to their ability to irritate tissue.

(d) Aspirin should not be retained in the mouth or placed on an oral lesion in an attempt to provide relief.

2. Cold sores (also called **fever blisters**) are primarily caused by the herpes simplex type I virus. An outbreak may be provoked by stress, minor infection, fever, or sunlight. Cold sores usually occur on the lips and are recurrent, often arising in the same location.

a. Presentation. An outbreak is preceded by burning, itching, or numbness. Red papules of fluid-containing vesicles then appear, and these eventually burst and form a crust. These sores are typically self-limited and heal in 10 to 14 days without scarring.

b. OTC products for cold sores include products that contain softening compounds (e.g., emollient creams, petrolatum, protectants), which keep the cold sore moist to prevent it from drying and fissuring. Local anesthetics in nondrying bases (e.g., Orabase®, with benzocaine) decrease pain. Highly astringent bases should be avoided. The ADA contraindicates caustic agents (e.g., phenol, silver nitrate), camphor and other counterirritants, and hydrocortisone for the treatment of cold sores.

(1) If a **secondary infection** develops, bacitracin or neomycin ointments should be recommended. If necessary, the patient should consult a physician for a systemic antibiotic prescription.

(2) Recommend a lip **sunscreen** for patients whose cold sores appear to be due to sun exposure.

(3) The essential amino acid L-lysine has been used in oral doses of 300 to 1200 mg daily to accelerate recovery or suppress recurrence of cold sores. However, studies have produced conflicting data regarding L-lysine and its effect on the duration, severity, and recurrence rate of cold sores.

D. Common oral infections and OTC products

1. Candidiasis (also called **thrush**) is caused by the fungus *Candida albicans,* which is the most common opportunistic pathogen associated with oral infections. Thrush has a milky curd appearance, and affected patients should contact a physician.

2. Oral cancer. The most common oral cancer is **squamous cell carcinoma,** which can appear as red or white lesions, ulcerations, or tumors.

a. Signs and symptoms include a color change in the tongue, a sore throat that does not heal, and persistent or unexplained bleeding. Patients with any of these signs should contact a physician or a dentist.

b. Risk factors include smoked and smokeless tobacco as well as alcohol.

c. Treatment consists of eliminating the use of tobacco and alcohol in any form (e.g., alcoholic beverages, mouth rinses with alcohol). Also, treatment generally includes **wide local excision** for small lesions and **en bloc excisions** for larger lesions (in continuity with radical neck dissection if lymph nodes are involved). Radiation, alone or combined with surgery, may be appropriate. Chemotherapy may be used as palliation or as an adjunct to surgery and radiation.

d. OTC medications should not be administered until after first checking with a physician. For example, OTC medication used for inflammation may increase the effects of methotrexate. Many possible side effects exist from chemotherapeutic agents, which require immediate medical attention (e.g., chest pain, inflammation, unusual bleeding). Some examples of side effects that usually do not require medical attention include nausea, vomiting, loss of appetite or hair, and trouble sleeping. OTC medications may be useful in these cases. However, nausea and vomiting are treated by prescription medications such as ondansetron or metoclopramide. Nonpharmacologic measures, such as avoiding disturbing environmental odors and vestibular disturbances, may be helpful in minimizing nausea and vomiting.

E. OTC denture products

1. **Denture cleansers** are either **chemical** or **abrasive** in respect to their cleansing ability.
   a. **Chemical denture cleansers** include alkaline peroxide, alkaline hypochlorite, or dilute acids.
      (1) **Alkaline peroxide** is the most commonly used chemical denture cleanser and is available as tablets or powder. It causes oxygen to be released, which creates a cleansing effect. Alkaline peroxide does not damage the surface of acrylic resins; however, it may bleach them.
      (2) **Alkaline hypochlorite** (i.e., bleach) dissolves the matrix of plaque but has no effect on calculus. It is both bactericidal and fungicidal. A **disadvantage** of alkaline hypochlorite is that it **corrodes metal denture components**. It may also bleach acrylic resin, therefore, it should not be used more than once a week.
   b. **Abrasive denture cleansers** are available as gel, paste, or powder (e.g., silicates, sodium bicarbonate, dicalcium phosphate, calcium carbonate).
      (1) Dentures should not be soaked in hot water, since the heat may distort or warp the appliances.
      (2) The ADA accepts the following denture cleansers as safe and effective: Complete®, Dentu-Gel®, Dentu-Creme®, Efferdent®, Polident®, and Fresh 'N' Brite®.
2. **Denture adherents** contain materials, such as karaya gum, pectin, or methylcellulose, that swell, gel, and become viscous in order to promote adhesion, which increases the denture attachment to underlying soft tissues.
   a. **Disadvantages.** As the use of denture adherents increases, the soft tissue deteriorates. Denture adherents can also provide a medium for bacterial and fungal growth. Daily use of denture adherents is not recommended.
   b. The ADA accepts the following denture adherents as safe and effective: Co-Re-Ga®, Perma-Grip®, Effergrip®, Firmdent®, Wernet's products, Orafix®, and Secure®.

F. Pharmacists' responsibilities to the patient using OTC oral products

1. Refer a patient to a dentist if the oral complaint involves an abscess with fever, swelling, malaise, lymphadenopathy, or purulent exudate.
2. Remind patients that cold and canker sores, with appropriate treatment, are usually a self-limiting problem.
3. Patients should be informed about how to use recommended products, the duration of use, the expectations of using the product, and the procedure to follow if the product is ineffective.
4. If a nonprescription product does not improve a condition, or if the condition worsens, use of the product should be discontinued and a physician or dentist should be contacted.

III. OPHTHALMIC PRODUCTS

A. Anatomy

1. **Eyelids** are folds of tissue that protect the eye and distribute tears.
2. The **external eye** is formed by the lacrimal apparatus and the conjunctival cul-de-sac.
3. **Internal eye**
   a. The **sclera** is the outer coating over the eyeball.
   b. The **iris** is the colored membrane that regulates the entrance of light through the pupil.
   c. **Aqueous humor** is the fluid derived from the blood by a process of secretion and ultrafiltration.
   d. The **lens,** which is a transparent refracting membrane, focuses rays to form an image on the retina.
   e. The **retina** receives the image formed by the lens.

f. The **conjunctiva** is the mucous membrane that lines the eyelids.
g. The **trabecular meshwork** and **Schlemm's canal** serve as exit pathways for aqueous humor.

B. Eye disorders

1. **Conditions affecting the eyelid** include irritation, inflammation, and infections (e.g., contusions (black eyes), styes).
   a. **Symptoms of a stye** include pain, tenderness, redness and swelling. A stye is defined as a localized, purulent, inflammatory infection of one or more sebaceous glands of the eyelid. Styes cannot be treated with OTC medications. Often, hot compresses applied four times a day are helpful. However, some patients may require treatment with an antibiotic.
   b. **Inflammation of the eyelid (blepharitis)** can be detected by redness of the lids, and burning, itching, and scaly skin. The underlying problem (e.g., seborrheic dermatitis, *Staphylococcus aureus*) should be treated, which often requires an antibiotic.
   c. **Black eyes** may be treated with cold compresses for the first 24 hours then warm compresses. Damage to the eyelid itself should be referred to a physician.
2. **External ocular disorders** include chemical burns, conjunctivitis, and lacrimal system disorders.
   a. **Symptoms of conjunctivitis** include redness, itching, and discharge.
      (1) **Familiar types of conjunctivitis** include bacterial, chlamydial, viral, and allergic.
      (2) **Treatment.** Antihistamines and decongestants can be used for symptomatic relief for allergic and bacterial conjunctivitis.
   b. **Dacryoadenitis** (i.e., swelling of the lacrimal gland) should be referred to a physician. Symptoms include red, burning eyes and the sensation of a foreign body in the eye.
   c. **Corneal edema** is the result of an underlying cause (e.g., damage to the eye). Hypertonic solutions and decongestants may be helpful treatments. However, if edema persists for more than 24 hours, a physician should be contacted.
   d. **Insufficient tearing** (e.g., Sjögren's syndrome) is generally successfully treated with artificial tear products (see III D 5).
   e. **Chemical burns** should be referred to a physician.
3. **Internal ocular disorders** include glaucoma (i.e., an increase in intraocular pressure), cataracts (i.e., opacity of the crystalline lens of the eye or its capsule) and uveitis (i.e., inflammation of the uvea). These internal ailments should be diagnosed and treated by a physician.

C. Treatment. The following **pharmaceutical agents** are included in ophthalmic products for the specific purposes listed below.

1. **Antioxidants and stabilizers** are used to delay or prevent deterioration of the drug. Examples include edetic acid, sodium bisulfite, sodium metabisulfite, sodium thiosulfate, and thiourea.

2. **Buffers** are designed to keep products within the appropriate pH range, which is 6.0 to 8.0 (tears are 7.4). Buffers include: acetic acid, boric acid, hydrochloric acid, phosphoric acid, potassium bicarbonate, potassium borate, potassium tetraborate, potassium bicarbonate, potassium citrate, the potassium phosphates, sodium acetate, sodium bicarbonate, sodium biphosphate, sodium borate, sodium carbonate, sodium citrate, sodium hydroxide, and sodium phosphate.

3. **Clarifying or wetting agents** reduce surface tension of the lens. Examples include polysorbate 20, polysorbate 80, poloxamer 282, and tyloxapol.

4. **Preservatives** destroy or inhibit the development of microorganisms. Examples of these agents are benzalkonium chloride and benzethonium chloride.

5. **Tonicity adjusters** include dextrose, glycerine (1%), potassium chloride, propylene glycol (1%), and sodium chloride. Agents considered to be isotonic should equal 0.9% ± 0.2% sodium chloride. When applied to the eye, these agents pull water from the middle of the cornea. Nonisotonic agents used in the eye may produce excessive blinking or cause damage.

6. **Viscosity-increasing agents** are used to increase the retention time for ophthalmic medications. These agents include cellulose derivatives, dextran 70, gelatin (0.01%) and liquid polyols.

D. Medicinal agents. There are no FDA-approved anti-infectives available for OTC ophthalmic use. The following compounds are medicinal agents used for ophthalmic therapy.

1. **Astringents.** The only FDA-recommended astringent is zinc sulfate (0.25%). This agent is relatively mild but still provides some relief from eye irritation, since it decreases inflammation. The recommended dose is 1 to 2 drops four times a day.

2. **Demulcents** are relatively free of side effects and are used to protect and lubricate the eye from dryness and irritation from sun exposure. Demulcents include carboxymethylcellulose sodium, dextran 70, gelatin, glycerin, hydroxyethyl cellulose, hydroxypropyl methylcellulose, methylcellulose, polyethylene glycol 300, polyethylene glycol 400, polysorbate 80, polyvinyl alcohol, povidone, and propylene glycol.

3. **Decongestants and vasoconstrictors**
   a. **Mechanism of action.** These agents work by producing a temporary constriction of the blood vessels located in the conjunctiva.
   b. **Products** include naphazoline hydrochloride (e.g., Clear Eyes®), phenylephrine hydrochloride (e.g., Isopto Frin®), tetrahydrozoline hydrochloride (e.g., Murine Plus®), and oxymetazoline hydrochloride (OcuClear®).
   c. **Rebound congestion** can occur with a long duration of use.
   d. **Contraindication.** The available OTC agents are useful in relieving eye redness and irritations, and are contraindicated in angle-closure glaucoma patients.

4. **Hypertonic agents** (e.g., sodium chloride 2% to 5%) are used for the relief of corneal swelling. Because of their concentration, these products should be used under the supervision of a physician, although they are available as nonprescription products.

5. **Artificial tears** (combination of hypertonic agent, buffer, viscosity agent and preservative) are used to lubricate the eye for relief of dry eyes or irritation.

E. General patient information

1. Patients should be counselled regarding appropriate administration of individual products. They should also be told to wash hands thoroughly before applying these products.

2. If a patient presents with a headache or vision abnormalities, has had symptoms persisting for more than 3 days, or a recommended OTC product has not abated symptoms during this time, a physician should be contacted. In general, OTC ophthalmic products should not be used for more than 3 days without physician supervision.

F. Contact lenses. Wearing contact lenses successfully depends on adequate tear production.

1. **General considerations**
   a. **Indications** include keratoconus (protrusion of the central part of the cornea), aphakia (absence of lens), visual aberrations, myopia (nearsightedness), hyperopia (farsightedness), astigmatism (improper focus of light rays), presbyopia (diminution of the accommodation of the lens) and monovision.
   b. **Contraindications** include occupations with exposure to excessive dust, wind, or smoke; chronic conjunctivitis or blepharitis; and recurrent bacterial, fungal, or viral infections.
   c. **Caution** should be taken by patients suffering from diseases that can affect the normal eye (e.g., epilepsy, high blood pressure, heart disease, diabetes mellitus). Similar cautions should be taken by patients using medications that can alter the eye (e.g., oral contraceptives). Certain diseases and drugs may have direct effects on the eye. For example, high blood pressure can produce retinal hemorrhage; diabetes mellitus produces an outgrowth of vessels in the iris and anterior chamber of the eye; and oral contraceptives have numerous possible effects on the eye (e.g., increased corneal sensitivity, color changes, decreased visual acuity).

2. **Types of contact lenses**
   a. **Hard lenses** are rigid, hydrophobic products. The most common plastic used is polymethylmethacrylate (PMMA) better known as lucite or plexiglas.
      (1) **Advantages** include the ability to mark the contact lens to identify for which eye the contact is intended. (Cost compared to soft lenses could be considered an advantage.)
      (2) **Disadvantages** include minimal wettability and limited oxygen permeability, which limits the length of patient wear and the ability to adapt to the lens.
   b. **Soft lenses** contain a hydroxyl group or a combination of hydroxyl and lactam groups, which allows the lens to hold water.
      (1) **Advantages.** Soft contact lenses are easier to apply, more comfortable to wear, and more difficult to dislodge than hard lenses.

(2) **Disadvantages** include the potential to absorb compounds (e.g., chemicals) from products, cost, the necessary extended care to keep the lens from deteriorating, and altered visual acuity due to hydration of the lens.

(3) With the exception of a small number of rewetting solutions, patients should be advised against the application of ophthalmic products when wearing soft lenses.

c. **Gas-permeable lenses** combine soft lens material and polymethylmethacrylate (PMMA).

(1) **Advantages** of the combined products include increased visual acuity and more comfort than with hard lenses.

(2) **Disadvantages** to gas-permeable lenses are that they accumulate protein and lipid deposits and are made of hydrophobic materials.

3. **Adverse effects of lenses**

a. **Corneal edema** can result from inadequate oxygenation.

b. **Medications** can affect the eye and potentiate problems (e.g., edema of the cornea). Examples include oral contraceptives, decongestants, antihistamines, tricyclic antidepressants, and diuretics.

4. **Contact lens care**

a. **Hard lens care** includes cleaning to remove oils and debris, soaking in a storage medium, wetting to produce a hydrophobic surface, and rewetting (cleaning and rewetting of lens).

b. **Soft lens care** includes cleaning (with surface-active or enzymatic cleaners), disinfecting (thermal and chemical) and rewetting.

c. **Gas-permeable lens care** involves cleaning, wetting, and soaking. Some of these lenses contain more silicone agents, requiring conditioning solutions, which are made especially for rewetting purposes.

d. **Solution ingredients**

(1) **Cleaning products** generally contain nonionic or amphoteric surfactants, which dislodge mucus, lipids, and proteins from the lens.

(2) **Wetting solutions** are applied directly to the lens before insertion into the eye. Wetting solutions are intended to lubricate, decrease lens surface tension, and change the lens surface from hydrophobic to hydrophilic.

(3) **Soaking and storage solutions** are used to provide an aseptic environment and to hydrate the lens.

(4) **Preservatives** used in these solutions include: benzalkonium chloride, thimerosal, phenylmercuric nitrate, sorbic acid and sodium edetate. Thimerosal causes a great deal of irritation to many soft contact lens wearers.

STUDY QUESTIONS

Directions: Each of the numbered items or incomplete statements in this section is followed by answers or by completions of the statement. Select the **one** lettered answer or completion that is **best** in each case.

1. Ophthalmic agents contraindicated in glaucoma patients include which one of the following substances?

(A) Antioxidants
(B) Antipruritics
(C) Decongestants
(D) Emollients

2. Which one of the following is the only Food and Drug Administration (FDA)-recommended astringent?

(A) Benzalkonium chloride
(B) Sodium chloride
(C) Zinc sulfate
(D) Edetic acid

3. Abrasives, ingredients in dentifrices, are noted for which of the following actions?

(A) Providing flavor
(B) Cleansing via a foaming detergent action
(C) Removing plaque and debris
(D) Preventing dental caries
(E) Adding thickness to the product

4. The appropriate pH range for ophthalmic products is

(A) 2.0 to 3.0
(B) 4.0 to 6.0
(C) 6.0 to 8.0
(D) 8.0 to 10.0

5. Which type of contact lens can most easily be ruined by the absorption of chemicals?

(A) Hard lenses
(B) Soft lenses
(C) Gas-permeable lenses

6. All of the following are true statements concerning the use of alkaline peroxide as a denture cleanser EXCEPT

(A) it may bleach the denture
(B) it is available as tablets or powders
(C) it acts by releasing oxygen
(D) it is fungicidal and bactericidal
(E) it does not damage the surface of acrylic resins

7. All of the following statements concerning teeth whitening products are true EXCEPT

(A) possible risks include tissue irritation and gingivitis
(B) most products contain 10% carbamide peroxide
(C) most products contain zinc to prevent calculus formation
(D) antiseptics (e.g., Proxigel®) have been used as bleaching agents
(E) calcium peroxide and sodium monofluorophosphate are teeth whitening agents

8. All of the following desensitizing agents are recommended for sensitive teeth EXCEPT

(A) 10% carbamide peroxide
(B) 5% potassium nitrate
(C) dibasic sodium citrate
(D) 10% strontium chloride hexahydrate

1-C	4-C	7-C
2-C	5-B	8-A
3-C	6-D	

Directions: Each item below contains three suggested answers of which **one or more** is correct. Choose the answer

- **A** if **I only** is correct
- **B** if **III only** is correct
- **C** if **I and II** are correct
- **D** if **II and III** are correct
- **E** if **I, II, and III** are correct

9. Which of the following compounds are considered a suspending agent, an ingredient in dentifrices?

I. Dicalcium phosphate
II. Karaya gum
III. Methylcellulose

10. Cold sore treatment may include which of the following ingredients?

I. Benzocaine
II. Dyclonine
III. Camphor

9-D
10-C

ANSWERS AND EXPLANATIONS

1. The answer is C *[III D 3].*
Decongestants may cause a slight pupillary dilation. Although this is not significant in open-angle glaucoma, these agents should be avoided in angle-closure patients. In angle-closure glaucoma, the blockage to outflow is more severe and directly involves the anterior chamber.

2. The answer is C *[III C 1, D].*
Zinc sulfate is the only ophthalmic astringent recommended by the Food and Drug Administration. Sodium chloride is a hypertonic agent. Benzalkonium chloride is a preservative used in contact lens solutions. Edetic acid is an antioxidant used to slow or prevent deterioration of ophthalmic drugs.

3. The answer is C *[II B 2 d (1) (a)].*
Abrasives are components in dentifrices that are responsible for physically removing plaque. Patients should use the least abrasive dentifrice, unless directed otherwise by the dentist.

4. The answer is C *[III C 2].*
The appropriate pH range for ophthalmic agents is 6.0 to 8.0, which is similar to the pH of tears (7.4).

5. The answer is B *[III F 2 b].*
Soft lenses allow for easier product absorption, and the absorption of chemicals from ophthalmic products may ruin the lenses. They also contain hydroxyl or hydroxyl and lactam groups, all of which are chemically reactive.

6. The answer is D *[II E 1 a (1)].*
The mechanism of action of alkaline peroxide is the release of oxygen for a mechanical cleaning effect. It can be used safely on acrylic appliances; however, it may bleach the appliance. It is available in tablet or powder form. Alkaline hypochlorite, not alkaline peroxide, is both bactericidal and fungicidal.

7. The answer is C *[II B 2 d (4)].*
Teeth whitening agents usually contain 10% carbamide peroxide, which is a white crystal that reacts with water to release hydrogen peroxide and, therefore, liberates free oxides. Cosmetic agents may alter the normal flora or cause tissue irritation, gingivitis, and teeth sensitivity. Antiseptics (e.g., Gly-Oxide®, Proxigel®) and calcium peroxide (e.g., calprox in EpiSmile®) have been used as teeth whitening agents. In addition, sodium monofluorophosphate is found in EpiSmile®.

8. The answer is A *[II B 2 d (5)].*
Desensitizing agents should not be abrasive or used on a chronic basis unless directed by a dentist. The products approved by the American Dental Association include the ingredients 5% potassium nitrate, 10% strontium chloride hexahydrate, and dibasic sodium citrate 2% in pluronic gel. The ingredient 10% carbamide peroxide is a whitening agent, which may cause teeth sensitivity and, therefore, should not be used by a patient with sensitive teeth.

9. The answer is D (II, III) *[II B 2 d (1) (c)].*
Suspending agents are products that add thickness to the dentifrices. Examples are tragacanth, karaya gum, and methylcellulose. Dicalcium phosphate is categorized as an abrasive product.

10. The answer is C (I, II) *[II C 1 c].*
Cold sore treatment involves keeping the lesion moist with emollient creams, petrolatum, or protectants. In addition, local anesthetics (e.g., benzocaine, dyclonine, salicyl alcohol) may be used. Topical counterirritants (e.g., camphor) and caustics or escharotic agents (e.g., phenol, menthol, silver nitrate) are not recommended since they may further irritate the tissue. Cold sores are usually self-limiting and heal within 10 to 14 days without scarring.

34

OTC Products: Pediculosis, Acne, Sunscreens, and Contact Dermatitis

Larry N. Swanson

I. PEDICULOSIS AND PEDICULICIDES

A. Introduction. Pediculosis is a skin infestation produced by blood-sucking lice. Lice are small, flat, wingless insects with stubby antennae and three pairs of legs which end in sharp, curved claws. Three **types of lice infest humans**:

1. *Pediculus humanus capitis* (i.e., the head louse)
2. *Pediculus humanus corporis* (i.e., the body louse)
3. *Phthirus pubis* (the pubic, or crab, louse)

B. Life cycles. The lice that infest humans pass through similar life cycles.

1. **Location.** All lice need human warmth to survive.
   a. **Head and pubic lice** spend their entire cycle on the skin of the human host.
   b. **Body lice** live in clothing, coming to the skin surface only to feed.
2. **Development**
   a. Each type of louse develops from **eggs (nits)** that incubate for about 1 week. When the small, grey–white, tear-shaped eggs hatch, the nymphs appear.
   b. In about 3 weeks, the **nymphs** mature; then, the females start to lay eggs.
   c. Each type of louse survives about 1 month as a **mature adult**. During this time, the females produce about five eggs daily. A female can lay as many as 150 eggs during her typical 30-day adulthood.
3. **Egg deposit**
   a. **Body lice** deposit their eggs on fibers of clothing, particularly in the seams. These lice can survive without food up to 10 days, and the eggs may remain viable for about 1 month.
   b. **Head and pubic lice** deposit their eggs on hair strands, about ¼ inch from the skin.

C. Incidence of infestation. The incidence of lice infestations increases each year.

1. As many as 12 million cases of head lice occur each year in the United States.
2. The bulk of these cases occur between September and November, when students are back in school.
3. In outbreaks of head lice, 70% of cases occur in children younger than age 12.
4. Infestations tend to be more common in girls, presumably because of their greater tendency to share grooming items.
5. Unlike the other two forms of lice, body lice are associated with improper hygiene and are often present in street people. This infestation is rare in the United States, especially when people follow proper hygiene routines.

D. The medical problem

1. Both the adult and nymph are blood-sucking; they feed on a human by piercing the skin and introducing a small amount of saliva (which contains an **anticoagulant**) into the feeding area.
   a. The attachment of lice to the body causes the **erythematous papule,** which may **itch**.
   b. The female louse produces a sticky **cement-like secretion** that holds the eggs in place on the hair shaft so securely that ordinary shampooing does not remove it.

2. Neither head nor crab lice transmit infections per se, but body lice transmit **typhus, relapsing fever,** and **trench fever**.

3. Lice and humans have a true **parasitic relationship;** lice depend on the human host for shelter, food, and reproductive success. Once hatched, nymphs must have access to the human host within the first 12- to 24-hour period, if they are to survive.

E. Methods of transmission

1. **Head lice** are most commonly spread by head-to-head contact with an infested person through hats, caps, scarves, pillowcases, communal combs and brushes, or clothing that is hung close together (e.g., on a coat rack).

2. **Pubic lice** are transmitted primarily through sexual contact, but also through shared undergarments, towels, or toilet seats.
   - **a.** The lice affect teens and young adults most often through sexual contact.
   - **b.** Lice frequently coexist with other sexually transmitted diseases.
   - **c.** Scratching in the genital areas may transmit pubic lice to other hairy regions, such as the eyelashes, eyebrows, sideburns, and mustaches.

F. Signs and symptoms

1. **Head lice**
   - **a.** The most common symptom is head-scratching.
   - **b.** Skin redness around the nape (i.e., back) of the neck and above the ears is usually seen.
   - **c.** The lice can be identified by direct examination using wooden applicator sticks or a comb to part the hair, then looking at the hair through a magnifying glass.
   - **d.** The lice appear as tiny brownish grey spots, that are often difficult to see. The shiny, whitish-silver eggs (nits), which appear almost as grains of sugar, are more likely to be seen than the lice. The nits usually reside about ¼ inch from the scalp on the hair shaft, and they may be confused with dandruff or hairspray droplets.

2. **Pubic lice.** The primary symptom is scratching in the genital area.

3. **Body lice.** The most common symptoms are bites and itching, which are commonly seen as vertical excoriations on the trunk area.

G. Treatment

1. There are **two goals** in the treatment of lice:
   - **a.** To kill the lice and nits
   - **b.** To control the symptoms of itching in order to prevent secondary infection

2. **Itching.** Pharmacists should advise patients that even after the causative organism and nits have been killed, itching may persist for several days. This aspect is very important because patients may decide to use pediculicides excessively, thinking that they have been ineffective when the itching continues. Excessive use of pediculicides may result in excessive drying, which can cause further itching.

3. **Home remedies.** Because of the social stigma attached to lice infestation, some individuals may resort to harmful home remedies. Examples of such uncomfortable, ineffective, and potentially dangerous approaches include the following:
   - **a.** Shaving the head and pubic area
   - **b.** Applying heat to the infested area with a hair dryer
   - **c.** Soaking the head in hot water for several minutes
   - **d.** Soaking the area of infestation with gasoline or kerosene

4. **Over-the-counter (OTC) pediculicide products** include:
   - **a. Pyrethrins 0.17%–0.33% with piperonyl butoxide 2%–4%.** This product is safe and effective for the treatment of head, pubic, and body lice. The combination of ingredients is an example of **pharmacologic synergism**.
     - **(1) Pyrethrins** kill by disrupting ion transport mechanisms at the nerve membranes. These natural insecticides are derived from a mixture of substances obtained from the flowers of the chrysanthemum plant. Because not all eggs (nits) may be killed with a single application of this agent or removed with a nit comb, it may be necessary to reapply the pyrethrin product within 7–10 days of the first application (since the usual hatching time of eggs is 7–10 days).

(2) **Piperonyl butoxide** enhances the pediculicide effect of pyrethrins by suppressing the oxidative degradation mechanisms of the lice. Therefore, the length of time that the pyrethrins contact the lice is increased.

(3) **Side effects** from either agent are uncommon.

(a) **Contact dermatitis** (see IV) is the most frequently reported side effect.

(b) **Allergic reactions.** Because pyrethrins are derived from a plant, they may produce hay fever (i.e., allergic rhinitis) and asthma attacks in susceptible individuals. Thus, patients who have known allergies to ragweed or chrysanthemum plants should use this product with caution.

(4) Common **trade names** for this product include A-200 Pediculicide Shampoo and Rid.

(5) **Directions for use**

(a) Apply the product, undiluted, to the infested area until it is entirely wet.

(b) Allow the product to remain on the area for 10 minutes.

(c) Wash the area thoroughly with warm, soapy water or shampoo.

(d) Dry the area, preferably with a disposable cloth.

(e) Comb hair in the previously infested area with a fine-toothed comb to remove dead lice and eggs.

(f) Do not exceed two applications within 24 hours.

b. Permethrin is a pyrethroid (i.e., a synthetic version of a pyrethrin). It is indicated only for head lice.

(1) **Mechanism of action.** Permethrin has the same mechanism of action as the pyrethrins.

(2) **Application.** Permethrin comes in the form of a creme rinse (Nix) and should be applied like a conventional hair conditioner after the hair has been shampooed, rinsed, and towel-dried. The hair should be thoroughly saturated with permethrin, which should remain on the hair for 10 minutes then rinsed.

(3) **Effectiveness.** A single application is 97%–99% effective in killing lice and eggs.

(a) Since the agent is retained on the hair shaft, the product provides **protection** for up to 14 days. This 2-week therapeutic effect persists regardless of normal shampooing.

(b) **Re-treatment** is required in less than 1% of cases.

(c) Because of this prolonged effect, **nits do not need to be removed**. However, for cosmetic reasons or school policy, they should be.

(d) Many people consider permethrin to be the **agent of choice** in treating lice infestations.

5. Prescription products

a. Lindane, or gamma benzene hexachloride, is available as a shampoo, cream, or lotion. It is indicated for head, pubic, and body lice.

(1) **Mechanism of action.** Lindane is neurotoxic to head lice and their eggs.

(2) **Application.** For head lice, the lindane shampoo should be applied to dry hair and thoroughly worked into the hair and scalp of the infested individual.

(a) The area should be shampooed for 4 minutes, then rinsed and towel-dried.

(b) The nits should be removed with a fine-toothed comb designed for this purpose.

(3) The **adverse effects** from this agent are rare if used properly. Severe central nervous system (CNS) toxicity has occurred in infants, with seizures and deaths reported, especially when the lotion is used or when the agent is ingested. Toxicity has been minimal when the shampoo is used properly to treat head lice.

b. Malathion is an organophosphate cholinesterase inhibitor that has been widely used as a lawn and garden insecticide. It is indicated only for head lice. Malathion kills both lice and nits in vitro.

(1) **Mechanism of action.** Sulfur atoms in the malathion bind with sulfur groups on the hair, giving a residual protective effect against reinfestation.

(2) **Application.** Malathion is prepared as a lotion in 78% alcohol; therefore, caution should be used near an open flame or a hair dryer. The product should be sprinkled on dry hair and left for 8–12 hours before rinsing. A fine-toothed comb should be used to remove the dead lice and eggs.

(3) No systemic **adverse effects** have been reported with topical use of this medication.

(a) The alcoholic vehicle may produce stinging.

(b) Although this agent is very effective, its unpleasant odor (due to sulfhydryl compounds) and the required time of 8–12 hours on the scalp represent two main drawbacks.

6. Adjunctive therapy

a. Nit removal

(1) The pediculicide products mentioned vary in their ability to kill the lice nits. To ensure successful therapy, after pediculicide application, the nits should be removed with a **fine-toothed comb**.

(2) Although various substances have been used in an effort to dislodge the nits from the hair shafts, most have been unsuccessful. A **formic acid formulation** (e.g., Step 2 Creme Rinse) softens the strong adhesive that binds the nits to the hair shaft. Indicated for use after pediculicide shampoo treatments, it comes packaged with a special fine-toothed comb.

b. Treatment of other household members. Once a lice infestation has been identified in one member of the household, all other members should be examined carefully. Everyone who is infested should be treated at the same time.

c. Adjunctive methods for controlling lice infestations

(1) Washable material items should be machine-washed in hot water (130°F) for 5–10 minutes.

(2) Nonwashable material goods should be dry-cleaned or sealed in a plastic bag for 35 days.

(3) Personal items (e.g., comb, brushes) should be soaked in hot water (130°F) for 5–10 minutes.

(4) Furniture and household items (e.g., carpets, chairs, couches, pillows) should be vacuumed thoroughly. OTC spray products that contain pyrethrins are no more effective than vacuuming in terms of removing the risk of reinfestation.

H. Head lice myths are numerous. The following additional facts may reassure and inform patients and parents of patients.

1. No significant difference in incidence occurs among the various socioeconomic classes or races.

2. Hygiene and hair length are not contributing factors.

3. Head lice do not fly or jump from person to person.

4. Head lice do not carry other diseases.

5. Head lice cannot be contracted from animals, and pets are not susceptible to *Pediculus humanus capitis*.

6. The head does not have to be shaved to get rid of lice.

7. Washing hair with "brown" soap is not effective.

8. Head lice are unrelated to ticks.

9. Hair does not fall out as a consequence of infestation.

10. Head lice infestations can occur at any time of the year.

II. ACNE AND ITS REMEDIES

A. General information

1. Definition. *Acne vulgaris* is a disorder of the pilosebaceous units, mainly of the face, chest, and back. The lesions usually start as open or closed comedones and evolve into inflammatory papules and pustules that either resolve as macules or become secondary pyoderma, which results in various sequelae.

2. Incidence

a. Acne vulgaris is the most common skin disease of adolescence.

b. It affects primarily adolescents in junior high and senior high, then decreases in adulthood.

c. More than 80% of the population is affected by age 17.

3. Importance

a. Acne vulgaris is usually **self-limiting**.

b. However, the condition is significant to adolescents because of heightened self-consciousness about appearance.

c. A great majority of people do not consult a physician for treatment of acne; therefore, a pharmacist can have a significant role.

B. Etiology and pathophysiology

1. The **pathogenesis** of acne vulgaris involves **three events**.
   a. **Increased sebum production**
      (1) Sebum secretion is regulated primarily by **androgens,** which are actively secreted in both sexes beginning at puberty.
      (2) One of these androgens, testosterone, is converted to **dihydrotestosterone (DHT)**.
      (3) DHT levels induce the sebaceous glands to increase in size and activity, resulting in increased amounts of sebum.
   b. **Abnormal clumping of epithelial horny cells within the pilosebaceous unit**
      (1) Normally, keratinized horny cells are sloughed from the epithelial lining of the pilosebaceous duct in the hair follicles and are carried to the skin surface with a flow of sebum.
      (2) In the acne patient, the keratinization process is abnormal, characterized by increased adherence and production of follicular epithelial cells. This process is called **retention hyperkeratosis,** and it results in obstruction of the outflow of the pilosebaceous unit.
   c. Presence of *Propionibacterium acnes* (a gram-positive anaerobe)
      (1) People with acne have skin colony counts of *P. acnes* that are significantly higher than the counts of those without acne.
      (2) *P. acnes* produces several enzymes, including lipases, which break down sebum triglycerides to short-chain free fatty acids (FFAs), which are irritating, cause comedones, and result in inflammation.

2. **Sequence of acne lesion development**
   a. Mechanical blockage of a pilosebaceous duct by clumped horny cells results in a closed comedo (i.e., a whitehead).
   b. Once a closed comedo develops, it can form either a papule or an open comedo (i.e., a blackhead). The color is attributed to melanin or oxidized lipid, not to dirt.
   c. The lesion may enlarge and fill with pus, which is then termed a pustule.
   d. In more severe cases of acne, papules may develop into nodules or cysts.
   e. The term "pimple" nonspecifically refers to whiteheads, blackheads, papules, and pustules.

C. Clinical features

1. **Location.** Acne vulgaris lesions usually occur on the face, neck, chest, upper back, and shoulders. Any or all types of lesions may be seen on a single patient.

2. **Symptoms.** This condition is usually asymptomatic; however, some patients may have pruritus or pain if large, tender lesions are present.

3. **Classification.** It is important to differentiate noninflammatory from inflammatory acne to determine the best treatment approach. There are many rating or grading scales for acne severity. One such classification follows.
   a. **Grade I** consists primarily of comedones.
   b. **Grade II** consists primarily of comedones and superficial papules and pustules.
   c. **Grade III** is marked by a predominance of papules and pustules.
   d. **Grade IV** shows cystic lesions with moderate to severe scarring. This grade is sometimes referred to as cystic acne—secondary infection involves cysts or pustules on the face, neck, or trunk. Scarring occurs with hypertrophic ridges, keloids, or atrophic "ice pick" pits.

D. Complicating factors. Other factors have been implicated in the exacerbation of acne.

1. **Drugs and hormones**
   a. Many topical and systemic medications (e.g., bromides, iodides, topical coal tar products, androgens, anticonvulsants, progestins, lithium, corticosteroids) can be comedogenic and can make acne worse or can induce acne-like eruptions (i.e., acneiform lesions).
   b. Acneiform eruptions differ from true acne lesions in that apparently no comedo forms, eruptions are usually acute, and the lesions usually are all in the same stage of development.

2. **Stress.** Some clinicians accept stress as an important contributory factor to acne. The mechanism probably involves the increased release of corticosteroids during times of stress and, thus, the increased sebum production.

3. **Diet** probably has a minimal role in acne. Allergies to foods (e.g., chocolate) may be misinterpreted as a worsening of acne. Anticipatory anxiety about "breakouts" after eating certain foods may produce acne flare-up because of the stress-related corticosteroid secretion. The majority of dermatologists today make the following recommendations regarding diet:
   a. The patient should be eating a well-balanced diet. As with most other human diseases, and as a matter of good health, excess fats and carbohydrates should be avoided.
   b. The patient who insists that certain foods cause exacerbation of acne should probably avoid those foods.
   c. Foods that may fall into the dubious role of worsening acne include: chocolate, shellfish, nuts, ice cream, eggs, milk, cream, fried foods, iodized salt, cheese, bacon, and pastry.

4. **Physical trauma or irritation** can promote the rupture of plugged follicles, which can produce more inflammatory reactions. Scrubbing the face, wearing headbands, and picking at the pimples can contribute to the primary inflammation process. Gentle, regular washing with soap and water can be beneficial.

5. **Cosmetics.** Some cosmetic bases and certain cosmetic ingredients are comedogenic (e.g., lanolins, petroleum bases, cocoa butter). Preparations such as cleansing creams, suntan oils, and heavy foundations should generally be avoided.

6. **Menstrual cycle.** Some women may notice flare-ups of acne during the premenstrual part of the cycle. Fluctuations in the level of progesterone are probably the cause.

7. **Environmental factors.** Very humid environments or heavy sweating lead to keratin hydration, swelling, and a decrease in the size of the pilosebaceous follicle orifice, which results in duct obstruction. The sun, as well as artificial ultraviolet (UV) light, can help acne by drying and peeling the skin, but both can also aggravate acne.

E. Treatment and care

1. **General**
   a. Most patients can be treated successfully with both topically and systemically administered medications. Acne often improves when patients reach their early twenties.
   b. Even the most effective treatment programs may take several weeks to produce any clinical improvement. This aspect must be emphasized.
   c. People affected with acne should avoid anything that seems to worsen the condition (e.g., certain foods, cosmetics, clothing, cradling the chin with the hand).
   d. The number and type of lesions should be roughly determined to assess further therapeutic responses.

2. **Cleansing recommendations**
   a. Since many acne patients have oily skin, gentle cleansing two to three times daily is recommended for removing excess oil.
   b. Acne lesions cannot be scrubbed away. Compulsive scrubbing may actually worsen the acne by disrupting the follicular walls and, thus, setting the stage for inflammation.
   c. Mild facial soaps, such as Dove, Neutrogena, and Purpose, should be used to cleanse the skin.
   d. Medicated soaps containing sulfur, resorcinol, or salicylic acid are of little value, because the medication rinses away rather than penetrating the follicle.
   e. Patients with mild comedonal acne may find benefit from cleansers containing pumice, polyethylene, or aluminum oxide particles (e.g., Brasivol). However, patients with inflammatory acne or sensitive skin should avoid these products.

3. **Approaches to treatment** depend on the severity of the condition. Although acne cannot be cured, most cases can be managed successfully with topical treatment alone. Based on the pathogenesis of the condition, potential methods include:
   a. Unblocking the sebaceous duct so that the contents can be easily expelled
   b. Decreasing the amount of sebum that is secreted
   c. Changing the composition of the sebum to make it less irritating by decreasing the population of *P. acnes*

4. Nonprescription topical medications

a. Benzoyl peroxide (Category III; 2.5%–10%) has traditionally been recognized as the most effective topical OTC agents for acne, and many OTC acne products contain it. However, the recently released final monograph from the Food and Drug Administration (FDA) changed the status of benzoyl peroxide from Category I to Category III, indicating that more data are needed to prove its safety with regards to long-term photocarcinogen effects. (see Chapter 32 II B for category descriptions).

(1) Effects. Benzoyl peroxide has irritant, drying, peeling, comedolytic, and antibacterial effects. A beneficial effect should be noticed within about 2 weeks, but the usual length of a therapeutic trial is 6 to 8 weeks. As for adverse effects, benzoyl peroxide may cause a burning or stinging sensation, which gradually disappears. The clinical response shows only minimal differences among the 2.5%, 5%, and 10% concentrations.

(a) Most of the **adverse effects** from this agent relate to its therapeutic effect of irritating and drying the skin. For this reason, the lowest concentration available should be chosen initially. From 1% to 3% of patients may be hypersensitive to benzoyl peroxide.

(b) The vehicle for the benzoyl peroxide is also important in its overall activity. The alcohol gel vehicle tends to be more effective than the lotion or cream formulations.

(c) Benzoyl peroxide may discolor certain types of fabric or clothing material and may also bleach hair.

(2) Mechanism of action. Benzoyl peroxide has a dual mode of action, so it is effective against both inflammatory and noninflammatory acne.

(a) Benzoyl peroxide decomposes to release oxygen, which is lethal to the *P. acnes* anaerobe.

(b) As an irritant, it increases the turnover rate of epithelial cells, resulting in increased sloughing and promoting of resolution of comedones.

(3) Application

(a) The affected area should be washed with mild soap and water, then gently patted dry.

(b) The product should be massaged gently into the skin, avoiding the eyes, mouth, lips, and inside of the nose.

(c) The product can be applied at night, left on for 15 or 20 minutes to test sensitivity, then washed off.

(d) If no excessive irritation develops, apply once daily for the first few days.

(e) If drying, redness, or peeling does not occur in 3 days, increase application to twice daily.

b. Salicylic acid (Category I; 0.5%–2%), an irritant keratolytic agent, results in increased turnover of the epithelial lining. Through this effect, salicylic acid probably promotes the penetration of other acne products.

c. Sulfur (3%–10%), sulfur 8% combined with resorcinol 2% or resorcinol monoacetate 3% (Category I)

(1) Sulfur is also a keratolytic agent, and it has antibacterial actions.

(2) Sulfur has traditionally been recognized as a less desirable product because it may be acnegenic with continued use, and it has an offensive color and odor.

d. Resorcinol (Category II; as a single agent) is a keratolytic agent that has been recognized as effective against acne when the agent is combined with sulfur.

F. Prescription medications, both topical and systemic, are included here to put into perspective how OTC agents fit into acne therapy.

1. Topical prescription agents

a. Tretinoin (Vitamin A acid, retinoic acid, Retin-A) increases the turnover rate of nonadhering horny cells in the follicular canal, which results in comedo clearing and inhibits new comedo development.

(1) Effectiveness. Tretinoin is probably the most effective topical agent for acne, especially acne characterized by comedones. It is best used for noninflammatory acne.

(2) Side effects. Because of its irritant properties, tretinoin can cause excessive irritation, erythema, peeling, and increased risk for severe sunburn. There may be an initial exacerbation of the acne, and a total of 12 weeks may be necessary to fully assess treatment efficacy.

(3) **Application.** The cream formulation of tretinoin, which is less irritating than the gel form (which is less irritating than the solution form), should be used initially. Because of the irritant properties, tretinoin should be applied 30 minutes after washing. Initially, it should be applied every other day, then daily. Other irritating substances, such as strong abrasive cleaners and astringents, should be avoided during treatment with tretinoin.

b. **Antibiotics: tetracycline** (Topicycline), **meclocycline sulfosalicylate** (Meclan), **erythromycin** (T-Stat, Eryderm), **clindamycin** (Cleocin-T)

(1) **Mechanism of action.** The mechanism of action apparently involves suppression of the *P. acnes* organism, which in turn minimizes the inflammatory response due to the acne.

(2) **Application.** These antibiotics are applied directly to acne sites, thus minimizing serious side effects from oral administration.

(3) **Side effects.** There are minimal side effects to these topically applied antibiotics. Mild burning or irritation may occur. Tetracycline may discolor the skin and fluoresce in black light. Clindamycin can be absorbed enough to result in pseudomembranous colitis.

2. **Systemic prescription agents**

a. **Isotretinoin** (Accutane) is a vitamin A derivative indicated for severe recalcitrant nodulocystic acne. A single course of therapy can result in a complete and prolonged remission period.

(1) **Mechanism of action.** Although the exact mechanism is unknown, isotretinoin decreases sebum production and keratinization, and it reduces the population of *P. acnes*.

(2) **Dosage.** Doses range from 0.5 mg/kg/day to 2 mg/kg/day given twice daily for 15 to 20 weeks.

(3) **Side effects** include the following.

(a) **Mucocutaneous dryness.** Cheilitis (i.e., inflammation of the lips), dryness of the nasal mucosa, and facial dermatitis may occur with tretinoin use. These effects can be treated with topical lubricants. Dryness of the eye can also occur, so people using isotretinoin should not wear contact lenses.

(b) **Elevated serum levels.** Isotretinoin may elevate serum triglycerides and cholesterol, as well as liver enzymes.

(c) **Birth defects.** Isotretinoin is a potent teratogen and should not be given to pregnant women.

b. **Oral antibiotics** are the most effective against inflammatory lesions, because they suppress *P. acnes*. Oral antibiotics have an onset of action of 3 to 4 weeks.

(1) **Tetracycline** is the most frequently used oral antibiotic for acne.

(a) **Initial doses** are 250 mg, two to four times daily, gradually reduced to a maintenance dose of about 250 mg per day.

(b) **Side effects.** The more common adverse effects include upset stomach, vaginal moniliasis, and photosensitivity.

(2) **Erythromycin** may be used as an alternative to tetracycline.

(a) **Initial doses** range from 500 mg to 2000 mg per day in divided doses. A maintenance dose ranges from 250 mg to 500 mg per day.

(b) **Side effects.** The primary side effect associated with erythromycin is gastrointestinal distress.

(3) **Clindamycin.** Rare cases of pseudomembranous colitis limit the use of clindamycin.

(4) **Minocycline.** Side effects including dizziness or vertigo and headache limit the use of this agent.

c. **Hormones**

(1) **Estrogens** can decrease sebum production through an antiandrogenic effect.

(2) Some **progestin agents** in oral contraceptives (e.g., norethindrone, norgestrel) have androgenic activity that can stimulate sebum secretion. **Norethynodrel** has the least androgenic activity among the available progestins. Therefore, it is favored as an ingredient in combination oral contraceptives used by people affected with or trying to treat acne.

(3) **Spironolactone (Aldactone)** is an androgen antagonist that may be used on a limited basis.

(4) **Prednisone** or its equivalent in doses of 20 mg per day or higher may be used for a short period of time.

III. SUNLIGHT, SUNSCREENS, AND SUNTAN PRODUCTS

A. Introduction. Overexposure to sunlight damages skin. A suntan, which has traditionally been associated with health, is actually a response to injury. Of the three types of solar radiation, only the UV spectrum produces sunburn and suntan.

1. The **UV spectrum** ranges from 200 to 400 nanometers (nm). Natural and artificial UV light is further subdivided into three bands.
   a. **UVA** (320–400 nm) can cause the skin to tan and it tends to be weak in causing the skin to redden.
      (1) **Advantages.** UVA is often used in tanning booths and in psoralen plus UVA (PUVA) treatment of psoriasis.
      (2) **Disadvantages.** UVA is responsible for many photosensitivity reactions, photoaging, and photodermatoses. UVA rays can also penetrate deeply into the dermis and augment the cancerous effects of UVB rays.
   b. **UVB** (290–320 nm) causes the usual sunburn reaction and stimulates tanning. It has long been associated with sunlight skin damage, including the various skin cancers.
   c. **UVC** (200–290 nm) does not reach the earth's surface since most of it is absorbed by the ozone layer. Artificial UVC sources (e.g., germicidal and mercury arc lamps) can emit this radiation.
2. The **visible spectrum** (400–770 nm) produces the brightness of the sun.
3. The **infrared spectrum** (770–1800 nm) produces the warmth of the sun.

B. Sunburn and suntanning

1. **Sunburn** is generally a superficial burn involving the epidermis. This layer is rapidly repaired while old cells are being sloughed off in a process called peeling. The newly formed skin is thicker and offers protection for the lower dermal layers.
   a. **Normal sequence after mild-to-moderate sunlight (UVR) exposure**
      (1) Erythema occurs within 20 to 30 minutes as a result of oxidation of bleached melanin and dilation of dermal venules.
      (2) The initial erythema rapidly fades, and true sunburn erythema begins from 2 to 8 hours after initial exposure to the sun.
      (3) Dilation of the arterioles results in increased vascular permeability, localized edema, and pain, which become maximal after 14 to 20 hours and last 24 to 72 hours.
   b. **Manifestations** range from mild (a slight reddening of the skin) to severe (formation of blisters and desquamation). If the effect is severe, the patient may experience pain, swelling, and blistering. Fever, chills, and nausea may also develop, as well as prostration, which is related to excessive synthesis and diffusion of prostaglandins.
2. **Suntan** is the result of two processes:
   a. **Oxidation of melanin,** which is already present in the epidermis
   b. **Stimulation of melanocytes** to produce additional melanin, which is subsequently oxidized upon further exposure to sunlight
      (1) With increased melanin production, the melanocytes introduce the pigment into keratin-producing cells, which gradually become darkened keratin and a full suntan in 2 to 10 days.
      (2) Tanning increases tolerance to additional sunlight and reduces the likelihood of subsequent burning. However, dark skin is not totally immune to sunburn.

C. Factors affecting exposure to UV radiation (UVR)

1. **Time of day and season.** The greatest exposure to harmful UVB rays occurs between 10 A.M. and 2 P.M. in midsummer. UVA rays are fairly continuous throughout the day and season.
2. **Altitude.** Sunburn is more likely to occur at high altitudes. UVB intensity increases 4% with each 1000-foot increase in altitude.
3. **Environmental factors.** Atmospheric conditions (e.g., smog, haze, smoke) may affect (i.e., decrease) the amount of UVR reaching the skin. Although direct sunlight greatly reduces the amount of UV exposure needed to produce a burn, sunburn can occur without it. For example, a sunburn can also develop on a cloudy day due to the percentage of UVR penetration through cloud layers (60%–80%). However, the **reflection of light rays** (e.g., by snow, sand, and water) greatly **increases** the amount of UV exposure to sunlight.

4. **Predisposing factors.** People with fair skin and light hair are at greater risk for developing sunburn and other UVR skin damage than their darker counterparts (Table 34-1).

D. Other reactions to sunlight (UVR) exposure

1. **Actinic keratosis** is a precancerous condition and may occur after many years of excessive exposure to sunlight. Typically arising during middle age or later, this disorder manifests as a sharply demarcated, roughened, or hardened growth, which may be flat or raised.

2. **Skin cancer.** Chronic overexposure to sunlight may lead to squamous cell carcinoma, basal cell carcinoma, or malignant melanoma. Malignant melanoma is the deadliest form of skin cancer, and its incidence has been increasing. Moles should be watched for indications of malignancy—the ABCDs are **a**symmetrical shape, **b**order irregularity, nonuniform **c**olor, and **d**iameter over 6 mm. Malignant melanoma formation may be associated with intense, intermittent overexposure to the sun (sunburning).

3. **Drug-induced photosensitivity reactions**
   a. **Types**
      (1) **Photoallergenic reactions** occur when light makes a drug become antigenic or act as a hapten (i.e., a photoallergen). These reactions also require previous contact with the offending drug. Photoallergenic reactions are relatively rare and are associated more frequently with topically applied agents than with oral medications.
         (a) **Occurrence** of these reactions is not dose-related: The patient is usually cross-sensitive with chemically related compounds.
         (b) **Rashes** are most prominent on light-exposed sites (i.e., face, neck, forearms, back of hands), and they usually occur, after an incubation period of 24 to 48 hours of combined drug and sun exposure, as discrete papules and plaques.
      (2) **Phototoxic reactions** occur when light alters a drug to a toxic form, which results in tissue damage that is independent of an allergic response.
         (a) **Occurrence.** These reactions are usually dose-related, and the patient usually has no cross-sensitivity to other agents.
         (b) **Rashes** often appear as an exaggerated sunburn and are usually confined to areas of combined chemical and light exposure.
      (3) **Implicated drugs.** Many drugs have been implicated in causing photoallergenic and phototoxic reactions: thiazides, tetracyclines, phenothiazines, sulfonamides, and even sunscreens. Some drugs may produce both types of reactions.
   b. **Prevention.** Standard sunscreens do not always prevent photosensitivity reactions caused by drugs. UV light above 320 nm (i.e., UVA light) has been implicated in inducing photosensitivity reactions, so a chemical or physical sunscreen must cover this spectrum [see III E 2].

4. **Photodermatoses** are skin conditions that are triggered or worsened by light within specific wavelengths. These conditions include polymorphous light eruption (PMLE), lupus erythematosus, and solar urticaria.

5. **Photoaging** is a skin condition that is not merely an acceleration of normal aging. UVA radiation is thought to be involved. The skin appears dry, scaly, yellow, and deeply wrinkled; it is also thinner and more fragile.

Table 34-1. Skin Types and Recommended Sun Protection Factor (SPF)

Skin Color/ Complexion	Skin Type	Susceptibility to Sunburn or Suntan*	Recommended SPF to Avoid Sunburn
Very fair	I	Always burns easily; never tans	15+
Fair	II	Always burns easily; tans minimally	15
Light	III	Burns moderately; tans eventually	10–15
Medium	IV	Burns minimally; always tans well	6–10
Dark	V	Rarely burns; tans readily	4–6
Black	VI	Rarely burns; becomes deeply pigmented	. . .

Reprinted with permission from Gossel TH: The skin and the sun—deadly enemies. *US Pharmacist* (suppl):10–16, June, 1991.

*Based on 45- to 60-minute exposure to midday summer sun without sunscreen protection or previous tan. SPF values relate to exposure to only ultraviolet B (UVB) rays.

E. Sunscreen agents. People can protect their skin from harmful UVR by avoiding exposure to sunlight and other sources of UVR, wearing protective clothing, and applying sunscreen.

1. **Application and general information.** All exposed areas should be covered evenly with sunscreen, optimally 1 to 2 hours before sun exposure.
   a. **Reapplication.** Perspiration, swimming, sand, towels, and clothing tend to remove sunscreen and may increase the need for reapplication.
   b. **Protection.** Sunscreen products vary widely in their ability to protect against sunburn; the sun protection factor (SPF) and UVA/UVB ray protection should be noted to determine the level of protection. Moreover, baby oil, mineral oil, olive oil, and cocoa butter are not sunscreens (but are often used in the process of seeking to attain a tan).
   c. **Sensitivity.** Some people may be hypersensitive to sunscreening agents.

2. The two basic **types of sunscreen agents** are physical sunblocks and chemical sunscreens.
   a. **Physical sunblocks** are opaque formulations that reflect and scatter up to 99% of light in both the UV and visible spectrums (290–700 nm). Examples include titanium dioxide and zinc oxide. These sunblocks are less cosmetically acceptable than chemical sunscreens, since they have a greasy appearance, but they may be useful for protecting small areas (e.g., the nose). These sunblocks are also useful for photosensitization protection. Newer, more dilute versions of titanium dioxide products are more cosmetically appealing. Red petrolatum covers a lesser spectrum (290–365 nm).
   b. **Chemical sunscreens** act by absorbing a specific portion of the UV light spectrum to keep it from penetrating the skin. They can be categorized on the basis of their spectra of UVR blockage and basic chemical classification. Five main groups of chemical sunscreens are available.
      (1) **PABA and PABA esters** primarily absorb UVB rays. Examples are *p*-aminobenzoic acid, padimate O, and glyceryl PABA.
      (2) **Cinnamates** primarily absorb UVB rays. Examples are cinoxate and octyl methoxycinnamate.
      (3) **Salicylates** primarily absorb UVB rays. Examples are ethylhexyl salicylate and homosalate.
      (4) **Benzophenones** absorb UVB rays and sometimes extend into the UVA range. Examples are oxybenzone and dioxybenzone. Because of their extension into the UVA range, they are somewhat protective against photosensitivity reactions.
      (5) **Miscellaneous.** The newest agent, butylmethoxydibenzoylmethane (Parsol 1789) provides coverage over the entire UVA range. In combination with padimate O, this agent offers protection in both the UVA and UVB ranges.
   c. **OTC sunscreen products.** Most sunscreen products on the market contain combinations of two or more of the classes of chemical sunscreen agents noted in the preceding paragraphs.

3. **SPF** gives the consumer a guide for determining how the product will protect the skin from UV rays, principally UVB rays.
   a. **Derivation.** SPF is defined as the minimal erythema dose (MED) of protected skin divided by the MED of unprotected skin. MED is the amount of solar radiation needed to produce minimal skin redness.
   b. **Example.** A person who usually gets red after 20 minutes in the sun and wants to stay in the sun for 2 hours (120 minutes) should apply a sunscreen with an SPF of 6 (120 minutes divided by 20 minutes = SPF 6). An SPF 6 product should provide adequate coverage provided it is not washed off (as from swimming) or dissolved by sweat. An SPF of 15 blocks 93% of the UVB rays. Although some products are marketed with SPFs higher than 15, little additional benefit is achieved.

4. **Phototoxic protection factor (PPF).** Because there is now evidence that both UVB and UVA radiation are involved in the development of skin cancer, attention has been given to the PPF. As previously stated, the SPF measures UVB protection. The PPF measures UVA protection.
   a. **Derivation.** PPF equals the minimal phototoxic dose (MPD) on protected skin divided by the MPD on unprotected skin. The MPD is the minimal phototoxic dose of UVA radiation that induces a uniform phototoxic reaction (i.e., in combination with a phototoxic drug).
   b. **Alternate term.** Some manufacturers of products that protect against UVA radiation use the term APP, which stands for UVA protection percent.

F. Special agents of interest

1. **Dihydroxyacetone (DHA)** is a chemical agent that darkens the skin by interacting with keratin in the stratum corneum to produce an artificial suntan. It provides no protection against UV rays and may not produce a natural-looking tan. DHA must be applied evenly. If an artificial suntan is achieved with this chemical, it wears off in a few days. In addition, it can discolor hair and clothing.
2. **Beta-carotene,** a vitamin A precursor, may produce skin coloration when ingested orally. While beta-carotene is protective against some forms of abnormal photosensitivity (e.g., erythropoietic protoporphyria), it has not been shown to protect against sunburn in normal individuals.
3. **Canthaxanthine** is a carotenoid (provitamin A). It has been used as a food coloring agent but has not been approved by the FDA for use as an oral tanning agent. It does not produce a true suntan, but is deposited into fatty tissues under the skin. It probably does not protect the skin from sunburn.
4. **Tyrosine** has been promoted as a tan accelerator or tan magnifier. Because melanin pigment is eventually synthesized from tyrosine, the theory is that topically applied tyrosine will enhance the formation of melanin. However, studies have not confirmed an enhanced tanning effect from this agent.

IV. CONTACT DERMATITIS AND ITS TREATMENT

A. Introduction

1. **Types of contact dermatitis.** Contact dermatitis is one of the most common dermatologic conditions encountered in clinical practice. It has traditionally been divided into **irritant contact dermatitis** and **allergic contact dermatitis** on the basis of the etiology and immunologic mechanism.
   a. **Irritant contact dermatitis** is caused by direct contact with a primary irritant. These irritants can be classified as absolute or relative primary irritants.
      (1) **Absolute primary irritants** are intrinsically damaging substances that injure, on first contact, any person's skin. Examples include strong acids, alkalis, and other industrial chemicals.
      (2) **Relative primary irritants** cause most cases of contact dermatitis seen in clinical practice. These irritants are less toxic than absolute primary irritants, and they require repeated or prolonged exposure to provoke a reaction. Examples of relative primary irritants include soaps, detergents, benzoyl peroxide, and certain plant and animal substances.
   b. **Allergic contact dermatitis.** Many plants, and almost any chemical, can cause allergic contact dermatitis. Poison ivy is a classic example of allergic contact dermatitis, which is classified as a type IV hypersensitivity reaction. This type of allergic reaction is T-cell–mediated, and the following **sequence of events** must occur to provoke it.
      (1) The epidermis must come in **contact** with the hapten (i.e., the specific allergen).
      (2) The **hapten–epidermal protein complex** (i.e., the complete antigen) must form.
      (3) The antigen must **enter the lymphatic system**.
      (4) **Immunologically competent lymphoid cells,** which are selective against the antigen, must form.
      (5) On **reexposure** to the hapten, the typical, local delayed hypersensitivity reaction (i.e., contact dermatitis) occurs.
      (6) The **induction period,** during which sensitivity develops, usually requires 14–21 days but may take as few as 4 days or more than several weeks. **Once sensitivity is fully developed:**
         (a) Reexposure to even minute amounts of the same material elicits an eczematous response, typically with an onset of 12 hours and a peak of 48–72 hours after exposure.
         (b) Sensitivity usually persists for life.
            (i) Most contact allergens produce sensitization in only a small percentage of exposed persons.
            (ii) Allergens or substances such as poison ivy, however, produce sensitization in more than 70% of the population.

2. **General phases of contact dermatitis**
   a. **Acute stage.** "Wet" lesions, such as blisters or denuded and weeping skin, are evident in well-outlined patches. Also evident are erythema, edema, vesicles, and oozing.
   b. **Subacute stage.** In this phase, crusts or "scabs" form over the previously wet lesions. Allergic contact dermatitis and irritant contact dermatitis caused by absolute primary irritants produce both the acute and subacute stages.
   c. **Chronic stage.** In this phase, the lesions become dry and thickened (i.e., lichenified). Initially, dryness and fissuring are the signs. Later, erythema, lichenification, and excoriations appear. The chronic phase of contact dermatitis usually occurs more often with irritant contact dermatitis caused by relative primary irritants.

B. **Toxic plants.** Poison ivy and poison oak are the most common causes of allergic contact dermatitis in North America. These plants were formerly known as the *Rhus* genus, but they are now properly referred to as the *Toxicodendron* genus.

1. **Poison ivy** (*Toxicodendron radicans*) may grow as a vine or as a bush. It is found in most parts of the United States, but is especially prevalent in the northeastern part of the country. Poison ivy is often identified by its characteristic growth pattern, described by the saying, "Leaves of three, let it be."

2. **Poison oak** (*T. diversilobum*) is found in the western United States and Canada. It grows as an upright shrub or a woody vine. *T. quercifolium* is found in the eastern United States.

3. **Poison sumac** (*T. vernix*) grows in woody or swampy areas as a coarse shrub or tree and is prevalent in the eastern United States and southeastern Canada.

C. **Toxicodendron dermatitis.** In order for dermatitis to develop, previous sensitization (a 5- to 21-day incubation period) caused by direct contact with a sensitizing agent is required (see IV A 1 b). An oleoresin, **urushiol oil,** which is a pentadecacatechol, is the active sensitizing agent in poison ivy, poison oak, and poison sumac.

1. **Release of the urushiol oil.** The plants must be bruised or injured to release the oleoresin. The urushiol oil may remain active on tools, toys, clothes, and pets, and under fingernails if those items have had contact with the broken plants.
   a. Urushiol oil does not volatilize, so one cannot get dermatitis from just being near a poison ivy plant—direct contact is necessary. **Burning plants,** however, can cause droplets of oil carried by smoke to enter the respiratory system, which can cause significant respiratory distress.
   b. A cut or damaged poison ivy, poison oak, or poison sumac plant yields a milky sap containing the oleoresin, which turns black within a few minutes. This change can be a means for confirming identification of these plants.
   c. Because the oleoresin can rapidly penetrate the skin, the affected area must be washed with soap and water within 10–15 minutes after exposure to prevent the dermatitis eruption.
2. If an individual has been **previously sensitized,** the lesions usually occur within 6–48 hours after contact with the allergen. If the patient becomes initially sensitized as a result of this contact, the lesions may not appear for 9–14 days.

3. Typically, the **initial eruption** exists as small patches of erythematous papules (usually streaks). Pruritus (itching) is the primary symptom.
   a. Papules may progress to vesicles, which may then ooze and bleed when they are scratched. Secondary infection may then develop. Often, the inflammation is severe, and a significant amount of edema occurs over the exposed area.
   b. The lesions may last from a few days to several weeks. Left untreated, the condition rarely persists longer than 2–3 weeks.

4. **Poison ivy dermatitis does not spread.** New lesions, however, may continue to appear for several days despite lack of further contact with the plant. This reaction may be due to the following facts.
   a. Skin that has been minimally exposed to the antigen begins to react only as the person's sensitivity heightens.
   b. Antigen is absorbed at varying rates through the skin of different parts of the body.
   c. The person inadvertently touches contaminated objects or may have residual oleoresin underneath the fingernails, for instance.

5. **Poison ivy is not contagious.** The serous fluid from the weeping vesicles are not antigenic. No one can "catch" poison ivy from another person.

D. Treatment. The treatment of irritant and allergic contact dermatitis focuses on therapy for the specific symptomatology.

1. A pharmacist should **refer a patient** with a poison ivy eruption to a physician if:
   a. The eruption involves more than 15% of the body
   b. The eruption involves the eyes, genital area, mouth, or respiratory tract (some patients may experience respiratory difficulties if they inhale the smoke of burning poison ivy plants)
2. The **severity of the eruption** depends on:
   a. The quantity of allergen that the patient has been exposed to
   b. The individual patient's sensitivity to the allergen
3. **For severe eruptions,** a patient should consult a physician, who may prescribe **systemic corticosteroids**.
   a. Systemic corticosteroids are the cornerstone of therapy. One should use sufficiently high doses to suppress this inflammation. Generally, it is recommended that prednisone be given in the dose of 60 mg/day for 5 days, then reduced to 40 mg/day for 5 days, then 20 mg/day for 5 days, then discontinued.
   b. Some blisters may be drained at their base. The skin on top of the blister should be kept intact. Draining the blister allows more topical medication to penetrate for an antipruritic effect. Baths and soaks (see IV D 4 b 1 (b)) may be beneficial as well.
4. **For a less severe eruption,** the principal goals are to relieve the itching and inflammation and to protect the integrity of skin.
   a. Several therapeutic classes of agents can be used **to relieve itching.**
      (1) The application of **local anesthetics** [e.g., benzocaine (5%–20%)] may relieve itching. Relief may be of short duration (30–45 minutes), but application of benzocaine may be especially useful at bedtime, when pruritus is most bothersome. There is some question about the frequency of the sensitizing ability of benzocaine (0.17%–5%). Certainly, treatment should be discontinued if the rash worsens.
      (2) **Oral antihistamines** may be helpful in alleviating pruritus mainly due to their sedating effect rather than a specific antipruritic effect. The principal concern with these agents involves the effect of CNS depression (drowsiness) and possible anticholinergic effects.
      (3) **Topical antihistamines** (e.g., diphenhydramine) provide relief of mild itching principally through a topical anesthetic effect rather than any antihistamine effect. The main concern with topical antihistamines is that they may also have a significant sensitizing potential.
      (4) **Counterirritants** include camphor (0.1%–3%), phenol (0.5%–1.5%), and menthol (0.1%–1%). These agents have an analgesic effect due to depression of cutaneous receptors. The exact antipruritic mechanism is not fully known, but a placebo effect may result from the characteristic "medicinal" odors of these agents.
      (5) **Astringents** are mild protein precipitants that result in contraction of tissue, which in turn decreases the local edema and inflammation.
         (a) The principal agent used is **aluminum acetate** (Burow's solution).
         (b) **Calamine** (zinc oxide with ferric oxide) is also used sometimes. Calamine contracts tissue and helps dry the area, but the formation of the thick dried paste may not be acceptable to some people.
      (6) **Topical hydrocortisone,** which is available in concentrations up to 1%, is useful for its antipruritic and anti-inflammatory effects. The antipruritic effect, however, may not be seen for 1–2 days.
   b. **Basic treatment**
      (1) **Acute (weeping) lesions** (see IV A 2 a)
         (a) **Wet dressings** work on the principle that water evaporating from the skin cools it and, thus, relieves itching. Wet dressings have an additional benefit of causing gentle debridement and cleansing of the skin.
         (b) **Burow's solution** in concentrations of 1:20–1:40 as a wet dressing or a cool bath of 15–30 minutes, three to six times per day provides a significant antipruritic effect.
         (c) **Colloidal oatmeal baths** may also provide an antipruritic effect.

(d) **Topical therapy that may hinder treatment**

(i) **Local anesthetics and topical antihistamines** may sensitize

(ii) **Alcohol** and **calamine** may irritate

(2) **Subacute dermatitis** (see IV A 2 b). A thin layer of hydrocortisone cream or lotion (0.5%–1%) may be applied three or four times a day to treat subacute dermatitis. Supplemental agents, such as oral antihistamines or topical anesthetics, may be used as well.

(3) **Chronic dermatitis** (see IV A 2 c) is best treated with hydrocortisone ointment. This stage is observed more frequently in forms of contact dermatitis that involve continuous exposure to the irritant or allergen.

E. Prevention

1. The best treatment for poison ivy contact dermatitis is to **prevent contact** with the offending cause. This approach involves avoiding the plant and wearing protective clothing.
2. **Barrier preparations.** Linoleic acid dimers (e.g., Stoko Gard) and organic clays have been used, with limited success, to prevent urushiol from binding to the dermis.
3. **Hyposensitization** using plant extracts of poison ivy has had mixed success. Maximal hyposensitization requires 3 to 6 months to develop, and it diminishes rapidly when administration of the extracts ceases.

STUDY QUESTIONS

Directions: Each of the numbered items or incomplete statements in this section is followed by answers or by completions of the statement. Select the **one** lettered answer or completion that is **best** in each case.

1. A woman, who has not been in the sun for 4 months, develops redness on her chest after lying in the sun for 20 minutes. The next day, she applies a suntan lotion and develops the same degree of redness on her back in 2 hours and 20 minutes. What is the sun protection factor (SPF) of the lotion she is using?

(A) 14
(B) 10
(C) 12
(D) 9
(E) 7

2. Which of the following cleansing products would a pharmacist recommend for a patient with inflammatory acne?

(A) An abrasive facial sponge and soap used four times daily
(B) Aluminum oxide particles used twice daily
(C) Sulfur 5% soap used twice daily
(D) Mild facial soap used twice daily

3. If a patient needs a second application of an OTC pediculicide shampoo, how many days after the eggs hatch should she wait to apply the product?

(A) 4–5
(B) 6
(C) 7–10
(D) 14–21
(E) 15–17

4. All of the following treatments for personal articles infested with head lice would be effective EXCEPT

(A) placing woolen hats in a plastic bag for 35 days
(B) using an aerosol of pyrethrins with piperonyl butoxide to spray all bathrooms
(C) machine-washing clothes in hot water and drying them using the hot setting on the dryer
(D) dry-cleaning woolen scarves
(E) soaking hair brushes in hot water for 5 to 10 minutes

5. All of the following sunscreen agents or combinations of agents help prevent a drug-induced photosensitivity reaction EXCEPT

(A) titanium dioxide
(B) glyceryl *p*-aminobenzoic acid (PABA) plus homosalate
(C) oxybenzone and padimate O
(D) zinc oxide
(E) padimate O plus butylmethoxydibenzoylmethane

6. All of the following would be appropriate recommendations for a patient in the acute stage (i.e., blistering, weeping) of poison ivy contact dermatitis EXCEPT

(A) two 25-mg capsules of diphenhydramine at night for itching
(B) 60 mg per day of prednisone initially, then tapered over 15 days
(C) Burow's solution; 1:20 wet dressing to area for 15 to 30 minutes, four times per day
(D) two soaks per day in Aveeno® Bath Treatment
(E) two applications of Stoko Gard®

7. All of the following nonprescription agents have been classified by the Food and Drug Administration (FDA) as safe and effective (Category I) for acne EXCEPT

(A) sulfur
(B) salicylic acid
(C) sulfur–resorcinol combination
(D) benzoic acid

8. Pharmacists educating patients about acne should mention all of the following EXCEPT

(A) eliminating all chocolate and fried foods from the diet
(B) cleansing skin gently two to three times daily
(C) using water-based noncomedogenic cosmetics
(D) not squeezing acne lesions
(E) keeping in mind that acne usually resolves by one's early twenties

---

1-E	4-B	7-D
2-D	5-B	8-A
3-C	6-E	

9. A 15-year-old male patient has been using benzoyl peroxide 5% cream faithfully every day for the past 2 months with no apparent side effects. All of the following can be said about this patient EXCEPT

(A) he has been using this product for a long enough time to determine if the dose and dosage form are going to have any benefit
(B) he should use this product no more frequently than every other day because of its irritating properties
(C) this starting dose and dosage form are useful, especially if he has dry skin or it is wintertime
(D) his scalp hair may look bleached if the product comes in contact with it
(E) the product would sting if it got into his eyes

10. All of the following descriptions match the therapeutic agent for poison ivy EXCEPT

(A) calamine—phenolphthalein gives it the pink color
(B) Stoko Gard—it contains linoleic acid dimer and has some effect in preventing poison ivy dermatitis
(C) benzocaine—data regarding incidence of hypersensitivity are conflicting
(D) hydrocortisone—it may take 1 to 2 days for an antipruritic effect

11. All of the following statements about sun protection factor (SPF) are true EXCEPT

(A) the sun's intensity increases 20% when going from sea level to an altitude of 5000 feet
(B) a patient with skin type I or II should use a product with an SPF of 15 or higher
(C) baby oil is not a sunscreen, but its application to the skin after tanning causes melanin to rise to the surface
(D) products now have SPFs greater than 20, but 15 is probably the highest SPF necessary
(E) the SPF is really only a measure of ultraviolet B (UVB) protection

12. All of the following statements about sunscreens are true EXCEPT

(A) malignant melanoma formation may be associated with intense, intermittent overexposure to the sun (sunburning)
(B) dihydroxyacetone (DHA) will not prevent sunburn
(C) canthaxanthine provides only minimal protection against sunburn in normal patients
(D) *p*-aminobenzoic acid (PABA) is best applied within 10 minutes before sun exposure
(E) tyrosine has been marketed as a tan accelerator

9-B
10-A
11-C
12-D

ANSWERS AND EXPLANATIONS

1. The answer is E *[III E 3].*
The sun protection factor (SPF) is the minimal erythema dose (MED) of protected skin divided by the MED of unprotected skin. Thus, 2 hours and 20 minutes (140 minutes) divided by 20 minutes equals an SPF of 7.

2. The answer is D *[II E 2 c, e].*
For patients with inflammatory acne, the best product is a mild facial soap used twice daily. The soap should be gently rubbed into the skin with only the fingertips. Cleansing products that irritate already inflamed skin should be avoided.

3. The answer is C *[I G 4 a (1)].*
Reapplication of pyrethrins with piperonyl butoxide should be within 7 to 10 days of the first application. Any lice nits that were not killed on the first application would have time to hatch and then be killed with the second application.

4. The answer is B *[I G 4 a, 6 c].*
Pyrethrins with piperonyl butoxide in an aerosol form can be sprayed directly on inanimate objects (e.g., chairs, headrests) to kill head lice, but the combination should not be sprayed in the air like an aerosol deodorizer. Moreover, vacuuming the furniture would probably be as effective as spraying it. The other selections are appropriate for personal articles infested with head lice.

5. The answer is B *[III E 2 b (1)].*
Glyceryl *p*-aminobenzoic acid (PABA) and homosalate protect against only ultraviolet B (UVB) exposure. Because photosensitivity reactions are often associated with UVA radiation exposure, people also need sunscreen protection for this portion of the UV radiation band. The other agents listed cover at least part of both UVA and UVB spectra.

6. The answer is E *[IV D 4 b].*
Stoko Gard is used as a barrier protectant for the prevention of poison ivy dermatitis, not for the treatment of an acute eruption. The other options are appropriate to recommend to someone suffering from the acute stage of poison ivy dermatitis.

7. The answer is D *[II E 4].*
Benzoic acid has not been shown to be effective for acne treatment, so it has been placed in Category III. The other agents—sulfur, salicylic acid, and a sulfur–resorcinol combination—are all safe and effective products for treating acne.

8. The answer is A *[II E].*
Evidence does not show that acne worsens from any particular type of food, including chocolate or fried foods. The other choices are pieces of information that the pharmacist should convey to a patient with acne.

9. The answer is B *[II E 4 a].*
Although the irritating properties of benzoyl peroxide would indicate applying it only every other day upon initiating treatment, this patient has tolerated the agent on a daily basis for 2 months. Thus, there would be no need to decrease the application frequency. All of the other choices do apply to this patient's use of benzoyl peroxide.

10. The answer is A *[IV D 4].*
Ferric oxide provides the pink color of calamine. All of the other descriptions match their associated agents.

11. The answer is C *[III C 2, E 1 b, c; 2 b; 3; Table 34-1].*
Baby oil is not a sunscreen, and it has no effect on melanin. SPF does measure ultraviolet B (UVB) protection, and an SPF higher than 15 is probably not necessary. People with skin type I or II (that is, very fair or fair) should use a product with an SPF of 15. The intensity of the sun does increase by 4% with each 1000 ft. elevation.

12. The answer is D *[III D 2, E 1, 2 b (1); F 1, 3, 4].*
Optimally, sunscreens should be applied 1 to 2 hours before exposure to the sun. This allows time for the product to bind to the stratum corneum, which provides better protection.

35

OTC Products: Weight Control and Sleep Aids

Larry N. Swanson

I. WEIGHT CONTROL

A. Obesity

1. **Definition.** Obesity is defined as surplus body fat that results in a weight that exceeds a person's ideal body weight by more than 20%.
2. **Statistics**
   a. Obesity afflicts more people in the United States than does any disease. As much as one-third of the United States population over the age of 30 may be obese.
   b. Yearly, over $10 billion is spent on the treatment of obesity, yet less is known about its cause than is known about the cause of almost any other medical condition.
   c. The medical management of obesity is almost universally unsuccessful. An estimated 90% of all patients who lose more than 25 pounds in a diet program regain that weight within 3 years.
3. **Cause of obesity.** Although many hypotheses, theories, and proposed mechanisms have been discussed, no uniform cause of obesity has been determined. Patients may become obese because they consistently ingest more calories than their body is able to metabolize. Observations about the cause of obesity include the following.
   a. Patients may have an **elevated body weight set point**. When these patients lose weight, compensatory adjustments in metabolism result in their regaining the weight, even with a decreased caloric intake.
   b. **Heredity** is accepted as an important factor in the etiology of obesity. Studies of identical twins raised apart show that each twin's weight does not vary significantly, which indicates that genetics has a more important role than environmental factors in determining obesity.
   c. Obese patients may be **more responsive to external food cues** (e.g., taste, smell, sight of food).
   d. Obese patients may have higher levels of **lipoprotein lipase,** an enzyme produced by adipose cells to help store calories as fat.
4. **Medical consequences.** Numerous studies have shown that a significant number of patients with hypertension, non–insulin-dependent diabetes mellitus, and osteoarthritis can significantly control their conditions through weight loss. People who are 20% or more over their ideal body weight are more likely to suffer from the following diseases or disorders:
   a. Amenorrhea
   b. Cancer of the cervix, colon, endometrium, gallbladder, prostate, and uterus
   c. Congestive heart failure
   d. Coronary heart disease
   e. Diabetes mellitus
   f. Fatty liver
   g. Gallbladder disease
   h. Hirsutism
   i. Hypertension
   j. Hypertriglyceridemia
   k. Respiratory tract infections and other problems
   l. Varicose veins
5. **Types of obesity**
   a. Overweight people with large abdomens are generally in worse health than equally obese people who have fat distributed around their hips and limbs.

b. Waist measurement to hip measurement ratios of greater than 0.95 for men and 0.80 for women are associated with higher death rates.

B. **Management of obesity.** Weight reduction involves an integrated program of diet, correct eating habits, exercise, patient follow-up, and, sometimes, medication. An approximate **weight loss goal** should be set when the patient and physician are establishing ideal body weight. Realistic goals about the frequency of weight loss should be established.

1. A weight loss goal of 1 to 2 pounds per week is appropriate.

2. To lose 1 pound in a week, a person must expend 3500 calories through physical work or decrease caloric intake by 3500 calories during that week.

3. For example, a patient who normally consumes 3000 calories per day must decrease that intake by 500 calories per day in order to lose 1 pound in 1 week (500×7 days = 3500 calories).

C. **Diets** are specific eating plans that provide a certain number of calories per day.

1. **Balanced diets** with calories derived from protein, carbohydrate, and fat are optimal. The caloric intake of fat should be minimized (i.e., < 30% of total calories, < 10% saturated fat) for general health reasons (e.g., incidence of ischemic heart disease and certain types of cancer). Also, fat contains 9 calories per gram; carbohydrate or protein contains 4 calories per gram. Recent evidence suggests that the proportion of fat in the diet may be more important than the total daily caloric intake.

2. **Fad diets** do not teach patients how to eat properly for long-range benefits. Weight maintenance is the key.

3. **Very low-calorie diets,** which provide 300 to 800 calories per day, may be useful in severely obese patients under strict medical supervision.
   a. Adequate protein must be present in these diets in order to preserve lean body mass.
   b. Patients must be monitored carefully for electrolyte imbalances, postural hypotension, and electrocardiogram (ECG) abnormalities.
   c. **Formula diets**
      (1) The **"Last Chance Diet,"** a liquid protein diet marketed over the counter in the mid-1970s, resulted in several deaths from cardiovascular problems, which were probably caused by a negative nitrogen balance due to the poor-quality protein in these products.
      (2) **Optifast, Medifast, and Health Management Resources (HMR)** are available through physicians or hospitals as part of a packaged weight-reduction program (approximately 400 to 800 calories per day) that uses high-quality (i.e., milk or egg, not vegetable) protein and variable proportions of carbohydrate and fat. These products appear to be safe, but maintenance of weight loss over the long term is still the main issue.
      (3) **Slimfast and Ultra Slimfast** are high-quality protein, over-the-counter (OTC) variations to formula diets. The consumer is instructed to mix the formula with milk (approximately 200 calories) and use it to replace one or two meals. For the third meal, the patient eats regular food.

D. **Eating habits.** Patients need to be trained in gaining self-control of their eating behavior if they are planning to lose weight and maintain the weight loss.

1. **Behavior modification programs,** which seek to eliminate improper eating behaviors (e.g., eating while watching television, eating too rapidly, eating when not hungry), may be beneficial.

2. **Self-help groups** (e.g., Weight Watchers, Nutri-System, Jenny Craig) use a program of diet, education, and positive emotional support to help patients lose weight.

E. **Exercise.** Because 3500 calories of work must be expended to lose 1 pound, exercise is clearly a difficult way to lose weight. However, an effective weight loss program incorporates exercise.

1. **Benefits of exercise**
   a. Exercise burns calories [e.g., walking (2 mph) burns 200 calories per hour; running (5.3 mph) burns 570 calories per hour].
   b. Exercise raises body metabolism, which can have an extended effect on weight loss.
   c. Exercise may decrease appetite.
   d. Patients usually feel better (mentally and emotionally) when they exercise regularly.
   e. Exercise helps to prevent the loss of muscle mass.

2. **Effective exercise expends energy.** Vibrating belts, continuous passive motion machines, and similar products do not result in increased weight loss because those using them are not expending energy.

F. Prescription weight loss products

1. **Amphetamines and related agents** have been prescribed for obesity for years.
   a. **Indication.** These drugs may be justified for someone who has lost weight on a diet and then reaches a plateau or, more rarely, for someone who is beginning a diet. These agents traditionally have been used for short-term therapy (8 to 12 weeks), and their use results in small, but statistically significant weight loss.
   b. The **mechanism of action** apparently involves suppression of the satiety center in the hypothalamic ventromedial nucleus. Other mechanisms may be involved as well.
   c. **Side effects.** In addition to the tolerance that develops to these drugs, there are the potentials for abuse and drug dependence, as well as other side effects.
   d. **Recent data.** A recent 4-year study that used two of these agents, **phentermine and fenfluramine,** concluded that prescription appetite suppressants can enable people to lose weight and keep it off. This study suggests that obesity should be viewed and treated like other chronic diseases, such as hypertension and arthritis.
2. **Other prescription products** that have been used for the treatment of obesity include thyroid hormone and human chorionic gonadotropin (hCG). However, these products have not proven to be effective in weight-loss treatment.

G. OTC weight-loss products

1. **Benzocaine and phenylpropanolamine (PPA)** are two OTC agents that have been considered Category I for weight control. However, considerable controversy has developed about the true effectiveness of these agents.
   a. **Benzocaine** appears to act topically on nerve endings in the oral cavity to decrease the ability to detect different degrees of sweetness. Through this numbing effect, the desire for food may be decreased in some people.
      (1) The **dosage form** must be a substance that remains in the mouth for an extended period of time, such as gum, a lozenge, or candy.
      (2) The **dose** is 3 to 15 mg just prior to food consumption.
      (3) The principal **adverse** effect with this medication is hypersensitivity.
      (4) **Examples** of products that contain benzocaine in this form include Ayds and Slim-Line.
   b. **PPA,** which is the active ingredient in Dexatrim, Accutrim, and Prolamine, is a sympathomimetic agent that is chemically related to amphetamines. It appears to have an appetite-suppressing effect similar to that of the amphetamines and amphetamine-related agents found in prescription medications for obesity.
      (1) **Dose and dosage form.** The approved dose is 37.5 mg in an immediate-releasing dosage form, which should be taken about 30 minutes before a meal. The approved dose for the sustained-release form is 75 mg, which is the maximum daily dose.
      (2) **Safety.** Because of its sympathomimetic properties, PPA should be used cautiously by patients with heart disease, hypertension, diabetes, and hyperthyroidism. When used in therapeutic doses, PPA has only minimal cardiovascular effects.
         (a) **Central nervous system (CNS) stimulation** may be a problem, producing such symptoms as insomnia, nervousness, and headache.
         (b) **Drug interactions.** Patients should exercise caution when using other OTC products containing PPA (e.g., cold and allergic rhinitis medications). PPA can antagonize the effects of antihypertensive agents through various mechanisms. Concurrent use of PPA and other sympathomimetic agents can also result in additive CNS and cardiovascular effects.
         (c) **Efficacy.** PPA-containing products show minimal efficacy, but modest weight loss is achieved. For example, in a 4-week, double-blind study, a group treated with PPA (combined with caffeine) had an average weight loss of 5.5 pounds versus 4 pounds in the placebo group. The OTC panel that originally reviewed these agents stated that each of the double-blind, placebo-controlled studies available at the time were defective in one way or another.
2. **Additional agents.** A number of other OTC agents have been proposed for the treatment of obesity, but support for their effectiveness is weak. For example, the bulk-producing laxatives

have been proposed to create a feeling of fullness in the stomach. However, x-ray studies have shown that the bulk leaves the stomach within 30 minutes.

II. SLEEP AIDS

A. Normal sleep and sleep requirements

1. **Length of sleep.** Sleep time and quality of sleep vary widely among individuals. The usual range of sleep time per night is 5 to 10 hours, with an average of about 7½ hours.
2. **Sleep requirements** change as a person ages. Newborns may sleep up to 18 hours. Preteens usually fall asleep within 5 or 10 minutes, sleep for 9½ hours, and spend 95% of their time in bed in solid, continuous, deep sleep. By adulthood, 7 or 8 hours usually provide adequate rest. In old age, 6 hours may suffice.
3. **Polysomnography** uses electroencephalogram (EEG), electro-oculogram (EOG), and electromyogram (EMG) recordings to note changes that occur during sleep.
   a. **Stages of sleep.** Using polysomnography, researchers have discovered five stages of sleep.
      (1) **One rapid eye movement (REM) stage** occupies about 25% of normal total sleep time.
      (2) **Four non–rapid eye movement (NREM) stages** make up the remaining 75% of normal total sleep time. Stages three and four of NREM sleep are considered to be the deepest sleep and are often referred to collectively as **delta sleep** or **restorative sleep**.
   b. Most **dreaming** occurs during the REM stage of sleep, and the degree of "restfulness" of sleep is associated with the amount of REM sleep.
   c. Most of the **medications** used to treat insomnia, including the OTC agents, interfere with some component of the sleep stages, especially the REM sleep.

B. Insomnia

1. **Definition.** Insomnia is an interruption of the natural sleep cycle that results in impaired daytime performance. Insomnia must be defined not only in terms of the amount of sleep but also with attention to the perceived quality of sleep.
2. **Diagnosis of insomnia.** Daytime performance deficits, not the number of hours slept, should be the primary determinant of an insomnia diagnosis.
   a. An occasional night of inadequate or no sleep is of little concern in healthy individuals. Apart from **extreme sleepiness** and the occurrence of **"microsleeps,"** remarkably little **pathology** is associated with extended sleeplessness.
   b. As long as patients awake each morning feeling fully refreshed and do not need an afternoon nap, they should be reassured that they do not have insomnia and that the full 8-hour sleep pattern at night is not absolutely necessary. Oftentimes, simple **reassurance** may be all that is needed to **"cure"** insomnia.
3. **Categories of insomnia.** Insomnias can generally be divided into three categories.
   a. **Transient insomnia,** which accounts for approximately 15% of insomnia cases, generally lasts less than 7 days. Causes of transient insomnia include **jet lag, shift work, or acute anxiety**.
   b. **Short-term insomnia** lasts from 1 to 3 weeks. Causes of short-term insomnia include usually identifiable, often self-limiting problems, such as **grief, pain, noise, or an anxiety-provoking situation**.
   c. **Long-term insomnia** (or chronic insomnia) lasts longer than 3 weeks, indicates an underlying pathology, and requires a thorough assessment of the patient's physical and emotional health. Long-term insomnia may stem from an underlying medical condition such as **hyperthyroidism or arthritis**. Often, treatment strategies that relieve the underlying physical disorder resolve the insomnia complaint.
4. **Causes of insomnia.** Patients who experience insomnia may have different causes for this condition.
   a. **Intrinsic sleep disorders**
      (1) **Psychophysiologic insomnia** is a conditioned form of sleep loss in which the patient associates increased wakefulness with the bedroom and the bedtime routine.
      (2) **Restless leg syndrome** is characterized by extremely uncomfortable sensations in leg muscles at rest, which are relieved only by getting up and moving around.

(3) **Sleep apnea** can be obstructive or centrally mediated. The hallmark is breathing that stops for short periods during sleep. Patients with sleep apnea should not use hypnotic or OTC sleep aids.
(4) **Sleep-related myoclonus** is the periodic, rhythmic curling or jumping of the feet during sleep.

b. Extrinsic sleep disorders
(1) **Adjustment sleep disorder** is prompted by a stressful life change.
(2) **Inadequate sleep hygiene** is caused by a lifestyle that reduces the amount of quality sleep.
(3) **Hypnotic-, stimulant-, or alcohol-dependent** sleep disorder is caused by dependence, tolerance, or overreliance on a given agent.

c. Circadian sleep disorders
(1) **Delayed sleep phase syndrome** occurs in people whose natural sleep times are altered due to work. For instance, a person who must be at work at 8 A.M., but naturally gets tired after 2 A.M. and wakes after 10 A.M., would be affected by this type of disorder.
(2) **Jet lag** is primarily a problem for people who travel across several time zones.

d. Psychiatric disorders, such as **major depressive disorder,** result in poor sleep that usually improves with specific antidepressant medication.

5. Treatment of insomnia is highly dependent on the type of insomnia. It is very important to distinguish among transient insomnia, short-term insomnia, and long-term insomnia (see II B 3).

a. Nondrug intervention and sleep-hygiene measures include the following lifestyle and environmental recommendations:
(1) Establishing a regular bedtime
(2) Going to bed when tired and ready to sleep
(3) If unable to sleep, getting out of bed
(4) Shortly before bedtime, engaging in a relaxing activity, such as taking a warm bath, eating a light snack, or doing relaxation exercises
(5) Avoiding strenuous exercise or other stimulating activity for several hours before bedtime
(6) Avoiding alcohol, since it may produce fragmented sleep
(7) Making sure that the bedroom and the bed are comfortable for sleeping
(8) Avoiding stimulants (e.g., caffeine, nicotine, PPA, pseudoephedrine) late in the day
(9) Avoiding naps during the day

b. Treatment of transient and short-term insomnia
(1) The **goal of therapy** for transient and short-term insomnia is:
(a) Restoring daytime functioning
(b) Avoiding the self-reinforcing pattern that may develop into chronic insomnia.
(2) **Prescription hypnotic agents** are reserved primarily for this type of insomnia. Sedative hypnotic agents should be used only as part of a plan that makes use of good sleep-hygiene techniques.
(a) **Benzodiazepines** are considered to be the drugs of choice for symptomatic relief of insomnia, and they are the closest to an ideal hypnotic sleep aid.
(i) **Selection of a benzodiazepine** is based on the specific pharmacokinetic profile that matches the particular sleep problem (Table 35-1).
(ii) **Contraindication.** The use of hypnotics for longer than a few weeks is contraindicated because of tolerance and physical dependence.
(iii) **Therapeutic contract.** A wise strategy for using hypnotics is to enter into a therapeutic contract with patients, limiting hypnotic use to no more than two or three nights in succession, followed by one or more medicine-free nights. In this way, hypnotics can serve as a safety net, and patients can be assured that they will have no more than one night of sleeplessness without obtaining relief.
(b) **Barbiturates** have lost popularity as a result of:
(i) Their narrow therapeutic index
(ii) Moderately high abuse potential
(iii) Potential drug–drug interactions (as a result of liver enzyme induction)
(iv) Suppression of delta and REM sleep with a REM rebound following abrupt discontinuation
(v) Loss of efficacy in inducing and maintaining sleep with consecutive-night use

Table 35-1. Examples of Short-, Intermediate-, and Long-acting Benzodiazepines

Agent (generic)	Rate of Elimination	Usual Adult Dose (mg)
Triazolam	Rapid	0.125–0.25
Estazolam	Intermediate	1–2
Temazepam	Intermediate	15–30
Flurazepam HCl	Slow	15–30
Quazepam	Slow	7.5–15

Reprinted with permission from Becker PM, Jamieson AO, Brown WD: Insomnia: Use of a decision tree to assess and treat. *Postgrad. Med.* 93(1):79, 1993.

(c) **Nonbarbiturate nonbenzodiazepines** were originally thought to be superior to the barbiturates because of their different chemical structures. However, they share many of the disadvantages of barbiturates, plus having additional disadvantages of their own (e.g., glutethimide can result in a more severe overdose or toxicity).

(3) **OTC drug therapy**

(a) The Food and Drug Administration (FDA) has deemed two antihistamines, **diphenhydramine** (e.g., Nytol, Sleep-Eze, Sominex II, and Compoz) and **doxylamine** (e.g., Unisom), safe and effective sleep aids. They are both ethanolamine antihistamines, which possess the highest sedative effects and the lowest gastrointestinal side effects of the various antihistamines.

(i) The **therapeutic use** of these agents capitalizes on the drowsiness side effect.

(ii) **Indications.** These OTC products are indicated for mild situational insomnia.

(iii) The usual **dose** for adults is 25 mg for doxylamine and 50 mg for diphenhydramine. Increasing the dose of diphenhydramine does not produce a linear increase in hypnotic effect. However, it does produce greater anticholinergic side effects, particularly in elderly people.

(iv) The most common **side effects** include dizziness, dry mouth, blurred vision, and upset stomach. Both doxylamine and diphenhydramine cause REM suppression and, therefore, some REM rebound after discontinuation. Anticholinergic effects include constipation and urinary retention. Central anticholinergic effects that also affect the elderly include confusion, disorientation, impaired short-term memory, and, at times, visual and tactile hallucinations.

(v) **Contraindications.** These agents should not be used by individuals under age 12 and should not be taken longer than 2 weeks. In addition, they should be used cautiously by patients who have asthma, narrow-angle glaucoma, and prostate enlargement.

(vi) **Efficacy.** Diphenhydramine and doxylamine are considered to be roughly equivalent in efficacy.

(b) The essential amino acid, **L-tryptophan,** has been recommended in the past for insomnia.

(i) L-tryptophan has never been approved by the FDA as a safe and effective drug.

(ii) L-tryptophan was withdrawn from the market in 1990 because of several deaths due to eosinophilia–myalgia syndrome, which was attributed to a contaminant in the manufacturing process at one plant.

STUDY QUESTIONS

Directions: Each of the numbered items or incomplete statements in this section is followed by answers or by completions of the statement. Select the **one** lettered answer or completion that is **best** in each case.

1. Based on the calorie decrease necessary to lose 1 pound of body fat, how many pounds will a woman likely lose in 20 days if she cuts her caloric intake from 2200 per day to 1600 per day but does not increase her physical activity?

(A) 10 pounds
(B) Approximately 5 pounds
(C) Almost 3.5 pounds
(D) Slightly less than 2 pounds
(E) Not enough data to calculate

2. All of the following statements about diphenhydramine are true EXCEPT

(A) a 50-mg dose that is ineffective should be doubled for the elderly patient
(B) it suppresses rapid eye movement (REM) sleep
(C) the sedation that it produces is considered unpleasant in comparison to sedation from alcohol or benzodiazepines
(D) it should not be taken with alcohol
(E) it is similar to doxylamine in efficacy as a sleep aid

3. All of the following statements about sleep stages are true EXCEPT

(A) a normal, young, healthy adult spends about 20%–25% of total sleep time in rapid eye movement (REM) sleep
(B) the degree of restfulness of sleep is associated with the amount of REM sleep
(C) dreaming appears to occur most often in the first stage of non-rapid eye movement (NREM) sleep
(D) ethanol and barbiturates suppress REM sleep
(E) stages three and four of NREM sleep are often referred to as delta sleep

4. All of the following would be useful sleep hygiene measures EXCEPT

(A) exercising intensely just before bedtime
(B) taking a warm bath just before bedtime
(C) reading until drowsy
(D) keeping the bedroom somewhat cool
(E) establishing a regular bedtime

5. All of the following statements about obesity are true EXCEPT

(A) an obese patient is generally defined as a person who has surplus body fat and is above their ideal body weight by at least 20%
(B) some evidence indicates that weight loss can come from simply cutting down on the amount of fat in the diet, even with no decrease in the total number of calories eaten per day
(C) very low-calorie diets initially result in a significant amount of water loss, as glycogen and protein are metabolized
(D) fad diets do not teach patients how to eat for long-term maintenance of the decreased weight
(E) a bulk laxative like Metamucil has been proven to be an effective weight loss agent

---

1-C 4-A
2-A 5-E
3-C

ANSWERS AND EXPLANATIONS

1. The answer is C *[I B].*
The woman would lose about 3.5 pounds. To lose 1 pound of fat, caloric intake must decrease by 3500 calories. This woman decreased her caloric intake from 2200 calories per day to 1600 calories per day, a decrease of 600 calories. Six hundred calories multiplied by 20 days equals a decrease of 12,000 calories. Twelve thousand divided by 3500 equals 3.43 pounds, or approximately 3.5 pounds.

2. The answer is A *[II B 5 b (3) (a)].*
Increasing the dose of diphenhydramine does not automatically bring a linear increase in hypnotic effect. However, it does produce greater anticholinergic side effects, which are particularly troublesome in the elderly. Diphenhydramine, which suppresses rapid eye movement (REM) sleep, produces a sedation more unpleasant than that of alcohol or benzodiazepines. Diphenhydramine should not be taken with alcohol. As a sleep aid, it is similar in efficacy to doxylamine.

3. The answer is C *[II A 3].*
Most dreaming appears to occur during rapid eye movement (REM) rather than non-REM (NREM) sleep. The average, young, healthy adult spends about one-quarter of the time sleeping in rapid eye movement (REM) sleep. The amount of REM sleep is associated with the degree of restfulness. Alcohol and barbiturates suppress REM sleep. Delta sleep consists of stages three and four of non-rapid eye movement (NREM) sleep.

4. The answer is A *[II B 5 a].*
Exercising intensely just before going to bed will usually have a stimulating effect. Taking a warm bath shortly before bedtime, reading until drowsy, keeping the bedroom cool, and establishing a regular bedtime are considered appropriate sleep hygiene measures.

5. The answer is E *[I A 1, C 1–3].*
Bulk laxatives produce a feeling of fullness, but x-ray studies show that the bulk leaves the stomach within 30 minutes. They may decrease appetite somewhat, but the effectiveness of bulk laxatives as a weight loss agent is weak. Obese people are those who have surplus body fat and are at least 20% above their ideal body weight. A person can lose weight simply by reducing the amount of fat in the diet and expending more calories than are consumed. Very low-calorie diets result in initial significant water loss, as glycogen and protein are metabolized. Fad diets do not teach people how to eat to maintain any achieved weight loss. Consequently, many people who follow fad diets usually regain weight.

36
OTC Products: Fever, Pain, Cough, Cold, and Allergic Rhinitis

Gerald E. Schumacher
Kim Poinsett-Holmes
Ronnie Chapman

I. ANALGESIC, ANTI-INFLAMMATORY, AND ANTIPYRETIC AGENTS. Over-the-counter (OTC) analgesics and antipyretics relieve mild-to-moderate pain and reduce inflammation and fever. These agents are effective for somatic pain (e.g., musculoskeletal pain arising from the joints, pain from headache, myalgia, dysmenorrhea, and discomfort resulting from generalized inflammation), but they are not effective in reducing discomfort from the visceral organs (e.g., stomach, lungs, heart). Salicylates and nonsteroidal anti-inflammatory drugs (NSAIDs) reduce pain, inflammation, and fever, but acetaminophen generally is effective for only pain and fever.*

A. Pathogenesis of pain. An intense stimulus (e.g., tissue injury) releases substances that sensitize pain receptors to mechanical, thermal, and chemical stimulation. This triggers pain receptors to send pain impulses over afferent nerve fibers to the central nervous system (CNS).

1. **Awareness of pain** occurs in the thalamus.
2. **Pain recognition and localization** occur in the cortex.
3. **Mechanism of analgesic, anti-inflammatory, and antipyretic action.** These agents inhibit (centrally, peripherally, or both) the biosynthesis of various **prostaglandins,** substances involved in the development of pain and inflammation as well as in the regulation of body temperature.

B. Salicylates

1. **Therapeutic uses.** Salicylates are used to relieve mild-to-moderate pain and reduce inflammation and fever. Aspirin (acetylsalicylic acid), specifically, is also used to reduce the incidence of:
   a. **Strokes** in men at risk
   b. **Myocardial infarction** in men and women who have had a previous infarction, stable and unstable angina pectoris, or coronary artery bypass surgery
2. **Mechanism of action**
   a. **Analgesic and anti-inflammatory actions.** The action of aspirin is due to both the acetyl and the salicylate portions of the drug. Actions of other salicylates (e.g., sodium salicylate, salicylsalicylic acid, choline salicylate) are due only to the salicylate portion of the agents.
      (1) These drugs **inhibit cyclooxygenase,** the enzyme that is responsible for the formation of precursors of prostaglandins and thromboxanes from arachidonic acid (Figure 36-1).
      (2) Analgesia is produced mainly by **blocking the peripheral generation of pain impulses** mediated by prostaglandins and other chemicals. Analgesia probably secondarily involves a reduction in the awareness of pain in the CNS.
   b. **Antipyretic action.** The principal antipyretic action occurs in the CNS. Salicylates act on the hypothalamic heat-regulating center to produce peripheral vasodilation, which results from the inhibition of prostaglandin synthesis.
   c. **Antiplatelet and antithrombotic actions**
      (1) **Antiplatelet.** Aspirin (but not other salicylates, acetaminophen, or NSAIDs) **irreversibly inhibits cyclooxygenase in platelets,** which prevents the formation of the aggregating agent thromboxane A_2.

---

*In some instances, aspirin is considered to be a nonsteroidal anti-inflammatory drug (NSAID), while in other instances it is not. For the purpose of demonstrating different dosage information, aspirin and NSAIDs are discussed separately in this chapter.

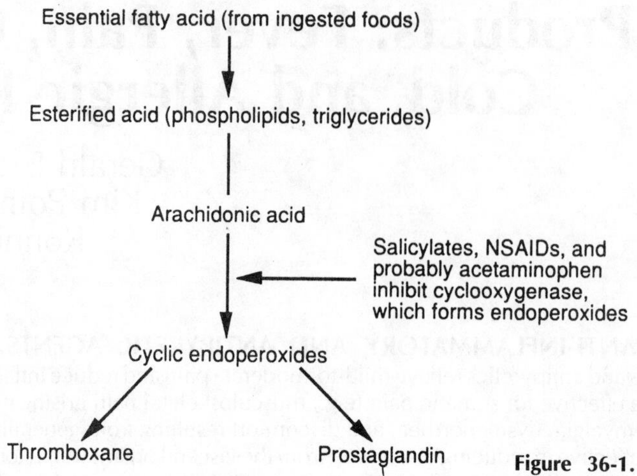

Figure 36-1. Inhibition of prostaglandin formation by aspirin, NSAIDs, and acetaminophen.

(2) **Antithrombotic.** Aspirin also **reversibly inhibits the formation of prostacyclin** [prostaglandin I_2 (PGI_2)], which is an aggregation inhibitor in blood vessels.

3. **Administration and dosage**
   a. **For analgesia or antipyresis in adults,** 325 mg to 650 mg every 4 hours or 650 mg to 1000 mg every 6 hours should be administered as needed. The maximum daily dose is 4000 mg for no longer than 10 days for pain or 3 days for fever, without consulting a physician.
   b. **Child dosage depends on age.** The dosages are 160 mg every 4 hours for children 2 to 4 years of age, 400 mg to 480 mg every 4 hours for children 9 to 12 years of age. Salicylates should be given for no longer than 5 days for pain, 3 days for fever, and 2 days for sore throat, without consulting a physician.
   c. The **antirheumatic dosage for adults** is 3600 mg to 4500 mg daily in divided doses.
   d. **For patients with ischemic heart disease,** a 325-mg dose given daily or every other day is recommended for individuals with stable angina, unstable angina, and evolving myocardial infarction. For patients without clinically apparent ischemic heart disease, the hemorrhagic complications associated with routine aspirin use may outweigh its benefit, unless subjects have established risk factors for atherosclerotic disease.
   e. **Anti-inflammatory dosages.** Although antipyretic and analgesic effects should appear within the first few doses, the anti-inflammatory effect may take 2 or more weeks to be observed, even at high doses. The usual anti-inflammatory dosage of aspirin is 4000 mg to 6000 mg per day. The usual anti-inflammatory dosage of ibuprofen is 1200 mg to 3200 mg per day.

4. **Precautions**
   a. **Hypersensitivity** to aspirin occurs in up to 0.5% of the population.
      (1) Allergic reactions resulting in bronchoconstriction occur most frequently in people with **nasal polyps.**
      (2) **Cross-reactivity** with other NSAIDs occurs in more than 90% of people. Cross-reactivity with acetaminophen occurs in 5% of people.
   b. **Contraindications.** Aspirin is contraindicated in patients with bleeding disorders or peptic ulcers. Also, aspirin should not be given to children or teenagers with a viral illness, because Reye's syndrome (i.e., fatty liver degeneration accompanied by encephalopathy) may occur.
   c. **Pregnancy.** Salicylates in chronic high doses are recommended with extreme caution during the last trimester of pregnancy because of:
      (1) Potential bleeding problems in the mother, fetus, or neonate
      (2) Prolonging or complicating delivery
   d. **Gastrointestinal disturbances** resulting from the inhibition of the gastric prostaglandins occur in 10% to 20% of people at analgesic and antipyretic dosages. Anti-inflammatory regimens affect up to 40% of people. These percentages decrease by using enteric-coated dosage forms and taking salicylates with food or large doses of antacids. Buffered aspirin products contain insufficient "buffers" to counteract the adverse gastrointestinal effects of aspirin.

e. **CNS disturbances** such as tinnitus, dizziness, or headache may occur at anti-inflammatory doses in some patients.

f. **Salicylism** (salicylate toxicity) may occur at anti-inflammatory doses. In addition to the CNS disturbances above, respiratory alkalosis, nausea, hyperthermia, confusion, and convulsions may occur.

5. **Significant interactions**
   a. Salicylates potentiate the effect of **anticoagulants** and **thrombolytic agents.**
   b. Salicylates potentiate (at anti-inflammatory doses) the effect of **hypoglycemics.**
   c. Salicylates potentiate the adverse gastrointestinal reactions resulting from chronic **alcohol** or **NSAID** use.
   d. Aspirin may competitively inhibit the metabolism of **zidovudine,** resulting in potentiation of zidovudine or aspirin toxicity.
   e. **Caffeine** taken in conjunction with salicylates appears to enhance the analgesic effect.

C. Acetaminophen

1. **Therapeutic uses.** Acetaminophen is used to relieve mild-to-moderate pain and reduce fever. Although it may be used to reduce the pain associated with mild osteoarthritis, it has minimal anti-inflammatory activity and cannot be used to treat the swelling or stiffness resulting from rheumatoid arthritis.

2. **Mechanism of action.** The analgesic and antipyretic actions of acetaminophen are the same as those for aspirin (see I B 2 a–b).

3. **Administration and dosage.** Available dosage forms are 325 mg and 500 mg.
   a. **For analgesia or antipyresis in adults,** the dosage is 500 mg to 1000 mg three times daily as needed. The maximum daily dose is 4000 mg for no longer than 10 days for pain or 3 days for fever, without consulting a physician.
   b. **For children 6 years of age or older,** 325 mg is administered every 4 to 6 hours as needed. The maximum daily dose is 1600 mg for no longer than 5 days for pain, 3 days for fever, and 2 days for sore throat, without consulting a physician.
   c. **Routine use.** Acetaminophen is routinely used in patients who:
      (1) Are sensitive to the gastrointestinal disturbances caused by salicylates and NSAIDs
      (2) Are prone to bleeding disorders
      (3) Are hypersensitive to salicylates

4. **Precautions.** Patients with active alcoholism, hepatic disease, or viral hepatitis are at risk from chronic administration of acetaminophen. Toxicity is rare, but chronic daily ingestion of 5 g or more for longer than 1 month is likely to result in liver damage. Acute doses of 10 g or more are hepatotoxic.

5. **Significant interactions.** Acetaminophen may competitively inhibit the metabolism of **zidovudine,** resulting in potentiation of zidovudine or acetaminophen toxicity.

D. NSAIDs.

NSAIDs. Currently, **ibuprofen** is the only NSAID available without a prescription. (Remember that aspirin and NSAIDs are separated in this chapter.)

1. **Therapeutic uses.** NSAIDs are used to relieve mild-to-moderate pain and reduce inflammation and fever. OTC use largely focuses on the analgesic and antipyretic indications of ibuprofen. Prescription level dosage is required for arthritic and other inflammatory diseases.

2. **Mechanism of action**
   a. **Analgesic and anti-inflammatory actions.** NSAIDs inhibit prostaglandin synthesis both peripherally and centrally. Like salicylates, these drugs inhibit cyclooxygenase (see Figure 36-1). NSAIDs produce analgesia mainly by blocking the peripheral generation of pain impulses that are mediated by prostaglandins and other chemicals. Secondarily, analgesia probably involves a reduction in the awareness of pain in the CNS.
   b. **Antipyretic action.** The principal antipyretic action is central. NSAIDs act on the hypothalamic heat-regulating center to produce peripheral vasodilation, which results from the inhibition of prostaglandin synthesis.

3. **Administration and dosage.** The available OTC dosage form of ibuprofen is 200 mg.
   a. **For analgesia or antipyresis in adults,** the dosage is 200 mg to 400 mg every 4 to 6 hours as needed. The maximum daily dose is 1200 mg for no longer than 10 days for pain or 3 days for fever, without consulting a physician.

b. The **antirheumatic dosage for adults** is 400 mg to 800 mg every 6 to 8 hours to a maximum daily dose of 3200 mg.
c. Ibuprofen is not recommended for children under 12 years of age.

4. **Precautions**
a. NSAIDS are contraindicated in patients with **bleeding disorders** or **peptic ulcers.**
b. NSAIDs are recommended with extreme caution during the last trimester of **pregnancy** because of:
(1) Potential adverse effects on fetal blood flow
(2) The possibility of prolonging pregnancy
c. **Gastrointestinal disturbances** resulting from the inhibition of the gastric prostaglandins occur in 5% to 10% of people at analgesic and antipyretic doses. Anti-inflammatory regimens (i.e., higher doses) affect up to 20% of people. These percentages decrease by taking NSAIDs with food or large doses of antacids. Ibuprofen is often preferred to aspirin by patients because ibuprofen causes fewer gastrointestinal disturbances and bleeding events occur less frequently.
d. **Renal toxicity** during chronic administration is a significant concern and may occur in the form of nephrotic syndrome, hyperkalemia, or interstitial nephritis.

5. **Significant interactions**
a. NSAIDs potentiate the effect of **anticoagulants** and **thrombolytic agents.**
b. NSAIDs potentiate (at anti-inflammatory doses) the effect of **hypoglycemics.**
c. NSAIDs potentiate the adverse gastrointestinal reactions resulting from chronic **alcohol** or **salicylate** use.
d. **Caffeine** taken in conjunction with ibuprofen appears to enhance the analgesic effect.
e. Hypersensitivity to **aspirin** can occur with NSAID use.

II. COUGH AND COLD PREPARATIONS

A. **The common cold.** Coughs and colds, self-limiting inflammatory viral infections of the upper respiratory tract (e.g., acute coryza, acute or infectious rhinitis, rhinorrhea, catarrh), cause more lost time from work and school than do all other diseases combined. Over 800 OTC cold preparations are on the market, resulting in annual sales in the United States of approximately 2 billion dollars.

1. **Primary anatomic sites of infection**
a. **Rhinitis** is inflammation of the nose.
b. **Pharyngitis** is inflammation of the pharynx, which commonly causes a sore throat.
c. **Laryngitis** is inflammation and soreness of the larynx, which leads to hoarseness or loss of the voice.
d. **Bronchitis** is inflammation of bronchi, which leads to a chest cold.
e. **Nasopharyngitis** is nasal congestion with possible postnasal drip and sore throat.

2. **Presentation.** Colds have a rapid onset with a short incubation period. Rhinorrhea, the hallmark of a cold, produces clear, watery, profuse secretions. Headache (due to congested sinuses), malaise, moderate throat symptoms (e.g., pharyngitis, laryngitis), and fever may occur. Muscle aches prevail in people affected by influenza.

3. **Progression.** A cold often begins as a nonproductive dry cough and progresses to a productive cough (with sputum). Mucus becomes tenacious secondary to bacterial infection, and discharge increases, which produces sneezing, postnasal drip, and congestion. Colds often last several weeks, possibly because of secondary infection, inflammation, mucus backup, and irritated bronchi.

4. **Transmission.** Colds are usually transmitted by direct person-to-person contact via infected airborne droplets. The average incubation period is approximately 1 to 4 days. Patients may be unaware that they are infectious.

5. **Peak seasons.** The incidence of colds peaks in early fall, when school begins, and in midwinter, when 50% of the population have colds. Approximately 20% of the population experience colds during the summer. Spring is usually associated with allergies but not colds.

6. **Occurrence.** Colds occur most often in children less than 6 years of age (i.e., an individual child may have approximately six to twelve colds per year). Women have 25% more colds than men, which may be associated with the larger amount of time that women spend around

children. Adults over 30 years who do not have children have an average of two to three colds per year. Adults with children have an average of five to six colds per year.

7. **Susceptibility.** Viral exposure, not just exposure to cold temperature, must occur. However, temperature changes can alter the character of mucus (i.e., cold temperature thickens mucus, which enables viruses to maintain longer contact with the mucosa and increases the chance of penetration). The mucosa can be altered by factors that increase the ability of a virus to penetrate. These factors include:
   - **a.** Poor nutrition
   - **b.** Fatigue
   - **c.** Emotional distress
   - **d.** Allergies, which cause antigen–antibody inflammatory reactions that facilitate viral invasion
8. **Etiology**
   - **a. Viruses,** such as rhinovirus, coronavirus, adenovirus, coxsackievirus, echovirus, influenza virus, parainfluenza virus, and respiratory syncytial virus, cause the common cold.
   - **b.** Viruses **differ from bacteria.** Because viruses exist within the host cell, they have a different chemical composition and mode of replication, and they respond to drug therapy differently than bacteria.
   - **c.** More than **200 different strains** of viruses can cause 75% of all respiratory illnesses. Immunity to a specific strain lasts for about 2 years. The **most prevalent strain is rhinovirus.**
     - **(1)** Rhinovirus is **responsible for one-half of all common colds,** with many colds being the result of a combination of viruses.
     - **(2)** More than **120 strains** of rhinovirus have been identified.
9. **Pathophysiology**
   - **a.** Initially, the **rhinorrhea** is clear, but it is followed by a thicker mucoid secretion composed of white blood cells. **Nasal congestion** results from the engorgement of the nasal vasculature and the swelling of turbinates and is characterized by sneezing, nasal irritation, and discharge.
   - **b. Nonbacterial pharyngitis** is characterized by dry, sore, or raspy throat or a tickling sensation when swallowing. The **early stages** are characterized by a nonproductive cough, irritation of the pharynx, and postnasal drip. The **later stages** are characterized by a productive cough, which results from cellular debris of local phagocytic activity combined with respiratory tract fluids. Headache and fever may occur; however, a fever is uncommon and, if present, is usually slight and transient.

B. Symptomatic pharmacologic treatment

1. **Antihistamines**
   - **a. Mechanism of action. Histamine (H_1) blockers** competitively inhibit the effects of histamine. They do not prevent histamine release, but if histamine concentration is greater than the drug concentration, histamine effects predominate. H_1 blockers inhibit smooth muscle response. They are structurally similar to anticholinergics, local anesthetics, ganglionic blocking agents, and adrenergic blocking agents. H_1 blockers do not prevent the common cold, but they decrease the amount of mucus secretion, relieving rhinorrhea with a drying effect.
   - **b. Precautions.** The anticholinergic effect of antihistamines is very weak with a high therapeutic index. Anticholinergic effects include dry mouth, blurred vision, constipation, and urinary retention.
     - **(1)** These medications must be used with caution in patients with an **enlarged prostate** or **narrow-angle glaucoma.**
     - **(2)** Antihistamines may have a paradoxical effect in **children,** causing CNS stimulation rather than depression.
     - **(3) Overdosing** produces excitement, ataxia, incoordination, muscular twitching, and generalized convulsions with pupillary dilation and flushing.
     - **(4) Side effects** include:
       - **(a)** CNS depression
       - **(b)** Local anesthesia
       - **(c)** Tolerance, which may require switching antihistamine classes
   - **c. Significant interactions.** Antihistamines must be used with caution with other **CNS depressants.**

d. Specific products

(1) Ethanolamines (e.g., diphenhydramine, doxylamine)

(a) Mechanism of action. Ethanolamines vary in potency, dosage, and side effects. They have the most potent sedative effect of any group of antihistamines. Ethanolamines are good antiemetics and have high anticholinergic activity (i.e., CNS activity is +3 and anticholinergic activity is +3).

(b) Administration and dosage. Diphenhydramine was previously administered by prescription only, but OTC preparations are now available in liquid, tablet, and capsule form. The **adult dosage** is 25 mg to 50 mg every 4 to 6 hours to a maximum daily dose of 300 mg. The dose for **children 2 to 6 years** of age is 6.25 mg. The dose for **children 6 to 12 years** of age is 12.5 mg to 25 mg.

(2) Ethylenediamines

(a) Mechanism of action. Ethylenediamines produce intermediate sedation and effective H_1 antagonist effects. **Pyrilamine** was used in many products in combination with pheniramine (25 mg to 50 mg every 6 to 8 hours). CNS activity is moderate (+1), and anticholinergic activity is mild (+/−).

(b) Administration and dosage. The **adult dosage** is 25 mg to 50 mg four times daily to a maximum daily dose of 200 mg. The dose for **children 2 to 6 years** of age is 6.25 mg. The dose for **children 6 to 12 years** of age is 12.5 mg to 25 mg.

(3) Alkylamines (e.g., brompheniramine, chlorpheniramine)

(a) Mechanism of action. Alkylamines produce the weakest amount of sedation of all antihistamines and, therefore, are most suitable for daytime use. They are also the most active H_1 blockers of the antihistamines. The degree of CNS activity (+1/+2) and anticholinergic activity (+2) can be significant.

(b) Administration and dosage. The dosage for brompheniramine and chlorpheniramine is 4 mg every 4 to 6 hours to a maximum daily dose of 24 mg. The **adult dosage** of chlorpheniramine (Chlor-Trimeton) is 4 mg every 4 to 6 hours to a maximum daily dose of 24 mg. The dose of chlorpheniramine for **children 2 to 6 years** of age is 1 mg. The dose of chlorpheniramine for **children 6 to 12 years** of age is 2 mg.

2. Topical decongestants. Topical decongestants are characterized by intensive symptomatic relief, rapid onset and short duration of action, and few systemic side effects. However, topical decongestants cause rebound congestion after more than 3 to 4 days of use.

a. Mechanism of action. Decongestants stimulate the α-adrenergic receptors in vascular smooth muscle, which results in vasoconstriction in the mucous membranes.

b. Administration and dosage. Decongestants are available as drops, sprays, inhalers, and gels. The sprays produce a fine mist when squeezed. If decongestants are swallowed, they can produce systemic effects. Drops should be used in children 2 to 6 years of age. For children under 6, there is no recommended dosage of ephedrine and naphazoline, except under the advice of a physician.

c. Precautions. Patients with **chronic rhinitis** should avoid topical decongestants because of the risk of rhinitis medicamentosa.

d. Products

(1) Arylalkylamines

(a) Ephedrine is not commonly used today.

(i) Mechanism of action. It is the prototype of the topical sympathomimetics and is a rapidly acting nasal decongestant with a short duration of action. It decomposes very rapidly in light or heat.

(ii) Administration and dosage. The **adult dosage** is 2 to 3 drops or sprays every 4 hours. The dosage for **children 6 to 12 years** of age is 1 to 2 drops or sprays every 4 hours. Ephedrine should not be used in **children younger than 6 years** of age.

(b) Phenylephrine (e.g., Neosynephrine) is one of the most effective nonprescription decongestants available.

(i) Precaution. Phenylephrine may cause rebound congestion because of nasal irritation.

(ii) Administration and dosage. Phenylephrine is used primarily by otorhinolaryngologists in concentrations of 0.125%, 0.250%, and 1%. The **adult dosage** is 2 to 3 drops or sprays (0.25% or 1%) every 4 hours. The dosage for **children 6 to 12 years** of age is 2 to 3 drops or sprays of the 0.25% concentration every 4 hours. The dosage for **children less than 6 years** of age is 2 to 3 drops or sprays of 0.125% concentration every 4 hours.

(2) **Naphazoline hydrochloride** is a potent decongestant.
(a) **Precautions.** It causes significant topical absorption, which may lead to CNS depression, decreased body temperature, coma, or death. Naphazoline hydrochloride is not recommended for children because of its potency. Side effects include irritation to the mucosa, burning, and stinging.
(b) **Administration and dosage.** Naphazoline is available in a 0.05% concentration. The **adult dosage** is 1 to 2 drops or sprays every 6 hours. The dosage for **children 6 to 12 years** of age is 1 to 2 drops or sprays of 0.025% concentration every 6 hours. Naphazoline is not recommended for children younger than 6 years of age.

(3) **Oxymetazoline** is found in Afrin, Neosynephrine Maximum Strength 12-Hour Nasal Spray, and Sinex LA. Oxymetazoline is long acting and is less likely to cause rebound congestion than other decongestants. Oxymetazoline is available in concentrations of 0.05% and 0.025%. The **adult dosage** is 2 to 3 drops or sprays of 0.05% concentration every 5 to 6 hours. The dosage for **children 6 to 12 years** of age is the same as the adult dosage. The dosage for **children younger than 6 years** of age is 2 to 3 drops or sprays in the morning and evening.

(4) **Xylometazoline** is found in Otrivin Nasal Drops. The decongestant effect may last 5 to 6 hours, with a gradual decline. Xylometazoline, which is available in concentrations of 0.1% and 0.05%, is administered twice daily because of the prolonged duration of action. The **adult dosage** is 2 to 3 drops or sprays of 0.1% concentration every 8 to 10 hours. The dosage for **children 6 to 12 years** of age is 2 to 3 drops or sprays of 0.05% concentration every 8 to 10 hours. The dosage for **children younger than 6 years** of age is 2 to 3 drops of 0.05% every 8 to 10 hours.

(5) **Propylhexedrine** (e.g., Benzedrex) **and levodesoxyephedrine** (e.g., Vicks Inhaler) are sympathomimetic amines. They are commonly used in inhalants that contain camphor and menthol. They lose their potency easily because of high aromaticity, and total nasal congestion limits their effectiveness.
(a) The **adult dosage** is two inhalations in each nostril every 2 hours.
(b) The dose for **children 6 years of age or older** is one inhalation.
(c) Propylhexedrine and levodesoxyephedrine are not approved for use in **children younger than 6 years** of age.

3. Oral decongestants provide less intensive symptom relief. They have a slow onset but a long duration of action. They have systemic side effects but do not cause rebound congestion or local irritation.

a. Mechanism of action. Oral decongestants distribute systemically to the nasal mucosa and have a longer duration of action with less vasoconstriction than the topical decongestants.

b. Precautions. Oral decongestants may produce changes in blood pressure, may induce arrhythmias, and may increase the blood glucose level, if β-adrenergic activity occurs (e.g., with ephedrine). They may produce α-adrenergic activity. Oral decongestants should be used with caution in patients with hypertension, hyperthyroidism, diabetes mellitus, or ischemic heart disease.

c. Significant interactions. Oral decongestants should be avoided in patients receiving monoamine oxidase (MAO) inhibitors to avoid a possible hypertensive crisis.

d. Specific products

(1) **Ephedrine** is effective as a bronchodilator for asthma but has questionable use as a decongestant. CNS stimulation may occur; effects appear within 30 minutes to 1 hour. Oral doses of 12.5 mg to 25 mg provide effective bronchodilator treatment of asthma in adults and children 12 years of age and older.

(2) **Phenylpropanolamine (PPA)** is found in Dimetapp and Alka Seltzer Plus Cold Medicine.
(a) **Mechanism of action.** PPA resembles ephedrine in action, but it causes more vasoconstriction and less CNS stimulation and bronchodilation.
(b) **Precautions.** Use of PPA is associated with transient hypertension, intracranial hemorrhage, severe headache, central retinal vein occlusion, atrioventricular conduction block, and death.
(c) **Significant interactions.** People at risk for adverse reactions to PPA include:
(i) Patients with hypertension
(ii) Overweight patients who may be using diet aids that contain PPA (see Chapter 35 I G 1 b)
(iii) Women taking oral contraceptives

(iv) The elderly
(v) Patients taking other sympathomimetic drugs

(d) **Administration and dosage.** The **adult dosage** is 25 mg every 4 hours to a daily maximum of 150 mg. Levels peak after 3 hours. The dosage for **children 6 to 12 years** of age is 12.5 mg every 4 hours to a daily maximum of 75 mg. For **children 2 to 6 years** of age, the dosage is 6.25 mg every 4 hours to a daily maximum of 37.5 mg.

(3) **Phenylephrine** is rapidly metabolized in the gastrointestinal tract. It is often present in "shotgun" (i.e., combination) products but in decreased amounts. The **adult dosage** is 10 mg every 4 hours to a daily maximum of 60 mg. The dosage for **children 6 to 12 years** of age is every 4 hours to a daily maximum of 30 mg. The dosage for **children 2 to 6 years** of age is 2.5 mg every 4 hours to a daily maximum of 15 mg.

(4) **Pseudoephedrine** (e.g., Sudafed) is considered safe and effective, especially in children. It is a vasoconstrictor with less vasopressor action than ephedrine, and it causes little CNS stimulation. The **adult dosage** is 60 mg every 6 hours to a daily maximum of 240 mg. The dosage for **children 6 to 12 years** of age is 30 mg to a daily maximum of 120 mg. The dosage for **children 2 to 6 years** of age is 15 mg every 6 hours to a daily maximum of 60 mg.

4. **Antitussives.** Three cough suppressants are approved by the Food and Drug Administration (FDA): **codeine** (Category I), **dextromethorphan** (Category I), and **diphenhydramine** (Category II). In addition, benzonatate, camphor, and menthol are antitussive agents.

a. **Mechanism of action.** Most antitussives act centrally to depress the medullary cough center (e.g., dextromethorphan, codeine). Others act peripherally by increasing the threshold of sensory nerve cough receptors within the respiratory tract (e.g., local anesthetics, menthol, camphor).

b. **Precautions.** Congestive and productive coughs are associated with chest congestion and phlegm expectoration. Congestive and nonproductive coughs are associated with chest congestion and scanty phlegm expectoration. Dry and nonproductive coughs are not associated with chest congestion. Some coughs may signify asthma.

c. **Specific products**

(1) **Codeine** is the standard by which all other antitussives are measured. It is found in Robitussin A-C and Robitussin-DAC.

(a) **Precautions.** There is a low incidence of dependency on codeine with the usual antitussive dose. The respiratory depressant effect of codeine is one-fourth that of morphine. In common OTC dosage in healthy adults, respiratory depression is not apparent. The most common adverse effects are drowsiness, lightheadedness, and constipation.

(b) **Administration and dosage.** The **adult dosage** is 10 mg to 20 mg every 4 to 6 hours to a daily maximum of 120 mg. The dosage for **children 6 to 12 years** of age is 5 mg to 10 mg every 4 to 6 hours to a daily maximum of 60 mg. The dosage for **children 2 to 6 years** of age is 2.5 mg to 5 mg every 4 to 6 hours to a daily maximum of 30 mg.

(2) **Dextromethorphan** (e.g., Delsym) is a dextrorotatory isomer of levorphanol. It lacks analgesic, respiratory depressive, and addictive properties. Approximately 15 mg to 30 mg of dextromethorphan is equivalent to 8 mg to 15 mg of codeine, when used as an antitussive. The **adult dosage** is 10 mg to 20 mg every 4 hours or 30 mg every 6 to 8 hours to a daily maximum of 120 mg. The dosage for **children 6 to 12 years** of age is 5 mg to 10 mg every 4 hours or 15 mg every 6 to 8 hours to a daily maximum of 60 mg. The dosage for **children 2 to 6 years** of age is 2.5 mg to 5 mg every 4 hours or 7.5 mg every 6 to 8 hours to a daily maximum of 30 mg.

(3) **Diphenhydramine**

(a) **Mechanism of action.** Diphenhydramine has strong antitussive activity because of its central action on the cough center and its anticholinergic activity. It has low abuse potential. A dose of approximately 25 mg to 50 mg of diphenhydramine is equivalent to 15 mg of codeine.

(b) **Administration and dosage.** The **adult dosage** is 25 mg every 4 hours to a daily maximum of 150 mg. The dosage for **children 6 to 12 years** of age is 12.5 mg every 4 hours to a daily maximum of 75 mg. The dosage for **children 2 to 6 years** of age is 6.25 mg every 4 hours to a daily maximum of 37.5 mg.

(4) **Benzonatate** (e.g., Tessalon perles) is related chemically to the local anesthetic procaine. It has been marketed for 24 years as a prescription antitussive.

(a) **Mechanism of action.** Benzonatate diminishes the cough reflex by anesthetizing stretch receptors in the respiratory passages, lungs, and pleura. The onset of action is 15 to 20 minutes, and the duration of action is 3 to 8 hours.

(b) **Precautions.** The perle should be swallowed whole because release of benzonatate in the mouth can cause temporary anesthesia of the oral mucosa, which could result in choking. The patient should be cautioned about biting or sucking on the perle.

(c) **Administration and dosage.** The dosage for both **adults and children (10 years of age and older)** is 100 mg three times daily.

(5) **Camphor and menthol** produce a sensation of coolness in the respiratory tract. Five to ten milligrams of menthol in a lozenge or compressed tablet is dissolved in the mouth.

5. Expectorants

a. Mechanism of action. Expectorants facilitate the removal of mucus and other irritants from the respiratory tract by increasing the volume and decreasing the viscosity of bronchial secretions (i.e., increasing the watery secretions of the cells of the respiratory tract to loosen phlegm). Inhaling water vapor provides a demulcent action, adding to and diluting respiratory tract fluid. Clinically, expectorants do not appear to have a well-defined role in therapy. However, their use is based on the fact that some patients feel that they provide some degree of therapeutic benefit.

b. Precautions. Guaifenesin is the only expectorant classified by the FDA as Category I (i.e., agents that are generally recognized as safe and effective). The most common adverse effect is gastric upset. Fluid intake (8 to 10 glasses daily) and adequate humidity of inspired air are important.

c. Specific products

(1) **Guaifenesin** (glyceryl guaiacolate)

(a) **Mechanism of action.** Guaifenesin acts by reflex gastric stimulation. It seldom produces gastric irritation at normal doses, but plenty of water is required to decrease stomach irritation and increase effectiveness.

(b) **Administration and dosage.** The effectiveness of guaifenesin is dose dependent. Excess dosing decreases platelet aggregation and increases bleeding time without further therapeutic benefit. OTC products typically contain 100 mg/5 ml (Robitussin) or 200 mg/5 ml (Naldecon-SR). Guaifenesin is also available as 300-mg, extended-release capsules and 600-mg, long-acting tablets (e.g., Humibid L.A.).

(i) The **adult dosage** is 200 to 400 mg every 4 hours to a daily maximum of 2400 mg.

(ii) The dosage for **children 6 to 12 years** of age is 100 to 200 mg every 4 hours to a daily maximum of 1200 mg.

(iii) The dosage for **children 2 to 6 years** of age is 50 to 100 mg every 4 hours to a daily maximum of 600 mg.

(2) **Ammonium chloride**

(a) **Mechanism of action.** The mechanism of action of ammonium chloride is not fully understood. It probably produces mild irritation of the stomach mucosa, which triggers reflex stimulation of mucous glands in the lungs, increasing respiratory secretions.

(b) **Precautions.** Ammonium chloride should be avoided in patients with renal disease, hepatic disease, and chronic heart disease because of the likelihood of metabolic acidosis. Ammonium chloride also acidifies the urine, which may affect excretion of other drugs.

(3) **Ipecac syrup**

(a) **Mechanism of action.** Ipecac syrup increases respiratory secretions by gastric irritation.

(b) **Precautions.** The primary toxicity of ipecac syrup is cardiac and neuromuscular, which may be fatal. Therefore, the FDA recommends limiting treatment with ipecac syrup to 1 week. Ipecac syrup used as an expectorant should be avoided in children younger than 6 years of age.

(c) **Administration and dosage.** Approximately 0.5 ml to 1 ml of ipecac syrup is administered 3 to 4 times daily.

6. **Vitamin C** is one of the most widely misused vitamins. At the onset of a cold, up to 20,000 mg of vitamin C have been recommended; during periods of health, 1000 mg to 2000 mg have been recommended. However, there is little evidence that large doses prevent colds or shorten the duration of a cold.
   a. The **recommended daily allowance for adults** is 60 mg/day.
   b. Potential **side effects** include:
      (1) Diarrhea
      (2) Inhibition of the ability of the white blood cells to kill bacteria
      (3) Urinary tract stones
      (4) Interference with urine glucose tests
      (5) Inhibition of the effectiveness of anticoagulant therapy

III. ALLERGIC RHINITIS

A. Etiology. There is a genetic predisposition to become sensitized after exposure to an allergen, and allergic rhinitis can begin at any age. The incidence of the first onset is greatest in children and young adults.

1. **Seasonal allergic rhinitis.** Allergens, or antigens, include pollen from plants and mold spores. Ragweed pollen typically is responsible for approximately 75% of all seasonal rhinitis that occurs in the United States. The seasonal appearance of symptoms reflects the pollen or spores in the air, which are most prevalent from mid-March to late November.
   a. **Trees** pollinate from late March to early June.
   b. **Grasses** pollinate from mid-May to mid-July.
   c. **Ragweed** pollinates from early August to early October (first frost).
2. **Chronic allergic rhinitis** is caused by house dust, animal dander, feathers, wheat, grains, cotton, paint, foods, and medications.

B. Immunology. Allergic rhinitis is precipitated by exposure of a sensitized patient to allergens (antigens). The nasal mucosa is vulnerable because antigen is deposited directly and can act locally.

1. **Histamine and slow reacting substance of anaphylaxis (SRS-A)** are released as a result.
2. **Vasodilators** become deposited in the sinuses, which may congest the turbinates by:
   a. Increasing vascular permeability
   b. Increasing fluid leakage
   c. Increasing swelling and edema
   d. Increasing mucus

C. Pathophysiology

1. Allergens, which are proteinaceous, are deposited onto the nasal mucosa to initiate an inflammatory response and symptoms.
2. The inflammatory process of allergic rhinitis develops in minutes after exposure in a sensitive patient.
3. Subsequent exposure to the same antigen produces an antigen–antibody reaction.
4. Sensitized host cells release vasoconstrictive chemical mediators (e.g., histamine, eosinophilic and neutrophilic chemotactic factors, and mast cell proteases).
5. Immediate effects include:
   a. Vasodilation
   b. Increased vascular permeability
   c. Increased mucus secretion, which produces symptoms

D. Symptoms. Major symptoms include edema, sneezing, rhinorrhea, nasal pruritus, and congestion. Symptoms of allergic rhinitis are more intense in the morning and on windy days because of the increased pollen. Symptoms decrease with rain when pollen is cleared from the air. Most common perennial antigens include dust and pet dander. Symptoms may overlap if patients are allergic to mold, grass, and ragweed. Symptoms tend to increase in severity for 2 to 3 years until they become stable; however, symptoms may increase or decrease in severity. Hypersensitivity may disappear after several years.

1. **Sneezing** attacks may occur.
2. **Rhinorrhea** (a clear, watery discharge) is continuous and, if purulent, produces secondary infection.
3. **Nasal congestion** is secondary to swollen turbinates and, if severe, produces headaches, earaches, dysgeusia (distorted taste), and loss of smell.
4. **Conjunctival symptoms** include itching and lacrimation caused by trapped pollen in the conjunctival sac and lacrimal ducts.

E. Complications include otitis media with hearing loss, sinusitis, loss of epithelial cilia, hyposmia (decreased smell sensation), nasal polyps, and vocal changes. These problems are more prevalent in children.

F. Conditions that mimic allergic rhinitis

1. **Infectious rhinitis** is similar. However, mucopurulent discharge, fever, systemic symptoms without pruritus, chronic sinusitis, and recurrent infectious rhinitis may be present.
2. **Abnormalities of nasal structures** (e.g., septal deviations). Nonseasonal, nonallergic, noninfectious rhinitis may occur.
3. **Rhinitis medicamentosa** resulting from overuse of topical decongestants may occur.
4. **Reserpine rhinitis** may develop where sympatholytics can cause nasal congestion. This effect is usually transient.
5. **Cerebrospinal rhinorrhea** may occur after a head injury.

G. Effective allergy treatment

1. **Avoiding allergens.** To avoid allergens, patients should be instructed to:
   - **a.** Avoid burning leaves
   - **b.** Sleep with the bedroom windows closed
   - **c.** Avoid driving through the country when the pollen count is high
   - **d.** Relocate to the Southwest
   - **e.** Use a dust mask
   - **f.** Close the house windows
   - **g.** Place mechanical filters in air conditioners
2. **Desensitization** may be effective for patients with severe reactivity problems (anaphylaxis). It is not a cure but simply decreases the symptoms. A physician must:
   - **a.** Identify the antigen with a skin test
   - **b.** Inject the extract in small amounts at frequent intervals
3. **Pharmaceutical intervention.** Sensitive patients should take an antihistamine before contact with an allergen or before a reaction. To avoid unnecessary side effects, specific agents should be used for specific symptomology. For instance, a decongestant should be used to relieve nasal congestion; an antitussive to control coughing; an antihistamine to control sneezing, watery eyes, and runny nose; an expectorant to relieve chest congestion; and an analgesic to relieve pain and fever. Combination products should be used by patients with multiple symptoms.

STUDY QUESTIONS

Directions: Each of the numbered items or incomplete statements in this section is followed by answers or by completions of the statement. Select the **one** lettered answer or completion that is **best** in each case.

1. Which one of the following agents can be used to prevent the signs and symptoms associated with allergic rhinitis?

(A) Chlorpheniramine
(B) Guaifenesin
(C) Oxymetazoline
(D) Phenylephrine
(E) Dextromethorphan

2. All of the following statements about the routine use of antihistamines in treating the common cold are correct EXCEPT

(A) they are safe for use both in adults and children
(B) they competitively inhibit histamine effects at the H_2 receptor sites
(C) they have a high therapeutic index
(D) they produce anticholinergic side effects
(E) they may lead to tolerance

3. Which of the following statements regarding the ethanolamine antihistamine group is correct?

(A) Of all antihistamines, they have the most active H_1 blocking activity
(B) They have poor antiemetic properties
(C) They are the most sedating antihistamine group
(D) The standard ethanolamine is chlorpheniramine

4. An advantage of using oral decongestants instead of topical decongestants to treat symptoms of the common cold is

(A) more intensive symptomatic relief
(B) a more rapid onset of action
(C) fewer systemic side effects
(D) no rebound congestion

5. The advantage of recommending dextromethorphan instead of codeine includes

(A) more analgesia for muscle aches and pain
(B) fifty percent as much respiratory depression
(C) fifty percent as much addiction
(D) peripheral action instead of central action
(E) none of the above

6. All of the following statements regarding guaifenesin are correct EXCEPT

(A) it is found in Robitussin
(B) it is also known as glyceryl guaicolate
(C) it produces reflex gastric stimulation to produce its therapeutic effects
(D) it requires large amounts of water to be effective
(E) it may cause an increase in platelet aggregation and a decrease in bleeding time with overdosing

---

1-A 4-D
2-B 5-E
3-C 6-E

ANSWERS AND EXPLANATIONS

1. The answer is A *[II B 1 d (3); 2 d (1) (b), (3); 4 c (2); 5 c (1)].*
Unlike the other products listed, chlorpheniramine blocks the effects of histamine, which is released during an allergic reaction and is primarily responsible for the signs and symptoms associated with allergic rhinitis. Guaifenesin, oxymetazoline, phenylephrine, and dextromethorphan are effective in treating the signs and symptoms after they have occurred but not in preventing them.

2. The answer is B *[II B 1 a–b].*
Antihistamines inhibit histamine effects at H_1 receptor sites not H_2 receptor sites. These agents can routinely be administered to children and adults. Antihistamines have a high therapeutic index, although there are minor side effects, such as anticholinergic activity, associated with their use. Chronic use of antihistamines can lead to tolerance, which may require switching to a different class of antihistamine.

3. The answer is C *[II B 1 d (1)].*
The ethanolamines (e.g., diphenhydramine, doxylamine) are the most sedating of the antihistamines, and they are good antiemetics. The alkylamines (e.g., chlorpheniramine) are the most potent H_1 blockers.

4. The answer is D *[II B 2–3].*
Oral decongestants provide less intensive symptomatic relief, have a slower onset of action, and produce more systemic side effects because they are absorbed systemically. However, there is no rebound congestion associated with oral medications because these products do not come into direct contact with the nasal mucosa.

5. The answer is E *[II B 4 c (1)–(2)].*
Dextromethorphan lacks analgesic, respiratory depressive, and addictive properties. Both dextromethorphan and codeine act centrally to depress the medullary cough center.

6. The answer is E *[II B 5 c (1)].*
Guaifenesin tends to cause a decrease in platelet aggregation, which results in an increase in bleeding time. Guaifenesin (glyceryl guaicolate) produces reflex gastric stimulation and requires plenty of water to be effective. It is found in the nonprescription product Robitussin.

37

OTC Products: Constipation, Diarrhea, and Hemorrhoids

Stephen H. Fuller
Larry N. Swanson

I. CONSTIPATION

A. General information

1. **Definition.** Constipation is the difficult or infrequent passage of stools. Normal stool frequency ranges from two to three times daily to two to three times per week. Patients may experience abdominal bloating, headaches, or a sense of rectal fullness from incomplete evacuation of feces.

2. **Causes.** Constipation can be caused by many factors, including:
   a. **Insufficient dietary fiber**
   b. **Lack of exercise**
   c. **Poor bowel habits,** such as failure to respond to the defecatory urge or hurried bowels (i.e., incomplete evacuation)
   d. **Medications,** such as narcotics, antacids, or anticholinergics (i.e., antidepressants, antihypertensives, antihistamines, phenothiazines, and antispasmodics)
   e. **Organic problems,** such as intestinal obstruction, tumor, inflammatory bowel disease, diverticulitis, hypothyroidism, or hyperglycemia

3. **Practitioners should question the patient about the following:**
   a. Normal stool frequency
   b. Duration of the constipation
   c. Frequency of constipation episodes
   d. Exercise routine
   e. Amount of dietary fiber consumed
   f. Presence of other symptoms
   g. Medications used currently
   h. Medications used to relieve constipation and their effectiveness

B. Treatment

1. **Nonpharmacologic**
   a. Increase intake of fluids and fiber (e.g., cereals, green vegetables, fruit, potatoes)
   b. Increase exercise to increase and maintain bowel tone
   c. Bowel training to increase regularity

2. **Pharmacologic.** Therapeutic agents are classified according to their mechanism of action. Laxatives should not be taken if nausea, vomiting, or abdominal pain is present.
   a. **Bulk-forming laxatives.** These medications are natural or synthetic polysaccharide derivatives that adsorb water to soften the stool and increase bulk, which stimulates peristalsis. Bulk-forming laxatives work in both the small and large intestines. The onset of action of these agents is slow (12 to 24 hours and up to 72 hours), which is why they are best used to prevent constipation rather than to treat severe acute constipation. There are both natural and synthetic products. All bulk-forming agents must be given with at least 8 ounces of water to minimize the possible constipation experienced by some patients. Some bulk-forming medications may contain sugar, so diabetics should use sugar-free products.
      (1) Natural bulk-forming laxatives
         (a) Psyllium (e.g., Metamucil, Konsyl, Fiberall). An **adult dose** is 3.5 to 7 g one to three times per day. A **child's dose** is half the adult dose one to three times per day.

(b) **Barley malt** (e.g., Maltsupex). An **adult dose** is 16 g two to four times per day. A **child's dose** is 16 g one to two times per day.

(2) **Synthetic bulk-forming laxatives**

(a) **Methylcellulose** (e.g., Citrucel). An **adult dose** is 1 to 2 g one to three times per day. A **child's dose** is 0.5 g one to three times per day.

(b) **Polycarbophil** (e.g., Mitrolan). An **adult dose** is 1 g one to four times per day. A **child's dose** is 0.5 g one to three times per day. Calcium polycarbophil may impair the absorption of tetracyclines if the drugs are taken concurrently.

b. **Saline and osmotic laxatives** work by creating an osmotic gradient to pull water into the small and large intestine. This increased volume results in distention of the intestinal lumen resulting in increased peristalsis and bowel motility. These laxatives also increase the activity of cholecystokinin–pancreozymin, which is an enzyme that increases the secretion of fluids into the gastrointestinal tract. The **onset of action varies** depending upon the ingredient and dosage form. Rectal formulations (e.g., enemas, suppositories) have an onset of action of 5 to 30 minutes, while oral preparations work within 4 hours.

(1) **Saline laxatives** include sodium and magnesium salts. As much as 20% of magnesium may be absorbed from these products, which may lead to hypermagnesemia in patients with preexisting renal impairment. Patients with hypertension or congestive heart failure should not receive saline laxatives on a prolonged basis due to fluid retention from sodium absorption. Products include:

(a) **Magnesium citrate** or citrate of magnesia

(b) **Magnesium hydroxide** (e.g., Phillips' Milk of Magnesia)

(c) **Magnesium sulfate** or Epsom salt

(d) **Sodium phosphate** (e.g., Fleet Phospho-soda)

(2) **Osmotic laxatives**

(a) **Glycerin** is available in rectal products in suppository or liquid form (e.g., Fleet Babylax). Rectal burning may occur with glycerin products. In addition to the osmotic effect, sodium stearate in these products can produce a local irritant effect. An **adult dose** is 3 g in suppository form or 5 to 15 ml as an enema. A **child's dose** is 1.5 g in suppository form or 2 to 5 ml as an enema.

(b) **Lactulose** (e.g., Chronulac) is available only by prescription and is used to decrease blood ammonia levels in hepatic encephalopathy. It may cause flatulence and cramping and should be taken with fruit juice, water, or milk to increase the palatability. An **adult dose** is 15 to 30 ml two to three times daily. A **child's dose** is 2.5 to 5 ml two to three times daily.

c. **Stimulant laxatives.** These medications work in the small and large intestine to stimulate bowel motility and increase the secretion of fluids into the bowel. All stimulant laxatives can cause abdominal cramping. Also, chronic use of stimulant laxatives can lead to **cathartic colon,** which results in a poorly functioning colon and resembles the symptoms of ulcerative colitis. The oral preparations usually have an onset of action within 6 to 10 hours. Rectal preparations usually have an onset of action within 30 to 60 minutes.

(1) **Anthraquinone laxatives** include senna, cascara sagrada, and casanthranol. **Melanosis coli,** which is a dark pigmentation of the colonic mucosa, can result with long-term use of anthraquinone laxatives. This usually disappears 6 to 12 months after discontinuing the medication. Discoloration (pink/red, yellow, or brown) of the urine may occur. Cascara sagrada is excreted into breast milk. Anthraquinone products include:

(a) **Senna** (e.g., Senokot, Fletcher's Castoria) is considered to be more potent than cascara products; however, senna causes more abdominal cramping.

(i) An **adult dose** is 300 to 1200 mg/day.

(ii) A **child's dose** is 100 to 600 mg/day.

(b) **Cascara sagrada.** Liquid preparations of cascara are more reliable than solid dosage forms. An **adult dose** is 300 to 1000 mg/day.

(c) **Casanthranol** is considered to be a mild stimulant laxative and is present in Peri-Colace, which also contains docusate.

(2) **Diphenylmethane derivatives** include the following:

(a) **Phenolphthalein** preparations (e.g., Ex-Lax, Feen-a-mint, Modane) have caused allergic reactions in some patients (e.g., a rash of pink-purple eruptions, itching, burning), which necessitates discontinuation of phenolphthalein products. An **adult dose** is 60 to 200 mg/day. Alkaline urine may be discolored pink/red, red/violet, or red/brown.

(b) **Bisacodyl** (e.g., Dulcolax). The tablet formulations of bisacodyl are enteric coated, so they should not be crushed or chewed. Also, bisacodyl-containing products should not be taken within 1 hour of ingesting antacids or milk.

(3) **Castor oil** (e.g., Purge, Neoloid) has an onset of action within 2 to 6 hours. Castor oil works primarily at the small intestine, which can result in strong cathartic effects (e.g., excessive fluid and electrolyte loss). These cathartic effects can lead to dehydration. Castor oil should not be used in pregnant patients, since it may induce premature labor. An **adult dose** is 15 to 60 ml; a **child's dose** is 5 to 15 ml.

d. **Emollient laxatives** act as surfactants by allowing absorption of water into the stool, which makes the softened stool easier to pass. These medications are particularly useful in patients who must avoid straining to pass hard stools, such as those who recently had a myocardial infarction or rectal surgery.

(1) **Onset of action.** Emollient laxatives have a slow onset of action (24 to 72 hours), which is why they are not considered the drug of choice for severe acute constipation, and they are more useful for preventing constipation.

(2) **Products.** Emollient laxatives are salts of the surfactant **docusate**. These products contain insignificant amounts of calcium, sodium, or potassium, and there are no specific guidelines for the selection of any one product. The products include:

(a) **Docusate sodium** (e.g., Colace, Doxinate)

(b) **Docusate calcium** (e.g., Surfak)

(c) **Docusate potassium** (e.g., Dialose)

(3) **Dosage information.** The **adult dose** is 100 to 300 mg per day. A **child's dose** is 50 to 150 mg per day. Each dose must be taken with at least 8 ounces of water. Liquid preparations should be taken in fruit juice or infant formula to increase palatability. Docusate products may facilitate the systemic absorption of mineral oil, so these agents should not be used concurrently.

e. **Lubricant laxative (mineral oil).** Mineral oil works at the colon to increase water retention in the stool to soften the stool. It has an **onset of action** of 6 to 8 hours.

(1) **Dosage information.** An **adult dose** is 15 to 45 ml per day. A **child's dose** is 10 to 15 ml per day.

(2) **Warnings**

(a) Mineral oil can **decrease absorption of fat-soluble vitamins** (i.e., vitamins A, D, E, K), so it should not be used on a chronic basis.

(b) Elderly, young, debilitated, and dysphagic patients are at the greatest risk of **lipid pneumonitis** from mineral oil aspiration.

(c) Emollients (e.g., docusate) may increase the systemic absorption of mineral oil, which can lead to **hepatotoxicity.**

(d) Mineral oil products may cause anal seepage, which results in itching (i.e., pruritus ani) and perianal discomfort.

(e) Mineral oil should be taken on an empty stomach.

C. Special patient populations

1. **Pediatric patients.** The bowel patterns of pediatric patients varies. During the first weeks of life, infants pass approximately four stools per day. As children get older, approximately 1 to 3 stools are passed per day. Constipation should be expected if there is a drastic change from a child's baseline bowel function.

a. **Nonpharmacologic methods** such as increasing the bulk content of the child's diet should be tried as the first form of treatment.

b. **If nonpharmacologic methods do not work,** rectal stimulation may be useful. Pharmacologic agents that can be used for acute relief include glycerin suppositories and magnesium laxatives. Stimulant laxatives and enemas should be administered as a last resort. Bulk-forming agents and stool softeners can be used if the constipation does not need immediate relief.

2. **Pregnant patients.** Constipation in pregnancy is common and is often due to compression of the colon by the enlarged uterus. Pregnant patients should avoid any preparation that may be absorbed systemically (e.g., stimulant laxatives), any preparation that can interfere with vitamin absorption (e.g., mineral oil), or any preparation that can induce premature labor (e.g., castor oil). Pregnant patients should use bulk-forming agents or stool softeners.

3. Geriatric patients should be evaluated to ensure that they do not have a primary disease state (e.g., hypothyroidism) that may cause constipation. Any medications that the geriatric patient is taking should be evaluated also, since drugs that possess anticholinergic effects may result in constipation.

a. Contraindications. A major concern with geriatric patients is the possible loss of fluid, which can be induced by aggressive laxative treatment (e.g., enemas and high-dose saline laxatives). Geriatric patients should not use stimulant laxatives on a chronic basis, and patients with renal impairment should not use magnesium products.

b. Treatment of acute constipation can include glycerin suppositories and lactulose (available by prescription), with bulk-forming agents and stool softeners as needed.

II. DIARRHEA.

Diarrhea is an abnormal increase in the frequency and looseness of stools. The overall weight and volume of the stool is increased (> 200 g or ml/day), and the water content is increased to 60% to 90%. In general, diarrhea results when some factor impairs the ability of the intestine to absorb water from the stool, which results in excess water in the stool. **Antidiarrheals** may serve to prevent an attack of diarrhea or to relieve existing symptoms.

A. Classification.

Diarrhea can be classified based on mechanisms or etiology.

1. Classification by mechanism

a. Osmotic diarrhea occurs when a nonabsorbable solute pulls excess water into the intestinal tract.

(1) Ingestion of large meals or certain osmotic substances (e.g., sorbitol, glycerin) can lead to diarrhea.

(2) Disaccharidase deficiency, which is a lack of enzymes needed to break down disaccharides in the gut for absorption (e.g., lactase deficiency), results in an increase in osmotic sugars (i.e., lactose, sucrose) in the intestinal tract.

(3) Medications that can induce osmotic diarrhea include lactulose and magnesium-containing antacids and laxatives.

b. Secretory diarrhea occurs when the intestinal wall is damaged, resulting in an increased secretion rather than absorption of electrolytes into the intestinal tract. Common sources include:

(1) **Bacterial endotoxins** (e.g., *Escherichia coli, Vibrio cholerae, Shigella, Staphylococcus aureus*)

(2) **Bacterial infections** (e.g., *Shigella, Salmonella*)

(3) **Viral infections** (e.g., rotavirus, Norwalk virus)

(4) **Protozoal infections** (e.g., *Giardia lamblia, Entamoeba histolytica*)

(5) **Miscellaneous causes** include inflammatory bowel disease and medications (e.g., prostaglandins, antibiotics, colchicine, chemotherapeutic agents)

c. Motility disorders. Diarrhea induced by motility disorders results from decreased contact time of the fecal mass with the intestinal wall, so less water is absorbed from the feces.

(1) Motility disorders include irritable bowel syndrome, scleroderma, diabetic neuropathy, gastric/intestinal resection, and vagotomy.

(2) Medications that can induce motility disorders include parasympathomimetic agents that enhance the effects of acetylcholine (e.g., metoclopramide, bethanechol), digitalis, quinidine, and antibiotics.

(a) Antibiotics cause diarrhea by causing intestinal irritation, increased bowel motility, and altered bowel microbial flora.

(b) Most antibiotic-induced diarrhea can be minimized by taking the agent with food.

2. Classification by etiology

a. Acute diarrhea (lasts less than 2 weeks)

(1) **Infection.** Most common sources include viral and bacterial, but protozoal diarrhea also occurs. Organisms include:

(a) **Viruses** that commonly cause diarrhea include rotaviruses and the Norwalk virus.

(i) **Rotaviruses** usually affect children under 2 years of age. The virus has an onset of 1 to 2 days and lasts 5 to 8 days. Patients usually have vomiting, a mild fever, and may experience severe dehydration. There is usually no blood or pus in the stool.

(ii) The **Norwalk virus** affects older children and adults. It has an onset of 1 to 2 days and lasts 24 to 48 hours (the "24-hour bug"). Like rotaviruses, there is mild fever but no blood or pus in the stool.

(b) Bacteria. Most bacterial diarrhea results from consumption of contaminated water or food with an onset of diarrhea in 2 hours to several days. Diarrhea due to consumption of contaminated food or water that occurs in a foreign country (e.g., Mexico, third world countries) is referred to as turista or traveler's diarrhea.

(i) Toxigenic bacteria. Diarrhea caused by toxigenic *E. coli, S. aureus, V. cholerae,* and *Shigella* results from the secretory effects of enterotoxins released by these organisms in the small intestine. Patients usually experience large-volume stools that are watery or greasy.

(ii) Invasive bacteria. Diarrhea caused by invasive *E. coli, Shigella, Salmonella, Campylobacter,* and *Clostridium difficile* results from mucosal invasion of the colon. This results in a dysentery-like diarrhea, which is characterized by an extreme urgency to defecate, abdominal cramping, tenesmus, fever, chills, and small-volume stools that contain blood or pus.

(c) Protozoa. *G. lamblia, E. histolytica,* and *Cryptosporidium* cause explosive, foul-smelling, large-volume, watery stools. This is thought to be caused by invasion of the small intestine, which causes damage to the microvilli and, therefore, decreases absorption of fluids. This type of diarrhea can result in large fluid losses, and patients are at risk for dehydration. Although protozoan-induced diarrhea is self-limiting, it may persist for several months, so therapy should be considered to eradicate the organism.

(2) Diet-induced diarrhea. Diarrhea induced by foods results from food allergies, high-fiber diets, fatty or spicy foods, large amounts of caffeine, or milk intolerance. The best treatment is prevention, by avoiding troublesome foods.

(3) Drug-induced diarrhea (see II A 1 a–c)

b. Chronic diarrhea (lasts longer than 2 weeks). If a patient suffers from diarrhea for long periods of time, or from recurrent episodes of diarrhea, the following causes must be considered: protozoal organisms, food-induced diarrhea (e.g., lactose intolerance), irritable bowel syndrome, malabsorption syndromes (e.g., celiac sprue, diverticulosis, short bowel syndrome), inflammatory bowel disease, pancreatic disease, and hyperthyroidism.

B. Patient evaluation

1. Pharmacists who are consulted by patients should ask the patient for the following information before recommending a therapy:
   - **a. Age** of the patient
   - **b. Onset and duration** of the diarrhea
   - **c. Description of stool** (i.e., frequency, volume, blood, pus, watery)
   - **d. Other symptoms** (e.g., abdominal cramping, fever, nausea, vomiting, weight loss)
   - **e. Medications** recently started or medications used to relieve the diarrhea
   - **f. Recent travel** (where and how long ago?)
   - **g. Medical history** (history of gastrointestinal disorders?)
2. **Referrals to a physician** should be made by the pharmacist who encounters a patient with diarrhea that meets the following criteria:
   - **a. Younger than 3 years** of age or **older than 60 years** of age (with multiple medical problems)
   - **b. Bloody stools**
   - **c. High fever**
   - **d. Dehydration or weight loss** greater than 5% of total body weight
   - **e. Duration of diarrhea longer than 5 days**
   - **f. Vomiting**

C. Treatment

1. Nonpharmacologic

a. Food. Patients should not receive solid food for 6 to 12 hours after an episode of diarrhea. However, fluids (at room temperature) may be given and may be necessary if the patient has lost a large amount of fluid through watery diarrhea. When foods are initiated, patients should receive soft foods. Many people use the BRAT diet (i.e., bananas, rice (or cereals), applesauce, toast) or gelatin, and continue fluids. Milk and other dairy products and fatty or spicy foods should be avoided for 7 to 10 days.

b. Fluids. When replenishing lost fluid and electrolytes, several commercial products are available and home remedies may be useful.

(1) **Fluid and electrolyte replacement.** Fluid and electrolyte therapy is aimed at replacing what the body has lost. During this situation, the patient's fluid input and output as well as weight should be monitored. The World Health Organization has established guidelines for oral replacement therapy (Table 37-1). Recommended doses are given in Table 37-2.

(2) **Fluids to be avoided** include hypertonic fruit juices and drinks (e.g., apple juice, powdered drink mixes, gelatin water) or carbonated beverages, which can make diarrhea worse and do not contain needed electrolytes (i.e., Na^+, K^+). Gatorade diluted in water (1:1) is adequate and provides the necessary combination of glucose, sodium, and potassium.

2. **Pharmacologic.** Based on the Food and Drug Administration (FDA) review of the various antidiarrheal products, three agents have been identified as Category I (i.e., safe and effective) ingredients: activated attapulgite, calcium polycarbophil, and loperamide. Several other agents are still marketed as Category III agents, pending final assessment of their status by the FDA. Antidiarrheal agents are classified in different categories on the basis of their chemical class or pharmacologic mechanism of action.

a. Antiperistaltic drugs

(1) **Mechanism of action.** Antiperistaltic drugs act directly on the circular and longitudinal musculature of the small and large intestine to normalize peristaltic intestinal movements. They slow intestinal motility and affect water and electrolyte movement through the bowel. The frequency of bowel movements is decreased, and the consistency of stools is increased.

(2) **Contraindication.** These agents should not be administered to patients with diarrhea secondary to invasive bacteria or pseudomembranous colitis, since these conditions may be worsened.

(3) **Prescription agents** in this class include the opiate and opiate-related agents including diphenoxylate/atropine (e.g., Lomotil) and difenoxin/atropine (e.g., Motofen).

(4) **Nonprescription agents. Loperamide** (e.g., Imodium A-D, Kaopectate II, Pepto Diarrhea Control) provides effective control of diarrhea as quickly as 1 hour after administration.

(a) **Side effects.** At recommended doses, loperamide is generally well tolerated. Side effects are infrequent and consist primarily of abdominal pain, distention, or discomfort; drowsiness; dizziness; and dry mouth.

(b) **Dosage information.** An **adult dose** is 4 mg followed by 2 mg after each unformed stool, not to exceed 16 mg/day. A **child's dose** is 1 mg to 2 mg up to three times per day, depending on weight and age.

b. Adsorbents. These medications adsorb toxins, bacteria, gases, and fluids. They are not absorbed systemically, so they produce few adverse effects. There are several products available; some are more effective than others, but none are very effective for severe acute diarrhea. These products are given for symptomatic relief, and are usually administered in large doses immediately following a loose stool.

(1) **Activated attapulgite** (e.g., Kaopectate Maximum Strength, Donnagel, Diar-Aid). Attapulgite is a naturally occurring aluminum magnesium silicate that absorbs eight times its weight in water. It is considered to be safe and effective in reducing the number of bowel movements, improving stool consistency, and relieving cramps associated with diarrhea.

(a) **Dosage information.** An **adult dose** is 1200 mg after each loose stool. A **child's dose** is 300 mg to 600 mg after each loose stool.

Table 37-1. Guidelines for Oral Replacement Therapy Established by the World Health Organization (WHO)

Ingredients	Dose
Sodium chloride (table salt)	90 mEq (0.5 teaspoon)
Potassium chloride (potassium salt)	20 mEq (0.25 teaspoons)
Sodium bicarbonate (baking soda)	30 mEq (0.5 teaspoons)
Glucose (sugar)	20 g (2 tablespoons)
Water	Enough to make 1 liter of solution

Table 37-2. Guidelines for Fluid and Electrolyte Replacement Therapy

Age Group	Dose
Adults (≥ 10 years)	2000–3000 ml/day
Children (5 to 10 years)	1000–2000 ml day
Children (< 5 years)	40–75 ml/kg for the first 6 hours **or** 5–10 ml every 10 to 15 minutes for 30 minutes then 15–20 ml every 10 to 15 minutes for 30 minutes then 30 ml (1 ounce) every 30 minutes to complete the first 6 hours 60 ml (2 ounces; ¼ cup) every 30 minutes for the next 12 hours Fluids as tolerated for the next 24 hours

(b) **Adverse effects.** Because activated attapulgite is inert and is not absorbed systemically, side effects are essentially nonexistent.

(2) **Calcium polycarbophil** (e.g., FiberCon, Mitrolan, Fiberall, Fiber-Lax) is a synthetic, hydrophilic polyacrylic resin that has the potential to absorb up to 60 times its weight in water. Polycarbophil has been shown to be safe and effective for the symptomatic treatment of diarrhea.

(a) **Side effects.** Like attapulgite, calcium polycarbophil is not systemically absorbed. It is metabolically inactive and essentially does not produce systemic side effects.

(b) **Dosage information.** An **adult dose** is 1 gram one to four times daily. A **child's dose** is 0.5 grams one to three times daily.

(3) **Additional adsorbents**

(a) **Kaolin/pectin.** Kaolin is a natural, hydrated aluminum silicate that is safe but has questionable efficacy. Pectin is a polymer extracted from citrus fruit rinds that also has questionable efficacy.

(i) An **adverse effect** is constipation.

(ii) **Dosage information.** An **adult dose** is 60 to 120 ml after each loose stool. A **child's dose** is 15 to 50 ml after each loose stool.

(b) **Activated charcoal** is a carbon residue powder that has been modified (i.e., activated) to increase its surface area and its adsorptive potency. Although this product is useful for adsorbing toxic substances (e.g., drug overdose), its effectiveness for the treatment of diarrhea is questionable since it can cause diarrhea or constipation.

c. **Miscellaneous agents**

(1) **Bismuth subsalicylate** (e.g., Pepto-Bismol). Bismuth salts work as adsorbents but also are believed to decrease secretion of water into the bowel. Bismuth preparations have moderate effectiveness against traveler's diarrhea, but doses required for relief are large and must be administered frequently so these preparations may be inconvenient.

(a) **Dose.** An **adult dose** is two tablets or 30 ml (524 mg) every hour as needed to a maximum of eight doses in a 24-hour period. A **child's dose** is ⅓ to ½ the adult dose. Bismuth subsalicylate can prevent traveller's diarrhea when two tablets are taken four times per day.

(b) **Adverse effects** may include harmless grayish-black stools or tongue and ringing in the ears, if high doses are taken or if the patient is simultaneously taking other salicylate products.

(c) **Contraindication.** Bismuth subsalicylate should not be given to children or teenagers during or after recovery from chicken pox or flu because of the possible association of salicylates with Reye syndrome.

(2) **Lactobacillus** (e.g., Bacid, Lactinex) products are intended to replace the normal bacterial flora that is lost during the administration of oral antibiotics. However, there is little information to show that these products are useful for antibiotic-induced diarrhea, so most clinicians do not recommend their use.

(3) **Lactase** (e.g., LactAid, Lactrase, Dairy Ease) is indicated for individuals who have insufficient amounts of lactase in the small intestine. Lactose (a disaccharide present in dairy products) must be broken down to glucose and galactose to be fully digested. If it is not, lactose draws water into the gastrointestinal tract and diarrhea results. Lactase is the enzyme responsible for digesting lactose. The dose is one to two capsules taken with milk or dairy products or added to milk prior to drinking. Titration of doses to higher levels may be required in some cases.

(4) **Anti-infectives.** Depending upon the suspected etiology of the infectious diarrhea, prescription antibiotics and antiprotozoal medications can be used to eradicate the organisms and decrease the duration of symptoms (Table 37-3). If antibiotics are used to prevent traveler's diarrhea, therapy should be started 1 day prior to arrival in high-incidence regions and continue until 2 days after departure. If diarrhea has occurred, antibiotic treatment should last for 7 days.

(5) **Anticholinergics** (e.g., atropine, hyoscyamine) decrease bowel motility, which results in an increase of fluid absorption from the intestinal tract and a decrease in abdominal cramping. These products are found in combination with adsorbents or opiates. However, the amount of anticholinergic found in most products is not considered to be enough to alter the course of severe acute diarrhea. **Adverse effects** include dry mouth, blurred vision, and tachycardia. These products should not be used in patients with narrow-angle glaucoma.

III. HEMORRHOIDS

III. HEMORRHOIDS have traditionally been defined as clusters of dilated blood vessels in the lower rectum (internal hemorrhoids) or anus (external hemorrhoids). Fairly recently, it has been determined that hemorrhoids simply represent downward displacement of anal cushions that contain arteriovenous anastomoses. Hemorrhoids are very common, and although they are considered a minor medical problem, they may cause considerable discomfort and anxiety. A proper diagnosis is important, however, since there are a number of conditions that may produce symptoms that mimic those of hemorrhoids (see III D). For example, colorectal cancer may produce bleeding, which is a common symptom of hemorrhoids. Fortunately, patient reassurance and the proper administration of a few simple treatments usually improves the condition.

A. Types of hemorrhoids are determined by their anatomic position and vascular origin.

1. An **internal hemorrhoid** is an exaggerated vascular cushion with an engorged internal hemorrhoidal plexus located above the dentate line and covered with a mucous membrane.

2. An **external hemorrhoid** is a dilated vein of the inferior hemorrhoidal plexus located below the dentate line and covered with squamous epithelium.

B. Causes of hemorrhoids. Although heredity may predispose a person to hemorrhoids, the exact cause is probably more clearly related to acquired factors.

1. Situations that result in **increased venous pressure in the hemorrhoidal plexus** (e.g., chronic straining during defecation; small, hard stools; prolonged sitting on the toilet; occupations that routinely require heavy lifting; and pregnancy) can transform an asymptomatic hemorrhoid into a problem.

2. The hemorrhoidal veins are pushed downward during defecation or straining, and, with increased venous pressure, they **dilate and become engorged**. Over time, the **fibers stretch** that anchor the hemorrhoidal veins to their underlying muscular coats, which results in **prolapse**.

Table 37-3. Drugs and Doses Used to Treat Infectious Diarrhea

Antibacterials	Antiprotozoals	Dose
Ciprofloxacin	N/A	500 mg twice daily
Doxycycline	N/A	100 mg twice daily
Norfloxacin	N/A	400 mg twice daily
Tetracycline	N/A	250 mg four times a day
Trimethoprim	N/A	1 tablet twice daily
N/A	Metronidazole	250 mg three times a day
N/A	Quinacrine	100 mg three times a day

C. Symptoms

1. The most common symptom of hemorrhoids is **painless bleeding** occurring during a bowel movement. The blood is usually bright red and may be visible on the stool, on the toilet tissue, or coloring the water in the toilet.

2. **Prolapse** is the second most common symptom of hemorrhoids. A temporary protrusion may occur during defection, and it may need to be replaced manually. A permanently prolapsed hemorrhoid may give rise to chronic, moist soiling of the underwear.

3. A less common presentation of hemorrhoids is **thrombosis,** and is the only time that a hemorrhoid should cause significant pain.

4. **Discomfort, pruritus, swelling, and discharge** may also occur with hemorrhoids.

D. Other conditions that may mimic hemorrhoids include the following, which usually require a physician.

1. An **anal abscess,** usually a *Staphylococcus* infection

2. **Cryptitis,** which is inflammation of the crypts (the small indentations at the mucocutaneous junction)

3. **Anal fissure,** which is a small tear in the lining of the anus

4. An **anal fistula,** which is an abnormal communication between the mucosa of the rectum and the skin adjacent to the anus

5. A **polyp,** which is a tumor of the large intestine

6. **Colorectal cancer**

E. Classification of hemorrhoids. Clinically, hemorrhoids are divided into four groups.

1. A **first-degree hemorrhoid** does not descend, or prolapse, during straining when defecating.

2. A **second-degree hemorrhoid** descends but returns spontaneously with relaxation.

3. A **third-degree hemorrhoid** requires manual replacement into the rectum after prolapse.

4. A **fourth-degree hemorrhoid** is permanently prolapsed.

F. Treatment. The symptoms of hemorrhoids are produced by a cycle of events: the protrusion of the vascular submucosal cushion through a tight anal canal, which becomes further congested and hypertrophic, which causes the cushion to protrude further. All treatments of hemorrhoids aim to break this cycle, and they fall into a number of broad groups.

1. **For first- and second-degree internal hemorrhoids that bleed minimally, a conservative approach can be taken.**
   a. To **reduce straining and downward pressure** on the hemorrhoids, patients should be told to avoid straining when defecating and to avoid sitting on the toilet longer than necessary.
   b. **Correction of constipation is of paramount importance.** This can be accomplished by eating a high-fiber diet and by increasing the intake of water. Bulk-forming laxatives, such as psyllium, and stool softeners, such as docusate, may be helpful.
   c. **Sitz baths** taken several times a day can soothe the anal mucosa. Warm (not hot) water should be used, and prolonged bathing should be avoided. Epsom salts (magnesium sulfate) added to the bath or the application of an ice pack can help reduce the swelling of an edematous or clotted hemorrhoid.
   d. **OTC hemorrhoidal ointments, creams, foams, and suppositories** may also help relieve symptoms (see III G).

2. If **chronic bleeding or repeated bouts of thrombosis** occur, a standard surgical hemorrhoidectomy or other surgical procedures may need to be performed.
   a. **Injection sclerotherapy** is used to affix the anal rectal mucosa and hemorrhoidal plexus to its underlying muscular coat and thereby reduce prolapse and bleeding.
   b. **Rubber band ligation** may be a useful procedure for treating second- and third-degree hemorrhoids, which involves placing a small rubber band around the base of these hemorrhoids. The ligated area sloughs off within a few days.
   c. **Photocoagulation, electrocoagulation, and cryotherapy** represent alternative methods of treating second- and third-degree hemorrhoids.

d. A traditional **hemorrhoidectomy** may ultimately be necessary. Disadvantages to this approach include a hospital stay of about 48 hours, use of an anesthetic, and post-operative pain.

3. An **external, thrombosed hemorrhoid** can be completely excised in an office setting, clinic, or operating room.

G. **Nonprescription medication for hemorrhoidal and other anorectal diseases.** The FDA has identified several ingredients as safe and effective to alleviate burning, discomfort, inflammation, irritation, itching, pain, and swelling. These products are simply palliative; they are not meant to cure hemorrhoids or other anorectal disease. Also, if these products do not improve symptoms within 7 days, a physician should be consulted. A physician should also be consulted if there is bleeding, prolapse of the hemorrhoid, seepage of feces, thrombosis, or severe pain.

1. **Ointments versus suppositories.** Generally, the ointment or cream dosage form is believed to be superior to a suppository, which may bypass the affected area. Patients should be advised to wash the anorectal area with mild soap and warm water and to pat (not wipe) the area dry before applying a product. Alternatively, they can use an OTC anal cleansing pad (e.g., Tucks).

2. **Local anesthetics** work by blocking nerve impulse transmission. They should be used for symptoms of pain, itching, burning, discomfort, and irritation in the perianal region or lower anal canal (not in the rectum).
   a. **Products** deemed safe and effective include benzocaine 5% to 20% (e.g., Americaine), pramoxine HCl 1% (e.g., Tronolane, Anusol), benzyl alcohol 1% to 4%, dibucaine and dibucaine HCl 0.25% to 1%, dyclonine HCl 0.5% to 1%, lidocaine 2% to 5% (e.g., Xylocaine), tetracaine and tetracaine HCl 0.5% to 1%.
   b. **Adverse effects.** These agents may produce a hypersensitivity reaction with burning and itching similar to that of anorectal disease.

3. **Vasoconstrictors** have been shown to decrease mucosal perfusion in the anorectal area after topical application. However, because bleeding in this area may be a sign of more serious disease, vasoconstrictors are not approved for control of minor bleeding. For temporary relief of itching and swelling, these agents have a local anesthetic effect of unknown mechanism.
   a. **Products** deemed safe and effective (although none of these agents are available in the dosage forms below) include ephedrine sulfate 0.1% to 0.125% in aqueous solution, epinephrine HCl 0.005% to 0.01% in aqueous solution, and phenylephrine HCl 0.25% in aqueous solution.
   b. **Contraindications** apply to people with cardiovascular disease, high blood pressure, hyperthyroidism, diabetes, and prostate enlargement because of the possibility of systemic absorption.

4. **Protectants** provide a physical barrier, forming a protective coating over skin or mucous membranes, for temporary relief of itching, irritation, discomfort, and burning. They prevent irritation of anorectal tissue and prevent water loss from the stratum corneum. Protectants are often the bases or vehicles for the other agents used for anorectal disease. Products include aluminum hydroxide gel, cocoa butter, kaolin, lanolin, mineral oil, white petrolatum, wood alcohols, glycerin (external), calamine, cod liver oil, shark liver oil, and zinc oxide in combination with one to three other protectants.
   a. **Absorbents** take up fluids that are on or secreted by skin or mucous membranes.
   b. **Adsorbents** attach to substances secreted by skin or mucous membranes.
   c. **Demulcents** combine with water to form a colloidal solution, which protects the skin in a way similar to mucus.
   d. **Emollients,** which are derived from animal or vegetable fats or petroleum products, soften or protect internal or external body surfaces.

5. **Astringents** lessen mucus and other secretions and protect underlying tissue through a local and limited protein coagulant effect. Action is limited to surface cells, but astringents provide temporary relief of itching, discomfort, irritation, and burning. Products considered to be safe and effective include calamine 5% to 25% (internal and external), witch hazel 10% to 50% (external), and zinc oxide 5% to 25%.

6. **Keratolytics** cause desquamation and debridement of the surface cells of the epidermis and provide temporary relief of discomfort and itching. It is theorized that keratolytics help expose underlying tissue to other therapeutic agents. Products considered to be safe and effective include aluminum chlorhydroxyallantoinate (alcloxa) 0.2% to 2.0% and resorcinol 1% to 3%.

7. **Analgesics, anesthetics, and antipruritics** provide temporary relief of burning, discomfort, itching, pain, and soreness. The FDA has redesignated several ingredients into this category that were formerly classified as counterirritants. Ingredients considered to be safe and effective for external use in the anorectal area include menthol 0.1% to 1%, juniper tar (1% to 5%), and camphor (0.1% to 3%).
8. **Wound-healing agents.** There are few ingredients that claim to be effective in promoting wound healing or tissue repair in the anorectal region. Live yeast cell derivative (skin respiratory factor), which is a water-soluble extract of brewer's yeast, is present in Preparation H and continues to undergo evaluation for effectiveness.
9. **Hydrocortisone and hydrocortisone acetate (0.25% to 1%)** work by causing vasoconstriction, stabilization of lysosomal membranes, and antimitotic activity. These agents have the potential to reduce itching, inflammation, and discomfort.

STUDY QUESTIONS

Directions: Each of the numbered items or incomplete statements in this section is followed by answers or by completions of the statement. Select the **one** lettered answer or completion that is **best** in each case.

1. All of the following are part of a standard conservative approach to the treatment of a first- or second-degree internal hermorrhoid EXCEPT

(A) Epsom salt sitz baths
(B) psyllium bulk laxatives
(C) avoiding prolonged sitting on the toilet
(D) a topical anesthetic/hemorrhoidal ointment
(E) injection sclerotherapy

2. All of the following agents are considered close to being ideal laxatives EXCEPT

(A) emollient laxatives
(B) bulk-forming laxatives
(C) fiber
(D) stimulant laxatives

3. All of the following rectal symptoms can be treated by over-the-counter (OTC) anorectal products EXCEPT

(A) bleeding
(B) itching
(C) burning
(D) discomfort
(E) irritation

4. All of the following statements about stool softeners are true EXCEPT

(A) there is minimal systemic absorption
(B) the onset of action is usually between 1–2 days
(C) they are useful in patients with constipation who have experienced an acute myocardial infarction
(D) they can be taken with little or no water

5. All of the following statements adequately describe bulk-forming laxatives EXCEPT

(A) they produce a much more complete evacuation of constipation than stimulant products
(B) they can cause constipation if not taken with water
(C) they are derived from polysaccharides, and they resemble fiber (bran) in the mechanism of action
(D) the onset of action is 24–72 hours

6. A patient suffering from acute infectious diarrhea caused by *Shigella* can be managed in all of the following ways EXCEPT

(A) not treating, since signs and symptoms usually resolve in 48 hours
(B) using solutions of glucose (e.g., soda, apple juice) to settle the stomach and decrease the number of stools
(C) avoiding food for at least 6 hours, then slowly increasing fluid intake
(D) using antibiotics (e.g., Bactrim, Doxycycline) for 7 days

---

1-E
2-D
3-A
4-D
5-A
6-B

Directions: Each item below contains three suggested answers of which **one or more** is correct. Choose the answer

A if **I only** is correct
B if **III only** is correct
C if **I and II** are correct
D if **II and III** are correct
E if **I, II, and III** are correct

7. Which of the following drugs most commonly cause constipation?

I. Ampicillin
II. Narcotic analgesics
III. Drugs possessing anticholinergic properties

8. Which of the following statements about stimulant laxatives is/are correct?

I. They produce a stool quicker than any other type of laxative
II. They are associated with more adverse effects than any other type of laxative
III. They work by irritating the lining of the colon wall to increase peristalsis and produce a stool

9. A patient experiencing diarrhea should be referred to a physician by a pharmacist

I. if the patient has pus or blood in the stool
II. if the patient also suffers from vomiting
III. if the patient has a fever

10. Which of the following statements about adsorbent drugs used for diarrhea are true?

I. They are safe because they are not absorbed systemically
II. Polycarbophil has been found to be the most effective agent
III. In general, small doses are enough to relieve diarrhea

7-D
8-D
9-E
10-C

ANSWERS AND EXPLANATIONS

1. The answer is E *[III F 1–2].*
A conservative approach to treatment includes sitz baths, the use of bulk laxatives to prevent straining when passing a stool, the avoidance of prolonged sitting on the toilet (as well as other good bowel habits), and the use of an anesthetic hemorrhoidal preparation. If improvement is not seen, more aggressive therapy may need to be pursued (e.g., injection sclerotherapy).

2. The answer is D *[I B 2].*
The ideal laxative is natural (i.e., similar to food) and produces a stool on a regular basis. The product produces a stool quickly (i.e., in several hours) without adverse effects such as abdominal cramping or the formation of a hard stool, which may be difficult to pass. Products such as fiber or bulk-forming agents produce a stool similar to a bolus of food, without adverse effects. Emollient laxatives (i.e., stool softeners) produce soft stools without difficult defecation. Stimulants produce a stool quickly, but patients often experience severe abdominal cramping and hard stools.

3. The answer is A *[III G 3].*
Because of the possibility that a serious anorectal condition (e.g., anorectal cancer) may cause bleeding, patients with this symptom should be referred to a physician for assessment. The vasoconstrictive agents that are present in some anorectal products may decrease bleeding, but these products cannot be labeled as doing so. Itching, burning, discomfort, and irritation may be abated by various over-the-counter products.

4. The answer is D *[I B 2 d].*
Stool softeners are safe and do not produce any adverse systemic effects. Since stool softeners work as surfactants, they allow absorption of water into the stool, which makes the stool softer and easier to pass. These products are useful in patients who should avoid straining to pass hard stools (e.g., post-myocardial infarction patients), since straining may be stressful to the patient. Each dose must be taken with 8 ounces of water.

5. The answer is A *[I B 2 a, c].*
Stimulant products result in a quicker, more complete, and often more violent evacuation of the bowel than do the bulk-forming agents. Bulk-forming agents are developed from complex sugars similar to fiber, which provide bulk to increase gastrointestinal motility and increase water absorption into the bowel. However, patients must drink plenty of water to facilitate the absorption of water into the bowel or they may become more constipated.

6. The answer is B *[II C; Table 37-3].*
Giving highly osmotic solutions of glucose (e.g., soda, fruit juice) can result in more water absorbed into the intestinal tract and, thus, further diarrhea. Many cases of diarrhea resolve within 48 hours without treatment. People with diarrhea can avoid food for at least 6 hours, then increase their fluid intake slowly. Severe cases of infectious diarrhea can be treated with antibiotics or antiprotozoals, depending on the organism that caused the episode.

7. The answer is D (II, III) *[I A 2 d].*
Opiate analgesics (e.g., narcotics) and drugs with anticholinergic properties decrease bowel motility, which results in increased water absorption from the intestinal tract. This can cause a harder, drier stool, which results in constipation. Ampicillin is often poorly absorbed from the intestinal tract and can alter the flora of the intestinal bowel. This destruction of bowel organisms causes increased secretions into the bowel, which results in diarrhea.

8. The answer is D (II, III) *[I B 2 c].*
Stimulant laxatives do have a quick onset of action, but not any quicker than the saline laxatives, which usually work in 4 to 6 hours. The mechanism of action for stimulant laxatives is that they irritate the lining of the colon wall, which increases peristalsis and produces a stool. These laxatives are associated with more adverse effects than other laxatives.

9. The answer is E (all) *[II B 2].*
Patients with pus or blood in the stool, vomiting, or fever may be suffering from severe bacterial diarrhea and may lose large amounts of fluid, which could result in severe dehydration.

10. The answer is C (I, II) *[II C 2 b].*
Large doses of adsorbents are needed to decrease symptoms slightly, but overall these agents are not very effective. Adsorbents are not effective for severe diarrhea because they cannot adsorb enough water and they do not eliminate the cause. Of all the adsorbents, polycarbophil has been found to be the most effective, probably because it can adsorb more water than other products. All adsorbents are safe since they are not adsorbed systemically.

38

OTC Products: Menstrual, Vaginal, and Contraceptive

Constance McKenzie Fleming
Larry N. Swanson

I. MENSTRUATION AND MENSTRUAL PRODUCTS

A. Introduction. Menstruation is a cyclic, physiologic discharge of blood and mucus through the vagina of a nonpregnant woman. The menstrual cycle eliminates a mature, unfertilized egg and prepares the endometrium for the possible implantation of a fertilized egg the following month. The **average duration** of the menstrual cycle is 28 days. The duration of menstrual flow is from 3 to 7 days.

B. Menstrual abnormalities

1. **Dysmenorrhea** is painful menstruation.
   a. **Types**
      (1) **Primary dysmenorrhea** is pain associated with menstruation with the absence of identifiable pelvic disease. It is prompted by increased levels of prostaglandins in the menstrual fluids.
      (2) **Secondary dysmenorrhea** is associated with an underlying pelvic disorder.
   b. **Symptoms** of dysmenorrhea often include nausea, vomiting, diarrhea, headache, dizziness, and lower abdominal cramping.
   c. **Treatment**
      (1) **Recommendation of therapy** should be based on the patient's assessment of the degree of pain. Pain associated with dysmenorrhea generally tapers within 2 days. Prolonged pain may be associated with an underlying problem, and patients should be referred to a physician.
      (2) **Agents** for the relief of dysmenorrhea include:
         (a) **Analgesics** are used as primary treatment of dysmenorrhea and for relief of cramping associated with premenstrual syndrome (PMS; see I B 4). Analgesic treatment with aspirin or acetaminophen may begin at the onset of the menstrual period and continue throughout the menstrual flow.
         (b) **Nonsteroidal anti-inflammatory** drugs (NSAIDs) have been approved for the treatment of primary dysmenorrhea. The dosage of ibuprofen is 200 mg every 4 to 6 hours with the maximum not exceeding 1200 mg per day. Other NSAIDs include aspirin and acetaminophen.
         (c) **Diuretics** are recommended by the Food and Drug Administration (FDA) for use in eliminating water during premenstrual and menstrual periods. When administered approximately 5 days before menses, diuretics help relieve bloating, excess water, cramps, and tension. Included in this category are ammonium chloride, caffeine, and pamabrom.
            (i) **Ammonium chloride** (NH_4Cl) is an acid-forming salt often used in combination with caffeine. Up to three grams of NH_4Cl per day can be administered in three divided doses per day. Larger doses are often associated with gastrointestinal symptoms. Over-the-counter (OTC) products include Aqua Ban and Aqua Ban Plus, which contains NH_4Cl and caffeine.
            (ii) **Caffeine,** a xanthine derivative, promotes diuresis by inhibiting tubular reabsorption of sodium and chloride. The **recommended dosage** is 100 to 200 mg every 3 to 4 hours. **Side effects** associated with caffeine use are gastrointestinal disturbances and sleeplessness.
            (iii) **Pamabrom** (Midol PMS and Pamprin) is a theophylline derivative often used in combination with analgesics and antihistamines. Dosages should not exceed 200 mg per day.

2. **Amenorrhea** is an absence of menstruation. The development of primary or secondary amenorrhea requires physician evaluation.

3. **Intermenstrual pain and bleeding** generally occurs at midcycle and may last from several hours to days. Pain is often associated with ovulation (mittelschmerz). Therapy consists of nonprescription analgesics. Patients with pain lasting longer than 2 days should be referred to a physician.

4. **Premenstrual syndrome (PMS)**
   a. **Symptoms** (e.g., marked mood swings, fatigue, appetite changes, bloating) begin 1 to 7 days before the onset of menses.
   b. **Nonpharmacologic therapy** includes regular exercise and reduction of stress factors. Patients experiencing symptoms abnormal to their cycle should be referred to a physician.
   c. **Pharmacologic treatment.** The efficacy and safety of pharmacologic treatment of PMS is aimed at the proposed etiologies (e.g., a drop in progesterone concentrations, high levels of prolactin, elevated estrogen concentrations, deficiencies of vitamin A or vitamin B_6, or an underlying disorder) and is not well studied.

C. **Toxic shock syndrome (TSS)** is a rare but sometimes fatal disease associated with the use of tampons during menstruation.

1. This condition usually affects women under 30 years of age who use tampons. Women between the ages of 15 and 19 years are at the highest risk.

2. TSS is characterized by an abrupt onset of flulike symptoms (e.g., high fever, myalgias, vomiting, diarrhea).

3. When TSS is suspected, patients should be hospitalized immediately. To lower the risk of TSS, women should use lower-absorbancy tampons and alternate the use of tampons with feminine pads.

II. VAGINAL PRODUCTS

A. Yeast infections

1. **General considerations**
   a. **Occurrence.** Approximately 75% of women will experience a yeast infection at least once, while 15% to 20% may have a recurrence.
   b. **Cause.** The most common cause of this type of vaginitis is *Candida albicans*.
   c. **Predisposing factors** for vaginal candidiasis include antibiotics, diabetes, pregnancy, and sexual intercourse.
   d. **Symptoms** include vaginal burning, discomfort, itching, or abnormal vaginal discharge.

2. **Pharmacologic treatment. Nonprescription agents** are recommended for patients who have had prior yeast infections and who can potentially accurately diagnose and self-medicate. **Imidazole antifungal agents** (e.g., Gyne-Lotrimin and Monistat 7) are available OTC.
   a. Infections should be treated for 7 consecutive days.
   b. Patients should refrain from intercourse during therapy.
   c. If medication causes burning, if symptoms worsen, or if there is no response to treatment, a physician should be contacted.

B. Feminine hygiene products

1. There are a variety of feminine hygiene products available for cleansing and controlling the odor associated with vaginal discharge.

2. Vaginal douches irrigate the vagina and can be used for cleansing, soothing and refreshing, as an astringent, or to produce a mucolytic effect.

3. Vaginal suppositories are used for soothing and refreshing, to relieve minor irritations, and to reduce the number of pathogenic microorganisms.

III. OTC CONTRACEPTIVES

A. Introduction. The **efficacy** and **pregnancy rates** for various means of contraception depend greatly upon the **degree of compliance**. The relative effectiveness of various contraceptive methods is reported in Table 38-1. The pregnancy rate is calculated as pregnancies per 100 woman years.

$$\text{Pregnancy rate per 100 woman years} = 1200 \times \frac{\text{total number of conceptions}}{\text{total months of exposure}}$$

B. Methods of contraception that may make use of nonprescription products or devices include:

1. Rhythm

a. The theory behind rhythm is calculation of the probable day of ovulation and abstinence from sexual intercourse for a period of time before and after.

b. To prevent pregnancy by the rhythm method, the patient must understand the significance of ovulation and that:

(1) It usually occurs 14 ± 2 days before the onset of menses.

(2) An ova is viable for approximately 24 hours, but can survive up to 72 hours; a sperm is viable for approximately 48 hours, but can survive for as long as 7 days. Thus, the span of fertility may last from 7 days before ovulation to 3 days after.

c. Disadvantages to the rhythm method (but necessary to ensure efficacy) include both the **long periods of abstinence** and the **charting of menses** that is required.

d. Three approaches may be used to calculate the period of abstinence—**basal temperature determination, calendar method,** and the **observation of cervical mucus change** (i.e., Billing's method).

(1) Basal temperature determination makes use of a **basal thermometer,** which can be purchased without a prescription. The thermometer covers the range of temperature from 96°F–100°F and has 0.1°F gradations.

(a) The significance of basal temperature determination lies in the fact that within 24

Table 38-1. Pregnancy Rates for Various Means of Contraception

Method of Contraception	Pregnancies/100 Woman Years
Oral contraceptives	
≥ 35 μg Ethinyl estradiol	< 1
≥ 50 μg Mestranol	< 1
≤ 35 μg or less Ethinyl estradiol	> 1
Progestin only	3
Mechanical/chemical	
Intrauterine device (IUD)	< 1–6
Levonorgestrel implants	< 1
Diaphragm (with spermicidal cream or gel)	2–20
Vaginal sponge	9–27*
Aerosol foams	2–29
Condoms	3–36
Gels and creams	4–36
Rhythm (all types)	< 1–47
Calendar method	14–47
Temperature method	1–20
Temperature method (intercourse in postovulatory phase only)	< 1–7
Mucus method	1–25
No contraception	60–80

Reprinted with permission from *Drug Facts and Comparisons*. St. Louis, Facts and Comparisons, Division of JB Lippincott, 1991.

*Highest failure rate in parous women.

hours preceding ovulation, there is a **moderate drop in the basal temperature** followed by a **noticeable rise in the body temperature,** usually about 24 hours after ovulation. This rise is usually maintained for the remainder of the cycle and is thought to be due to the thermogenic properties of **progesterone,** the hormone indicative of the transition from the ovulatory phase to the luteal phase. Therefore, ovulation is represented by the transition of the falling temperature to the rising temperature.

(b) For many women, abstinence should be practiced from approximately 5 days after the onset of menses until 3 days after the transition in temperature.

(c) To minimize any fluctuation nonreflective of basal temperature, the thermometer should be shaken down the evening before and kept at bedside. Because the basal temperature reflects the amount of heat radiation when the body is at its metabolic low, the temperature should be taken first thing in the morning (i.e., before any activity). The thermometer may be placed under the tongue, in the rectum, or in the vagina (the temperature should always be taken from the same place) and should be left undisturbed for at least 5 minutes. Infections, tension, a restless night, or any type of excessive movement can cause variations nonreflective of the basal temperature.

(2) The calendar method estimates the possible day of ovulation. Abstinence should be practiced during the period around ovulation when there may be a fertilizable egg present.

(a) For a span of approximately 1 year, the patient records her menstruation dates on a calendar.

(b) The calendar is then reviewed to determine the length of her shortest and longest cycle.

(i) Eighteen days should be subtracted from the number of days of the shortest cycle. This number should correspond with the first possible fertile day in any given cycle [see III B 1 b—14 + 2 = 16 days; 16 + 2 = 18 days (viability of sperm)].

(ii) Eleven days should be subtracted from the number of days of the longest cycle. This number should correspond with the last possible fertile day in any given cycle [see III B 1 b—14 − 2 = 12 days; 12 − 1 = 11 days (viability of ova)].

(c) Abstinence should be practiced from the first possible fertile day through the last possible fertile day.

(d) Example. Assume the shortest number of days between two consecutive menses is 25 and the longest number of days between two consecutive menses is 32. Eighteen days subtracted from 25 days (the shortest cycle) equals 7 (or day 7). Eleven days subtracted from 32 days (the longest cycle) equals 21 (or day 21). Therefore, abstinence should be practiced from day 7 through and including day 21 of each cycle.

(3) The Billings method of rhythm is based on the principle that the normal, thick, creamy white vaginal mucus becomes clear and tenacious around the time of ovulation—much like a raw egg white.

(a) The woman should watch for this change in mucus consistency and practice abstinence around the time of ovulation.

(b) The woman should consider herself fertile for 3–4 days after the peak change.

(4) The sympto—thermal method, rather than relying on a single physiologic index, uses several indices to determine the fertile period.

(a) The most common calendar calculations and **changes in the cervical mucus** are used to estimate the **onset of the fertile period.**

(b) Changes in the mucus or basal temperature are used to estimate the end of the fertile period.

(c) Because several indices need to be monitored, this method is more difficult to learn than the single-index method, but it is more effective than the cervical-mucus method alone.

2. Spermicidal agents are composed of an **active spermicidal chemical,** which immobilizes or kills sperm, and an **inert base** (e.g., foam, cream or jelly), which localizes the spermicidal chemical in proximity to the cervical os.

a. Mode of action. These agents work by disrupting the sperm membrane and by decreasing the ability of sperm to metabolize fructose.

b. Active ingredients (i.e., **nonoxynol-9** or **octoxynol-9**)
   (1) Both are considered safe and effective by the FDA.
   (2) Side effects (e.g., sensation of warmth, rare allergic reactions) are minimal.
   (3) There are no significant differences in birth-defect rates between users and nonusers.

c. Effects against sexually transmitted diseases (STDs). These agents have some effects on several STDs, as summarized below:
   (1) In vitro inactivation of human immunodeficiency virus (HIV)
   (2) In vitro inactivation and decreased infection rate of gonorrhea
   (3) In vitro inactivation and decreased infection rate of chlamydia
   (4) Reduced risk of bacterial vaginosis
   (5) Reduced risk of trichomoniasis
   (6) Evidence lacking of effectiveness against herpes, hepatitis B, syphilis, and cytomegalovirus

d. Dosage forms. Contraceptive spermicides offer the greatest variety within one specific method of contraception, being available in various forms, including the following.
   (1) Creams and jellies are used with a diaphragm. The concentration of spermicide is less than the necessary 8% to be employed as a single contraceptive method.
   (2) Foams disperse better into the vagina and over the cervical opening. They usually contain a higher concentration of spermicide (i.e., they contain the optimal concentration of 8% or higher). Volume differences among brands may require various dosage amounts. If vaginal or penile irritation develops, another brand should be tried.
      (a) The can should be shaken vigorously 20 times before use.
      (b) The foam should be inserted intravaginally about two-thirds the length of the applicator, and the contents should be discharged.
      (c) Foam should be reapplied during prolonged intercourse (e.g., that lasting longer than 1 hour) and before every subsequent act of intercourse.
      (d) In order to ensure efficacy, at least 8 hours should pass before douching.
   (3) Suppositories and foaming tablets. These agents are both small and convenient. Although solid at room temperature, suppositories melt at body temperature while foaming tablets effervesce.
      (a) The tablets should be wetted prior to insertion, which may create a sensation of warmth.
      (b) The tablet or suppository should be inserted high into the vagina, and approximately 10–15 minutes should pass before intercourse.
      (c) Intercourse must occur within 1 hour, or the dose must be repeated.
      (d) Another tablet or suppository should be inserted before each repeated act of intercourse.
      (e) In order to ensure efficacy, 6–8 hours after the last act of intercourse should pass before douching.
   (4) The **vaginal contraceptive sponge** is a disposable polyurethane sponge that contains 1 g of nonoxynol-9. It is smaller and thicker than a diaphragm and has an indentation on one side.
      (a) Mode of action. The vaginal sponge acts as a contraceptive in three ways: It releases spermicide; blocks the cervical os; and absorbs seminal fluid.
      (b) Use
         (i) The sponge is moistened with 2 tablespoonfuls of water.
         (ii) It is folded and inserted high into the vagina.
         (iii) Once inserted, the sponge is protective immediately, as well as for the next 24 hours.
         (iv) To ensure efficacy, the sponge should be left in place for at least 6 hours after intercourse.
      (c) Precautions. To reduce the risk of TSS, women should wash their hands before insertion, refrain from using the products during menstruation or during the postpartum period, and avoid retention of the sponge for more than 24 hours.
   (5) Film comes as small paper-thin sheets. It is inserted into the vagina; 5 minutes must pass before intercourse.

3. Condoms are used to prevent transmission of sperm into the vagina.

a. Types. They are made either of latex rubber or of processed collagenous lamb caecum sheaths (lambskin).

(1) **Latex** condoms may help prevent the transmission of many STDs. They are usually packaged with the following label "when used properly, the latex condom may prevent the transmission of many STDs such as syphilis, gonorrhea, chlamydia infections, genital herpes, and AIDS."
   (a) Latex affords greater elasticity than lambskin, and latex condoms are more likely to remain in place on the penis.
   (b) Various types are available (e.g., lubricated, ribbed, colored) including some with spermicide. There is a standard size, but recently smaller and larger versions were put on the market.
      (i) Latex condoms are available with a plain end or with a reservoir tip (sometimes designated as "enz"). The reservoir tip provides room for the ejaculate; however, a space may be left when using the plain-end condom, which accommodates the fluid just as effectively.
      (ii) The prelubricated condom helps prevent dyspareunia in a couple with insufficient natural lubrication. Prelubrication decreases the risk of tearing the condom. However, the extra lubrication may be excessive, to the extent of lessening sexual fulfillment in a couple who have adequate natural lubrication or when contraceptive foam is also used.
      (iii) Latex rubber may cause an allergic reaction, especially with continued exposure.

(2) **Lambskin** condoms are not considered as effective as latex condoms (and cannot be labelled as such) in preventing the transmission of STDs, including acquired immune deficiency syndrome (AIDS). The lambskin condoms are structured to consist of membranes that reveal layers of fibers crisscrossing in various patterns. This gives the lambskin strength, but also allows for an occasional pore. Therefore, lambskin may allow HIV, which is smaller than a sperm, to pass through.
   (a) Lambskin has less elasticity than latex, and lambskin condoms may slip off the penis.
   (b) Lambskin affords greater sensitivity than latex.
   (c) Lambskin condoms are more expensive than latex condoms.

b. **Advantages and disadvantages.** The relative accessibility, ease of transport, and low cost make condoms an attractive method of contraception. However, the coital act must be interrupted to apply the condom, and often one or both partners complain of a partial or complete decrease in sensation.

c. **Use**

(1) The female external genitalia should not be touched with the exposed penis, and the vagina should not be penetrated, until the condom is unrolled onto the erect penis.
(2) The condom should be unrolled onto the penis as far as it will go. With the plain-end condom, a space between the tip of the penis and the tip of the condom should be allowed to catch the ejaculate.
(3) With either reservoir-tip or plain-end condoms, the tip of the condom must be held between the thumb and index finger to avoid trapping air while unrolling the condom onto the penis. (The space will decrease the likelihood both of rupture secondary to pressure and regurgitation of the ejaculate onto the external genitalia.)
(4) Proper lubrication to minimize the possibility of tearing can be ensured by using either a lubricated condom or by applying K-Y jelly, spermicidal cream or jelly to either the condom or the woman's genitalia. [Petroleum jelly (Vaseline®) should never be used since it causes deterioration of the rubber; it is also a poor lubricant.] Spermicidal foam, cream, or jelly is an excellent adjunctive contraceptive.
(5) **Before the penis becomes flaccid,** it must be withdrawn from the vagina and the condom eased off. The condom should be handled with special care so as not to lose it into the vagina or spill any of the ejaculatory fluid onto the external genitalia.
(6) A condom should never be reused.
(7) Condoms should not be stored near excessive heat.
(8) If the condom should break or leak, spermicide should be immediately inserted vaginally.

4. **The condom for women** is a **disposable polyurethane sac** that fits into the vagina and provides protection from pregnancy and STDs. The sac resembles a **plastic vaginal pouch** and **consists of an inner ring and an outer ring**. The inner ring is inserted near the cervix, much like a diaphragm, while the outer ring is spread over the front of the vaginal area.

5. **The diaphragm** is a contraceptive device that is self-inserted into the vagina to block access of sperm to the cervix. It requires a prescription but must be used in conjunction with a nonprescription spermicide to seal off crevices between the vaginal wall and the device.
   - **a.** The diaphragm is held in place by the spring tension of a wire rim encased by rubber. When positioned properly, the diaphragm forms a flexible dome to cover the cervix, the sides pressing against the vaginal muscle wall and the pubic bone.
   - **b.** There are **four types of diaphragms** including the **coil spring,** the **flat spring, the arcing spring** and a **wide-seal rim**. The tone of vaginal muscles as well as the position of the uterus and adjacent organs usually determine the type of diaphragm necessary.
   - **c.** Sizes of the diaphragm range from 50 mm to 105 mm in diameter, in 5-mm gradations.
   - **d. Use**
     - **(1)** Prior to inserting the diaphragm one teaspoonful (2″–3″ ribbon) of spermicidal cream or jelly is spread over the inside of the rubber dome.
     - **(2)** Also, spermicide is spread around the rim to permit a good seal between the diaphragm and the vaginal wall. (For added protection, it is applied outside of the dome.)
     - **(3)** To ensure efficacy, the diaphragm should not be removed for 6–8 hours after intercourse.
   - **e. Proper care of the diaphragm**
     - **(1)** The diaphragm should be washed with soap and water, rinsed thoroughly, and dried with a towel.
     - **(2)** It should be dusted with cornstarch and kept in its original container (away from heat).
6. **The cervical cap** is the prescription rubber device smaller than a diaphragm, that fits over the cervix like a thimble. It is more difficult to fit than the diaphragm.
   - **a.** The cap should be filled one-third full of spermicide cream or jelly; the spermicide is then applied to the rim.
   - **b.** The cervical cap may be left in place for a maximum of 48 hours and should be left in place at least 8 hours after intercourse.

STUDY QUESTIONS

Directions: The numbered item in this section is followed by answers or by completions of the statement. Select the **one** lettered answer or completion that is **best**.

1. For how many consecutive days should a yeast infection be treated?

(A) 3
(B) 5
(C) 7
(D) 10

Directions: The question below contains three suggested answers of which **one or more** is correct. Choose the answer

A if **I only** is correct
B if **III only** is correct
C if **I and II** are correct
D if **II and III** are correct
E if **I, II, and III** are correct

2. True statements about the vaginal sponge include which of the following?

I. It acts as a physical barrier to sperm
II. It is impregnated with a nonionic spermicide
III. It may be inserted up to 24 hours prior to intercourse

Directions: The group of items in this section consists of lettered options followed by a set of numbered items. For each item, select the **one** lettered option that is most closely associated with it. Each lettered option may be selected once, more than once, or not at all.

Questions 3–4

Match the following primary nonprescription treatments with the correct drug.

(A) Diuretics
(B) Salicylates
(C) Nonsteroidal anti-inflammatory drugs (NSAIDs)
(D) Narcotic analgesics

3. The primary nonprescription pharmacologic treatment for pain associated with dysmenorrhea

4. Recommended by the Food and Drug Administration (FDA) for elimination of water prior to and during menstruation

---

1-C
2-E
3-C
4-A

ANSWERS AND EXPLANATIONS

1. The answer is C *[II A 2].*
The recommended length of therapy with imidazole antifungal agents, which are the primary treatment for yeast infections, is 7 days. A physician should be contacted for those patients who do not respond to nonprescription therapy.

2. The answer is E (all) *[III B 2 d (4)].*
The vaginal sponge is a relatively new contraceptive device. Made of polyurethane and impregnated with a nonionic surfactant spermicide, the vaginal sponge serves both as a physical barrier and as a spermicidal agent. It may be inserted as early as 24 hours before intercourse, and intercourse may be repeated during that time period without the need for a new sponge or additional spermicide.

3–4. The answers are: 3-C *[I B 1 c (2) (b)],* **4-A** *[I B 1 c (2) (c)].*
Nonsteroidal anti-inflammatory drugs (NSAIDs) are approved by the Food and Drug Administration (FDA) for the treatment of primary dysmenorrhea. For premenstrual and menstrual relief of water retention, bloating, and tension, the FDA has approved over-the-counter (OTC) diuretics.

Part IV
Clinical Pharmacy and Therapeutics

Alan H. Mutnick
Paul F. Souney

39
Therapeutic Drug Monitoring

Lyndon D. Braun

I. INTRODUCTION

A. Basic pharmacokinetic terms

1. **Bioavailability** is the fraction of an administered dose that reaches the systemic circulation.
2. **Volume of distribution** is the amount of drug in the body relative to the concentration of drug in the blood (or plasma).

$$V_D = D/C_p,$$

where V_D is the apparent volume of distribution, D is the drug dose, and C_p is the plasma concentration of the drug.

3. **Clearance** is the volume of blood (or plasma) that can be completely cleared of a drug per unit of time (units = volume/time).
4. **Half-life** is the time required for the drug concentration in the plasma to be reduced by 50%, provided no drug absorption occurs during the decline. Half-life is also a measure of the time required for the drug concentration in the plasma to reach a steady-state concentration with a new dosing regimen.
5. **Steady-state concentration** is the drug concentration at which the body is in equilibrium (i.e., the rate of drug absorption equals drug elimination).
6. **Loading dose** is the amount of drug that must be administered to bring the drug concentration in the blood (or plasma) into the therapeutic range rapidly when initiating therapy or when increasing the dosing rate after inadequate therapy.
7. **Maintenance dose** is the amount of drug that must be administered to maintain a steady-state concentration.
8. **Dosing interval** is the amount of time between consecutive doses of a regularly administered drug. This is usually a multiple of 24 hours or a number that is easily divided into 24 hours.
9. **Trough or minimum concentration** is the lowest concentration of a drug within a dosing interval. This typically is reached at the end of the dosing interval, immediately before the next dose is administered.
10. **Peak or maximum concentration** is the highest drug concentration within a dosing interval. Peak concentration usually is reached within 2 hours of dose administration, but it depends on the route of administration.

B. Drug criteria for therapeutic drug monitoring (Tables 39-1 and 39-2)

1. **Serum drug concentration** and the **concentration at the receptor site** must be in equilibrium.
2. **Intensity** and **duration of the pharmacodynamic effect (efficacy** and **toxicity)** must be correlated with the timing of the sampling and drug concentration at the receptor site.

C. Benefits of therapeutic drug monitoring

1. At the initiation of drug therapy when rapid and effective treatment is needed, as in antibiotic therapy or anticonvulsant therapy, drug monitoring quickly determines the proper dose and dosing rate.

Table 39-1. Drugs Commonly Monitored Through Plasma Levels

Antibiotics	Cardiovascular Agents
Amikacin	Digoxin
Chloramphenicol	Disopyramide
Gentamicin	Lidocaine
Tobramycin	Procainamide
Vancomycin	Quinidine
Anticonvulsants	**Other Drugs**
Carbamazepine	Cyclosporine
Ethosuximide	Lithium
Phenobarbital	Salicylic acid
Phenytoin	Theophylline
Primidone	
Valproic acid	

2. During maintenance therapy in stable, chronically ill patients, such as those requiring antiarrhythmic therapy or antimanic therapy, drug monitoring determines the best possible dosage regimen—one that provides a therapeutic outcome while avoiding toxicity.
3. When interacting drugs are added to or removed from a dosage regimen, drug monitoring maintains optimal therapy.
4. Patients with altered physiologic and pharmacokinetic parameters may benefit from therapeutic drug monitoring.
   a. **Impaired renal function**
      (1) Dosage modification may be necessary, depending on the extent of renal impairment and the amount of drug normally excreted unchanged in the urine.
      (2) Renal function normally declines with increasing age; therefore, middle-aged and older patients, in addition to patients with nephrotoxicity or acute or chronic renal failure, may require therapeutic monitoring.
      (3) Measurement of creatinine clearance can estimate renal function, using the **Cockcroft and Gault equation**:

$$\frac{(140 - \text{age in years})\ (\text{body weight in kg})\ (0.85 \text{ for females})}{(72)\ (\text{serum creatinine in mg/dl})} = \text{creatinine clearance in ml/min.}$$

   b. **Impaired hepatic function**
      (1) Dosage modification may be necessary in patients with impaired hepatic function, depending on the:
         (a) Extent of hepatic impairment, which is often difficult to determine

Table 39-2. Drugs Occasionally Monitored Through Plasma Levels

Anticonvulsants	Cardiovascular Agents
Clonazepam	N-acetylprocainamide
Mephenytoin	Amiodarone
	Encainide
Antidepressants	Flecainide
Amitriptyline	Mexiletine
Doxepin	Propranolol
Fluoxetine	Tocainide
Imipramine	Verapamil
Maprotiline	
Trazodone	**Other Drugs**
	Fluphenazine
Toxic Agents	Methotrexate
Acetaminophen	
Ethanol	
Cocaine	

(b) Amount of drug normally metabolized
(c) Contribution of metabolites to therapeutic efficacy or toxicity

(2) Impaired hepatic albumin production may necessitate a dosage change for drugs that are highly protein-bound.

(3) Unlike renal function tests, liver function tests measure the presence of hepatic injury, not the extent of hepatic function.

c. **Congestive heart failure (CHF)** can impair absorption, distribution, and elimination of many drugs.

d. Disease states and other changes that affect **protein binding** are discussed in IV D.

II. ROUTES OF DRUG ADMINISTRATION

A. Intravenous administration. This route delivers 100% of the drug directly into the circulation (bioavailability = 100%).

1. **Bolus.** The entire dose is administered rapidly, producing a high plasma concentration and, usually, the most rapid effect. **Injection volume** is limited only by the size of the patient (i.e., plasma volume) and the properties (i.e., toxicities) of the drug or fluid administered.

2. **Infusion.** The drug is administered at a constant rate. At steady state, the rate of drug administration is equal to the rate of drug elimination. After 1 half-life, plasma concentration is 50% of the way to steady-state concentration; after 2 half-lives, 75%; and after 3.3 half-lives, 90%. **Injection volume** is unlimited.

B. Subcutaneous administration. The drug is injected into subcutaneous tissue (bioavailability ≤ 100%).

1. **Entry of the drug** into the circulation is slower than with intravenous administration and is limited by drug solubility, drug lipophilicity, and subcutaneous circulation.

2. The **peak effect** is generally much less than with intravenous administration; however, the **duration of effect** is generally longer than with intravenous administration, owing to slower release into the circulation.

3. The **maximum injection volume** is approximately 1 ml.

C. Intramuscular administration. The drug is administered into muscle tissue, usually deep muscle, such as the gluteus or deltoid (bioavailability ≤ 100%).

1. **Entry of the drug** into the circulation is slower than with intravenous administration and is limited by drug solubility, drug lipophilicity, and muscular circulation.

2. The **peak effect** is generally much less than with intravenous administration; however, the **duration of effect** is generally longer than with intravenous administration, owing to slower release into the circulation.

3. **Administration into a depot site** of a minimally soluble drug or vehicle can produce therapeutic levels of some drugs for up to 2–4 weeks.

4. The **maximum injection volume** is approximately 2–5 ml.

D. Intradermal administration. The drug is injected into dermal tissue. This route is generally used for local effects (e.g., allergy testing) and only rarely, if ever, for systemic effects, due to poor distribution into the systemic circulation. The **maximum injection volume** is approximately 1 ml.

E. Oral administration. The drug is swallowed (bioavailability ≤ 100%). Entry of the drug into the circulation is slower than with intravenous administration and limited by many factors.

1. **First-pass effect.** Orally administered drugs must pass through the portal circulation and the liver before entering the systemic circulation. This reduces the bioavailability of many drugs because they are significantly metabolized before reaching the bloodstream. Some drugs must be administered in much larger doses orally than intravenously (e.g., propranolol requires an oral dose 20–40 times larger than its intravenous dose).

2. **Metabolic activation.** Some drugs are activated on passage through the liver before entering the systemic circulation. Drugs that are administered in inactive form (e.g., clorazepate, sulindac) must be metabolically altered to a physiologically active and available form. This type

of drug would have a much smaller effect if administered intravenously since only a small fraction of the systemic circulation passes through the liver. This situation contrasts with gastrointestinal absorption in which virtually all of the portal circulation passes through the liver.

F. Sublingual administration. The drug is administered by placement under the tongue (**bioavailability is ≤ 100%** but often greater than with oral administration). The advantages of this administration route include rapid absorption, due to the vascularity of sublingual tissues, and increased bioavailability, because sublingual circulation passes directly into the systemic circulation rather than into the portal circulation. The usual sublingual form is a tablet, but some agents are commercially available in a spray.

G. Rectal administration. The drug is administered rectally, usually in suppository form, but otherwise as a liquid (**bioavailability ≤ 100%**). **Absorption** is slow, erratic, and often incomplete. Bioavailability may be greater than with oral administration because only one (the superior hemorrhoidal vein) of the three rectal veins empties into the portal circulation.

H. Vaginal administration. The drug is administered vaginally as a suppository, tablet, cream, or foam. **Drug effects** are usually local, but systemic absorption does occur through the vaginal mucosa. Systemic effects are usually side effects, rather than the desired therapeutic goal.

I. Topical administration. The drug is applied to the skin and absorbed into the systemic circulation after passing through all five layers of the stratum corneum (the outermost epidermis).

1. **Bioavailability** is variable and depends on the thickness of the skin surface, circulation in the local area, drug lipophilicity, and skin condition (see III D).
2. **Advantages** of topical drug administration include a long duration of action and the ability to remove the dosage form once it has been administered.
3. **Absorption** is generally slower than with most other routes of administration.

J. Inhalation. The drug is inhaled into the lungs, where the site of action may be local (e.g., beclomethasone) or systemic (e.g., enflurane, other inhalational anesthetics).

1. **Absorption** is generally rapid, due to the vascular nature of the pulmonary capillary system, but it also depends on drug lipophilicity, droplet or particle size, pulmonary function, and respiratory status.
2. **Excretion.** Most systemic inhaled drugs are generally short-acting (minutes to hours) and may be eliminated by the lungs. Locally acting inhaled drugs generally have longer durations of action and may last from 2 to 12 hours or more.

K. Buccal administration. The drug is absorbed through the oral mucosa, after being placed between the cheek and the gums. Absorption is usually rapid, and bioavailability is similar to that of sublingual administration (see II F).

L. Intranasal administration. The drug is inhaled nasally and then absorbed through the nasal mucosa. Onset is generally rapid, but bioavailability can be variable and dependent on the condition of nasal membranes. Drugs may be administered for a local (e.g., phenylephrine) or systemic (e.g., desmopressin) effect. The duration of action may be from minutes to hours, depending on the drug.

M. Ophthalmic administration. The drug is administered onto the conjunctiva. The effect is usually local with systemic side effects occasionally occurring. Absorption into the central nervous system (CNS) is sometimes a problem because of the proximity of the eyes to the brain and the lipophilic nature of ophthalmically active medications.

N. Otic administration. The drug is administered into the auditory canal, usually for local results, such as an anti-inflammatory or anti-infective effect.

III. DRUG ABSORPTION

A. Dissolution. Drugs administered in solid dosage forms must be dissolved so that they can be absorbed across membranes. Determinants of the dissolution rate are particle size, coating, or protective layer (e.g., tablets), and drug solubility. Some tablets owe their sustained-release properties to slow dissolution. Most highly bioavailable oral dosage forms are readily soluble in gastric juices.

B. Membrane transport. Drug molecules must cross the membrane of absorption to enter the systemic circulation.

1. Most drugs cross the membrane by **simple diffusion,** which depends on the lipophilicity of the drug molecule (i.e., highly lipophilic drugs cross the membrane more rapidly and more easily) and the drug concentration gradient existing across the membrane (i.e., a larger gradient causes faster transport).

2. Some drugs (e.g., vitamins) are carried across the absorption membrane by enzymes; such **carrier-mediated transport** may be passive or active and can move drugs against a concentration gradient as well as with the gradient.

C. Blood flow to the absorbing organ. Rapid and extensive blood flow to the organ or membrane of absorption:

1. Facilitates rapid and complete absorption of the drug
2. Reduces the drug concentration on the systemic side of the absorption membrane, thereby increasing the concentration gradient across which the drug molecule is absorbed
3. Facilitates more rapid drug entry into the systemic circulation, enabling the drug to exert its effect at the intended site of action

D. Skin condition is a concern only for topically administered medications. Highly vascular skin (e.g., scrotum, eyelid), broken skin (e.g., burned, eczematous), or hydrated skin (e.g., occluded) leads to a more rapid and complete systemic absorption of topically applied drugs. Thick and highly keratinized skin areas (e.g., calluses, soles of feet) are poor sites for systemic drug absorption because the thickened stratum corneum retards the passage of drug molecules. Drugs applied to such sites should be intended for local not systemic effects.

E. pH-Dependence. Some drugs (e.g., weak acids, weak bases) carry a molecular charge at different pHs. Weak bases become positively charged at low pH, such as that in the stomach. Charged molecules cannot cross the lipid membranes easily. Such molecules can be absorbed only when they are uncharged, as occurs lower in the gastrointestinal tract, where the pH is higher. Weak acids are more easily absorbed in acidic environments, where they are uncharged.

F. Bioavailability. Some drugs are incompletely absorbed from the administration site. Oral drugs are most commonly mentioned, but intramuscular, topical, and rectal administration sites are also common sites where incomplete absorption occurs. In addition to the first-pass effect discussed in II E 1, incomplete absorption is the other leading cause of low bioavailability.

1. Some sustained-release tablets may pass through the gastrointestinal tract and leave the body before their enteric coatings dissolve.
2. Sustained-release tablets may also retain some active drug in their wax matrices.

G. Compliance. If drugs are not actually taken in prescribed amounts or at planned intervals, plasma levels may be subtherapeutic. Therapeutic drug monitoring is sometimes used to monitor the compliance of patients.

H. Food co-administration. Many oral agents are incompletely absorbed if they are taken with food. Food can increase the gastric pH and hinder the dissolution of some medications.

1. Although high plasma levels are usually achieved with most drugs (particularly antibiotics) when taken on an empty stomach, many drugs can achieve therapeutic concentrations if taken with food.
2. Certain foods contain specific products that interfere with absorption. Tetracycline, for example, chelates calcium ions if taken with dairy products and forms a complex that cannot be absorbed.

IV. DRUG DISTRIBUTION to various body tissues and compartments is affected by many factors, such as body composition and binding propensities. Measuring drug concentrations (most commonly in plasma) assesses drug distribution, a key element in therapeutic effect. Plasma concentrations may or may not reflect drug concentration at the site of action or the site of toxicity.

A. Therapeutic concentration and therapeutic index

1. For many drugs, the concentrations at which most patients begin to experience therapeutic effects [**minimum effective concentration** (MEC)] and toxic effects [minimum toxic concentration (MTC)] are known. These concentrations are generally used as the upper and lower limits of the therapeutic concentration range or window. The science of clinical pharmacokinetics is concerned with designing dosage regimens to keep a drug concentration in a specific patient within the therapeutic window.

2. The **therapeutic index** of a drug is the **ratio of the MTC to the MEC.**
   a. If the **therapeutic index is small,** the patient is more likely to experience toxicity or ineffective therapy.
   b. If the **therapeutic index is large,** the therapeutic window is usually larger, and it is easier to achieve an effective, nontoxic dosage regimen.

B. Tissue binding. Some drugs are bound to extravascular tissues, such as muscle or fat. Such drugs have low concentrations in the plasma compartment and a large apparent volume of distribution. Some drugs preferentially distribute to specific body tissues, depending on blood flow, pH conditions, and the lipophilicity of the tissue. Other drugs remain largely in the plasma compartment, have a small apparent volume of distribution, and produce higher plasma concentrations for any given dose of drug.

C. Body composition. The composition of the body, which changes with certain disease states and with age, is an important consideration for the distribution of certain drugs. The examples of obesity and edema are discussed here, but similar principles are true for other abnormal physiologic conditions.

1. **Obesity.** The apparent volume of distribution is usually based on a patient's weight.
   a. In addition to increased adipose tissue, obese patients have excess fluid in comparison to patients with a lean body mass.
   b. Some drugs preferentially leave the plasma in favor of adipose tissue; thus, plasma concentrations for these drugs are lower, resulting in a larger volume of distribution in obese patients.
   c. Drugs that have a low solubility in fat remain in the plasma and produce higher plasma concentrations. In obese patients, therefore, the volume of distribution is smaller (per weight unit) than in thinner patients. Doses for drugs that distribute poorly to adipose tissues (e.g., aminoglycosides) are usually based on a patient's lean body weight, rather than total body weight. This consideration is important because the relative proportion of adipose and lean tissue mass changes with age, with fat comprising a larger percentage of the body weight with increasing age.

2. **Edema.** Some hydrophilic drugs (e.g., lithium, aminoglycosides) remain largely in the plasma compartment. Patients with edema or ascites may distribute a large percentage of such drugs into the extra body fluid rather than into the target tissue (e.g., infected muscle tissue). If doses of such drugs are based on the patient's weight, the plasma concentration is lower because of the large plasma compartment relative to the patient's weight, and the observed concentration may be subtherapeutic.

D. Protein binding

1. **Free and bound concentrations.** Many drugs are bound to plasma proteins. In the plasma, these drugs exist in a state of equilibrium with some of the drug free (unbound) and some bound to proteins. Drug plus protein is referred to as a **drug–protein complex**.
   a. Only the free drug can cross membranes to enter body tissues, and only the free drug can interact with receptors to produce therapeutic or toxic effects.
   b. Clinical laboratories generally report total plasma drug concentrations (free plus bound drug). For most patients and most drugs, this report provides sufficient information because standard therapeutic concentrations reflect such factors as drug affinity for protein and free-drug concentrations. Special circumstances exist, however, in which data on total drug concentrations prove insufficient or misleading. Information about the free-drug concentration in a blood sample is obtainable for some drugs, notably, phenytoin, but the test is expensive, difficult to perform, and not always available.

Table 39-3. Some Drugs That Bind to Albumin

Clofibrate	Salicylic acid
Ethacrynic acid	Sulfa drugs
Flufenamic acid	Sulfinpyrazone
Oxyphenbutazone	Warfarin
Phenylbutazone	

2. **Displacement.** Drugs are generally considered highly protein-bound when over 90% of the total drug in plasma is protein-bound. These drugs can sometimes be displaced by other substances that bind the same protein. In such instances, the second drug *pushes* the first drug off the protein. This causes a much higher free-drug concentration of the first drug while the total concentration remains unchanged.
   a. **Example.** If a patient has been stabilized on aspirin, which binds albumin, and then begins taking phenylbutazone, which also binds albumin, the phenylbutazone may displace some salicylic acid and increase the free salicylate concentration. This previously stable patient may now experience some symptoms of salicylate toxicity due to an increased plasma concentration of free salicylate, despite an apparently normal salicylic acid (free plus bound) concentration. Eventually, the higher free salicylic acid concentration causes more salicylic acid to be excreted, and a new equilibrium (steady state) is reached.
   b. **Albumin**
      (1) The main plasma and drug-binding protein, albumin, is an abundant protein that occurs in a concentration of 3.5–5.5 g/dl (0.6 mmol) in the plasma.
      (2) Most drugs bound to albumin are acidic, including those listed in Table 39-3; some of them are also capable of displacing drugs bound to albumin.
      (3) For a drug to be an effective displacer, it must occupy a large number of binding sites on albumin (i.e., it must accumulate to high concentrations or be given in large doses).
      (4) Drugs such as aspirin, phenylbutazone, and sulfa drugs are the most common displacers. Other substances, such as bilirubin, may bind albumin and may be displaced. For example, sulfa drugs displace albumin-bound bilirubin, which can cause free bilirubin to increase to toxic concentrations. Because kernicterus can result, sulfa drugs should not be administered to neonates.
      (5) Albumin levels may also be altered by certain disease states listed in Table 39-4. Increases in albumin concentration decrease the free concentration of drugs that bind to albumin; conversely, decreases in albumin concentration increase the free concentration of albumin-binding drugs.
   c. **Alpha$_1$-acid glycoprotein (AAG)**
      (1) After albumin, AAG is the second most important drug-binding plasma protein. AAG occurs in much smaller concentrations [2–4 mg/L (0.01–0.02 mmol)] than albumin and primarily binds the basic drugs listed in Table 39-5.

Table 39-4. Conditions That May Change Plasma Albumin Concentrations

Decrease Plasma Albumin	Increase Plasma Albumin
Acute infection	Benign tumor
Bone fractures	Gynecologic disorders
Burns	Myalgia
Cystic fibrosis	Schizophrenia
Inflammatory disease	
Liver disease	
Malnutrition	
Myocardial infarction	
Neoplastic disease	
Nephrotic syndrome	
Pregnancy	
Renal disease	
Surgical procedures	

Table 39-5. Some Drugs That Bind to $Alpha_1$-Acid Glycoprotein (AAG)

Amitriptyline	Lidocaine
Chlorpromazine	Meperidine
Dipyridamole	Nortriptyline
Disopyramide	Propranolol
Erythromycin	Quinidine
Imipramine	

(2) Circumstances affecting AAG concentrations are listed in Table 39-6.

(3) The same basic protein-binding principles discussed for albumin are true for AAG. Conditions that increase AAG concentrations decrease free concentrations of drugs that bind AAG; those that decrease AAG increase free-drug concentrations. One notable exception, however, is that few drugs are nearly totally bound to AAG, as some are to albumin. AAG exists in much smaller concentrations in the blood and is, therefore, unlikely to bind most of a drug, unless that drug is given in very small doses.

(4) Drug binding to AAG is not likely to be as clinically significant as drug–albumin-binding.

E. Sample timing. Objectives of monitoring include assessing a drug in its steady state and anticipating drug clearance (particularly for toxic agents); thus, sampling should take into account approximate distribution time and the half-life of the drug.

1. **Distribution.** The rate and pattern of distribution vary widely among drugs and require estimation when considering a monitoring plan.
   a. Certain drugs, such as aminoglycosides, reside in the plasma compartment prior to distribution to target tissues. This initial residence may last up to 30 minutes for an aminoglycoside. Therefore, a plasma aminoglycoside sample should not be drawn within 30 minutes of administration as it would appear to be too high because the drug would not have distributed to the tissues.
   b. The probable location of receptor sites for specific drugs is important for sample planning. Digoxin, for example, exerts its therapeutic and toxic effects through receptor sites that reside in the tissue compartments of the heart. Thus, concentrations only become relevant after the drug has had a chance to redistribute from the plasma to the tissue compartment (about 6 hours for digoxin). Samples should not be drawn within 6–8 hours after administration of an intravenous dose of digoxin (longer for an oral dose).

2. **Half-lives.** When a change in administration rate is considered, the patient should be at or near steady state when the sample is taken for evaluation. Steady state is usually achieved after the passage of four half-lives with constant dosage.
   a. If the sample is taken before steady state has been reached and the infusion rate is raised based on the results of the premature sample, the patient begins to accumulate drug from the new infusion while continuing to accumulate drug from the initial dose. This accumulation could result in toxic concentrations.
   b. Administration of toxic agents (or those with narrow therapeutic indices) make it prudent to sample sooner than usual (e.g., after one half-life). In this way, progress toward steady state can be determined while it is still possible to exert control, such as by reducing the dosage rate.

Table 39-6. Circumstances That May Change Plasma $Alpha_1$-Acid Glycoprotein (AAG) Concentrations

Decrease Plasma AAG	Increase Plasma AAG
Nephrotic syndrome	Burns
	Chronic pain
	Inflammatory disease (e.g., Crohn's disease, rheumatoid arthritis)
	Myocardial infarction
	Neoplastic disease
	Surgical procedures
	Trauma injury

V. DRUG ELIMINATION

A. Metabolism. The liver is the site of metabolism for most drugs, but other organs and tissues (e.g., lungs, kidneys, intestines) may also metabolize drugs. Lipophilic drugs, for example, require chemical modification (e.g., acetylation, conjugation) by the liver to render them more water-soluble and, thus, more readily removable by renal filtration.

1. Extraction ratio

a. Drugs that are extensively metabolized during a single pass through the liver are said to have a high extraction ratio (i.e., the proportion of extracted drug to total drug that entered the liver is high). If a significant proportion of the drug has been extracted (rendered inactive) before entering systemic circulation—the **first-pass effect** (see II E 1)—then the amount of active drug left to produce the desired effect is significantly reduced.

b. The difference in extraction ratios among drugs accounts for the differences in magnitude of the first-pass effect from drug to drug.

c. Oral agents traverse the liver before entering the systemic circulation. If a drug is administered orally and has a high extraction ratio (e.g., propranolol), then most of the drug is eliminated before reaching the systemic circulation. Therefore, the effective dose for such a drug given orally may be much higher than for the same drug administered intravenously.

2. Hepatic blood flow changes

a. Changes in hepatic blood flow affect the rate at which the liver is presented with a drug. Since the liver effectively processes drugs as they arrive, a change in the presentation rate changes the rate at which drugs with a high extraction ratio are metabolized. (Most drugs with low-extraction ratios are affected only minimally or not at all by changes in hepatic flow rate.)

b. Some drugs [e.g., most histamine$_2$ (H_2)-antagonists] reduce hepatic blood flow. Therefore, close monitoring of plasma drug concentrations is required if H_2-antagonists are administered to a patient already stabilized on a drug with high-extraction ratio (e.g., theophylline, propranolol, lidocaine).

3. Changes in enzyme activity

a. Metabolic enzyme activity, rather than hepatic blood flow, determines the removal rate of drugs with low-extraction ratios.

b. Drugs and other substances can affect this activity, enhancing or inhibiting it by altering the amount of enzymes or influencing their function.

(1) Induction of enzyme metabolism

(a) Phenobarbital can stimulate hepatic enzymes to speed metabolism and change the effect of the other drugs metabolized by the liver. Thus, a patient who has been stabilized on rifampin (a drug with a low-extraction ratio) may experience subtherapeutic rifampin concentrations once phenobarbital is added to the regimen.

(b) Smoking can also increase enzyme activity, as the theophylline clearance rate is higher in smokers than in nonsmokers.

(2) Inhibition of enzyme metabolism may allow drug concentrations to build up to toxic levels. For example, less theophylline is removed if cimetidine is added to the regimen because cimetidine inhibits cytochrome P-450, a key element of the oxidative enzyme system.

4. Metabolites. Many metabolites are inactive and are simply removed by the kidneys. In some circumstances, however, drug metabolites must be considered in therapeutic drug monitoring. Like their parent drugs, metabolites may contribute both therapeutic and toxic effects.

a. Efficacy. Some metabolites actually contribute to the therapeutic effectiveness of a drug. For instance, N-acetylprocainamide has antiarrhythmic properties that contribute to the effectiveness of procainamide, the parent drug. Other drugs with metabolites that enhance their therapeutic effectiveness include primidone, diazepam, flurazepam, and imipramine.

b. Toxicity. Some metabolites may be more toxic than the parent drug. An example of a toxic metabolite is normeperidine, which is produced from meperidine. In most patients, normeperidine is quickly removed, but in patients with impaired renal function, it may build up to toxic levels and produce seizures. Other drugs with toxic metabolites include ethanol and acetaminophen.

c. Prodrugs. Some drugs are inactive when they are administered and must be *activated,* usually by the metabolic process, to be effective. Examples of prodrugs include sulindac, clorazepate, and aspirin.

d. Assay interference. Drug metabolites may be misinterpreted by the clinical laboratory as active drugs. Most clinical laboratories and commercially available assays distinguish between parent drugs and metabolites, but mistakes occur. This is particularly relevant if a patient has impaired renal function and metabolites have built up to significant levels. If necessary, plasma concentration for drug metabolites, such as N-acetylprocainamide or desipramine, can be obtained from the clinical laboratory.

B. Excretion

1. Urinary excretion. Most drugs are removed by the kidneys, either as unchanged drug or as a metabolite; therefore, renal function greatly influences drug concentration and, thus, figures prominently in adjustments of drug regimens.

a. Renal function is usually estimated using the **Cockcroft and Gault equation** [see I C 4 a (3)]. Generally, all aspects of renal function are assumed to rise or fall together; thus, filtration, secretion, and reabsorption are considered impaired to the same degree in a patient with renal failure. However, the effect of an individual drug may rely more heavily on one of these three aspects. The individual processes are discussed in VI.

b. Dose adjustment. Many nomograms have been developed to determine dosage adjustments (i.e., amount or frequency) in given circumstances. Generally, the greater the degree of renal impairment and the larger the fraction of drug excreted unchanged, the greater the dosage adjustment necessary to maintain drug concentrations in the plasma within the therapeutic range.

2. Biliary and fecal excretion

a. Some drugs undergo biliary excretion and enterohepatic recycling. These drugs may be eliminated in the feces, even though they were administered intravenously. This is an important consideration for some drugs. For example, a patient who has taken an overdose of theophylline may be saved if activated charcoal is administered. The charcoal works, even if the theophylline was not administered orally, because it adsorbs the theophylline on contact in the gastrointestinal tract, promotes gastrointestinal trapping of the theophylline, and hastens its elimination.

b. Biliary elimination is only a consideration if a patient has impaired biliary function because some drugs may accumulate.

3. Other routes. Several other minor routes of drug elimination exist, but these are insignificant for purposes of therapeutic drug monitoring.

a. Some volatile anesthetics (e.g., halothane) are eliminated primarily on exhalation.

b. A few drugs are eliminated through perspiration, saliva, tears, and breast milk.

VI. PHARMACOKINETIC DRUG INTERACTIONS.

Co-administration of drugs can enhance, inhibit, or negate the effect each drug should achieve when administered alone. These interactions occur when one drug alters, opposes, or potentiates the basic pharmacokinetics of the other drug.

A. Absorption

1. Rate

a. The **absorption rate decreases** when drugs that decrease local blood flow, such as topically administered drugs, or that slow stomach emptying, such as orally administered drugs, are administered.

(1) With the co-administration of propantheline and acetaminophen, propantheline slows stomach emptying; therefore, acetaminophen is absorbed more slowly.

(2) Vasoconstriction caused by epinephrine when it is co-administered with lidocaine for topical anesthesia reduces blood flow to and from the affected area, prolonging the effect of lidocaine and reducing the need for subsequent injections.

b. The **absorption rate increases** if the drug that speeds stomach emptying is co-administered. For example, metoclopramide, which speeds stomach emptying, increases the absorption rate of co-administered oral acetaminophen.

2. Extent. Co-administration can affect drug availability.

a. Increased bioavailability of digoxin, for example, is achieved through oral co-administration of digoxin and propantheline. The propantheline slows stomach emptying and improves the availability of the slow-dissolving digoxin tablets.

b. Decreased absorption (bioavailability) results from co-administration in many instances. Co-administration of heavy metal ions and tetracyclines results in the formation of nonabsorbable complexes; kaolin–pectin adsorbs co-administered digoxin and results in less digoxin absorption.

c. Only nonionized molecules cross lipid absorption membranes. For this reason, drugs that alter the ionic status of other drug molecules affect their absorption. For example, ketoconazole is only absorbed from an acidic stomach; co-administration of antacids greatly impairs ketoconazole absorption.

B. Volume of distribution. Changes in protein binding (see IV D) are generally the cause of altered volumes of distribution. For example, the volume of distribution increases for salicylic acid when phenylbutazone is co-administered because the concentration of free (unbound) salicylic acid is the same as it was prior to phenylbutazone administration; however, the total concentration (free plus bound) is lower. Since the volume of distribution is based upon total concentration, a lower salicylic acid concentration produces a larger apparent volume of distribution.

C. Clearance

1. Metabolic clearance. Several factors influence metabolic clearance (see V A).

a. For drugs with a high-extraction ratio, metabolism is inhibited by co-administration of a drug that reduces hepatic blood flow. For example, co-administration of lidocaine and cimetidine inhibits the elimination of lidocaine (a drug with a high-extraction ratio) and produces higher-than-expected lidocaine concentrations.

b. Metabolic clearance may be increased for a drug with a low-extraction ratio by co-administration of an enzyme inducer. For example, warfarin (a drug with a low-extraction ratio) metabolism is increased when phenobarbital is also administered. If a patient has been stabilized on warfarin and phenobarbital is introduced, close monitoring is required to maintain the appropriate anticoagulant status.

2. Renal clearance. Drugs eliminated by glomerular filtration are only affected by drugs that modify renal function, a pharmacodynamic interaction (e.g., nephrotoxic cisplatin impairs renal elimination of gentamicin). Secretion and reabsorption are subject to pharmacokinetic interactions.

a. Secretion. Some drugs, such as penicillins, are actively secreted. Co-administration of a drug that competes for secretion, such as probenecid, inhibits the secretion of penicillin and results in sustained blood levels of penicillin. This is sometimes used to improve the therapeutic outcome in patients with a history of poor compliance.

b. Reabsorption. Drugs that are filtered or secreted and then reabsorbed are also subject to drug interactions.

(1) If a drug becomes ionized in the renal tubule due to a change in pH, it is impossible for it to be reabsorbed, because only nonionized molecules can cross biologic membranes. For example, ammonium chloride decreases urinary pH. Amphetamine becomes positively charged at the lower pH and cannot be reabsorbed. More amphetamine is, thus, eliminated.

(2) Urine acidification or alkalinization is often used in cases of overdoses and poisonings.

STUDY QUESTIONS

Directions: The numbered item or incomplete statement in this section is followed by answers or by completions of the statement. Select the **one** lettered answer or completion that is **best**.

1. All of the following statements about intramuscular drug administration are true EXCEPT

(A) entry of the drug into the circulation is affected by the drug's degree of lipophilicity
(B) peak effect is generally less than with intravenous administration
(C) bioavailability equals 100%
(D) maximum injection volume is 2–5 ml
(E) drug effects generally last longer than with intravenous administration

Directions: Each item below contains three suggested answers of which **one or more** is correct. Choose the answer

A if **I only** is correct
B if **III only** is correct
C if **I and II** are correct
D if **II and III** are correct
E if **I, II, and III** are correct

2. True statements about protein binding include which of the following?

I. Only bound drug can interact with receptors to produce therapeutic or toxic effects
II. Drugs are considered highly protein-bound when over 90% of the total drug in plasma is protein-bound
III. Albumin is the main plasma protein that binds drugs

3. Which of the following patients should have therapeutic drug monitoring?

I. An 80-year-old man with congestive heart failure
II. A 6-year-old boy with kidney disease
III. A 3-month-old girl with acute gastroenteritis

4. Conditions that may decrease plasma albumin include

I. malnutrition
II. pregnancy
III. myalgia

1-C
2-D
3-E
4-C

ANSWERS AND EXPLANATIONS

1. The answer is C *[II C].*
With intramuscular administration, bioavailability is not always 100%. Only intravenous administration consistently provides 100% bioavailability. The other statements listed in the question are correct. The entry of an intramuscularly injected drug into the circulation is limited by the drug's solubility and lipophilicity and by the blood supply in the muscle. Because an intramuscular drug enters the blood more slowly and gradually than an intravenous drug, the peak effect of an intramuscular drug is not as great, but its duration of action is generally longer than with intravenous administration. Not more than 2–5 ml should be injected into any one intramuscular site.

2. The answer is D (II, III) *[IV D].*
Only free drug can interact with receptors to produce a therapeutic (or toxic) effect. A drug that is bound to plasma protein cannot cross membranes to enter body tissues and cannot interact with receptors to produce an effect. Albumin, one of the major proteins of blood plasma, is the main plasma protein that binds drugs. The second most important drug-binding plasma protein is alpha$_1$-acid glycoprotein (AAG). Albumin binds acidic drugs; AAG binds basic drugs.

3. The answer is E (all) *[I C 1, 4].*
Patients who need rapidly effective treatment and patients with altered physiologic and pharmacokinetic parameters, would benefit from therapeutic drug monitoring. Also, extremes of age affect drug absorption, distribution, metabolism, and excretion, so that elderly patients and very young patients require special care in dosage determinations. Congestive heart failure can impair absorption, distribution, and elimination of many drugs. Impaired renal function often requires dosage modification. Acute gastroenteritis in an infant can rapidly cause dehydration and electrolyte imbalance and, therefore, calls for rapid, effective treatment and close monitoring.

4. The answer is C (I, II) *[Table 39-4].*
Albumin levels may be altered by a variety of disease states. Infections, malnutrition, myocardial infarction, and renal disease are among the numerous diseases that can lower the plasma albumin levels. Pregnancy can also cause a decrease in plasma albumin. Conditions that may increase plasma albumin levels include myalgia and some gynecologic disorders. A decrease in plasma albumin increases the free concentration of a drug that binds to albumin and, thus, increases the effects of the drug. Conversely, an increase in plasma albumin lowers the concentration of free drug and, thus, reduces its effects.

40
Common Clinical Laboratory Tests

Larry N. Swanson

I. GENERAL PRINCIPLES

A. Monitoring drug therapy

1. **Laboratory test results** are monitored by pharmacists to:
   a. **Assess the therapeutic and adverse effects of a drug** (e.g., monitoring the serum uric acid level after allopurinol is administered or checking for elevated liver function test values after administration of isoniazid)
   b. **Determine the proper drug dose** (e.g., assessment of the serum creatinine value before use of a renally excreted drug)
   c. **Assess the need for additional or alternate drug therapy** [e.g., assessment of white blood cell (WBC) count after penicillin is administered]
   d. **Prevent test misinterpretation resulting from drug interference** (e.g., determination of a false positive for a urine glucose test after cephalosporin administration)
2. These tests can be **very expensive** and requests for them must be balanced against potential benefits for patients.

B. Definition of normal values

1. **Normal laboratory test results** fall within a predetermined range of values, and **abnormal values** fall outside that range.
   a. **Normal limits may be defined somewhat arbitrarily;** thus, values outside the normal range may not necessarily indicate disease or the need for treatment (e.g., asymptomatic hyperuricemia).
   b. Many factors (e.g., age, sex, time since last meal) must be taken into account when evaluating test results.
   c. **Normal values also vary among institutions** and may depend on the method used to perform the test.
   d. Attempts have been made in recent years to standardize the presentation of laboratory data by using the International System of Units (SI units). Controversy surrounds this issue in the United States, and resistance to adopt this system continues.
2. **Laboratory error** must always be considered when **test results do not correlate with expected results for a given patient**. If necessary, the test should be repeated. Common sources of laboratory error include spoiled specimens, incomplete specimens, specimens taken at the wrong time, faulty reagents, technical errors, incorrect procedures, and failure to take diet or medication into account.
3. During hospital admission or routine physical examination, a **battery of tests** is usually given to augment the history and physical examination. Basic tests may include an electrocardiogram (ECG), a chest x-ray, a sequential multiple analyzer (SMA) profile, electrolyte tests, a hemogram, and urinalysis.

II. HEMATOLOGIC TESTS.

II. HEMATOLOGIC TESTS. Blood contains three types of formed elements; red blood cells (RBCs), WBCs, and platelets (Figure 40-1). A complete blood count (CBC) includes hemoglobin (Hb), hematocrit (Hct), total WBCs, total RBCs, mean cell volume (MCV), and mean cell hemoglobin concentration (MCHC).

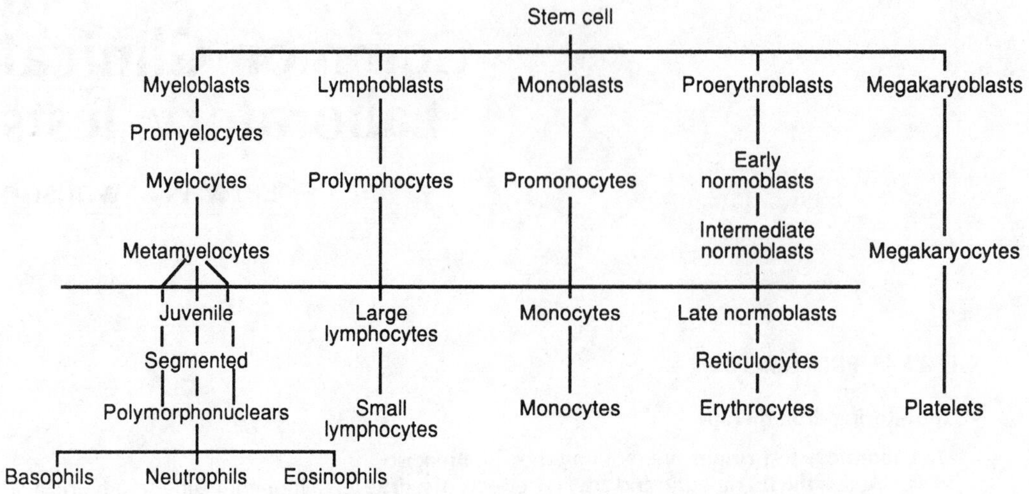

Figure 40-1. Derivation of blood elements from stem cells. Cells located below the *horizontal line* are found in normal peripheral blood with the exception of the late normoblasts.

A. Red blood cells (erythrocytes)

1. The **RBC count,** which reports the number of RBCs found in a cubic millimeter (mm^3) of whole blood, provides an indirect estimate of the blood's Hb content. **Normal values** are:
   a. 4.3–5.9 million/mm^3 of blood for men
   b. 3.5–5.0 million/mm^3 of blood for women

2. The **Hct or packed cell volume (PCV)** measures the percentage by volume of packed RBCs in a whole blood sample after centrifugation. The Hct value is usually three times the Hb value (see II A 3) and is given as a percent.
   a. **Low Hct** values indicate such conditions as anemia or overhydration.
   b. **High Hct** values indicate such conditions as polycythemia or dehydration.

3. The **Hb test** measures the grams of Hb contained in 1 dl of whole blood and provides an estimate of the oxygen-carrying capacity of the RBCs. The Hb value depends on the **number of RBCs** and the **amount of Hb in each RBC.**
   a. **Normal values** are 14–18 g/dl for men and 12–16 g/dl for women.
   b. **Low Hb** values indicate anemia.

4. **RBC indices** (also known as **Wintrobe indices**) provide important information regarding RBC size, Hb concentration, and Hb weight. They are used primarily to categorize anemias, although they may be affected by average cell measurements. A peripheral blood smear can provide most of the information obtained through RBC indices. Observations of a smear may show variation in RBC shape (**poikilocytosis**), as might occur in sickle cell anemia, or it may show a variation in RBC size (**anisocytosis**), as might occur in a mixed anemia (folic acid and iron deficiency).
   a. **Mean cell volume (MCV)** is the ratio of the Hct to the RBC count. It essentially assesses average RBC size and reflects any anisocytosis.

$$\frac{\text{Hct (\%)} \times 10}{\text{RBC count (in millions)}} = \text{MCV}$$

      (1) **Low MCV** indicates **microcytic** (undersized) **RBCs,** as occurs in iron deficiency.
      (2) **High MCV** indicates **macrocytic** (oversized) **RBCs,** as occurs in a vitamin B_{12} or folic acid deficiency.
      (3) Normal range for MCV is 90 ± 10.

   b. **Mean cell hemoglobin (MCH)** assesses the amount of Hb in an average RBC.
      (1) MCH is defined as:

$$\frac{\text{Hb} \times 10}{\text{RBC count (in millions)}} = \text{MCH}$$

      (2) **Normal range for MCH** is 30 ± 4.

c. **Mean cell hemoglobin concentration (MCHC)** represents the average concentration of Hb in an average RBC, defined as:

$$\frac{\text{Hb} \times 100}{\text{Hct}} = \text{MCHC}$$

(1) **Normal range for MCHC** is 34 ± 3.
(2) **Low MCHC** indicates **hypochromia** (pale RBCs resulting from decreased Hb content), as occurs in iron deficiency.

d. **RBC distribution width (RDW)** is a relvlh new index of RBCs. Normally, most RBCs are approximately equal in size, so that only one bell-shaped histogram peak is generated. Disease may change the size of some RBCs—for example, the gradual change in size of newly produced RBCs in folic acid or iron deficiency. The difference in size between the abnormal and less abnormal RBCs produces either more than one histogram peak or a broadening of the normal peak.
(1) **Elevated RDW** is seen in factor deficiency anemia (e.g., iron, folate, vitamin B_{12}).
(2) **Normal RDW** is seen in such conditions as anemia of chronic disease.
(3) The **RDW index** is never decreased.

5. The **reticulocyte count** provides a measure of immature RBCs (reticulocytes), which contain remnants of nuclear material (reticulum). Normal RBCs circulate in the blood for about 1–2 days in this form. Hence, this test provides an index of bone marrow production of mature RBCs.
   a. Reticulocytes normally comprise 0.1%–2.4% of the total RBC count.
   b. **Increased reticulocyte count** occurs with such conditions as hemolytic anemia, acute blood loss, and response to the treatment of a factor deficiency (e.g., an iron, vitamin B_{12}, or folate deficiency). **Polychromasia** (the tendency to stain with acidic or basic dyes) noted on a peripheral smear laboratory report, usually indicates increased reticulocytes.
   c. **Decreased reticulocyte count** occurs with such conditions as drug-induced aplastic anemia.

6. The **erythrocyte sedimentation rate (ESR)** measures the rate of RBC settling of whole, uncoagulated blood over time, and primarily reflects plasma composition. Most of the sedimentation effect results from alterations in plasma proteins.
   a. **Normal ESR rates** range from 0 mm/hr to 20 mm/hr for males and from 0 mm/hr to 30 mm/hr for females.
   b. **ESR values increase** with acute or chronic infection, tissue necrosis or infarction, well-established malignancy, and rheumatoid collagen diseases.
   c. **ESR values** are used to:
   (1) Follow the clinical course of a disease
   (2) Demonstrate the presence of occult organic disease
   (3) Differentiate conditions with similar symptomatology [e.g., angina pectoris (no change in ESR value) as opposed to a myocardial infarction (increase in ESR value)]

B. White blood cells (leukocytes)

1. The **WBC count** reports the number of WBCs in a cubic millimeter of whole blood.
   a. **Normal values** range from 4,000 WBC/mm^3 to 11,000 WBC/mm^3
   b. **Increased WBC count (leukocytosis)** usually signals infection; it may also result from leukemia or from tissue necrosis. It is most often seen with **bacterial infection**.
   c. **Decreased WBC count (leukopenia)** indicates bone marrow depression, which may result from metastatic carcinoma, lymphoma, or toxic reactions to substances such as antineoplastic agents.

2. The **WBC differential** evaluates the distribution and morphology of the five major types of WBCs— the **granulocytes** (i.e., **neutrophils, basophils, eosinophils**) and the **nongranulocytes** (i.e., **lymphocytes, monocytes**). A certain percentage of each type comprises the total WBC count (Table 40-1).
   a. **Neutrophils** may be mature (**polymorphonuclear leukocytes,** also known as PMNs, "polys," segmented neutrophils, or "segs") or immature (**"bands"** or "stabs").
   (1) **Chemotaxis.** Neutrophils, which **phagocytize and degrade many types of particles,** serve as the body's first line of defense when tissue is damaged or foreign material gains entry. They congregate at sites in response to a specific stimulus, through a process known as chemotaxis.

Table 40-1. Normal Percentage Values for White Blood Cell (WBC) Differential

Cell Type	Normal Percentage Value
Polymorphonuclear leukocytes	50%–70%
Bands	3%–5%
Lymphocytes	20%–40%
Monocytes	0%–7%
Eosinophils	0%–5%
Basophils	0%–1%

(2) **Neutrophilic leukocytosis** describes a response to an appropriate stimulus in which the total neutrophil count rises, often with an increase in the percentage of immature cells (**a shift to the left**). This may represent a systemic bacterial infection, such as pneumonia (Table 40-2).

(a) **Certain viruses** (e.g., chicken pox, herpes zoster); some **rickettsial diseases** (e.g., Rocky Mountain spotted fever); some **fungi;** and **stress** (e.g., physical exercise, acute hemorrhage or hemolysis, acute emotional stress) may also cause this response.

(b) Other causes include **inflammatory diseases** (e.g., acute rheumatic fever, rheumatoid arthritis, acute gout); **hypersensitivity reactions to drugs; tissue necrosis** (e.g., from myocardial infarction, burns, certain cancers); **metabolic disorders** (e.g., uremia, diabetic ketoacidosis); **myelogenous leukemia;** and **use of certain drugs** (e.g., epinephrine, lithium).

(3) **Neutropenia,** a decreased number of neutrophils, may occur with an **overwhelming infection of any type** (bone marrow is unable to keep up with the demand). It may also occur with **certain viral infections** (e.g., mumps, measles) and with **idiosyncratic drug reactions.**

b. **Basophils** stain deeply with blue basic dye. Their function in the circulation is not clearly understood; in the tissues they are referred to as **mast cells.**

(1) **Basophilia,** an increased number of basophils, may occur with chronic myelogenous leukemia as well as other conditions.

(2) A decrease in basophils is generally not apparent because of the small numbers of these cells in the blood.

c. **Eosinophils** stain deep red with acid dye and are classically associated with immune reactions. **Eosinophilia,** an increased number of eosinophils, may occur with such conditions as **acute allergic reactions** (e.g., asthma, hay fever, drug allergy) and **parasitic infestations** (e.g., trichinosis, amebiasis).

Table 40-2. Examples of Changes in Total White Blood Cell (WBC) Count and WBC Differential in Response to Bacterial Infection

	WBC Count	
Cell Type	**Normal**	**With Bacterial Infection**
Total WBCs	8000 (100%)	15,500 (100%)
Neutrophils		
Polymorphonuclear leukocytes	60%	82%
Bands	3%	6%
Lymphocytes	30%	10%
Monocytes	4%	1%
Eosinophils	2%	1%
Basophils	1%	0%

d. **Lymphocytes** play a dominant role in immunologic activity and appear to produce antibodies. They are classified as B lymphocytes or T lymphocytes; T lymphocytes are further divided into helper-inducer cells (T_4 cells) and suppressor cells (T_8 cells).

(1) **Lymphocytosis,** an increased number of lymphocytes, usually accompanies a normal or decreased total WBC count and is most commonly caused by **viral infection.**

(2) **Lymphopenia,** a decreased number of lymphocytes, may result from **severe debilitating illness, immunodeficiency,** or from **acquired immune deficiency syndrome (AIDS),** which has a propensity to attack T_4 cells.

(3) **Atypical lymphocytes** (i.e., T lymphocytes in a state of immune activation) are classically associated with **infectious mononucleosis.**

e. **Monocytes** are phagocytic cells. **Monocytosis,** an increased number of monocytes, may occur with **tuberculosis, subacute bacterial endocarditis,** and during the recovery phase of some **acute infections.**

C. **Platelets (thrombocytes),** the smallest formed elements in the blood, are involved in **blood clotting** and are vital to the formation of a hemostatic plug after vascular injury.

1. **Normal values for a platelet count** are 150,000 mm^3–300,000/mm^3.

2. **Thrombocytopenia,** a decreased platelet count, can occur with a variety of conditions, such as idiopathic thrombocytopenic purpura or, occasionally, from such drugs as quinidine and sulfonamides.

a. Thrombocytopenia is **moderate** when the platelet count is less than 100,000/mm^3.

b. Thrombocytopenia is **severe** when the platelet count is less than 50,000/mm^3.

III. COMMON SERUM ENZYME TESTS.

Small amounts of enzymes (catalysts) circulate in the blood at all times and are released into the blood in larger quantities when tissue damage occurs. Thus, serum enzyme levels can be used to **aid in the diagnosis of certain diseases.**

A. Creatine kinase (CK)

1. CK, known formerly as creatine phosphokinase (CPK), is found primarily in heart muscle, skeletal muscle, and brain tissue.

2. CK levels are used primarily to **aid in the diagnosis of acute myocardial** (Figure 40-2) **or skeletal muscle damage.** However, vigorous exercise, a fall, or deep intramuscular injections can cause significant elevations in CK levels.

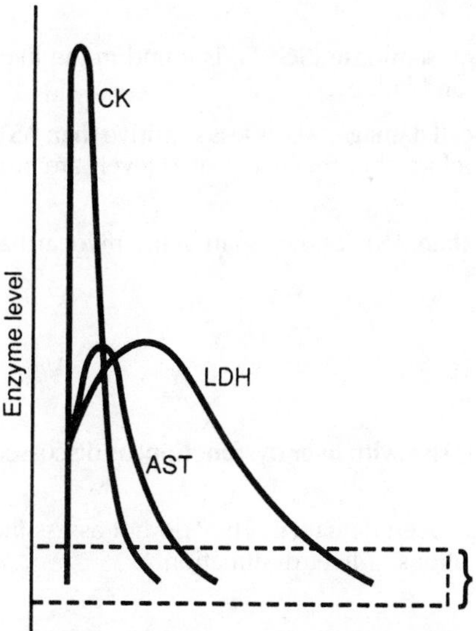

Figure 40-2. The graph shows the elevation of serum creatine kinase (CK), lactate dehydrogenase (LDH), and aspartate aminotransferase (AST) levels following a myocardial infarction.

3. The **isoenzymes** of CK–**CK-MM,** found in skeletal muscle; **CK-BB,** found in brain tissue; and **CPK-MB,** found in heart muscle can be used to differentiate the source of damage.
   a. Normally serum CK levels are virtually all the **CK-MM isoenzyme**.
   b. Increases in **CK-MB** levels provide a sensitive indicator of myocardial necrosis.

B. Lactate dehydrogenase (LDH)

1. LDH catalyzes the interconversion of lactate and pyruvate and represents a group of enzymes present in almost all metabolizing cells.
2. Five individual **isoenzymes** make up the total LDH serum level.
   a. **LDH_1** and **LDH_2** appear primarily in the heart.
   b. **LDH_3** appears primarily in the lungs.
   c. **LDH_4** and **LDH_5** appear primarily in the liver and in skeletal muscles.
3. The **distribution pattern** of LDH isoenzymes aids in diagnosing myocardial infarction, hepatic disease, and lung disease.

C. Alkaline phosphatase (ALP)

1. ALP is produced primarily in the **liver** and in the **bones**.
2. Serum ALP levels are **particularly sensitive to partial or mild biliary obstruction**—either extrahepatic (e.g., caused by a stone in the bile duct) or intrahepatic, both of which cause levels to rise.
3. **Increased osteoblastic activity,** as occurs in Paget's disease, hyperparathyroidism, osteomalacia, and others, also increases serum ALP levels.

D. Aspartate aminotransferase (AST)

1. **AST,** formerly known as **serum glutamic-oxaloacetic transaminase (SGOT),** is found in a number of organs, primarily in heart and liver tissues and, to a lesser extent, in skeletal muscle, kidney tissue, and pancreatic tissue.
2. **Damage to the heart** (e.g., from **myocardial infarction;** see Figure 40-2) results in elevated AST levels about 8 hours after the injury.
   a. Levels are **elevated markedly** with **acute hepatitis;** they are **elevated mildly** with **cirrhosis** and a **fatty liver**.
   b. Levels are also **elevated** with **passive congestion of the liver** [as occurs in congestive heart failure (CHF)].

E. Alanine aminotransferase (ALT)

1. ALT, formerly known as **serum glutamic-pyruvic transaminase (SGPT),** is found in the liver with lesser amounts in the heart, skeletal muscles, and kidney.
2. Although ALT values are **relatively specific for liver cell damage,** ALT is **less sensitive than AST,** and extensive or severe liver damage is necessary before abnormally elevated levels are produced.
3. ALT also **rises less consistently and less markedly than AST** following an **acute myocardial infarction**.

IV. LIVER FUNCTION TESTS

A. Liver enzymes

1. **Levels of certain enzymes** (e.g., LDH, ALP, AST, ALT) **rise with liver dysfunction,** as discussed in III.
2. These **enzyme tests indicate only that the liver has been damaged**. They do not assess the liver's ability to function. Other tests provide indications of liver dysfunction.

B. Serum bilirubin

1. Bilirubin, a breakdown product of Hb, is the **predominant pigment in bile**. Effective bilirubin conjugation and excretion depend on **hepatobiliary function** and on the **rate of RBC turnover**.

2. Serum bilirubin levels are reported as **total bilirubin** (conjugated and unconjugated) and as **direct bilirubin** (conjugated only).
   a. Bilirubin is released by Hb breakdown and is bound to albumin as water-insoluble **indirect bilirubin** (unconjugated bilirubin), which is not filtered by the glomerulus.
   b. **Unconjugated bilirubin** travels to the liver, where it is separated from albumin, conjugated with diglucuronide, and then actively secreted into the bile as **conjugated bilirubin** (direct bilirubin), which is filtered by the glomerulus (Figure 40-3).

3. **Normal values of total serum bilirubin** are 0.1 mg/dl–1.0 mg/dl; of **direct bilirubin,** 0.0 mg/dl–0.2 mg/dl.

4. **Increase in serum bilirubin** results in **jaundice** from bilirubin deposition in the tissues. There are three major causes of increased serum bilirubin.
   a. **Hemolysis** increases total bilirubin; direct bilirubin (conjugated) is usually normal or slightly elevated. Urine color is normal, and no bilirubin is found in the urine.
   b. **Biliary obstruction,** which may be intrahepatic (as with a chlorpromazine reaction) or extrahepatic (as with a biliary stone) increases total bilirubin and direct bilirubin; intrahepatic cholestasis (e.g., from chlorpromazine) may increase direct bilirubin as well. Urine color is dark, and bilirubin is present in the urine.
   c. **Liver cell necrosis,** as occurs in viral hepatitis, may cause an increase in both direct bilirubin (because inflammation causes some bile sinusoid blockage) and indirect bilirubin (because the liver's ability to conjugate is altered). Urine color is dark, and bilirubin is present in the urine.

C. Serum proteins

1. **Primary serum proteins** measured are **albumin** and the **globulins** (i.e., alpha, beta, gamma).
   a. **Albumin** (4.0–6.0 g/dl) maintains serum oncotic pressure and serves as a transport agent. Because it is primarily manufactured by the liver, liver disease can decrease albumin levels.
   b. **Globulins** (2.3–3.5 g/dl) function as transport agents and play a role in certain immunologic mechanisms. A decrease in albumin levels usually results in a compensatory increase in globulin production.

2. **Normal values** for total serum protein levels are 6.0–8.0 g/dl.

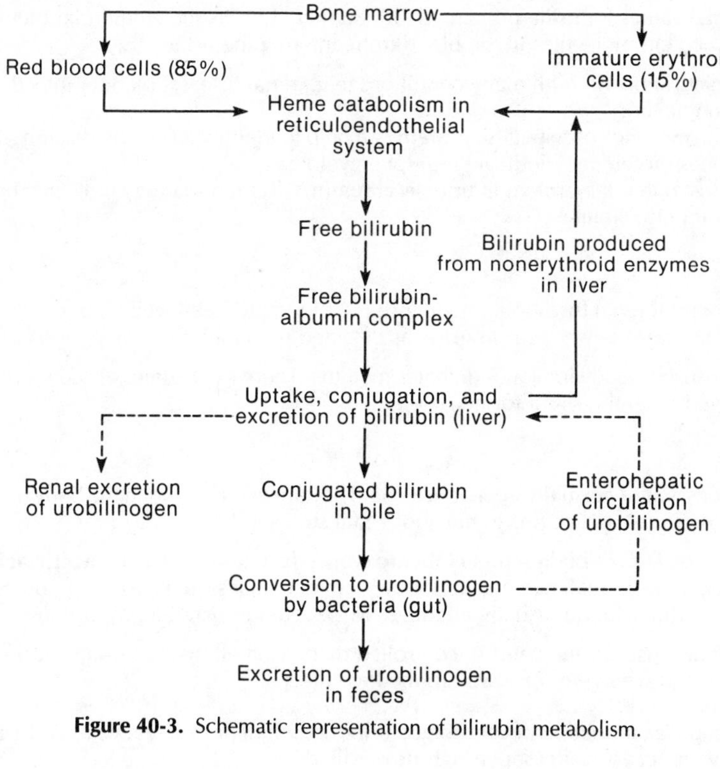

Figure 40-3. Schematic representation of bilirubin metabolism.

V. URINALYSIS. Standard urinalysis provides basic information regarding renal function, urinary tract disease, and the presence of certain systemic diseases. Components of a standard urinalysis include appearance, pH, specific gravity, protein level, glucose level, ketone level, and microscopic examination.

A. Appearance. Normal urine is **clear** and ranges in color from **pale yellow to deep gold. Changes in color** can result from drugs, diet, or disease.

1. A **red color** may indicate, among other things, the presence of blood or phenolphthalein (a laxative).
2. A **brownish-yellow color** may indicate the presence of conjugated bilirubin.
3. **Other shades of red, orange, or brown** may be caused by ingestion of various drugs.

B. pH

1. **Normal pH** ranges from 4.5 to 9 but is typically **acid** (around 6).
2. **Alkaline pH** may indicate such conditions as alkalosis, a *Proteus* infection, or acetazolamide use. It may also reflect changes caused by leaving the urine sample at room temperature.

C. Specific gravity

1. **Normal range** for specific gravity is 1.003–1.035; it is usually between 1.010 and 1.025.
2. Specific gravity is influenced by the number and nature of solute particles in the urine.
   a. **Elevated specific gravity** may occur with such conditions as diabetes mellitus (excess glucose in the urine) or nephrosis (excess protein in the urine).
   b. **Decreased specific gravity** may occur with diabetes insipidus, which decreases urine concentration.
   c. **Specific gravity, fixed at 1.010** (the same as plasma), occurs when the kidneys lose their power to concentrate or dilute.

D. Protein

1. **Normal values** for urine protein are 50–80 mg/24 hr, as the glomerular membrane prevents most protein molecules in the blood from entering the urine.
2. **Proteinuria** occurs with many conditions (e.g., renal disease, bladder infection, venous congestion, fever).
   a. The presence of a **specific protein** can help to identify a specific disease state (e.g., Bence Jones protein may indicate multiple myeloma).
   b. Most often, the protein in urine is **albumin**. Albuminuria may indicate abnormal glomerular permeability.

E. Glucose

1. The normal **renal threshold** for glucose is a blood glucose level of about 180 mg/dl; **glucose does not normally appear in urine** as detected by popular testing methods.
2. **Glycosuria** usually indicates diabetes mellitus. There are certain less common causes (e.g., a lowered renal threshold for glucose).

F. Ketones

1. Ketones **do not normally appear in urine**. They are excreted when the body has used available glucose stores and begins to metabolize fat stores.
2. The **three ketone bodies** are **betahydroxybutyric acid** (80%), **acetoacetic acid** (about 20%), and **acetone** (a small percentage). Some commercial tests (e.g., Ames products) measure only acetoacetic acid, but usually all three are excreted in parallel proportions.
3. **Ketonuria** usually indicates uncontrolled diabetes mellitus, but it may also occur with starvation and with zero- or low-carbohydrate diets.

G. Microscopic examination of centrifuged urine sediment normally reveals 0–1 RBC, 0–4 WBCs, and only an occasional cast per high-power field.

1. **Hematuria** (i.e., the presence of RBCs) may indicate such conditions as trauma, a tumor, or a systemic bleeding disorder. In women, a significant number of **squamous cells** suggests vaginal contamination (menstruation).
2. **Casts** (i.e., protein conglomerations outlining the shape of the renal tubules in which they were formed) may or may not be significant. Excessive numbers of certain types of casts indicate renal disease.
3. **Crystals,** which are pH-dependent, may occur normally in acid or alkaline urine. **Uric acid crystals** may form in acid urine; **phosphate crystals** may form in alkaline urine.
4. **Bacteria** do not normally appear in urine. The finding of 20 or more bacteria per high-power field may indicate a urinary tract infection; smaller values may indicate urethral contamination.

VI. COMMON RENAL FUNCTION TESTS

A. Introduction

1. Renal function may be assessed by measuring **blood urea nitrogen (BUN)** and **serum creatinine**. Renal function decreases with age, which must be taken into account when interpreting test values.
   a. These tests primarily evaluate glomerular function by assessing the **glomerular filtration rate (GFR)**.
   b. In many **renal diseases,** urea and creatinine accumulate in the blood because they are not excreted properly.
   c. These tests also aid in determining **drug dosage** for drugs excreted through the kidneys.
2. **Azotemia** describes excessive retention of nitrogenous waste products (BUN and creatinine) in the blood. The clinical syndrome resulting from decreased renal function and azotemia is called **uremia**.
   a. **Renal azotemia** results from renal disease, such as glomerulonephritis and chronic pyelonephritis.
   b. **Prerenal azotemia** results from such conditions as severe dehydration, hemorrhagic shock, and excessive protein intake.
   c. **Postrenal azotemia** results from such conditions as ureteral or urethral stones or tumors and prostatic obstructions.
3. **Clearance**—a theoretical concept defined as the volume of plasma from which a measured amount of substance can be completely eliminated, or cleared, into the urine per unit time—can be used to estimate glomerular function.

B. Blood urea nitrogen (BUN)

1. **Urea,** an end product of protein metabolism, is produced in the liver. From there, it travels through the blood and is excreted by the kidneys. Urea is **filtered at the glomerulus,** where the tubules reabsorb approximately 40%. Thus, under normal conditions, **urea clearance** is about 60% of the true GFR.
2. **Normal values for BUN** range from 8 mg/dl to 18 mg/dl.
   a. **Low BUN levels** occur with **significant liver disease**.
   b. **Elevated BUN levels** may indicate **renal disease**. However, factors other than glomerular function (e.g., protein intake, reduced renal blood flow, blood in the gastrointestinal tract) readily affect BUN levels, making interpretation of results sometimes difficult.

C. Serum creatinine

1. Creatinine, the metabolic breakdown product of muscle creatine phosphate, has a relatively constant level of daily production. Blood levels vary little in a given individual.
2. Creatinine is **excreted** by glomerular filtration and tubular secretion. **Creatinine clearance** parallels the GFR within a range of ± 10% and is a **more sensitive indicator of renal damage than BUN levels,** because renal impairment is almost the only cause of serum creatinine elevation.

3. Normal values for serum creatinine range from 0.6 mg/dl to 1.2 mg/dl.

a. Values vary with the **amount of muscle mass**—a value of 1.2 mg/dl in a muscular athlete may represent normal renal function, whereas the same value in a small, sedentary person with little muscle mass may indicate significant renal impairment.

b. Generally, the **serum creatinine value doubles with each 50% decrease in GFR**. For example, if a patient's normal serum creatinine is 1 mg/dl, 1 mg/dl represents 100% renal function, 2 mg/dl represents 50% function, and 4 mg/dl represents 25% function.

D. Creatinine clearance

1. Creatinine clearance, which represents the **rate at which creatinine is removed from the blood by the kidneys,** roughly approximates the GFR.

a. The value is given in units of ml/min, representing the volume of blood (in milliliters) cleared of creatinine by the kidney per minute.

b. Normal values for men range from 75 ml/min to 125 ml/min.

2. Calculation requires knowledge of **urinary creatinine excretion** (usually over 24 hours) and concurrent **serum creatinine levels. Creatinine clearance is calculated** as follows:

$$Cl_{CR} = \frac{C_U V}{C_{CR}}$$

Here, Cl_{CR} is the creatinine clearance in ml/min, C_U is the concentration of creatinine in the urine, V is the urine volume (in ml/min of urine formed over the collection period), and C_{CR} is the serum creatinine concentration.

3. Suppose the serum creatinine concentration is 1 mg/dl, and 1440 ml of urine were collected in 24 hours (1440 min) for a urine volume of 1 ml/min. The urine contains 100 mg/dl of creatinine. Creatinine clearance is calculated as:

$$\frac{100 \text{ mg/dl} \times 1 \text{ ml/min}}{1 \text{ mg/dl}} = 100 \text{ ml/min.}$$

4. Incomplete bladder emptying and other problems may interfere with obtaining an accurate timed urine specimen. Thus, **estimations of creatinine clearance** may be necessary. These estimations require only a serum creatinine value. One estimation uses the method of **Cockroft and Gault,** which is based on body weight, age, and gender.

a. This formula provides an **estimated value,** calculated for **males** as:

$$Cl_{CR} = \frac{(140 - \text{age in years})(\text{body weight in kg})}{72\ (C_{CR} \text{ in mg/dl})}$$

Again, Cl_{CR} is the creatinine clearance in ml/min, and C_{CR} is the serum creatinine concentration.

b. For **females,** use 0.85 of the value calculated for males.

c. Example: A 20-year-old male weighing 72 kg has a Cl_{CR} = 1.0 mg/dl; thus,

$$Cl_{CR} = \frac{(140 - 20)(72)}{72(1)}$$

$$Cl_{CR} = 120 \text{ ml/min.}$$

STUDY QUESTIONS

Directions: Each of the numbered items or incomplete statements in this section is followed by answers or by completions of the statement. Select the **one** lettered answer or completion that is **best** in each case.

1. Hematologic testing of a patient with acquired immune deficiency syndrome (AIDS) is most likely to show which of the following abnormalities?

(A) Basophilia
(B) Eosinophilia
(C) Lymphopenia
(D) Reticulocytosis
(E) Agranulocytosis

2. Hematologic studies are most likely to show a low reticulocyte count in a patient with

(A) aplastic anemia secondary to cancer chemotherapy
(B) acute hemolytic anemia secondary to quinidine treatment
(C) severe bleeding secondary to an automobile accident
(D) iron deficiency anemia, one week after treatment with ferrous sulfate
(E) megaloblastic anemia due to folate deficiency, one week after treatment with folic acid

3. All of the following findings on a routine urinalysis would be considered normal EXCEPT

(A) pH: 6.5
(B) glucose: negative
(C) ketones: negative
(D) WBC: 3 per high-power field, no casts
(E) RBC: 5 per high-power field

4. A 12-year-old boy is treated for otitis media with cefaclor (Ceclor). On the seventh day of therapy, he "spikes" a fever and develops an urticarial rash on his trunk. Which of the following laboratory tests could best confirm the physician's suspicion of a hypersensitivity (allergic) reaction?

(A) Complete blood count (CBC) and differential
(B) Serum hemoglobin (Hb) and reticulocyte count
(C) Liver function test profile
(D) Lactate dehydrogenase (LDH) isoenzyme profile
(E) Red blood cell (RBC) count and serum bilirubin

5. An elevated hematocrit (Hct) is a likely finding in all of the following individuals EXCEPT

(A) a man who has just returned from a 3-week skiing trip in the Colorado Rockies
(B) a woman who has polycythemia vera
(C) a hospitalized patient who mistakenly received 5 L of intravenous dextrose 5% in water over the last 24 hours
(D) a man who has been rescued from the Arizona desert after spending 4 days without water
(E) a woman who has chronic obstructive pulmonary disease

6. A 29-year-old white man is seen in the emergency room. His white blood cell (WBC) count is 14,200 with 80% "polys." All of the following conditions could normally produce these laboratory findings EXCEPT

(A) a localized bacterial infection on the tip of the index finger
(B) acute bacterial pneumonia caused by *Streptococcus pneumoniae*
(C) a heart attack
(D) a gunshot wound to the abdomen with a loss of 2 pints of blood
(E) an attack of gout

7. A 52-year-old male construction worker who drinks "fairly heavily" when he gets off work is seen in the emergency room with, among other abnormal laboratory results, an elevated creatine kinase (CK) level. All of the following circumstances could explain this elevation EXCEPT

(A) he fell against the bumper of his car in a drunken stupor and bruised his right side
(B) he is showing evidence of some liver damage due to the heavy alcohol intake
(C) he has experienced a heart attack
(D) he received an intramuscular injection a few hours before the blood sample was drawn
(E) he pulled a muscle that day in lifting a heavy concrete slab

---

1-C	4-A	7-B
2-A	5-C	
3-E	6-A	

8. A 45-year-old man with jaundice has spillage of bilirubin into his urine. All of the following statements could apply to this patient EXCEPT

(A) his total bilirubin is elevated
(B) his direct bilirubin is increased
(C) he may have viral hepatitis
(D) he may have hemolytic anemia
(E) he may have cholestatic hepatitis

Directions: Each item below contains three suggested answers of which **one or more** is correct. Choose the answer

A if **I only** is correct
B if **III only** is correct
C if **I and II** are correct
D if **II and III** are correct
E if **I, II, and III** are correct

9. Factors likely to cause an increase in the blood urea nitrogen (BUN) level include

I. intramuscular injection of diazepam (Valium)
II. severe liver disease
III. chronic kidney disease

10. A patient who undergoes serum enzyme testing is found to have an elevated aspartate aminotransferase (AST) level. Possible underlying causes of this abnormality include

I. methyldopa-induced hepatitis
II. congestive heart failure (CHF)
III. pneumonia

11. Serum enzyme tests that may aid in the diagnosis of myocardial infarction include

I. alkaline phosphatase
II. creatinine kinase (CK)
III. lactate dehydrogenase (LDH)

8-D
9-B
10-C
11-D

Directions: The group of items in this section consists of lettered options followed by a set of numbered items. For each item, select the **one** lettered option that is most closely associated with it. Each lettered option may be selected once, more than once, or not at all.

Questions 12–14

A 70-year-old black man weighing 154 lb complains of chronic fatigue. Several laboratory tests were performed with the following results:

BUN: 15 mg/dl
AST: within normal limits
WBC: 7500/mm^3
RBC: 4.0 million/mm^3
Hct: 29%
Hb: 9.0 g/dl

12. This patient's mean cell hemoglobin concentration (MCHC) is

(A) 27.5
(B) 28.9
(C) 31.0
(D) 33.5
(E) 35.4

13. His mean cell volume (MCV) is

(A) 61.3
(B) 72.5
(C) 77.5
(D) 90.2
(E) 93.5

14. From the data provided above and from the calculations in questions 12 and 13, this patient is best described as

(A) normal except for a slightly elevated BUN
(B) having normochromic, microcytic anemia
(C) having sickle cell anemia
(D) having hypochromic, normocytic anemia
(E) having folic acid deficiency

12-C
13-B
14-B

ANSWERS AND EXPLANATIONS

1. The answer is C *[II B 2 d (2)].*
Valuable diagnostic information can be obtained through quantitative and qualitative testing of the cells of the blood. A finding of lymphopenia (i.e., decreased number of lymphocytes) suggests an attack on the immune system or some underlying immunodeficiency. Acquired immune deficiency syndrome (AIDS) attacks the T_4 population of lymphocytes and thus may result in lymphopenia.

2. The answer is A *[II A 5].*
The reticulocyte count measures the amount of circulating immature red blood cells (RBCs), which provides information about bone marrow function. A low reticulocyte count is a likely finding in a patient with aplastic anemia—a disorder characterized by a deficiency of all cellular elements of the blood due to a lack of hematopoietic stem cells in bone marrow. A variety of drugs (e.g., those used in anticancer therapy) and other agents produce marrow aplasia. A high reticulocyte count would likely be found in a patient with hemolytic anemia or acute blood loss or in a patient who has been treated for an iron, vitamin B_{12}, or folate deficiency.

3. The answer is E *[V B, E–G].*
Microscopic examination of the urine sediment normally shows fewer than 1 red blood cell (RBC) and from 0–4 white blood cells (WBCs) per high-power field. Other normal findings on urinalysis include an acid pH (i.e., around 6) and an absence of glucose and ketones.

4. The answer is A *[II B 2 c].*
An allergic drug reaction will usually produce an increase in the eosinophil count (eosinophilia). This could be determined by ordering a white blood cell (WBC) differential.

5. The answer is C *[II A 2].*
Overhydration with an excess infusion of dextrose 5% in water produces a low hematocrit (Hct). The other situations described in the question result in elevations of the Hct.

6. The answer is A *[II B 2 a].*
The patient has leukocytosis with an elevated neutrophil count (neutrophilia). A localized infection does not normally result in an increase in the total leukocyte count or neutrophil count. The other situations given in the question can produce a neutrophilic leukocytosis.

7. The answer is B *[III A].*
Because creatine kinase (CK) is not present in the liver, alcoholic liver damage would not result in an elevation of this enzyme. CK is present primarily in cardiac and skeletal muscle. The other situations described in the question could all result in the release of increased amounts of CK into the bloodstream.

8. The answer is D *[IV B].*
The patient with jaundice (deposition of bilirubin in the skin) usually has an increase in the total bilirubin serum level. Spillage of bilirubin into the urine requires an elevated direct bilirubin, which is likely with viral hepatitis or cholestatic hepatitis. In hemolytic anemia, direct bilirubin is not usually increased, and therefore, there would be no spillage of bilirubin into the urine.

9. The answer is B (III) *[VI B 2].*
Chronic kidney disease can cause an increase in the blood urea nitrogen (BUN) level; a heavy protein diet and bleeding into the gastrointestinal tract are other factors that can produce this finding. Severe liver disease can prevent the formation of urea and, therefore, is likely to cause a decrease in the BUN level. Although an intramuscular injection of diazepam (Valium) may cause an increase in the serum creatine kinase (CK) or aspartate aminotransferase (AST) level, it would have no effect on the BUN.

10. The answer is C (I, II) *[III D].*
A lung infection, such as pneumonia, normally would not cause an increase in the release of aspartate aminotransferase (AST), an enzyme primarily found in the liver and heart. In acute hepatitis, a marked elevation of AST is a likely finding. AST levels also can be elevated with passive congestion of the liver, as occurs in congestive heart failure (CHF).

11. The answer is D (II, III) *[III A–C].*
Usually, the creatine kinase (CK), alanine aminotransferase (ALT), aspartate aminotransferase (AST), and lactate dehydrogenase (LDH) enzyme levels are elevated after a myocardial infarction. Alkaline phosphatase is not present in cardiac tissue and, therefore, would not be useful in the diagnosis of a myocardial infarction.

12–14. The answers are: 12-C *[II A 4 c],* **13-B** *[II A 4 a],* **14-B** *[II A 4; VI B 2].*
The mean cell hemoglobin concentration (MCHC) is calculated as follows:

$$\text{MCHC} = \frac{\text{Hemoglobin (Hb)} \times 100}{\text{Hematocrit (Hct)}} = \frac{9 \times 100}{29} = 31.0$$

The mean cell volume (MCV) is calculated as follows:

$$\text{MCV} = \frac{\text{Hct (\%)} \times 10}{\text{RBC count (in millions)}} = \frac{29 \times 10}{4} = 72.5$$

The patient described in the question is anemic, since his Hb is 9 (normal: 14–18). The anemia is normochromic, since the patient's MCHC of 31 is normal (normal range: 31–37), but the anemia is microcytic, since the patient's MCV is 72.5 (normal: 80–100). The patient's blood urea nitrogen (BUN), 15 mg/dl, is within the normal range of 10–20 mg/dl.

41
Ischemic Heart Disease

Barbara Szymusiak-Mutnick

I. INTRODUCTION

A. Definition. Ischemic heart disease (IHD) is a condition in which there is an insufficient supply of oxygen to the myocardium (cardiac tissue) so that oxygen demand exceeds the oxygen supply.

B. Manifestations

1. **Angina pectoris,** an episodic, reversible oxygen insufficiency, is the most common form of IHD (see II).

2. **Acute myocardial infarction** occurs with a severe, prolonged deprivation of oxygen to a portion of the myocardium, resulting in irreversible myocardial tissue necrosis (see III).

3. **Sudden death.** Myocardial ischemia or infarction can trigger the abrupt onset of ventricular fibrillation (the most disorganized arrhythmia), which can stop cardiac output. Without immediate intervention—such as precordial thump, cardiopulmonary resuscitation, or defibrillation countershock—the result is death. Episodic recurrences of ventricular fibrillation, sudden death, and resuscitation are known as the **sudden death syndrome**.

C. Etiology. The processes, singly or in combination, that produce IHD include decreased blood flow to the myocardium, increased oxygen demand, and decreased oxygenation of the blood.

1. **Decreased blood flow.** (Coronary blood flow is illustrated in Figure 41-1.)
   a. **Atherosclerosis,** with or without coronary thrombosis, is the most common cause of IHD. In this condition, the coronary arteries are progressively narrowed by smooth muscle cell proliferation and the accumulation of lipid deposits (plaque) along the inner lining (intima) of the arteries.
   b. **Coronary artery spasm,** a sustained contraction of one or more coronary arteries, can occur spontaneously or be induced by irritation (e.g., by coronary catheter or intimal hemorrhage), exposure to the cold, or ergot-derivative drugs. These spasms can cause Prinzmetal's angina and even myocardial infarction.
   c. **Traumatic injury,** whether blunt or penetrating, can interfere with myocardial blood supply (e.g., the impact of a steering wheel on the chest causing a myocardial contusion in which the capillaries hemorrhage).
   d. **Embolic events,** even in otherwise normal coronary vessels, can abruptly restrict the oxygen supply to the myocardium.

2. **Increased oxygen demand** can occur with exertion (e.g., exercise, shoveling snow) and emotional stress, which increases sympathetic stimulation and, thus, the heart rate. Some factors affecting cardiac workload, and therefore myocardial oxygen supply and demand, are listed in Table 41.1.
   a. **Diastole.** Under normal circumstances, almost all of the oxygen is removed (during diastole) from the arterial blood as it passes through the heart. Thus, little remains to be extracted if oxygen demand increases. To increase the coronary oxygen supply, blood flow has to increase. The normal response mechanism is for the blood vessels, particularly the coronary arteries, to dilate, thereby increasing blood flow.
   b. **Systole.** The two phases of systole—**contraction** and **ejection**—strongly influence oxygen demand.
      (1) The **contractile (inotropic) state of the heart** influences the amount of oxgen it requires to perform.

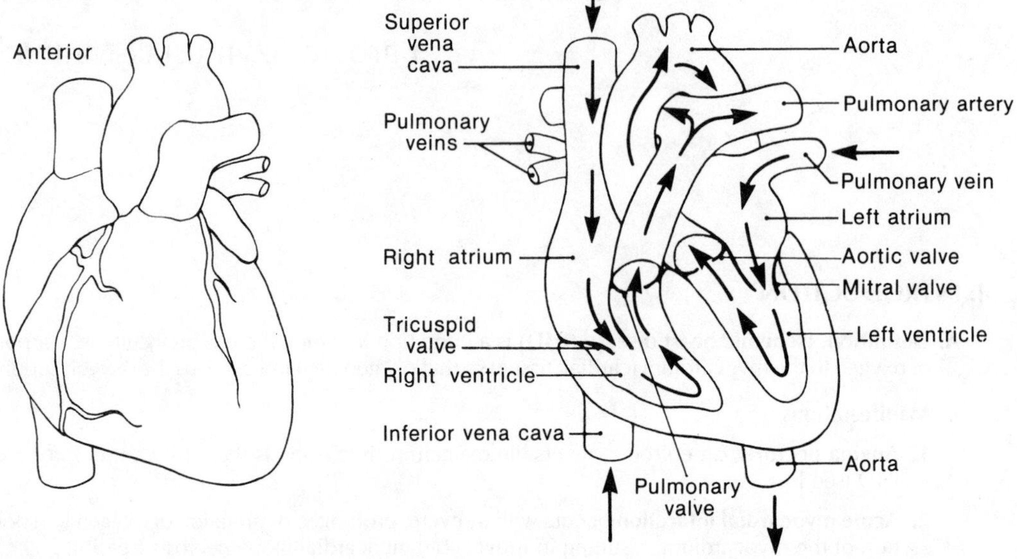

Figure 41-1. Oxygen and other nutrients are borne to the myocardium through the two major coronary arteries (the left and right) and their tributaries. The hemodynamic consequences of ischemic heart disease (IHD) depend on which of the coronary vessels is involved and what part of the myocardium that vessel supplies.

(2) **Increases in systolic wall tension,** influenced by left ventricular volume and systolic pressure, increases oxygen demand.

(3) **Lengthening of ejection time** (i.e., the duration of systolic wall tension per cardiac cycle) also increases oxygen demand.

(4) **Changes in heart rate** influence oxygen consumption by changing the ejection time.

3. **Reduced blood oxygenation.** The oxygen-carrying capacity of the blood may be reduced, as occurs in various anemias.

D. **Risk factors** for IHD appear in Table 41-2.

E. **Therapeutic considerations.** As most IHD occurs secondary to atherosclerosis, which is a long-term, cumulative process, medical efforts focus on reducing risk factors through individual patient education and media campaigns. Once manifestations occur, treatment addresses their variables.

II. ANGINA PECTORIS

A. **Definition.** The term, angina pectoris, is applied to varying forms of transient chest discomfort that are attributable to insufficient myocardial oxygen.

Table 41-1. Factors Affecting Cardiac Parameters That Control Myocardial Oxygen Demand

Factors	Heart Rate	Blood Pressure	Ejection Time	Ventricular Volume	Inotropic Effect
Exercise	Increase	Increase	Decrease	Increase or decrease	Increase
Cold	Increase	Increase	. . .	. . .	. . .
Smoking	Increase	Increase	Increase	. . .	Increase
Nitroglycerin	Increase	Decrease	Decrease	Decrease	Increase
β-Blockers	Decrease	Decrease	Increase	Increase	Decrease

Table 41-2. Risk Factors for Ischemic Heart Disease

Hyperlipidemia
Excess serum cholesterol
Increased ratio of low-density lipoproteins (LDLs) to high-density lipoproteins (HDLs)
Excess triglycerides
Hypertension
Smoking
Diabetes mellitus
Obesity
Family history of ischemic heart disease (IHD)
Sedentary life-style
Chronic stress or type A personality (i.e., aggressive, ambitious, chronically impatient, competitive)
Age and sex (i.e., prevalence is higher among men than among premenopausal women and increases for both sexes with age)
Oral contraceptive use
Gout

B. Common etiologies. Atherosclerotic lesions that produce a narrowing of the coronary arteries is the major cause of angina. However, tachycardia, anemia, hyperthyroidism, hypotension, and arterial hypoxemia are all capable of causing an oxygen imbalance.

C. Types

1. Stable (classic) angina

a. In this most common form, exertion, emotional stress, or a heavy meal usually precipitates chest discomfort, which is relieved by rest, nitroglycerin, or both.

b. Characteristically, the discomfort builds to a peak, radiating to the jaw, neck, shoulder, and arms, and then subsides without residual sensation. If the angina is related to physical exertion, the discomfort usually subsides quickly (i.e., in 3–5 minutes) with rest; if precipitated by emotional stress, the episode tends to last longer (i.e., about 10 minutes).

c. Stable angina is characteristically due to a fixed obstruction in a coronary artery.

2. Unstable angina

a. Angina is considered unstable and requires further evaluation if patients experience:

(1) New-onset angina

(2) Pattern changes (i.e., an increase in intensity, duration, frequency)

(3) Occurrences at rest for the first time

(4) Decreased response to rest or nitroglycerin

b. Progressive, unstable angina may signal incipient myocardial infarction and should be reported promptly to a physician.

3. Angina decubitus (nocturnal angina)

a. This angina occurs in the recumbent position and is not specifically related to either rest or exertion.

b. Increased ventricular volume, causing increased oxygen needs, produces this angina, which may indicate cardiac decompensation.

c. Diuretics alone or in combination are effective in reducing left ventricular volume and may aid the patient.

d. Nitrates such as nitroglycerin, by reducing preload and improving left ventricular dysfunction, may relieve the paroxysmal nocturnal dyspnea associated with angina decubitus.

4. Prinzmetal's angina (vasospastic or variant angina)

a. Coronary artery spasm that reduces blood flow precipitates this angina. The spasm may be superimposed on a coronary artery that already has a fixed obstruction due to thrombi or plaque formation.

b. It usually occurs at rest (i.e., pain may disrupt sleep) rather than with exertion or emotional stress.

c. Characteristically, an electrocardiogram (ECG) taken during an attack reveals a transient ST-segment elevation.

d. Calcium-channel blockers, rather than β-blockers, are most effective for this form of angina. Nitroglycerin may not provide relief, depending on the cause of vasospasm.

D. Characteristic patient complaints. Patients' descriptions of angina include squeezing pressure, sharp pain, burning, aching, bursting, and indigestion-like discomfort, sensations that commonly radiate or move to the arms, legs, neck, shoulders, and back.

E. Physical examination is usually not revealing, especially between attacks. However, the patient's history, risk factors, and full description of attacks—precipitation pattern, intensity, duration, relieving factors—usually prove diagnostic.

F. Diagnostic test results

1. The **ECG** is normal in 50%–70% of patients at rest and who are asymptomatic. During chest pain, the ST segment is usually depressed, except in Prinzmetal's angina (see II C 4 c).
2. **Stress testing (exercise ECG)** aids the diagnosis in patients who have normal resting ECGs. ST-segment depression of more than 1 mm is fairly indicative of a vascular abnormality, but the degree of positivity is most indicative of the degree of abnormality.
3. **Coronary arteriography** and **cardiac catheterization** are very specific and sensitive but are also invasive, expensive, and risky (the mortality rate is about 1%–2%); therefore, they must be used judiciously when trying to confirm suspected angina and to differentiate its etiology.

G. Treatment goals

1. To reduce the risk of sudden death
2. To prevent myocardial infarction
3. To increase myocardial oxygen supply or reduce oxygen demand
4. To reduce discomfort and anxiety associated with an angina attack
5. To remove or reduce **risk factors**
   - **a. Hyperlipidemia** should be reduced through diet, drugs, or both, with serum monitoring and feedback to the patient at regular intervals.
     - **(1)** Cholesterol-lowering drugs such as cholestyramine (Questran), clofibrate (Atromid-S), colestipol (Colestid), niacin, probucol (Lorelco), gemfibrozil (Lopid), lovastatin (Mevacor), pravastatin (Pravachol), and simvastatin (Zocor) have been shown most recently to have a favorable effect in reducing total cholesterol levels, LDL cholesterol levels, triglyceride levels, or increasing HDL levels. However, controversy still exists as to the long-term effect of these agents on patient mortality.
     - **(2)** Recent evidence suggests that coronary lesions may actually regress over time with appropriate antilipidemic therapy.
     - **(3)** Despite the controversies, these agents have been used in an attempt to reduce the incidence of nonfatal myocardial infarction.
   - **b. Hypertension** should be controlled (see Chapter 43).
   - **c. Smoking** should be stopped unless increased anxiety offsets the benefits. Quitting is associated with a 50% decline in cardiovascular mortality within 2 years up until the age of 65.
     - **(1)** Transdermal use of nicotine-containing patches has become one strategy for aiding the cessation of smoking.
     - **(2)** Products such as Nicotrol, Habitrol, Nicoderm, and others are available in varying strengths to wean patients off the use of cigarettes over a 4–8 week period.
   - **d. Obesity** should be reduced through diet and an appropriate exercise program.

H. Therapeutic agents

1. **Nitrates (e.g., nitroglycerin)**
   - **a. Mechanism of action**
     - **(1)** The primary value of nitrates is venous dilation, which reduces left ventricular volume (preload) and myocardial wall tension, decreasing oxygen requirements (demand).
     - **(2)** Nitrates may also reduce arteriolar resistance, helping to reduce afterload, which decreases myocardial oxygen demand.
     - **(3)** By reducing pressure in cardiac tissues, nitrates also facilitate collateral circulation, which increases blood distribution to ischemic areas.

b. Indications

(1) Acute attacks of angina pectoris can be managed with sublingual, transmucosal (spray or buccal tablets), or intravenous delivery.

(2) Indications include the prevention of anticipated attacks, using tablets (oral or buccal) or transdermal paste or patches. Sublingual nitrates can be used prior to eating, sexual activity, or a known stressful event.

c. Choice of preparation should be based on onset of action, duration of action, and patient compliance and preference because all nitrates have the same mechanism of action.

d. Precautions and monitoring effects

(1) To maximize the therapeutic effect, patients should thoroughly understand the use of their specific dosage forms (e.g., sublingual tablets, transdermal patches or pastes, tablets, capsules).

(2) Blood pressure and heart rate should be monitored because all nitrates can increase heart rate while lowering blood pressure.

(3) Preload reduction can be assessed through reduction of pulmonary symptoms such as shortness of breath, paroxysmal nocturnal dyspnea, or dyspnea.

(4) Nitrate-induced headaches are the most common side effect.

(a) Patients should be warned of the nature, suddenness, and potential strength of these headaches to minimize the anxiety that might otherwise occur.

(b) Compliance can be enhanced if the patient understands that the effect is transient and that the headaches usually disappear with continued therapy.

(c) Acetaminophen ingested 15–30 minutes before nitrate administration may prevent the headache.

e. Effective therapy should result in a reduction in the number of anginal attacks without inducing significant adverse effects (e.g., postural hypotension, hypoxia). If maximal doses are reached and the patient still experiences attacks, additional agents should be administered.

2. β-Adrenergic blockers

a. Mechanism of action. β-Blockers reduce oxygen demand, both at rest and during exertion, by decreasing the heart rate and myocardial contractility, which also decreases arterial blood pressure.

b. Indications. These agents reduce the frequency and severity of exertional angina that is not controlled by nitrates.

c. Precautions and monitoring effects

(1) Doses should be increased until the anginal episodes have been reduced or until unacceptable side effects occur.

(2) β-Blockers should be avoided in Prinzmetal's angina (caused by coronary vasospasm) because they increase coronary resistance.

(3) Asthma is a relative contraindication because all β-blockers increase airway resistance and have the potential to induce bronchospasm in susceptible patients.

(4) Diabetic patients and others predisposed to hypoglycemia should be warned that β-blockers mask tachycardia, which is a key sign of developing hypoglycemia.

(5) Patients should be monitored for excessive negative inotropic effects. Findings such as fatigue, shortness of breath, edema, and paroxysmal nocturnal dyspnea may signal developing cardiac decompensation, which also increases the metabolic demands of the heart.

(6) Sudden cessation of β-blocker therapy may trigger a withdrawal syndrome that can exacerbate anginal attacks (especially in patients with coronary artery disease) or cause myocardial infarction.

d. Choice of preparations. All β-blockers are likely to be equally effective for stable (exertional) angina. For further review of β-adrenergic blockers, see Chapter 43 III B 3 a.

3. Calcium-channel blockers

a. Mechanism of action. Two actions are most pertinent in the treatment of angina.

(1) These agents prevent and reverse coronary spasm by inhibiting calcium influx into vascular smooth muscle and myocardial muscle. This results in increased blood flow, which enhances myocardial oxygen supply.

(2) Calcium-channel blockers decrease total peripheral vascular resistance through dilation of peripheral arterioles and reduce myocardial contractility, resulting in decreased oxygen demand.

b. Indications

(1) Calcium-channel blockers are used in stable (exertional) angina that is not controlled by nitrates and β-blockers and in patients for whom β-blocker therapy is inadvisable. Combination therapy—with nitrates, β-blockers, or both—may be most effective.

(2) These agents, alone or with a nitrate, are particularly valuable in the treatment of Prinzmetal's angina.

c. Individual agents

(1) Diltiazem, verapamil, and bepridil

(a) These drugs produce negative inotropic effects, and patients must be monitored closely for signs of developing cardiac decompensation (i.e., fatigue, shortness of breath, edema, paroxysmal nocturnal dyspnea). When co-administered with β-blockers or other agents that produce negative inotropic effects (e.g., disopyramide, quinidine, procainamide, flecainide), the negative effects are additive.

(b) Patients should be monitored for signs of developing bradyarrhythmias and heart block because these agents have negative chronotropic effects.

(c) Verapamil frequently causes constipation, which must be treated as needed to prevent straining at stool, which could cause an increased oxygen demand (Valsalva maneuver).

(d) Doses of diltiazem for the treatment of angina are 30–60 mg every 6–8 hours initially, up to 360 mg/day or 180–300 mg once a day using Cardizem.

(e) Doses of verapamil are 80–120 mg three times a day initially, up to a maximum of 480 mg/day.

(2) Nifedipine

(a) This calcium-channel blocker does not seem to have a strongly negative inotropic effect; therefore, it is preferred for combination therapy with agents that do.

(b) Because nifedipine increases the heart rate somewhat, it can produce tachycardia, which would increase oxygen demand. Co-administration of a β-blocker should prevent reflex tachycardia.

(c) Its potent peripheral dilatory effects can decrease coronary perfusion and produce excessive hypotension, which can aggravate myocardial ischemia.

(d) Dizziness, lightheadedness, and lower extremity edema are the most common adverse effects, but these tend to disappear with time or dose adjustment.

(e) Doses of nifedipine are 10–20 mg three times a day (up to a maximum dose of 20–30 mg three to four times a day or 30–90 mg once a day).

(3) Nicardipine (Cardene) doses are 20–40 mg three times a day or 30–60 mg every 12 hours.

(4) Bepridil (Vascor) and amlodipine (Norvasc). These newly released calcium-channel blockers represent the second-generation agents; they have been used effectively as once a day agents due to their long activity.

(a) Bepridil doses are 200–400 mg/day.

(b) Amlodipine doses are 2.5–10 mg/day.

III. MYOCARDIAL INFARCTION

A. Definition. In myocardial infarction, a portion of the cardiac muscle suffers a severe and prolonged restriction of oxygenated coronary blood. This results in cellular ischemia, tissue injury, and tissue necrosis.

1. Recently, the introduction of thrombolytic agents for the acute management of myocardial infarction has removed thrombus formation in coronary vessels.

2. However, the damage on myocardial tissue is not reversible as it is in angina pectoris, because the myocardial tissue dies.

B. Signs and symptoms

1. The foremost characteristic of a myocardial infarction is persistent, severe chest pain or pressure, commonly described as crushing, squeezing, or heavy (likened to having an elephant sitting on the chest). The pain generally begins in the chest and, like angina, may radiate to the left arm, the abdomen, back, neck, jaw, or teeth. The onset of pain generally occurs at rest or with normal daily activities; it is not commonly associated with exertion.

2. Unlike an angina attack, sensations associated with a myocardial infarction usually persist—longer than 30 minutes—and are unrelieved by nitroglycerin. However, it has been estimated that 20%–30% of heart attacks are associated with no pain (silent myocardial infarction).

3. Other common complaints include a sense of impending doom, sweating, nausea, vomiting, and difficulty breathing. In some patients, fainting and sudden death may be the initial presentation of an acute myocardial infarction.
4. Observable findings include extreme anxiety, restless, agitated behavior, and ashen pallor.
5. Some patients, particularly diabetics or the elderly, may experience only mild or indigestion-like pain or a clinically silent myocardial infarction, which may only manifest in worsening congestive heart failure (CHF), loss of consciousness, a sudden drop in blood pressure, or a lethal arrhythmia.

C. Diagnostic test results. Because a myocardial infarction is a life-threatening emergency, diagnosis is presumed—and treatment is instituted—based on the patient's complaints and the results of an immediate 12-lead ECG. Laboratory tests and further diagnostic tests can rule out or provide confirmation of a myocardial infarction and help to identify the locale and extent of myocardial damage.

1. **Serial 12-lead ECG.** Abnormalities may be absent or inconclusive during the first few hours after a myocardial infarction and may not aid the diagnosis in about 15% of the cases. When present, characteristic findings show progressive changes.
   - **a.** First, ST-segment elevation (injury current) appears in the leads, reflecting the injured area.
   - **b.** Then T waves invert (reflecting ischemia), and Q waves develop (indicating necrosis) in those leads where the ST-segment was elevated.
   - **c.** Unequivocal diagnosis can only be made in the presence of all three abnormalities. However, the manifestations depend on the area of injury. For example, in the non–Q-wave infarction only ST-segment depression may appear.
   - **d.** The most serious arrhythmic complication of an acute myocardial infarction is ventricular fibrillation, which may occur without warning.
   - **e.** Ventricular premature beats (VPBs) are the most commonly encountered arrhythmias and may require treatment.
2. **Chest x-ray** findings are commonly normal unless CHF is developing, indicated by cardiomegaly, pulmonary vascular congestion, or pleural effusion.
3. **Myocardial scanning** with technetium 99m (^{99m}Tc) pyrophosphate for example, is useful in confirming or localizing damage; a "hot spot" on the film indicates the area of uptake by damaged tissue. This is usually positive between 1 day and 1 week after the myocardial infarction.
4. **Cardiac enzyme studies.** Changes in some of the laboratory values do not appear until 6–24 hours after the myocardial infarction (Table 41-3).

D. Treatment goals

1. To relieve chest pain and anxiety
2. To reduce cardiac workload and stabilize cardiac rhythm

Table 41-3. Serum Cardiac Enzyme Values in Myocardial Infarction

Test	Approximate Post-Myocardial Infarction Appearance Time	Comments
CPK (creatine phosphokinase) or CK (creatine kinase)	4–8 hours	MB isoenzyme elevation is particularly telling as it derives almost exclusively in the myocardiam
SGOT (serum glutamic-oxaloacetic transaminase) or AST (aspartate aminotransferase)	8–12 hours	Activity peaks in 24–48 hours; returns to normal in 3–5 days
LDH (lactate dehydrogenase)	24–48 hours	LDH_1 exceeds LDH_2
WBC (white blood cells)	24 hours	A count of 12,000–15,000/μl indicates necrosis

3. To reduce myocardial infarction by limiting the area affected and preserving pump function
4. To prevent or arrest complications, such as lethal arrhythmias, CHF, or sudden death
5. To reopen (or reperfuse) closed coronary vessels with thrombolytic drugs

E. Therapeutic agents. Intramuscular drug administration in myocardial infarction therapy can invalidate the results of cardiac enzyme studies; therefore, this route should be avoided if possible.

1. Nitrates (e.g., nitroglycerin)

a. Mechanism of action. The nitrates decrease oxygen demand and facilitate coronary blood flow, as detailed in II H 1 a.

b. Indications. These agents help to relieve chest pain. Control of pain is crucial to relieve anxiety and to prevent the release of catecholamines, which may be triggered when pain persists. Catecholamines can produce coronary spasm and increased oxygen demand.

2. Morphine

a. Mechanism of action. Morphine causes venous pooling and reduces preload, cardiac workload, and oxygen consumption. Morphine should be administered intravenously, starting with 2 mg and titrating at 5–15-minute intervals until the pain is relieved or toxicity becomes evident.

b. Indications. Morphine is the drug of choice for myocardial infarction pain and anxiety.

c. Precautions and monitoring effects

(1) Because morphine increases peripheral vasodilation and decreases peripheral resistance, it can produce orthostatic hypotension and fainting.

(2) Patients should be monitored for hypotension and signs of respiratory depression.

(3) Morphine has a vagomimetic effect that can produce bradyarrhythmias. If ECG monitoring reveals excess bradycardia, it should be reversed by the administration of atropine (0.5–1 mg).

(4) Nausea and vomiting may occur, especially with initial doses, and patients must be protected against aspiration of stomach contents.

(5) Severe constipation is a potential problem with ongoing morphine administration. The patient may use a Valsalva maneuver while straining at the stool, which can produce a bradycardia or can overload the cardiac system and trigger cardiac arrest. Docusate (100 mg twice daily) is a useful prophylactic.

3. Oxygen. Current **advanced cardiac life support recommendations** require the institution of oxygen therapy in any patient who is suffering from chest pain and who may be ischemic. Increasing the oxygen content of the blood, thus improving oxygenation of the myocardium, is a top priority as continuing hypoxia rapidly increases myocardial damage.

4. Lidocaine

a. Mechanism of action. This antiarrhythmic agent has a rapid effect and is highly controllable because its effects diminish rapidly once infusion is withdrawn. Usual doses begin with a 100-mg loading dose intravenously, followed by a continuous infusion at 2.0–4.0 mg/min.

b. Indications. In recent years, the routine use of lidocaine has become controversial. Some cardiologists elect to treat patients prophylactically with lidocaine, while others believe that the ventricular premature beats (VPBs) mentioned at III C 1 e can be observed cautiously without treatment.

c. Precautions and monitoring effects

(1) Only lidocaine preparations without sympathomimetic amines or other vasoconstrictors should be used in myocardial infarction. Other forms can cause lethal arrhythmias and are, therefore, contraindicated.

(2) The risk of lidocaine toxicity increases with an increased rate of infusion.

d. Significant interactions. Co-administration of a **β-blocker** diminishes the metabolism of lidocaine and may result in lidocaine toxicity. At the first signs of toxicity (e.g., dizziness, somnolence, confusion, paresthesias, convulsions), the lidocaine should be withdrawn.

5. Thrombolytic agents

a. Indications

(1) Thrombolytic agents are used in patients with suspected myocardial infarction with chest pain for 6–8 hours. Successful early reperfusion has been shown to reduce infarct size, improve ventricular function, and improve mortality.

(2) Intravenous administration of streptokinase (SK), recombinant tissue-type plasminogen activator (t-PA), or anisoylated plasminogen streptokinase activator complex (APSAC) may restore blood flow in an occluded artery if administered within 6–8 hours of an acute myocardial infarction.

(a) These agents promote thrombus dissolution by working on plasminogen either directly or indirectly, resulting in clot lysis.

(b) t-PA is relatively fibrin-specific and is able to lyse clots without depleting fibrinogen. SK activates the fibrinolytic system and has a greater likelihood of causing systemic effects than t-PA. This effect may result in a greater degree of systemic bleeding as compared to t-PA.

(c) Though it is still controversial as to which agent—t-PA or SK—is the best, most studies have shown that both drugs, when used early, can re-open (reperfusion) occluded coronary arteries and reduce mortality from myocardial infarction.

b. Individual agents

(1) Streptokinase (SK)

(a) Absolute contraindications to SK include active internal bleeding, recent cerebrovascular accident (CVA), intracranial or intraspinal surgery, intracranial neoplasm, pregnancy, arteriovenous malformation, aneurysm, bleeding diathesis, and severe uncontrolled hypertension or hemorrhagic ophthalmic conditions.

(b) Precautions and monitoring effects

(i) Patients who have received SK within the previous 6 months have an added predisposition to allergic reactions as well as a refractory response to SK due to systemic antibody formation.

(ii) Patients must be monitored for bleeding, arrhythmias, anaphylactoid reactions, and hypotension,. Many patients develop arrhythmias, which do not require treatment, within 30–45 minutes of SK administration; these arrhythmias are called **reperfusion arrhythmias,** referring to a clot that has been removed and resulted in coronary reperfusion.

(c) Dosage. An intravenous dose of 1.5 million IU is infused over 60 minutes. Other treatments are currently being used, including bolus doses followed by continuous infusions, as well as combination therapy with t-PA.

(2) Recombinant tissue-type plasminogen activator (t-PA)

(a) Absolute contraindications to t-PA include active internal bleeding; recent CVA; intracranial neoplasm; aneurysm; pregnancy; arteriovenous malformations; recent (within 2 months) intracranial surgery, spinal surgery, or trauma; and severe uncontrolled hypertension, bleeding diathesis, or hemorrhagic ophthalmic conditions.

(b) Dosage for patients over 65 kg. A total of 100 mg of t-PA is generally administered to all patients over 65 kg over a 3-hour period. Though many regimens have been used, generally speaking, 6–10 mg of t-PA is given as an intravenous bolus dose over 1–2 minutes, followed by the remaining infusion rates over the next 3 hours:

(i) A 54-60 mg intravenous infusion over the first hour

(ii) A 20-mg intravenous infusion over the second hour

(iii) A 20-mg intravenous infusion over the third hour

(c) Dosage for patients under 65 kg. For patients less than 65 kg, a dose of 1.25 mg/kg is given over a 3-hour period with 10% of the total dose given initially as a bolus dose over 1–2 minutes.

(3) Anisoylated plasminogen streptokinase activator complex (APSAC)

(a) APSAC is the newest thrombolytic agent to be approved in the United States. It is effective in the treatment of acute myocardial infarction and has many properties similar to that of SK.

(b) The **major advantage** of APSAC over the other agents is its ease of administration as a rapid intravenous bolus dose of 30 units over a short time (less than 5 minutes).

(c) Further evaluation is needed to identify its place in the treatment of acute myocardial infarction.

c. Adjunctive therapy

(1) Aspirin administered 160–325 mg during acute thrombolytic therapy has been shown to effect thrombolysis positively by preventing platelet aggregation. Though the data are not totally conclusive at this time, most cardiologists favor the early use of aspirin after a myocardial infarction and continue doses of 160–325 mg daily thereafter.

(2) Heparin has been administered along with the thrombolytics to prevent re-occlusion once a coronary artery has been opened. In the United States, heparin has been given intravenously as a 5000-unit bolus, followed by a continuous infusion of 1000 units/hour; the goal is to maintain the activated partial thromboplastin time (APTT) between 1½–2½ times normal. Heparin has also been administered subcutaneously in some centers but that seems to be the exception rather than the rule at this time.

6. **β-Adrenergic blockers**
   a. If administered early in the acute phase, β-blockers (e.g., propranolol, metoprolol, atenolol, timolol) have been shown to reduce the potential zone of infarction, decrease oxygen demands, and decrease cardiac workload.
   b. β-Blocker therapy has also been shown to reduce significantly postmyocardial infarction mortality due to sudden death.
   c. **Precautions and monitoring effects** (see II H 2 c).

F. Complications. Myocardial infarction potentiates many complications; the most common of these include:

1. **Lethal arrhythmias.** Arrhythmias refractory to lidocaine may respond to procainamide, and bretylium.
2. **Congestive heart failure.** (See Chapter 44 for a more detailed discussion.)
   a. Left ventricular failure causes pulmonary congestion. Diuretics, especially furosemide, help reduce the congestion.
   b. Digitalis glycosides have a positive inotropic effect, which improves myocardial contractility, helping to compensate for myocardial damage.
3. **Cardiogenic shock**
   a. In this life-threatening complication, cardiac output is decreased and pulmonary artery and pulmonary capillary wedge pressures are increased. This typically occurs when the area of infarction exceeds 40% of muscle mass and compensatory mechanisms only strain the already compromised myocardium.
   b. Vasopressors [e.g., norepinephrine, epinephrine, dopamine (high doses)] enhance blood pressure through α-receptor stimulation and may be indicated.
   c. Inotropic drugs [e.g., epinephrine, dopamine (middle doses), dobutamine, isoproterenol, digitalis] are rapidly acting agents used to increase myocardial contractility and improve cardiac output.
   d. Vasodilators (e.g., nitroprusside) reduce preload by lowering pulmonary capillary wedge pressure through venous dilation while reducing afterload by decreasing resistance to left ventricular ejection.
   e. Additional treatment may include invasive procedures such as intra-aortic balloon pumping.

G. Recent advances in adjunctive therapy

1. The role of warfarin is currently being explored for its beneficial effects postmyocardial infarction. Initial effects seem promising.
2. Magnesium sulfate has been shown in preliminary trials to protect the myocardium against ischemia-induced reperfusion injury, to limit CHF, and to reduce early mortality.
3. Angiotensin-converting enzyme (ACE) inhibitors have been used in clinical trials after myocardial infarctions and have been shown to be effective in preventing and treating CHF. Further studies are ongoing.

STUDY QUESTIONS

Directions: Each of the numbered items or incomplete statements in this section is followed by answers or by completions of the statement. Select the **one** lettered answer or completion that is **best** in each case.

1. Exertion-induced angina, which is relieved by rest, nitroglycerin, or both, is referred to as

(A) Prinzmetal's angina
(B) unstable angina
(C) classic angina
(D) variant angina
(E) preinfarction angina

2. Myocardial oxygen demand is increased by all of the following factors EXCEPT

(A) exercise
(B) smoking
(C) cold temperatures
(D) isoproterenol
(E) propranolol

3. Which of the following agents used in Prinzmetal's angina has spasmolytic actions, which increase coronary blood supply?

(A) Nitroglycerin
(B) Nifedipine
(C) Timolol
(D) Isosorbide dinitrate
(E) Propranolol

4. For what adverse drug effect must angina pectoris patients receiving propranolol plus diltiazem be monitored?

(A) Decreased cardiac output
(B) Decreased heart rate
(C) Increased heart rate
(D) Decreased cardiac output and decreased heart rate
(E) Decreased cardiac output and increased heart rate

5. Maximal medical therapy for treating angina pectoris is represented by which of the following choices?

(A) Diltiazem, verapamil, nitroglycerin
(B) Atenolol, isoproterenol, diltiazem
(C) Verapamil, nifedipine, propranolol
(D) Isosorbide, atenolol, diltiazem
(E) Nitroglycerin, isosorbide, atenolol

6. The term ischemic heart disease (IHD) is used to designate all of the following conditions EXCEPT

(A) angina pectoris
(B) sudden cardiac death
(C) congestive heart failure (CHF)
(D) arrhythmias
(E) myocardial infarction

7. The development of ischemic pain occurs when the demands for oxygen exceed the supply. Determinants of oxygen demand include all of the following choices EXCEPT

(A) contractile state of the heart
(B) myocardial ejection time
(C) left ventricular volume
(D) right atrial pressure
(E) systolic pressure

8. The use of morphine in the myocardial infarction patient centers around three distinct pharmacologic properties. Which of the following choices includes these properties?

(A) Relief of pain, relief of anxiety, and increased oxygen supply
(B) Relief of anxiety, afterload reduction, increased preload
(C) Relief of anxiety, preload reduction, and relief of pain
(D) Vagomimetic effect, relief of anxiety, respiratory depression
(E) Bradycardia, preload reduction, and increased afterload

1-C	4-D	7-D
2-E	5-D	8-C
3-B	6-C	

Directions: Each item below contains three suggested answers of which **one or more** is correct. Choose the answer

A if **I only** is correct
B if **III only** is correct
C if **I and II** are correct
D if **II and III** are correct
E if **I, II, and III** are correct

Questions 9–10

A 55-year-old white man is seen in the emergency room of a local hospital with the signs and symptoms of an acute myocardial infarction. This is the second such attack within the last 4 months, and the patient has not altered his life-style to eliminate important risk factors. Previous therapy included a thrombolytic agent (name unknown), a blood thinner, and daily aspirin.

9. Which of the following thrombolytic agents would be appropriate at this time?

I. Anisoylated plasminogen streptokinase activator complex (APSAC)
II. Streptokinase (SK)
III. Recombinant tissue-type plasminogen activator (t-PA)

10. Which of the following agents should be recommended during the acute myocardial infarction to help prevent sudden death?

I. Atenolol
II. Metoprolol
III. Propranolol

9-B
10-E

ANSWERS AND EXPLANATIONS

1. The answer is C *[II C 1 a].*
Classic, or stable, angina refers to the syndrome in which physical activity or emotional excess causes chest discomfort, which may spread to the arms, legs, neck, and so forth. This type of angina is relieved promptly (within 1–10 minutes) with rest, nitroglycerin, or both.

2. The answer is E *[I C 2; Table 41-1].*
Due to the β-adrenergic blocking effects of propranolol (e.g., decreased heart rate, decreased blood pressure, decreased inotropic effect), there is a net decrease in myocardial oxygen demand. This is directly opposite of the effects seen with the β-agonist isoproterenol. Exercise, cigarette smoking, and exposure to cold temperatures have all been shown to increase myocardial oxygen demand.

3. The answer is B *[II C 4, H 3 c (2)].*
Due to the calcium-channel blocking properties of nifedipine, primarily coronary dilation and spasmolytic effects, there is proven benefit of this agent in the treatment of Prinzmetal's angina, a syndrome believed due more to a spastic event rather than to a fixed coronary occlusion.

4. The answer is D *[II H 2, 3].*
As propranolol (a β-adrenergic blocker) and diltiazem (a calcium-channel blocker) both reduce heart rate (a negative chronotropic effect) and reduce cardiac contractility (negative inotropic effect), patients receiving both drugs must be monitored for signs of decompensation (reduced cardiac output) and bradyarrhythmias.

5. The answer is D *[II H 3 b (1)].*
The use of a nitrate (isosorbide) in conjunction with a β-adrenergic blocker (atenolol) and a calcium-channel blocker (diltiazem) represents the maximal medical regimen that presently could be used in a nonresponsive angina patient. Venous dilation and coronary dilation due to nitrates reduces oxygen demand while increasing oxygen supply, respectively. The addition of diltiazem further reduces oxygen demand by decreasing the heart rate and cardiac contractility. The use of a β-blocker such as atenolol reduces oxygen demand even more, resulting in a total net reduction in myocardial oxygen demand.

6. The answer is C *[I B].*
Ischemic heart disease (IHD) is a clinical condition that exists when there is a lack of oxygen to the heart. This may be due to increased demands of or decreased supplies to the heart. Angina pectoris, sudden cardiac death due to toxic ventricular arrhythmias, and myocardial infarction represent the various conditions associated with IHD.

7. The answer is D *[I C 2].*
As with most muscles in the body, the contractile force of the heart dictates the amount of oxygen that the heart needs to perform. Consequently, as contractility decreases, the oxygen needs of the heart increase. As contractility continues to decrease, the volume of fluid in the left ventricle increases due to poor muscle performance and increasing tension within the ventricle, resulting in additional oxygen requirements. As the amount of tension within the ventricle increases per cardiac cycle, there is again an added requirement for oxygen by the heart muscle.

8. The answer is C *[III E 2].*
Venous dilation (preload reduction) along with relief of pain and anxiety make morphine a very helpful agent in the myocardial infarction patient. In the clinical situation, pain and anxiety in the myocardial infarction patient represent an added stress, which only increases myocardial oxygen demands further, thus adding potential insult to the already compromised myocardium. Venous dilation would help in reducing venous return to the heart and, therefore, reduce oxygen demands placed on the myocardium. Both of these physiologic responses aid in re-establishing the balance between myocardial oxygen supply and demand.

9 and 10. The answers are: 9-B (III) *[III E 5 b],* **10-E (all)** *[III E 6 a, b].*
Streptokinase (SK) and anisoylated plasminogen streptokinase activator complex (APSAC) are derived from exogenous substances, which initiate antibody formation after initial exposure. A patient receiving either agent within 6 months of previous exposure may have a refractory response to them due to excess antibody production. It has also been speculated that such patients may have an increased likelihood

of developing an allergic reaction. Recombinant tissue-type plasminogen activator (t-PA) represents recombinant DNA technology where exogenous substances are not introduced into the body. The likelihood for antibody formation is nil, and therefore, this agent, barring any absolute contraindications, would be the agent of choice.

Recent studies have made it relatively clear that when atenolol, metoprolol, and propranolol are given during the acute phases of a myocardial infarction, there is a significant reduction in sudden death and overall mortality in the patients treated. Each of these β-adrenergic blockers is given intravenously, followed by oral therapy, in an attempt to eliminate sudden death as a consequence of myocardial infarction. Due to the negative inotropic, chronotropic effects, it is still imperative to monitor the patient closely for signs of cardiac decompensation and bradyarrhythmias.

42
Cardiac Arrhythmias

Alan H. Mutnick

I. INTRODUCTION

A. Definition. Cardiac arrhythmias are deviations from the normal heartbeat pattern. They include **abnormalities of impulse formation,** such as heart rate, rhythm, or site of impulse origin, and **conduction disturbances,** which disrupt the normal sequence of atrial and ventricular activation.

B. Electrophysiology

1. **Conduction system**
   a. **Two electrical sequences** that cause the heart chambers to fill with blood and contract are initiated by the conduction system of the heart.
      (1) **Impulse formation,** the first sequence, takes place when an electrical impulse is generated automatically.
      (2) **Impulse transmission,** the second sequence, occurs once the impulse has been generated, signaling the heart to contract.
   b. **Four main structures** composed of tissue that can generate or conduct electrical impulses comprise the conduction system of the heart.
      (1) The **sinoatrial (SA) node,** in the wall of the right atrium, contains cells that spontaneously initiate an action potential. Serving as the main pacemaker of the heart, the SA node initiates 60–100 beats/min.
         (a) Impulses generated by the SA node trigger atrial contraction.
         (b) Impulses travel through internodal tracts—the anterior tract, middle tract (Wenckebach's bundle), posterior tract (Thorel's bundle), and anterior interatrial tract (Bachmann's bundle) [Figure 42-1].
      (2) At the **atrioventricular (AV) node,** situated in the lower interatrial septum, the impulses are delayed briefly to permit completion of atrial contraction before ventricular contraction begins.
      (3) At the **bundle of His**—muscle fibers arising from the AV junction—impulses travel along the left and right bundle branches, located on either side of the intraventricular septum.
      (4) The impulses reach the **Purkinje fibers,** a diffuse network extending from the bundle branches and ending in the ventricular endocardial surfaces. Ventricular contraction then occurs.
   c. **Latent pacemakers.** The AV junction, bundle of His, and Purkinje fibers are latent pacemakers; they contain cells capable of generating impulses. However, these regions have a slower firing rate than the SA node. Consequently, the SA node predominates except when it is depressed or injured, which is known as **overdrive suppression**.

2. **Myocardial action potential.** Before cardiac contraction can take place, cardiac cells must depolarize and repolarize.
   a. **Depolarization** and **repolarization** result from changes in the electrical potential across the cell membrane, caused by the exchange of sodium and potassium ions.
   b. **Action potential,** which reflects this electrical activity, has five phases (Figure 42-2).
      (1) **Phase 0 (rapid depolarization)** takes place as sodium ions enter the cell through fast channels; the cell membrane's electrical charge changes from negative to positive.
      (2) **Phase 1 (early rapid repolarization).** As fast sodium channels close and potassium ions leave the cell, the cell rapidly repolarizes (i.e., returns to resting potential).

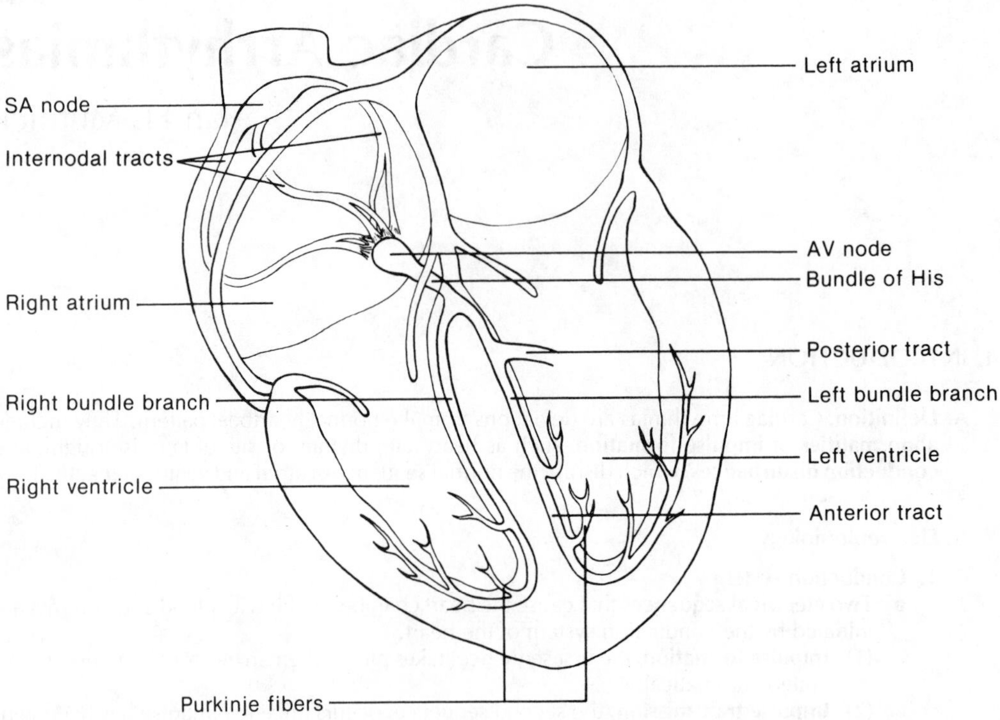

Figure 42-1. Electrical pathways of the heart. *SA* = sinoatrial; *AV* = atrioventricular.

(3) **Phase 2 (plateau).** Calcium ions enter the cell through slow channels while potassium ions exit. As the cell membrane's electrical activity temporarily stabilizes, the action potential reaches a plateau (represented by the notch at the beginning of this phase in Figure 42-2).

(4) **Phase 3 (final rapid repolarization).** Potassium ions are pumped out of the cell as the cell rapidly completes repolarization and resumes its initial negativity.

(5) **Phase 4 (slow depolarization).** The cell returns to its resting state with potassium ions inside the cell and sodium and calcium ions outside.

c. During both depolarization and repolarization, a cell's ability to initiate an action potential varies.

(1) The cell cannot respond to any stimulus during the **absolute refractory period** (beginning during phase 1 and ending at the start of phase 3).

(2) A cell's ability to respond to stimuli increases as repolarization continues. During the **relative refractory period,** occurring during phase 3, the cell can respond to a strong stimulus.

(3) When the cell has been completely repolarized, it can again respond fully to stimuli.

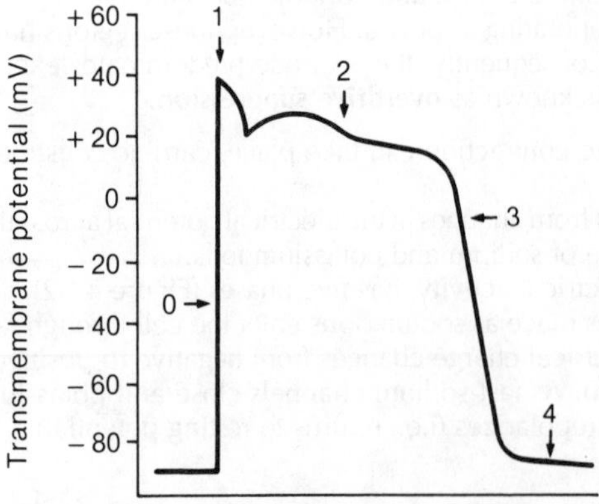

Figure 42-2. Myocardial action potential curve. This curve represents ventricular depolarization/repolarization. *0* = phase 0 (rapid depolarization); *1* = phase 1 (early rapid repolarization); *2* = phase 2 (plateau); *3* = phase 3 (final rapid repolarization; *4* = phase 4 (slow depolarization).

d. Cells in different cardiac regions depolarize at various speeds, depending on whether fast or slow channels predominate.
  (1) Sodium flows through fast channels; calcium flows through slow channels.
  (2) Where fast channels dominate (e.g., in cardiac muscle cells), depolarization occurs quickly. Where slow channels dominate (e.g., in the electrical cells of the SA node and AV junction), depolarization occurs slowly.

3. Electrocardiography. The electrical activity occurring during depolarization–repolarization can be transmitted through electrodes attached to the body and transformed by an **electrocardiograph (ECG) machine** into a series of waveforms (ECG waveform). Figure 42-3 shows a normal ECG waveform.
  a. The **P wave** reflects atrial depolarization.
  b. The **PR interval** represents the spread of the impulse from the atria through the Purkinje fibers.
  c. The **QRS complex** reflects ventricular depolarization.
  d. The **ST segment** represents phase 2 of the action potential—the absolute refractory period (part of ventricular repolarization).
  e. The **T wave** shows phase 3 of the action potential—ventricular repolarization.

C. Classification. Arrhythmias generally are classified by origin (i.e., supraventricular or ventricular).

1. Supraventricular arrhythmias stem from enhanced automaticity of the SA node (or another pacemaker region) or from re-entry conduction.

2. Ventricular arrhythmias occur when an ectopic (abnormal) pacemaker triggers a ventricular contraction before the SA node fires (e.g., from a conduction disturbance or ventricular irritability).

D. Etiology

1. Precipitating causes. Arrhythmias result from various conditions, including:
  a. Heart disease (e.g., infection, coronary artery disease, valvular heart disease, rheumatic heart disease, ischemic heart disease)
  b. Myocardial infarction
  c. Toxic doses of cardioactive drugs (e.g., digitalis preparations)
  d. Increased sympathetic tone
  e. Decreased parasympathetic tone
  f. Vagal stimulation (e.g., straining at stool)
  g. Increased oxygen demand (e.g., from stress, exercise, fever)
  h. Metabolic disturbances
  i. Cor pulmonale
  j. Systemic hypertension
  k. Hyperkalemia
  l. Chronic obstructive pulmonary disease (COPD) [e.g., chronic bronchitis, emphysema]
  m. Thyroid disorders

2. Mechanisms of arrhythmias. Abnormal impulse formation, abnormal impulse conduction, or a combination of both may give rise to arrhythmias.
  a. Abnormal impulse formation may stem from:
    (1) Depressed automaticity, as in escape beats and bradycardia
    (2) Increased automaticity, as in premature beats, tachycardia, and extrasystole
    (3) Depolarization and triggered activity, leading to sustained ectopic firing
  b. Abnormal impulse conduction results from:
    (1) A conduction block or delay
    (2) **Re-entry,** which occurs when an impulse is re-routed through certain regions in which it has already traveled. The impulse, thus, depolarizes the same tissue more than once,

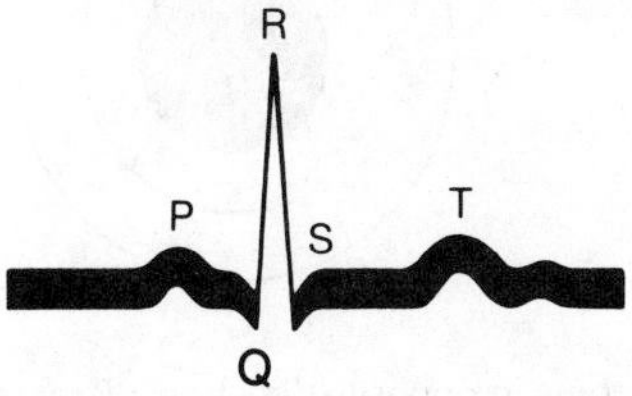

Figure 42-3. Normal ECG waveform.

producing an additional impulse (Figures 42-4 and 42-5). Re-entry sites include the SA and AV nodes as well as various accessory pathways in the atria and ventricles (Figure 42-6). For re-entry to occur, the following conditions must exist:

(a) Markedly shortened refractoriness or a slow conduction area that allows an adequate delay so that depolarization recurs

(b) Unidirectional conduction

E. Pathophysiology. Arrhythmias may decrease cardiac output, reduce blood pressure, and disrupt perfusion of vital organs. Specific pathophysiologic consequences depend on the arrhythmia present (see III).

F. Clinical evaluation

1. **Physical findings.** Although some arrhythmias are silent, most produce signs and symptoms. Only an ECG can definitively identify an arrhythmia. However, physical findings may suggest which arrhythmia is present; they also yield information about the patient's clinical status and may help to identify associated complications. **Signs and symptoms** that typically accompany arrhythmias include:
   - **a.** Chest pain
   - **b.** Anxiety and confusion (from reduced brain perfusion)
   - **c.** Dyspnea
   - **d.** Skin pallor or cyanosis
   - **e.** Abnormal pulse rate, rhythm, or amplitude
   - **f.** Reduced blood pressure
   - **g.** Palpitations
   - **h.** Syncope
   - **i.** Weakness
   - **j.** Convulsions
   - **k.** Hypotension
   - **l.** Decreased urinary output

2. **Diagnostic test results**
   - **a.** An **ECG** can identify a specific arrhythmia; usually, a 12-lead ECG is used. (For ECG findings in specific arrhythmias, see III.)
   - **b. Electrophysiologic (EP) testing.** This intracardiac procedure determines the location of ectopic foci and bypass tracts and may help assess therapeutic response to antiarrhythmic drug therapy. It also can determine the need for a pacemaker or surgical intervention.
     - **(1)** Intracardiac catheters and pacing wires are placed transvenously or transarterially.
     - **(2)** The heart is divided into imaginary sections, and each section is stimulated until an arrhythmia is induced. The section in which the arrhythmia occurs is identified as the origin of the ectopic foci.
   - **c. His bundle study,** a type of EP testing, can locate the origin of a heart block or re-entry pattern.
   - **d. Laboratory findings.** Some arrhythmias result from electrolyte abnormalities—most commonly, hyperkalemia and hypocalcemia.
     - **(1)** A serum potassium level above 5 mEq/L reflects hyperkalemia; a serum calcium level below 4.5 mEq/L signifies hypocalcemia.
     - **(2)** An ECG tracing may suggest an electrolyte abnormality. For example, prolonged QRS complexes, tented T waves, and lengthened PR intervals may signal hyperkalemia; prolonged QT intervals and flattened, or inverted, T waves suggest hypocalcemia.

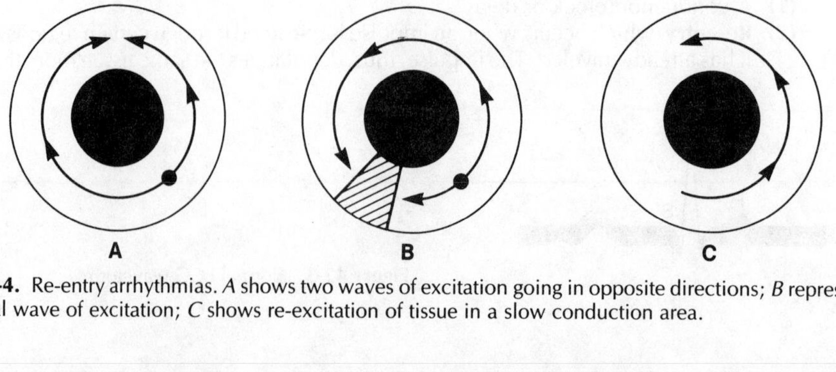

Figure 42-4. Re-entry arrhythmias. *A* shows two waves of excitation going in opposite directions; *B* represents a unidirectional wave of excitation; *C* shows re-excitation of tissue in a slow conduction area.

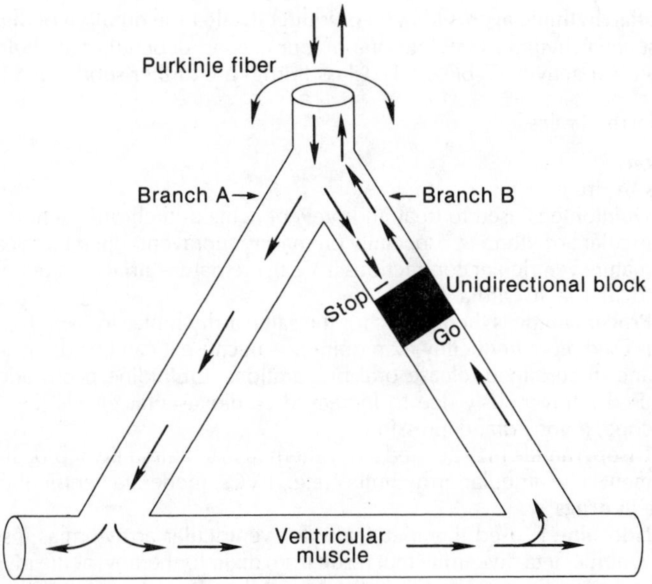

Figure 42-5. Ventricular re-entry. This diagram shows a branched Purkinje fiber joining ventricular muscle. The *darkened area* represents the site of a unidirectional block; in this depolarized region, the impulse heading toward the AV node continues upward while the impulse traveling toward the muscle is blocked. Because retrograde conduction in *branch B* is slow, cells in *branch A* have time to recover and respond to the re-entrant impulse.

G. Treatment objectives

1. **Terminate or suppress the arrhythmia,** if it causes hemodynamic compromise or disturbing symptoms.
2. **Maintain adequate cardiac output and tissue perfusion.**
3. **Correct or maintain fluid balance** (some arrhythmias cause hypervolemia).

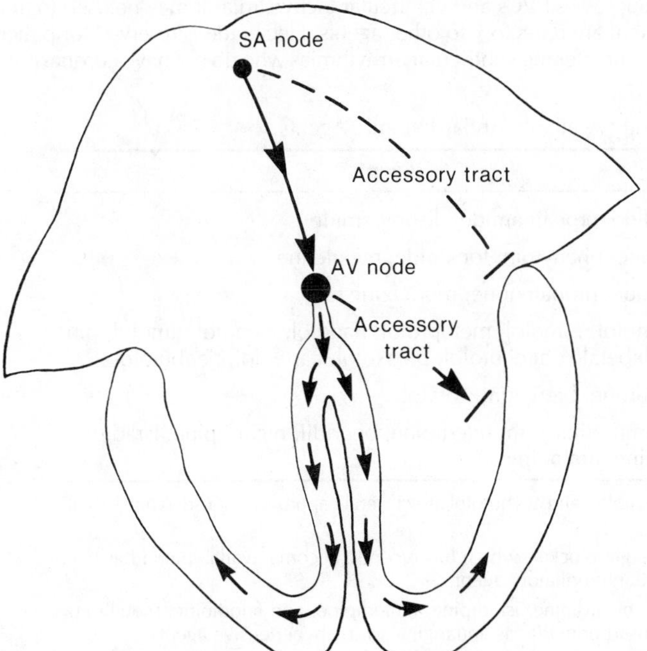

Figure 42-6. Re-entry sites.

II. THERAPY. Antiarrhythmic agents directly or indirectly alter the duration of the myocardial action potential. Most antiarrhythmics fall into one of four classes, depending on their specific effects on the heart's electrical activity (Table 42-1). Class I drugs are further subdivided into three groups.

A. Class I antiarrhythmics

1. Indications

a. Class IA drugs

(1) Quinidine is used to treat and prevent acute and chronic ventricular and supraventricular arrhythmias, especially premature supraventricular tachycardias (PSVTs), premature ventricular contractions (PVCs), premature atrial contractions (PACs), and ventricular tachycardia.

(2) Procainamide is therapeutic for the same arrhythmias for which quinidine is given. It is used more frequently than quinidine because it can be administered intravenously and in sustained-release oral preparations. Quinidine poses added concern when used intravenously due to increased cardiovascular effects (i.e., hypotension, syncope, myocardial depression).

(3) Disopyramide may be used as an alternative to quinidine or procainamide in the treatment of ventricular arrhythmias (e.g., PVCs, moderate ventricular tachycardia).

b. Class IB drugs

(1) Lidocaine is used therapeutically for ventricular arrhythmias (especially PVCs and ventricular tachycardia) that result from digitalis therapy, acute myocardial infarction, and open-heart surgery. Controversy still exists as to the benefits of lidocaine when used prophylactically in patients with acute myocardial infarction to prevent ventricular fibrillation.

(2) Tocainide, closely related to lidocaine, is used to treat and prevent ventricular arrhythmias, including frequent PVCs and ventricular tachycardia. It may be given after an acute myocardial infarction.

(3) Phenytoin most commonly is used to treat digitalis-induced ventricular and supraventricular arrhythmias. It is also given to suppress ventricular arrhythmias associated with acute myocardial infarction, open-heart surgery, or ventricular arrhythmias that are refractory to lidocaine or procainamide, but its efficacy is less significant for these indications than it is for digitalis-induced arrhythmias.

(4) Mexiletine, another drug that closely resembles lidocaine, is used to suppress ventricular arrhythmias, including those following an acute myocardial infarction. It is effective against ventricular tachycardia that has not responded to other antiarrhythmics.

c. Class IC drugs

(1) Flecainide suppresses PVCs and ventricular tachycardia; it may be used to treat some arrhythmias that are refractory to other agents. Flecainide is reserved for patients with refractory life-threatening ventricular arrhythmias who do not have coronary artery disease.

Table 42-1. Currently Available Antiarrhythmic Agents

Class	Agents
IA	Quinidine, procainamide, disopyramide
IB	Lidocaine, phenytoin, tocainide, mexiletine
IC	Flecainide, propafenone, moricizine
II*	Propranolol, esmolol, metoprolol, nadolol, atenolol, timolol, pindolol, labetalol, acebutolol, betaxolol, carteolol, penbutolol
III†	Amiodarone, bretylium, sotalol
IV‡	Verapamil, diltiazem, nifedipine, bepridil, nicardipine, isradipine, felodipine, amlodipine

*Only propranolol, esmolol, and acebutolol are currently approved for use as antiarrhythmics.

†Sotalol is a β-adrenergic blocker, which has recently become available and has been classified as a type III antifibrillatory agent.

‡Nifedipine, bepridil, nicardipine, isradipine, amlodipine, and felodipine, though currently available, are used primarily as antianginal or antihypertensive agents.

(2) **Propafenone** also suppresses PVCs and ventricular tachycardia and has been used successfully in the treatment of sustained ventricular tachycardia when the arrhythmia is life-threatening.

(3) **Moricizine** is a difficult antiarrhythmic to classify based on the fact that it has properties of all three class I antiarrhythmic groups. Because it prolongs the QRS interval like other class IC agents, it has been classified as a class IC agent throughout this discussion. Moricizine is effective for suppression of PVCs, and may offer some benefits over other agents due to a lower incidence of proarrhythmia effects.

2. **Mechanism of action.** Class I antiarrhythmics slow impulse conduction through the AV node by depressing the flow of sodium ions into cells during phase 0 of the action potential. Class I subgroups (i.e., IA, IB, IC) differ in the degree and onset of their myocardial depressant actions and in their effects on the duration of the action potential and repolarization phase.
   a. **Class IA drugs** moderately reduce the depolarization rate and prolong repolarization (refractory period).
   b. **Class IB drugs** shorten repolarization (refractory period); they also weakly affect the repolarization rate.
   c. **Class IC drugs** strongly depress depolarization but have a negligible effect on the duration of repolarization or refractoriness.

3. **Administration and dosage**
   a. **Quinidine** is administered orally, usually in three or four daily doses of 200–300 mg. Sustained-release products may be given every 8–12 hours, depending on the salt form. (In special circumstances, it cautiously can be given intravenously or intramuscularly.) To achieve an effective plasma concentration rapidly, a loading dose of 600–1000 mg may be administered in doses of 200 mg every 2 hours to a maximum of 1000 mg.
   b. **Procainamide** is available for oral, intravenous, or intramuscular use.
      (1) For **acute therapy,** intravenous administration is preferred.
         (a) Intermittent intravenous administration calls for infusion of 100 mg over 2–4 minutes, repeated every 5 minutes until the arrhythmia is abolished, side effects occur, or 1 g has been given. The usual effective dose is 500–1000 mg.
         (b) Rapid intravenous administration calls for infusion of 1–1.5 g at a rate of 20–50 mg/min.
         (c) Once the arrhythmia is terminated, 2–6 mg/min are given as a continuous infusion.
      (2) For **long-term therapy,** oral administration is used. The usual daily dosage is 3–6 g, given at intervals of 4–6 hours or less frequently with the sustained-release form of the drug (every 6–8 hours).
   c. **Disopyramide** is available in oral form. Usually, 400–800 mg/day are administered in divided doses or less frequently with the controlled-release product. (A loading dose of 300–400 mg may be given to attain an effective plasma level rapidly.
   d. **Lidocaine** may be administered intravenously or intramuscularly.
      (1) An intravenous loading dose rapidly achieves a therapeutic plasma level.
         (a) Initially, 1–1.5 mg/kg are administered.
         (b) A second injection of half the initial dose may be required 5 minutes later.
      (2) Continuous intravenous infusion of 1–4 mg/min produces an effective plasma level in 7–10 hours.
      (3) In an emergency, an intramuscular injection rapidly achieves an effective plasma level. The usual dosage is 300–400 mg injected into the deltoid muscle.
   e. **Tocainide** is administered orally. Initially, 400 mg are given every 8 hours; then, 1200–1800 mg/day are given in two or three divided doses.
   f. **Phenytoin** is given orally or in intermittent intravenous doses.
      (1) For oral administration, a loading dose of 1 g is divided over the first 24 hours; for the next 2 days, 300–500 mg/day are administered. The maintenance dosage is 300–400 mg/day.
      (2) For intermittent intravenous administration, 100 mg are given every 5 minutes at a rate not exceeding 25–50 mg/min, until the arrhythmia disappears, adverse effects develop, or 1 g has been given. The usual effective dosage is 700 mg.
   g. **Mexiletine** is given orally in an initial dosage of 200–400 mg, followed by 200 mg every 8 hours. If this fails to control the arrhythmia, the dosage may be increased to 400 mg every 8 hours. (Alternatively, doses may be given every 12 hours.)

h. **Flecainide** is administered orally in a dosage of 50–100 mg every 12 hours. To obtain satisfactory arrhythmia control, the dosage may be increased in twice-daily increments of 50 mg every 4 days to a maximum of 400–600 mg/day.

i. **Propafenone** is administered orally in an initial dose of 150 mg every 8 hours. This dose may be slowly increased at 3–4-day intervals to a maximum dose of 300 mg every 8 hours.

j. **Moricizine** is administered orally in doses ranging from 600–900 mg divided into three equal doses throughout the day.

4. Precautions and monitoring effects

a. Quinidine

(1) This drug is contraindicated in patients with:

(a) Complete AV block unless a ventricular pacemaker is in place

(b) Marked prolongation of the QT interval or prolonged QT syndrome because ventricular tachyarrhythmia (torsades de pointes) may arise, resulting in quinidine syncope (i.e., syncope or sudden death)

(2) An increase of 50% or more in the duration of the QRS complex necessitates dosage reduction.

(3) Quinidine has a narrow therapeutic index. Toxicity may cause acute cardiac effects, such as pronounced slowing of conduction in all heart regions; this, in turn, may lead to SA block or arrest, ventricular tachycardia, or asystole.

(4) The ECG should be monitored during quinidine therapy to detect signs of cardiotoxicity. To counteract quinidine-induced ventricular tachyarrhythmias, catecholamines, glucagon, or sodium lactate may be given.

(5) In patients receiving quinidine for atrial tachyarrhythmias, vagolytic effects may increase impulse conduction at the AV node, resulting in an accelerated ventricular response. To prevent this, agents that slow AV nodal conduction (e.g., verapamil, digoxin) may be administered.

(6) The dosage should be reduced in elderly patients (over 60 years) and in patients with hepatic dysfunction or congestive heart failure (CHF).

(7) Embolism may occur upon restoration of normal sinus rhythm after prolonged atrial fibrillation. To prevent or minimize this complication, anticoagulants may be administered before quinidine therapy begins.

(8) Quinidine may cause cinchonism at high serum concentrations, manifested by tinnitus, hearing loss, blurred vision, and gastrointestinal disturbances. In severe cases, nausea, vomiting, diarrhea, headache, confusion, delirium, photophobia, diplopia, and psychosis may occur.

(9) Gastrointestinal reactions are the most common adverse reactions to quinidine. About 30% of patients experience diarrhea; nausea and vomiting may also occur. Arising almost immediately after the first dose, these symptoms sometimes warrant drug discontinuation. However, aluminum hydroxide or use of the polygalacturonate salt may reverse this.

(10) Hypersensitivity reactions include anaphylaxis, thrombocytopenia, respiratory distress, and vascular collapse.

(11) Plasma quinidine levels of 2–6 μg/ml are therapeutic.

b. Procainamide

(1) This drug is contraindicated in patients with hypersensitivity to procaine and related drugs, myasthenia gravis, second- or third-degree AV block with no pacemaker, a history of procainamide-induced systemic lupus erythematosus (SLE), prolonged QT syndrome, or torsades de pointes.

(2) An increase of 50% or more in the duration of the QRS complex necessitates dosage reduction.

(3) Procainamide has a narrow therapeutic index. Toxicity may cause acute cardiac effects (e.g., pronounced slowing of conduction in all heart regions), which, in turn, may lead to SA block or arrest, ventricular tachycardia, or asystole.

(4) High serum procainamide levels may induce ventricular arrhythmias (e.g., PVCs, ventricular tachycardia or fibrillation). The ECG should be monitored continuously to detect these problems. Catecholamines, glucagon, or sodium lactate may be administered to counteract these arrhythmias.

(5) Hypotension may occur with rapid intravenous administration.

(6) Gastrointestinal effects are less common than with quinidine therapy.

(7) Hypersensitivity reactions are the most severe adverse effects of procainamide. These reactions include drug fever, agranulocytosis, and an SLE–like syndrome.

(a) An SLE-like syndrome is manifested by fatigue, arthralgia, myalgia, and low-grade fever.

(b) Antinuclear antibody titer is positive in 50%–80% of patients receiving procainamide. However, only 20%–30% of these patients develop symptoms of the SLE-like syndrome.

(c) Drug discontinuation usually is necessary when symptomatic SLE-like syndrome occurs.

(8) N-Acetylprocainamide (NAPA), an active procainamide metabolite, may accumulate in patients with renal dysfunction, increasing the risk of drug toxicity.

(9) The dosage should be reduced and given over 6 hours to patients with renal or hepatic impairment, as the drug half-life is increased in these patients.

(10) Lower doses may be needed in patients with CHF to adjust for the lower volume of distribution.

(11) Embolism may occur upon restoration of normal sinus rhythm after prolonged atrial fibrillation. An anticoagulant is frequently administered before procainamide therapy begins to prevent this complication.

(12) Plasma levels of both procainamide and NAPA should be monitored. Generally, a procainamide level of 4–8 μg/ml and a NAPA level of 15–25 μg/ml are considered therapeutic. Controversy still exists as to the routine monitoring of both of these levels.

c. Disopyramide

(1) This drug may cause marked hemodynamic compromise and ventricular dysfunction. It is contraindicated in patients with cardiogenic shock or second- or third-degree AV block with no pacemaker.

(2) Disopyramide should be avoided or used with extreme caution in patients with CHF. It should also be used cautiously in patients with urinary tract disorders, myasthenia gravis, and renal or hepatic dysfunction.

(3) In patients receiving this drug for atrial tachyarrhythmias, vagolytic effects may increase impulse conduction at the AV node, resulting in an accelerated ventricular response. To prevent this, agents that slow AV nodal conduction (e.g., verapamil, digoxin) may be given.

(4) Anticholinergic effects of this drug include dry mouth, constipation, urinary hesitancy or retention, and blurred vision.

(5) Therapeutic plasma levels range from 2 μg/ml to 4 μg/ml.

d. Lidocaine

(1) This drug may cause hemodynamic compromise in patients with severe cardiac dysfunction. Generally, however, it has few untoward cardiovascular effects.

(2) Lidocaine should be used cautiously and in reduced dosage in patients with CHF or renal or hepatic impairment.

(3) Central nervous system (CNS) reactions are the most pronounced adverse effects of lidocaine. These reactions may range from light-headedness and restlessness to confusion, tremors, stupor, and convulsions.

(4) Tinnitus, blurred vision, and anaphylaxis have been reported.

(5) Plasma lidocaine levels of 1.5–6.5 μg/ml are therapeutic.

(6) Lidocaine's metabolites—glycinexylidide and monoethylglycinexylidide—may have neurotoxic as well as antiarrhythmic effects.

e. Tocainide

(1) This drug is contraindicated in patients with hypersensitivity to lidocaine and related agents.

(2) Tocainide must be used cautiously in patients with CHF or reduced cardiac reserve.

(3) Neurologic effects, including light-headedness, paresthesias, restlessness, confusion, and tremors, are encountered in 30%–50% of patients.

(4) Nausea, vomiting, epigastric pain, and diarrhea occur frequently.

(5) Other adverse effects of tocainide include hypotension, blurred vision, aplastic anemia, hepatitis, skin rash, and pulmonary fibrosis.

(6) Dosage reduction may be necessary in patients with renal or hepatic impairment.

(7) Plasma tocainide levels of 3–10 μg/ml are therapeutic.

f. Phenytoin

(1) This drug is contraindicated in patients with sinus bradycardia or heart block.

(2) Phenytoin must be used cautiously in patients with CHF, renal or hepatic impairment, myocardial insufficiency, respiratory depression, or hypotension.
(3) During acute therapy, this drug may cause CNS reactions (e.g., drowsiness, vertigo, nystagmus, ataxia, nausea). Cardiotoxicity also may occur, especially with fast intravenous infusion rates.
(4) Chronic phenytoin may lead to vestibular and cerebellar effects, behavioral changes, gastrointestinal distress, gingival hyperplasia, megaloblastic anemia, and osteomalacia.
(5) Hypersensitivity reactions may be manifested by liver, skin, and hematologic problems.
 (a) Toxic hepatitis may occur.
 (b) Skin reactions include exfoliative dermatitis, Stevens-Johnson syndrome, scarlatiniform or morbilliform rash, SLE, toxic epidermal necrolysis, eosinophilia, and erythema multiforme.
 (c) Hematologic reactions include agranulocytosis, megaloblastic anemia, leukopenia, thrombocytopenia, and pancytopenia.
(6) Therapeutic plasma phenytoin levels range from 10 μg/ml to 20 μg/ml.

g. Mexiletine
(1) This drug is contraindicated in patients with cardiogenic shock or second- or third-degree AV block with no pacemaker.
(2) Tremor is an early sign of mexiletine toxicity. Dizziness, ataxia, and nystagmus indicate an increasing plasma drug concentration.
(3) Hypotension, bradycardia, and widened QRS complexes may develop during mexiletine therapy.
(4) Adverse gastrointestinal effects include nausea and vomiting.
(5) Therapeutic serum levels range from 0.50 μg/ml to 2.0 μg/ml.

h. Flecainide
(1) This drug is contraindicated in patients with cardiogenic shock or second- or third-degree AV block with no pacemaker.
(2) The ECG should be monitored during flecainide therapy because this drug may exacerbate existing arrhythmias or precipitate new ones.
(3) This drug has a significant negative inotropic effect and may bring on or worsen CHF and cardiomyopathy.
(4) Adverse CNS effects (e.g., dizziness, headache, tremor) and gastrointestinal effects (e.g., nausea, abdominal pain) may occur.
(5) Blurred vision and dyspnea have been reported.

i. Propafenone
(1) This drug, like other antiarrhythmic agents, may cause new or worsened arrhythmias. Such proarrhythmic properties range from an increased frequency of PVCs to the development of severe ventricular tachycardia, ventricular fibrillation, and torsades de pointes. This proarrhythmic effect has been under discussion for the class IC agents, and, thus, this agent should be monitored closely. Most recently, encainide, was taken off the market in the United States due to significant arrhythmogenic properties in the completed Cardiac Arrhythmia Suppression Trial (CAST). The findings from this trial must be weighed against the benefits of using these agents for the treatment of significant ventricular arrhythmias.
(2) Dizziness is a side effect that has been reported in as many as 10%–15% of patients taking the drug.
(3) Other associated side effects include vomiting, a metallic, bitter taste in the mouth, constipation, headache, and new or worsening CHF and asthma.

j. Moricizine
(1) This drug has been reported to have proarrhythmic properties. However, it has been reported that the incidence of this effect may be less than with other antiarrhythmics. Patients predisposed to the development of such proarrhythmic effects include those with a history of coronary artery bypass surgery, pacemakers, coronary artery disease, CHF, and conduction abnormalities. As most patients receiving this agent have at least one of the above-mentioned risk factors, this agent must be used cautiously. The benefits of using this agent must be weighed against its associated risks.
(2) Dizziness is the most commonly reported adverse effect associated with the drug and has been reported in up to 15% of all patients.
(3) Other associated side effects include nausea, intraventricular conduction delays, headache, fatigue, palpitations, and shortness of breath.

5. Significant interactions

a. Quinidine

(1) Quinidine may increase serum levels of **digoxin** and increase the effects of **digitalis** on the heart with a resultant increase in toxicity.

(2) Severe orthostatic hypotension may occur with concomitant administration of **vasodilators** (e.g., **nitroglycerin**).

(3) **Phenytoin, rifampin,** and **barbiturates** may antagonize quinidine activity and reduce its therapeutic efficacy.

(4) **Nifedipine** may reduce plasma quinidine levels.

(5) **Antacids, sodium bicarbonate,** and **sodium acetazolamide** may increase plasma quinidine levels, possibly resulting in toxicity.

(6) Quinidine may produce additive hypoprothrombinemic effects with **coumarin** anticoagulants.

b. Amiodarone and **cimetidine** may increase plasma procainamide levels, possibly leading to drug toxicity.

c. Phenytoin accelerates disopyramide metabolism, possibly reducing its therapeutic efficacy.

d. Lidocaine

(1) **Phenytoin** may increase the cardiodepressant effects of lidocaine.

(2) **β-Blockers** (class II antiarrhythmics) may reduce lidocaine metabolism, possibly leading to drug toxicity.

e. Phenytoin

(1) The risk of phenytoin toxicity increases with concomitant administration of **diazepam, antihistamines, isoniazid, chloramphenicol, dicumarol, cimetidine, salicylates, sulfisoxazole, phenylbutazone, amiodarone,** and **valproate**.

(2) **Carbamazepine** may enhance phenytoin metabolism and, thus, reduce plasma phenytoin levels and therapeutic efficacy. (Phenytoin has the same effect on carbamazepine.)

f. Mexiletine. Phenobarbital, rifampin, and **phenytoin** reduce plasma mexiletine levels and may decrease therapeutic efficacy.

B. Class II antiarrhythmics

1. Indications. These drugs—**β-adrenergic blockers**—are used mainly to treat systemic hypertension. Among the drugs in this class, propranolol and esmolol are approved for antiarrhythmic use. (The use of class II drugs in the treatment of hypertension is discussed in Chapter 43.)

a. Propranolol may be given to:

(1) Control supraventricular arrhythmias (e.g., atrial fibrillation or flutter, PSVTs)

(2) Treat tachyarrhythmias caused by catecholamine stimulation (e.g., in hypothyroidism, during anesthesia)

(3) Suppress severe ventricular arrhythmias in **prolonged QT syndrome**

(4) Treat digitalis-induced ventricular arrhythmias

(5) Terminate certain ventricular arrhythmias (e.g., PVCs in patients without structural heart disease)

b. Esmolol is used to treat supraventricular tachycardias; it possesses a very short (9-minute) half-life and has been used to control the ventricular response to atrial fibrillation or flutter during or after surgery.

2. Mechanism of action. Class II antiarrhythmics reduce sympathetic stimulation of the heart, decreasing impulse conduction through the AV node and lengthening the refractory period. As a result, the heart rate slows, with a decrease in myocardial oxygen demand.

3. Administration and dosage

a. Propranolol may be given intravenously or orally when used as an antiarrhythmic.

(1) Emergency therapy calls for slow intravenous administration of 1–3 mg diluted in 50 ml dextrose 5% in water or normal saline solution. This dose is infused slowly (no faster than 1 mg/min). A second dose of 1–3 mg may be given 2 minutes later.

(2) For oral therapy, 10–80 mg/day are given in three or four doses. (However, 1000 mg or more may be required for resistant ventricular arrhythmias.)

b. Esmolol is given intravenously. A loading dose of 500 μg/kg/min is infused over 1 minute, followed by a 4-minute maintenance infusion of 50 μg/kg/min. If a satisfactory response is not achieved within 5 minutes, the loading dose is repeated and followed by a maintenance infusion of 100 μg/kg/min.

4. **Precautions and monitoring effects**
   a. **Propranolol**
      (1) This drug is contraindicated in patients with sinus bradycardia, second- or third-degree AV block, cardiogenic shock, severe CHF, or asthma.
      (2) The β-blocking effects of this drug may lead to marked hypotension, exacerbation of CHF and left ventricular failure, or cardiac arrest.
      (3) Blood pressure, heart rate, and the ECG should be monitored during intravenous infusion.
      (4) Embolism may occur upon restoration of normal sinus rhythm after sustained atrial fibrillation. An anticoagulant may be given before propranolol therapy begins to prevent this complication.
      (5) Propranolol may depress AV node conduction and ventricular pacemaker activity, resulting in AV block or asystole.
      (6) This drug may mask the signs and symptoms of hypoglycemia. It also may mask signs of shock.
      (7) Fatigue, lethargy, increased airway resistance, and skin rash have been reported.
      (8) Nausea, vomiting, and diarrhea may occur.
      (9) Sudden withdrawal of propranolol may lead to acute myocardial infarction, arrhythmias, or angina in cardiac patients. Drug therapy is discontinued by tapering the dose over 4–7 days.
   b. **Esmolol**
      (1) This drug is contraindicated in patients with severe CHF or sinus bradycardia.
      (2) Hypotension occurs in approximately 30% of patients receiving esmolol. This effect can be reversed by reducing the dosage or stopping the infusion.
      (3) This drug is for short-term use only and should be replaced by a long-acting antiarrhythmic once the patient's heart stabilizes.
      (4) Dizziness, headache, fatigue, and agitation may occur.
      (5) Other adverse effects include nausea, vomiting, and bronchospasm.

5. **Significant interactions**
   a. **Propranolol**
      (1) Severe vasoconstriction may occur with concomitant **epinephrine** administration.
      (2) **Digitalis** preparations can cause excessive bradycardia.
      (3) **Calcium-channel blockers** (e.g., **diltiazem, verapamil**) and other negative **inotropic** and **chronotropic drugs** (e.g., **disopyramide, quinidine**) add to the myocardial depressant effects of propranolol.
   b. **Esmolol. Morphine** may raise plasma esmolol levels.

C. **Class III antiarrhythmics**

1. **Indications**
   a. **Amiodarone** is given to control refractory ventricular arrhythmias and may be used prophylactically against ventricular tachycardia and fibrillation. It usually is reserved as a last-line agent for arrhythmias that are unresponsive to first- and second-line agents.
   b. **Bretylium** is used solely to treat life-threatening ventricular arrhythmias, including ventricular tachycardia and ventricular fibrillation, that have not responded to other agents. It should be given only in intensive care facilities.
   c. **Sotalol** is used to treat supraventricular and ventricular tachyarrhythmias. It does not have nonselective β-blocking activity and works by delaying atrial and ventricular repolarization. This property is its main distinguishing factor and is the reason why it is classified as a type III antiarrhythmic drug rather than a type II agent (β-blocker).

2. **Mechanism of action.** Class III antiarrhythmic drugs prolong the refractory period and action potential; they have no effect on myocardial contractility or conduction time.

3. **Administration and dosage**
   a. **Amiodarone** is available for oral use, where 800–1600 mg are given daily for 1–3 weeks until a satisfactory response occurs; a maintenance dose (200–600 mg/day) is then given.
   b. **Bretylium** is used for short-term intravenous or intramuscular therapy.
      (1) For ventricular fibrillation, 5 mg/kg are given by rapid intravenous injection. As needed, the dosage may be increased to 10 mg/kg and repeated every 15–30 minutes up to a total of 30 mg/kg.
      (2) For other ventricular arrhythmias, 500 mg are diluted to 50 ml with dextrose 5% or

normal saline solution and infused intravenously at 5–10 mg/kg over more than 8 minutes. The dose may be repeated in 1–2 hours, then given every 6–8 hours.
(3) Bretylium has also been used successfully as a continuous infusion at a rate of 1–2 mg/min, after diluting 500 mg in 50 ml dextrose 5% in water or normal saline solution.
(4) Intramuscular therapy calls for administration of 5–10 mg/kg undiluted. As needed, the dose may be repeated in 1–2 hours, then given every 6–8 hours.

c. Sotalol
(1) Sotalol is available commercially as an oral tablet in two divided doses of 160–480 mg/day.
(2) An intravenous preparation has been used in the acute treatment of arrhythmias with doses of 0.2–1.0 mg/kg.

4. Precautions and monitoring effects

a. Amiodarone
(1) Life-threatening pulmonary toxicity may occur during amiodarone therapy, especially in patients receiving more than 400 mg/day. Baseline as well as routine pulmonary function tests reveal relevant pulmonary changes.
(2) Most patients develop corneal microdeposits 1–4 months after amiodarone therapy begins. However, this reaction rarely causes visual disturbance, but the patient should be monitored with routine ophthalmologic examinations.
(3) Blood pressure and heart rate and rhythm should be monitored.
(4) Patients should be monitored routinely for the possible development of hepatic dysfunction, thyroid disorders (e.g., hyperthyroidism, hypothyroidism) and photosensitivity.
(5) CNS reactions include fatigue, malaise, peripheral neuropathy, and extrapyramidal effects.
(6) Nausea and vomiting have been reported.
(7) This drug has an extremely long half-life (up to 50 days). Therapeutic response may be delayed for weeks after oral therapy begins; adverse reactions may persist up to 4 months after therapy ends.

b. Bretylium
(1) This drug is contraindicated in digitalis-induced arrhythmias.
(2) Severe hypotension, especially orthostatic hypotension, may develop when bretylium is administered intravenously for the treatment of acute arrhythmias.
(3) Rapid intravenous injection may cause severe nausea and vomiting.
(4) Patients with renal impairment may require dosage reduction.

c. Sotalol
(1) Side effects of this drug are directly related to β-blockade and prolongation of repolarization.
(2) Transient hypotension, bradycardia, myocardial depression, and bronchospasm have all been associated with this drug.
(3) This drug carries all the contraindications associated with other β-blockers along with those due to its electrophysiologic properties.

5. Significant interactions

a. Amiodarone
(1) Amiodarone may increase the plasma levels of **quinidine, procainamide, diltiazem, digitalis,** and **flecainide**.
(2) It may increase the pharmacologic effect of **β-blockers, calcium-channel blockers,** and **warfarin**.

b. Bretylium. Antihypertensives may potentiate bretylium-induced hypotension.

c. Sotalol
(1) Sotalol must be used cautiously in those patients receiving agents with cardiac depressant properties.
(2) Agents such as sotalol, which prolong the QT interval, may induce malignant arrhythmias when used in combination with other type IA antiarrhythmics, especially in the presence of low potassium levels.

D. Class IV antiarrhythmics

1. Indications

a. Calcium-channel blockers (e.g., verapamil, diltiazem) are used mainly to treat and prevent supraventricular arrhythmias.

(1) They are first-line agents for the suppression of PSVTs stemming from AV nodal reentry.
(2) They can rapidly control the ventricular response to atrial flutter and fibrillation.

b. Other calcium-channel blockers available include nicardipine, nifedipine, bepridil, amlodipine, and felodipine, but these agents have primarily been used in the treatment of angina pectoris and hypertension. For information on these agents see Chapters 41 and 43.

2. **Mechanism of action.** Class IV antiarrhythmics are calcium-channel blockers. They inhibit AV node conduction by depressing the SA and AV nodes, where calcium channels predominate.

3. **Administration and dosage**
   a. To control atrial arrhythmias, verapamil usually is administered intravenously. A dose of 5–10 mg is given over at least 2 minutes and may be repeated in 30 minutes, if necessary. A 5–10 mg/hr continuous intravenous infusion has also been used in treating arrhythmias.
   b. To prevent PSVTs, verapamil may be given orally in four daily doses of 80–120 mg each.
   c. To control atrial arrhythmias, diltiazem usually is administered intravenously. A dose of 20 mg (0.25 mg/kg) is given over 2 minutes. If an adequate response is not obtained, a second dose of 25 mg (0.35 mg/kg) is administered after 15 minutes. A 5–15 mg/hr intravenous continuous infusion has also been used in treating arrhythmias.

4. **Precautions and monitoring effects**
   a. Verapamil and diltiazem are contraindicated in patients with AV block, left ventricular dysfunction, severe hypotension, concomitant intravenous, β-blocking, and atrial fibrillation with an accessory AV pathway.
   b. These drugs must be used cautiously in patients with CHF, sick sinus syndrome, myocardial infarction, and hepatic or renal impairment.
   c. Because of the negative chronotropic effect, verapamil and diltiazem must be used cautiously in patients who have slow heart rates or who are receiving digitalis glycosides.
   d. The ECG (especially the RR interval) should be monitored during therapy.
   e. Patients over age 60 should receive reduced dosages and slower injection rates.
   f. Constipation and nausea have been reported with verapamil.

5. **Significant interactions**
   a. Concomitant administration of **β-blockers** or **disopyramide** may precipitate heart failure.
   b. **Quinidine** may increase the risk of calcium-channel blocker–induced hypotension.
   c. Verapamil may increase serum **digoxin** concentrations, and diltiazem may do the same to a lesser extent.
   d. **Rifampin** may enhance the metabolism of calcium-channel blockers with a resultant decrease in pharmacologic effect.
   e. Verapamil and diltiazem may inhibit **theophylline** metabolism and may require reductions in theophylline dosage.
   f. Diltiazem and verapamil inhibit the metabolism of **cyclosporine** and may require reductions in cyclosporine dosages.

E. Unclassified antiarrhythmics

1. **Atropine**
   a. **Indications.** Atropine is therapeutic for symptomatic sinus bradycardia and junctional rhythm.
   b. **Mechanism of action.** An anticholinergic, atropine blocks vagal effects on the SA node, promoting conduction through the AV node and increasing the heart rate.
   c. **Administration and dosage.** For antiarrhythmic use, atropine is administered in a dose of 0.4–1 mg by intravenous push; the dose is given every 5 minutes to a maximum of 2 mg.
   d. **Precautions and monitoring effects**
      (1) Thirst and dry mouth are the most common adverse effects of atropine.
      (2) CNS reactions (e.g., restlessness, headache, disorientation, dizziness) may occur with doses greater than 5 mg.
      (3) Tachycardia and ophthalmic disturbances (e.g., mydriasis, blurred vision, photophobia) may occur with doses of 1 mg or more.
      (4) Initial doses may induce a reflex bradycardia due to incomplete suppression of vagal impulses.

2. **Adenosine**
   a. **Indications.** Adenosine is indicated for the conversion of acute supraventricular tachycardia to normal sinus rhythm.

b. Mechanism of action. Adenosine is a naturally occurring nucleoside, which is normally present in all cells of the body. It has been shown to:
(1) Slow conduction through the AV node.
(2) Interrupt re-entry pathways through the AV node.
(3) Restore normal sinus rhythm in patients with PSVTs.

c. Administration and dosage. For antiarrhythmic effects, adenosine is given as a rapid bolus intravenous injection in a 6-mg dose over 1–2 seconds. If the first dose does not result in elimination of the arrhythmia within 1–2 minutes, the dose should be increased to 12 mg and again given as a rapid intravenous dose. An additional 12 mg dose may be repeated if necessary.

d. Precautions and monitoring effects
(1) The effects of adenosine are antagonized by methylxanthines, such as caffeine and theophylline. Theophylline has been successfully used for the treatment of adenosine-induced side effects, such as hypotension, sweating, and palpitations. If side effects are encountered, aggressive therapy is not required because of the ultra-short half-life of the drug (10 seconds or less).
(2) The main side effect associated with adenosine use in up to 18% of patients is facial flushing, but this effect is normally very short-lived.
(3) Other side effects associated with adenosine use include shortness of breath, chest pressure, nausea, headache, and a metallic taste.

e. Additional use. Adenosine has recently been used as an adjunctive agent in patients undergoing various types of pharmacologic stress testing (e.g., with thallium). In this situation, adenosine is given as a continuous infusion over a period of about 4–6 minutes and is able to provide a form of exercise tolerance test in patients not able to exert themselves due to age, fatigue, and other various physical handicaps.

III. MAJOR ARRHYTHMIAS

A. Supraventricular arrhythmias

1. Sinus bradycardia

a. Description. This arrhythmia occurs when the heart rate is less than 60 beats/min and impulses originate in the SA node. Signs and symptoms include light-headedness, palpitations, fatigue, hypotension, and ventricular ectopy.

b. Causes include hyperkalemia, drugs, vagal stimulation, severe pain, and myocardial infarction. (In well-conditioned athletes, sinus bradycardia is considered normal.)

c. Therapy
(1) Asymptomatic sinus bradycardia usually requires no treatment.
(2) When this arrhythmia leads to hemodynamic compromise, atropine may be administered intravenously in a dose of 0.4–1.0 mg every 5–10 minutes until the desired heart rate is attained.
(3) Artificial pacing may be indicated in some cases.

2. Sinus tachycardia

a. Description. This arrhythmia occurs when the heart rate ranges from 100 beats/min to 160 beats/min; impulses originate from the SA node. Sinus tachycardia commonly causes palpitations but is usually benign.

b. Causes include decreased vagal tone, increased sympathetic tone, digitalis toxicity, and increased myocardial oxygen demand as well as fever, stress, and inflammation. Nonpathologic causes include caffeine and alcohol consumption.

c. Therapy. A class II antiarrhythmic (e.g., propranolol) may be given if treatment is required and if heart failure is not present. Digitalis may be helpful in the patient with heart failure.

3. Sinus arrest

a. Description. This arrhythmia occurs when the SA node fails to initiate an electrical impulse. On ECG, the P wave is dropped or absent, and the PP interval is not a multiple of the sinus rhythm.

b. Causes include myocardial infarction, digitalis toxicity, increased vagal tone, and degenerative heart disease.

c. Therapy. The underlying cause should be treated if symptomatic bradycardia develops. Drug therapy has not shown long-term benefits, and a permanent pacemaker may be indicated in the symptomatic patient.

4. Sick sinus syndrome

a. Description. In this conduction disturbance (also known as Stokes-Adams syndrome), tachycardia and bradycardia alternate; these arrhythmias are interrupted by a long sinus pause. Symptoms include dizziness and syncope.

b. Causes include cardiomyopathy, atherosclerosis, myocardial infarction, neuromuscular disorders, and drug therapy.

c. Therapy. Chronic sick sinus syndrome may warrant drugs (digitalis or propranolol), permanent pacing, or both.

5. Premature atrial contractions (PACs)

a. Description. PACs occur when an ectopic pacemaker generates premature beats before the SA node fires again. On the ECG, the P wave is premature and abnormal (possibly buried in the preceding T wave); PR intervals are abnormally short or long. Nonconducted PACs, which occur when the impulse reaches the ventricles during the absolute refractory period, cause absent QRS complexes. PACs typically produce an irregular pulse and palpitations.

b. Causes include coronary heart disease, valvular heart disease, drug therapy (e.g., procainamide, digitalis), infection, and inflammation. Nonpathologic causes include fatigue, stress, caffeine or alcohol consumption, and nicotine.

c. Therapy. Usually, PACs are clinically insignificant and do not require treatment. However, when they occur frequently or lead to prolonged tachycardia, therapy with digitalis, propranolol, or another drug that prolongs the atrial refractory period (e.g., quinidine or procainamide) may be given.

6. Paroxysmal supraventricular tachycardias (PSVTs)

a. Description. This category includes two tachyarrhythmias originating above the bundle of His bifurcation: paroxysmal atrial tachycardia (PAT) and paroxysmal junctional tachycardia (PJT). These arrhythmias result from AV nodal re-entry mechanism.

(1) The heart rate is from 140 beats/min to 240 beats/min; the rhythm is regular.

(2) On the ECG, PSVTs are manifested by aberrant QRS complexes and a P wave contour that deviates from that of sinus beats.

(3) PSVTs may cause no symptoms or may produce mild chest pain, palpitations, nausea, and dyspnea.

b. Causes include digitalis toxicity, primary cardiac disease (e.g., myocardial infarction, congenital heart disease), hyperthyroidism, and cor pulmonale.

c. Therapy. Most PSVTs subside spontaneously.

(1) In patients with underlying cardiac disease or if PSVTs cause hemodynamic compromise, an emergency mechanical measure (e.g., Valsalva maneuver, carotid sinus massage, synchronized cardioversion) or drug therapy (e.g., adenosine, digitalis, diltiazem, verapamil) may be needed.

(2) Chronic PSVTs may warrant maintenance therapy with digitalis, propranolol, verapamil, diltiazem, quinidine, or procainamide.

7. Atrial flutter

a. Description. This arrhythmia occurs when ectopic impulses are at a rate of 220 beats/min to 350 beats/min. However, a protective mechanism of the AV node allows only some of these impulses to reach the ventricles. The ventricular rate determines how much danger this arrhythmia poses. On the ECG, sawtoothed F (flutter) waves appear; the ratio of atrial to ventricular contractions may be constant or variable.

b. Causes include myocardial infarction, valvular heart disease, cor pulmonale, coronary artery disease, cardiac infection, CHF, COPD, thyrotoxicosis, and quinidine therapy.

c. Therapy

(1) Atrial flutter, causing a rapid ventricular rate and decreased cardiac output, calls for emergency measures, such as:

(a) Synchronized cardioversion, if hypotension, severe heart failure, and angina are present with a rapid ventricular rate

(b) A class IV antiarrhythmic (e.g., verapamil, diltiazem)

(2) Digoxin (used for chronic atrial flutter) possibly can be given in combination with verapamil or a β-blocker

8. Atrial fibrillation

a. Description. In this arrhythmia, many ectopic foci fire at different times. However, the AV node blocks many impulses from reaching the ventricles.

(1) The atrial rate is 400 beats/min to 600 beats/min.

(2) The atrial rhythm is chaotic.

b. Causes include valvular, ischemic, or rheumatic heart disease; coronary artery disease; systemic hypertension; cardiomyopathy; thyrotoxicosis; COPD; CHF; and myocardial infarction.

c. Therapy. The goal of treatment is to control the ventricular response.

(1) Immediate synchronized cardioversion is necessary in hemodynamically unstable patients.

(2) Verapamil or diltiazem (administered intravenously) is the drug of choice in acute atrial fibrillation.

(3) Digoxin frequently is used in chronic atrial fibrillation. It may be administered in combination with a calcium-channel blocker or a β-blocker.

(4) Type I antiarrhythmics may be useful in converting atrial fibrillation to sinus rhythm or preventing recurrence.

B. Preexcitation syndromes. This arrhythmia category includes **Wolff-Parkinson-White (WPW)** syndrome and **Lown-Ganong-Levine (LGL)** syndrome.

1. Description. In these arrhythmias, early ventricular depolarization occurs.

a. In **WPW syndrome,** the ECG shows a PR interval of less than 0.12 second and a QRS complex greater than 0.12 second.

(1) The ventricular rate may be as high as 300 beats/min. At rates of 180 beats/min or more, atrial fibrillation may develop.

(2) Delta waves, the hallmark of WPW, appear as a slurring of the initial portion of the QRS complex.

b. In **LGL syndrome,** the ECG shows short but constant PR intervals and normal P waves and QRS complexes.

2. Cause. Preexcitation syndromes result from abnormal conduction of impulses from the atria to the ventricles. Impulses travel along accessory pathways, which connect the atria and ventricles at abnormal locations and provide a re-entry route for impulses.

3. Therapy

a. In an emergency, vagotonic maneuvers or drugs (e.g., propranolol, procainamide, verapamil, diltiazem, lidocaine) may be necessary. If no response occurs, cardioversion may be used.

b. Long-term management may involve administration of a class IA antiarrhythmic (to increase refractoriness in the bypass tract), a class II or IV antiarrhythmic, or digoxin.

c. In resistant cases, electrophysiologic testing, surgical ablation of the bypass tract, or therapy with amiodarone, flecainide or propafenone may be necessary.

C. Ventricular arrhythmias

1. Premature ventricular contractions (PVCs)

a. Description. These common arrhythmias, when associated with frequent or complex ventricular ectopy in patients with heart disease may be associated with an increased risk of sudden death.

(1) A premature heart beat occurs, followed by a compensatory pause (as evidenced on heart auscultation or radial pulse palpation).

(2) On the ECG, PVCs appear as wide, bizarre QRS complexes; absent P waves; and large, wide T waves pointing in the direction opposite the QRS complexes.

(3) PVCs occur in the following patterns:

(a) Couplet, consisting of two consecutive PVCs

(b) Salvo (run of ventricular tachycardia), consisting of three or more consecutive PVCs

(c) Ventricular bigeminy, consisting of a PVC following each normal beat

(d) Ventricular trigeminy, consisting of two normal beats followed by a PVC

(4) PVCs may be **unifocal** or **multifocal.**

(a) In **unifocal PVCs,** QRS complexes are identical in configuration, reflecting a single ectopic ventricular pacemaker.

(b) In **multifocal PVCs,** QRS complexes have varying configurations, reflecting two ectopic ventricular pacemakers.

(5) The **R-on-T phenomenon** occurs when the PVC falls on the T wave of the preceding beat.

b. Causes include cardiomyopathy, coronary artery disease, and mitral valve prolapse. In people with normal hearts, PVCs may arise from caffeine or alcohol consumption or tobacco use. The mechanism underlying this arrhythmia is unknown.

c. **Therapy**
 (1) Treatment is always required for the following types of PVCs:
  (a) Multifocal PVCs
  (b) Frequent (> 6 beats/min) PVCs
  (c) Couplets or salvos
  (d) R-on-T phenomenon
 (2) Treatment may involve a class IA, IB, or IC antiarrhythmic agent (lidocaine is commonly given).
 (3) Asymptomatic patients with benign PVC types and no underlying heart disease do not require treatment.
 (4) Benefits of treatment need to be weighed against the risks associated with antiarrhythmic agents (e.g., flecainide), which may increase mortality.

2. **Ventricular tachycardia**
 a. **Description.** This dangerous arrhythmia, which may be brief or sustained, is defined as three or more consecutive PVCs.
  (1) Uncoordinated atrial and ventricular activity may lead to a drastic reduction in cardiac output; ventricular fibrillation may occur.
  (2) The ventricular rate is 150 beats/min to 240 beats/min; the rhythm is fairly regular.
  (3) On the ECG, QRS complexes are wide and bizarre, P waves are absent, T waves appear in the direction opposite the QRS complexes, and RR intervals are regular or slightly irregular.
 b. **Causes.** Ventricular tachycardia results from myocardial irritability or ischemia (e.g., from myocardial infarction, valvular heart defects, cardiomyopathy, or heart failure).
 c. **Therapy**
  (1) Immediate intervention is necessary to prevent acute ventricular tachycardia from evolving into ventricular fibrillation.
   (a) In unconscious patients, cardiopulmonary resuscitation (CPR) and defibrillation are warranted.
   (b) In less acute cases, lidocaine is given.
  (2) Long-term drug therapy may include quinidine, procainamide, disopyramide, tocainide, mexiletine, flecainide, propafenone, moricizine, and finally amiodarone.

3. **Ventricular fibrillation**
 a. **Description.** This deadly arrhythmia is the most common cause of cardiac arrest after an acute myocardial infarction. The ventricles quiver rather than contract; as a result, cardiac output is interrupted, and death may ensue.
  (1) Typically, the patient does not register a pulse, is apneic, and may have seizures. Acidosis and hypoxemia develop.
  (2) The ECG shows a rapid, chaotic ventricular rhythm and an undulating baseline; P waves, T waves, and QRS complexes cannot be discerned.
 b. **Causes.** PVCs and ventricular tachycardia most commonly cause this arrhythmia. Rarely, it arises spontaneously.
 c. **Therapy.** Ventricular fibrillation calls for immediate emergency measures, such as CPR and defibrillation. Emergency intravenous drug therapy may include epinephrine, lidocaine, bretylium, procainamide, or propranolol.

D. **AV blocks.** These arrhythmias reflect disturbances in impulse conduction from the atria to the ventricles. AV block occurs in three major variations—first degree, second degree, and third degree.

1. **Description**
 a. **First-degree AV block.** All supraventricular impulses are delayed. On the ECG, the PR interval is prolonged (greater than 0.20 second) but constant, QRS complexes are normal, and the rhythm is regular.
 b. **Second-degree AV block.** Some impulses are blocked at the AV node. Second-degree AV block occurs in two types.
  (1) **Type I** (also called **Mobitz I** or **Wenckebach**). Each successive impulse is conducted at an earlier stage of the refractory period, until one impulse arrives during the absolute refractory period and cannot be conducted. The next impulse, arriving during the relative refractory period, is conducted normally. The dropped ventricular beats have a

predictable pattern. ECG evidence of this arrhythmia includes grouped beating, an irregular rhythm, progressively lengthening PR intervals, progressively shortening RR intervals, and constant PP intervals.

(2) Type II (also called **Mobitz II**). Abnormal conduction in the bundle of His and the bundle branches causes dropped ventricular beats at unpredictable times. ECG manifestations include a sudden dropped beat with normal PR intervals and QRS complexes.

c. Third-degree AV block (also known as **complete heart block**). All supraventricular impulses are blocked at the AV junction. As a result, the atria and ventricles beat independently of one another.

(1) An ectopic pacemaker in the AV junction or the ventricles stimulates ventricular contractions.

(2) On the ECG, QRS complexes may be wide or narrow, depending on the location of the secondary pacemaker, PP intervals are constant, and P waves have no relationship to QRS complexes.

(3) Usually, the ventricular rate exceeds 45 beats/min.

2. Causes. AV heart block typically results from drug toxicity (e.g., digitalis, quinidine), degenerative disease of myocardial conductive tissue, acute myocardial infarction, rheumatic fever, or severe coronary artery disease. In some cases, this arrhythmia is congenital.

3. Therapy

a. First- and second-degree AV blocks usually do not require treatment. If the underlying cause is drug toxicity, the offending drug is withdrawn. If the arrhythmia reduces cardiac output, atropine may be given.

b. Type II second-degree AV block may warrant drug therapy to maintain cardiac output if the patient is hypotensive. Long-term management may involve artificial pacing to prevent ventricular standstill.

c. Third-degree AV block may warrant drug therapy (e.g., atropine, isoproterenol) if the arrhythmia has compromised cardiac output. Artificial pacing frequently is necessary.

STUDY QUESTIONS

Directions: Each of the numbered items or incomplete statements in this section is followed by answers or by completions of the statement. Select the **one** lettered answer or completion that is **best** in each case.

1. Strong anticholinergic effects limit the antiarrhythmic use of

(A) quinidine
(B) procainamide
(C) tocainide
(D) flecainide
(E) disopyramide

2. A pronounced slowing of phase 0 of the myocardial action potential would be reflected on the electrocardiogram (ECG) as a

(A) shortened QRS complex
(B) shortened P wave
(C) prolonged QRS complex
(D) flipped T wave
(E) ST segment depression

3. Which of the following class I antiarrhythmics would be most capable of inducing the torsades de pointes type of ventricular tachycardia?

(A) Lidocaine
(B) Amiodarone
(C) Quinidine
(D) Flecainide
(E) Diltiazem

4. A patient receiving a class I antiarrhythmic agent on a chronic basis complains of fatigue, low-grade fever, and joint pain suggestive of systemic lupus erythematosus (SLE). The patient is most likely receiving

(A) lidocaine
(B) procainamide
(C) quinidine
(D) flecainide
(E) propranolol

5. Class IA antiarrhythmics do all of the following to the cardiac cell's action potential EXCEPT

(A) slow the rate of rise for phase 0 of depolarization
(B) delay the fast-channel conductance of sodium ions
(C) prolong phases 2 and 3 of repolarization
(D) inhibit the slow-channel conductance of calcium ions
(E) prolong the refractory period of the action potential

6. Which of the following drugs is a class IV antiarrhythmic that is primarily indicated for the treatment of supraventricular tachyarrhythmias?

(A) Nifedipine
(B) Mexiletine
(C) Diltiazem
(D) Quinidine
(E) Propranolol

7. Sinus tachycardia is characterized by a heart rate

(A) in excess of 100 with impulses initiated by the AV node
(B) in excess of 60 with impulses initiated by the SA node
(C) less than 60 with impulses initiated by the AV node
(D) less than 60 with impulses initiated by the SA node
(E) in excess of 100 with impulses initiated by the SA node

8. Which of the following agents has a direct effect on the AV node, delaying calcium-channel depolarization?

(A) Lidocaine
(B) Verapamil
(C) Bretylium
(D) Quinidine
(E) Nifedipine

1-E	4-B	7-E
2-C	5-D	8-B
3-C	6-C	

9. Which of the following drugs is a class III antiarrhythmic agent that is effective in the acute management of ventricular tachycardia, including ventricular fibrillation?

(A) Bretylium
(B) Lidocaine
(C) Metoprolol
(D) Disopyramide
(E) Diltiazem

10. All of the following problems represent concerns when patients are started on amiodarone EXCEPT

(A) extremely long elimination half-life
(B) need for multiple daily doses
(C) development of hyper- or hypothyroidism
(D) development of pulmonary fibrosis
(E) interactions with other antiarrhythmic drugs

Directions: The group of items in this section consists of lettered options followed by a set of numbered items. For each item, select the **one** lettered option that is most closely associated with it. Each lettered option may be selected once, more than once, or not at all.

Questions 11–15

For each description of a phase of an action potential in Purkinje fibers, choose the corresponding letter in the accompanying diagram.

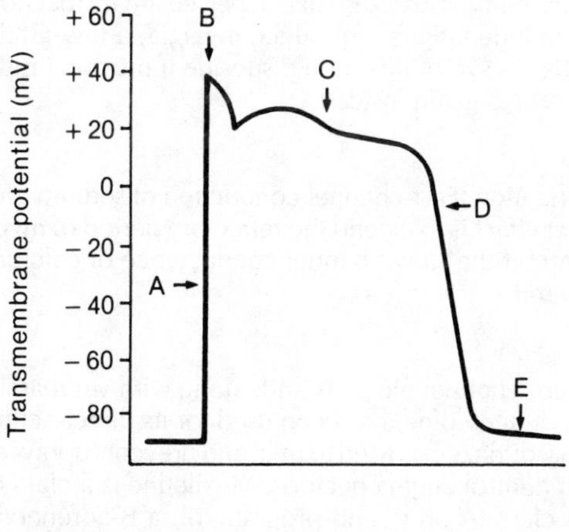

11. Slow-channel depolarization—calcium influx
12. Resting phase—diastole
13. Rapid repolarization
14. Fast-channel depolarization—sodium influx
15. Early repolarization

9-A 12-E 15-B
10-B 13-D
11-C 14-A

ANSWERS AND EXPLANATIONS

1. The answer is E *[II A 4 c (4)].*
Disopyramide has anticholinergic actions about one-tenth the potency of atropine. Effects include dry mouth, constipation, urinary retention, and blurred vision. Therefore, it cannot be used in patients with glaucoma or with conditions causing urinary retention. Moreover, disopyramide has a negative inotropic effect and must, therefore, be used with great caution, if at all, in patients with preexisting ventricular failure.

2. The answer is C *[I B 2 b, 3].*
A slowing in phase 0 of the myocardial action potential corresponds to a slowing down of depolarization within the myocardium. This results in a prolongation of either atrial depolarization [causing a prolonged P wave on the electrocardiogram (ECG)] or ventricular depolarization (causing a prolonged QRS complex).

3. The answer is C *[II A 4 a (1) (b)].*
Torsades de pointes is a form of ventricular tachyarrhythmia characterized by electrocardiographic (ECG) changes, which include a markedly prolonged QT interval. This potentially fatal reaction to quinidine causes syncopal episodes (quinidine syncope) or sudden death. Therefore, quinidine should not be used in patients whose QT interval is long or shows a marked prolongation in response to quinidine administration.

4. The answer is B *[II A 4 b (7)].*
The patient's complaints are typical of a systemic lupus erythematosus (SLE)–like hypersensitivity reaction to procainamide. Symptoms of an SLE-like syndrome include fatigue, arthralgia, myalgia, a low-grade fever, and a positive antinuclear antibody titer. The patient's symptoms should subside if procainamide therapy is stopped and an alternative antiarrhythmic agent is given instead.

5. The answer is D *[II A 2].*
Class IA antiarrhythmic agents delay phase 0 of depolarization. Fast-channel conduction of sodium and phases 2 and 3 of repolarization are also slowed. The net effect is to extend the refractory period of myocardial tissue. Class IA antiarrhythmic agents do not inhibit the slow-channel conductance of calcium ions; that is an action of class IV agents such as verapamil.

6. The answer is C *[II D 1 a].*
Of the agents listed, diltiazem and nifedipine are calcium-channel blockers and, along with verapamil, represent the class IV antiarrhythmics. Diltiazem, but not nifedipine, has been used for its direct-acting effects on impulse conduction throughout the heart. Thus, diltiazem is used to treat and prevent supraventricular arrhythmias, while nifedipine is used mainly to control angina pectoris. Mexiletine is a class IB drug that closely resembles lidocaine. Quinidine is a class IA drug, and propranolol, a β-adrenergic blocker, is class II. Mexiletine, quinidine, and propranolol are all also effective for supraventricular arrhythmias.

7. The answer is E *[III A 2].*
The term sinus tachycardia denotes a rapid heart rate with impulses originating in the sinoatrial (SA) node. In sinus tachycardia, the heart rate ranges from 100–160 beats/min. Though a sinus tachycardia commonly causes palpitations, it is usually a benign condition.

8. The answer is B *[II D 2].*
Verapamil, a calcium-channel blocker, inhibits calcium influx through slow channels into myocardial cells. Verapamil's direct actions on the slow-channel–dependent SA node and AV node, along with its availability in injection form, make it an ideal agent for the acute intravenous treatment of such re-entry arrhythmias as paroxysmal supraventricular tachyarrhythmias.

9. The answer is A *[II C 1 b].*
Bretylium, amiodarone, and sotalol are class III antiarrhythmic agents. Class III agents prolong the refractory period and myocardial action potential; they are used to treat ventricular arrhythmias. Bretylium is considered a second-line drug for controlling ventricular fibrillation. When used intravenously, bretylium requires close monitoring for hypotension, especially orthostatic hypotension, and may cause severe nausea and vomiting.

10. The answer is B *[II C 3 a, 4 a, 5 a].*
Amiodarone, like bretylium and sotalol, is a class III antiarrhythmic agent and acts by prolonging repolarization of cardiac cells. Amiodarone is given orally, often in once-a-day or twice-a-day maintenance dosage. Because of its very long elimination half-life, therapeutic response may be delayed for weeks. Therefore, an initial loading phase is often advisable. This requires hospitalization with close monitoring for desired effects, untoward reactions, and adjustments in dosage. Amiodarone may increase the plasma levels of quinidine, procainamide, diltiazem, and digitalis. During therapy with amiodarone, patients may develop hypo- or hyperthyroidism, pulmonary disorders, hepatic dysfunction, and various other unwanted effects. Because of amiodarone's extremely long half-life, adverse reactions may persist for months after therapy ends.

11–15. The answers are: 11-C, 12-E, 13-D, 14-A, 15-B *[I B 2 b].*
The action potential of cardiac Purkinje fibers reflects the depolarization and repolarization of the cardiac cells. This electrical activity involves the transport of sodium, calcium, and potassium ions across the cell membrane. The action potential has five phases. Phase 0 (rapid depolarization) is primarily dependent on the conduction of sodium ions into the cell through fast channels. Phase 0 is followed by phase 1 (early repolarization), which precedes phase 2, a slight notch that represents the inward flow of calcium ions into the cardiac cell via slow channels. Phase 3 (rapid repolarization) represents the inward flow of potassium ions. Phase 4 (slow repolarization), ending the action potential, represents electrical diastole.

43
Systemic Hypertension

Alan H. Mutnick

I. GENERAL CONSIDERATIONS

A. Definition. Hypertension is an elevation of the blood pressure necessary to perfuse tissues and organs. Elevated systemic blood pressure is usually defined as a systolic reading greater than or equal to 140 mm Hg and a diastolic reading greater than or equal to 90 mm Hg.

B. Classification of hypertension is shown in Table 43-1. This table reflects the latest recommendations of the Fifth Report of the Joint National Committee on Detection, Evaluation, and Treatment of HIgh Blood Pressure (JNC-V).

C. Incidence. Hypertension is the most common cardiovascular disorder. Approximately 50 million Americans have blood pressure measurements exceeding 140/90 mm Hg. Incidence increases with age—that is, 54%–65% of people over age 60 have hypertension.

1. **Primary (or essential) hypertension,** in which no specific cause can be identified, constitutes approximately 90% of all cases of systemic hypertension. The average age of onset is about 35 years.
2. **Secondary hypertension,** resulting from an identifiable cause, such as renal disease, accounts for the remaining 10% of cases of systemic hypertension. This type usually develops before age 35 or after age 55.

D. Physiology

Blood pressure = (stroke volume × heart rate) × systemic vascular resistance.

Altering any of the factors on the right side of the blood pressure equation results in a change in blood pressure, as shown in Figure 43-1.

1. **Sympathetic nervous system. Baroreceptors** (pressure receptors) in the carotids and aortic arch respond to changes in blood pressure and influence vasodilation or vasoconstriction. When stimulated to vasoconstriction, the contractile force strengthens, increasing the heart rate and augmenting peripheral resistance, thus increasing cardiac output. If pressure remains elevated, then baroreceptors reset at the higher levels, sustaining the hypertension.

Table 43-1. Classification of Hypertension Based on the Fifth Report of the Joint National Committee on Detection, Evaluation, and Treatment of High Blood Pressure (JNC-V)

Category	Systolic Blood Pressure (mm Hg)	Diastolic Blood Pressure (mm Hg)
High normal	130–139	85–89
Stage 1 (mild)	140–159	90–99
Stage 2 (moderate)	160–179	100–109
Stage 3 (severe)	180–209	110–119
Stage 4 (very severe)	> 210	> 120

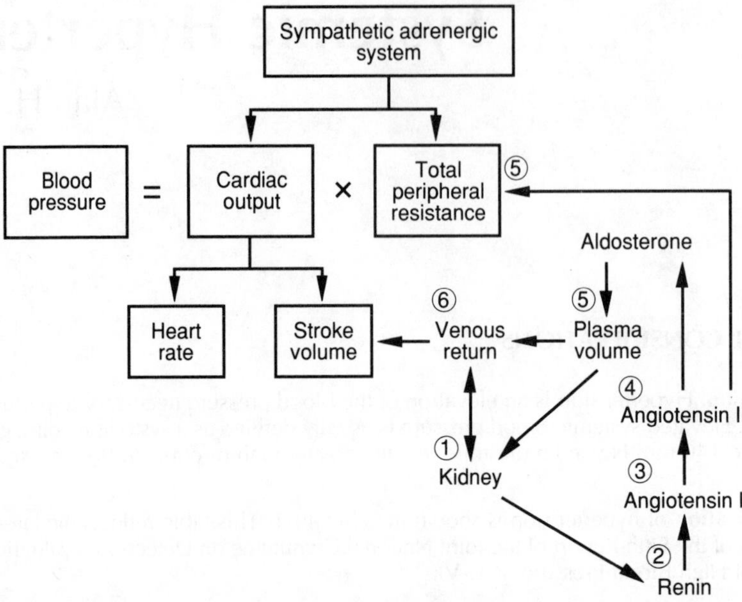

Figure 43-1. Blood pressure regulation. This figure depicts the various determinants of blood pressure as they relate to cardiac output and total peripheral resistance. Angiotensin II, a potent vasopressor, not only increases total peripheral resistance but, by stimulating aldosterone release, leads to an increase in plasma volume, venous return, stroke volume, and ultimately an increase in cardiac output.

2. **Renin–angiotensin–aldosterone system.** Decreased renal perfusion pressure in afferent arterioles stimulates the release of renin from juxtaglomerular cells. The renin reacts with circulating angiotensinogen to produce angiotensin I (a weak vasoconstrictor). This, in turn, is hydrolyzed to form angiotensin II (a very potent natural vasoconstrictor). This vasopressor stimulates aldosterone release, with a resulting increase in sodium reabsorption and fluid volume.

3. **Fluid volume regulation. Increased fluid volume** increases venous system distention and venous return, affecting cardiac output and tissue perfusion. These changes lead to **alterations in vascular resistance,** increasing the blood pressure.

E. Complications. Untreated systemic hypertension, regardless of cause, results in inflammation and necrosis of the arterioles, narrowing of the blood vessels, and restriction of the blood flow to major body organs (Table 43-2). When blood flow is severely compromised, target organ damage ensues.

1. **Cardiac effects**
   a. Left ventricular hypertrophy compensates for the increased cardiac work load. Signs and symptoms of heart failure occur, and the increased oxygen requirements of the enlarged heart may produce angina pectoris.
   b. Hypertension can be caused by accelerated atherosclerosis. Atheromatous lesions in the coronary arteries lead to decreased blood flow, resulting in angina pectoris. Myocardial infarction and sudden death may ensue.

2. **Renal effects**
   a. Decreased blood flow leads to an increase in renin–aldosterone secretion, which heightens the reabsorption of sodium and water and increases blood volume.
   b. Accelerated atherosclerosis causes a decreased oxygen supply, leading to renal parenchymal damage with decreased filtration capability and to azotemia. The atherosclerosis also causes decreased blood flow to the renal arterioles, leading to nephrosclerosis and, ultimately, renal failure (acute as well as chronic).

3. **Cerebral effects.** Decreased blood flow, decreased oxygen supply, and weakened blood vessel walls lead to transient ischemic attacks, cerebral thromboses, and the development of aneurysms with hemorrhage. There are alterations in mobility, weakness, paralysis, and memory deficits.

Table 43-2. Findings in Hypertension

Findings	Basis of Findings
Cardiovascular	
Blood pressure persistently ≥ 140 mm Hg systolic and/or 90 mm Hg diastolic	Constricted arterioles, causing abnormal resistance to blood flow
Angina pain	Insufficient blood flow to coronary vasculature
Dyspnea on exertion	Left-sided heart failure
Edema of extremities	Right-sided heart failure Decrease in blood supply
Neurologic	
Severe occipital headaches with nausea and vomiting; drowsiness; giddiness; anxiety; mental impairment	Vessel damage within the brain characteristic of severe hypertension, resulting in transient ischemic attacks or strokes
Renal	
Polyuria, nocturia, and diminished ability to concentrate urine; protein and red blood cells in urine; elevated serum creatinine	Arteriolar nephrosclerosis (hardening of arterioles within the kidney)
Ocular	
Retinal hemorrhage and exudates	Damage to arterioles that supply the retina
Peripheral vascular	Absence of pulses in extremities with or without intermittent claudication; development of an aneurysm

4. **Retinal effects.** Decreased blood flow with retinal vascular sclerosis and increased arteriolar pressure with the appearance of exudates and hemorrhage result in visual defects (e.g., blurred vision, spots, blindness).

II. SECONDARY HYPERTENSION

A. Clinical evaluation. Since most patients presenting with high blood pressure have primary rather than secondary hypertension, extensive screening is unwarranted. A thorough history and physical examination followed by an evaluation of common laboratory tests should rule out most causes of secondary hypertension. If a secondary cause is not found, the patient is considered to have essential hypertension.

1. A patient's **history and other physical findings** suggest an underlying cause of hypertension. These include the following.
   - **a.** Weight gain, moon face, truncal obesity, hirsutism, hypokalemia, diabetes, and increased plasma cortisol may signal Cushing syndrome.
   - **b.** Weight loss, episodic flushing, diaphoresis, increased urinary catecholamines, headaches, intermittent hypertension, tremors, and palpitations suggest pheochromocytoma.
   - **c.** Steroid or estrogen intake, including oral contraceptives, nonsteroidal anti-inflammatory drugs (NSAIDs), nasal decongestants, tricyclic antidepressants, appetite suppressants, cyclosporine, erythropoietin, and monoamine oxidase (MAO) inhibitors, suggest drug-induced hypertension.
   - **d.** Repeated urinary tract infections, nocturia, hematuria, and pain on urinating may signal renal involvement.
   - **e.** Abdominal bruits, recent onset, and accelerated hypertension indicate renal artery stenosis.
   - **f.** Muscle cramps, weakness, excess urination, and hypokalemia may suggest primary aldosteronism.

2. **Laboratory findings**
   - **a.** Blood urea nitrogen (BUN) and creatinine elevations suggest renal disease.
   - **b.** Increased urinary excretion of catecholamine or its metabolites (e.g., vanillylmandelic acid, metanephrine) confirms pheochromocytoma.
   - **c.** Serum potassium evaluation revealing hypokalemia suggests primary aldosteronism or Cushing syndrome.

3. **Diagnostic tests**
   a. Renal arteriography or renal venography may show evidence of renal artery stenosis.
   b. Electrocardiography (ECG) may reveal left ventricular hypertrophy or ischemia.

B. Etiology

1. **Primary aldosteronism.** Hypersecretion of aldosterone by the adrenal cortex yields increased distal tubular sodium retention, expanding the blood volume, which increases total peripheral resistance.

2. **Pheochromocytoma.** A tumor of the adrenal medulla stimulates hypersecretion of epinephrine and norepinephrine, which results in increased total peripheral resistance.

3. **Renal artery stenosis.** Decreased renal tissue perfusion results in the activation of the renin–angiotensin–aldosterone system (see I D 2).

C. Treatment. Secondary hypertension requires treatment of the underlying cause (e.g., surgical intervention accompanied by supplementary control of hypertensive effects) [see III B].

III. ESSENTIAL (PRIMARY) HYPERTENSION

A. Clinical evaluation requires a thorough history and physical examination followed by a careful analysis of common laboratory test results.

1. **Objectives**
   a. To rule out uncommon secondary causes of hypertension
   b. To determine the presence and extent of target organ damage
   c. To determine the presence of other cardiovascular risk factors in addition to high blood pressure
   d. To lower blood pressure with minimal side effects

2. **Predisposing factors**
   a. **Family history** of essential hypertension, stroke, and premature cardiac disease
   b. **Patient history** of intermittent blood pressure elevations
   c. **Racial predisposition.** Hypertension is more common among blacks than whites.
   d. **Obesity.** Weight reduction has been shown to reduce blood pressure in a large proportion of hypertensive patients who are more than 10% above ideal body weight.
   e. **Smoking,** resulting in vasoconstriction and activation of the sympathetic nervous system. Smoking is a major risk factor for cardiovascular disease.
   f. Stress
   g. High dietary intake of saturated fats or sodium
   h. Sedentary life-style
   i. Diabetes mellitus
   j. Hyperlipidemia

3. **Physical findings**
   a. Serial blood pressure readings equal to or above 140 mm Hg systolic and 90 mm Hg diastolic should be obtained on at least two occasions before specific therapy is begun, unless the initial blood pressure levels are markedly elevated (i.e., ≥ 210 mm Hg systolic, ≥ 120 mm Hg diastolic, or both) or are associated with target organ damage. A single elevated reading is an insufficient basis for a diagnosis.
   b. Essential hypertension usually does not become clinically evident—other than through serial blood pressure elevations—until vascular changes affect the heart, brain, kidneys, or ocular fundi.
   c. Examination of the ocular fundi is valuable; their condition can indicate the duration and severity of the hypertension.
      (1) **Early stages.** Hard shiny deposits, tiny hemorrhages, and elevated arterial blood pressure occur.
      (2) **Late stages.** Cotton–wool patches, exudates, retinal edema, papilledema due to ischemia and capillary insufficiency, hemorrhages, and microaneurysms become evident.

B. Treatment (Table 43-3; Figure 43-2)

1. **General principles.** Treatment primarily aims to lower blood pressure toward "normal" with minimal side efects and to prevent or reverse organ damage.

Table 43-3. Common Antihypertensive Drugs

Diuretics	Sympatholytics
Thiazide diuretics	β-Adrenergic blocking agents
Chlorothiazide	Acebutolol
Chlorthalidone	Atenolol
Hydrochlorothiazide	Betaxolol
Methyclothiazide	Carteolol
Loop diuretics	Esmolol
Bumetanide	Labetalol
Ethacrynic acid	Metoprolol
Furosemide	Nadolol
Potassium-sparing diuretics	Penbutolol
Amiloride	Pindolol
Spironolactone	Propranolol
Triamterene	Timolol
Quinazoline diuretics	Centrally acting α-agonists
Metolazone	Clonidine
Indoline diuretics	Guanabenz
Indapamide	Guanfacine
	Methyldopa
Vasodilators	Postganglionic adrenergic neuron blockers
Diazoxide	Guanadrel
Hydralazine	Guanethidine
Minoxidil	Reserpine
Nitroprusside	α-Adrenergic blocking agents
Angiotensin-converting enzyme (ACE) inhibitors	Doxazosin
	Prazosin
Benazepril	Terazosin
Captopril	Calcium-channel blockers
Enalapril	Amlodipine
Enalaprilat	Diltiazem
Fosinopril	Felodipine
Lisinopril	Isradipine
Quinapril	Nicardipine
Ramipril	Nifedipine
	Verapamil

a. Candidates for treatment

(1) All patients with a diastolic pressure of 90 mm Hg or above, a systolic pressure of 140 mm Hg or above, or a combination of both should receive antihypertensive drug therapy.

(2) For those patients with a diastolic pressure of 85–90 mm Hg or a systolic pressure of 130–139 mm Hg (high normal), treatment should be individualized with risk factors considered.*

b. Nonspecific measures. Prior to initiating antihypertensive drug therapy, patients are encouraged to eliminate or minimize controllable risk factors (see III A 2).

c. Pharmacologic treatment

(1) The recent recommendations of the JNC-V reveal that:

(a) Diuretics and β-adrenergic blocking agents are the only drugs that have been shown to lower morbidity and mortality rates.

(b) β-Blockers and diuretics should be considered as initial agents for treatment unless a contraindication exists for a given patient.

(c) Agents such as angiotensin-converting enzyme (ACE) inhibitors, α-blockers, α–β-blockers, and calcium-channel blockers have all been recommended for patients not able to receive a diuretic or a β-blocker as initial therapy.

*The risks associated with certain antihypertensive agents (e.g., β-blockers, diuretics) may outweigh or partially cancel the treatment benefits. However, treatment to reduce risk factors through nonpharmacologic intervention should be initiated.

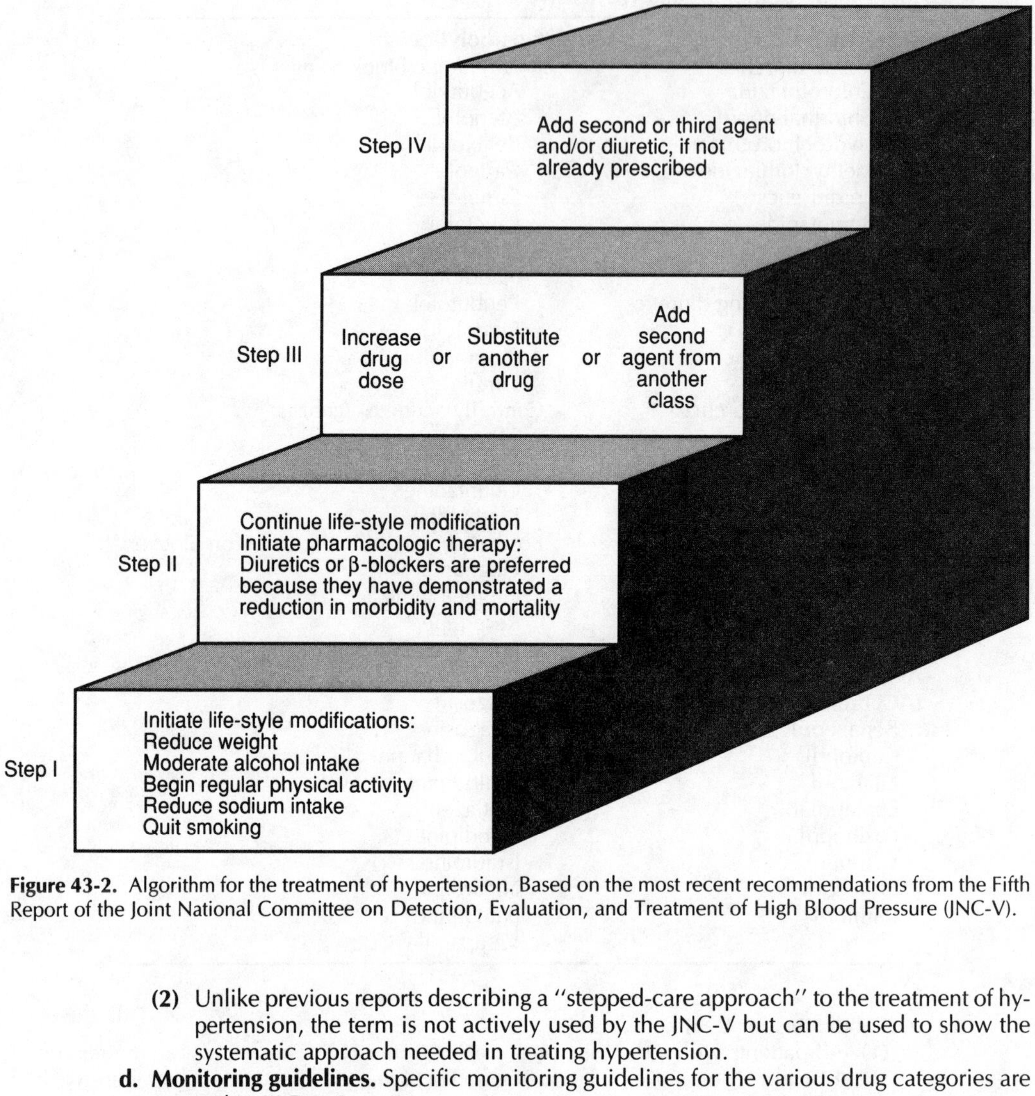
Step IV
Add second or third agent and/or diuretic, if not already prescribed
Step III
Increase drug dose
or
Substitute another drug
or
Add second agent from another class
Step II
Continue life-style modification
Initiate pharmacologic therapy:
Diuretics or β-blockers are preferred because they have demonstrated a reduction in morbidity and mortality
Step I
Initiate life-style modifications:
Reduce weight
Moderate alcohol intake
Begin regular physical activity
Reduce sodium intake
Quit smoking

Figure 43-2. Algorithm for the treatment of hypertension. Based on the most recent recommendations from the Fifth Report of the Joint National Committee on Detection, Evaluation, and Treatment of High Blood Pressure (JNC-V).

(2) Unlike previous reports describing a "stepped-care approach" to the treatment of hypertension, the term is not actively used by the JNC-V but can be used to show the systematic approach needed in treating hypertension.

d. Monitoring guidelines. Specific monitoring guidelines for the various drug categories are covered in III B 2–6.

(1) Blood pressure should be monitored routinely to determine the therapeutic response and to encourage patient compliance.

(2) Clinicians must be alert to indications of adverse drug effects. Many patients do not link side effects to drug therapy or are embarrassed to discuss them, especially effects related to sexual function or effects that appear late in therapy.

e. Patient compliance

(1) Because hypertension is usually a symptomless disease, "how the patient feels" does not reflect the blood pressure level. In fact, the patient may actually report "feeling normal" with an elevated blood pressure and "abnormal" during a hypotensive episode, because of the lightheadedness associated with a sudden drop in blood pressure. Because essential hypertension requires a lifelong drug regimen, it is difficult to impress on patients the need for compliance.

(2) Recognition of the seriousness of the consequences of noncompliance is key. Patients should be told that prolonged, untreated hypertension, known as the "silent killer," can affect the heart, brain, kidneys, and ocular fundi.

2. Diuretics

a. Thiazide diuretics and their derivatives are currently recommended as initial therapy for hypertension.

(1) **Actions.** Antihypertensive effects are produced by direct dilation of the arterioles and reduction of the total fluid volume. Thiazide diuretics increase:
   (a) Urinary excretion of sodium and water by inhibiting sodium and chloride reabsorption in the distal renal tubules
   (b) Urinary excretion of potassium and, to a lesser extent, bicarbonate
   (c) The effectiveness of other antihypertensive agents by preventing re-expansion of extracellular and plasma volumes

(2) **Significant interactions. NSAIDs,** such as the now common over-the-counter forms of ibuprofen, interact to diminish the antihypertensive effects of the thiazide diuretics.

(3) **Usual effective doses**
   (a) **Hydrochlorothiazide,** 12.5–50 mg daily
   (b) **Chlorothiazide,** 125–500 mg daily
   (c) **Chlorthalidone,** 12.5–50 mg daily
   (d) **Methyclothiazide,** 2.5–5.0 mg daily
   (e) **Metolazone,** 0.5–5.0 mg daily
   (f) **Indapamide,** 2.5–5.0 mg daily

(4) **Precautions and monitoring effects**
   (a) Potassium ion (K^+) depletion may require supplementation, increased dietary intake, or the use of a potassium-sparing diuretic.
   (b) Uric acid retention may occur; this is potentially significant in patients who are predisposed to gout and related disorders.
   (c) Blood glucose levels may increase, which may be significant in the diabetic patient.
   (d) Calcium levels may increase due to the potential for calcium ion retention.
   (e) Patients with known allergies to sulfa-type drugs should be questioned to determine the significance of the allergy.
   (f) Other common effects include fatigue, headache, palpitations, rash, vertigo, and transitory impotence.
   (g) Hyperlipidemia, including **hypertriglyceridemia,** hypercholesterolemia, increased low-density lipoprotein (LDL) cholesterol, and decreased high-density lipoprotein (HDL) cholesterol must be evaluated routinely to prevent an added risk for coronary artery disease.
   (h) Fluid losses must be evaluated and monitored to prevent dehydration, postural hypotension, and even hypovolemic shock.
   (i) Alterations in fluid and electrolytes (e.g., hypokalemia, hypomagnesemia, hypercalcemia) may predispose patients to cardiac irritability, with a resultant increase in cardiac arrhythmias. Electrocardiograms (ECGs) are performed routinely to prevent the development of life-threatening arrhythmias.

b. Loop (high-ceiling) diuretics

(1) **Indications.** These agents are indicated when patients are unable to tolerate thiazides, experience a loss of thiazide effectiveness, or have impaired renal function (clearance < 30 ml/min).

(2) **Actions. Furosemide, ethacrynic acid,** and **bumetanide** act primarily in the loop of Henle; hence they are called "loop" diuretics. Their action is more intense but of shorter duration (1–4 hours) than that of the thiazides; they may also be more expensive.

(3) **Significant interactions.** As with the thiazides, the antihypertensive effect of loop diuretics may be diminished by **NSAIDs.**

(4) **Precautions and monitoring effects.** Loop diuretics have the same effects as thiazides [see III B 2 a (4)] in addition to the following.
   (a) Loop diuretics have a complex influence on renal hemodynamics; thus, patients must be monitored closely for signs of hypovolemia.
   (b) Because these agents should be used cautiously in patients with episodic or chronic renal impairment, BUN and serum creatinine levels should be checked routinely.
   (c) Transient deafness has been reported. If the patient is taking a potentially ototoxic drug (e.g., an aminoglycoside antibiotic), another class of diuretic (e.g., a thiazide diuretic) should be substituted.

(5) **Usual effective doses**
   (a) **Bumetanide,** 0.5–5.0 mg daily
   (b) **Ethacrynic acid,** 25–100 mg daily
   (c) **Furosemide,** 20–320 mg daily

c. **Potassium-sparing diuretics**

(1) **Indications.** The diuretics in this group—**spironolactone, amiloride,** and **triamterene**—are indicated for patients in whom potassium loss is significant and supplementation is not feasible. These agents are often used in combination with a thiazide diuretic because they potentiate the effects of the thiazide while minimizing potassium loss. **Spironolactone** is particularly useful in patients with hyperaldosteronism as it has direct antagonistic effects on aldosterone.

(2) **Actions.** Potassium-sparing diuretics achieve their diuretic effects differently and less potently than the thiazides and loop diuretics. Their most pertinent shared feature is promotion of potassium retention.

(3) **Significant interactions.** Co-administration with **ACE inhibitors** or **potassium supplements** significantly increases the risk of hyperkalemia.

(4) **Precautions and monitoring effects**

(a) Potassium-sparing diuretics should be avoided in patients with acute renal failure and used with caution in patients with impaired renal function due to their ability to retain potassium.

(b) **Triamterene** should not be used in patients with a history of kidney stones or hepatic disease.

(c) **Hyperkalemia** is a major risk, requiring routine monitoring of serum electrolytes. BUN and serum creatinine levels should be checked routinely to signal incipient excess potassium retention and impaired renal function.

(5) **Usual effective doses**

(a) **Amiloride,** 5–10 mg daily

(b) **Spironolactone,** 25–100 mg daily and 100–400 mg daily to treat hyperaldosteronism

(c) **Triamterene,** 50–150 mg daily

d. **Combination products.** Four agents combine a thiazide and a potassium-sparing diuretic.

(1) **Aldactazide,** 25 mg spironolactone/25 mg hydrochlorothiazide (2–4 tablets daily)

(2) **Moduretic,** 5 mg amiloride/50 mg hydrochlorothiazide (1–2 tablets daily)

(3) **Dyazide,** 50 mg triamterene/25 mg hydrochlorothiazide (1–2 capsules daily)

(4) **Maxzide,** 75 mg triamterene/50 mg hydrochlorothiazide (1/2–1 tablet daily)

3. **Sympatholytics**

a. **β-Adrenergic blockers**

(1) **Indications.** These agents are used for the initial treatment of hypertension. β-Blockers are particularly effective in patients with rapid resting heart rates or concomitant ischemic heart disease.

(2) **Actions.** Proposed mechanisms of action include the following.

(a) Stimulation of renin secretion is blocked.

(b) Cardiac contractility is decreased, thus diminishing cardiac output.

(c) Sympathetic output is decreased centrally.

(d) Reduction in heart rate decreases cardiac output.

(e) β-Blocker action may combine all of the above mechanisms.

(3) **Epidemiology.** Young (< 45 years) whites with high cardiac output and heart rate and normal vascular resistance respond best to β-blocker therapy.

(4) **Precautions and monitoring effects**

(a) Patients must be monitored for signs and symptoms of **cardiac decompensation** (i.e., increasingly reduced cardiac output) because decreased contractility can trigger compensatory mechanisms, leading to congestive heart failure (CHF).

(b) ECGs should be monitored routinely because all β-blockers have the ability to decrease electrical conduction within the heart.

(c) Relative cardioselectivity is dose-dependent and is lost as dosages are increased. Therefore, no β-blocker is totally safe in patients with bronchospastic disease [e.g., asthma, chronic obstructive pulmonary disease (COPD)].

(d) Sudden cessation of β-blocker therapy puts the patient at risk for a **withdrawal syndrome** that may produce:

(i) Exacerbated anginal attacks, particularly in patients with coronary artery disease

(ii) Myocardial infarction

(iii) A life-threatening rebound of blood pressure to levels exceeding pretreatment readings

(e) β-Blocker therapy should be used with caution in patients with the following conditions:

(i) **Diabetes.** β-Blockers can mask hypoglycemic symptoms, such as tachycardia.

(ii) **Raynaud's phenomenon or peripheral vascular disease.** Vasoconstriction can occur.

(iii) **Neurologic disorders.** Several β-blockers enter the central nervous system (CNS), potentiating related side effects (e.g., fatigue, lethargy, poor memory, weakness, or mental depression).

(f) Hypertriglyceridemia, reduced HDL cholesterol, or increased LDL cholesterol have been reported as major consequences of β-blockers, which require routine lipid evaluations with chronic therapy.

(g) Impotence and decreased libido may result in reduced patient compliance.

(5) **Significant interactions.** β-Adrenergic blockers interact with numerous agents, requiring cautious selection, administration, and monitoring.

(6) **β-Blocker terms**

(a) **Relative cardioselective activity.** Relative to propranolol, β-blockers have a greater tendency to occupy the β_1-receptor in the heart, rather than the β_2-receptors in the lungs.

(b) **Intrinsic sympathomimetic activity.** These agents have the ability to release catecholamines and to maintain a satisfactory heart rate. Intrinsic sympathomimetic activity may also prevent bronchoconstriction and other direct β-blocking actions.

(7) **Specific agents**

(a) **Propranolol** was the first β-blocking agent shown to block both β_1- and β_2-receptors. The **average daily dose** is 80–240 mg.

(b) **Metoprolol** was the first β-blocking agent with relative cardioselective blocking activity. The **average daily dose** is 50–200 mg.

(c) **Nadolol** was the first β-blocking agent that allowed once-daily dosing. It blocks both β_1- and β_2-receptors. The **average daily dose** is 20–240 mg.

(d) **Atenolol** was the first β-blocking agent to combine once-daily dosing with relative cardioselective, blocking activity. The **average daily dose** is 25–100 mg.

(e) **Timolol** was the first β-blocking agent shown to be effective after an acute myocardial infarction for the prevention of sudden death. It blocks both β_1- and β_2-receptors. The **average daily dose** is 20–40 mg.

(f) **Pindolol** was the first β-blocking agent shown to have high intrinsic sympathomimetic activity. The **average daily dose** is 10–60 mg.

(g) **Labetalol** was the first β-blocking agent shown to possess both α- and β-blocking activity. The **average daily dose** is 200–1200 mg. Labetalol is also effective for the treatment of hypertensive crisis (Table 43-4).

(h) **Acebutolol** was the first β-blocking agent that combined efficacy with once-daily dosing, possessing intrinsic sympathomimetic activity and having relative cardioselective blocking activity. The **average daily dose** is 200–1200 mg.

(i) **Esmolol** was the first β-blocking agent to have an ultrashort duration of action. This agent is not used routinely in treating hypertension due to its duration of action and the need for intravenous administration.

(j) **Betaxolol** is a new β-blocker, which possesses relative cardioselective blocking activity similar to metoprolol but has a half-life that allows for once-daily dosing. The **average daily dose** is 5–40 mg.

(k) **Carteolol** is a new β-blocking agent, which has low lipid solubility so less drug penetrates the CNS, has moderate intrinsic sympathomimetic activity like pindolol, and allows for once-daily dosing. The **average daily dose** is 2.5–10.0 mg.

(l) **Penbutolol** is a new β-blocking agent, which has weak intrinsic sympathomimetic activity like pindolol and allows for once-daily dosing. The **average daily dose** is 20–80 mg.

b. **Peripheral α_1-adrenergic blockers** (e.g., prazosin, terazosin, doxazosin)

(1) **Actions.** The α_1-blockers (indirect vasodilators) block the peripheral postsynaptic α_1-adrenergic receptor, causing vasodilation of both arteries and veins. Also, the incidence of reflex tachycardia is lower with these agents than with the vasodilator hydralazine. These hemodynamic changes reverse the abnormalities in hypertension and preserve organ perfusion. Recent studies have also shown that these agents have no adverse effect on serum lipids and other cardiac risk factors.

Table 43-4. Rapid-Acting Parenteral Antihypertensive Agents for Hypertensive Crisis

Drug	Mode of Administration	Dose	Onset of Action	Duration of Action	Precautions	Side Effects
Diazoxide	IV bolus (usually 10–30 seconds)	50–150 mg or 15–30 mg/min as infusion	1–2 minutes	1–18 hours	Use with care in cerebral vascular disease, coronary artery disease, aortic dissections; blood glucose monitoring is necessary	Hyperglycemia; hyperuricemia; hypotension, tachycardia; chest pain; nausea; vomiting; sodium retention
Enalaprilat	IV	0.625–1.25 every 6 hours	15 minutes	4–6 hours		Hypotension; declining renal function; potential renal failure
Hydralazine	IM or IV	IV 10–20 mg	10 minutes	4–6 hours	Relatively contraindicated in patients with angina pectoris; aortic dissections	Flushing; headache; tachycardia; nausea; vomiting; possible aggravation of angina
		or IM 10–40 mg	20–30 minutes			
Labetalol	IV	20–80 mg every 10 minutes or 2 mg/min as infusion	5–10 minutes	2–4 hours		Dizziness; fatigue; nausea; dyspnea; congestive heart failure (CHF); bradycardia; bronchoconstriction
Methyldopate	IV	250–500 mg every 6 hours as infusion	30–60 minutes	10–16 hours		Drowsiness; headache; nasal stuffiness; weight gain
Sodium nitroprusside	IV drip	Titration 0.25–10 μg/kg/min	Instantaneous	2–3 minutes after cessation of drip	Use fresh solution every 4–8 hours; shield solution from light; constant monitoring is needed	Nausea; vomiting; hypotension; thiocyanate intoxication; sodium retention
Trimethaphan camsylate	IV drip	1–4 mg/min as infusion	2–5 minutes	5 minutes after cessation of drip	Requires constant monitoring; resistance develops in 24–48 hours; not advised for postoperative patients or those with a history of allergies	Paresis of the bowel, bladder; hypotension; visual blurring; dry mouth; sodium retention

(2) **Indications.** This group of drugs has been added to the current recommendations for initial therapy in hypertensive patients as alternatives for those who cannot take diuretics or β-blockers.

(3) **Precautions and monitoring effects**

(a) **First-dose phenomenon.** A syncopal episode may occur within 30–90 minutes of the first dose; similarly associated are postural hypotension, nausea, dizziness, headache, palpitations, and sweating. To minimize these effects, the first dose should be limited to 1.0 mg of each agent and administered just before bedtime.

(b) Additional adverse effects include diarrhea, weight gain, peripheral edema, dry mouth, urinary urgency, constipation, and priapism.

(4) The **average daily doses** are:

(a) Prazosin, 1–20 mg

(b) Terazosin, 1–20 mg

(c) Doxazosin, 1–16 mg

c. **Centrally active α-agonists** have been used in the past as alternatives to initial antihypertensives, but they are currently recommended as "supplemental" agents in patients not responding to initial antihypertensive agents. They act primarily within the CNS on α_2-receptors to decrease sympathetic outflow to the cardiovascular system.

(1) **Methyldopa**

(a) **Actions.** Methyldopa decreases total peripheral resistance through the above mechanism while having little effect on cardiac output or heart rate (except in older patients).

(b) **Precautions and monitoring effects**

(i) Common untoward effects include orthostatic hypotension, fluid accumulation (in the absence of a diuretic), and rebound hypertension upon abrupt withdrawal. Sedation is a common finding upon initiating therapy and when increasing doses; however, the sedative effect usually decreases with continued therapy.

(ii) Fever and other flulike symptoms occasionally occur and may represent hepatic dysfunction, which should be monitored by liver function tests.

(iii) A positive Coombs' test develops in 25% of patients with chronic use (longer than 6 months). Fewer than 1% of these patients develop a hemolytic anemia. (Red blood cells, hemoglobin, and blood count indices should be checked.) The anemia is reversible with discontinuation of the drug.

(iv) Other effects include dry mouth, subtly decreased mental activity, sleep disturbances, depression, impotence, and lactation in either sex.

(c) The **average daily dose** is 250 mg–2.0 g.

(2) **Clonidine**

(a) **Indications.** Clonidine is effective in patients with renal impairment, although they may require a dose reduction or prolongation of the dosing interval.

(b) **Actions.** Clonidine stimulates α_2-receptors centrally and results in a decrease in vasomotor tone and heart rate.

(c) **Precautions and monitoring effects**

(i) Intravenous administration causes an initial paradoxical increase in pressure (diastolic and systolic), which is followed by a prolonged drop. As with methyldopa, abrupt withdrawal can cause rebound hypertension.

(ii) Sedation and dry mouth are common but usually disappear with continued therapy.

(iii) Clonidine has a tendency to cause or worsen depression, and it heightens the depressant effects of alcohol and other sedating substances.

(d) The **average daily dose** is 0.1–1.2 mg.

(e) Patient compliance is a major issue for most hypertensive patients. The recently released once-weekly patch, which provides 0.1–0.3 mg/24-hr period, may improve compliance.

(3) **Guanabenz and guanfacine**

(a) **Actions.** Guanabenz and guanfacine are centrally active α_2-agonists, which have actions similar to clonidine.

(b) **Indications.** These agents are recommended as adjunctive therapy with other antihypertensives for additive effects when initial therapy has failed.

(c) **Precautions and monitoring effects.** These agents should be used cautiously with other sedating medications and in patients with severe coronary insufficiency, recent myocardial infarction, cerebrovascular accident (CVA), and hepatic or renal disease. Side effects include sedation, dry mouth, dizziness, and reduced heart rate.

(d) The **average daily doses** are 4–64 mg for guanabenz and 1–3 mg for guanfacine.

d. Postganglionic adrenergic neuron blockers. This class of antihypertensive drugs is best avoided unless it is necessary to treat severe refractory hypertension that is unresponsive to all other medications, as agents in this class are poorly tolerated by most patients.

(1) Reserpine

(a) **General considerations.** Due to the high incidence of adverse effects, other agents are usually chosen first. When used, reserpine is given in low doses and in conjunction with other antihypertensive agents. Reserpine in very low doses (0.05 mg) combined with a diuretic such as chlorothiazide (50–100 mg) may be an alternative to traditional doses of 0.1–0.25 mg/day.

(b) **Actions.** Reserpine acts centrally as well as peripherally by depleting catecholamine stores in the brain and in the peripheral adrenergic system.

(c) **Precautions and monitoring effects**

(i) A history of depression is a contraindication for reserpine. Even low doses, such as 0.25 mg/day, can trigger a range of psychic responses, from nightmares to suicide attempts. Drug-induced depression may linger for months after the last dose.

(ii) Peptic ulcer is also a contraindication for reserpine use. Even a single dose of reserpine tends to increase gastric acid secretion.

(iii) Common adverse effects include drowsiness, dizziness, weakness, lethargy, memory impairment, sleep disturbances, and weight gain. Nasal congestion is also common but may decrease with continued therapy.

(d) The **average daily dose** is 0.05–0.25 mg.

(2) Guanethidine

(a) **Actions.** Guanethidine acts in peripheral neurons, where it first produces a sympathetic blockade. With chronic administration, its cumulative effect reduces tissue concentrations of norepinephrine. This lasts several days after discontinuation of the drug.

(b) **Significant interactions**

(i) Patients should avoid **over-the-counter preparations** that contain sympathomimetic substances (e.g., cold medicines) because the combination may potentiate an acute hypertensive effect.

(ii) **Tricyclic antidepressants** and **chlorpromazine** antagonize the therapeutic effect of guanethidine.

(c) **Precautions and monitoring effects**

(i) Pheochromocytoma is a contraindication for guanethidine use due to the risk of a severe hypertensive reaction.

(ii) Postural and exercise hypotension are common side effects, which may be heightened by heat (e.g., hot weather, hot showers) and alcohol ingestion. The patient should be warned of these effects with changes in body position, particularly upon standing.

(iii) Fluid retention can occur, diminishing the antihypertensive effect and usually requiring a diuretic.

(iv) Sexual dysfunction (primarily inhibition of ejaculation) can occur and should be considered before initiating therapy.

(v) Bradycardia, CHF, and exacerbation of angina are possible side effects for which the patient should be monitored.

(d) The **average daily dose** is 10–100 mg.

(3) Guanadrel

(a) **Actions.** Guandrel decreases adrenergic neuronal activity like guanethidine and does not cross into the CNS.

(b) **Significant interactions** are similar to those of guanethidine.

(c) **Precautions and monitoring effects.** Guanadrel should be avoided in patients with CHF, angina, and cerebrovascular disease. Side effects include faintness, orthostatic hypotension, diarrhea, and severe volume depletion.

(d) The **average daily dose** is 10–75 mg.

4. Vasodilators. These drugs are used as alternative agents in patients refractory to initial therapy with diuretics, β-blockers, α-blockers, ACE inhibitors, or calcium-channel blockers. Vasodilators directly relax peripheral vascular smooth muscle—arterial, venous, or both. The direct vasodilators should not be used alone due to increases in plasma renin activity, cardiac output, and heart rate.

a. Hydralazine

(1) Actions. Hydralazine directly relaxes arterioles, decreasing systemic vascular resistance. It is also used intravenously or intramuscularly in hypertensive crisis management.

(2) Precautions and monitoring effects

(a) Because hydralazine triggers compensatory reactions that counteract its antihypertensive effects, it is most useful when combined with a β-blocker, central α-agonist, or diuretic as a latter-step agent.

(b) Reflex tachycardia is common and should be considered prior to initiating therapy.

(c) Hydralazine may induce angina, especially in patients with coronary artery disease and those not receiving a β-blocker.

(d) Drug-induced systemic lupus erythematosus (SLE) may occur.

(i) Baseline and serial complete blood counts (CBCs) with antinuclear antibody titers should be followed routinely to detect SLE.

(ii) Slow acetylators of this drug have an increased incidence of SLE; their risk may be reduced by administering doses of less than 200 mg/day.

(iii) Fatigue, malaise, low-grade fever, and joint aches may signal SLE.

(e) Other adverse effects may include headache, peripheral neuropathy, nausea, vomiting, fluid retention, and postural hypotension.

(3) The **average daily dose** is 50–300 mg.

b. Minoxidil

(1) Actions. A more potent vasodilator than hydralazine, minoxidil relaxes arteriolar smooth muscle directly, decreasing peripheral resistance. It also decreases renal vascular resistance while preserving renal blood flow. Effective in most patients, minoxidil is commonly used to treat patients with severe hypotension that has been refractory to conventional drug regimens.

(2) Precautions and monitoring effects

(a) Peripheral dilation results in a reflex activation of the sympathetic nervous system and an increase in heart rate, cardiac output, and renin secretion.

(b) Because this agent promotes sodium and water retention, particularly in the presence of renal impairment, patients should be monitored for fluid accumulation and signs of cardiac decompensation. Administering minoxidil along with a sympatholytic agent and a potent diuretic (e.g., furosemide) minimizes increased sympathetic stimulation and fluid retention.

(c) Hypertrichosis (i.e., excessive hair growth) is a common side effect, particularly if the drug is continued for more than 4 weeks.

(3) The **average daily dose** is 2.5–80 mg.

c. Nitroprusside

(1) Actions. A direct-acting peripheral dilator, this agent has potent effects on both the arterial and venous systems. It is usually used only in short-term emergency treatment of acute hypertensive crisis, when a rapid effect is required. Onset of action is almost instantaneous and is maximal in 1–2 minutes. Nitroprusside is administered intravenously with continuous blood pressure monitoring.

(2) Precautions and monitoring effects. To prevent acute hypotensive episodes, initial doses should be very low, followed by slow titration upward until the desired effect is achieved.

(a) Once the solution is prepared, it should be protected from light. Color changes are a signal that replacement is needed.

(b) Thiocyanate toxicity may develop with long-term treatment—particularly in patients with reduced renal activity—but can be treated with hemodialysis. Symptoms may include fatigue, anorexia, disorientation, nausea, psychotic behavior, or muscle spasms.

(c) Cyanide toxicity can occur (rarely) with long-term, high-dose administration. It may present as altered consciousness, convulsions, tachypnea, or even coma.

(3) The **average daily dose** is 0.25–10 μg/kg/min as a continuous intravenous infusion.

d. Diazoxide

(1) Indications. Diazoxide exerts a direct action on the arterioles but has little effect on venous capacity. It is used intravenously in the emergency treatment of acute hypertensive crisis.

(2) Administration

(a) Because the antihypertensive effect of diazoxide increases with the speed of infusion, recent recommendations suggest that a slow infusion spread over 15–30 minutes may achieve more predictable, controllable, hypotensive effects than rapid, high-dose administration.

(b) Alternatively, maximal reductions in mean arterial pressure may be obtained after 2 minutes through bolus injections of 50–150 mg for 5–10 seconds, with repetition of this dose every 5–10 minutes, if needed. Additionally, the drug may be administered as a continuous infusion of 15–30 mg/min.

(3) Precautions and monitoring effects

(a) Diazoxide is closely related to the thiazides chemically; therefore, patients with thiazide sensitivity cross-react to diazoxide. In patients with impaired cerebral or cardiac function, the risks may outweigh the benefits of diazoxide administration.

(b) Diazoxide also produces transient hyperglycemia, requiring caution if administered to diabetic patients.

(c) Hypotensive reactions may be severe.

(d) Unlike the thiazides, this agent promotes sodium and water retention, potentiating edema.

5. ACE inhibitors

a. General considerations. The ACE inhibitors (e.g., benazepril, captopril, enalapril, lisinopril, ramipril, quinapril, fosinopril) are a rapidly growing group of drugs, which most recently have been recommended for the initial treatment of hypertension in those patients who cannot take diuretics or β-blockers. Seven agents are currently available for use, but as the number of agents continues to grow, the differences among them must be considered.

b. Indications. Although the use of ACE inhibitors was initially restricted to patients with refractory hypertension, they currently are indicated as first-line alternatives in the treatment of hypertension. This has been primarily due to studies documenting their clinical efficacy as well as minimal impact on patients' abilities to maintain normal function. However, as reported by the JNC-V, ACE inhibitors have not been tested and shown to reduce morbidity and mortality.

c. Actions

(1) These agents inhibit the conversion of angiotensin I (a weak vasoconstrictor), to angiotensin II (a potent vasoconstrictor), which decreases the availability of angiotensin II.

(2) ACE inhibitors indirectly inhibit fluid volume increases when interfering with angiotensin II by inhibiting angiotensin II–stimulated release of aldosterone, which promotes sodium and water retention. The net effect appears to be a decrease in fluid volume, along with peripheral vasodilation.

d. Significant interactions

(1) The antihypertensive effect of ACE inhibitors may be diminished by **NSAIDs** (e.g., over-the-counter forms of ibuprofen).

(2) **Potassium-sparing diuretics** cause an increase in serum potassium levels when used with ACE inhibitors.

e. Precautions and monitoring effects

(1) Neutropenia is rare (especially with **enalapril**) but serious; there is an increased incidence in patients with renal insufficiency or autoimmune disease.

(2) Proteinuria occurs, particularly in patients with a history of renal disease. Urinary proteins should be monitored regularly.

(3) Serum potassium levels should be monitored regularly for hyperkalemia. The mechanism of action tends to increase potassium levels somewhat. Patients with renal impairment are at increased risk.

(4) Renal insufficiency can occur in patients with predisposing factors, such as renal stenosis, and when ACE inhibitors are administered with thiazide diuretics. Renal function should be monitored [e.g., through monitoring levels of serum creatinine and BUN].

(5) A dry cough may occur but disappears within a few days after the ACE inhibitor is discontinued. All ACE inhibitors have the potential to cause this side effect, but switching to an alternative agent may improve the symptoms.

(6) Other untoward effects include rashes, alteration in sense of taste (dysgeusia), vertigo, headache, fatigue, first-dose hypotension, and minor gastrointestinal disturbances.

f. Specific agents

(1) **Captopril.** The original ACE inhibitor is given initially as a 6.25-mg dose three times daily and is increased to an **average daily dose** of 12.5–150 mg.

(2) **Enalapril** is a prodrug, which is rapidly converted to its active metabolite enalaprilat. Initial doses are 5.0 mg daily, with an **average daily dose** of 2.5–40 mg. Additionally, the enalaprilat form of the drug has been used effectively in the treatment of acute hypertensive crisis (see Table 43-4).

(3) **Lisinopril** is a long-acting analog of enalapril, given initially as a 5–10 mg daily dose and adjusted to an **average daily dose** of 5–40 mg.

(4) **Ramipril, fosinopril, benazepril,** and **quinapril** are four recently released ACE inhibitors whose major benefit currently is once-daily dosing. Currently, ramipril as a 1.25–20-mg daily dose, fosinopril as a 10–40-mg daily dose, benazepril as a 10–40-mg daily dose, and quinapril as a 10–80-mg daily dose represent current usual dose ranges for these new agents. Further study is needed to determine the specific benefits of each agent in the hypertensive patient.

6. Calcium-channel blockers

a. Indications. Similar to the ACE inhibitors, the calcium-channel blockers have rapidly become alternative drugs for the initial treatment of hypertensive patients who cannot take diuretics or β-blockers. Currently, seven agents (e.g., amlodipine, diltiazem, felodipine, isradipine, nicardipine, nifedipine, verapamil) are available, but as the number of agents continues to grow, the differences among them must be considered.

b. Actions

(1) Calcium-channel blockers inhibit the influx of calcium through slow channels in vascular smooth muscle and cause relaxation. Low-renin hypertensive patients, blacks, and elderly individuals respond well to these agents.

(2) Although the calcium-channel blockers share a similar mechanism of action, each agent produces different degrees of systemic and coronary arterial vasodilation, sinoatrial (SA) and atrioventricular (AV) nodal depression, and a decrease in myocardial contractility.

c. Significant interactions. β-Adrenergic blockers when used with calcium-channel blockers may have an additive effect on inducing CHF and bradycardia. Electrical conduction to the AV node may be further depressed when patients are given agents such as verapamil and diltiazem along with **β-blockers**.

d. Precautions and monitoring effects

(1) Diltiazem and verapamil must be used with extreme caution or not at all in patients with conductive disturbances involving the SA or AV node, such as second- or third-degree AV block, sick sinus syndrome, and digitalis toxicity.

(2) Nifedipine use has been associated with flushing, headache, and peripheral edema, which the patient may find very troublesome, thus jeopardizing compliance. The use of the sustained-release product once daily has been shown to reduce these effects effectively.

(3) Verapamil use has been associated with a significant degree of constipation, which must be treated to prevent stool straining and noncompliance.

e. Specific agents

(1) **Diltiazem.** The release of an extended-release product has greatly increased this agent's role in the treatment of hypertension. Daily doses of 90–360 mg are effective in the treatment of mild-to-moderate hypertension. Diltiazem has already proven efficacy as an antiarrhythmic and an antianginal agent. This product contrasts with a previously released sustained-released product, which required two daily doses for maximal effects.

(2) **Nifedipine.** The release of a once-daily sustained-release preparation has made this agent very effective in the long-term treatment of hypertension. A previously reported long list of side effects has been reduced with the use of the sustained-release product at a daily dose of 30–120 mg.

(3) **Verapamil.** This drug is similar to diltiazem in its actions (though with more potent effects on electrical conduction depression). A sustained-release product at doses of

80–480 mg daily has been shown to be efficacious in the long-term management of mild-to-moderate hypertension, while side effects such as dizziness, constipation, and hypotension are reduced. An additional form of verapamil (Verelan) has recently been released with the hope of providing 24-hour blood pressure control.

(4) **Amlodipine, isradipine, felodipine, and nicardipine** are newly released second-generation calcium-channel blockers. These agents have been developed to produce more selective effects on specific target tissues than the first-generation agents, diltiazem, nifedipine, and verapamil. These agents are similar chemically to nifedipine and are referred to as dihydropyridine derivatives. The daily dose ranges are:

(a) **Amlodipine,** 2.5–10.0 mg
(b) **Isradipine,** 2.5–10.0 mg
(c) **Felodipine,** 5.0–20 mg
(d) **Nicardipine,** 60–120 mg

IV. HYPERTENSIVE EMERGENCIES

A. Definition. A hypertensive emergency is a severe elevation of blood pressure (i.e., >200 mm Hg systolic or >140 mm Hg diastolic) that demands either immediate (within minutes) or prompt (within hours) reduction.

1. Conditions requiring immediate reduction include hypertensive encephalopathy, acute left ventricular failure with pulmonary edema, dissecting aortic aneurysm, acute myocardial infarction, and intracranial hemorrhage.

2. Conditions requiring prompt reduction include malignant or accelerated hypertension.

B. Treatment

1. The **reduction in blood pressure must be gradual** (e.g., a 15–mm Hg decrease in mean arterial pressure over the first hour) rather than precipitous to avoid compromising perfusion of critical organs, particularly cerebral perfusion.

2. **Diuretics should be avoided initially,** as they may exacerbate hypovolemia and induce severe vasoconstriction, unless intravascular fluid overload has been demonstrated. They may be introduced later to treat sodium and fluid retention resulting from drug therapy with agents such as diazoxide or sodium nitroprusside.

3. **Specific agents** used in hypertensive crisis are shown in Table 43-4; for further information on vasodilators, see III B 4.

STUDY QUESTIONS

Directions: Each of the numbered items or incomplete statements in this section is followed by answers or by completions of the statement. Select the **one** lettered answer or completion that is **best** in each case.

1. Which of the following β-adrenergic blockers would be the best treatment for a hypertensive patient suffering from sinus bradycardia?

(A) Propranolol
(B) Atenolol
(C) Nadolol
(D) Pindolol
(E) Metoprolol

2. Reflex tachycardia, headache, and postural hypotension are adverse effects that limit the use of which of the following antihypertensive agents?

(A) Prazosin
(B) Captopril
(C) Methyldopa
(D) Guanethidine
(E) Hydralazine

3. A 60-year-old man presents with moderate hypertension that is refractory to diuretics, β-blockers, and methyldopa. He has renovascular hypertension with elevated renin levels confirmed on laboratory evaluation. This patient's antihypertensive regimen would be enhanced best by the addition of which of the following agents?

(A) Prazosin
(B) Hydralazine
(C) Enalapril
(D) Nitroprusside
(E) Clonidine

4. A hypertensive patient who is asthmatic and very noncompliant would be best treated with which of the following β-blocking agents?

(A) Timolol
(B) Penbutolol
(C) Esmolol
(D) Acebutolol
(E) Propranolol

5. Long-standing hypertension leads to tissue damage in all of the following organs EXCEPT the

(A) heart
(B) lungs
(C) kidneys
(D) brain
(E) eyes

6. According to the Fifth Report of the Joint National Committee on Detection, Evaluation, and Treatment of High Blood Pressure (JNC-V), all of the following agents are suitable as initial therapy for the treatment of hypertension EXCEPT

(A) isradipine
(B) fosinopril
(C) betaxolol
(D) guanadrel
(E) lisinopril

1-D
2-E
3-C
4-D
5-B
6-D

Directions: Each question below contains three suggested answers, of which **one or more** is correct. Choose the answer

A if **I only** is correct
B if **III only** is correct
C if **I and II** are correct
D if **II and III** are correct
E if **I, II, and III** are correct

7. A patient treated with a thiazide diuretic should be monitored regularly for altered plasma levels of

I. potassium
II. glucose
III. uric acid

8. Before antihypertensive therapy begins, secondary causes of hypertension should be ruled out. Laboratory findings that suggest an underlying cause of hypertension include

I. a decreased serum potassium level
II. an increased urinary catecholamine level
III. an increased blood cortisol level

9. In an otherwise healthy adult with mild hypertension, appropriate initial antihypertensive therapy would be

I. hydrochlorothiazide
II. furosemide
III. hydralazine

Directions: Each group of items in this section consists of lettered options followed by a set of numbered items. For each item, select the **one** lettered option that is most closely associated with it. Each lettered option may be selected once, more than once, or not at all.

Questions 10–14

Match the adverse effects with the antihypertensive agent that is most likely to cause them.

(A) Captopril
(B) Methyldopa
(C) Nitroprusside
(D) Terazosin
(E) Carteolol

10. Thiocyanate intoxication, hypotension, and convulsions

11. Bradycardia, bronchospasm, and cardiac decompensation

12. Dysgeusia, skin rash, and proteinuria

13. Postural hypotension, fever, and a positive Coombs' test

14. First-dose syncope, postural hypotension, and palpitations

Questions 15–19

Match each description of a β-blocker with the most appropriate β-adrenergic blocking agent.

(A) Esmolol
(B) Labetalol
(C) Betaxolol
(D) Nadolol
(E) Pindolol

15. A β-blocker with intrinsic sympathomimetic activity

16. A β-blocker that also blocks α-adrenergic receptors

17. A β-blocker with an ultrashort duration of action

18. A β-blocker with a long duration of action and nonselective blocking activity

19. A β-blocker with relative cardioselective blocking activity

---

7-E	10-C	13-B	16-B	19-C
8-E	11-E	14-D	17-A	
9-A	12-A	15-E	18-D	

ANSWERS AND EXPLANATIONS

1. The answer is D *[III B 3 a (7) (a)–(f)].*
Pindolol is a nonselective β–adrenergic blocking agent with intrinsic sympathomimetic activity, as evidenced by a lesser decrease in cardiac output and heart rate than is seen with other β-blockers (e.g., propranolol, atenolol, nadolol, metoprolol). As a result, pindolol would be a good choice of treatment for a hypertensive patient with sinus bradycardia.

2. The answer is E *[III B 4 a].*
Hydralazine is a vasodilator that works by directly relaxing arterioles, thereby reducing peripheral vascular resistance. Its effectiveness as an antihypertensive agent is compromised, however, by the compensatory reactions it triggers (i.e., reflex tachycardia) and by its other adverse effects (e.g., headache, postural hypotension, nausea, palpitations). Fortunately, the unwanted effects of hydralazine are minimized when it is used in combination with a diuretic agent and a β-blocker. Thus, hydralazine is most effective as a supplemental antihypertensive drug in combination with first-line therapy.

3. The answer is C *[III B 5 f].*
Enalapril, an angiotensin-converting enzyme (ACE) inhibitor, acts by inhibiting the conversion of angiotensin I (a weak vasoconstrictor) to angiotensin II (a potent vasoconstrictor). As this patient has renovascular hypertension, a response would be expected from an ACE inhibitor such as enalapril; enalapril works directly on the renin–angiotensin system, which is activated by renal artery stenosis. ACE inhibitors are indicated as initial therapy for hypertension if the patient is unable to take diuretics or β-blockers.

4. The answer is D *[III B 3 a (7)].*
The β-adrenergic blocking agents are employed as initial agents in the treatment of hypertension. A major feature of some of these agents is their relative selectivity for β_1-receptors (in the heart) rather than for β_2-receptors (in the lung), which provides advantages in the treatment of certain (e.g., asthmatic) patients. Of the β-blockers listed in the question, acebutolol is less likely than the rest to block β_2-receptors, due to its relative cardioselective blocking activity. Acebutolol also has a long duration of action, which could be helpful in the noncompliant patient by requiring fewer doses per day. Penbutolol is a new β-blocker, which has weak intrinsic sympathomimetic activity like pindolol but lacks relative cardioselectivity despite its long duration of action.

5. The answer is B *[I E; Table 43-2].*
Left untreated, hypertension can be lethal due to its progressively destructive effects on major organs, such as the heart, kidneys, and brain. The eyes also suffer damage; the lungs, however, do not. End-organ damage caused by hypertension includes left ventricular hypertrophy, congestive heart failure (CHF), angina pectoris, myocardial infarction, renal insufficiency due to atherosclerotic lesions, nephrosclerosis, cerebral aneurysm and hemorrhage, retinal hemorrhage, and papilledema.

6. The answer is D *[III B 6; Figure 43-2].*
Calcium-channel blockers such as isradipine, β-adrenergic blockers such as betaxolol, angiotensin-converting enzyme (ACE) inhibitors such as fosinopril and lisinopril, and diuretics are considered initial agents in the treatment of mild-to-moderate hypertension. Due to adverse drug reactions, guanadrel, a postganglionic adrenergic neuronal blocker, like reserpine and guanethidine, should be reserved for those patients who do not respond to all other antihypertensive drugs. Strictly speaking, diuretics and β-blockers are initial agents for the treatment of hypertension because they have been shown to reduce mortality and morbidity rates, while ACE inhibitors, calcium-channel blockers, and α_1-blockers are considered initial therapy only if the patient cannot take diuretics or β-blockers.

7. The answer is E (all) *[III B 2 a].*
Thiazide diuretics act directly on the kidneys by increasing the excretion of sodium and water and, to a lesser extent, the excretion of potassium. Patients who are treated with thiazides should be monitored for hypokalemia, which may require potassium supplementation or the addition of a potassium-sparing diuretic to the antihypertensive regimen. Thiazide diuretics have the opposite effect on uric acid and glucose excretion. Thus, patients receiving these drugs also should be monitored for increased plasma levels of uric acid (especially if they are predisposed to gout) and glucose (especially if they are predisposed to diabetes).

8. The answer is E (all) *[II A 1].*
Low serurm potassium levels in a hypertensive patient suggest primary aldosteronism. Elevated urinary catecholamines suggest a pheochromocytoma; other signs and symptoms of this tumor include weight loss, episodic flushing, and sweating. Elevated serum cortisol levels suggest Cushing syndrome; the patient is also likely to have a round face and truncal obesity. Secondary hypertension requires treatment of the underlying cause; supplementary antihypertensive drug therapy may also be needed.

9. The answer is A (I) *[III B 2 a, b (1), 4 a (1); Figure 43-2].*
Thiazide diuretics, such as hydrochlorothiazide, are indicated as initial antihypertensive agents for the treatment of hypertension. Furosemide is a diuretic that acts primarily in the loop of Henle with a shorter but more intense action than that of thiazide diuretics; it is reserved for patients who cannot tolerate thiazides, who have experienced a loss of thiazide function, or who have impaired renal clearance. Hydralazine is a vasodilator that is used as a supplemental agent for patients not responding to initial agents.

10–14. The answers are: 10-C *[III B 4 c (2)],* **11-E** *[III B 3 a (4), (7) (k)],* **12-A** *[III B 5 e (6), f (1)],* **13-B** *[III B 3 c (1) (b)],* **14-D** *[III B 3 b (3)].*
The goal of treatment in hypertension is to lower blood pressure toward "normal" with minimal side effects. All antihypertensive drugs can cause adverse effects. Therefore, the stepped-care approach has evolved on the principle that combination therapy allows the use of lower doses of each drug and, thus, reduces the risk of adverse effects while providing optimal therapeutic benefits.

15–19. The answers are: 15-E, 16-B, 17-A, 18-D, 19-C *[III B 3 a (7)].*
The β-adrenergic blocking agents are valuable in the management of hypertension and are used as initial antihypertensives. The β-blockers are sympathetic antagonists: They act by blocking various receptors of the sympathetic nervous system. They differ in their selectivity for these sympathetic receptors. For example, β_1-blockers have relative cardioselective activity; that is, they block β_1-receptors (in the heart) rather than β_2-receptors (in bronchial smooth muscle) and, therefore, are highly useful antihypertensive agents. Intrinsic sympathomimetic activity also appears to reduce the problem of bronchoconstriction; moreover, drugs with this property also have the ability to maintain a satisfactory heart rate.

44
Congestive Heart Failure

Alan H. Mutnick

I. INTRODUCTION

A. Definition. Congestive heart failure (CHF) is a condition in which an abnormality in myocardial function results in the inability of the ventricles to deliver adequate quantities of blood to the metabolizing tissues during normal activity or at rest. The condition is termed **congestive because of the edematous state** commonly produced by the fluid backup resulting from poor pump function.

B. Mortality rate. According to the Framingham Heart Disease Epidemiology Study, of those who were diagnosed as having CHF, less than 50% of the men and less than 60% of the women survived 5 years after the initial diagnosis.

C. Etiology

1. Although the disease occurs most commonly among the elderly, it may appear at any age as a consequence of underlying cardiovascular disease (Table 44-1).
2. CHF should not be considered an independent diagnosis, as it is superimposed on an underlying cause.
   a. Hypertension and coronary artery disease are the two major underlying causes of CHF development.
   b. Myocardial stress may be caused by trauma, disease, or other abnormal state (e.g., pulmonary embolism, infection, anemia, pregnancy, drug use or abuse, fluid overload, and arrhythmias).

D. Forms of heart failure

1. **Low-output versus high-output failure**
   a. If metabolic demands are within normal limits but the heart is unable to meet them, the failure is designated **low output** (the most common type).
   b. If metabolic demands increase (e.g., hyperthyroidism, anemia), and the heart is unable to meet them, the failure is designated **high output**.
2. **Left-sided versus right-sided failure**
   a. **General symptomatology**
      (1) The signs and symptoms of heart failure usually result from the effects of blood backing up behind the failing ventricle (except in heart failure due to increased body demands).
      (2) Initially, the signs and symptoms tend to be specific to failure of one side of the heart, but eventually bilateral involvement is evidenced.

Table 44-1. Cardiac Diseases Commonly Underlying Congestive Heart Failure

Age Range (Years)	Common Underlying Causes
20–40	Rheumatic fever, rheumatic heart disease
40–50	Myocardial infarction, hypertension, pulmonary disease
Over 50	Calcific aortic stenosis

(3) This progression occurs because the cardiovascular system is a closed system (Figure 44-1); thus, over time, right-sided failure causes left-sided failure and vice versa.

b. **Left-sided failure**

(1) If blood cannot be adequately pumped from the left ventricle to the peripheral circulation and it accumulates within the left ventricle, the failure is designated **left-sided**.

(2) Given this accumulation, the left ventricle is unable to accept blood from the left atrium and lung; therefore, the fluid portion of the blood backs up into the pulmonary alveoli, producing pulmonary edema.

c. **Right-sided failure**

(1) When blood cannot be pumped from the right ventricle into the lungs and it accumulates within the right ventricle, the failure is designated **right-sided**.

(2) When blood is not pumped from the right ventricle, the fluid portion of the blood backs up throughout the body (e.g., in the veins, liver, legs, bowels), producing systemic edema.

E. Treatment goals. CHF requires a two-pronged therapeutic approach, the overall goals of which are:

1. **To remove or mitigate the underlying cause;** for example, by eliminating ingestion of certain drugs or other substances (Table 44-2) that can produce or exacerbate CHF or by correcting an anemic syndrome, which can increase cardiac demands

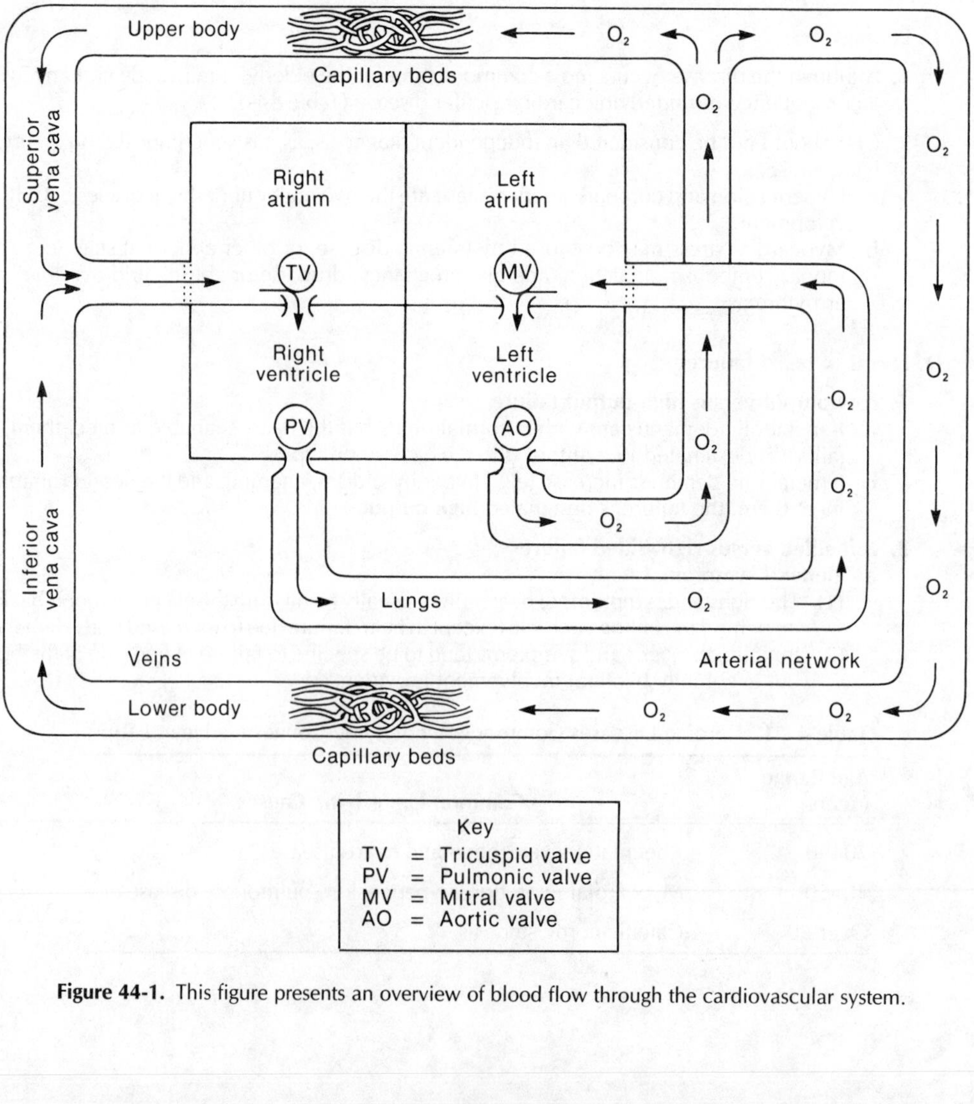

Figure 44-1. This figure presents an overview of blood flow through the cardiovascular system.

Table 44-2. Substances that May Exacerbate Congestive Heart Failure

Promote Sodium Retention	Produce Osmotic Effect	Decrease Contractility
Androgens	Albumin	Antiarrhythmic agents (e.g., quinidine, disopyramide, procainamide, flecainide)
Corticosteroids	Glucose	β-Adrenergic blocking agents
Diazoxide	Mannitol	Calcium channel blockers (e.g.,verapamil, diltiazem)
Estrogens	Saline	Doxorubicin hydrochloride
Guanethidine	Urea	
Licorice		
Lithium carbonate		
Methyldopa		
Phenylbutazone		
Salicylates		

2. **To relieve the symptoms and improve pump function by:**
   - **a.** Reducing metabolic demands through rest, relaxation, and pharmaceutical controls
   - **b.** Reducing fluid volume excess through dietary and pharmaceutical controls
   - **c.** Administering digitalis and other inotropic substances
   - **d.** Promoting patient compliance and self-regulation through education
   - **e.** Select appropriate patients for cardiac transplantation

II. PATHOPHYSIOLOGY. Heart failure and decreased cardiac output trigger a complex scheme of compensatory mechanisms designed to normalize cardiac output (cardiac output = stroke volume × heart rate).

A. Compensation. These mechanisms are represented schematically in Figure 44-2.

1. **Sympathetic responses.** Inadequate cardiac output stimulates reflex activation of the sympathetic nervous system and an increase in circulating catecholamines. The heart rate increases, and blood flow is redistributed to ensure perfusion of the most vital organs (the brain and the heart).

2. **Hormonal stimulation.** The redistribution of blood flow results in reduced renal perfusion, which decreases the glomerular filtration rate (GFR). Reduction in GFR results in:
   - **a.** Sodium and water retention
   - **b.** Activation of the renin–angiotensin–aldosterone system, which further enhances sodium retention and, thus, volume expansion

3. **Concentric cardiac hypertrophy** describes a mechanism that thickens cardiac walls, providing larger contractile cells and diminishing the capacity of the cavity in an attempt to precipitate expulsion at lower volumes.

4. **Frank-Starling mechanism.** The premise of this response is that increased fiber dilation heightens the contractile force, which then increases the energy released.
   - **a.** Within physiologic limits, the heart pumps all the blood it receives without allowing excessive accumulation within the veins or cardiac chambers.
   - **b.** As blood volume increases, the various cardiac chambers dilate (stretch) and enlarge in an attempt to accommodate the excess fluid.
   - **c.** As these stretched muscles contract, the contractile force increases in proportion to their distention. Then the extended fibers "snap back" (as a rubber band would), expelling the extra fluid into the arteries.

B. Decompensation. Over time, the compensatory mechanisms become exhausted and increasingly ineffective, entering a vicious spiral of decompensation in which the mechanisms surpass their limits and become self-defeating—as they work harder, they only exhaust the system's capacity to respond.

1. As the strain continues, total peripheral resistance and afterload increase, thereby decreasing the percentage of blood ejected per unit of time. Afterload is determined by the amount of contractile force needed to overcome intraventricular pressure and eject the blood.
   - **a. Afterload** is the tension in ventricular muscles during contraction. In the left ventricle, this tension is determined by the amount of force needed to overcome pressure in the aorta.

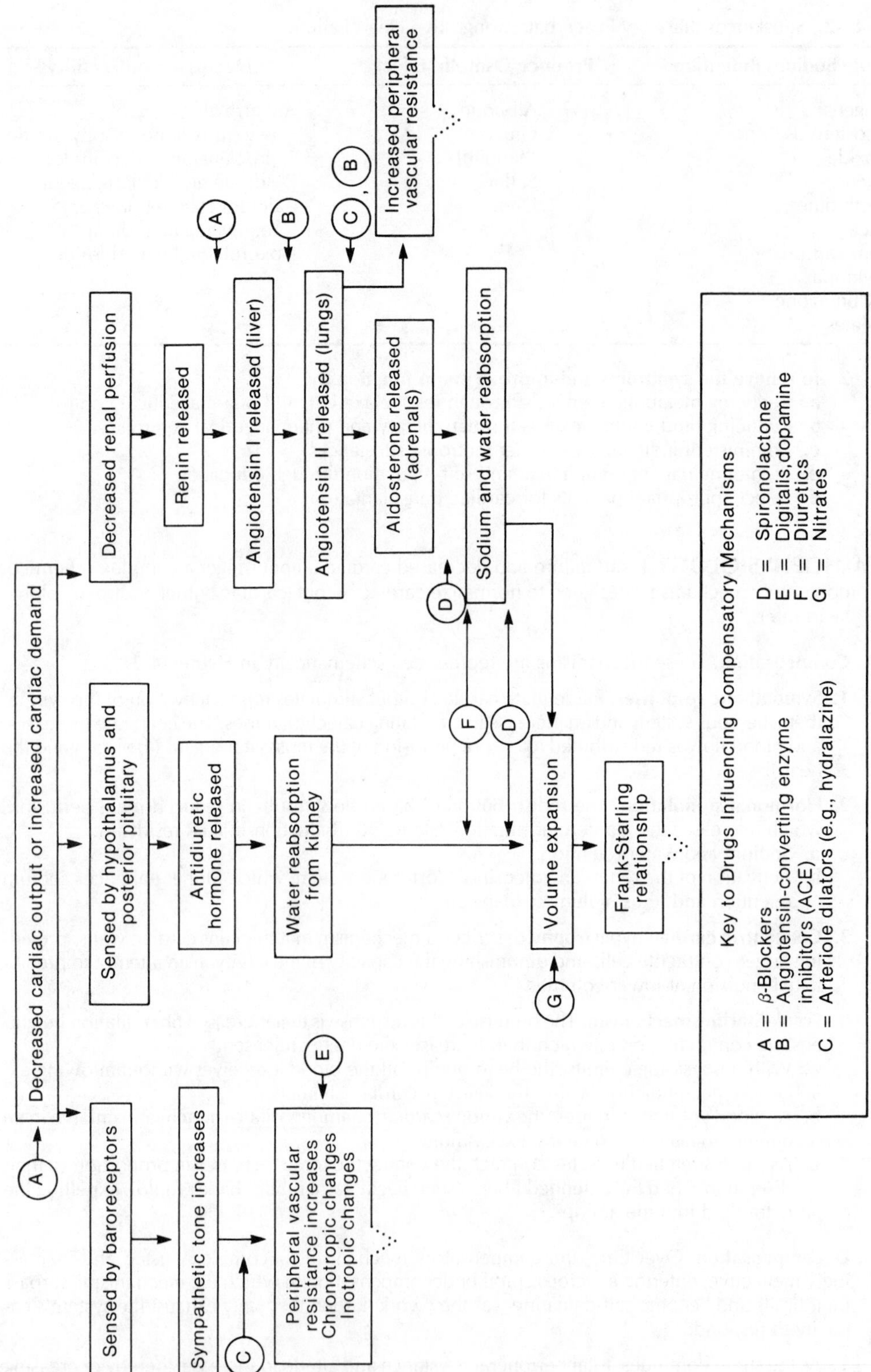

Figure 44-2. Compensatory mechanisms in congestive heart failure (CHF).

Afterload (also known as intraventricular systolic pressure) is sometimes used to describe the amount of force needed in the right ventricle to overcome pressure in the pulmonary artery.

b. Preload is the force exerted on the ventricular muscle at the end of diastole that determines the degree of muscle fiber stretch. This concept is also known as ventricular end-diastolic pressure. Preload is a key factor in contractility because the more these muscles are stretched in diastole, the more powerfully they contract in systole.

2. As the fluid volume expands, so do the demands on an already exhausted pump, allowing increased volume to remain in the ventricle.

3. The resulting fluid backup (from the left ventricle into the lungs; from the right ventricle into peripheral circulation) produces the signs and symptoms of CHF.

III. CLINICAL EVALUATION

A. Left-sided heart failure

1. Signs and symptoms

a. Dyspnea

(1) As CHF progresses, the amount of effort required to trigger **exertional dyspnea** lessens.

(2) Both paroxysmal nocturnal dyspnea and orthopnea result from volume pooling in the recumbent position and can be relieved by propping with pillows or sitting upright. (Orthopnea is often gauged by the number of pillows the patient needs to sleep comfortably.)

b. Dry, wheezing cough

c. Exertional fatigue and weakness

d. Nocturia. Edematous fluids that accumulate during the day migrate from dependent areas when the patient is in a recumbent position and renal perfusion increases.

2. Physical findings

a. Rales (or crackles) indicate the movement of air through fluid-filled passages.

b. Tachycardia is an early compensatory response detected through an increased pulse rate.

c. S_3 ventricular gallop is a vibration produced by rapid filling of the left ventricle early in diastole.

d. S_4 atrial gallop is a vibration produced by increased resistance to sudden, forceful ejection of atrial blood in late diastole; it does not vary with inspiration in left-sided failure.

3. Diagnostic test results

a. Cardiomegaly (heart enlargement), left ventricular hypertrophy, and pulmonary congestion may be evidenced by chest x-ray, electrocardiogram (ECG), and echocardiography.

b. Arm-to-tongue circulation time is prolonged.

c. Transudative pleural effusion may be suggested by x-ray and confirmed by analysis of aspirated pleural fluid.

B. Right-sided heart failure

1. Signs and symptoms

a. Complaints by the patient of tightness and swelling (e.g., "My ring is too tight"; "My skin feels too tight") suggest edema.

b. Nausea, vomiting, anorexia, bloating, or abdominal pain on exertion may reflect hepatic and visceral engorgement, resulting from venous pressure elevation.

2. Physical findings

a. Jugular vein distention reflects increased venous pressure and is a cardinal sign of CHF.

b. S_3 ventricular gallop is described in III A 2 c.

c. S_4 atrial gallop intensifies on inspiration in right-sided failure.

d. Hepatomegaly (a tender, enlarged liver) is revealed when pushing on the edge of the liver results in a fluid reflux into the jugular veins, causing bulging (positive hepatojugular reflux).

e. Bilateral leg edema is an early sign of right-sided heart failure; pitting ankle edema signals more advanced heart failure. However, edema is common to many disorders, and a pattern of associated findings, such as concurrent neck vein distention, is required for differential diagnosis.

3. **Laboratory findings. Elevated levels of hepatic enzymes** [e.g., alanine aminotransferase (ALT)] reflect hepatic congestion.

IV. THERAPY

A. Bed rest

1. **Advantages**
   a. Bed rest decreases metabolic needs, which reduces cardiac workload.
   b. Reduced workload, in turn, reduces pulse rate and dyspnea.
   c. Bed rest also helps decrease excess fluid volume by promoting diuresis.

2. **Disadvantages.** The risk of venous stasis increases with bed rest and can result in thromboembolism. Antiembolism stockings help minimize this risk, as do passive or active leg exercises, when the patient's condition permits.

3. **Progressive ambulation** should follow adequate bed rest.

B. Dietary controls

1. **Consuming small, but frequent meals** (4–6 daily) that are low in calories and residue provide nourishment without unduly increasing metabolic demands.

2. **Sodium restriction** is a primary tool in reducing central volume in CHF.
   a. Renal function should be evaluated to assess sodium conservation if severe sodium restriction is contemplated.
   b. Moderate sodium restriction (2–4 g of dietary sodium/day) can be achieved with relative ease by limiting the addition of salt during cooking and at the table.
   c. The patient should be advised about medications and common products that contain sodium and cautioned about their use (e.g., antacids, sodium bicarbonate or baking soda, commercial diet food products, water softeners). Table 44-2 lists other substances that promote sodium retention.

C. Digitalis glycosides.

Digitalis usually is considered a mainstay of CHF treatment, but its use, particularly in chronic CHF, has become somewhat controversial. Some authorities feel that digitalis use should be reserved for cases refractory to therapy combining rest, dietary controls, diuretics, and vasodilators.

1. **Therapeutic effects**
   a. **Positive inotropic effects** provide most of the benefits:
      (1) Increased cardiac output
      (2) Decreased cardiac filling pressure
      (3) Decreased venous and capillary pressure
      (4) Decreased heart size
      (5) Increased renal blood flow
      (6) Deactivation of renin–angiotensin–aldosterone compensation, promoting diuresis
      (7) Decreased fluid volume
      (8) Diminished edema
   b. **Negative chronotropic effects** accrue from the effect of digitalis on the sinoatrial (SA) node when given in doses that produce high total body stores (e.g., 15–18 μg/kg).

2. **Choice of agent.** All of the digitalis glycosides have similar properties; thus, selection is based on absorption, elimination kinetics, speed of onset, and duration of effect. Overall, digoxin is the most versatile and widely used and is, therefore, used as the therapeutic prototype.
   a. Digoxin is available in tablet, injection, elixir, and capsule forms.
   b. Calculation of doses must factor in the differences in systemic availability among these forms. For example, digoxin solution in capsules is more bioavailable than digoxin tablets; therefore, 0.125-mg tablets are equivalent to 0.1-mg capsules.

3. **Dosage and administration.** The range between therapeutic and toxic doses is extremely narrow. There is no "magic threshold" level for digitalis therapy, but serum concentrations of 0.8–2.0 ng/ml for digoxin (10–35 ng/ml for digitoxin) have been associated with therapeutic response and minimal toxicity.
   a. **Rapid digitalization**

(1) In this method, the effects (and steady-state levels) are achieved within 24 hours, but the actual administration rate is usually slow and delivered in divided doses.
(2) In the presence of an acute need for an immediate effect, intravenous digitalization with digoxin may be required—if the patient has not received any digitalis in the previous 2 weeks. Intravenous digitoxin is not usually used in acute situations because it has a long latency period.

b. **Slow digitalization.** When urgency is not the driving force, oral administration of maintenance doses should achieve steady-state levels in 7–8 days for the average patient (3–4 weeks in a patient with renal dysfunction).

4. **Precautions and monitoring effects**

a. **Potassium** seems to antagonize digitalis preparations.
(1) Decreased potassium levels favor digoxin binding to cardiac cells and increase its effect, thus increasing the likelihood of digitalis toxicity. This antagonism is particularly significant for the CHF patient who is receiving a diuretic (many of which decrease potassium levels).
(2) Conversely, increased potassium levels seem to decrease digoxin binding and decrease its effect. This is likely in patients taking potassium or a captopril-like agent (which increases potassium reabsorption).

b. **Calcium** ions act synergistically with digoxin, and increased levels increase the force of myocardial contraction. At excessive levels, arrhythmias and systolic standstill can develop.

c. **Magnesium** levels are inversely related to digoxin activity. As magnesium levels decrease, the predisposition to toxicity increases and, within reason, vice versa.

d. **Serum digoxin levels**
(1) In cardiac glycoside therapy, the patient's clinical state is the most practical barometer of a successful regimen. However, should questions arise as to compliance, absorption, or a drug–drug interaction, serum digoxin levels may be helpful.
(2) After oral ingestion of digoxin, serum levels rise rapidly, then drop sharply as the drug enters the myocardium and other tissues. Therefore, a meaningful evaluation requires a determination of the relationship between serum digoxin levels and myocardial tissue levels.
(3) The most meaningful results are obtained if serum samples are taken after steady-state has been reached and 6–8 hours after an oral dose (3–4 hours after an intravenous dose).

e. **Renal function studies.** Because the kidney is the primary metabolic route for **digoxin,** renal function studies such as serum creatinine levels aid the evaluation of elimination kinetics for digoxin. (For **digitoxin,** which is eliminated primarily through the liver, evaluation of metabolizing capabilities is more difficult.)

5. **Digitalis toxicity** is a fairly common occurrence because of the narrow therapeutic range and can be fatal in a significant percentage of patients experiencing a toxic reaction.

a. **Risk of toxicity** increases with coadministration of quinidine, verapamil, and amiodarone and is influenced by the electrolyte effects described in IV C 4 a–c.

b. **Signs of toxicity** include:
(1) Anorexia, a common and early sign
(2) Fatigue, headache, malaise
(3) Nausea and vomiting
(4) Mental confusion and disorientation
(5) Alterations in visual perception (e.g., blurring, yellowing, or a halo effect)
(6) Cardiac effects, which include:
(a) Premature ventricular contractions; ventricular tachycardia and fibrillation
(b) SA and atrioventricular (AV) block
(c) Atrial tachycardia with AV block

c. **Treatment of toxicity**
(1) Digitalis is discontinued immediately, as is any potassium-depleting diuretic.
(2) If the patient is hypokalemic, potassium supplements are administered and serum levels are monitored to avoid hyperkalemia through overcompensation. However, potassium supplements are contraindicated in a patient with severe AV block.
(3) Arrhythmias are treated with lidocaine (usually a 100-mg bolus, followed by infusion at 2–4 mg/min) or phenytoin (as a slow intravenous infusion of 25–50 mg/min, to a maximum of 1.0 g.

(4) Cholestyramine, which binds to digitalis glycosides, may help prevent absorption and reabsorption of digitalis in the bile.
(5) Patients with very high serum digoxin levels (such as those resulting from a suicidal overdose) may benefit from the use of purified digoxin-specific Fab fragment antibodies. One vial (40 mg) will bind 0.6 mg of digitalis. The dosage is calculated based on the estimated total body store of digitalis.

D. Diuretics (see Chapter 43 III B 2) All diuretics reduce excess sodium and water. Thus, they reduce preload by decreasing venous return, which is essential in managing CHF.

1. **Thiazide diuretics** are effective and commonly used, but they deplete potassium stores in the process.
2. The **loop diuretic furosemide** is the most frequently used diuretic and has the effect plus the added advantage of reducing venous return independent of diuresis. Also, because furosemide's action is more intense, it is useful as a rapid-acting intravenous agent in reversing acute pulmonary edema, due to its direct dilating effects on pulmonary vasculature.
3. **Potassium-sparing diuretics** may help avoid the exacerbating effects of hypokalemia, but they have a weaker diuretic effect than the other diuretics.

E. Vasodilators (see Chapter 43 III B 4)

1. These agents reduce pulmonary congestion and increase cardiac output by reducing preload and afterload.
2. Because of the complexity of vasodilator actions in patients with CHF, their use requires close hemodynamic monitoring and individualized adjustments to avoid excessive vasodilation and its adverse effects.
3. Some vasodilators exert their action primarily on the veins (preload reduction) or on the arteries (afterload reduction); others act on venous and arterial beds almost equally, providing a balanced effect (preload–afterload reduction).
4. **Individual agents**
   a. **Nitroprusside** (see Chapter 43 III B 4 c) is administered intravenously in doses of 0.5–10 μg/kg/min to provide potent dilation of both arteries and veins.
   b. **Hydralazine** (see Chapter 43 III B 4 a)
      (1) This arteriole dilator decreases afterload and increases cardiac output in patients with CHF.
      (2) Effective long-term therapy has been achieved with doses of 50–75 mg taken orally up to four times daily.
   c. **Prazosin**
      (1) This α-adrenergic blocker acts as a balanced arteriovenous dilator.
      (2) It has been shown to be effective in long-term therapy in doses of 2–10 mg taken up to four times daily.
   d. **Nitrates**
      (1) Venous dilation by nitrates increases venous pooling, which decreases preload.
      (2) Their arterial effects seem to result in decreased afterload with continued therapy.
      (3) Nitrates are available in many forms and doses. Because individual reactions vary widely, dosages have to be adjusted, but, in general, they are higher for CHF than for angina. Table 44-3 provides examples of nitrate doses used in CHF patients.
   e. **Combination therapy.** Hydralazine has been used with isosorbide dinitrate to reduce afterload (or with nitroglycerin to reduce preload) in the treatment of chronic CHF. A recently completed multicenter study within the Veterans Administration Hospitals has shown that combination therapy with hydralazine and isosorbide dinitrate significantly reduced mortality in patients unresponsive to digitalis and diuretics.
   f. **Angiotensin-converting enzyme (ACE) inhibitors** [see Chapter 43 III B 5 f (1), (2)]
      (1) **Captopril** and **enalapril** inhibit the conversion of angiotensin I to angiotensin II (a potent vasoconstrictor). This action significantly decreases total peripheral resistance, which aids in reducing afterload.
      (2) Inhibiting the production of angiotensin II interferes with stimulation of aldosterone release, thus indirectly reducing retention of sodium and water, which decreases venous return and preload.

Table 44-3. Examples of Nitrate Use in Congestive Heart Failure

Form	Typical Dose	Interval
Intravenous nitroglycerin	5–20 μg/min	Continuous infusion
Nitroglycerin buccal tablets	1–3 mg	4–6 hours
Nitroglycerin capsules (sustained-release)	6.5–19.5 mg	4–6 hours
Nitroglycerin ointment	1–3 inches	4–6 hours
Sublingual nitroglycerin	0.4 mg	1–2 hours
Oral isosorbide dinitrate	10–60 mg	4–6 hours
Sublingual isosorbide dinitrate	5–10 mg	4 hours

(3) Captopril (50–100 mg three times daily) and enalapril (2.5–10 mg twice daily) have been used effectively for the treatment of heart failure.

(4) Though not conclusive, current data support the use of these agents in heart failure to help reduce mortality rates, which are currently high.

(5) The list of available agents continues to grow (see Chapter 43).

F. Inotropic agents have been used in the emergency treatment of patients with CHF and in patients refractory to, or unable to take, digitalis.

1. Dopamine (intravenous)

a. Low doses of 2–5 μg/kg/min stimulate specific dopamine receptors within the kidney to increase renal blood flow, and thus increase urine output.

b. Moderate doses of 5–10 μg/kg/min increase cardiac output in CHF patients.

c. High doses

(1) As doses are raised above 10 μg/kg/min, alpha peripheral activity increases, resulting in increased total peripheral resistance and pulmonary pressures.

(2) When the infusion exceeds 8–9 μg/kg/min, the patient should be monitored for tachycardia. If the infusion is slowed or interrupted, the adverse effect should disappear, as dopamine has a very short half-life in plasma.

2. Dobutamine (intravenous)

a. Patients who are unresponsive to, or adversely affected by, dopamine may benefit from dobutamine in doses of 5–20 μg/kg/min.

b. Although dobutamine resembles dopamine chemically, its actions differ somewhat. For example, dobutamine does not have a direct effect on renal receptors and, therefore, does not act as a renal vasodilator. It only increases urinary output through increased cardiac output.

c. Serious arrhythmias are a potential occurrence, although less likely to occur than with dopamine. Slowing or interrupting the infusion usually reverses this effect, as it does for dopamine.

d. Dobutamine and dopamine have been used together to treat cardiogenic shock, but similar use in CHF has yet to be accepted.

3. Amrinone (intravenous) is the first of a class of drugs referred to as nonglycoside, nonsympathomimetic inotropic agents.

a. A derivative of bipyridine, amrinone has both a positive inotropic effect and a vasodilating effect.

b. By inhibiting phosphodiesterase located specifically in the cardiac cells, it increases the amount of cyclic adenosine monophosphate (cAMP).

c. Amrinone has been used in patients with heart failure that has been refractory to treatment with other inotropic agents.

d. Effective regimens have used loading intravenous infusions of 0.75 mg/kg over 3–4 minutes followed by maintenance infusions of 5–10 μg/kg/min.

e. Precautions and monitoring effects

(1) Amrinone is unstable in dextrose solutions and should be added to saline solutions instead. Because of fluid balance concerns, this may be a potential problem in patients with CHF.

(2) Because of the peripheral dilating properties, patients should be monitored for hypotension.
(3) Thrombocytopenia has occurred and is dose-dependent and asymptomatic.
(4) Ventricular rates may increase in patients with atrial flutter or fibrillation.

4. **Milrinone (intravenous)** is the newest inotropic agent released and is similar to amrinone. It possesses both inotropic and vasodilatory properties.
   a. This agent has been used to treat patients with heart failure as short-term management.
   b. Most milrinone patients in clinical trials have also been receiving digoxin and diuretics.
   c. Effective dosing regimens have used a loading dose of 50 μg/kg, administered slowly over 10 minutes intravenously, followed by maintenance doses of 0.59–1.13 mg/kg/day by continuous infusion based on the clinical status of the patient.
   d. **Precautions and monitoring effects**
      (1) Renal impairment significantly prolongs the elimination rate of milrinone, and infusions need to be reduced accordingly.
      (2) Monitoring is necessary for the potential arrhythmias occurring in CHF, which may be increased by drugs such as milrinone and other inotropic agents.
      (3) Blood pressure and heart rate should be monitored when administering milrinone, due to its vasodilatory effects and its potential to induce arrhythmias.
      (4) Additional side effects include mild-to-moderate headache, tremor, and thrombocytopenia.

G. Patient education

1. The patient should be made aware of the importance of taking the digitalis glycoside (and any other medications) exactly as prescribed and should be advised to watch for signs of toxicity (see IV C 5 b).

2. Dietary sodium restrictions should be emphasized.

3. The patient should understand the need for regular checkups and be able to recognize symptoms that require immediate physician notification; for example, an unusually irregular pulse rate, palpitations, shortness of breath, swollen ankles, visual disturbances, or weight gain exceeding 3–5 lb in 1 week.

STUDY QUESTIONS

Directions: Each of the numbered items or incomplete statements in this section is followed by answers or by completions of the statement. Select the **one** lettered answer or completion that is **best** in each case.

1. Which of the following groups of symptoms is most often associated with a patient who has right-sided heart failure?

(A) Nocturia, rales, paroxysmal nocturnal dyspnea
(B) Paroxysmal nocturnal dyspnea, pedal edema, jugular venous distention, hepatojugular reflux
(C) Jugular venous distention, hepatojugular reflux, pedal edema, shortness of breath
(D) Hepatojugular reflux, jugular venous distention, pedal edema, abdominal distention
(E) Paroxysmal nocturnal dyspnea, jugular venous distention, abdominal distention, shortness of breath

2. Which of the following combinations of drugs, when used together, reduce both preload and afterload?

(A) Nitroglycerin and isosorbide dinitrate
(B) Hydralazine and isosorbide dinitrate
(C) Captopril and methyldopa
(D) Prazosin and angiotensin II
(E) Hydralazine and methyldopa

3. When digitalis glycosides are used in the patient with congestive heart failure (CHF), they work by exerting a positive effect on

(A) stroke volume
(B) total peripheral resistance
(C) heart rate
(D) blood pressure
(E) venous return

Questions 4–5

A 60-year-old hypertensive woman is currently being treated with atenolol, nitroglycerin, nifedipine, aspirin, and dipyridamole. She is admitted with a diagnosis of congestive heart failure (CHF).

4. Which agent is most likely to be discontinued in this patient?

(A) Nifedipine
(B) Atenolol
(C) Aspirin
(D) Nitroglycerin
(E) Dipyridamole

5. It is later found that the patient has developed CHF as a result of a serious anemia due to aspirin-induced bleeding. What type of heart failure does the patient have?

(A) High-output
(B) Low-output
(C) Left-sided
(D) Right-sided
(E) Low-output, left-sided

6. Because of direct dilating effects on the lung, certain agents aid in the treatment of congestive heart failure (CHF) patients suffering from pulmonary congestion. Which of the following agents is in this category?

(A) Hydrochlorothiazide
(B) Triamterene
(C) Furosemide
(D) Metolazone
(E) Spironolactone

7. Which of the following vasodilators is an orally effective preload–afterload reducer in the patient with congestive heart failure (CHF)?

(A) Hydralazine
(B) Diltiazem
(C) Isosorbide dinitrate
(D) Prazosin
(E) Nitroprusside

1-D
2-B
3-A
4-B
5-A
6-C
7-D

8. For treating the patient with congestive heart failure (CHF), which of the following dosages of dopamine is selected for its positive inotropic effects?

(A) 2.0 μg/kg/min
(B) 5–10 μg/kg/min
(C) 10–20 μg/kg/min
(D) 40 μg/kg/min
(E) > 40 μg/kg/min

9. The use of angiotensin-converting enzyme (ACE) inhibitors in congestive heart failure (CHF) centers around their ability to cause

(A) direct reduction in renin levels with a resultant decrease in angiotensin II and aldosterone levels
(B) indirect reduction in angiotensin II and aldosterone levels due to inhibition of ACE
(C) direct reduction in aldosterone secretion and angiotensin I production by inhibiting ACE
(D) increase in afterload due to an indirect decrease in angiotensin II as well as a decrease in preload due to an indirect reduction in aldosterone secretion
(E) indirect increase in renin levels, secondary to a secondary hyperaldosteronism

10. All of the following have been shown to be effective in the acute management of digitalis toxicity EXCEPT

(A) cholestyramine resin
(B) lidocaine or phenytoin
(C) potassium administration
(D) digoxin-specific Fab fragment antibodies
(E) calcium

Directions: Each item below contains three suggested answers of which **one or more** is correct. Choose the answer

A if **I only** is correct
B if **III only** is correct
C if **I and II** are correct
D if **II and III** are correct
E if **I, II, and III** are correct

11. Situations that predispose a digitalis-treated patient to toxicity include

I. hypercalcemia
II. hyperkalemia
III. hypermagnesemia

12. Guidelines necessary for monitoring the patient with congestive heart failure (CHF) include which of the following questions?

I. Does the patient have therapeutic blood levels of digoxin in the range of 0.8–2.0 ng/ml?
II. Is the patient taking a product that may decrease the effectiveness of therapy (e.g., antacids, baking soda)?
III. Does the patient have signs of digitalis toxicity or a digoxin–drug interaction?

8-B
9-B
10-E
11-A
12-E

13. Correct statements about dobutamine include which of the following?

I. Doses of 5–20 μg/kg/min have been associated with a positive inotropic effect in treating the patient with congestive heart failure (CHF)
II. Patients receiving dobutamine should be monitored for increases in peripheral vascular resistance
III. Dobutamine is considered a nonglycoside, nonsympathomimetic positive inotropic agent

---

13-A

ANSWERS AND EXPLANATIONS

1. The answer is D *[III B 2].*
A patient with right-sided heart failure would present with symptoms and signs of peripheral edema, due to the backup of fluid behind the failing right ventricle. The patient's symptoms and signs result from the peripheral accumulation of fluid within the liver, the legs, the abdomen, and the venous system in general. Pulmonary signs (e.g., rales, shortness of breath, paroxysmal nocturnal dyspnea) are more the consequence of the backup of fluid behind the failing left ventricle, characteristically seen in left-sided heart failure.

2. The answer is B *[IV E 4 d–e].*
The venous dilating properties of isosorbide dinitrate (preload) in conjunction with the arteriolar dilating effects of hydralazine (afterload) make this combination of agents effective in reducing both preload and afterload. The Veterans Administration Cooperative Vasodilator–Heart Failure Trial demonstrated that, as compared to placebo, the combination of the vasodilators hydralazine and isosorbide dinitrate reduced mortality in patients with mild-to-moderate heart failure previously treated with digoxin and diuretics.

3. The answer is A *[IV C 1 a].*
Digitalis glycosides are used in congestive heart failure (CHF) as positive inotropic agents to increase stroke volume. By increasing stroke volume, digitalis glycosides increase the cardiac output by increasing the right side of the following equation:

$$\text{Cardiac output} = \text{stroke volume} \times \text{heart rate}.$$

4–5. The answers are: 4-B *[I E 1, 2; Table 44-2],* **5-A** *[I D 1 b].*
Because they produce negative inotropic effects, β-adrenergic receptor blockers, such as atenolol must be used very cautiously in patients who develop congestive heart failure (CHF). All β-blockers have the potential to reduce cardiac output. The physician must determine whether the benefit of such therapy for a patient with angina, hypertension, arrhythmia, and so forth is worth the risk of inducing heart failure. In many situations, the risk is worth taking; in other situations, it may not be if alternative therapy is available.

In anemia, the lack of oxygen-carrying capacity by the red blood cells puts an added stress on the heart, which must work harder to provide better oxygenation to the metabolizing tissues. Initially, the heart may be able to compensate, either by increasing the heart rate or by increasing stroke volume through cardiac dilation and hypertrophy. However, if the anemia is allowed to continue, the heart is unable to meet the metabolic demands placed on it, resulting in the signs and symptoms of heart failure.

6. The answer is C *[IV D 2].*
Furosemide has been shown to possess direct pulmonary dilating effects, which are independent of a diuretic effect and which occur prior to the diuretic effect.

7. The answer is D *[IV E 4 c].*
Prazosin acts as an α-adrenergic blocking agent. The physiologic response seen includes both arteriolar and venous dilation. Prazosin has been shown to produce a balanced dilating effect, making it a useful agent in the ambulatory setting. Unlike hydralazine (which produces afterload reduction), isosorbide dinitrate (producing preload reduction), and nitroprusside (a parenteral agent), prazosin is effective orally in reducing both preload and afterload when used alone.

8. The answer is B *[IV F 1].*
Dopamine has shown great versatility in its effects. At doses of 2–5 μg/kg/min, it increases renal blood flow through its dopaminergic effects. At doses of 5–10 μg/kg/min, it increases cardiac output through its β-adrenergic stimulating effect. At doses of 10–20 μg/kg/min, it increases peripheral vascular resistance through its α-adrenergic stimulating effects. There is no specific cutoff for any of these effects, so close titration is required to provide for individual response.

9. The answer is B *[IV E 4 f (2); Figure 44-2].*
By directly inhibiting the angiotensin-converting enzyme (ACE), production of angiotensin II is reduced, as is angiotensin II–mediated secretion of aldosterone from the adrenal gland.

10. The answer is E *[IV C 5 c].*
Cholestyramine resin has been used in the acute situation to decrease the absorption of digoxin within the gastrointestinal tract. This results in lower digoxin levels if the resin is administered before all the digoxin has been absorbed. Digoxin-specific antibodies have been shown to be effective in binding free digoxin in the blood, thereby reducing the potential for digoxin toxicity. Potassium administration has been shown to be effective in protecting the myocardium from the toxic effects of digoxin while toxic levels return to normal. Both lidocaine and phenytoin have been shown to be useful in preventing and treating toxic arrhythmias associated with digitalis toxicity. Calcium ions are expected to work synergistically with digitalis to increase the myocardial force of contractions. This effect would work to increase the toxic effects of digitalis.

11. The answer is A (I) *[IV C 4 a–c].*
Calcium ions act synergistically with digitalis. Therefore, when hypercalcemia occurs, digitalis exerts an added pharmacologic effect on the heart. This may present itself as toxic arrhythmias, cardiac standstill, and even death. Elevated potassium levels or elevated magnesium levels seem to aid in the prevention of digitalis-induced toxicity. There is building evidence that digitalis preparations need calcium ions to work, and consequently low calcium levels may negate the pharmacologic potential of digitalis.

12. The answer is E (all) *[IV B 2 c; C 3, 5 a–b; G 1–3].*
Digitalis has a narrow therapeutic range; serum levels of 0.8–2.0 ng/ml provide a therapeutic response with minimal toxicity. Monitoring serum digoxin levels is especially helpful during initial dosage titrations and when questions arise as to compliance, absorption, or a drug–drug interaction. Patients with congestive heart failure (CHF) must be informed of the need to take their medication appropriately and accurately so that blood levels for all drugs will be within the therapeutic range. Patients must also be told to inform their pharmacist of any additional drugs they are taking since these could aggravate the disease or interact with digoxin or with other drugs. Patients should also be monitored for those symptoms related to CHF that effective therapy should prevent. Reporting symptoms such as swollen legs or shortness of breath enables the physician to add different drugs or increase the dosage of current medications.

13. The answer is A (I) *[IV F 2 a].*
Dobutamine in doses of 5–20 μg/kg/min is an inotropic agent that is useful in the treatment of congestive heart failure (CHF). Dobutamine does not have the versatility that dopamine offers, lacking comparable effects on renal blood flow or peripheral vascular resistance. Rather, dobutamine has a peripheral dilating effect that offers a benefit to patients who have reduced cardiac output due to elevated peripheral resistance.

45
Infectious Diseases

Paul F. Souney
Cheryl A. Stoukides

I. PRINCIPLES OF ANTI-INFECTIVE THERAPY

A. Definition. Anti-infective agents treat infection by suppressing or destroying the causative microorganisms—bacteria, mycobacteria, fungi, protozoa, or viruses. Anti-infective agents derived from natural substances are called **antibiotics;** those produced from synthetic substances are called **antimicrobials**. These two terms are now used interchangeably.

B. Indications. Anti-infective agents should be used only when:

1. A significant infection has been diagnosed or is strongly suspected
2. An established indication for prophylactic therapy exists

C. Gram stain, microbiologic culturing, and susceptibility tests. These tests should be performed before anti-infective therapy is initiated. Test materials must be obtained by a method that avoids contamination of the specimen by the patient's own flora.

1. **Gram stain.** Performed on all specimens except blood cultures, the Gram stain helps to identify the cause of infection immediately. By determining if the causative agent is gram-positive or gram-negative, the test allows a better choice of drug therapy, especially when an anti-infective regimen must begin without delay.
   a. **Gram-positive** microorganisms stain **blue** or **purple**.
   b. **Gram-negative** microorganisms stain **red** or **rose-pink**.
   c. **Fungi** may also be identified by Gram stain.

2. **Microbiologic cultures.** To identify the specific causative agent, specimens of body fluids or infected tissue are collected for analysis.

3. **Susceptibility tests.** Different strains of the same pathogenic species may have widely varying susceptibility to a particular anti-infective agent. Susceptibility tests determine microbial susceptibility to a given drug and, thus, can be used to predict whether the drug will combat the infection effectively.
   a. **Microdilution method.** The drug is diluted serially in various media containing the test microorganism.
      (1) The lowest drug concentration that prevents microbial growth after 18–24 hours of incubation is called the **minimum inhibitory concentration (MIC)**.
      (2) The lowest drug concentration that reduces bacterial density by 99.9% is called the **minimum bactericidal concentration (MBC)**.
   b. **Kirby-Bauer disk diffusion technique.** This test is less expensive but less reliable than the microdilution method; however, it provides qualitative susceptibility information.
      (1) Filter paper disks impregnated with specific drug quantities are placed on the surface of agar plates streaked with a microorganism culture. After 18 hours, the size of a clear inhibition zone is determined; drug activity against the test strain is then correlated to zone size.
      (2) The Kirby-Bauer technique does not reliably predict therapeutic effectiveness against certain microorganisms (e.g., *Staphylococcus aureus, Shigella*).

D. Choice of agent. An anti-infective agent should be chosen on the basis of its pharmacologic properties and spectrum of activity as well as on various host (patient) factors.

1. **Pharmacologic properties** include the drug's ability to reach the infection site and to attain a desired level in the target tissue.

2. **Spectrum of activity.** To treat an infectious disease effectively, an anti-infective drug must be active against the causative pathogen. Susceptibility testing or clinical experience in treating a given syndrome may suggest the effectiveness of a particular drug.

3. **Patient factors.** Selection of an anti-infective drug regimen must take various patient factors into account to determine which type of drug should be administered, the correct drug dosage and administration route, and the potential for adverse drug effects.

   a. **Immunologic status.** A patient with impaired immune mechanisms may require a drug that rapidly destroys pathogens (i.e., **bactericidal agent**) rather than one that merely suppresses a pathogen's growth or reproduction (i.e., **bacteriostatic agent**).

   b. **Presence of a foreign body.** The effectiveness of anti-infective therapy is reduced in patients who have prosthetic joints or valves, cardiac pacemakers, and various internal shunts.

   c. **Age.** A drug's pharmacokinetic properties may vary widely in patients of different ages. In very young and very old patients, drug metabolism and excretion commonly decrease. Elderly patients also have an increased risk of suffering ototoxicity when receiving certain antibiotics.

   d. **Underlying disease**

      (1) Preexisting **kidney or liver disease** increases the risk of nephrotoxicity or hepatotoxicity during the administration of some antibacterial drugs.

      (2) Patients with **central nervous system (CNS) disorders** may suffer neurotoxicity (motor seizures) during penicillin therapy.

      (3) Patients with **neuromuscular disorders** (e.g., myasthenia gravis) are at increased risk for developing neuromuscular blockade during aminoglycoside or polymyxin B therapy.

   e. **History of drug allergy or adverse drug reactions.** Patients who have had previous allergic or other untoward reactions to a particular antibiotic have a higher risk of experiencing the same reaction during subsequent administration of that drug. Except in life-threatening situations, patients who have had serious allergic reactions to penicillin, for example, should not receive the drug again.

   f. **Pregnancy and lactation.** Because drug therapy during pregnancy and lactation can cause unwanted effects, the mother's need for the antibiotic must be weighed against the drug's potential harm.

      (1) Pregnancy can increase the risk of adverse drug effects—for both mother and fetus. Also, plasma drug concentrations tend to decrease in pregnant women, reducing a drug's therapeutic effectiveness.

      (2) Most drugs, including antibiotics, appear in the breast milk of nursing mothers and may cause adverse effects in infants. For example, sulfonamides may lead to toxic bilirubin accumulation in a newborn's brain.

   g. **Genetic traits**

      (1) Sulfonamides may cause hemolytic anemia in patients with glucose-6-phosphate dehydrogenase (G6PD) deficiency.

      (2) Patients who rapidly metabolize drugs (i.e., rapid acetylators) may develop hepatitis when receiving the antitubercular drug isoniazid.

E. **Empiric therapy.** In serious or life-threatening disease, anti-infective therapy must begin before the infecting organism has been identified. In this case, the choice of drug (or drugs) is based on clinical experience suggesting that a particular agent is effective in a given setting.

1. A **broad-spectrum antibiotic** usually is the most appropriate choice until the specific organism has been determined.

2. In all cases, **culture specimens must be obtained before therapy begins**.

F. **Multiple antibiotic therapy.** A combination of drugs should be given only when clinical experience has shown such therapy to be more effective than single-agent therapy in a particular setting. A multiple-agent regimen can increase the risk of toxic drug effects and, in a few cases, may result in drug antagonism and subsequent therapeutic ineffectiveness. Indications for multiple-agent therapy include:

1. **Need for increased antibiotic effectiveness.** The **synergistic** (intensified) effect of two or more agents may allow a dosage reduction or a faster or enhanced drug effect.

2. **Treatment of an infection caused by multiple pathogens** (e.g., intra-abdominal infection)
3. **Prevention of proliferation of drug-resistant organisms** (e.g., during treatment of tuberculosis)

G. **Duration of anti-infective therapy.** To achieve the therapeutic goal, anti-infective therapy must continue for a sufficient duration.

1. **Acute uncomplicated infection.** Treatment generally should continue until the patient has been afebrile and asymptomatic for at least 72 hours.
2. **Chronic infection** (e.g., endocarditis, osteomyelitis). Treatment may require a longer duration (4–6 weeks) with follow-up culture analyses to assess therapeutic effectiveness.

H. **Monitoring therapeutic effectiveness.** To assess the patient's response to anti-infective therapy, appropriate specimens should be cultured and the following parameters monitored:

1. **Fever curve.** An important assessment tool, the fever curve may be a reliable indication of response to therapy. Defervescence usually indicates favorable response.
2. **White blood cell (WBC) count.** In the initial stage of infection, the neutrophil count from a peripheral blood smear may rise above normal (neutrophilia) and immature neutrophil forms ("bands") may appear ("left shift"). In patients who are elderly, debilitated, or suffering overwhelming infection, the WBC count may be normal or subnormal.
3. **Radiographic findings.** Small effusions, abscesses, or cavities may appear on x-ray and indicate the focus of infection.
4. **Pain and inflammation** (as evidenced by swelling, erythema, and tenderness) may occur when the infection is superficial or within a joint or bone, also indicating a possible focus of infection.

I. **Lack of therapeutic effectiveness.** When an antibiotic drug regimen fails, other drugs should not be added indiscriminately or the regimen otherwise changed. Instead, the situation should be reassessed and diagnostic efforts intensified. Causes of therapeutic ineffectiveness include:

1. **Misdiagnosis.** The isolated organism may have been misidentified by the laboratory or may not be the causative agent for infection (e.g., the patient may have an unsuspected infection).
2. **Improper drug regimen.** The drug dosage, administration route, dosing frequency, or duration of therapy may be inadequate or inappropriate.
3. **Inappropriate choice of antibiotic agent.** As discussed in I D, patient factors and the pharmacologic properties and spectrum of activity of a given drug must be considered when planning anti-infective drug therapy.
4. **Microbial resistance.** By acquiring resistance to a specific antibiotic, microorganisms can survive in the drug's presence. Many gonococcal strains, for instance, now resist penicillin. Drug resistance is especially common in geographic areas where a particular drug has been used excessively (and perhaps improperly).
5. **Unrealistic expectations.** Antibiotics are ineffective in certain circumstances.
   a. Patients with conditions that require **surgical drainage** frequently cannot be cured by anti-infective drugs until the drain has been removed. For example, the presence of necrotic tissue or pus in patients with pneumonia, empyema, or renal calculi is a common cause of antibiotic failure.
   b. **Fever** should not be treated with anti-infective drugs unless infection has been identified as the cause. Although fever frequently signifies infection, it sometimes stems from non-infectious conditions (e.g., drug reactions, phlebitis, neoplasms, metabolic disorders, arthritis). These conditions do not respond to antibiotics.
6. **Infection by two or more types of microorganisms.** If not detected initially, an additional cause of infection may lead to therapeutic failure.

J. **Perioperative antibiotic prophylaxis**

1. **Definition.** Perioperative antibiotic prophylaxis is a short course of antibiotic administered before there is clinical evidence of infection.

2. **General considerations**
   a. **Timing.** Antibiotic should be administered at the site of contamination prior to incision. Initiation of prophylaxis is often at induction of anesthesia, just prior to surgical incision. This ensures peak serum and tissue antibiotic levels.
   b. **Duration.** Prophylaxis should be maintained for the duration of surgery. Long surgical procedures (e.g., > 3 hours) may require additional doses. There is little evidence to support continuation of prophylaxis beyond 24 hours.
   c. **Antibiotic spectrum** should be appropriate for the usual pathogens.
      (1) In general, first-generation cephalosporins (e.g., cefazolin) are the drugs of choice for most procedures and patients. These agents have an appropriate spectrum, a low frequency of side effects, a favorable half-life, and a low cost.
      (2) Vancomycin is a suitable alternative in penicillin-sensitive patients and in situations where methicillin-resistant *S. aureus* is a concern.
   d. **Route of administration.** Intravenous or intramuscular routes are preferred to guarantee good serum and tissue levels at the time of incision.

II. ANTIBACTERIAL AGENTS

A. **Definition and classification.** Used to treat infections caused by **bacteria,** antibacterial agents fall into several major categories: **aminoglycosides, cephalosporins, erythromycins, penicillins** (including various subgroups), **sulfonamides, tetracyclines, fluoroquinolones, urinary tract antiseptics** and **miscellaneous antibacterials** (Table 45–1).

B. **Aminoglycosides.** These drugs, containing amino sugars, are used primarily in infections caused by gram-negative enterobacteria and in suspected sepsis. They have little activity against anaerobic and facultative organisms. The toxic potential of these drugs limits their use. Major aminoglycosides include **amikacin, kanamycin, gentamicin, neomycin, netilmicin, streptomycin,** and **tobramycin.**

1. **Mechanism of action.** Aminoglycosides are **bactericidal;** they inhibit bacterial protein synthesis by binding to and impeding the function of the 30S ribosomal subunit. (Some aminoglycosides also bind to the 50S ribosomal subunit.) Their mechanism of action is not fully known.

2. **Spectrum of activity**
   a. **Streptomycin** is active against both gram-positive and gram-negative bacteria. However, widespread resistance to this drug has restricted its use to the organisms that cause plague and tularemia; gram-positive streptococci (given in combination with penicillin); and *Mycobacterium tuberculosis* (given in combination with other antitubercular agents, as described in V C).
   b. **Amikacin, kanamycin, gentamicin, tobramycin, neomycin,** and **netilmicin** are active against many gram-negative bacteria (e.g., *Proteus, Serratia,* and *Pseudomonas* organisms).
      (1) **Gentamicin** is active against some *Staphylococcus* strains; it is more active than tobramycin against *Serratia* organisms.
      (2) **Amikacin** is the broadest spectrum aminoglycoside with activity against most aerobic gram-negative bacilli as well as many anaerobic gram-negative bacterial strains that resist gentamicin and tobramycin. It is also active against *M. tuberculosis.*
      (3) **Tobramycin,** as compared to gentamicin, may be more active against *Pseudomonas aeruginosa.*
      (4) **Netilmicin** may be active against gentamicin-resistant organisms; it appears to be less ototoxic than other aminoglycosides.
      (5) **Neomycin,** in addition to its activity against such gram-negative organisms as *Escherichia coli* and *Klebsiella pneumoniae,* is active against several gram-positive organisms (e.g., *S. aureus, M. tuberculosis*). *P. aeruginosa* and most streptococci are now neomycin-resistant.

Table 45-1. Some Important Parameters of Anti-Infective Drugs

Agent	Elimination Route	Half-Life	Administration Route	Common Dosage Range (Adults)
Aminoglycosides				
Amikacin	Renal	2–3 hours	IV, IM	15 mg/kg/day
Gentamicin	Renal	2 hours	IV, IM	3 mg/kg/day
Kanamycin	Renal	2–4 hours	Oral, IV	15 mg/kg q 8–12 hours
Neomycin	Renal	2–3 hours	Oral, topical	50–100 mg/kg/day (oral); 10–15 mg/day (topical)
Netilmicin	Renal	2–7 hours	IV, IM	3–6 mg/kg/day
Streptomycin	Renal	2–3 hours	IM	15 mg/kg/day[†]
Tobramycin	Renal	2–5 hours	IV, IM	3–5 mg/kg/day
Cephalosporins				
First-generation				
Cefadroxil	Renal	1.5 hours	Oral	1–2 g/day
Cefazolin	Renal	1.4–2.2 hours	IV	250 mg–1 g q 8 hours
Cephalexin	Renal	0.9–1.3 hours	Oral	250–500 mg q 6 hours
Cephalothin	Renal (H)	0.5–0.9 hours	IV, IM	500 mg–2 g q 4–6 hours
Cephapirin	Renal (H)	0.6–0.8 hours	IV, IM	500 mg–2 g q 4–6 hours
Cephradine	Renal	1.3 hours	Oral, IV	250–500 mg q 6 hours
Second-generation				
Cefaclor	Renal (H)	0.8 hours	Oral	250–500 mg q 8 hours
Cefamandole	Renal	1 hour	IV	500 mg–1 g q 4–8 hours
Cefmetazole	Renal	72 minutes	IV	2 g q 6–12 hours
Cefonicid	Renal	4 hours	IV	1–2 g/day
Ceforanide	Renal	2.2–3 hours	IV	0.5 mg–1 g q 12 hours
Cefotetan	Renal	2.8–4.6 hours	IV, IM	1–2 g q 12 hours
Cefoxitin	Renal	0.8 hours	IV	1–2 g q 6–8 hours
Cefpodoxime	Renal	2.5 hours	Oral	100–400 mg q 12 hours
Cefprozil	Renal	78 minutes	Oral	250–500 mg q 12–24 hours
Cefuroxime	Renal	1.5–2.2 hours	IV, IM	750 mg–1.5 g q 8 hours
Loracarbef	Renal	1 hour	Oral	200 mg q 12 hours or 400 mg/day
Third-generation				
Cefixime	Renal	3–4 hours	Oral	400 mg/day
Cefoperazone	Hepatic	1.6–2.4 hours	IV	2–4 g q 12 hours
Cefotaxime	Renal (H)	1.5 hours	IV	1–2 g q 6–8 hours
Cefotetan	Renal	4.2 hours	IV, IM	1–2 g q 12 hours
Ceftazidime	Renal	1.8 hours	IV, IM	1–2 g q 8–12 hours
Ceftizoxime	Renal	1.7 hours	IV	1–2 g q 8–12 hours
Ceftriaxone	Renal	8 hours	IV, IM	1–2 g/day
Moxalactam	Renal	2.2 hours	IV, IM	2–4 g q 8–12 hours
Erythromycins and other macrolides				
Azithromicin	Hepatic	68 hours	Oral	250 mg/day
Clarithromycin	Renal	3–7 hours	Oral	250–500 mg q 12 hours

(continued on next page)

Table 45-1. (continued) Some Important Parameters of Anti-Infective Drugs

Agent	Elimination Route	Half-Life	Administration Route	Common Dosage Range (Adults)
Erythromycin base, estolate, ethylsuccinate, and stearate	Hepatic	1.2–2.6 hours	Oral	250–500 mg q 6 hours
Erythromycin gluceptate and lactobionate			IV	0.5–2 g q 6 hours
Troleandomycin	Hepatic (R)	1.05 hours	Oral	250–500 mg q 12 hours
Natural penicillins				
Penicillin G	Renal (H)	0.5 hours	Oral, IV, IM	200,000–500,000 units q 6–8 hours
Penicillin V	Renal	1 hour	Oral	500 mg–2 g/day
Penicillin G procaine	Renal	24–60 hours	IM	300,000–600,000 units/day
Penicillin G benzathine	Renal	24–60 hours	IM	300,000–600,000 units/day
Penicillinase-resistant penicillins				
Cloxacillin	Renal (H)	0.5 hours	Oral	250–500 mg q 6 hours
Dicloxacillin	Renal (H)	0.5–0.9 hours	Oral	500 mg–1 g/day
Methicillin	Renal (H)	0.5–1 hour	IV, IM	1–2 g q 4–6 hours
Nafcillin	Hepatic (R)	0.5 hours	Oral, IV, IM	0.25–2 g q 6 hours
Oxacillin	Renal (H)	0.5 hours	Oral, IV, IM	500 mg–2 g q 4–6 hours
Aminopenicillins				
Amoxicillin	Renal (H)	0.9–2.3 hours	Oral	250–500 mg q 8 hours
Amoxicillin/clavulanic acid	Renal	1 hour	Oral	250–500 mg q 8 hours
Ampicillin	Renal (H)	0.8–1.5 hours	Oral, IV, IM	250 mg–2 g q 4–6 hours
Ampicillin/sulbactam	Renal	1–1.8 hours	IV, IM	1.5–3 g q 6 hours
Bacampicillin	Renal	1 hour	Oral	400–800 mg q 12 hours
Cyclacillin	Renal (H)	0.5 hours	Oral	250–500 mg q 6 hours
Extended-spectrum penicillins				
Azlocillin	Renal (H)	0.8–1.5 hours	IV	100–300 mg/kg/day
Carbenicillin	Renal (H)	1.5 hours	IM, IV	1–5 g q 4–6 hours
Carbenicillin indanyl	Renal (H)	1.5 hours	Oral	382–764 mg qid
Mezlocillin	Renal (H)	0.6–1.2 hours	IV, IM	1–3 g q 4–6 hours
Piperacillin	Renal (H)	0.8–1.4 hours	IV, IM	1–1.5 mg/kg q 6–12 hours
Ticarcillin	Renal	0.9–1.5 hours	IV, IM	1–3 g q 4–6 hours
Ticarcillin/clavulanic acid	Renal	1–1.5 hours	IV	3.1 g q 4–6 hours
Sulfonamides				
Sulfacytine	Renal	4–4.5 hours	Oral	250 mg q 6 hours
Sulfadiazine	Renal (H)	6 hours	Oral, IV	2–4 g/day
Sulfamethoxazole	Hepatic (R)	9–11 hours	Oral	1–3 g/day
Sulfisoxazole	Renal (H)	3–7 hours	Oral, IV	2–8 g/day
Tetracyclines				
Demeclocycline	Renal	10–17 hours	Oral	300 mg–1 g/day
Doxycycline	Hepatic	14–25 hours	Oral, IV	100–200 mg q 12 hours
Methacycline	Renal	16 hours	Oral	150 mg q 6 hours to 300 mg q 12 hours
Minocycline	Hepatic	12–15 hours	Oral, IV	100–200 mg q 12 hours

Table 45-1. (continued) Some Important Parameters of Anti-Infective Drugs

Agent	Elimination Route	Half-Life	Administration Route	Common Dosage Range (Adults)
Oxytetracycline	Renal	6–12 hours	Oral, IM	250–500 mg q 6 hours 250–500 mg qid or 300 mg/day in one or two divided doses
Tetracycline[‡]	Renal	6–12 hours	Oral, IV, IM	1–2 g/day
Fluoroquinolones				
Ciprofloxacin	Renal (H)	5–6 hours 3–5 hours	IV Oral	200–600 mg q 12 hours 250–750 mg q 12 hours
Enoxacin	Renal (H)	6.2 hours	Oral	200 mg/day–600 mg q 12 hours
Lomefloxacin	Renal	6.35–7.77 hours	Oral	400 mg/day
Ofloxacin	Renal	5–7.5 hours	IV, Oral	100 mg/day–400 mg q 12 hours
Urinary tract antiseptics				
Cinoxacin	Renal	1–1.5 hours	Oral	250 mg q 6 hours or 500 mg q 12 hours
Methenamine hippurate and mandelate	Renal	1–3 hours	Oral	0.5–2 g qid
Nalidixic acid	Renal	8 hours	Oral	4 g/day
Nitrofurantoin	Renal	0.3–1 hour	Oral	5–7 mg/kg/day
Norfloxacin	Hepatic	3–4 hours	Oral	400 bid
Miscellaneous anti-infectives				
Aztreonam	Renal	1.7 hours	IV, IM	500 mg–2 g q 8–12 hours
Chloramphenicol	Hepatic	1.5–4.1 hours	Oral, IV	50–100 mg/kg/day
Ciprofloxacin	Hepatic (R)	3–5 hours	Oral	250–750 mg q 12 hours
Clindamycin	Hepatic	2–4 hours	Oral, IM, IV	300–900 mg q 6–8 hours
Clofazimine	Hepatic	70 days	Oral	100 mg/day
Dapsone	Hepatic (R)	28 hours	Oral	50–100 mg/day
Imipenem	Renal	1 hour	IV	250 mg–1 g q 6 hours
Lincomycin	Hepatic (R)	4.4–6.4 hours	IV, IM	600 mg–1 g q 8–12 hours
Mupirocin	Renal	19–35 minutes	Topical	Apply q 8–12 hours
Spectinomycin	Renal	1.2–2.8 hours	IM	2–4 g (single dose)
Trimethoprim	Renal (H)	8–15 hours	Oral	100–200 mg/day
Vancomycin	Renal	6–8 hours	Oral, IV	500 mg q 6 hours
Antifungal agents				
Amphotericin B	Unknown	24 hours	IV	1–1.5 mg/kg/day
Fluconazole	Renal	30 hours	IV, Oral	100–200 mg/day
Flucytosine	Renal	3–6 hours	Oral	50–150 mg/kg/day
Griseofulvin	Hepatic (R)	9–24 hours	Oral	300–375 mg/day
Intraconazole	Hepatic	34–42 hours	Oral	200–400 mg/day
Ketoconazole	Hepatic	1.5–3.3 hours	Oral	200–400 mg/day
Miconazole	Hepatic	20–24 hours	IV	600 mg–3 g/day
Nystatin	Fecal	. . .	Oral	500,000–1,000,000 units tid

(continued on next page)

Table 45-1. (continued) Some Important Parameters of Anti-Infective Drugs

Agent	Elimination Route	Half-Life	Administration Route	Common Dosage Range (Adults)
Antiprotozoal agents				
Atovaquone	Hepatic	2.9 days	Oral	750 mg/day for 21 days
Chloroquine hydrochloride phosphate	Renal	3 days	IM, Oral	160–200 mg/day[§] 500 mg–1 g/day
Diloxanide furoate	Renal	. . .	Oral	500 mg tid
Eflornithine	Renal	3 hours	IV	100 mg/kg/dose q 6 hours
Emetine	Renal	4–7 days	SC, IM	1 mg/kg/day to 60 mg/day maximum
Fansidar	Hepatic (R)	150 hours	Oral	3 tablets for one dose
Iodoquinol	Fecal	. . .	Oral	650 mg tid for 20 days
Mefloquine	Hepatic	15–33 days	Oral	5 tablets for one dose
Metronidazole	Hepatic (R)	6–14 hours	Oral	250–500 mg q 6–8 hours
Paramomycin	Fecal	. . .	Oral	25–35 mg/kg/day
Pentamidine	Renal	6–9 hours	IV	4 mg/kg qid for 14 days (treatment IV) 300 mg q 4 weeks (prophylaxis INH)
Primaquine phosphate	Renal	3–6 hours	Oral	15 mg (base)/day
Pyrimethamine	Renal	4 days	Oral	25 mg/week
Quinacrine	. . .	5 days	Oral	100 mg/day
Quinine sulfate	Renal	12 hours	Oral	650 q 8 hours[‖]
Antitubercular agents				
Aminosalicylic acid	Renal	1 hour	Oral	10–12 g/day
Capreomycin	Renal	4–6 hours	IM	15 mg/kg/day to 1 g/day maximum
Cycloserine	Renal	10 hours	Oral	500 mg/day to 1 g/day maximum
Ethambutol	Hepatic	3.3 hours	Oral	15 mg/kg/day
Ethionamide	Hepatic	3 hours	Oral	500 mg–1 g/day
Isoniazid	Hepatic	1–4 hours	Oral, IM	5 mg/kg/day to 300 mg/day maximum
Pyrazinamide	Hepatic	9–10 hours	Oral	20–35 mg/kg/day to 3 g/day maximum
Rifampin	Hepatic	3 hours	Oral	600 mg/day
Antiviral agents				
Acyclovir	Renal	2.1–3.8 hours	Oral, IV, topical	200 mg q 4 hours (oral); 5 mg/kg q 8 hours (IV)
Amantadine	Renal	12 hours	Oral	100–200 mg/day
Didanosine	Hepatic (R)	1.6 hours	Oral	125–300 mg q 12 hours
Foscarnet	Renal	2–8 hours	IV	60 mg/kg q 8 hours
Ganciclovir	Renal	2.9 hours	IV	5 mg/kg q 12 hours
Ribavirin	Renal	9.5 hours	Aerosol	6 g q 24 hours
Vidarabine	Renal (H)	1.5 hours	IV, topical	15 mg/kg/day
Zalcitabine	Renal	1–3 hours	Oral	0.75 mg q 8 hours
Zidovudine	Renal (H)	1 hour	Oral	200 mg q 4 hours
Anthelmintics				
Diethylcarbamazine	Renal	30 hours	Oral	25 mg/day for 3 days, then 50 mg/day for 5 days, then 100 mg/day for 3 days, then 150 mg/day for 12 days
Mebendazole	Hepatic	0.83–11.5 hours	Oral	100 mg q 12 hours

Table 45-1. (continued) Some Important Parameters of Anti-Infective Drugs

Agent	Elimination Route	Half-Life	Administration Route	Common Dosage Range (Adults)
Niclosamide	Fecal	. . .	Oral	2 g/day
Praziquantel	Renal	0.8–1.5 hours	Oral	20 mg/kg for 3 doses
Pyrantel	Hepatic	. . .	Oral	11 mg/kg for 1 dose (maximum, 1 g)
Oxamniquine	Renal	1–2.5 hours	Oral	12–15 mg/kg for 1 dose
Thiabendazole	Renal	. . .	Oral	$<$ 70 kg, 25 mg/kg $>$ 70 kg, 1.5 g

(H) = secondary hepatic elimination; IM = intramuscular; IV = intravenous; (R) = secondary renal elimination; and SC = subcutaneous.

[*]Dosage applies to infections other than tuberculosis; for tuberculosis, dosage is 1 g/day.

[†]Intravenous agent withdrawn from U.S. market.

[§]For short-term therapy.

[‖]For initial therapy.

3. Therapeutic uses

a. Streptomycin is used to treat plague, tularemia, acute brucellosis (given in combination with tetracycline), bacterial endocarditis caused by *Streptococcus viridans* (given in combination with penicillin), and tuberculosis (given in combination with other antitubercular agents, as described in V C 2).

b. Gentamicin, tobramycin, amikacin, and **netilmicin** are therapeutic for serious gram-negative bacillary infections (e.g., those caused by *Enterobacter, Serratia, Klebsiella, P. aeruginosa*), pneumonia (given in combination with a cephalosporin or penicillin), meningitis, complicated urinary tract infections, osteomyelitis, bacteremia, and peritonitis.

c. Neomycin is used for preoperative bowel sterilization; hepatic coma (as adjunctive therapy); and, in topical form, for skin and mucous membrane infections (e.g., burns).

4. Precautions and monitoring effects. Aminoglycosides can cause serious adverse effects. To prevent or minimize such problems, blood drug concentrations and blood urea nitrogen (BUN) and serum creatinine levels should be monitored during therapy.

a. Ototoxicity. Aminoglycosides can cause vestibular or auditory damage.

(1) Gentamicin and streptomycin cause primarily **vestibular** damage (manifested by tinnitus, vertigo, and ataxia). Such damage may be bilateral and irreversible.

(2) Amikacin, kanamycin, and neomycin cause mainly **auditory** damage (hearing loss).

(3) Tobramycin can result in both vestibular and auditory damage.

b. Nephrotoxicity. Because aminoglycosides accumulate in the proximal tubule, mild renal dysfunction develops in up to 25% of patients receiving these drugs for several days or more. Usually, this adverse effect is reversible.

(1) Neomycin is the most nephrotoxic aminoglycoside; streptomycin, the least nephrotoxic. Gentamicin and tobramycin are nephrotoxic to about the same degree.

(2) Risk factors for increased nephrotoxic effects include:

(a) Preexisting renal disease

(b) Previous or prolonged aminoglycoside therapy

(c) Concurrent administration of another nephrotoxic drug

(3) Trough levels above 2 μg/ml for gentamicin and tobramycin and above 10 μg/ml for amikacin are associated with nephrotoxicity.

c. Neuromuscular blockade. This problem may arise in patients receiving high-dose aminoglycoside therapy.

(1) Risk factors for neuromuscular blockade include:

(a) Concurrent administration of a neuromuscular blocking agent or an anesthetic

(b) Preexisting hypocalcemia or myasthenia gravis

(c) Intraperitoneal or rapid intravenous drug administration

(2) Apnea and respiratory depression may be reversed with administration of calcium or an anticholinesterase.

d. **Hypersensitivity and local reactions** are rare adverse effects of aminoglycosides.

e. **Therapeutic levels**

(1) Gentamicin and tobramycin peak at 6–10 μg/ml. Their trough level is 0.5–1.5 μg/ml.

(2) Amikacin peaks at 25–30 μg/ml. The trough level is 5–8 μg/ml.

5. **Significant interactions**

a. **Intravenous loop diuretics** can result in increased ototoxicity.

b. **Other aminoglycosides, cephalothin, cisplatin, amphotericin B,** and **methoxyflurane** can cause increased nephrotoxicity when given concurrently with streptomycin.

C. **Cephalosporins.** These agents are known as **β-lactam antibiotics** because their chemical structure consists of a β-lactam ring adjoined to a thiazolidine ring. Cephalosporins generally are classified in three major groups based mainly on their spectrum of activity (Table 45-2).

1. **Mechanism of action.** Cephalosporins are **bactericidal;** they inhibit bacterial cell wall synthesis, reducing cell wall stability, thus causing membrane lysis.

2. **Spectrum of activity**

a. **First-generation cephalosporins** are active against most gram-positive cocci (except enterococci) as well as enteric aerobic gram-negative bacilli (e.g., *E. coli, K. pneumoniae, Proteus mirabilis*).

b. **Second-generation cephalosporins** are active against the organisms covered by first-generation cephalosporins and have extended gram-negative coverage, including β-lactamase-producing strains of *Haemophilus influenzae.*

c. **Third-generation cephalosporins** have wider activity against most gram-negative bacteria; for example, *Enterobacter, Citrobacter, Serratia, Providencia, Neisseria,* and *Haemophilus* organisms, including β-lactamase-producing strains.

d. Each generation of cephalosporin has shifted toward increased gram-negative activity but has lost activity toward gram-positive organisms.

Table 45-2. Classification of Cephalosporins

First-Generation	Second-Generation	Third-Generation
Cefadroxil* (Duricef, Ultracef)	Cefaclor* (Ceclor)	Cefixime* (Suprax)
Cefazolin Ancef, Kefzol)	Cefamandole (Mandol)	Cefoperazone (Cefobid)
Cephalexin* (Keflex)	Cefmetazole (Zefazone)	Cefotaxime (Claforan)
Cephalothin (Keflin)	Cefonicid (Monocid)	Ceftazidime (Fortax, Taxicef, Tazidime)
Cephapirin (Cefadyl)	Ceforanide (Precef)	Ceftizoxime (Cefizox)
Cephradine* (Anspor, Velosef)	Cefotetan (Cefotan)	Ceftriaxone (Rocephin)
	Cefoxitin (Mefoxin)	Moxalactam (Moxam)
	Cefuroxime (Zinacef)	
	Cefuroxime axetil* (Ceftin)	
	Cefpodoxime* (Vantin)	
	Cefprozil* (Cefzil)	
	Loracarbef* (Lorabid)	

*Oral agents

3. Therapeutic uses

a. First-generation cephalosporins commonly are administered to treat serious *Klebsiella* infections and gram-positive and some gram-negative infections in patients with mild penicillin allergy. They also are used widely in perioperative prophylaxis. For most other indications, they are not the preferred drugs.

b. Second-generation cephalosporins are valuable in the treatment of urinary tract infections resulting from *E. coli* organisms and gonococcal disease caused by organisms that resist other agents.

(1) Cefaclor is useful in otitis media and sinusitis in patients who are allergic to ampicillin and amoxicillin.

(2) Cefoxitin is therapeutic for mixed aerobic–anaerobic infections, such as intra-abdominal infection. **Cefprozil, cefotetan, cefpodoxime,** and **loracarbef** are second-generation cephalosporins that can be administered twice daily but offer no important spectrum differences.

(3) Cefamandole and **cefuroxime** are commonly administered for community-acquired pneumonia.

c. Third-generation cephalosporins penetrate the cerebrospinal fluid (CSF) and, thus, are valuable in the treatment of meningitis caused by such organisms as meningococci, pneumococci, *H. influenzae,* and enteric gram-negative bacilli.

(1) These agents also are used to treat sepsis of unknown origin in immunosuppressed patients and to treat fever in neutropenic immunosuppressed patients (given in combination with an aminoglycoside).

(2) Third-generation cephalosporins are useful in infections caused by many organisms resistant to older cephalosporins.

(3) These agents frequently are administered as empiric therapy for life-threatening infection in which resistant organisms are the most likely cause.

(4) Initial therapy of mixed bacterial infections (e.g., sepsis) commonly involves third-generation cephalosporins.

4. Precautions and monitoring effects

a. Because all cephalosporins (except cefoperazone) are eliminated renally, doses must be adjusted for patients with renal impairment.

b. Cross-sensitivity with penicillin has been reported in up to 10% of patients receiving cephalosporins. More recent information indicates that true cross-reactivity is rare.

c. Cephalosporins can cause hypersensitivity reactions similar to those resulting from penicillin [see II E 1 e (1)]. Manifestations include fever, maculopapular rash, anaphylaxis, and hemolytic anemia.

d. Other adverse effects include nausea, vomiting, diarrhea, superinfection, and nephrotoxicity; with cefoperazone, moxalactam, and cefamandole, bleeding diastheses may occur. Bleeding can be reversed by vitamin K administration.

e. Cephalosporins may cause false–positive glycosuria results on tests using the copper reduction method.

5. Significant interactions

a. Probenicid may impair the excretion of cephalosporins (except ceftazidime and moxalactam), causing increased cephalosporin levels and possible toxicity.

b. Alcohol consumption may result in a disulfiram-type reaction in patients receiving moxalactam, cefoperazone, and cefamandole.

c. Aminoglycosides may cause additive toxicity when administered with cephalothin.

D. Erythromycins. The chemical structure of these macrolide antibiotics is characterized by a lactone ring to which sugars are attached. Erythromycin base and the estolate, ethylsuccinate, and stearate salts are given orally; erythromycin lactobionate and gluceptate are given parenterally.

1. Mechanism of action. Erythromycins may be **bactericidal** or **bacteriostatic;** they bind to the 50S ribosomal subunit, inhibiting bacterial protein synthesis.

2. Spectrum of activity. Erythromycins are active against many gram-positive organisms, including streptococci (e.g., *Streptococcus pneumoniae*), and *Corynebacterium* and *Neisseria* species as well as some strains of *Mycoplasma, Legionella, Treponema,* and *Bordetella*. Some *S. aureus* strains that resist penicillin G are susceptible to erythromycins.

3. Therapeutic uses

a. Erythromycins are the preferred drugs for the treatment of *Mycoplasma pneumoniae* and *Campylobacter* infections, legionnaires' disease, chlamydial infections, diphtheria, and pertussis.

b. In patients with penicillin allergy, erythromycins are important alternatives in the treatment of pneumococcal pneumonia, *S. aureus* infections, syphillis, and gonorrhea.

c. Erythromycins may be given prophylactically before dental procedures to prevent bacterial endocarditis.

4. Precautions and monitoring parameters

a. Serious adverse effects from erythromycins are rare.

b. Gastrointestinal distress (nausea, vomiting, diarrhea, epigastric discomfort) may occur with all erythromycin forms.

c. Allergic reactions (rare) may present as skin eruptions, fever, and eosinophilia.

d. Cholestatic hepatitis may arise in patients treated for 1 week or longer with erythromycin estolate; symptoms usually disappear within a few days after drug therapy ends. There have been infrequent reports of hepatotoxicity with other salts of erythromycin.

e. Intramuscular injections of over 100 mg produce severe pain persisting for hours.

f. Transient hearing impairment may develop with high-dose erythromycin therapy.

5. Significant interactions

a. Erythromycin inhibits the hepatic metabolism of **theophylline,** resulting in toxic accumulation.

b. Erythromycin interferes with the metabolism of **digoxin, corticosteroids, carbamazepine, cyclosporin,** and **lovastatin,** possibly potentiating the effect and toxicity of these drugs.

6. Alternatives to erythromycin

a. Clarithromycin and **azithromycin** are expensive but well-tolerated alternatives to erythromycin. Their greatest utility may be for treatment of opportunistic infections and other difficult-to-treat infections in patients with acquired immunodeficiency syndrome (AIDS).

(1) Clarithromycin is more active than erythromycin against staphylococci and streptococci. In addition to activity against other organisms covered by erythromycin, it is also active in vitro against *Mycobacterium avium–intracellulare* (MAI), *Toxoplasma gondii,* and *Cryptosporidium* species.

(2) Azithromycin is less active than erythromycin against gram-positive cocci but more active against *H. influenzae* and other gram-negative organisms. Azithromycin concentrates within cells, and tissue levels are higher than serum levels.

b. Troleandomycin is similar to erythromycin in most respects, but generally is less active against susceptible organisms.

E. Penicillins

1. Natural penicillins. Like cephalosporins and all other penicillins, natural penicillins are β-lactam antibiotics. Among the most important antibiotics, natural penicillins are the preferred drugs in the treatment of many infectious diseases.

a. Available agents

(1) Penicillin G sodium and potassium salts can be administered orally, intravenously, or intramuscularly.

(2) Penicillin V, a soluble drug form, is administered orally.

(3) Penicillin G procaine and penicillin G benzathine are repository drug forms. Administered intramuscularly, these insoluble salts allow slow drug absorption from the injection site and, thus, have a longer duration of action (12–24 hours).

b. Mechanism of action. Penicillins are **bactericidal;** they inhibit bacterial cell wall synthesis in a manner similar to that of the cephalosporins.

c. Spectrum of activity

(1) Natural penicillins are highly active against gram-positive cocci and against some gram-negative cocci.

(2) Penicillin G is five to ten times more active than penicillin V against gram-negative organisms and some anaerobic organisms.

(3) Because natural penicillins are readily hydrolyzed by penicillinases (β-lactmases), they are ineffective against *S. aureus* and other organisms that resist penicillin.

d. Therapeutic uses

(1) Penicillin G is the preferred agent for all infections caused by *S. pneumoniae* organisms, including:

(a) Pneumonia
(b) Arthritis
(c) Meningitis
(d) Peritonitis
(e) Pericarditis
(f) Osteomyelitis
(g) Mastoiditis

(2) Penicillins G and V are highly effective against other streptococcal infections, such as pharyngitis, otitis media, sinusitus, and bacteremia.

(3) Penicillin G is the preferred agent in gonococcal infections, syphilis, anthrax, actinomycosis, gas gangrene, and *Listeria* infections.

(4) Administered when an oral penicillin is needed, penicillin V is most useful in skin and soft-tissue infections and mild respiratory infections.

(5) Penicillin G procaine is effective against syphilis and uncomplicated gonorrhea.

(6) Used to treat syphilis infections outside the CNS, penicillin G benzathine also is effective against group A β-hemolytic streptococcal infections.

(7) Penicillins G and V may be used prophylactically to prevent streptococcal infection, rheumatic fever, and neonatal gonorrhea ophthalmia. Patients with valvular heart disease may receive these drugs preoperatively.

e. Precautions and monitoring effects

(1) Hypersensitivity reactions. These occur in up to 10% of patients receiving penicillin. Manifestations range from mild rash to anaphylaxis.

(a) The rash may be urticarial, vesicular, bullous, scarlatiniform, or maculopapular. Rarely, thrombopenic purpura develops.

(b) Anaphylaxis is a life-threatening reaction that most commonly occurs with parenteral administration. Signs and symptoms include severe hypotension, bronchoconstriction, nausea, vomiting, abdominal pain, and extreme weakness.

(c) Other manifestations of hypersensitivity reactions include fever, eosinophilia, angioedema, and serum sickness.

(d) Before penicillin therapy begins, the patient's history should be evaluated for reactions to penicillin. A positive history places the patient at heightened risk for a subsequent reaction. In most cases, such patients should receive a substitute antibiotic. (However, hypersensitivity reactions may occur even in patients with a negative history.)

(2) Other adverse effects of natural penicillins include gastrointestinal distress (e.g., nausea, diarrhea); bone marrow suppression (e.g., impaired platelet aggregation, agranulocytosis); and superinfection. With high-dose therapy, seizures may occur, especially in patients with renal impairment.

f. Significant interactions

(1) Probenecid increases blood levels of natural penicillins and may be given concurrently for this purpose.

(2) Antibiotic antagonism occurs when **erythromycins, tetracyclines,** or **chloramphenicol** is given within 1 hour of the administration of penicillin. The clinical significance of such antagonism is not clear.

(3) With penicillin G procaine and benzathine, precaution must be used in patients with a history of hypersensitivity reactions to penicillins since prolonged reactions may occur. Intravascular injection should be avoided. Procaine hypersensitivity is a contraindication to the use of procaine penicillin G.

(4) Parenteral products contain either potassium (1.7 mEq/million units) or sodium (2 mEq/million units).

2. Penicillinase-resistant penicillins. These penicillins are not hydrolyzed by staphylococcal penicillinases (β-lactamases). These agents include **methicillin, nafcillin,** and the **isoxazolyl penicillins—cloxacillin, dicloxacillin,** and **oxacillin**.

a. Mechanism of action (see II E 1 b)

b. Spectrum of activity. Because these penicillins resist penicillinases, they are active against staphylococci that produce these enzymes.

c. **Therapeutic uses**
   (1) Penicillinase-resistant penicillins are used solely in staphylococcal infections resulting from organisms that resist natural penicillins.
   (2) They are less potent than natural penicillins against organisms susceptible to natural penicillins and, thus, make poor substitutes in the treatment of infections caused by these organisms.
   (3) **Nafcillin** is excreted by the liver and, thus, may be useful in treating staphylococcal infections in patients with renal impairment.
   (4) **Oxacillin, cloxacillin,** and **dicloxacillin** are most valuable in long-term therapy of serious staphylococcal infections (e.g., endocarditis, osteomyelitis) and in the treatment of minor staphylococcal infections of the skin and soft tissues.

d. **Precautions and monitoring effects**
   (1) Like all penicillins, the penicillinase-resistant group can cause hypersensitivity reactions [see II E 1 e (1)].
   (2) Methicillin may cause nephrotoxicity and interstitial nephritis.
   (3) Oxacillin may be hepatotoxic.
   (4) Complete cross-resistance exists among the penicillinase-resistant penicillins.

e. **Significant interactions. Probenecid** increases blood levels of these penicillins and may be given concurrently for that purpose.

3. **Aminopenicillins.** This penicillin group includes the semisynthetic agents **ampicillin** and **amoxicillin** and their derivatives, **bacampicillin** and **cyclacillin.** Because of their wider antibacterial spectrum, these drugs are also known as **broad-spectrum penicillins**.

a. **Mechanism of action** (see II E 1 b)

b. **Spectrum of activity.** Aminopenicillins have a spectrum that is similar to but broader than that of the natural and penicillinase-resistant penicillins. Easily destroyed by staphylococcal penicillinases, aminopenicillins are ineffective against most staphylococcal organisms. Against most bacteria sensitive to penicillin G, aminopenicillins are slightly less effective than this agent.

c. **Therapeutic uses.** Aminopenicillins are used to treat gonococcal infections, upper respiratory infections, uncomplicated urinary tract infections, and otitis media caused by susceptible organisms.
   (1) For infections resulting from penicillin-resistant organisms, **ampicillin** may be given in combination with sulbactam.
   (2) **Amoxicillin** is less effective than ampicillin in shigellosis.
   (3) **Amoxicillin** is more effective against *S. aureus, Klebsiella,* and *Bacteroides fragilis* infections when administered in combination with clavulanic acid (amoxicillin/potassium clavulanate) because clavulanic acid inactivates penicillinases.

d. **Precautions and monitoring effects**
   (1) Hypersensitivity reactions may occur [see II E 1 e (1)].
   (2) Diarrhea is most common with ampicillin.
   (3) In addition to urticarial hypersensitivity rash seen with all penicillins, ampicillin and amoxicillin frequently cause a generalized erythematous, maculopapular rash. (This occurs in 5%–10% of patients receiving ampicillin.)

e. **Significant interactions** (see II E 2 e)

4. **Extended-spectrum penicillins.** These agents have the widest antibacterial spectrum of all penicillins. Also called **antipseudomonal penicillins,** this group includes the **carboxypenicillins** (e.g., **carbenicillin, carbenicillin indanyl, ticarcillin**) and the **ureidopenicillins** (e.g., **azlocillin, mezlocillin, piperacillin**).

a. **Mechanism of action** (see II E 1 b)

b. **Spectrum of activity.** These drugs have a spectrum similar to that of the aminopenicillins but also are effective against *Klebsiella* and *Enterobacter* species, some *B. fragilis* organisms, and indole-positive *Proteus* and *Pseudomonas* organisms.
   (1) **Carbenicillin** frequently is active against ampicillin-resistant *Proteus* strains and some other gram-negative organisms.
   (2) **Ticarcillin** is two to four times as active as carbenicillin against *P. aeruginosa*. Combined with clavulanic acid, ticarcillin has enhanced activity against organisms that resist ticarcillin alone.
   (3) **Azlocillin** and **piperacillin** are 10 times as active as carbenicillin against *Pseudomonas* organisms and are more active than carbenicillin against streptococcal organisms.

(4) **Mezlocillin** and **piperacillin** are more active than carbenicillin against *Klebsiella* organisms.

c. **Therapeutic uses.** Extended-spectrum penicillins are used mainly to treat serious infections caused by gram-negative organisms (e.g., sepsis; pneumonia; infections of the abdomen, bone, and soft tissues).

d. **Precautions and monitoring effects**

(1) Hypersensitivity reactions may occur [see II E 1 e (1)].

(2) Carbenicillin and ticarcillin may cause hypokalemia.

(3) The high sodium content of carbenicillin and ticarcillin may pose a danger to patients with congestive heart failure (CHF).

(4) All inhibit platelet aggregation, which may result in bleeding.

e. **Significant interactions** (see II E 2 e)

F. Sulfonamides. Derivatives of sulfanilamide, these agents were the first drugs to prevent and cure human bacterial infection successfully. Although their current usefulness is limited by the introduction of more effective antibiotics and the emergence of resistant bacterial strains, sulfonamides remain the drugs of choice for certain infections. The major sulfonamides are **sulfadiazine, sulfamethoxazole, sulfisoxazole, sulfacytine,** and **sulfamethizole**.

1. **Mechanism of action.** Sulfonamides are **bacteriostatic;** they suppress bacterial growth by triggering a mechanism that blocks folic acid synthesis, thereby forcing bacteria to synthesize their own folic acid.

2. **Spectrum of activity.** Sulfonamides are broad-spectrum agents with activity against many gram-positive organisms (e.g., *Streptococcus pyrogenes, S. pneumoniae*) and certain gram-negative organisms (e.g., *H. influenzae, E. coli, P. mirabilis*). They also are effective against certain strains of *Chlamydia trachomatis, Nocardia, Actinomyces,* and *Bacillus anthracis.*

3. **Therapeutic uses**

a. Sulfonamides most often are used to treat urinary tract infections caused by *E. coli,* including acute and chronic cystitis, and chronic upper urinary tract infections.

b. These agents have value in the treatment of nocardiosis, trachoma and inclusion conjunctivitis, and dermatitis herpetiformis.

c. **Sulfadiazine** may be administered in combination with pyrimethamine to treat toxoplasmosis.

d. **Sulfamethoxazole** may be given in combination with trimethoprim to treat such infections as *Pneumocystis carinii* pneumonia, *Shigella* enteritis, *Serratia* sepsis, urinary tract infections, respiratory infections, and gonococcal urethritis (see II J 7 c).

e. **Sulfisoxazole** is sometimes used in combination with erythromycin ethylsuccinate to treat acute otitis media caused by *H. influenzae* organisms. For the initial treatment of uncomplicated urinary tract infections, sulfisoxazole may be given in combination with phenazopyridine for relief of symptoms of pain, burning, or urgency.

f. Prophylactic sulfonamide therapy has been used successfully to prevent streptococcal infections and rheumatic fever recurrences.

4. **Precautions and monitoring effects**

a. Sulfonamides may cause blood dyscrasias (e.g., hemolytic anemia—especially in patients with G6PD deficiency, aplastic anemia, thrombocytopenia, agranulocytosis, eosinophilia).

b. Hypersensitivity reactions to sulfonamides probably result from sensitization and most commonly involve the skin and mucous membranes. Manifestations include various types of skin rash, exfoliative dermatitis, and photosensitivity. Drug fever and serum sickness also may develop.

c. Crystalluria and hematuria may occur, possibly leading to urinary tract obstruction. (Adequate fluid intake and urine alkalinization can prevent or minimize this risk.) Sulfonamides should be used cautiously in patients with renal impairment.

d. Life-threatening hepatitis caused by drug toxicity or sensitization is a rare adverse effect. Signs and symptoms include headache, nausea, vomiting, and jaundice.

5. **Significant interactions.** Sulfonamides may potentiate the effects of **phenytoin, oral anticoagulants,** and **sulfonylureas.**

G. Tetracyclines. These broad-spectrum agents are effective against certain bacterial strains that resist other antibiotics. Nonetheless, they are the preferred drugs in only a few situations. The major tetracyclines include **demeclocycline, doxycycline, methacycline, minocycline,** and **chlortetracycline**.

1. **Mechanism of action.** Tetracyclines are **bacteriostatic;** they inhibit bacterial protein synthesis by binding to the 30S ribosomal subunit.

2. **Spectrum of activity.** Tetracyclines are active against gram-negative and gram-positive organisms, spirochetes, *Mycoplasma* and *Chlamydia* organisms, rickettsial species, and certain protozoa.
   a. *Pseudomonas* and *Proteus* organisms are now resistant to tetracyclines. Many coliform bacteria, pneumococci, staphylococci, streptococci, and *Shigella* strains are increasingly resistant.
   b. Cross-resistance within the tetracycline group is extensive.

3. **Therapeutic uses**
   a. Tetracyclines are the agents of choice in rickettsial, chlamydial, and mycoplasmal infections; amebiasis; and bacillary infections (e.g., cholera, brucellosis, tularemia, some *Salmonella* and *Shigella* infections).
   b. Tetracyclines are useful alternatives to penicillin in the treatment of anthrax, syphilis, gonorrhea, Lyme disease, nocardiosis, and *H. influenzae* respiratory infections.
   c. Oral or topical tetracycline may be administered as a treatment for acne.
   d. **Doxycycline** is highly effective in the prophylaxis of "traveler's diarrhea" (commonly caused by *E. coli*). Because the drug is excreted mainly in the feces, it is the safest tetracycline for the treatment of extrarenal infections in patients with renal impairment.
   e. **Demeclocycline** is commonly used as an adjunctive agent to treat the **syndrome of inappropriate antidiuretic hormone (SIADH)** secretion.

4. **Precautions and monitoring effects**
   a. Gastrointestinal distress (e.g., diarrhea, abdominal discomfort, nausea, anorexia) is a common adverse effect of tetracyclines. This problem can be minimized by administering the drug with food or temporarily decreasing the dosage.
   b. Skin rash, urticaria, and generalized exfoliative dermatitis signify a hypersensitivity reaction. Rarely, angioedema and anaphylaxis occur.
   c. Cross-sensitivity within the tetracycline group is common.
   d. Phototoxic reactions (severe skin lesions) can develop with exposure to sunlight. This reaction is most common with demeclocycline and doxycycline.
   e. Tetracyclines may cause hepatotoxicity, especially in pregnant women. Manifestations include jaundice, acidosis, and fatty liver infiltration.
   f. Patients with renal impairment may suffer nephrotoxicity.
   g. Tetracyclines may induce permanent tooth discoloration, tooth enamel defects, and retarded bone growth in infants and children.
   h. Use of outdated and degraded tetracyclines can lead to renal tubular dysfunction, possibly resulting in renal failure.
   i. Minocycline can cause vestibular toxicity (e.g., ataxia, dizziness, nausea, vomiting).
   j. Intravenous tetracyclines are irritating and may cause phlebitis.

5. **Significant interactions**
   a. **Dairy products** and other foods, **iron preparations,** and **antacids** and **laxatives** containing aluminum, calcium, or magnesium can cause reduced tetracycline absorption. Absorption of doxycycline is not inhibited by these factors.
   b. **Methoxyflurane** may exacerbate the tetracyclines' nephrotoxic effects.
   c. **Barbiturates** and **phenytoin** decrease the antibiotic effectiveness of tetracyclines.
   d. Demeclocycline antagonizes the action of **antidiuretic hormone (ADH)** and may be given as a diuretic in patients with SIADH.

H. **Fluoroquinolones** are agents related to nalidixic acid [see II I 1 c, 2 c (1), 4 c (1)] and include **amifloxacin, ciprofloxacin, enoxacin, lomefloxacin, norfloxacin, ofloxacin,** and **befloxacin**. They are bactericidal for growing bacteria.

1. **Mechanism of action.** Fluoroquinolones inhibit DNA gyrase.

2. **Spectrum of activity.** Fluoroquinolones are highly active against enteric gram-negative bacilli, *Salmonella, Shigella, Campylobacter, Haemophilus,* and *Neisseria.*
   a. **Ciprofloxacin** has good activity against *P. aeruginosa,* but the fluoroquinolones as a group

have variable activity against non–*P. aeruginosa.* Ciprofloxacin is active against many anaerobes; it has moderate activity against *M. tuberculosis.*

b. Gram-positive organisms are less susceptible than gram-negative organisms but usually are sensitive except for *Streptococcus faecalis* and methicillin-resistant staphylococci.

c. Ofloxacin has the greatest activity against *Chlamydia.*

3. Therapeutic uses

a. Norfloxacin is indicated for the oral treatment of urinary tract infections. Unapproved indications include therapy for gonorrhea and prostatitis, treatment and prophylaxis of traveler's diarrhea and bacterial gastroenteritis, and prophylaxis of neutropenic patients.

b. Ciprofloxacin and **ofloxacin** are available orally and intravenously. In addition to the indications described for norfloxacin, these agents are useful for the treatment of bone and joint infections, respiratory tract infections, and soft tissue infections.

c. Lomefloxacin and **enoxacin** are approved for the treatment of urinary tract infections (lomefloxacin may be given once a day), but they offer no improvement in the spectrum of activity as compared to other fluoroquinolones.

d. Pefloxacin and **Amifloxacin** are currently under investigation.

4. Precautions and monitoring effects.

a. Occasional adverse effects include nausea, dyspepsia, headache, dizziness, and insomnia.

b. Infrequent adverse effects include rash, urticaria, leukopenia, and elevated liver enzymes.

c. Crystalluria occurs with high doses at alkaline pH.

d. Cartilage erosion has been observed in young animals; thus, fluoroquinolones should not be used in children or in women who are pregnant or nursing.

5. Significant interactions

a. Ciprofloxacin has been shown to increase **theophylline** levels. Variable effects on theophylline levels have been reported from other members of the group. In patients requiring fluoroquinolones, theophylline levels should be monitored.

b. Antacids and **sucralfate** may significantly decrease the absorption of fluoroquinolones.

c. Fluoroquinolones may increase prothrombin times in patients receiving **warfarin**.

d. Concurrent use with **nonsteroidal anti-inflammatory drugs** (NSAIDs) may increase the risk of CNS stimulation (seizures).

I. Urinary tract antiseptics. Concentrating in the renal tubules and bladder, these agents exert local antibacterial effects; most do not achieve blood levels high enough to treat systemic infections. [However, some new quinolone derivatives, such as ciprofloxacin and ofloxacin, are valuable in the treatment of certain infections outside the urinary tract (see II H 3 b).]

1. Mechanism of action

a. Methenamine is hydrolyzed to ammonia and formaldehyde in acidic urine; formaldehyde is antibacterial against gram-positive and gram-negative organisms. Mandelic and hippuric acids, with which methenamine is combined, provide supplementary antibacterial action.

b. Nitrofurantoin is **bacteriostatic;** in high concentrations, it may be **bactericidal**. Presumably, it disrupts bacterial enzyme systems.

c. Quinolones. Nalidixic acid and its analogues and derivatives—**oxolinic acid, norfloxacin, cinoxacin, ciprofloxacin, pefloxacin,** and others—interfere with DNA gyrase and inhibit DNA synthesis during bacterial replication.

2. Spectrum of activity

a. Methenamine is active against both gram-positive and gram-negative organisms (e.g., *Enterobacter, Klebsiella, Proteus, P. aeruginosa, S. aureus*).

b. Nitrofurantoin is active against many gram-positive and gram-negative organisms, including some strains of *E. coli, S. aureus, Proteus, Enterobacter,* and *Klebsiella.*

c. Quinolones (see II H)

(1) Nalidixic acid and **oxolinic acid** are active against most gram-negative organisms that cause urinary tract infections, including *P. mirabilis, E. coli, Klebsiella,* and *Enterobacter* organisms. These drugs are not effective against *Pseudomonas* organisms.

(2) Norfloxacin is active against *E. coli, Enterobacter, Klebsiella, Proteus, P. aeruginosa, S. aureus, Citrobacter,* and some *Streptococcus* organisms.

(3) Cinoxacin is active against *E. coli, Klebsiella, P. mirabilis, Proteus vulgaris, Proteus morganii, Serratia,* and *Citrobacter* organisms.

3. **Therapeutic uses**
   a. **Methenamine** and **nitrofurantoin** are used to prevent and treat urinary tract infections.
   b. **Quinolones** are administered to treat urinary tract infections; some also are used in such diseases as osteomyelitis and respiratory tract infections.

4. **Precautions and monitoring effects**
   a. **Methenamine** may cause nausea, vomiting, and diarrhea; in high doses, it may lead to urinary tract irritation (e.g., dysuria, frequency, hematuria, albuminuria). Skin rash also may develop.
   b. **Nitrofurantoin** may cause various adverse effects.
      (1) Gastrointestinal distress (e.g., nausea, vomiting, diarrhea) is relatively common.
      (2) Hypersensitivity reactions to nitrofurantoin may involve the skin, lungs, blood, or liver; manifestations include fever, chills, hepatitis, jaundice, leukopenia, granulocytopenia, and pneumonitis.
      (3) Adverse CNS effects include headache, vertigo, and dizziness. Polyneuropathy may develop with high doses or in patients with renal impairment.
   c. **Quinolones**
      (1) **Nalidixic acid** and **oxolinic acid** may cause nausea, vomiting, abdominal pain, urticaria, pruritus, skin rash, fever, eosinophilia, and CNS effects, such as headache, dizziness, confusion, vertigo, drowsiness, and weakness.
      (2) **Cinoxacin** may induce nausea, vomiting, diarrhea, headache, insomnia, skin rash, pruritus, and urticaria.

5. **Significant interactions**
   a. The effects of methenamine are inhibited by **alkalinizing agents** and are antagonized by **acetazolamide**.
   b. Nitrofurantoin absorption is decreased by **magnesium-containing antacids**. Nitrofurantoin blood levels are increased and urine levels decreased by **sulfinpyrazone** and **probenicid,** leading to increased toxicity and reduced therapeutic effectiveness.
   c. **Quinolones**
      (1) Cinoxacin urine levels are decreased by **probenecid,** reducing therapeutic effectiveness.
      (2) Norfloxacin is rendered less effective by **antacids**.

J. Miscellaneous antibacterial agents

1. **Aztreonam.** This agent was the first commercially available monobactam (monocyclic β-lactam compound). It resembles the aminoglycosides in its efficacy against many gram-negative organisms but does not cause nephrotoxicity or ototoxicity. Other advantages of this drug include its ability to preserve the body's normal gram-positive and anaerobic flora, activity against many gentamicin-resistant organisms, and lack of cross-allergenicity with penicillin.
   a. **Mechanism of action.** Aztreonam is **bactericidal;** it inhibits bacterial cell wall synthesis.
   b. **Spectrum of activity.** This drug is active against many gram-negative organisms, including *Enterobacter* and *P. aeruginosa*.
   c. **Therapeutic uses.** Aztreonam is therapeutic for urinary tract infections, septicemia, skin infections, lower respiratory tract infections, and intra-abdominal infections resulting from gram-negative organisms.
   d. **Precautions and monitoring effects**
      (1) Aztreonam sometimes causes nausea, vomiting, and diarrhea.
      (2) Liver enzymes may increase transiently during aztreonam therapy.
      (3) This drug may induce skin rash.

2. **Chloramphenicol.** A nitrobenzene derivative, this drug has broad activity against rickettsia as well as many gram-positive and gram-negative organisms. It also is effective against many ampicillin-resistant strains of *H. influenzae*.
   a. **Mechanism of action.** Chloramphenicol is primarily **bacteriostatic,** although it may be bactericidal against a few bacterial strains.
   b. **Spectrum of activity.** This agent is active against rickettsia and a wide range of bacteria, including *H. influenzae, Salmonella typhi, Neisseria meningitidis, Bordetella pertussis, Clostridium, B. fragilis, S. pyogenes,* and *S. pneumoniae*.

c. **Therapeutic uses.** Because of its toxic side effects, chloramphenicol is used only to suppress infections that cannot be treated effectively with other antibiotics. Such infections typically include:
   (1) Typhoid fever
   (2) Meningococcal infections in cephalosporin-allergic patients
   (3) Serious *H. influenzae* infections, especially in cephalosporin-allergic patients
   (4) Anaerobic infections (e.g., those originating in the pelvis or intestines)
   (5) Anaerobic or mixed infections of the CNS
   (6) Rickettsial infections in pregnant patients, tetracycline-allergic patients, and renally impaired patients

d. **Precautions and monitoring effects**
   (1) Chloramphenicol can cause bone marrow suppression (dose-related) with resulting pancytopenia; rarely, the drug leads to aplastic anemia (non–dose-related).
   (2) Hypersensitivity reactions may include skin rash and, in extremely rare cases, angioedema or anaphylaxis.
   (3) Chloramphenicol therapy may lead to gray baby syndrome in neonates (especially premature infants). This dangerous reaction, which stems partly from inadequate liver detoxification of the drug, is manifested by vomiting, gray cyanosis, rapid and irregular respirations, vasomotor collapse, and, in some cases, death.

e. **Significant interactions**
   (1) Chloramphenicol inhibits the metabolism of **phenytoin, tolbutamide, chlorpropamide,** and **dicumarol,** leading to prolonged action and intensified effect of these drugs.
   (2) **Phenobarbital** shortens chloramphenicol's half-life, thereby reducing its therapeutic effectiveness.
   (3) **Penicillins** can cause antibiotic antagonism.
   (4) **Acetaminophen** elevates chloramphenicol levels and may cause toxicity.

3. **Clindamycin.** This agent has essentially replaced lincomycin, the drug from which it is derived. It is used to treat skin, respiratory tract, and soft-tissue infections caused by staphylococci, pneumococci, and streptococci.

a. **Mechanism of action.** Clindamycin is **bacteriostatic;** it binds to the 50S ribosomal subunit, thereby suppressing bacterial protein synthesis.

b. **Spectrum of activity.** This agent is active against most gram-positive and many anaerobic organisms, including *B. fragilis.*

c. **Therapeutic uses.** Because of its marked toxicity, clindamycin is used only against infections for which it has proven to be the most effective drug. Typically, such infections include abdominal and female genitourinary tract infections caused by *B. fragilis.*

d. **Precautions and monitoring effects**
   (1) Clindamycin may cause rash, nausea, vomiting, diarrhea, and pseudomembranous colitis as evidenced by fever, abdominal pain, and bloody stools.
   (2) Blood dyscrasias (e.g., eosinophilia, thrombocytopenia, leukopenia) may occur.

e. **Significant interactions.** Clindamycin may potentiate the effects of **neuromuscular blocking agents**.

4. **Dapsone.** A member of the sulfone class, this drug is the primary agent in the treatment of all forms of leprosy.

a. **Mechanism of action.** Dapsone is **bacteriostatic** for *Mycobacterium leprae;* its mechanism of action probably resembles that of the sulfonamides.

b. **Spectrum of activity.** This drug is active against *M. leprae;* however, drug resistance develops in up to 40% of patients. Dapsone also has some activity against *P. carinii* organisms and the malarial parasite *Plasmodium.*

c. **Therapeutic uses**
   (1) Dapsone is the drug of choice for treating leprosy.
   (2) This agent may be used to treat dermatitis herpetiformis, a skin disorder.
   (3) Maloprim, a dapsone–pyrimethamine product, is valuable in the prophylaxis and treatment of malaria.

d. **Precautions and monitoring effects**
   (1) Hemolytic anemia can occur with daily doses above 200 mg. Other adverse hematologic effects include methemoglobinemia and leukopenia.
   (2) Nausea, vomiting, and anorexia may develop.

(3) Adverse CNS effects include headache, dizziness, nervousness, lethargy, paresthesias, and psychosis.
(4) Dapsone occasionally results in a potentially lethal mononucleosis-like syndrome.
(5) Paradoxically, this drug sometimes exacerbates leprosy.
(6) Other adverse effects include skin rash, peripheral neuropathy, blurred vision, tinnitus, hepatitis, and cholestatic jaundice.

e. **Significant interactions. Probenecid** elevates blood levels of dapsone, possibly resulting in toxicity.

5. **Imipenem.** Formerly known as thienamycin, imipenem is the first carbapenem compound introduced in the United States. A β-lactam antibiotic, it resists destruction by most β-lactamases. Because it is inhibited by renal dipeptidases, imipenem must be combined with cilastatin sodium, a dipeptidase inhibitor.
a. **Mechanism of action.** Imipenem is **bactericidal;** it inhibits bacterial cell wall synthesis.
b. **Spectrum of activity.** This drug has the broadest spectrum of all β-lactam antibiotics. It is active against most gram-positive cocci (including many enterococci), gram-negative rods (including many *P. aeruginosa* strains), and anaerobes. It has good activity against many bacterial strains that resist other antibiotics.
c. **Therapeutic uses.** Imipenem has most value in the treatment of severe infections caused by drug-resistant organisms susceptible only to imipenem.
d. **Precautions and monitoring effects**
(1) Imipenem may cause nausea, vomiting, diarrhea, and pseudomembranous colitis.
(2) Seizures, dizziness, and hypotension may develop.
(3) Patients who are allergic to penicillin or cephalosporins may suffer cross-allergy during imipenem therapy.

6. **Spectinomycin.** An aminocyclitol agent related to the aminoglycosides, this antibiotic is useful against penicillin-resistant strains of gonorrhea.
a. **Mechanism of action.** Spectinomycin is **bacteriostatic;** it selectively inhibits protein synthesis by binding to the 30S ribosomal subunit.
b. **Spectrum of activity.** This agent is active against various gram-negative organisms.
c. **Therapeutic uses.** Spectinomycin is used only to treat gonococcal infections in patients with penicillin allergy or when such infection stems from penicillinase-producing gonococci (PPNG).
d. **Precautions and monitoring effects.** Because spectinomycin is given only as a single-dose intramuscular injection, it causes few adverse effects. Nausea, vomiting, urticaria, chills, dizziness, and insomnia occur rarely.

7. **Trimethoprim.** A substituted pyrimidine, trimethoprim is most commonly combined with sulfamethoxazole (a sulfonamide discussed in II F) in a preparation called co-trimoxazole. However, it may be used alone for certain urinary tract infections.
a. **Mechanism of action.** Trimethoprim inhibits dihydrofolate reductase, thus blocking bacterial synthesis of folic acid.
b. **Spectrum of activity.** This agent is active against various gram-negative organisms.
(1) Trimethoprim is active against most gram-negative and gram-positive organisms. However, drug resistance may develop when this drug is used alone.
(2) Trimethoprim–sulfamethoxazole is active against a variety of organisms, including *S. pneumoniae, N. meningitidis,* and *Corynebacterium diphtheriae* and some strains of *S. aureus, Staphylococcus epidermidis, P. mirabilis, Enterobacter, Salmonella, Shigella, Serratia,* and *Klebsiella* species, and *E. coli*.
(3) The trimethoprim–sulfamethoxazole combination is synergistic; many organisms resistant to one component are susceptible to the combination.
c. **Therapeutic uses**
(1) Trimethoprim may be used alone or in combination with sulfamethoxazole to treat uncomplicated urinary tract infections caused by *E. coli, P. mirabilis,* and *Klebsiella* and *Enterobacter* organisms.
(2) Trimethoprim–sulfamethoxazole is therapeutic for acute gonococcal urethritis, acute exacerbation of chronic bronchitis, shigellosis, and *Salmonella* infections.
(3) Trimethoprim–sulfamethoxazole may be given as prophylactic or suppressive therapy in *P. carinii* pneumonia.
d. **Precautions and monitoring effects**
(1) Most adverse effects involve the skin (possibly from sensitization). These include rash, pruritus, and exfoliative dermatitis.

(2) Rarely, trimethoprim–sulfamethoxazole causes blood dyscrasias (e.g., acute hemolytic anemia, leukopenia, thrombocytopenia, methemoglobinemia, agranulocytosis, aplastic anemia).
(3) Adverse gastrointestinal effects including nausea, vomiting, and epigastric distress glossitis may occur.
(4) Neonates may develop kernicterus.
(5) Patients with AIDS sometimes suffer fever, rash, malaise, and pancytopenia during trimethoprim therapy.

8. **Vancomycin.** This glycopeptide destroys most gram-positive organisms.
   a. **Mechanism of action.** Vancomycin is **bactericidal:** It inhibits bacterial cell wall synthesis.
   b. **Spectrum of activity.** This drug is active against most gram-positive organisms, including methicillin-resistant strains of *S. aureus*.
   c. **Therapeutic uses.** Vancomycin usually is reserved for serious infections, especially those caused by methicillin-resistant staphylococci. It is particularly useful in patients who are allergic to penicillin or cephalosporins. Typical uses include endocarditis, osteomyelitis, and staphylococcal pneumonia.
      (1) Oral vancomycin is valuable in the treatment of antibiotic-induced pseudomembranous colitis caused by *Clostridium difficile* or *S. aureus* enterocolitis. Since vancomycin is not absorbed after oral administration, it is not useful for systemic infections.
      (2) Because 1 g provides adequate blood levels for 7–10 days, intravenous vancomycin is especially useful in the treatment of anephric patients with gram-positive bacterial infections.
   d. **Precautions and monitoring effects**
      (1) Ototoxicity may arise; nephrotoxicity is rare but can occur with high doses.
      (2) Vancomycin may cause hypersensitivity reactions, manifested by such symptoms as anaphylaxis or skin rash.
      (3) Therapeutic levels peak at 20–40 μg/ml. The trough is less than 10 μg/ml.
      (4) "Red neck syndrome" may occur. This is facial flushing and hypotension due to too rapid infusion of the drug. Infusion should be over a minimum of 60 minutes for a 1-g dose.
      (5) Intravenous solutions are very irritating to the vein.

9. **Clofazimine** is phenazine dye with antimycobacterial and anti-inflammatory activity.
   a. **Mechanism of action.** Clofazimine appears to bind preferentially to mycobacterial DNA, inhibiting replication and growth. It is **bactericidal** against *M. leprae,* and it appears to be **bacteriostatic** against *M. avium–intracellulare.*
   b. **Spectrum of activity.** Clofazimine is active against various *Mycobacterium,* including *M. leprae, M. tuberculosis,* and *M. avium–intracellulare.*
   c. **Therapeutic uses.** Clofazimine is used to treat leprosy and a variety of atypical *Mycobacterium* infections.
   d. **Precautions and monitoring effects**
      (1) Pigmentation (pink to brownish) occurs in 75%–100% of patients within a few weeks. This skin discoloration has led to severe depression (and suicide).
      (2) Urine, sweat, and other body fluids may be discolored.
      (3) Other effects include ichthyosis and dryness of skin (8%–28%), rash and pruritus (1%–5%), and gastrointestinal intolerance (e.g., abdominal/epigastric pain, diarrhea, nausea, vomiting) in 40%–50% of patients. Clofazimine should be taken with food.

III. ANTIFUNGAL AGENTS

A. Definition. These agents treat systemic and local fungal (mycotic) infections—diseases that resist treatment with antibacterial drugs.

B. Amphotericin B. This polyene antibiotic is therapeutic for various fungal infections that frequently proved fatal before the drug became available. It is used increasingly in the empiric treatment of severely immunocompromised patients in certain clinical situations.

1. **Mechanism of action.** Amphotericin B is both **fungicidal** and **fungistatic;** it binds to sterols in the fungal cell membrane, thereby increasing membrane permeability and permitting leakage of intracellular contents. Other mechanisms may be involved as well.

2. **Spectrum of activity.** Amphotericin B is a broad-spectrum antifungal agent with activity against *Histoplasma capsulatum, Cryptococcus neoformans, Coccidioides immitis,* and *Candida* species. Many strains of *Aspergillus* and *Sporothrix schenckii* also are susceptible.

3. **Therapeutic uses.** Amphotericin B is the most effective antifungal agent in the treatment of systemic fungal infections, especially in immunocompromised patients.
   a. It is therapeutic for meningitis, histoplasmosis, coccidiodomycosis, blastomycosis, cryptococcosis, disseminated moniliasis, aspergillosis, and phycomycosis.
   b. This agent may be used to treat coccidioidal arthritis.
   c. Topical preparations are given to eradicate cutaneous and mucocutaneous candidiasis.

4. **Precautions and monitoring effects.** Because amphotericin B can cause many serious adverse effects, it should be administered in a hospital setting—at least during the initial therapeutic stage.
   a. Nephrotoxicity occurs in most patients; those with serious preexisting renal impairment may require dosage reduction or temporary drug discontinuation.
   b. Adverse CNS effects include headache, peripheral neuropathy, convulsions, and seizures.
   c. Adverse gastrointestinal effects include nausea, vomiting, diarrhea, anorexia, and cramps.
   d. Fever, malaise, and chills may be minimized by pretreatment with aspirin, acetaminophen, or diphenhydramine or by the addition of hydrocortisone to the intravenous infusion.
   e. Parenteral administration may cause local pain, thrombophlebitis, burning, stinging, irritation, and tissue damage with extravasation. Addition of heparin (100 units/infusion) helps minimize these effects.

5. **Significant interactions.** Other nephrotoxic drugs may cause additive nephrotoxicity.

C. **Flucytosine.** This fluorinated pyrimidine usually is given in combination with amphotericin B.

1. **Mechanism of action.** Flucytosine penetrates fungal cells and is converted to fluorouracil, a metabolic antagonist. Incorporated into the RNA of the fungal cell, flucytosine causes defective protein synthesis.

2. **Spectrum of activity.** This drug is active against some strains of *Cryptococcus, Candida, Aspergillus, Torulopsis,* and certain other fungal species. In combination with amphotericin B, flucytosine results in synergistic activity against *C. neoformans* and some strains of *Candida tropicalis* and *Candida albicans.*

3. **Therapeutic uses.** Flucytosine is therapeutic for systemic infections (e.g., septicemia, endocarditis, pulmonary and urinary tract infections, meningitis). In most cases, it is given with amphotericin B.

4. **Precautions and monitoring effects**
   a. Although flucytosine is less toxic than amphotericin B, it may cause serious adverse effects, including bone marrow suppression, severe enterocolitis, and hepatomegaly.
   b. Nausea, vomiting, diarrhea, dizziness, drowsiness, and skin rash also may occur.
   c. Flucytosine may increase serum creatinine values on tests using the EKTACHEM method.

D. **Griseofulvin.** Produced from *Penicillium griseofulvum dierckx,* this drug is deposited in the skin, bound to keratin.

1. **Mechanism of action.** This agent is **fungistatic;** it inhibits fungal cell activity by interfering with mitotic spindle structure.

2. **Spectrum of activity.** Griseofulvin is active against various strains of *Microsporum, Epidermophyton,* and *Trichophyton.*

3. **Therapeutic uses.** Griseofulvin is effective in tinea infections of the skin, hair, and nails (including athlete's foot) caused by *Microsporum, Epidermophyton,* and *Trichophyton.*
   a. Generally, it is given only for infections that do not respond to topical antifungal agents.
   b. Griseofulvin is available only in oral form.

4. **Precautions and monitoring effects**
   a. Griseofulvin rarely results in serious adverse effects. However, the following problems have been reported:
      (1) Headache, fatigue, confusion, impaired performance, syncope, and lethargy
      (2) Leukopenia, neutropenia, and granulocytopenia
      (3) Serum sickness, angioedema, urticaria, erythema, and hepatotoxicity

b. The dosage is dependent on the particle size of the product: 250 mg of ultramicrosize is equivalent in therapeutic effects to 500 mg of microsize.

5. Significant interactions

a. Griseofulvin may increase the metabolism of **warfarin,** leading to decreased prothrombin time.

b. Barbiturates may reduce griseofulvin absorption.

c. Alcohol consumption may cause tachycardia and flushing.

E. Imidazoles. The substituted imidazole derivatives **ketoconazole, miconazole, fluconazole,** and **itraconazole** are valuable in the treatment of a wide range of systemic fungal infections.

1. Mechanism of action. Imidazoles inhibit sterol synthesis in fungal cell membranes and increase cell wall permeability; this, in turn, makes the cell more vulnerable to osmotic pressure. These agents are **fungistatic**.

2. Spectrum of activity. These agents are active against many fungi, including yeasts, dermatophytes, actinomycetes, and some *Phycomycetes*.

3. Therapeutic uses

a. Ketoconazole, an oral agent, successfully treats many fungal infections that previously yielded only to parenteral agents.

(1) It is therapeutic for systemic and vaginal candidiasis, mucocandidiasis, candiduria, oral thrush, histoplasmosis, coccidioidomycosis, chromomycosis, and paracoccidioidomycosis.

(2) Because ketoconazole is slow-acting and requires a long duration of therapy (up to 6 months for some chronic infections), it is less effective than other antifungal agents for the treatment of severe and acute systemic infections.

b. Miconazole, primarily administered as a topical agent, also is available in parenteral form.

(1) Topical miconazole is highly effective in vulvovaginal candidiasis, ringworm, and other skin infections.

(2) Parenteral miconazole serves as a second-line agent in severe systemic fungal infections only when other antifungal drugs are ineffective or cannot be tolerated.

c. Fluconazole. Available in oral and parenteral forms, fluconazole can be used against systemic and CNS infections involving *Cryptococcus* and *Candida. Candida* oropharyngeal infection and esophagitis may also be treated with fluconazole. *Aspergillus, coccidioides,* and *Histoplasma* have demonstrated in vitro sensitivity.

d. Itraconazole is available as an oral agent with activity against systemic and invasive pulmonary aspergillosis without the hematologic toxicity of amphotericin B. Other deep mycotic infections susceptible to itraconazole include blastomycosis, coccidioidomycosis, cryptococcosis, and histoplasmosis.

4. Precautions and monitoring effects

a. Ketoconazole may cause nausea, vomiting, diarrhea, abdominal pain, and constipation. Rarely, it leads to headache, dizziness, gynecomastia, and fatal hepatotoxicity.

b. Parenteral miconazole therapy frequently induces nausea, vomiting, diarrhea, phlebitis, pruritic rash, anaphylactoid reaction, CNS toxicity, and hyponatremia. Dose-related anemia and thrombocytosis may also occur.

c. Fluconazole commonly causes gastrointestinal disturbances (e.g., nausea, vomiting, epigastric pain, diarrhea). Reversible elevations in serum aminotransferase, exfoliative skin reactions, and headaches have been reported.

d. Itraconazole may cause nausea, vomiting, hypertriglyceridemia, hypokalemia, rash, and elevations in liver enzymes.

5. Significant interactions

a. Both ketoconazole and miconazole may enhance the anticoagulant effect of **warfarin**.

b. Ketoconazole may antagonize the antibiotic effects of **amphotericin B**.

c. Fluconazole has been shown to elevate serum levels of **phenytoin, cyclosporine, warfarin,** and **sulfonylureas**. Concurrent hepatic enzyme inducers, such as **rifampin,** have resulted in increased elimination of both fluconazole and itraconazole.

d. Coadministration of itraconazole or ketoconazole with **astemizole** or **terfenadine** may result in increased astemizole or terfenadine levels, possibly leading to life-threatening dysrhythmias and death.

F. Nystatin. A polyene antibiotic, nystatin has a chemical structure similar to that of amphotericin B.

1. **Mechanism of action.** Nystatin is **fungicidal** and **fungistatic;** binding to sterols in the fungal cell membrane, it increases membrane permeability and permits leakage of intracellular contents.
2. **Spectrum of activity.** Nystatin is active against *Candida, Cryptococcus, Histoplasma,* and *Blastomyces* organisms.
3. **Therapeutic uses**
   a. This drug is used primarily as a topical agent in vaginal and oral *Candida* infections.
   b. Oral nystatin is therapeutic for *Candida* infections of the gastrointestinal tract, especially oral and esophageal infections.
4. **Precautions and monitoring effects.** Oral nystatin occasionally causes gastrointestinal distress (e.g., nausea, vomiting, diarrhea). Rarely, hypersensitivity reactions occur.

IV. ANTIPROTOZOAL AGENTS

A. Classification. These drugs fall into two main categories: **antimalarial agents,** used to treat malaria infection; and **amebicides** and **trichomonacides,** used to treat amebic and trichomonal infections.

B. Antimalarial agents. Still a leading cause of illness and death in tropical and subtropical countries, malaria results from infection by any of four species of the protozoal genus *Plasmodium*. Antimalarial agents are selectively active during different phases of the protozoan life cycle. Major antimalarial drugs include **chloroquine, primaquine, pyrimethamine, quinine, fansidar,** and **mefloquine.**

1. **Mechanism of action**
   a. **Chloroquine** binds to and alters the properties of microbial and mammalian DNA.
   b. The mechanism of action of **primaquine, quinine, fansidar,** and **mefloquine** is unknown.
   c. **Pyrimethamine** impedes folic acid reduction by inhibiting the enzyme dihydrofolate reductase.
2. **Spectrum of activity**
   a. **Chloroquine,** a suppressive agent, is active against the asexual erythrocyte forms of *Plasmodium vivax* and *Plasmodium falciparum* and gametocytes of *P. vivax, Plasmodium malariae,* and *Plasmodium ovale.*
   b. **Primaquine,** a curative agent, is active against liver forms of *P. vivax* and *P. ovale* and the primary exoerythrocyte forms of *P. falciparum.*
   c. **Pyrimethamine** is active against chloroquine-resistant strains of *P. falciparum* and some strains of *P. vivax.*
   d. **Quinine,** a generalized protoplasmic poison, is toxic to a wide range of organisms. In malaria, this drug has both suppressive and curative action against chloroquine-resistant strains.
   e. **Fansidar** is a blood **schizonticidal** agent that is active against the erythrocytic forms of susceptible plasmodia. It is also active against *T. gondii.*
   f. **Mefloquine** is a blood schizonticidal agent that is active against *P. falciparum* (both chloroquine-susceptible and resistant strains) and *P. vivax.*
3. **Therapeutic uses**
   a. **Chloroquine** is used to suppress malaria symptoms and to terminate acute malaria attacks resulting from *P. falciparum* and *P. malariae* infections.
      (1) It is more potent and less toxic than quinine.
      (2) Except where drug-resistant *P. falciparum* strains are prevalent, chloroquine is the most useful antimalarial agent.
   b. **Primaquine** is used to cure relapses of *P. vivax* and *P. ovale* malaria and to prevent malaria in exposed persons returning from regions where malaria is endemic.
   c. **Pyrimethamine** is effective in the prevention and treatment of chloroquine-resistant strains of *P. falciparum.* It is now used almost exclusively in combination with a sulfonamide or sulfone.
   d. **Quinine**
      (1) Quinine sulfate, an oral form, is therapeutic for acute malaria caused by chloroquine-resistant strains.

(2) Quinine dihydrochloride, a parenteral form, is used in severe cases of chloroquine-resistant malaria. (It is available only from the Centers for Disease Control in Atlanta.)
(3) Quinine is almost always given in combination with another antimalarial agent.

e. Fansidar

(1) Fansidar is used for the suppression or prophylaxis of chloroquine-resistant *P. falciparum* malaria.
(2) It has been used for the prophylaxis of *P. carinii* infections in AIDS patients unable to tolerate co-trimoxazole (trimethoprim–sulfarmethoxazole).

f. Mefloquine is indicated for the treatment of acute malaria and the prevention of *P. falciparum* and *P. vivax* infections.

4. Precautions and monitoring effects

a. Chloroquine

(1) Because this drug concentrates in the liver, it should be used cautiously in patients with hepatic disease.
(2) Chloroquine must be administered with extreme caution in patients with neurologic, hematologic, or severe gastrointestinal disorders.
(3) Visual disturbances, headache, skin rash, and gastrointestinal distress have been reported.

b. Primaquine

(1) This agent is contraindicated in patients with rheumatoid arthritis and lupus erythematosus and in those receiving other potentially hemolytic drugs or bone marrow suppressants.
(2) Primaquine may cause agranulocytosis, granulocytopenia, and mild anemia; in patients with G6PD deficiency, it may cause hemolytic anemia.
(3) Abdominal cramps, nausea, vomiting, and epigastric distress sometimes occur.

c. Pyrimethamine

(1) In high doses, this drug may cause agranulocytosis, megaloblastic anemia, aplastic anemia, and thrombocytopenia.
(2) Erythema multiforme (Stevens-Johnson syndrome), nausea, vomiting, and anorexia may develop during pyrimethamine therapy.

d. Quinine

(1) Quinine is contraindicated in patients with G6PD deficiency, tinnitus, and optic neuritis.
(2) Quinine overdose or hypersensitivity reactions may be fatal. Manifestations of quinine poisoning include visual and hearing disturbances; gastrointestinal symptoms (e.g., nausea, vomiting); hot, flushed skin; headache; fever; syncope; confusion; shallow, then depressed, respirations; and cardiovascular collapse.
(3) Quinine must be used cautiously in patients with atrial fibrillation.
(4) Renal damage and anuria have been reported.

e. Fansidar

(1) Severe, sometimes fatal, hypersensitivity reactions have occurred. In most cases, death resulted from severe cutaneous reactions, including erythema multiforme, Stevens-Johnson syndrome, and toxic epidermal necrolysis.
(2) Adverse hematologic and hepatic effects as seen with sulfonamides have been reported.

f. Mefloquine

(1) Concomitant use of mefloquine with quinine, quinidine, or β-adrenergic blockade may produce electrocardiographic (ECG) abnormalities or cardiac arrest.
(2) Concomitant use of mefloquine and quinine or chloroquine may increase the risk of convulsions.

C. Amebicides and trichomonacides. These agents are crucial in the treatment of amebiasis, giardiasis, and trichomoniases—the most common protozoal infections in the United States. The major amebicides include **diloxanide, emetine, iodoquinol, metronidazole, paromomycin,** and **quinacrine**.

1. Mechanism of action

a. Diloxanide, a dichloroacetamide derivative, is **amebicidal;** its mechanism of action is unknown. (It is available only from the Centers for Disease Control in Atlanta.)

b. Emetine, an alkaloid obtained from ipecac, is **amebicidal;** it kills amebae by inhibiting amebic protein synthesis.

c. **Metronidazole** is a synthetic compound with direct **amebicidal** and **trichomonacidal** action; it works at both intestinal and extraintestinal sites. Its mechanism of action involves disruption of the helical structure of DNA.
d. **Quinacrine** is an acridine derivative that inhibits DNA metabolism.
e. **Iodoquinol** is a luminal or contact amebicide that is effective against the trophozoites of *Entamoeba histolytica* located in the lumen of the large intestines.
f. **Paromomycin** is a poorly absorbed amebicidal aminoglycoside whose mechanism of action parallels other aminoglycosides (i.e., protein synthesis inhibitor). It is also effective against enteric bacteria *Salmonella* and *Shigella*.

2. Spectrum of activity and therapeutic uses

a. Diloxanide
(1) This drug is used to treat asymptomatic carriers of amebic and giardiac cysts.
(2) Diloxanide is therapeutic for invasive and extraintestinal amebiasis (given in combination with a systemic or mixed amebicide).
(3) Diloxanide is not effective as single-agent therapy for extraintestinal amebiasis.

b. Emetine
(1) This drug is widely used to treat severe invasive intestinal amebiasis, amebic abscess, and amebic hepatitis.
(2) Because of its toxicity, emetine generally is used only when other drugs are contraindicated or have proven to be ineffective.
(3) Usually, emetine is administered in combination with another amebicidal agent.

c. Metronidazole
(1) This agent is the preferred drug in amebic dysentery, giardiasis, and trichomoniasis.
(2) Metronidazole also is active against all anaerobic cocci and gram-negative anaerobic bacilli.

d. **Quinacrine** is useful in the treatment of giardiasis and tapeworms (see VII G).
e. **Iodoquinol** is indicated for treatment of intestinal amebiasis. It is active against the protozoa *Entamoeba histolytica*.
f. **Paromomycin** is indicated for acute and chronic intestinal amebiasis; it is not useful for extraintestinal amebiasis, since it is not absorbed. Paromomycin has been used for *Dientamoeba fragilis, Taenia saginata, Dipylidium caninum,* and *Hymenolepis nana*.

3. Precautions and monitoring effects

a. **Diloxanide** rarely causes serious adverse effects. Vomiting, flatulence, and pruritus have been reported.

b. Emetine
(1) This drug may induce potentially lethal systemic toxicity. Manifestations may be cardiovascular (e.g., ECG abnormalities, tachycardia, hypotension, CHF), gastrointestinal (e.g., nausea, vomiting, diarrhea), or neurologic (e.g., dizziness, headache, changes in central or peripheral nerve function).
(2) Emetine usually is contraindicated in patients with cardiac disease, renal impairment, muscle disease, and polyneuropathy; in children; and in patients who have taken the drug in the past 6–8 weeks.
(3) Intravenous injection is contraindicated.
(4) Deep subcutaneous administration (preferred over the intramuscular route) may cause muscle weakness at the injection site.

c. Metronidazole
(1) The most common adverse effects of this drug are nausea, epigastric distress, and diarrhea.
(2) Metronidazole is carcinogenic in mice and should not be used unnecessarily.
(3) Headache, vomiting, metallic taste, and stomatitis have been reported.
(4) Occasionally, neurologic reactions (e.g., ataxia, peripheral neuropathy, seizures) develop.
(5) A disulfiram-type reaction may occur with concurrent ethanol use.

d. **Quinacrine** (see VII G 4)
(1) This drug frequently causes dizziness, headache, nausea, and vomiting. Nervousness and seizures also have been reported.
(2) Quinacrine should not be taken in combination with primaquine because this may increase primaquine toxicity.
(3) Quinacrine should be administered with extreme caution in patients with psoriasis because it may cause marked exacerbation of this disease.

e. **Iodoquinol** may produce optic neuritis or atrophy or peripheral neuropathy with high-dose, long-term use. Protein-bound iodine levels may be increased during treatment and may interfere with the results of thyroid tests for 6 months after treatment. Iodoquinol should not be used in patients who are hypersensitive to 8-hydroxyquinolone (e.g., iodoquinol, iodochlorhydroxyquin) or iodine-containing agents or in patients with hepatic disorders.

f. Paromomycin may cause nausea, cramping, and diarrhea at high doses (> 3g/day). Inadvertent absorption through ulcerative bowel lesions may result in ototoxicity or renal damage.

D. Pentamidine isethionate is an aromatic diamide antiprotozoal agent. It can be administered intramuscularly, intravenously, and by inhalation.

1. **Mechanism of action** is not fully understood, but in vitro studies indicate interference with nuclear metabolism and inhibition of DNA, RNA, phospholipid, and protein synthesis.

2. **Therapeutic uses**
   - **a.** Pentamidine is indicated for the prevention and treatment of infections due to *P. carinii.*
   - **b.** Unlabeled uses include treatment of trypanosomiasis and visceral leishmaniasis.

3. **Precautions and monitoring effects**
   - **a.** This agent must be used cautiously in patients with hypertension, hypotension, hypoglycemia, hyperglycemia, hypocalcemia, leukopenia, thrombocytopenia, anemia, hepatic or renal dysfunction, ventricular tachycardia, or pancreatitis.
   - **b.** Inhalation of pentamidine may produce bronchospasm.
   - **c.** Laboratory tests before and during therapy include BUN, serum creatinine, complete blood count (CBC) and platelets, liver function tests (LFTs), serum calcium, blood glucose, and ECG.

E. Atovaquone is a hydroxynaphthoquinone initially synthesized as an antimalarial drug.

1. **Mechanism of action.** Atovaquone blocks mitochondrial electron transport at complex III of the respiratory chain of protozoa, resulting in inhibition of pyrimidine species.

2. **Spectrum of activity.** It is active against *P. carinii* with potential activity against *T. gondii* and *Cryptosporidium parvum.*

3. **Therapeutic uses.** Atovaquone is used for second-line treatment of mild-to-moderate *P. carinii* pneumonia in patients intolerant to co-trimoxazole or other sulfonamides, or nonresponsive to co-trimoxazole.

4. **Precautions and monitoring effects**
   - **a.** Oral absorption significantly increases when administered with food.
   - **b.** Rash, nausea, diarrhea, and headache are common.

5. **Significant interactions.** Atovaquone is highly bound to plasma protein. It should be used with caution when administered with other highly protein-bound drugs with a narrow therapeutic range.

F. Eflornithine HCl is an intravenous antiprotozoal agent. Its activity has been attributed to the inhibition of the enzyme ornithine decarboxylase.

1. **Mechanism of action** is a specific, enzyme-activated, irreversible inhibitor of ornithine decarboxylase.

2. **Spectrum of activity and therapeutic uses.** Eflornithine is active in the treatment of the meningoencephalitic stage of *Trypanosoma brucei gambiense* (sleeping sickness).

3. **Precautions and monitoring effects**
   - **a.** Myelosuppression is the most frequent serious side effect.
   - **b.** Seizures occur in about 8% of treated patients.
   - **c.** Cases of hearing impairment have been reported.

V. ANTITUBERCULAR AGENTS

A. Definition and classification. Drugs used to treat tuberculosis suppress or kill the slow-growing mycobacteria that cause this disease. Antitubercular agents fall into two main categories: **first-line** (primary) and **second-line** (secondary). Because the causative organisms tend to develop resistance to any single drug, combination drug therapy has become standard in the treatment of tuberculosis.

B. First-line antitubercular agents. These drugs—**isoniazid, rifampin,** and **ethambutol**—usually offer the greatest effectiveness with the least toxicity; they are successful in most tuberculosis patients. Frequently, two or three are administered together; in most cases, the combination of isoniazid and rifampin proves the most effective. In life-threatening or renal tuberculosis, initial therapy may include three antitubercular drugs (typically, a combination of first- and second-line agents) to ensure that the causative organism is susceptible to at least two.

1. **Ethambutol** is a synthetic water-based compound.
   a. **Mechanism of action.** This drug is **bacteriostatic;** its precise mechanism of action is unknown.
   b. **Spectrum of activity and therapeutic uses.** Ethambutol is active against many *M. tuberculosis* strains. However, drug resistance develops fairly rapidly when it is used alone. In most cases, ethambutol is given adjunctively in combination with isoniazid or rifampin.
   c. **Precautions and monitoring effects.** Rarely, ethambutol causes such adverse effects as reversible dose-related ($\geq$ 15 mg/kg/day) optic neuritis, drug fever, abdominal pain, headache, dizziness, and confusion.

2. **Isoniazid** is a hydrazide of isonicotinic acid. The mainstay of antitubercular therapy, this drug should be included (if tolerated) in all therapeutic regimens.
   a. **Mechanism of action.** Isoniazid is **bacteriostatic** for resting bacilli and **bactericidal** for rapidly dividing organisms. Its mechanism of action is not fully known; the drug probably disrupts bacterial cell wall synthesis by inhibiting mycolic acid synthesis.
   b. **Spectrum of activity.** Isoniazid is active against most tubercle bacilli; some atypical mycobacteria are resistant.
   c. **Therapeutic uses**
      (1) The most widely used antitubercular agent, isoniazid should be given in combination with another antitubercular drug (such as rifampin or ethambutol) to prevent drug resistance.
      (2) For uncomplicated pulmonary tuberculosis, isoniazid therapy may last 9 months to 2 years.
      (3) Prophylactic isoniazid may be administered alone for 1 year in children who have a positive tuberculin test result but lack active lesions.
   d. **Precautions and monitoring effects**
      (1) The most common adverse effects of isoniazid are skin rash, fever, jaundice, and peripheral neuritis.
      (2) Hepatitis, an occasional reaction, can be severe and, in some cases, fatal. The risk of hepatitis increases with the patient's age and rises with alcohol abuse.
      (3) Blood dyscrasias (e.g., agranulocytosis, aplastic or hemolytic anemia, thrombocytopenia) may occur.
      (4) Adverse gastrointestinal effects include nausea, vomiting, and epigastric distress.
      (5) CNS toxicity may result from pyridoxine deficiency. Signs and symptoms include insomnia, restlessness, hyperreflexia, and convulsions.
   e. **Significant interactions**
      (1) With concurrent **phenytoin** therapy, blood levels of both phenytoin and isoniazid may increase, possibly causing toxicity.
      (2) **Aluminum-containing antacids** may reduce isoniazid absorption.
      (3) Concurrent **carbamazepine** therapy may increase the risk of hepatitis.

3. **Rifampin** is a complex macrocyclic agent.
   a. **Mechanism of action.** This drug is **bactericidal;** it impairs bacterial RNA synthesis by binding to DNA-dependent RNA polymerase.
   b. **Spectrum of activity.** Rifampin is active against most gram-negative and many gram-positive organisms.
   c. **Therapeutic uses**
      (1) The combination of rifampin and isoniazid is the most effective therapy for tuberculosis. Rifampin should not be administered alone because this can lead to the emergence of highly drug-resistant organisms.
      (2) Prophylactic rifampin is effective when administered to carriers of meningococcal disease caused by *H. influenzae* organisms.
   d. **Precautions and monitoring effects**
      (1) Serious hepatotoxicity may result from rifampin therapy.
      (2) In rare cases, this drug induces an influenza-like syndrome.

(3) Other adverse effects include skin rash, drowsiness, headache, fatigue, confusion, nausea, vomiting, and abdominal pain.
(4) Rifampin colors urine, sweat, tears, saliva, and feces orange–red.

e. **Significant interactions**
(1) Rifampin induces hepatic microsomal enzymes and, thus, may decrease the therapeutic effectiveness of **corticosteroids, warfarin, oral contraceptives, quinidine, digitoxin,** and **barbiturates**.
(2) **Probenecid** may increase blood levels of rifampin.

4. **Rifabutin** is an antimycobacterial agent that is similar to rifampin with activity against both tubercular and nontubercular mycobacterium.
a. **Mechanism of action.** In addition to its antimycobacterial activity against tubercular and nontubercular mycobacterium, rifabutin has been reported to inhibit reverse transcriptase and block the in vitro infectivity and replication of human immunodeficiency virus (HIV).
b. **Therapeutic uses.** Rifabutin is indicated for the prevention of disseminated *M.* avium–intracellulare complex disease in patients with advanced HIV infections.
c. **Precautions and monitoring effects.** The use of rifabutin has resulted in mild elevation of liver enzymes and thrombocytopenia.
d. **Significant interactions**
(1) Rifabutin antagonizes and potentially negates the immune response mediated by the bacillus Calmette-Guérin (BCG) vaccine.
(2) Rifabutin may increase the clearance of **cyclosporine**. Serum cyclosporine levels should be monitored in patients receiving both agents.

C. **Second-line antitubercular agents.** This category includes **aminosalicylic acid, capreomycin, cycloserine, ethionamide, pyrazinamide,** and **streptomycin**.

1. **Mechanism of action**
a. **Aminosalicylic acid** is **bacteriostatic;** it probably inhibits the enzymes responsible for folic acid synthesis.
b. **Cycloserine** can be **bacteriostatic** or **bactericidal,** depending on its concentration at the infection site; it impairs amino acid utilization, thereby inhibiting bacterial cell wall synthesis.
c. The mechanism of action of capreomycin (**bacteriostatic**), ethionamide (**bactericidal**), and pyrazinamide (**bactericidal**) is unknown.
d. **Streptomycin** (see II B 2 a)

2. **Spectrum of activity and therapeutic uses.** Second-line antitubercular agents are active against various microorganisms, including *M. tuberculosis*. They generally are reserved for patients with extensive extrapulmonary or drug-resistant disease or for patients who need retreatment. These drugs are almost always administered in combination.

3. **Precautions and monitoring effects**
a. Adverse effects of **aminosalicylic acid** include leukopenia, agranulocytopenia, thrombocytopenia, hemolytic anemia, mononucleosis-like syndrome, malaise, joint pain, fever, and skin rash.
b. **Capreomycin** and **streptomycin** are ototoxic and nephrotoxic; they should not be administered together.
c. **Cycloserine** may cause adverse CNS effects, including headache, suicidal and psychotic tendencies, hyperirritability, confusion, paranoia, and nervousness.
d. **Ethionamide** may induce nausea, vomiting, orthostatic hypotension, metallic taste, epigastric distress, and peripheral neuropathy.
e. **Pyrazinamide** may result in hepatotoxicity and, rarely, hepatic necrosis resulting in death. Anorexia, nausea, vomiting, malaise, and fever have been reported.
f. **Streptomycin** (see II B 4, 5)

VI. ANTIVIRAL AGENTS

A. **Definition.** These drugs alleviate viral disease by influencing viral replication. Because viruses lack independent metabolic activity and can replicate only within living host cells, antiviral agents tend to injure host as well as viral cells. Consequently, few antiviral drugs have been introduced; most are active against only one virus.

1. **DNA viruses.** Currently approved antiviral therapy against the *Herpesviridae* family of DNA viruses [herpes simplex virus (HSV) 1 and 2, varicella-zoster virus (VZV), cytomegalovirus (CMV)] are virustatic and arrest DNA synthesis by inhibiting viral DNA polymerase. With the exception of the broad-spectrum antiviral drug **foscarnet,** these agents are prodrugs and require viral and host cellular enzymes (e.g., thymidine, deoxyguanosine kinase) to phosphorylate them into the active triphosphate form before being incorporated. Hence, a common mechanism of resistance is a deficiency or structural alteration in viral thymidine kinase (Table 45-3).

2. **RNA viruses.** Currently approved antiretroviral agents active against human immunodeficiency virus-1 (HIV-1) are limited to the reverse transcriptase inhibitors **zidovudine, didanosine,** and **zalcitabine**. These agents are virustatic and involve life-long therapy.

B. Acyclovir is a synthetic purine nucleoside analogue that is therapeutic for various herpes infections. It is the least toxic antiviral agent.

1. **Mechanism of action.** Acyclovir becomes incorporated into viral DNA and inhibits viral replication.

2. **Spectrum of activity.** This agent is active against herpes viruses, especially HSV-1.
   a. Acyclovir is used to treat mucocutaneous HSV infections in immunocompromised patients and to reduce pain and speed healing of herpes zoster, genital herpes, and neonatal herpes.
   b. This agent is available in topical, oral, and intravenous forms. Topical acyclovir is applied directly on herpes lesions in primary herpes infection and in non–life-threatening mucocutaneous HSV infection in immunocompromised patients.
   c. Acyclovir may be administered intravenously in the treatment of initial and recurrent mucocutaneous HSV infection in immunocompromised patients and in the treatment of severe initial herpes infection in patients with normal immunity.

3. **Precautions and monitoring effects**
   a. Oral acyclovir may induce nausea, vomiting, diarrhea, and headache.
   b. Intravenous administration may cause nephrotoxicity, neurologic effects (e.g., lethargy, confusion, tremors, agitation, seizures, coma, obtundation), hypotension, rash, itching, and inflammation and phlebitis at the injection site.
   c. Local discomfort and pruritus may result from topical administration.
   d. Acyclovir is removed in hemodialysis. Doses should be adjusted in renal impairment and hemodialysis.

4. **Significant interactions. Probenecid** may increase blood concentrations of acyclovir, possibly causing toxicity.

C. Amantadine, a synthetic tricyclic amine with a unique chemical structure, serves as a valuable agent against influenza A viral infection.

1. **Mechanism of action.** Amantadine inhibits replication of the influenza A virus by interfering with viral attachment and uncoating.

2. **Spectrum of activity and therapeutic uses**
   a. Amantadine is effective in the prophylaxis and treatment of influenza A virus.
   b. Clinicians recommend that all nonimmunized high-risk patients receive this drug at the first sign of community influenza A activity.
   c. Suppressive therapy should continue for 24–48 hours after influenza symptoms disappear or, if necessary, up to 90 days for repeated exposure to the virus.
   d. This drug may be used to treat some patients with parkinsonism.

Table 45-3. Activity of Anti-DNA Viral Agents

Agent	HSV-1	HSV-2	VZV	CMV	Influenza A
Ribavirin	+	+	...	...	...
Vidarabine*	+	+	+	...	...
Acyclovir*	+	+	+	...	...
Ganciclovir*	...	...	...	+	...
Amantadine	...	...	...	...	+
Foscarnet	+	+	+	+	...

*Requires activation into triphosphate form.

3. **Precautions and monitoring effects**
   a. The most pronounced adverse effects of amantadine are ataxia, nightmares, and insomnia. Other CNS effects include depression, confusion, dizziness, fatigue, anxiety, and headache. Patients with a history of epilepsy and psychiatric disorders should be monitored closely during therapy.
   b. Anticholinergic reactions (e.g., dry mouth, blurred vision, tachycardia) have been reported.

D. **Ribavirin** is a synthetic nucleoside analogue that plays a key role in the treatment of respiratory syncytial virus.

1. **Mechanism of action.** Ribavirin may inhibit RNA and DNA synthesis by depleting intracellular nucleotide reserves.

2. **Spectrum of activity.** This agent is active in vitro against RNA and DNA viruses, such as influenza A and B, respiratory syncytial virus, and herpes simplex.

3. **Therapeutic uses.** Administered in aerosol form, ribavirin is used to relieve symptoms and speed recovery in young adults with influenza A and B and in children with respiratory syncytial virus.

4. **Precautions and monitoring effects**
   a. Ribavirin must be administered only with a specific small-particle aerosol generator (Viratek SPAG-2).
   b. This agent is contraindicated in patients using respirators because it may precipitate on respirator valves and tubing, causing lethal malfunction. (However, use of a prefilter may permit ribavirin therapy in such patients.)
   c. Serious adverse effects include cardiac arrest, deterioration of pulmonary function, bacterial pneumonia, and apnea.
   d. Rash, conjunctivitis, and reticulocytosis have been reported.

E. **Vidarabine,** an adenosine analogue, is useful in the treatment of serious herpes infections.

1. **Mechanism of action.** Vidarabine inhibits viral multiplication by becoming incorporated into viral DNA.

2. **Spectrum of activity and therapeutic uses.** Vidarabine is effective against herpes simplex encephalitis (administered intravenously) and herpes simplex keratoconjunctivitis (administered as a topical ophthalmic agent). In immunocompromised patients, it is given intravenously to treat herpes zoster infection.

3. **Precautions and monitoring effects**
   a. The most common adverse effects of vidarabine are nausea, diarrhea, and rash.
   b. Dose-related CNS toxicity (manifested by tremors, dizziness, confusion, and ataxia) may develop.
   c. Intravenous administration requires dilution in a large volume of fluid, posing a danger to patients with cardiac or renal disease.
   d. Vidarabine may be carcinogenic and mutagenic.

4. **Significant interactions. Allopurinol** increases the risk of CNS toxicity.

F. **Ganciclovir** is a synthetic purine nucleoside analogue that is used for CMV infections.

1. **Mechanism of action.** Ganciclovir triphosphate is incorporated into viral DNA, inhibits viral DNA polymerase, and, thus, terminates viral replication.

2. **Spectrum of activity.** Ganciclovir has in vitro activity against HSV-1 and -2, VZV, and Epstein-Barr viruses, but due to its enhanced ability to penetrate host cells, it is indicated for CMV infections, such as colitis, pneumonia, and retinitis. However, ganciclovir use in CMV infections of the CNS has not been successful even though it is capable of CNS penetration.
   a. Conversion into the triphosphate form is greater in infected host cells, even though drug penetration occurs in both uninfected and infected cells.
   b. Inhibitory concentrations for the viral DNA polymerase are lower than those of the host cellular polymerase.
   c. In cases of CMV pneumonia or bone marrow transplant patients, CMV immune globulin is added to the regimen.
   d. Maintenance therapy for 75 days after the initial 14 days of therapy is required to prevent relapse.

3. **Precautions and monitoring effects**
   a. The main side effects of intravenous ganciclovir are neutropenia and thrombocytopenia. Phlebitis and pain may occur at the site of infusion.
   b. Since ganciclovir is cleared by glomerular filtration and tubular secretion, renal function and adequate hydration should be monitored. The drug is removed in hemodialysis. Doses should be adjusted in cases of renal impairment and hemodialysis.

4. **Significant interactions**
   a. **Probenecid** may increase ganciclovir levels and possibly toxicity.
   b. **Zidovudine** and **cytotoxic agents** in combination with ganciclovir may result in neutropenia; careful monitoring of granulocyte levels is required when they are taken concurrently with ganciclovir.
   c. **Imipenem–cilastatin** in combination with ganciclovir may induce generalized seizures.

G. **Foscarnet** (trisodium phosphonoformate hexahydrate, PFA) is a synthetic pyrophosphate analogue, which directly inhibits enzymes involved in viral DNA synthesis without incorporation into viral DNA. It is a broad-spectrum antiviral agent and is the drug of choice in cases of acyclovir or ganciclovir resistance.

1. **Mechanisms of action**
   a. Viral DNA replication requires the addition of deoxynucleoside triphosphates at the end of the DNA strand by DNA polymerase and the subsequent cleavage of pyrophosphate from the newly attached nucleotide. Foscarnet competitively binds directly to DNA polymerase to form an inactive complex and prevents pyrophosphate cleavage. Viral DNA chain elongation is thus terminated.
   b. Foscarnet is also active against HIV-1, an RNA retrovirus. It is a noncompetitive, reversible inhibitor of HIV reverse transcriptase, the enzyme responsible for converting viral RNA to viral DNA.

2. **Spectrum of activity and therapeutic uses.** Foscarnet has in vitro activity against HSV-1 and -2, CMV, VZV, and Epstein-Barr DNA polymerases, influenza polymerase, and HIV reverse transcriptase. Therapeutically, the drug may be used in HSV-1 and -2, VZV, CMV, and HIV-1 infections.
   a. The most experience with foscarnet is in the treatment of CMV retinitis in immunocompromised patients. An initial induction therapy lasts 2–4 weeks. Maintenance therapy within 1 month after induction may be needed to prevent relapse.
   b. Foscarnet may be used with zidovudine either synergistically in HIV therapy or concurrently in CMV infections in AIDS patients where neutropenia contraindicates ganciclovir therapy.
   c. Foscarnet is able to cross the blood–brain barrier.

3. **Precautions and monitoring effects**
   a. Intravenous foscarnet is highly nephrotoxic, causing acute tubular necrosis. Renal failure can be prevented if adequate hydration is maintained throughout therapy and with daily renal function monitoring.
   b. Other common adverse effects include hypercalcemia, hypocalcemia, hypomagnesemia, and hyperphosphatemia.
   c. Foscarnet is removed by hemodialysis.

4. **Significant interactions**
   a. Intravenous **pentamidine** increases the risk of renal toxicity and severe hypocalcemia.
   b. Foscarnet is exclusively eliminated by glomerular filtration and tubular secretion. **Probenecid** may prolong elimination and possibly cause toxicity.
   c. Other concurrent nephrotoxic agents should be avoided whenever possible.

H. **Zidovudine** is a synthetic thymidine analogue. Formerly called azidothymidine (AZT), this agent is the first available drug for the treatment of HIV infection in patients with AIDS and AIDS-related complex (ARC).

1. **Mechanism of action.** Zidovudine is phosphorylated by human cellular kinases to a triphosphate and then incorporated into viral DNA, where it can terminate viral DNA synthesis by inhibiting the viral enzyme reverse transcriptase or terminating DNA strand elongation. HIV replication is thus prevented.

2. **Spectrum of activity and therapeutic uses**
   a. Zidovudine has been shown to slow HIV-1 production, alleviate symptoms, and prolong life in some patients with AIDS.
   b. More recent clinical trials have revealed that maintenance doses of 500–600 mg/day are as efficacious as the higher and potentially more toxic dose of 800 mg/day.
   c. There is evidence that treating HIV-1–positive patients with $CD4^+$ lymphocyte counts of less than 500 cells/mm^3 (early in the natural history of the disease before the definitive AIDS diagnosis of $CD4^+$ count <200), using maintenance doses, prolongs survival. Further testing on the use of zidovudine early in the disease is likely.
   d. Zidovudine can cross the blood–brain barrier.
3. **Precautions and monitoring effects**
   a. Zidovudine can cause severe bone marrow suppression leading to anemia, granulocytopenia, and thrombocytopenia. Patients may require blood transfusions to reverse anemia.
   b. The use of erythropoietin or granulocyte colony-stimulating factor (G-CSF) is an alternative adjunctive therapy in zidovudine-induced anemia. There is a theoretical but yet unproven risk of activating latent HIV-1 in monocyte/macrophages when granulocyte/macrophage CSF (GM-CSF) is used. Studies using GM-CSF have not observed increased viremia.
   c. Other adverse effects include headache, agitation, confusion, anxiety, insomnia, rash, and itching.
4. **Significant interactions**
   a. **Co-trimoxazole** may impair zidovudine metabolism, causing increased zidovudine toxicity.
   b. Other **cytotoxic drugs** can cause additive bone marrow suppression.
   c. Fatigue and lethargy may develop with concurrent **acyclovir** therapy.

I. Dideoxyinosine (Didanosine DDI), a synthetic purine analogue, inhibits HIV-1 replication and is unique in having a long intracellular half-life (> 12 hours versus 3 hours for zidovudine) and rare hematologic toxicities. This agent is approved for patients who have failed or are intolerant of zidovudine therapy.

1. **Mechanism of action.** DDI is phosphorylated in human cells by the enzyme 5′-nucleotidase and other cellular kinases before it competitively inhibits the viral enzyme reverse transcriptase. This results in viral DNA synthesis termination and prevention of HIV-1 replication.
2. **Spectrum of activity.** DDI has demonstrated a dose-dependent activity against HIV-1, resulting in lower virus production (p24 antigens); increases in peripheral blood $CD4^+$ cell counts; and increases in appetite, weight, and energy without significant neutropenia.
   a. Clinical trials are assessing synergy, alternating therapy, or equivalent efficacy with zidovudine.
   b. DDI is well absorbed orally but is acid unstable, requiring administration with buffers or antacids.
   c. DDI is able to cross the blood–brain barrier.
3. **Precautions and monitoring effects**
   a. DDI can cause reversible peripheral neuropathy and acute, potentially lethal pancreatitis. Serum triglycerides should be monitored, and DDI should be withheld when potential pancreatitis-inducing agents (e.g., intravenous pentamidine, sulfonamides) are given. Transiently elevated serum amylase may not reflect pancreatitis.
   b. Other adverse effects include headaches, insomnia, hepatitis, and hyperuricemia (since DDI is catalyzed to uric acid).
4. **Significant interactions.** Pancreatitis-inducing drugs, such as **cimetidine, ranitidine, sulfonamides, pentamidine** and **alcohol,** should not be used with DDI.

J. Zalcitabine is a synthetic pyrimidine nucleoside analogue that is active against HIV.

1. **Mechanism of action.** Within cells, zalcitabine is converted to the active metabolite dideoxycytidine-5′-triphosphate (ddCTP) by cellular enzymes. ddCPT serves as an alternate substrate to deoxycytidine triphosphate (dCTP) for HIV reverse transcriptase and inhibits in vitro replication of HIV-1 by inhibition of viral DNA synthesis.
2. **Spectrum of activity and therapeutic uses.** Zalcitabine is indicated for combination therapy with zidovudine in advanced HIV infection; that is, for the treatment of adult patients with advanced infection ($CD4^+$ cell count <300/mm^3) who have demonstrated significant clinical or immunologic deterioration.

3. **Precautions and monitoring effects**
   a. The major clinical toxicity of zalcitabine is peripheral neuropathy, which occurs in up to 31% of patients.
   b. Documented pancreatitis has occurred alone or in combination with zidovudine. Serum amylase must be monitored.
   c. Other adverse effects include esophageal ulcers, cardiomyopathy/CHF, anaphylactoid reactions, and impaired renal or hepatic function.
4. **Significant interactions**
   a. Drugs that have the potential to cause peripheral neuropathy should be avoided. These include **chloramphenicol, cisplatin, dapsone, disulfiram, ethionamide, glutethimide, gold, hydralazine, iodoquinol, isoniazid, metronidazole, nitrofurantoin, phenytoin, ribavirin,** and **vincristine**.
   b. Zalcitabine treatment should be interrupted when a drug with the potential to cause pancreatitis is needed (i.e., **pentamidine**).

VII. ANTHELMINTICS

A. **Definition.** These drugs are used to rid the body of worms (**helminths**). These agents may act locally to rid the gastrointestinal tract of worms or work systemically to eradicate worms that are invading organs or tissues.

B. **Mebendazole** is a synthetic benzimidazole derivative anthelmintic.

1. **Mechanism of action.** Mebendazole interferes with reproduction and survival of helminths by inhibiting the formation of microtubules and irreversibly blocking glucose uptake, thereby depleting glycogen stores in the helminth.
2. **Spectrum of activity.** Mebendazole is active against *Trichuris trichiura* (whipworm), *Enterobius vermicularis* (pinworm), *Ascaris lumbricoides* (roundworm), *Ancylostoma duodenale* (common hookworm), and *Necator americanus* (American hookworm).
3. **Therapeutic uses.** Mebendazole is used for the treatment of single or mixed infections. Immobilization and subsequent death of helminths is slow with complete gastrointestinal clearance up to 3 days after therapy.
4. **Precautions and monitoring effects**
   a. In cases of massive infection, abdominal pain and nausea may result.
   b. If the patient is not cured in 3 weeks, retreatment is necessary.
5. **Significant interactions.** Agents that may reduce the blood levels and subsequent efficacy of mebendazole include **carbamazepine** and **hydantoins**.

C. **Diethylcarbamazine citrate**

1. **Mechanism of action.** Diethylcarbamazine citrate is a synthetic organic compound highly specific for several common parasites.
2. **Spectrum of activity.** This agent is active against *Wuchereria bancrofti, Onchocerca volvulus, Loa loa,* and *Ascaris lumbricoides.*
3. **Therapeutic uses.** Diethylcarbamazine citrate is used for the treatment of Bancroft's filariasis, onchocerciasis, ascariasis, tropical eosinophilia, and loiasis.
4. **Precautions and monitoring effects**
   a. Patients treated for *W. bancrofti* infection often present with headache and general malaise. Severe allergic phenomena in conjunction with a skin rash have been reported.
   b. Patients treated for onchocerciasis present with pruritos and facial edema. Severe reaction may be noted after a single dose.
   c. Children who are undernourished or are suffering from debilitating ascariasis infection may experience giddiness, malaise, nausea, and vomiting after treatment.

D. **Pyrantel** is a pyrimidine derivative anthelmintic.

1. **Mechanism of action.** Pyrantel is a depolarizing neuromuscular blocking agent that causes a spastic paralysis of the helminth.

2. **Spectrum of activity.** Pyrantel is active against *A. lumbricoides* (roundworm) and *E. vermicularis* (pinworm).

3. **Therapeutic uses.** Pyrantel is used for the treatment of ascariasis (roundworm) and enterobiasis (pinworm).

4. **Precautions and monitoring effects**
   a. Most commonly reported reactions include anorexia, nausea, vomiting, diarrhea, headache, and rash.
   b. A single dose may be taken with food, milk, juice, or on an empty stomach.

5. **Significant interactions**
   a. When **piperazine** is used with pyrantel, the agents are antagonistic.
   b. **Theophylline** serum levels may increase with concomitant pyrantel administration.

E. **Thiabendazole,** a pyrazinoisoquinolone derivative, is a synthetic heterocyclic anthelmintic.

1. **Mechanism of action.** Thiabendazole has both **vermicidal** and **vermifungal** activity.

2. **Spectrum of activity.** It is active against *A. lumbricoides* (roundworm), *E. vermicularis* (pinworm), *Strongyloides stercoralis* (threadworm), *N. americanus* (American hookworm), *A. duodenale* (common hookworm), *T. trichiura* (whipworm), *Ancylostoma braziliense* (dog and cat hookworm), *Toxocara canis,* and *Toxocara cati* (ascarides).

3. **Therapeutic uses.** Thiabendazole is used for the treatment of strongyloidiasis (threadworm), cutaneous larva migrans (creeping eruption), and visceral larva migrans. It is used for the treatment of uncinariasis (hookworm), *N. americanus, A. duodenale,* trichuriasis (whipworm), and ascariasis (large roundworm) when more specific therapy is unavailable or further treatment is required with a second agent.

4. **Precautions and monitoring effects**
   a. If hypersensitivity develops, the drug should be discontinued. Erythema multiforme (including Stevens-Johnson syndrome) has been reported.
   b. **CNS effects** related to therapy have been reported. Activities requiring mental alertness should be avoided.

5. **Significant interactions**
   a. Serum **xanthine** levels may increase.
   b. Serum **theophylline** levels may increase.

F. **Piperazine**

1. **Mechanism of action.** Piperazine causes flaccid paralysis of the helminth by blocking the response of ascaris muscle to acetylcholine.

2. **Spectrum of activity.** It is active against *A. lumbricoides* (roundworm) and *E. vermicularis* (pinworm).

3. **Therapeutic uses.** Piperazine is used for the treatment of enterobiasis (pinworm) and ascariasis (roundworm).

4. **Precautions and monitoring effects**
   a. The most commonly reported reactions include gastrointestinal and CNS effects. If these effects become significant, therapy should be discontinued.
   b. Piperazine should be taken on an empty stomach.
   c. Prolonged, repeated, and excessive therapy (especially in children) should be avoided due to potential neurotoxicity.

G. **Quinacrine** (see also IV)

1. **Mechanism of action.** Quinacrine erradicates intestinal cestodes.

2. **Spectrum of activity.** Quinacrine is active against *Taenia saginata* (beef tapeworm), *Taenia solium* (pork tapeworm), *Hymenolepis nana* (dwarf tapeworm), *Diphyllobothrium latum* (fish tapeworm), and the protozoa, *Giardia lamblia*.

3. **Therapeutic uses.** Quinacrine is used for the treatment of *giardiasis* and *cestodiasis.*

4. **Precautions and monitoring effects**
   a. This agent should be used with caution in patients with hepatic disease.

b. It may cause a transitory psychosis and should, therefore, be used with caution in those individuals over 60 years of age or with a history of psychosis.

H. Niclosamide

1. **Mechanism of action.** Niclosamide inhibits the oxidative phosphorylation in the mitochondria of cestodes.

2. **Therapeutic uses.** Niclosamide is used against *T. saginata* (beef tapeworm), *D. latum* (fish tapeworm), and *H. nana* (dwarf tapeworm).

3. **Precautions and monitoring effects**
   a. This agent may cause nausea, vomiting, dizziness, and drowsiness.
   b. It is not active against cysticercosis as it affects the cestodes of the intestine only.

I. Oxamniquine

1. **Mechanism of action.** Oxamniquine eradicates male and female schistosomes. Although it is less effective against female schistosomes, the residual females cease to lay eggs and lose the parasitologic activity.

2. **Therapeutic uses.** This agent is active against *Schistosoma mansoni* infection, including the acute and chronic phases with hepatosplenic involvement.

3. **Precautions and monitoring effects**
   a. Convulsions may occur within a few hours of the first dose in patients with a previous seizure history.
   b. Transitory dizziness, drowsiness, nausea, vomiting, and urticaria may occur.
   c. Oxamniquine should be taken with food to increase gastrointestinal tolerance.

J. Praziquantel

1. **Mechanism of action.** Praziquantel increases cell membrane permeability in susceptible helminths with loss of intracellular calcium and paralysis of their musculature. Vacuolization and disintegration of the schistosome tegument results, followed by attachment of phagocytes to the parasite and death.

2. **Therapeutic uses.** Praziquantel is active against *Schistosoma mekongi, S. japonicum, S. haematobium,* and infections due to liver flukes (*Clonorchis sinensis/Opisthorchis viverrin*).

3. **Precautions and monitoring effects**
   a. Treatment of ocular cysticercosis should be avoided since parasite destruction within the eyes may cause irreparable lesions.
   b. CNS effects are related to therapy, and activities requiring mental alertness should be avoided.
   c. Side effects are transient and may include malaise, headache, dizziness, and abdominal discomfort.

STUDY QUESTIONS

Directions: Each of the numbered items or incomplete statements in this section is followed by answers or by completions of the statement. Select the **one** lettered answer or completion that is **best** in each case.

1. Isoniazid is a primary antitubercular agent that

(A) requires pyridoxine supplementation
(B) may discolor the tears, saliva, urine, or feces orange-red
(C) causes ocular complications that are reversible if the drug is discontinued
(D) may be ototoxic and nephrotoxic
(E) should never be used due to hepatotoxic potential

2. All of the following factors may increase the risk of nephrotoxicity from gentamicin therapy EXCEPT

(A) age over 70 years
(B) prolonged courses of gentamicin therapy
(C) concurrent amphotericin B therapy
(D) trough gentamicin levels below 2 μg/ml
(E) concurrent cisplatin therapy

3. In which of the following groups do all four drugs warrant careful monitoring for drug-related seizures in high-risk patients?

(A) Penicillin G, imipenem, amphotericin B, metronidazole
(B) Penicillin G, chloramphenicol, tetracycline, vancomycin
(C) Imipenem, tetracycline, vancomycin, sulfadiazine
(D) Cycloserine, metronidazole, vancomycin, sulfadiazine
(E) Metronidazole, imipenem, doxycycline, erythromycin

4. Spectinomycin is an aminoglycoside-like antibiotic indicated for the treatment of

(A) gram-negative bacillary septicemia
(B) tuberculosis
(C) penicillin-resistant gonococcal infections
(D) syphilis
(E) gram-negative meningitis due to susceptible organisms

5. A man has an *Escherichia coli* bacteremia with a low-grade fever (101.6°F). Appropriate management of his fever would be to

(A) give acetaminophen 650 mg orally every 4 hours
(B) give aspirin 650 mg orally every 4 hours
(C) give alternating doses of aspirin and acetaminophen every 4 hours
(D) withhold antipyretics and use the fever curve to monitor his response to antibiotic therapy
(E) use tepid water baths to reduce the fever

6. A woman has an upper respiratory infection. Six years ago she experienced an episode of bronchospasm following penicillin V therapy. The cultures now reveal a strain of *Streptococcus pneumoniae* that is sensitive to all of the following drugs. Which of these drugs would be the best choice for this patient?

(A) Amoxicillin/clavulanate
(B) Erythromycin
(C) Ampicillin
(D) Cefaclor
(E) Cyclacillin

7. All of the following drugs are suitable oral therapy for a lower urinary tract infection due to *Pseudomonas aeruginosa* EXCEPT

(A) norfloxacin
(B) trimethoprim–sulfamethoxazole
(C) ciprofloxacin
(D) carbenicillin
(E) methenamine mandelate

8. A woman's neglected hangnail has developed into a mild staphylococcal cellulitis. Which of the following regimens would be appropriate oral therapy?

(A) Dicloxacillin 125 mg q 6h
(B) Vancomycin 250 mg q 6h
(C) Methicillin 500 mg q 6h
(D) Cefazolin 1g q 8h
(E) Penicillin V 500 mg q 6h

1-A	4-C	7-B
2-D	5-D	8-A
3-A	6-B	

9. Which of the following drugs has demonstrated in vitro activity against *Mycobacterium avium–intracellulare* (MAI)?

(A) Azithromycin
(B) Clarithromycin
(C) Erythromycin base
(D) Troleandomycin
(E) Erythromycin estolate

10. All of the following statements regarding pentamidine isethionate are true EXCEPT

(A) it is indicated for treatment or prophylaxis of infection due to *Pneumocystis carinii*
(B) it may be administered intramuscularly, intravenously, or by inhalation
(C) it has no clinically significant effect on serum glucose
(D) it is effective in the treatment of leishmaniasis

Directions: Each item below contains three suggested answers of which **one or more** is correct. Choose the answer

A if **I only** is correct
B if **III only** is correct
C if **I and II** are correct
D if **II and III** are correct
E if **I, II, and III** are correct

11. Drugs usually active against penicillinase-producing *Staphylococcus aureus* include which of the following?

I. Timentin (ticarcillin–clavulanate)
II. Augmentin (amoxicillin–clavulanate)
III. Oxacillin

12. Antiviral agents that are active against cytomegalovirus (CMV) include which of the following?

I. Ganciclovir
II. Foscarnet
III. Acyclovir

Directions: The group of items in this section consists of lettered options followed by a set of numbered items. For each item, select the **one** lettered option that is most closely associated with it. Each lettered option may be selected once, more than once, or not at all.

Questions 13–15

Match the following statements about effects or dosages with the appropriate drug.

(A) Clofazimine
(B) Itraconazole
(C) Lomefloxacin
(D) Neomycin

13. It may be administered once per day for the treatment of urinary tract infections

14. It may cause pink-to-brownish skin pigmentation within a few weeks of the initiation of therapy

15. Co-administration with astemizole or terfenadine may lead to life-threatening cardiac dysrhythmias

---

9-B
10-C
11-E
12-C
13-C
14-A
15-B

ANSWERS AND EXPLANATIONS

1. The answer is A *[V B 2 d (5)].*
Isoniazid increases the excretion of pyridoxine, which can lead to peripheral neuritis, especially in poorly nourished patients. Pyridoxine (a form of vitamin B_6) deficiency may cause convulsions as well as the neuritis, involving synovial tenderness and swelling. Treatment with the vitamin can reverse the neuritis and prevent or cure the seizures.

2. The answer is D *[II B 4 b].*
Trough serum levels below 2 μg/ml are considered appropriate for gentamicin and are recommended to minimize the risk of toxicity from this aminoglycoside. Because aminoglycosides accumulate in the proximal tubule of the kidney, nephrotoxicity can occur.

3. The answer is A *[II E 1 e (2), J 5 d (2); III B 4 b; IV C 3 c].*
Seizures have been attributed to the use of penicillin G, imipenem, amphotericin B, and metronidazole. Seizures are especially likely with high doses in patients with a history of seizures and in patients with impaired drug elimination.

4. The answer is C *[II J 6].*
Although active against various gram-negative organisms, spectinomycin is approved only for the treatment of gonorrhea and is particularly recommended for treatment of uncomplicated forms of the disease.

5. The answer is D *[I H 1].*
The fever curve is very useful for monitoring a patient's response to antimicrobial therapy. Antipyretics can be used to reduce high fever in patients at risk for complications (e.g., seizures) or, in some cases, to make the patient more comfortable.

6. The answer is B *[II D 3 b].*
Amoxicillin, ampicillin, and cyclacillin are all penicillins and should be avoided in patients with histories of hypersensitivity to other penicillin compounds. While the risk of cross-reactivity with cephalosporins (e.g., cefaclor) is now considered very low, most clinicians avoid the use of these agents in patients with histories of type I hypersensitivity reactions (anaphylaxis, bronchospasm, giant hives).

7. The answer is B *[II E 4, H 3 a, b, I 2 a, 3 a, J 7].*
Norfloxacin, ciprofloxacin, carbenicillin, and methenamine mandelate achieve urine concentrations high enough to treat urinary tract infection due to *Pseudomonas aeruginosa.* Trimethoprim–sulfamethoxazole is not useful for infection due to this organism, although the combination is useful for certain other urinary tract infections.

8. The answer is A *[II C, E 1 c (3), 2 b, J 8].*
Although vancomycin, methicillin, and cefazolin have excellent activity against staphylococci, they are not effective orally for systemic infections. Vancomycin is prescribed orally for infections limited to the gastrointestinal tract, but because it is poorly absorbed orally, it is not effective for systemic infections. Most hospital- and community-acquired staphylococci are currently resistant to penicillin V. Thus, of the drugs listed in the question, the most appropriate for oral therapy of staphylococcal cellulitis is dicloxacillin.

9. The answer is B *[II D 6 a, b].*
Clarithromycin, an alternative to erythromycin, has demonstrated in vitro activity against MAI. Clarithromycin is also used against *Toxoplasma gondii* and *Cryptosporidium* species, and it is more active than erythromycin against staphylococci and streptococci. Azithromycin is also an alternative to erythromycin, but it is more active against gram-negative organisms. Troleandomycin is similar to erythromycin but is generally less active against these organisms.

10. The answer is C *[IV D].*
Pentamidine isethionate is indicated for both treatment and prophylaxis of infection due to *Pneumocystis carinii.* It can be administered intramuscularly, intravenously, or by inhalation. Inhalation may produce bronchospasm. Blood glucose should be carefully monitored, since pentamidine may produce either hyperglycemia or hypoglycemia.

11. The answer is E (all) *[II E 2–4].*
Timentin and Augmentin each include a β-lactamase inhibitor, combined with ticarcillin and amoxicillin, respectively. These combinations offer activity against *Staphylococcus aureus* similar to that of the penicillinase-resistant penicillins, such as oxacillin.

12. The answer is C (I and II) *[VI B, F, G].*
Only ganciclovir and foscarnet are active against CMV infections. These agents are virustatic, and they arrest DNA synthesis by inhibiting viral DNA polymerase. Although ganciclovir can penetrate the central nervous system (CNS), the use of ganciclovir in the treatment of CMV infections in the CNS has not been successful. Foscarnet is a broad-spectrum antiviral agent, and is used in patients with ganciclovir resistance. Acyclovir is not clinically useful for the treatment of CMV infections, since CMV is relatively resistant to acyclovir in vitro.

13–15. The answers are: 13-C *[II H 3 c],* **14-A** *[II J 9],* **15-B** *[III E 5 d].*
Lomefloxacin may be administered once a day for treating urinary tract infections. Enoxacin is another fluoroquinolone used to treat urinary tract infections. As compared to other fluoroquinolones, neither lomefloxacin or enoxacin improve the spectrum of activity.

Since clofazimine contains phenazine dye, it can cause pink-to-brown skin pigmentation. This change in pigmentation occurs in 75%–100% of patients taking clofazimine, and it occurs within a few weeks of the initiation of therapy. The discoloration of skin has reportedly led to severe depression and even suicide in some patients. Clofazimine is used in the treatment of leprosy and several atypical *Mycobacterium* infections.

Administration of itraconazole or ketoconazole with astemizole or terfenadine may increase the level of astemizole or terfenadine, which can lead to life-threatening dysrhythmias and death. Itraconazole, which is an imidazole, is a fungistatic agent. Specifically, itraconazole can be taken orally to treat aspergillosis infections and other deep fungal infections, such as blastomycosis, coccidioidomycosis, cryptococcosis, and histoplasmosis.

46
Seizure Disorders

Azita Razzaghi

I. INTRODUCTION

A. Definitions

1. **Seizures** are characterized by an excessive, hypersynchronous discharge of cortical neuron activity, which can be measured by the electroencephalogram (EEG). In addition, there may be disturbances in consciousness, sensory motor systems, subjective well-being, and objective behavior; seizures are usually brief with a beginning and an end and may produce post-seizure impairment.

2. **Epilepsy** is defined as a chronic disorder, or group of disorders, characterized by seizures that usually recur unpredictably in the absence of a consistent provoking factor. The term epilepsy is derived from the Greek word meaning "to seize upon" or "taking hold of." It was first described by Hughlings Jackson in the nineteenth century as an intermittent derangement of the nervous system due to a sudden, excessive, disorderly discharge of cerebral neurons.

3. **Convulsions** are violent, involuntary contractions of the voluntary muscles. A patient may have epilepsy or a seizure disorder without convulsions.

B. Classification. There are two systems of classification: The first system is based on the seizure type and the characteristics of the seizures (Table 46-1), and the second system is based on the characteristics of the epilepsy, including age at onset, etiology, and frequency, as well as the characteristics of the seizures as in the first classification system (Table 46-2).

1. **Partial seizures** are the most common seizure type, occurring in approximately 80% of epileptic patients.
   a. **Clinical and electroencephalographic (EEG) changes** indicate initial activation of a system of neurons limited to part of one cerebral hemisphere, which may extend to other or all brain areas. Manifestations of the seizures depend on the site of the epileptogenic focus in the brain.
   b. **Types.** Partial seizures are subclassified as **simple** (usually unilateral involvement) and **complex** (usually bilateral involvement). Loss of consciousness is seen in complex seizures. Consciousness is defined as the degree of awareness and responsiveness of the patient to externally applied stimuli.
      (1) **Simple partial seizures** generally do not cause loss of consciousness. **Signs and symptoms** of simple partial seizures may be primarily motor, sensory, somatosensory, autonomic, or psychic. These signs and symptoms may help pinpoint the site of the abnormal brain discharge; for example, localized numbness or tingling reflects a dysfunction in the sensory cortex, located in the parietal lobe.
         (a) **Motor signs** include convulsive jerking, chewing motions, and lip smacking.
         (b) **Sensory and somatosensory manifestations** include paresthesias and auras.
         (c) **Autonomic signs** include sweating, flushing, and pupil dilation.
         (d) **Psychic manifestations,** which are sometimes accompanied by impaired consciousness, include dejá vu experiences, structured hallucinations, and dysphasia.
      (2) **Complex partial seizures** are accompanied by impaired consciousness; however, in some cases, the impairment precedes or follows the seizure. These seizures have variable manifestations.
         (a) Purposeless behavior is common.

Table 46-1. International Classification of Epileptic Seizures

- **I. Partial seizures** (seizures beginning locally)
  - **A. Simple partial seizures** (consciousness not impaired)
    - **1.** With motor symptoms
    - **2.** With somatosensory or special sensory symptoms
    - **3.** With autonomic symptoms
    - **4.** With psychic symptoms
  - **B. Complex partial seizures** (with impairment of consciousness)
    - **1.** Beginning as simple partial seizures and progressing to impairment of consciousness
      - **a.** Without automatisms
      - **b.** With automatisms
    - **2.** With impairment of consciousness at onset
      - **a.** With no other features
      - **b.** With features of simple partial seizures
      - **c.** With automatisms
  - **C. Partial seizures** (simple or complex), secondarily generalized
- **II. Generalized seizures** (bilaterally symmetric, without localized onset)
  - **A. Absence seizures**
    - **1. True absence seizures (petit mal)**
    - **2. Atypical absence seizures**
  - **B. Myoclonic seizures**
  - **C. Clonic seizures**
  - **D. Tonic seizures**
  - **E. Tonic–clonic seizures** (grand mal)
  - **F. Atonic seizures**
- **III. Unclassified seizures**

Reprinted from Commission on Classification and Terminology of the International League Against Epilepsy: Proposal for classification of epilepsies and epileptic syndomes. *Epilepsia* 26(3):268–278, 1985.

(b) The affected person may have a glassy stare, may wander about aimlessly, and may speak unintelligibly.

(c) Psychomotor (temporal lobe) epilepsy may lead to aggressive behavior (e.g., outbursts of rage or violence).

(d) Postictal confusion usually persists for 1–2 minutes after the seizure ends.

(e) Automatism (e.g., picking at clothes) is common and may follow visual, auditory, or olfactory hallucinations.

2. Generalized seizures are diffuse, affecting both cerebral hemispheres.

a. Clinical and EEG changes indicate initial involvement of both hemispheres.

(1) Consciousness may be impaired, and this impairment may be the initial manifestation.

(2) Motor manifestations are bilateral.

(3) The ictal EEG patterns initially are bilateral and presumably reflect neuronal discharge, which is widespread in both hemispheres.

b. Types

(1) Idiopathic epilepsies have an age-related onset, typical clinical and EEG characteristics, and a presumed genetic etiology.

(2) Symptomatic epilepsies are considered the consequence of a known or suspected disorder of the central nervous system (CNS).

(3) Cryptogenic epilepsy refers to a disorder whose cause is hidden or occult; it is presumed to be symptomatic, but the etiology is unknown. It is age-related, but often does not have well-defined clinical and EEG characteristics.

c. Signs and symptoms of generalized seizures may be minor or major.

(1) Absence (petit mal) seizures present as alterations of consciousness (absences) lasting 10–30 seconds.

(a) Staring (with occasional eye blinking) and loss or reduction in postural tone are typical. If the seizure takes place during conversation, the individual may break off in midsentence.

Table 46-2. Proposed International Classification of Epilepsies and Epileptic Syndromes

I. **Localized-related (focal, local, partial) epilepsies** and **syndromes**
  A. **Idiopathic** (with age-related onset)
    1. Benign childhood epilepsy with centrotemporal spikes (rolandic epilepsy)
    2. Childhood epilepsy with occipital paroxysms
  B. **Symptomatic**
    1. Chronic progressive epilepsia partialis continua of childhood
    2. Syndromes characterized by specific modes of precipitation
    3. Temporal lobe epilepsies
    4. Frontal lobe epilepsies
    5. Parietal lobe epilepsies
    6. Occipital lobe epilepsies
  C. **Cryptogenic**

II. **Generalized epilepsies and syndromes**
  A. **Idiopathic** (with age-related onset)
    1. Benign neonatal familial convulsions
    2. Benign neonatal convulsions
    3. Benign myoclonic epilepsy in infancy
    4. Childhood absence epilepsy (pyknolepsy)
    5. Juvenile absence epilepsy
    6. Juvenile myoclonic epilepsy
    7. Epilepsy with generalized tonic–clonic seizures on awakening
    8. Other generalized idiopathic epilepsies not defined above
    9. Epilepsies with seizures precipitated by specific modes of activation
  B. **Cryptogenic or symptomatic** (in order of age)
    1. West syndrome (infantile spasms)
    2. Lennox-Gastaut syndrome
    3. Epilepsy with myoclonic–astatic seizures
    4. Epilepsy with myoclonic absences
  C. **Symptomatic**
    1. **Nonspecific etiology**
      a. Early myoclonic encephalopathy
      b. Early infantile epileptic encephalopathy with suppression burst
      c. Other symptomatic generalized epilepsies not defined above
    2. **Specific syndromes** and generalized seizures complicating other disease states

III. **Epilepsies and syndromes undetermined whether focal or generalized**
  A. **With both focal and generalized seizures**
    1. Neonatal seizures
    2. Severe myoclonic epilepsy in infancy
    3. Epilepsy with continuous spike-waves during slow-wave sleep
    4. Acquired epileptic aphasia (Landau-Kleffner syndrome)*
    5. Other undetermined epilepsies not defined above
  B. **Without unequivocal generalized or focal features**

IV. **Special situations**
  A. Febrile convulsions
  B. Isolated seizures or isolated status epilepticus
  C. Seizures occurring only when there is an acute metabolic or toxic event due to such factors as alcohol, drugs, eclampsia, and nonketotic hyperglycemia

*Believed to be a localized-related epilepsy.

Reprinted from Bleck TP: Convulsive disorders: the use of anticonvulsant drugs. *Clin Neuropharmacol* 13(3):198–209, 1990.

(b) Enuresis and other autonomic components may occur during absence seizures.

(c) Some patients experience 100 or more absences daily.

(d) Onset of this seizure type occurs from ages 3–16 years; in most patients, absence seizures disappear by age 40.

(2) Myoclonic (bilateral massive epileptic myoclonus) seizures present as involuntary jerking of the facial, limb, or trunk muscles, possibly in a rhythmic manner.

(3) Clonic seizures are characterized by sustained muscle contractions alternating with relaxation.

(4) **Tonic seizures** involve sustained tonic muscle extension (stiffening).

(5) **Generalized (grand mal) tonic–clonic seizures** cause sudden loss of consciousness.

(a) The individual becomes rigid and falls to the ground. Respirations are interrupted. The legs extend, and the back arches; contraction of the diaphragm may induce grunting. This tonic phase lasts for about 1 minute.

(b) A clonic phase follows, marked by rapid bilateral muscle jerking, muscle flaccidity, and hyperventilation. Incontinence, tongue biting, tachycardia, and heavy salivation sometimes occur.

(c) During the postictal phase, the individual may experience headache, confusion, disorientation, nausea, drowsiness, and muscle soreness. This phase may last for hours.

(d) Some epileptics have serial grand mal seizures, regaining consciousness briefly between attacks. In some cases, grand mal seizures occur repeatedly with no recovery of consciousness between attacks (**status epilepticus**); this disorder is discussed in III A.

(6) **Atonic seizures (drop attacks)** are characterized by a sudden loss of postural tone so that the individual falls to the ground. They occur primarily in children.

C. Epidemiology

1. Epilepsy has a prevalence of approximately 1% (i.e., 500,000 cases per 50 million persons worldwide).

2. In the United States, the prevalence of epilepsy is 6.42 cases per 1000 population.

3. The onset of seizures is greatest during the first year of life; this probability decreases each decade after the first year until age 60.

4. Approximately 70% of epileptics have only one seizure type; the remainder have two or more seizure types.

D. Etiology.

Some seizures arise secondary to other conditions. However, in most cases, the cause of the seizure is unknown.

1. **Primary (idiopathic) seizures** have no identifiable cause.
   a. This type of seizure affects about 75% of epileptics.
   b. The onset of primary seizures typically occurs before age 20.
   c. Birth trauma, hereditary factors, and unexplained metabolic disturbances have been proposed as possible causes.

2. **Secondary seizures** (**symptomatic** or **acquired seizures**) occur secondary to an identifiable cause.
   a. Disorders that may lead to secondary seizures include:
      (1) Intracranial neoplasms
      (2) Infectious diseases, such as meningitis, influenza, toxoplasmosis, mumps, measles, and syphilis
      (3) High fever (in children)
      (4) Head trauma
      (5) Congenital diseases
      (6) Metabolic disorders, such as hypoglycemia and hypocalcemia
      (7) Alcohol or drug withdrawal
      (8) Lipid storage disorders
      (9) Developmental abnormalities
   b. Age at seizure onset suggests the precipitating cause (Table 46-3).

E. Pathophysiology.

Seizures reflect a sudden, abnormal, excessive neuronal discharge in the cerebral cortex. Any abnormal neuronal discharge could precipitate a seizure (Figure 46-1).

1. **Normal firing of neurons,** which usually originate from the gray matter of one or more cortical or subcortical areas, requires the following elements.
   a. **Voltage-dependent ion channels** are involved in action potential propagation or burst generation.

Table 46-3. Probable Causes of Recurrent Seizures by Age-Group

Age at Seizure Onset	Probable Cause of Seizure
Birth–1 month	Birth injury or anoxia, congenital or hereditary diseases, and metabolic disorders
1–6 Months	As above, plus infantile spasms
6 Months–2 years	Infantile spasms, febrile convulsions, birth injury or anoxia, meningitis, and head trauma
3–10 Years	Birth injury or anoxia, meningitis, cerebral vessel thrombosis, and idiopathic epilepsy
10–18 Years	Idiopathic epilepsy and head trauma
18–25 Years	Idiopathic epilepsy, trauma, neoplasm, and withdrawal from alcohol or drugs
35–60 Years	Trauma, neoplasm, vascular disease, and withdrawal from alcohol or drugs
Over 60 years	Vascular disease, neoplasm, degenerative disease, and trauma

b. **Neurotransmitters** control neuronal firing, including excitatory neurotransmitters, acetylcholine, norepinephrine, histamine, corticotropin-releasing factors (CRF), inhibitory neurotransmitters, γ-aminobutyric acid (GABA), and dopamine; therefore, for normal neuronal activity, there is a need for adequate ions (e.g., sodium, potassium, calcium); excitatory and inhibitory neurotransmitters; and glucose, oxygen, amino acids, and adequate systemic pH.

c. **Genetic factors.** Epileptics may be genetically predisposed to a **lower seizure threshold**.

d. **Deficient diencephalic nerves.** A diencephalic nerve group that normally suppresses excessive brain discharge may be deafferentated, hypersensitive, and vulnerable to activation by various stimuli in epileptics.

e. **Lack of oxygen in the brain.** During seizures, there is an increased use of energy, oxygen, and consequently, an increased production of carbon dioxide. Because of the limited capacity to increase the blood flow to the brain, the blood supply may be deficient. The ratio of supply and demand decreases when the seizure episode is prolonged, leading to increased ischemia and neuronal destruction. Thus, it is crucial to diagnose seizures and treat them as soon as possible.

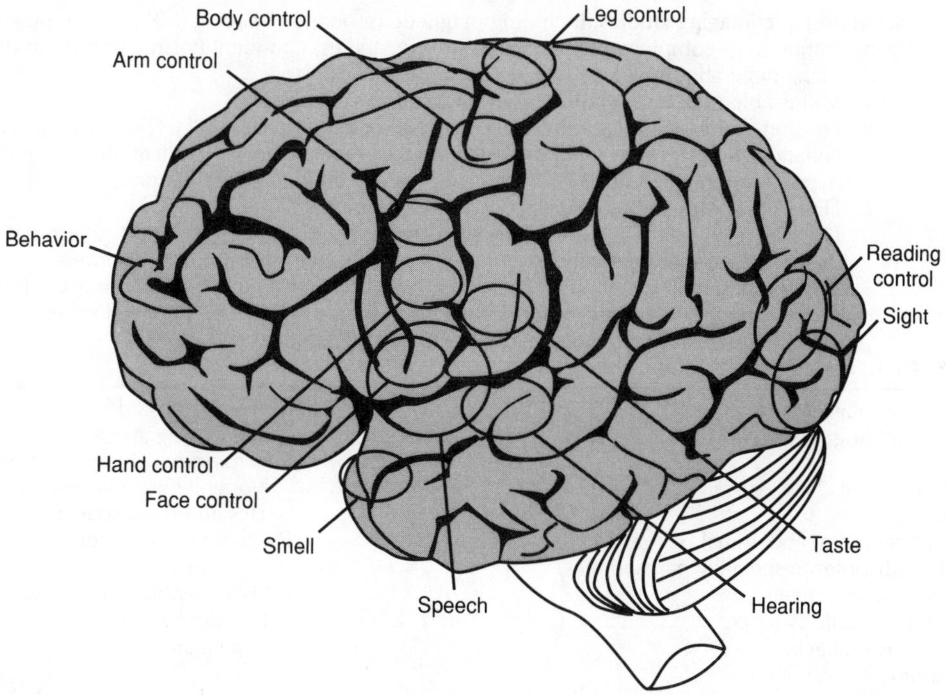

Figure 46-1. Gross anatomy of the brain. Clinical presentation of seizures depends on the area of the cortex that is affected and its function, the degree of irritability, and the identity of the impulse.

2. **Abnormal electrical brain activity** occurring during a seizure usually produces **characteristic changes on the EEG**. Each part of the cortical area has its own function, and the clinical presentation of a seizure depends on the site, the degree of irritability of the area, and the intensity of the impulse.

3. **Seizure phases.** Seizure activity may include three major phases.
   a. A **prodrome** may precede the seizure by hours or days.
      (1) Changes in behavior or mood typically occur during the prodrome.
      (2) This phase may include an aura—a subjective sensation, such as an unusual smell or flashing light.
   b. The **ictal phase** is the seizure itself. In some cases, its onset is heralded by a scream or cry.
   c. The **postictal phase** takes place immediately after the seizure.
      (1) Extensor plantar reflexes may appear.
      (2) The patient typically exhibits lethargy, confusion, and behavioral changes.

F. Clinical evaluation

1. **History** includes an evaluation of the seizure, including interviews of the patient's family and eyewitness accounts to establish:
   a. The frequency and duration of the episodes
   b. Precipitating factors
   c. The times at which episodes occur
   d. The presence or absence of an aura
   e. Ictal activity
   f. Postictal state

2. **Physical and neurologic examinations** are the tools with which to identify an underlying etiology to rule out diseases that manifest as seizures (Table 46-4).

3. **Laboratory tests** may also identify an underlying etiology.
   a. Liver and kidney function tests, complete blood count (CBC), urinalysis, serum drug levels (e.g., antidepressants and amphetamines may precipitate seizures) are necessary.
   b. Lumbar puncture may be required for the patient with a fever who has seizures for evidence of cerebrospinal fluid (CSF) infection.

4. **Neurologic imaging studies,** including magnetic resonance imaging (MRI) or computed tomography (CT)–complement electrophysiologic studies, can identify structural brain disorders (anatomic abnormalities).
   a. MRI is able to detect cerebral lesions related to epilepsy.
   b. Positron-emission tomography (PET), single-photoemission CT (SPECT), and stable xenon-enhanced x-ray CT offer functional views of the brain to detect hypometabolism or relative hypoperfusion. PET and SPECT scans are not available in all institutions.
   c. EEG studies measure the electrical activity of the brain.
      (1) EEG is useful for classifying the seizure, but the EEG by itself cannot rule seizures in or out, as there are patients with normal EEGs who have seizure disorders.
      (2) The best time to obtain an EEG is *during* a seizure episode. The EEG may be done in a sleep-induced state under normal conditions or in a sleep-deprived state.

Table 46-4. Disorders That Mimic Epilepsy

Gastroesophageal reflux	Movement disorders
Breath-holding spells	Shuddering attacks
Migraine	Paroxysmal choreoathetosis
Confusional	Nonepileptic myoclonus
Basilar	Tics and habit spasms
With recurrent abdominal pain and cyclic vomiting	Psychological disorders
Sleep disorders (especially parasomnias)	Panic disorder
Cardiovascular events	Hyperventilation attacks
Pallid infantile syncope	Pseudoseizures
Vasovagal attacks	Rage attacks
Vasomotor syncope	
Cardiac arrhythmias	

Reprinted from Scheurer ML, Pedley TA: The evaluation and treatment of seizures. *N Eng J Med* 323:1469, 1990.

G. Treatment objectives

1. To prevent or suppress seizures or reduce their frequency through drug therapy
2. To control or eliminate the factors that cause or precipitate seizures
3. To prevent serious consequences of seizures, such as anoxia, airway occlusion, or injury, by protecting the tongue and placing a pillow under the victim's head
4. To encourage a normal life-style and prevent an invalid attitude

II. THERAPY

A. Principles of drug therapy

1. **Seizure control.** Approximately 50% of epileptics achieve complete seizure control through drug therapy. In another 25%, drugs reduce the frequency of seizures. Epileptics generally require continuous drug therapy for at least 4 seizure-free years before the drug can be discontinued.

2. **Initial treatment**
   a. Before any drug treatment is instituted, remedial causes of the seizure activity should be excluded.
   b. A single primary drug that is most appropriate for the seizure type must be selected. If there is more than one appropriate primary drug, age, sex, and compliance of the patient must be considered.
   c. Approximately ¼–⅓ of the maintenance dose of a single medication is used to begin therapy; it is then increased over 3–4 weeks, except phenytoin or phenobarbital, which can be started with the loading or maintenance dose. The dose should be titrated until seizure control or intolerable side effects occur.
   d. With the initiation of therapy, blood concentrations of medications should be measured:
      (1) To establish therapeutic ranges and dosage regimens based on symptomatic toxicity or seizure frequency
      (2) To assess the patient's compliance with therapy
      (3) To control the correlation between the dose, blood levels, and clinical therapeutic levels or toxicity
         (a) Phenytoin follows nonlinear kinetics as drug levels increase dramatically (more than onefold) with only a small increase in the dose; however, prior to this dose increase, there is a predictable linear increase with dose increases. Thus, the maximum rate of hepatic enzyme clearance is reached, and the body can no longer clear the drug as fast as it is introduced into the body.
         (b) If physical examination reveals a new onset of nystagmus (except with phenytoin in which nystagmus develops before clinical intoxication), ataxia, and unsteady, wide gait, the next dose increase should be minimal.
         (c) Carbamazepine has an autoinduction metabolism property, which means that if the dose is increased twofold, blood levels increase less than twofold because of increased metabolism.
      (4) To determine the free drug level, which is helpful in patients who are in the therapeutic range but have side effects or no response. The plasma protein binding may be altered in these patients by some other disease state or medication. Because of this alteration, there is more free drug available in the system than the total level shows, especially with phenytoin, valproic acid, and carbamazepine.

3. **Additional therapy.** If seizures recur after the maximal tolerated dose is reached, a second anticholinergic drug is added at a low dose.
   a. The dose of the second drug is increased until a therapeutic level is reached.
   b. The first drug is maintained until the optimal dose of the second drug is determined, then the first drug is discontinued gradually to avoid triggering seizure activity.

4. **Diseases and conditions that alter antiepileptic drug–protein bindings**
   a. Liver disease
   b. Hypoalbuminemia
   c. Burns
   d. Pregnancy

e. High protein–binding drugs or antiepileptic agents. (Most important interactions are discussed under individual agents.)

5. Medications that decrease levels of phenytoin, carbamazepine, phenobarbital, and primidone by enhancing their metabolism. These drugs also cause false decreases in thyroid function tests.

a. Oral contraceptives
b. Oral hypoglycemics
c. Glucocorticoids
d. Tricyclic antidepressants
e. Azathioprine
f. Cyclosporine
g. Quinidine
h. Theophylline
i. Warfarin
j. Doxycycline
k. Levodopa

B. Specific antiseizure agents. Table 46-5 lists the uses of antiepileptic medications based on seizure type.

1. Carbamazepine

a. Mechanisms of action. Carbamazepine is chemically related to the tricyclic antidepressants. It was originally used to control the pain of trigeminal neuralgia. Its mechanism of action is unknown in the treatment of seizure disorders, but it is thought to act by reducing polysynaptic responses and blocking the post-tetanic potentiation. Carbamazepine is the drug of choice for simple partial and complex partial seizures.

b. Administration and dosage (Table 46-6)

(1) Adults and children over age 12. The initial oral dose is 200 mg twice daily. This may be increased gradually to 800–2000 mg/daily (usually given in divided doses).

(2) Children under age 12 usually receive 10–20 mg/kg/day in two or three divided doses.

c. Precautions and monitoring effects

(1) Carbamazepine should be used with caution in patients with bone marrow depression. A complete blood count should be taken and platelets measured to determine baseline levels before therapy and levels should be monitored during therapy.

(2) Tricyclic antidepressants should be avoided if there is a history of hypersensitivity to tricyclics. Monoamine oxidase (MAO) inhibitors should be discontinued 2 weeks prior to carbamazepine therapy.

(3) Carbamazepine should be used cautiously in patients with glaucoma due to its mild anticholinergic effects.

(4) Carbamazepine is an enzyme inducer; therefore, the half-life decreases over 3–4 weeks ($t_{1/2}$ = 18–54 hours; $t_{1/2}$ = 10–25 hours); for maximal enzyme induction, levels should be rechecked to avoid breakthrough seizures.

Table 46-5. Uses of Antiepileptic Medications Based on Seizure Type

	Choices of Drug Therapy			
Seizure Type	**1**	**2**	**3**	**4**
Simple partial	Carbamazepine	Phenytoin	Primidone	Valproic acid (phenytoin, phenobarbital)
Complex partial	Carbamazepine	Phenytoin	Phenobarbital	Valproic acid (primidone)
Primary generalized tonic–clonic	Valproic acid	Carbamazepine	Phenytoin (valproic acid)	Phenobarbital
Absence	Ethosuximide	Valproic acid		
Myoclonic	Valproic acid	Clonazepam		
Atonic	Valproic acid	Clonazepam		

Table 46-6. Dosages Characteristic of Antiepileptic Medications

Drug	Loading Dose	Usual Adult Dose (mg/day)	Half-life (hours)	Therapeutic Range of Total Plasma Concentration (µg/ml)	Major Mode of Elimination	Protein Binding Level
Carbamazepine	No	800–2000	11*–22	8–12	Hepatic	40%–90%
Phenytoin	Yes	300–700	22–72	10–20 1–2 (free)	Hepatic	90%
Phenobarbital	Yes	90–300	100	15–40	Hepatic > renal	50%
Primidone	No	750–3000	15*†	5–12	Hepatic	80%
Valproic acid	No	1000–3000	15–20	50–120	Hepatic	90%–95%
Ethosuximide	No	750–1000	50	40–100	Hepatic > renal	0%

*The half-life decreases autometabolism after chronic use.
†Metabolized in part to phenobarbital.
Adapted from Commission on Classification and Terminology of the International League Against Epilepsy: Proposal for classification of epilepsies and epileptic syndromes. *Epilepsia* 26(3):268–278, 1985.

(5) **Adverse effects.** The physician should be notified if any of the following signs or symptoms occur: jaundice, abdominal pain, pale stool, darkened urine, unusual bruising and bleeding, fever, sore throat, or an ulcer in the mouth.
   (a) **CNS effects** include, dizziness, ataxia, and diplopia. If diplopia and ataxia are common and occur after a dose, the schedule could be adjusted to include more frequent administration or a larger proportion of the dose at night. CNS side effects may decrease with chronic administration.
   (b) **Gastrointestinal effects** include most commonly nausea, vomiting, and anorexia.
   (c) **Metabolic effects.** Hyponatremia occurs after several weeks to months of therapy, and the incidence increases with age. The antidiuretic hormone (ADH) level may be low. Levels of 125–135 mEq/L without symptoms should be monitored. Fluid restriction should be instituted when levels fall below 125 mEq/L with or without symptoms. Another agent should be used if fluid dose reduction does not help or the seizures recur.
   (d) **Hematopoietic effects.** Aplastic anemia is rare. Thrombocytopenia and anemia have a 5% incidence and they respond to a cessation of drug therapy. Leukopenia is the most common hematopoietic side effect: 10% of cases are transient, and about 2% of patients have persistent leukopenia but do not seem to have increased infections even with white blood cell counts of 3000/ml.
   (e) **Dermatologic effects.** Pruritic and erythematous rashes, the Stevens-Johnson syndrome, and lupus erythematosus have been reported.

d. Significant interactions
(1) **Antiepileptic drugs,** such as **phenytoin, primidone,** and **phenobarbital,** decrease the level of carbamazepine (increase metabolism). **Valproic acid** increases the level of carbamazepine (decreases metabolism).
(2) **Other medications,** such as **erythromycin, isoniazid, cimetidine, propoxyphene, diltiazem,** and **verapamil** increase the level of carbamazepine (decrease metabolism).

2. Phenytoin

a. Mechanism of action
(1) Phenytoin inhibits the spread of seizures at the motor cortex and blocks post-tetanic potentiation by influencing synaptic transmission. There is an alternation of ion fluxes in depolarization, repolarization, and membrane stability phase and alternating calcium uptake in presynaptic terminals.
(2) Phenytoin is effective for the treatment of generalized tonic–clonic (grand mal) seizures and for partial seizures, both simple and complex. It is not effective for absence seizures.

b. Administration and dosage (see Table 46-6)
(1) **Adults.** The usual daily dose for adults is 300–700 mg, with adjustments made as needed.
   (a) Regular daily doses above 500 mg are poorly tolerated.

(b) A loading dose of 900 mg to 1.5 g may be given intravenously. The infusion rate should not exceed 50 mg/min. (Alternatively, an oral loading dose may be given.)

(2) **Children.** The usual daily dose for children is 4–7 mg/kg divided every 12 hours. An intravenous loading dose of 15 mg/kg may be given.

(3) Phenytoin sodium is available as capsules and parenteral solution. Phenytoin is available as tablets and oral suspension.

c. Precautions and monitoring effects

(1) Intravenous phenytoin should not be used in patients with sinus bradycardia, sinoatrial block, second- and third-degree atrioventricular (AV) block, or Adams-Stokes syndrome.

(2) Phenytoin should be used cautiously in patients with myocardial insufficiency and hypotension.

(3) Elimination of phenytoin converts from first-order elimination (proportional to its concentration) to zero-order elimination (a fixed amount per unit time), usually at high therapeutic levels. The daily dose of phenytoin can be increased 100 mg daily until therapeutic blood levels are attained after which increases of 30–50 mg will avoid two- to threefold increases in blood levels.

(4) It is necessary to measure free drug levels or correct the total level when aluminum levels are abnormal or the patient has renal failure.

(5) **Adverse effects.** The physician should be notified if any of the following occur: swollen or tender gums, skin rash, nausea and vomiting, swollen glands, bleeding, jaundice, fever, or sore throat (i.e., signs of infection or bleeding).

(a) **CNS effects** include, ataxia (limiting side effect), dysarthria, and insomnia. Transient hyperkinesia may follow intravenous phenytoin infusion. Alcoholic beverages should be avoided while on this medication.

(b) **Gastrointestinal effects** most commonly include nausea and vomiting. Phenytoin should be taken with food to enhance absorption and decrease gastrointestinal upset.

(c) **Dermatologic effects** include maculopapular rashes sometimes with fever, Stevens-Johnson syndrome, and lupus erythematosus. Gingival hyperplasia may be reduced by frequent brushing and appropriate oral care.

(d) **Connective tissue disorders** include a coarsening of the facial features.

(e) **Hematopoietic effects** include thrombocytopenia, leukopenia, and granulocytopenia.

(f) **Miscellaneous effects** include hyperglycemia and increased body hair.

d. Significant interactions

(1) **Antiepileptic drugs,** such as **carbamazepine, valproic acid, clonazepam,** and **phenobarbital** decrease the level of phenytoin (increase metabolism). **Phenytoin** increases the conversion of primidone to phenobarbital (increases metabolism).

(2) **Other medications** such as **disulfiram, isoniazid, chloramphenicol,** and **propoxyphene** increase the level of phenytoin (decrease metabolism). **Ethanol, folic acid, vitamin D,** and enteral nutritional therapy decrease the level of phenytoin (increase metabolism).

3. Valproic acid

a. Mechanism of action

(1) Increases levels of GABA

(2) Potentiates a postsynaptic GABA response by inhibiting the enzymatic response for the catabolism of GABA

(3) Affects the potassium channel, creating a direct membrane-stabilizing effect

b. Administration and dosage (see Table 46-6)

(1) **Adults.** Valproic acid is administered orally in a usual dose of 1000–3000 mg daily in divided doses.

(2) **Children.** Valproic acid is administered orally in a dose of 15–60 mg/kg/day divided into two or three doses.

(3) Medication should be taken with food to reduce gastrointestinal upset.

(4) Tablets or capsules should be swallowed, not chewed, to avoid irritation of the mouth and throat.

c. Precautions and monitoring effects. There are some reports of hepatotoxicity and increased liver function tests, which are mostly reversible. The severity and incidence of hepatotoxicity increase when the patient is less than 2 years old.

d. **Adverse effects**
   (1) **CNS effects** include tremor, ataxia, diplopia, lethargy, drowsiness, behavioral changes, and depression.
   (2) **Gastrointestinal effects** include nausea and increased appetite. Enteric-coated divalproex sodium may reduce these side effects.
   (3) **Dermatologic effects** include alopecia and petechiae.
   (4) **Hematopoietic effects** include thrombocytopenia, bruising, hematoma, and bleeding.
   (5) **Hepatic effects** include minor elevations of aspartate aminotransferase (AST), alanine aminotransferase (ALT), and lactate dehydrogenase (LDH).
   (6) **Endocrine effects** include decreased levels of prolactin, resulting in irregular menses, and secondary amenorrhea.
   (7) **Pancreatic effects** include acute pancreatitis.
   (8) **Metabolic effects** include hyperammonemia due to renal origin. Discontinuation may be considered if lethargy develops.

e. **Significant interactions**
   (1) **Antiepileptic drugs**
      (a) **Primidone** decreases valproic acid clearance (increases metabolism).
      (b) **Phenobarbital** and **phenytoin** displace protein binding, resulting in an increased total phenytoin level and an increase or no change of free phenytoin.
      (c) **Clonazepam** increases CNS toxicity in patients on valproic acid.
   (2) **Other medications**
      (a) **Aspirin** increases the level of valproic acid.
      (b) **Warfarin** inhibits the secondary phase of platelet aggregation.
      (c) **Antacids** increase the level of valproic acid.
   (3) **Laboratory tests**
      (a) False-positive urine ketone tests may result in patients taking valproic acid; thus, diabetic patients must use caution when using urine tests.
      (b) Thyroid function tests may be altered by antiepileptic drugs.

4. Phenobarbital

a. **Mechanism of action.** Phenobarbital increases the seizure threshold by decreasing postsynaptic excitation by stimulating postsynaptic GABA-A receptor inhibitor responses as a CNS depressant.

b. **Administration and dosage** (see Table 46-6).
   (1) **Adults.** In the treatment of seizures, phenobarbital is administered orally at 90–300 mg daily (in three divided doses or as a single dose at bedtime).
   (2) **Children** typically receive 3–6 mg/kg/day in two divided doses. Adjustment is made as needed.

c. **Precautions and monitoring effects**
   (1) Phenobarbital produces respiratory depression, especially with parenteral administration.
   (2) Phenobarbital should be used with caution in patients with hepatic disease who may need dose adjustments.
   (3) Phenobarbital has sedative effects in adults and produces hyperactivity in children.
   (4) Abrupt discontinuation of phenobarbital produces withdrawal convulsions. If the drug must be discontinued, another GABA-A agonist (e.g., benzodiazepine, paraldehyde) should be substituted.
   (5) **Adverse effects.** The physician should be notified if any of the following symptoms occur: sore throat, mouth sores, easy bruising or bleeding, and any signs of infection.
      (a) **CNS effects** include agitation, confusion, lethargy, and drowsiness. Patients should avoid alcohol and other CNS depressants.
      (b) **Respiratory effects** include hypoventilation and apnea.
      (c) **Cardiovascular effects** include bradycardia and hypotension.
      (d) **Gastrointestinal effects** include nausea, diarrhea, and constipation. If gastrointestinal upset is experienced, phenobarbital should be taken with food.
      (e) **Hematologic effects** include megaloblastic anemia after chronic use (a rare side effect).
      (f) **Miscellaneous effects** include osteomalacia and Stevens-Johnson syndrome, both of which are rare.

d. Significant interactions

(1) **Antiepileptic drugs,** such as **valproic acid** and **phenytoin,** increase the level of phenobarbital (decrease metabolism).

(2) **Other drugs,** such as **acetazolamide, chloramphenicol, cimetidine,** and **furosemide** increase the level of phenobarbital (decrease metabolism). **Rifampin, pyridoxine,** and **ethanol** decrease the level of phenobarbital (increase metabolism).

5. Primidone

a. Mechanism of action. Primidone is a metabolite of phenobarbital and phenylethylmalonamide (PEMA), which have some anticonvulsive effects. It has drug characteristics similar to phenobarbital with some differences in dose and half-life.

b. Administration and dosage

(1) Primidone has a short half-life of 7 hours, which may require three times daily dosing.

(2) Primidone is tolerated better if started at 50 mg at night for 3 days until the target daily dose is reached.

6. Ethosuximide

a. Mechanism of action

(1) Ethosuximide may inhibit the sodium-potassium adenosine triphosphatase (Na^+-K^+–ATPase) system and the reduced form of nicotinamide-adenine dinucleotide phosphate (NADPH)–linked aldehyde reductase (which is necessary for the formation of γ-hydroxybutyrate, which is associated with the induction of absence seizures).

(2) Ethosuximide reduces or eliminates the EEG abnormality; however, absence seizures are the only seizures in which the normal EEG has clinical value (i.e., when the EEG abnormality is corrected, the seizures are also controlled).

(3) Ethosuximide is a relatively benign anticonvulsant with minimum protein binding.

b. Administration and dosage (see Table 46-6). Ethosuximide is usually given orally in an initial dose of 500 mg/day in adults and older children and 250 mg/day in children ages 3–6. The dose may be raised by 250 mg every week to a maximum of 1.5 g/day in adults.

c. Precautions and monitoring effects

(1) Blood dyscrasias have been reported, making periodic blood counts necessary.

(2) There have been reports of hepatic and renal toxicity, thus periodic renal and liver function monitoring is necessary.

(3) Cases of systemic lupus erythematosus have been reported.

(4) **Adverse effects**

(a) **Gastrointestinal effects** include nausea and vomiting. Small doses may lessen these effects. Ethosuximide should be taken with food if gastrointestinal upset occurs.

(b) **CNS effects** include drowsiness, blurred vision, fatigue, lethargy, hiccups, and headaches. Alcoholic beverages should be avoided with this medication.

(c) **Miscellaneous effects** include skin rashes, lupus, and blood dyscrasias (all rare).

d. Significant interactions. Antiepileptic drugs, such as **carbamazepine,** decrease the level of ethosuximide (increase metabolism), and **valproic acid** increases the level of ethosuximide (decreases metabolism).

7. Clonazepam

a. Mechanism of action. Clonazepam is a potent GABA-A agonist, but its efficacy decreases over several months of treatment.

b. Administration and dosage

(1) **Adults.** Clonazepam is an oral agent that may be given in an initial dose of 1.5 mg/day divided two or three times. The dose may be increased to a maximum of 20 mg/day.

(2) **Children** should receive 0.01–0.03 mg/day divided two or three times. The dosage may be increased to a maximum of 0.2 mg/kg/day.

c. Precautions and monitoring effects

(1) Patients with psychoses, acute narrow-angle glaucoma, and significant liver disease should use this medicine cautiously.

(2) **Adverse effects**

(a) **CNS effects** include drowsiness, ataxia, and behavior disturbances seen in children, which may be corrected by dose reduction.

(b) **Respiratory effects** include hypersalivation and bronchial hypersecretion.

(c) **Miscellaneous effects** include anemia, leukopenia, thrombocytopenia, and respiratory depression.

d. Significant interactions

(1) Antiepileptic drugs, such as **phenytoin,** increase the level of clonazepam (decrease metabolism).

(2) Other drugs. Clonazepam decreases the efficacy of **levodopa** and increases the serum level of **digoxin.**

C. Surgery. If seizures do not respond to drug therapy, surgery may be performed to remove the epileptogenic brain region.

1. **Indications** for surgery are intractable or disabling seizures recurring for 6–12 months.

2. **Stereotaxic surgery.** In this technique, the surgeon uses three-dimensional coordinates to guide a needle through a hole drilled in the skull, then destroys abnormal pathways via small intracerebral incisions.

3. **Other surgical approaches** include temporal lobe resection, removal of the temporal lobe tip, and cerebral hemispherectomy.

III. COMPLICATIONS

A. Convulsive status epilepticus. This disorder is characterized by rapid repetition of generalized tonic–clonic seizures with no recovery of consciousness between seizures. This life-threatening condition may persist for hours or even days; if it lasts longer than 1 hour, severe permanent brain damage may result.

1. **Causes** of status epilepticus include poor therapeutic compliance, intracranial infection or neoplasm, alcohol withdrawal, drug overdose, and metabolic imbalance.

2. **Management**

a. A patent airway must be maintained.

b. If the cause of the condition is unknown, 50% dextrose in water (25–30 ml) is given intravenously in case hypoglycemia is the cause.

c. If the seizures persist, **diazepam** (10 mg) is administered intravenously at a rate not exceeding 2 mg/min until the seizures stop or 20 mg have been given.

d. Phenytoin is then administered intravenously no faster than 50 mg/min to a maximum dose of 11–18 mg/kg. Blood pressure is monitored to detect hypotension.

e. If these measures do not stop the seizures, **one** of the following drugs is given.

(1) Diazepam is given as an intravenous drip of 50–100 mg diluted in 500 ml dextrose 5% in water, infused at 40 ml/hr until the seizures stop.

(2) Phenobarbital is given as an intravenous infusion of 8–20 mg/kg no faster than 100 mg/min.

f. If seizures continue despite these measures, **one** of the following steps is then taken.

(1) Paraldehyde is given intravenously in a dosage of 0.10–0.15 ml/kg diluted to a 4% solution in normal saline solution.

(2) Lidocaine is given in an intravenous loading dose of 50–100 mg, followed by an infusion of 1–2 mg/min.

(3) General anesthesia is induced with ventilatory assistance and neuromuscular junction blockade.

B. Nonconvulsive status epilepticus. This condition presents as repeated absence seizures or complex partial seizures. The patient's mental state fluctuates; confusion, impaired responses, and automatisms are prominent. **Initial management** typically involves intravenous diazepam. Complex partial status epilepticus may also necessitate administration of such drugs as phenytoin or phenobarbital.

STUDY QUESTIONS

Directions: Each of the numbered items or incomplete statements in this section is followed by answers or by completions of the statement. Select the **one** lettered answer or completion that is **best** in each case.

1. Phenytoin is effective for the treatment of all of the following types of seizures EXCEPT

(A) generalized tonic–clonic
(B) simple partial
(C) complex partial
(D) absence
(E) grand mal

2. Which of the following anticonvulsants is contraindicated in patients with a history of hypersensitivity to tricyclic antidepressants?

(A) Phenytoin
(B) Ethosuximide
(C) Acetazolamide
(D) Carbamazepine
(E) Phenobarbital

3. Which anticonvulsant drug requires therapeutic monitoring of phenobarbital serum levels as well as its own serum levels?

(A) Phenytoin
(B) Primidone
(C) Clonazepam
(D) Ethotoin
(E) Carbamazepine

4. A 23-year-old patient is diagnosed with simple partial seizures. What would the drug of choice be in this patient?

(A) Carbamazepine
(B) Phenytoin
(C) Primidone
(D) Clonazepam
(E) Ethosuximide

1-D
2-D
3-B
4-A

ANSWERS AND EXPLANATIONS

1. The answer is D *[I B 2 c (1); II B 2].*
Phenytoin (diphenylhydantoin) is the most commonly prescribed hydantoin for seizure disorders. It is one of the preferred drugs for generalized tonic–clonic (grand mal) seizures and for partial seizures, both simple and complex. However, phenytoin is not effective for absence (petit mal) seizures.

2. The answer is D *[II B 1 c (2)].*
Carbamazepine is structurally related to the tricyclic antidepressants (e.g., amitriptyline, desipramine, imipramine, nortriptyline, protriptyline) and should not be administered to patients with hypersensitivity to any of the tricyclic antidepressants.

3. The answer is B *[II B 5].*
Primidone's antiseizure activity may be partly attributable to phenobarbital. In patients receiving primidone, serum levels of both primidone and phenobarbital should be measured.

4. The answer is A *[I B 1 b (1); II B 1 a].*
For simple partial seizures, the drug of choice is carbamazepine, especially in young individuals because it has fewer side effects. The patient should begin with a low dose; if the patient continues to have seizures without limiting side effects, the dose is increased until therapeutic effects are seen or the patient develops side effects. In the case of limiting side effects or a lack of response, a second drug (phenytoin) should be added. Optimally, the carbamazepine dose may be tapered as the patient responds to the second therapy.

47
Parkinson's Disease

Azita Razzaghi

I. DISEASE STATE AND PATHOLOGY

A. Definition. Parkinson's disease is a slowly progressive degenerative neurologic disease characterized by tremor, rigidity, bradykinesia (sluggish neuromuscular responsiveness), and postural instability. Parkinson's disease was first described by Dr. James Parkinson in 1817 as "shaking palsy."

B. Incidence

1. It is one of the most common neurologic disorders that occur after age 50 (with an incidence of 100–150/100,000 population).
2. Onset generally occurs between ages 50 and 65; usually in the 60s.

C. Pathogenesis. Parkinson's disease is a neurodegenerative disease associated with **depigmentation of the substantia nigra** and the **loss of dopaminergic input to the basal ganglia** (extrapyramidal system); it is characterized by distinctive **motor disability** (Figure 47-1).

D. Etiology. Several forms of Parkinson's disease have been recognized.

1. **Primary (idiopathic) Parkinson's disease**
   - **a.** This is also called classic Parkinson's disease or **paralysis agitans**.
   - **b.** The cause is unknown, and while treatment may be palliative, the disease is incurable.
   - **c.** Most patients suffer from this type of parkinsonism.
   - **d. Hypotheses of neuronal loss** in idiopathic Parkinson's disease are:
     - **(1) Absorption of highly potent neurotoxins,** such as carbon monoxide, manganese, solvents, and N-methyl-4-phenyl-1,2,3,6-tetrahydropyridine (MPTP), which is a product of improper synthesis of a synthetic heroin-like compound. Exposure to these agents, alone or in combination with the neuronal loss of age, may be the cause of Parkinson's disease.
     - **(2) Exposure to the free radicals.** Normally, dopamine is catabolized by monoamine oxidase (MAO). Hydrogen peroxide and production of free radicals are products of catabolism that are toxic to cells. Protective mechanisms, enzymes, and free radical scavengers, such as vitamins E and C, protect cells from damage. It is proposed that either a decrease in these protective mechanisms or an increase in the production of dopamine causes a destruction of the neurons by free radicals.
2. **Secondary parkinsonism—due to a known cause**
   - **a.** Only a small percentage of cases are secondary, and many of these are curable.
   - **b.** Secondary parkinsonism may be caused by drugs, including dopamine antagonists, such as:
     - **(1)** Phenothiazines (e.g., chlorpromazine, perphenazine)
     - **(2)** Butyrophenones (e.g., haloperidol)
     - **(3)** Reserpine
   - **c.** Poisoning by chemicals or toxins may be the cause, including:
     - **(1)** Carbon monoxide poisoning
     - **(2)** Heavy metal poisoning, such as that by manganese or mercury
     - **(3)** MPTP, a commercial compound used in organic synthesis and found (as a side product) in an illegal meperidine analogue

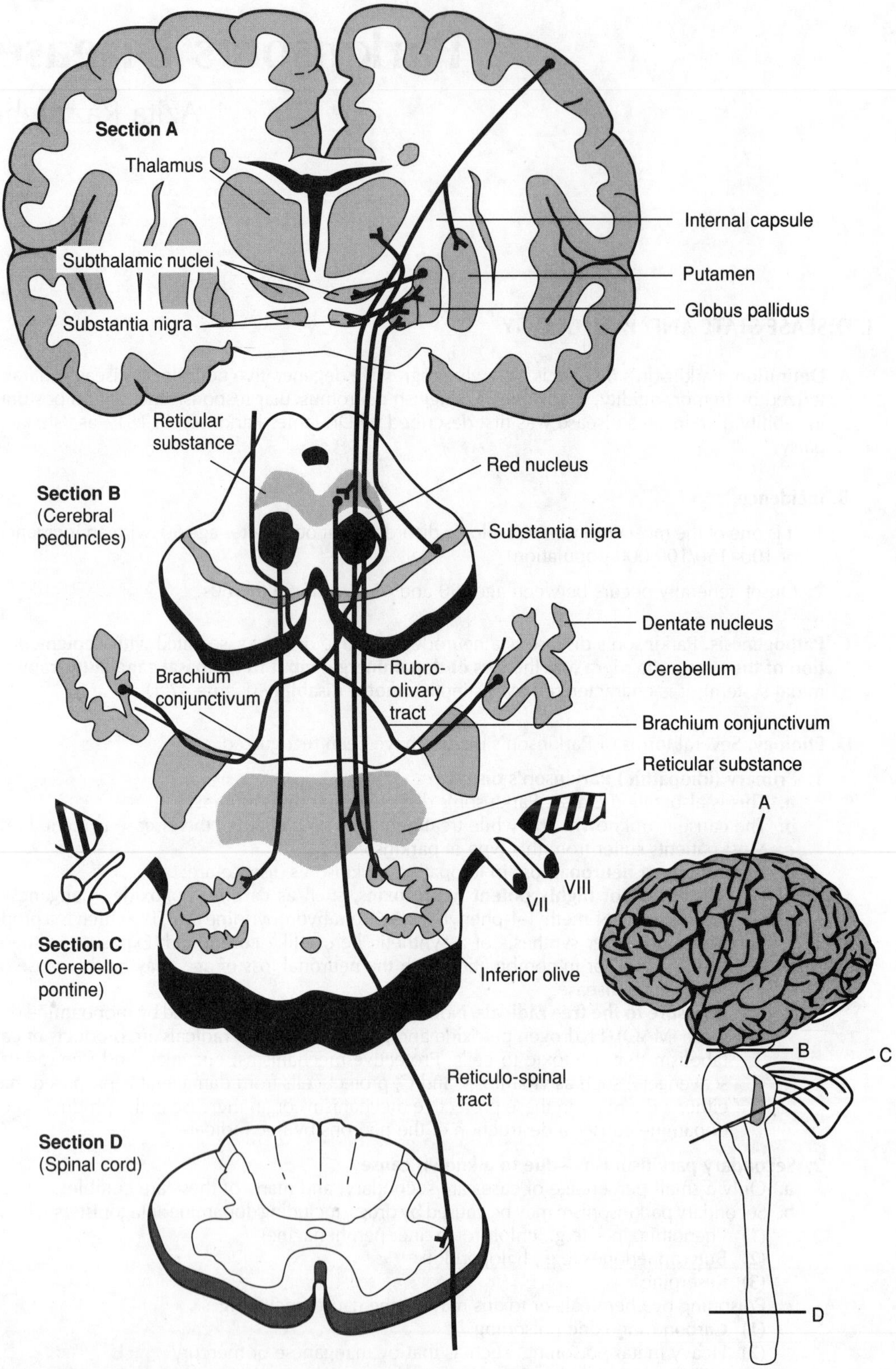

Figure 47-1. Extrapyramidal system involved in Parkinson's disease. (Reprinted from Netter F: *Ciba Collection of Medical Illustrations.* West Caldwell, NJ, Ciba Geigy Pharmaceuticals, 1983, p 69.)

d. Infectious causes include:
  (1) Encephalitis (viral)
  (2) Syphilis
e. Other causes include:
  (1) Arteriosclerosis
  (2) Degenerative diseases of the central nervous system (CNS), such as progressive supranuclear palsy
  (3) Metabolic disorders, such as Wilson's disease

E. Signs and symptoms

1. Tremor

a. Tremor may be the initial complaint in some patients. It is most evident at rest (**resting tremor**) and with low-frequency movement. When the thumb and forefinger are involved, it is known as the **pill-rolling tremor**. Before pills were made by machine, pharmacists made tablets (pills) by hand, which is how this action was named (Figure 47-2).

b. Some patients experience **action tremor** (most evident during activity), which can exist with or prior to the development of resting tremor.

2. Limb rigidity is present in almost all patients. It is detected clinically when the arm responds with a ratchet-like (i.e., cogwheeling) movement when the limb is moved passively. This is due to a tremor that is superimposed on the rigidity.

3. Akinesia or bradykinesia. Akinesia is characterized by difficulty in initiating movements, and bradykinesia is a slowness in performing common voluntary movements, including standing, walking, eating, writing, and talking. The lines of the patient's face are smooth, and the expression is fixed (**masked face**) with little evidence of spontaneous emotional responses (Figure 47-3).

4. Gait and postural difficulties. Characteristically, patients walk with a stooped, flexed posture; a small shuffling stride; and a diminished arm swing in rhythm with the legs. There may be a tendency to accelerate or festinate (Figure 47-4).

5. Changes in mental status. Mental status changes, including depression (50%), dementia (25%), and psychosis, are associated with the disease and may be precipitated or worsened by drugs.

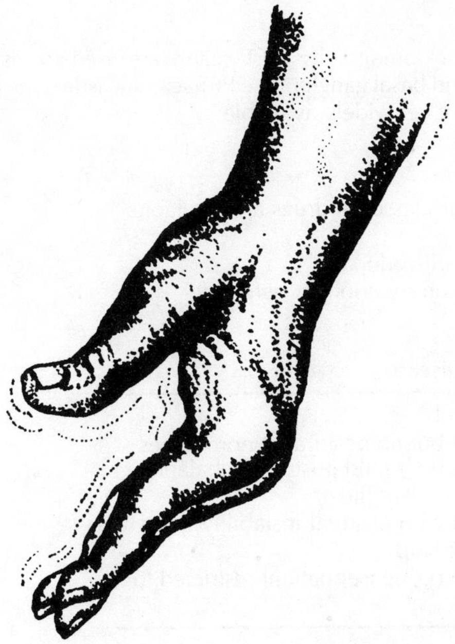

Figure 47-2. Resting (or static) tremors. (Adapted from Bates B: *A Guide to Physical Examination and History Taking,* 5th ed. Philadelphia, JB Lippincott, 1991, p 554.)

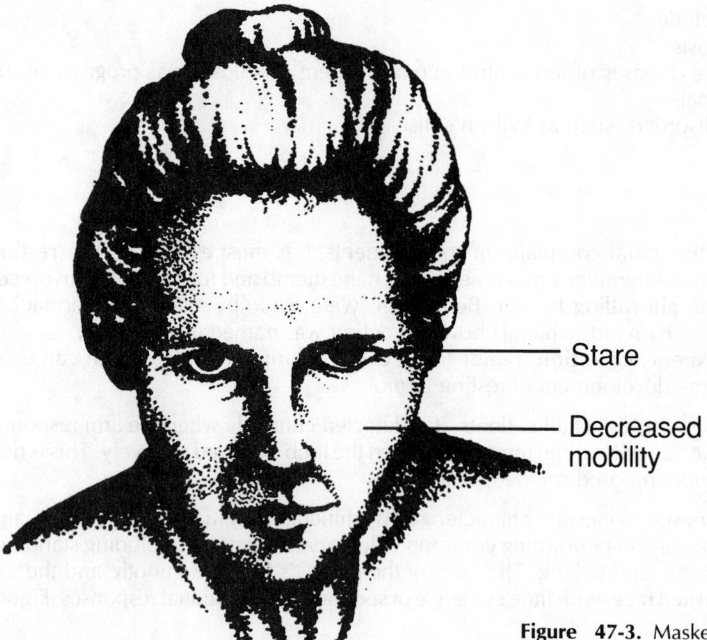

Figure 47-3. Masked face of Parkinson's disease. (Adapted from Bates B: *A Guide to Physical Examination and History Taking,* 5th ed. Philadelphia, JB Lippincott, 1991, p 197.)

F. Stages of Parkinson's disease (Table 47-1)

G. Diagnosis

1. Diagnosis depends on clinical findings.
2. Tests (including imaging) are mostly used to rule out an etiology of secondary Parkinson's disease.
3. New technologies [e.g., positron emission tomography (PET scan)] are used to visualize dopamine uptake in the substantia nigra and basal ganglia. The PET scan measures the extent of neuronal loss in these areas, but it is not yet widely available.

H. Treatment

1. **Drug therapy for symptomatic relief.** Four classes of drugs are available.
   a. Anticholinergics (for resting tremor)
   b. Precursor of dopamine (e.g., carbidopa/levodopa)
   c. Direct-acting dopamine agonists (e.g., bromocriptine, pergolide)
   d. Indirect-acting dopamine agonists

Table 47-1. Stages of Parkinson's Disease

Stage I	Unilateral involvement
Stage II	Bilateral involvement but no postural abnormalities
Stage III	Bilateral involvement with mild postural imbalance; patient leads independent life
Stage IV	Bilateral involvement with postural instability; patient requires substantial help
Stage V	Severe, fully developed disease; patient restricted to bed or chair

Reprinted from Hoehn MM, Yahr MD: Parkinsonism: onset, progression, and mortality. *Neurology* 17:427, 1967.

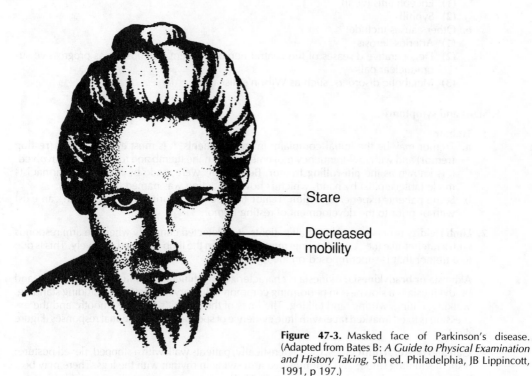

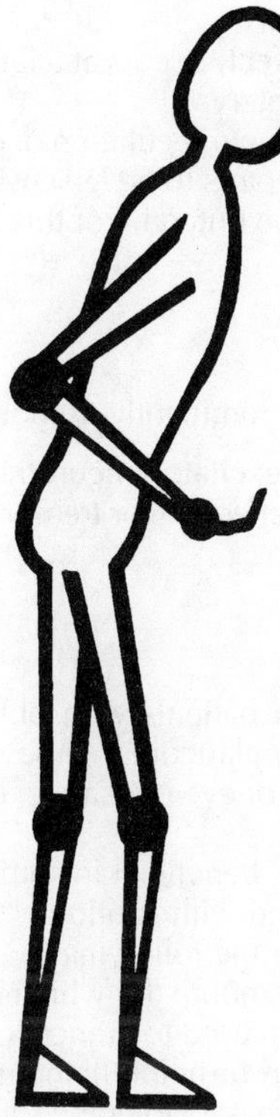

Figure 47-4. Characterisitc walk of patients with Parkinson's disease. (Adapted from Bates B: *A Guide to Physical Examination and History Taking,* 5th ed. Philadelphia, JB Lippincott, 1991, p 553.)

(1) Decrease re-uptake (e.g., amantadine)
(2) Decrease metabolism (e.g., selegiline)

2. Drug therapy for the treatment of associated symptoms

a. Tricyclic antidepressants are used to treat **depression**. They exhibit some dopaminergic and anticholinergic effects.

b. β-Blockers, especially **propranolol** with its high lipophilicity **benzodiazepines,** and **primidone** are medications used for **action tremor**. Usually patients show a clinical response in low doses.

3. General principles of drug therapy

a. If a patient does not respond to an agent in one class then another class should be tried. The two dopamine agonists, bromocriptine and pergolide, are two exceptions. Studies show that some patients respond to one agent when they fail to respond to another. This could be due to their different potency or the limited information available on pergolide.

b. Therapy should be started with a low dose and titrated up. Response usually is seen within a few days after the initiation of therapy.

c. If a second agent is added to the drug therapy, the dose of the first medication should be decreased to minimize side effects.

d. Drug therapy should never be discontinued suddenly as withdrawal may exacerbate the symptoms.

4. Definitions concerning drug therapy

a. Dyskinesias are typically oral–facial movements, grimacing, or jerky and writhing movements of the trunk and extremities. They are always reversible with the use of antiparkinsonian medications, and they decrease or diminish with dose reduction. Symptoms of Parkinson's disease may reappear with a reduction of the dose, and it is the clinical judgment of the physician or the preference of the patient whether or not to continue with the drug regimen or tolerate the side effects.

b. On–off effect describes oscillations in response (at the receptor site) and sudden changes in mobility from no symptoms to full parkinsonian symptoms in a matter of minutes. No direct relationship between the on–off effect and drug levels has been found. Usually, a second drug is added to the therapy regimen to correct the effect. Reducing the dose of one drug and adding a second drug may also be useful.

c. **End-dose effect,** known also as the **wearing off effect,** occurs at a latter part of dosing interval; it may improve by shortening the dosing interval.

d. **Drug holiday.** Long-term levodopa use results in down regulation of dopamine receptors. A drug holiday allows striatal nigra dopamine receptors to be re-sensitized, although controversy exists regarding the consequences and the outcome of this "holiday."

II. INDIVIDUAL DRUGS

A. **Anticholinergic agents** are used for mild symptoms, predominantly tremors.

1. **Mechanism of action.** This class of drugs blocks the excitatory neurotransmitter cholinergic influence in the basal ganglia. These drugs are more effective for tremor and rigidity than for bradykinesia, and less effective for postural imbalance.

2. **Administration and dosage** (Table 47-2)

3. **Precautions and monitoring effects**
   a. Anticholinergics should be used with caution in patients with obstruction of the gastrointestinal or genitourinary tracts, narrow-angle glaucoma, or severe cardiac disease. Physicians should be notified if a rapid heart beat or eye pain are experienced. (Frequent ophthalmology visits are recommended.)
   b. The sedative side effects of antihistamines may be beneficial in some patients.
   c. Alcohol and other CNS depressants should be used with caution.
   d. **Adverse effects** of anticholinergic therapy include the following:
      (1) **Peripheral anticholinergic effects** include dry mouth (for which hard candies may be helpful); decreased sweating, resulting in decreased tolerance to heat; urinary retention; constipation (for which stool softeners may be helpful); increased intraocular tension; and nausea. Because of patients' decreased tolerance to heat, these agents should be used with caution in hot weather. They should also be taken with food to minimize gastrointestinal upset.
      (2) **CNS effects** include dizziness, delirium, disorientation, anxiety, agitation, hallucinations, and impaired memory. The incidence of CNS effects increases in elderly individuals.
      (3) **Cardiovascular effects** include hypotension and orthostatic hypotension.

4. **Significant interactions**
   a. Side effects may be potentiated by other drugs with anticholinergic activity such as **antihistamines, antidepressants,** and **phenothiazines**.
   b. Anticholinergic agents increase **digoxin** levels.
   c. When anticholinergic agents are taken with **haloperidol,** the following occurs:
      (1) Schizophrenic symptoms may increase.
      (2) Haloperidol levels may decrease.

Table 47-2. Dosage Range and Characteristics of Drug Treatment

Drugs	Time to Peak Concentration (hours)	Half-Life (hours)	Daily Dosage Range (mg/day)
Anticholinergic agents			
Benztropine	Not available	Not available	1–6
Biperiden	1–1.5	18.4–24.3	2–8
Procyclidine	1.1–2	11.5–12.6	6–20
Trihexyphenidyl	1–1.3	5.6–10.2	2–15
Amantadine	4–8	9.7–14.5	100–400
Levodopa/carbidopa	1	1–1.75	10/100–25/100 tid q 3 hours
Dopaminergic agents			
Bromocriptine	1–3	48	2.50–25
Pergolide	2	8	0.1–5
Selegiline	0.5–2	2–20.5	5–10

(3) The severity of (not the risk of) tardive dyskinesia may increase.

d. When **phenothiazines** are taken with anticholinergic drugs, the effects of the phenothiazines decrease and the anticholinergic symptoms increase.

e. Patients on high doses of anticholinergics in combination with **levodopa** should be watched for decreased levodopa activity due to a delayed gastric empting time.

B. Dopamine precursor. Levodopa/carbidopa is the most effective drug in the management of Parkinson's disease; however, prolonged use decreases its therapeutic effects and increases adverse drug reactions. Dopamine does not cross the blood–brain barrier; therefore, a precursor is used. Peripheral conversion of levodopa to dopamine causes adverse reactions like nausea, vomiting, cardiac arrhythmias, and postural hypotension. To decrease the peripheral conversion and peripheral adverse effects, a peripheral dopa decarboxylase inhibitor (carbidopa) is added to levodopa (Sinemet).

1. **Mechanism of action.** Levodopa is converted to dopamine by the enzyme dopa decarboxylase, which results in elevation of CNS levels of dopamine.

2. **Administration and dosage** (see Table 47-2)

a. It is necessary to give at least 100 mg daily of carbidopa to decrease the incidence of the peripheral conversion of levodopa and gastrointestinal side effects (e.g., nausea) and increase the bioavailability of levodopa for the CNS.

b. If carbidopa is given in a separate dosage form, the dose of levodopa can be decreased by 75%.

c. If patients still complain of gastrointestinal side effects after combination levodopa/carbidopa, plain carbidopa (supplied by Merck & Co., Inc.) can be given.

3. **Precautions and monitoring effects**

a. Levodopa must be used with caution in patients with narrow-angle glaucoma.

b. Levodopa may activate a malignant melanoma in patients with suspicious undiagnosed skin lesions or a history of melanoma.

c. The efficacy of levodopa declines with long-term therapy by desensitizing the receptors or because of the decreased number of receptors, resulting from the progression of the disease.

d. **Adverse drug reactions**

(1) **Gastrointestinal effects** include anorexia, nausea and vomiting, and abdominal distress. Levodopa should be taken with food to minimize stomach upset.

(2) **Cardiovascular effects** include postural hypotension and tachycardia.

(3) **Musculoskeletal effects** include dystonia or choreiform muscle movement.

(4) **CNS effects** include confusion, memory changes, depression, hallucinations, and psychosis. Physicians should be notified if any of these symptoms occur.

(5) **Hematologic effects** include hemolytic anemia, leukopenia, and agranulocytosis (rare).

4. **Significant interactions**

a. **Antacids** cause rapid and complete intestinal levodopa absorption (by decreasing gastric emptying time).

b. **Hydantoin** decreases the effectiveness of levodopa.

c. **Methionine** increases the clinical signs of Parkinson's disease.

d. **Metoclopramide** increases the bioavailability of levodopa, which decreases the effects of metoclopramide on gastric emptying and on lower esophageal pressure. As a dopamine blocker, it may also precipitate parkinsonian symptoms.

e. False-positive results are seen with the Coombs test.

f. The uric acid test increases with the colorimetric method but not with the uricase method.

g. Hypertensive reactions may occur if levodopa is administered to patients receiving **MAO inhibitors** and **furazolidone**. MAO inhibitors must be discontinued 2 weeks prior to initiating levodopa.

h. Administration of **papaverine** may decrease the effect of levodopa.

i. **Tricyclic antidepressants** decrease the rate and extent of absorption of levodopa; hypertensive episodes have been reported when levodopa is administered in combination with tricyclic antidepressants.

j. **Food** decreases the rate and extent of absorption and transport to the CNS across the blood–brain barrier. A **protein-restricted diet** may also help to minimize the "fluctuations" (i.e., the decreased response to levodopa) at the end of each day or at various times of the day.

C. Direct-acting dopamine agonists

1. Bromocriptine

a. Mechanism of action. Bromocriptine is responsible for the direct stimulation of postsynaptic dopamine receptors; it is most commonly used as an adjunct to levodopa therapy in patients:

(1) With a deteriorating response to levodopa

(2) In patients with a limited clinical response to levodopa secondary to an inability to tolerate higher doses

(3) In patients who are experiencing fluctuations in response to levodopa

b. Administration and dosage (see Table 47-2)

(1) Initially, patients are given one-half tablet twice daily, which is then increased to one tablet twice daily every 2–3 days.

(2) Patients' responses are extremely variable. Many patients show a dopamine antagonist response at both low and high doses with the desirable agonist response in the mid-range.

(3) Because postural hypotension may result from the first few doses of bromocriptine, the first dose should be administered with the patient lying down, and sudden changes in posture should be avoided.

c. Precautions and monitoring effects

(1) Bromocriptine may cause a first-dose phenomenon that can trigger sudden cardiovascular collapse. It should be used with caution in patients with a history of myocardial infarction or arrhythmias.

(2) Early in therapy, dizziness, drowsiness, and fainting may occur, so patients should be cautious about driving or operating machinery. A physician should be notified if these symptoms appear.

(3) **Other adverse effects**

(a) **Gastrointestinal effects,** including anorexia, nausea, vomiting, and abdominal distress, may be decreased by taking bromocriptine with food.

(b) **Cardiovascular effects** include postural hypotension (to which tolerance develops) and tachycardia. Blood pressure must be monitored, particularly for patients taking antihypertensive medication.

(c) **Pulmonary effects,** including reversible infiltrations, pleural effusions, and pleural thickening, may develop after long-term treatment, so pulmonary function should be monitored in patients treated for longer than 6 months.

(d) **CNS effects,** including confusion, memory changes, depression, and hallucinations, and psychosis, may be exacerbated by bromocriptine; thus, patients with psychiatric illnesses must be monitored.

d. Significant interactions

(1) A combination of **antihypertensive drugs** and bromocriptine could result in a decrease in blood pressure.

(2) **Dopamine antagonists** increase the effect of bromocriptine.

2. Pergolide

a. Mechanism of action. Pergolide is a semisynthetic ergoline derivative. In Parkinson's disease, it exerts its effect by directly stimulating postsynaptic dopamine receptors in the nigrostriatal system, with D_1-agonist properties.

(1) It is 10 times more potent than bromocriptine on a milligram basis.

(2) It inhibits the secretion of prolactin, increases the serum concentration of growth hormone, and decreases the serum concentration of luteinizing hormone.

(3) It is most commonly used as adjunctive treatment to levodopa/carbidopa.

b. Administration and dosage (see Table 47-2)

c. Precautions and monitoring effects

(1) Hypersensitivity reactions to pergolide and other ergot derivatives can occur.

(2) Caution must be used with patients who are at high risk for ventricular arrhythmia, especially when doses higher than 3 mg/day are used.

(3) Adverse effects are similar to those experienced with bromocriptine [see II C 1 c (3)].

(4) **CNS effects** include dyskinesia, hallucinations, somnolence, and insomnia.

(5) **Gastrointestinal effects** include nausea, constipation, diarrhea, and dyspepsia.

(6) **Cardiovascular effects** include premature atrial contractions and sinus tachycardia (alone or in combination with levodopa).

(7) **Miscellaneous effects** include transient elevations of aspartate aminotransferase, alanine aminotransferase, and alkaline phosphatase, and pleural thickening.

d. **Significant interactions**

(1) Because pergolide is 90% protein bound, it must be used with caution with other highly **protein-bound drugs**.

(2) **Antipsychotic agents** (e.g., phenothiazines, haloperidol, metoclopramide) given in combination with dopamine agonists decrease the dopamine action and decrease the therapeutic action of the antipsychotic agent.

D. Indirect-acting dopamine agonists

1. Selegiline

a. **Mechanism of action**

(1) MAO catabolizes various catecholamines (e.g., dopamine, norepinephrine, epinephrine), serotonin, and various exogenous amines (e.g., tyramines) found in foods (e.g., aged cheese, beer, wine, smoked meat) and drugs. Lack of MAO in the intestinal tract causes absorption of these amines, causing a hypertensive crisis. MAO type A is predominantly found in the intestinal tract, and MAO type B, in the brain. They differ in their substrate specificity and tissue distribution. This specificity decreases with selegiline as the dose increases. Most patients experience side effects at doses of selegiline higher than 30–40 mg/day.

(2) Selegiline is a selective inhibitor of MAO type B, which prevents the breakdown of dopamine selectively in the brain at recommended doses.

(3) Selegiline is most commonly used as an adjunct with levodopa/carbidopa when patients experience a "wearing-off" phenomenon; it decreases the amount of "off" time and decreases the dose needed of levodopa/carbidopa by 10%–30%.

(4) Results of some studies show that selegiline delays the time before which treatment with a more potent dopaminergic drug like levodopa is needed; the proposed mechanism of action is that an oxidation mechanism contributes to the emergence and progression of Parkinson's disease.

b. **Administration and dosage** (see Table 47-2). Exceeding the recommended dose of 10 mg/day increases the risk of losing MAO selectivity. The precise selectivity dose is unknown but seems to be above 30–40 mg/day.

c. **Precautions and monitoring effects.** The adverse effects are similar to those listed for levodopa (see II B 3 d).

(1) **Gastrointestinal effects** include nausea, abdominal pain, and dry mouth. Selegiline should be used with caution in patients known to have ulcers because of its potential to inhibit MAO-mediated gastric histamine catabolism.

(2) **CNS effects** include dizziness, confusion, headache, hallucinations, vivid dreams, and dyskinesias. Patients who experience insomnia should avoid taking the drug late in the day.

(3) **Hepatic effects** include mild and transient elevations in liver function tests.

(4) Patients should be educated about foods and drugs containing tyramine and the signs and symptoms of hypertensive reactions.

d. **Significant interactions.** MAO inhibitors are contraindicated with **meperidine** and other opioids. Because the mechanism of action is unknown, administration with opioids should be avoided.

2. Amantadine

a. **Mechanism of action.** Amantadine is an antiviral agent (used for the prevention of influenza).

(1) Amantadine increases dopamine levels at postsynaptic receptor sites by decreasing presynaptic re-uptake and enhancing dopamine synthesis and release.

(2) It may also have some anticholinergic effects. It decreases tremor, rigidity, and bradykinesia.

(3) It can be given in combination with levodopa as Parkinson's disease progresses.

(4) Clinical effects of amantadine can be seen within the first few weeks of therapy unlike the other antiparkinsonian medications (e.g., carbidopa/levodopa) that need weeks to months to show their full clinical effect.

b. **Administration and dosage** (see Table 47-2)

(1) Amantadine should be started at 100 mg/day. This may be increased to 200–300 mg/day as a maintenance dose.

(2) Patients experiencing a decline in response may benefit from the following:
   (a) Discontinuing the drug for a few weeks, then restarting it
   (b) Using the drug episodically, only when the patient's condition most needs a therapeutic boost
(3) Amantadine is also available in liquid form for patients with dysphagia.

c. **Precautions and monitoring effects**
   (1) Amantadine should be used with caution in patients with renal disease, congestive heart failure (CHF), peripheral edema, history of seizures, and mental status changes. Dosage modification may be necessary in patients with renal failure.
   (2) Tolerance usually develops within 6–12 months. If tolerance occurs, another drug from a different class can be added, or the dose may be increased.
   (3) Patients should be informed about the side effect profile.
      (a) **Peripheral anticholinergic effects** include those mentioned in II A 3 d (1).
      (b) **CNS effects** include seizures as well as those mentioned in II A 3 d (2).
      (c) **Cardiovascular effects.** Patients may develop CHF. Periodic blood pressure monitoring and electrocardiograms (ECGs) are necessary in patients with myocardial infarction or arrhythmias.
      (d) **Dermatologic effects** include **livedo reticularis,** a diffuse rose color mottling of the skin, which is reversible upon discontinuation of the drug.
      (e) **Hematologic effects.** Periodic complete blood counts (CBCs) should be done for patients with long-term therapy.

d. **Significant interactions**
   (1) Amantadine increases the anticholinergic effects of **anticholinergic drugs,** necessitating a decrease in the dosage of the anticholinergic drug.
   (2) **Hydrochlorothiazide** plus **triamterene** decrease the urinary excretion of amantidine and increase its plasma concentration.

III. SURGICAL TREATMENT includes autologous adrenal medullar or fetal substantia nigra transplants, but the validity, applicability, and long-term benefits of surgery are unknown at the present time.

STUDY QUESTIONS

Directions: Each of the numbered items or incomplete statements in this section is followed by answers or by completions of the statement. Select the **one** lettered answer or completion that is **best** in each case.

1. The maximum recommended daily dose of levodopa is

(A) 500 mg
(B) 1 g
(C) 2 g
(D) 4 g
(E) 8 g

2. When administered with carbidopa, the dosage of levodopa is usually decreased by

(A) 75%
(B) 50%
(C) 40%
(D) 20%
(E) 10%

3. Which of the following agents should not be used concurrently with levodopa?

(A) Diphenhydramine
(B) Benztropine
(C) Amantadine
(D) Monoamine oxidase (MAO) inhibitors
(E) Carbidopa

Directions: Each item below contains three suggested answers of which **one or more** is correct. Choose the answer

A if **I only** is correct
B if **III only** is correct
C if **I and II** are correct
D if **II and III** are correct
E if **I, II, and III** are correct

4. Levodopa is associated with which of the following problems?

I. Gastrointestinal side effects
II. Involuntary movements
III. A decline in efficacy after 3–5 years

5. Amantadine has which of the following advantages over levodopa?

I. More rapid relief of symptoms
II. Higher success rate
III. Better long-term effects

1-E
2-A
3-D
4-E
5-A

ANSWERS AND EXPLANATIONS

1. The answer is E *[II B 2; Table 47-2].*
The maximum total daily dose of levodopa should be 8 g, administered in divided doses at least three times a day. Levodopa is used in the treatment of Parkinson's disease to replenish the brain's supply of dopamine, the neurotransmitter that is deficient in this disorder. Dopamine itself does not cross the blood–brain barrier, and therefore its precursor, levodopa, is administered. Levodopa is metabolized to dopamine in the body by dopa decarboxylase. Dosage of levodopa must be carefully titrated for each patient to produce the maximum improvement with the least side effects.

2. The answer is A *[II B 2 b].*
Administering carbidopa in combination with levodopa reduces the required dose of levodopa by about 75%. When levodopa is given alone, much of the dose is metabolized before the drug reaches the brain. Therefore, large doses are required, and these are apt to cause unwanted side effects. Carbidopa inhibits the peripheral decarboxylation of levodopa. This action simultaneously reduces the likelihood of peripheral side effects and allows more levodopa to reach the brain. Since carbidopa does not cross the blood–brain barrier, the levodopa in the brain is converted there to dopamine. Thus, coadministration of carbidopa plus levodopa allows a significant reduction of levodopa dosage without reducing the desired effects.

3. The answer is D [II B 4 g].
Levodopa causes a significant rise in blood pressure as well as flushing and palpitations when given to patients receiving monoamine oxidase (MAO) inhibitors. Levodopa can be used in combination with any of the other agents listed in the question without adverse interactions. Amantadine causes an increase in the body's dopamine supply, and carbidopa prevents decarboxylation of levodopa. Diphenhydramine (an antihistamine) and benztropine have anticholinergic effects; they are used to treat Parkinson's disease because they decrease the body's acetylcholine supply.

4. The answer is E (all) *[II B 3 c, d].*
Levodopa can cause gastrointestinal side effects such as nausea and vomiting, particularly on initiation of treatment. Bowel irregularity and gastrointestinal bleeding can also occur. With long-term levodopa therapy, involuntary choreiform movements can develop, and the efficacy of the drug declines. Other unwanted effects of levodopa include tachycardia and cardiac arrhythmias, postural hypotension, and psychiatric disturbances such as confusion or depression.

5. The answer is A (I) *[II D 2 a (4), c (2)].*
Amantadine is most efficacious within the first few weeks, while benefits from levodopa may not be seen for weeks to months. Amantadine is more beneficial than the anticholinergics, but is less effective than levodopa. Unfortunately, the efficacy of amantadine declines after 6–12 months of therapy. The efficacy of levodopa declines after 3–5 years of therapy.

48
Schizophrenia

Helen L. Figge

I. INTRODUCTION

A. Definition. Schizophrenia is a group of disorders involving disruption of thought and disintegration of personality. Symptoms involve alterations in behavior, thought, affect, and perception. Schizophrenia is characterized by all of the following disturbances in the content and form of thought:

1. Hallucinations
2. Delusions
3. Flat or grossly inappropriate affect
4. Catatonic behavior
5. Incoherence or marked loosening of associations

B. Incidence. Schizophrenia occurs in about 0.5%–1% of the general population. Onset is usually between the ages of 15 and 45 years with an equal distribution between men and women.

C. Etiology. Although the actual cause of schizophrenia is unproven, theorized etiologies can be categorized broadly as genetic, neurophysiologic, and psychosocial.

1. **Genetic studies** have provided significant data supporting a genetic basis for schizophrenia. The risk factor in the general population is 0.5%–1% but increases to 5%–10% if one parent has a history of schizophrenia. It may be as high as 46% if both parents are affected.
2. **Neurophysiologic theories** focus on a possible imbalance of brain neurotransmitter physiology. The predominant theory, the **dopamine hypothesis,** suggests that overactivity of dopamine in the brain is responsible. However, the recent introduction of clozapine, an antipsychotic agent with little effect on the dopamine system but marked efficacy, seriously challenges the dopamine hypothesis. Additional theories in this category focus on other neurotransmitters.
3. **Psychosocial theories,** though largely unproven, do exist. Among the proposed causes are stress, lack of interpersonal skills, conflicting and contradictory family communication, and socioeconomic influences. Each theory has its supporters, but none is definitive.

D. Clinical presentation. Characterization of the disorder has not been standardized.

1. **Four A's.** Swiss psychiatrist Eugen Bleuler (1857–1939) described the four A's of schizophrenia; however, these have been criticized as nonspecific symptoms because they are also seen in nonschizophrenics.
   - a. **Association defect** entails impaired thinking as evidenced by illogical or idiosyncratic thought processes. One idea is not obviously connected with the next, and verbalization ranges from subtly confusing to grossly disorganized.
   - b. **Affect.** The patient experiences an alteration of mood or feelings; the affect may be flat with no emotional responsiveness or inappropriate.
   - c. **Ambivalence.** Opposing attitudes may exist simultaneously, or there may be rapid fluctuations among contradictory emotions.
   - d. **Autism.** The patient may withdraw into a private world, absorbed in inner thoughts.
2. **Additional features** of importance include the following:
   - a. **Hallucinations.** Sensory perceptions may be abnormal, occurring without external stimuli. Any sense may be affected, but **auditory hallucinations** are the most common.

b. **Delusions.** Firmly held but false beliefs are expressed that have absolutely no basis in fact. These may be simple or multiple, poorly or well organized, and bizarre or seemingly realistic. Often they feature persecutory content. Patients may complain that their thoughts are being read by others or are being broadcast to others, that people are spying on them or talking about them, or that they are being controlled.

E. **Diagnostic criteria.** The current approach to diagnostic criteria is based on the *Diagnostic and Statistical Manual of Mental Disorders,* 3rd ed. (revised) [*DSM-III-R*]*, as summarized below.

1. During a phase of the illness, at least one of the following symptoms must be present for at least 1 week:
   a. Two of the following:
      (1) Delusions
      (2) Prominent hallucinations
      (3) Incoherence or marked loosening of associations
      (4) Catatonic behavior
      (5) Flat or grossly inappropriate affect
   b. Bizarre delusions
   c. Prominent hallucinations of a voice with content having no apparent relation to depression or elation, or a voice keeping up a running commentary on the person's behavior or thoughts
2. During the course of the disturbance, functioning in areas such as work, social relations, and self-care is markedly impaired.
3. Other disorders, such as schizoaffective disorders and mood disorders with psychotic features, must be ruled out.
4. Continuous signs of the disturbance must be present for at least 6 months.
5. An organic factor cannot be established that initiates or maintains the disturbance.
6. If there is a history of autistic disorder, prominent delusions or hallucinations must be present.

F. **Classification** of schizophrenia is based on the symptoms predominating at the time of evaluation, but these syndromes may change over time.

1. **Disorganized (hebephrenic) schizophrenia** is characterized by marked incoherence with inappropriate responses or unresponsiveness. Delusions or hallucinations are disorganized and fragmented. The patient may giggle, grimace, and act in an incongruous or silly manner. Hypochondriacal behavior may be present.
2. **Catatonic schizophrenia** is distinguished by marked psychomotor disturbances. The patient may demonstrate rigidity, immobility, or posturing and may also be withdrawn and silent. At the other extreme is characteristic excitement, such as pacing and shouting. Fluctuations between these behavioral extremes may occur.
3. **Paranoid schizophrenia** is identified by its most prominent characteristics: delusions of grandeur or persecution, during which the patient may be extremely aggressive and argumentative, even violent. Many of these patients are intensely concerned with homosexual impulses in themselves or others.
4. **Undifferentiated schizophrenia** may incorporate prominent delusions, hallucinations, incoherence, or grossly disorganized behavior, but the overall picture either does not meet the criteria for one of the specific types or meets the criteria for more than one type.
5. **Residual schizophrenia** designates a patient who, while not currently acutely psychotic, has a history of at least one prior episode of prominent psychotic symptoms. Residual symptoms such as loose or vague associations, illogical thinking, withdrawal, or inappropriate affect may be present, and daily living skills may be impaired.

G. **Treatment objectives.** Because there is no known cure for schizophrenia, treatment is primarily aimed at relieving symptoms. The two major therapeutic approaches—psychotherapy and pharmacotherapy with antipsychotic (neuroleptic) agents—share the following goals:

1. Bring the patient's thoughts and behavior under control

---

*American Psychiatric Association: *Diagnostic and Statistical Manual of Mental Disorders,* 3rd ed. (revised). Washington, DC, 1987.

2. Prevent self-inflicted harm
3. Restore contact with reality
4. Return the patient to society
5. Prevent a relapse

II. THERAPY: ANTIPSYCHOTIC AGENTS

A. Choice of agent. With the exception of clozapine, all antipsychotic agents are therapeutically equivalent when administered in appropriate doses, but responses vary from patient to patient and drug to drug. Consideration should be given prior to medical experience, if applicable. A patient who has failed to respond to a particular drug in the past is not likely to respond to that drug at any time. The major difference among these agents is their adverse effects (see II F).

B. Mechanism of action is not understood. It has been thought that the drugs work by antagonizing dopamine action; however, this view has been challenged by the introduction of clozapine, which appears to be more therapeutically effective than other agents; yet, it has only weak antidopaminergic effects. The dopamine theory has rested on the premise that most neuroleptics have antidopaminergic activity.

C. Specific agents (Table 48-1)

D. Administration and dosage

1. **General guidelines**
   - **a.** A drug-response history should be obtained, and potential side effects should be considered.
   - **b.** Therapy should be initiated, using a single drug administered in divided doses.
   - **c.** The first symptoms to respond are usually aggressiveness, paranoia, and irritability; later symptoms to be reduced are hallucinations and changes in social skills.
   - **d.** Once the patient has been stabilized, attempts should be made to lower the dose. The lowest possible dose should be used for maintenance.
   - **e.** When discontinuing therapy, withdrawal should be tapered.
2. **Gradual control method.** This is the standard therapeutic method.
   - **a.** Initial doses should be at the lower end of the usual daily dose schedule (see Table 48-1), such as 300–400 mg of chlorpromazine daily. Doses should be divided initially to allow for observation of effect and toxicity.

Table 48-1. Currently Available Antipsychotic Agents

Agent	Nonproprietary Name	Brand Name	Approximate Equivalent Dose	Usual Daily Dose Range (mg/day)	
				Acute	Maintenance
Phenothiazines					
Aliphatics	Chlorpromazine	Thorazine	100	300–800	100–300
Piperidines	Mesoridazine	Serentil	50	25–400	30–150
	Thioridazine	Mellaril	100	300–800	100–300
Piperazines	Acetophenazine	Tindal	25	40–120	20–40
	Fluphenazine	Prolixin	2	6–60	2–8
	Perphenazine	Trilafon	6–10	16–24	8–24
	Trifluoperazine	Stelazine	3–5	15–60	5–15
Thioxanthenes	Chlorprothixene	Taractan	100	300–600	75–400
	Thiothixene	Navane	3–5	10–60	4–30
Butyrophenones	Haloperidol	Haldol	2	1–100	1–15
Dihydroindolones	Molindone	Moban	10	15–225	15–100
Dibenzoxazepines	Loxapine	Loxitane	15	20–100	60–100
Dibenzodiazepines	Clozapine	Clozaril	ND	ND	250–450

ND = not determined

b. If no improvement is noted after 1 week, doses may be increased by 25%–33% weekly, if necessary. Increases should be smaller in the elderly and in other individuals known to be at particular risk for adverse effects. For patients who are acutely psychotic and agitated, increases may be larger.
c. Maximal improvement may take 6–8 weeks or longer if this is not initial therapy.
d. Once a patient's response and tolerance have been determined, the drug may be administered in one or two daily doses.

3. **Rapid control method.** This approach usually is reserved for patients who are acutely psychotic with agitation.
a. High-potency agents, such as fluphenazine or haloperidol, usually are injected intramuscularly; for example, haloperidol may be initiated at a dose of 5–10 mg every hour until the acute symptoms are controlled, adverse effects occur, or the patient falls asleep.
b. Once control has been established, therapy should be converted to oral administration. The physician may elect to administer the same agent, but in oral form, at a dose appropriate for initial therapy. Dosage may then be adjusted in accordance with the patient's response.

4. **Maintenance therapy** to prevent relapse has less clear guidelines.
a. Some practitioners suggest that therapy be continued for 6 months after an acute episode before drug withdrawal is considered. Signs favoring discontinuation of therapy include the following:
(1) Continued control of symptoms during maintenance therapy
(2) No history of relapse ensuing from drug withdrawal
(3) Willingness of the patient to discontinue therapy
b. Other practitioners suggest that therapy be continued for 6 months in a patient who has had one episode, for 1 year after a second episode, and indefinitely after a third episode.
c. **Long-acting (depot) preparations** are primarily for maintenance therapy and are administered intramuscularly. Depot preparations may improve compliance and help to prevent relapse.
(1) While the three preparations currently available are therapeutically equivalent, they differ in duration of action and in therapeutic dose.
(a) **Fluphenazine decanoate** has a longer duration of action than fluphenazine enanthate and may produce fewer extrapyramidal effects. A dose may last 3–4 weeks.
(b) **Fluphenazine enanthate** may require administration every 2 weeks.
(c) **Haloperidol decanoate** may be administered every 4 weeks.
(2) Therapy should be initiated at low doses to minimize adverse effects.
(3) If the patient has been receiving oral therapy, continuing the oral medication for the first few weeks of depot therapy may be beneficial while the blood levels of the depot preparation accumulate to steady-state levels.
(4) Before converting to long-acting preparations, it would be helpful if the patient were first converted to oral fluphenazine or haloperidol. Several formulas are available to guide the conversion, but they are only rough guidelines for initiation of therapy.
(5) Once depot therapy has begun, the patient must be monitored carefully to facilitate dosage adjustments.

E. **Evaluation of patient response** should focus on target symptoms to determine therapeutic effectiveness.

1. **Positive symptoms,** such as hallucinations, delusions, hostility, and hyperactivity, are most likely to respond to antipsychotic agents.

2. **Negative symptoms,** such as poor judgment, apathy, social incompetence, and withdrawal, are less likely to respond.

F. **Precautions and monitoring effects** (Table 48-2 lists the association of major side effects with specific antipsychotic agents.)

1. **Sedative effects** are common, particularly with the **phenothiazines**.

2. **Extrapyramidal effects**
a. **Dystonic reactions** involve sudden muscle spasms of the neck, face, or trunk. These reactions include torticollis (neck twisting), trismus (clenched jaw), and oculogyric crisis (fixed upward gaze). The risk of dystonias is highest during the first 24–48 hours of therapy

Table 48-2. Likelihood of Adverse Effects with Antipsychotic Agents

Agent	Sedative	Extrapyramidal	Anticholinergic	Cardiovascular (Alpha Blockade)
Acetophenazine	Medium	High	Medium	Low
Chlorpromazine	High	Medium	High	High
Chlorprothixene	High	Medium	Medium	Medium
Clozapine	High	Very low	High	High
Fluphenazine	Low	High	Low	Low
Haloperidol	Medium	High	Low	Low
Loxapine	Medium	High	Low	Medium
Mesoridazine	High	Low	Medium	Medium
Molindone	Low	High	Low	Low
Perphenazine	Low	High	Medium	Low
Thioridazine	High	Low	High	High
Thiothixene	Low	High	Low	Low
Trifluoperazine	Low	High	Low	Low

and when the dose is increased; they are most likely to occur in young patients, in men, and in patients receiving high doses. Dystonias can be managed initially through intramuscular or intravenous administration of anticholinergic agents, such as diphenhydramine or benztropine mesylate. Further reactions may be prevented by a short course of oral anticholinergic therapy.

b. Akathisia is associated with an inner tension or agitation that is relieved by activity. Patients usually manifest this restlessness in an inability to keep their legs and feet still. This side effect most commonly appears within the first few weeks of therapy and may respond to anticholinergic agents or diazepam. If not, a change in neuroleptic agent or discontinuation of therapy may be necessary.

c. Drug-induced parkinsonism includes parkinsonian symptoms such as akinesia, rigidity, resting tremor, shuffling gait, mask-like facial expression, and slowed speech. The onset of symptoms may occur within weeks or months. A related but less common effect, known as the **rabbit syndrome,** compels the patient to movements resembling the chewing motions typical of rabbits. Anticholinergic agents should manage these effects.

d. Tardive dyskinesia

(1) This disorder is characterized by abnormal facial movements with chewing, tongue protrusion, and puckering of the mouth. The reaction may progress to the extremities and trunk, producing involuntary movements, disturbance of the gag reflex, or respiratory distress.

(2) A late-onset effect, tardive dyskinesia usually does not appear for months or years. It is thought to be due to prolonged dopamine receptor blockade, which leads to increased receptor sensitivity, so that dopamine stimulation tends to produce movement disorders. The syndrome may begin when drugs are discontinued; in fact, a short drug holiday may reveal symptoms, allowing early detection.

(3) Treatment. Anticholinergics do not alleviate the syndrome and may even worsen it. Treatment attempts have been aimed at increasing cholinergic activity, using such compounds as physostigmine, lecithin, and choline, or decreasing dopamine activity. Agents that increase γ-aminobutyric acid (GABA) activity have had some success. No definitive treatment has been identified; the emphasis is on prevention.

(a) Antipsychotics and anticholinergics should be used only when needed and in the lowest possible doses.

(b) Patients should be examined for early signs of dyskinesia (e.g., fine worm-like movements when the tongue is at rest, facial tics, increased frequency of blinking). If any are discovered, antipsychotics should be discontinued gradually, if feasible. Nevertheless, symptoms may persist for months to years and may be irreversible.

(c) If the patient's condition necessitates continuing the medication, the lowest therapeutic dosage should be used.

3. Anticholinergic effects include dry mouth, blurred vision, constipation, and urinary retention. Administering the dose at night or reducing the dosage may reduce significant or persistent effects.

4. Cardiovascular effects include orthostatic hypotension resulting from alpha blockade. Other potential effects include reflex tachycardia and electrocardiogram abnormalities, specifically S-T depression, flattened T waves, Q-T prolongation, and the appearance of U waves.
5. **Ocular effects**
   a. **Degenerative pigmentary retinopathy** may occur with high doses of **thioridazine** (the maximum daily dose should be 800 mg).
   b. **Corneal lens opacities** have been associated with antipsychotic therapy, especially with **chlorpromazine**. Slit-lamp examination helps detect deposits in the cornea or lens. These deposits usually do not affect vision and may resolve within months after discontinuation of the drug.
6. Decreased seizure threshold may occur with neuroleptics, and they should be used cautiously in a patient with a seizure disorder. Anticonvulsant dose increases may be necessary.
7. **Neuroleptic malignant syndrome** is an uncommon but serious and potentially life-threatening complication of therapy. It is a complex of extrapyramidal effects, hyperthermia, altered consciousness, and autonomic changes (e.g., tachycardia, unstable blood pressure, diaphoresis, incontinence). The onset is sudden, and recovery may take 5–10 days after discontinuation of therapy. Specific management includes discontinuation of the drug; supportive measures, such as temperature control; and drug therapy with dantrolene or bromocriptine.
8. **Additional effects**
   a. **Temperature regulation** may be impaired, causing the patient to assume the environmental temperature; this can result in hyperthermia or hypothermia.
   b. **Sexual dysfunction** may include impotence, inability to ejaculate, retrograde ejaculation, diminished libido, amenorrhea, galactorrhea, and gynecomastia. These effects are seen most commonly with **thioridazine**.
   c. **Photosensitivity** in the form of gray to purple pigmentation has been reported with chlorpromazine, thioridazine, and the thiothixenes. A correlation has been noted between skin and ocular pigmentation; patients with a photosensitive reaction should have an ocular examination.

G. Clozapine therapy

1. **Overview.** Clozapine is one of the first effective antipsychotic agents to have few of the extrapyramidal side effects that are typical of nearly all of the neuroleptic agents in clinical use today.
   a. It can be effective in treating some patients who are unresponsive to standard neuroleptic drugs.
   b. It has only weak dopaminergic activity.
   c. In 14 double-blind studies, clozapine produced superior clinical results in 79% of subjects as compared to a standard neuroleptic agent.
2. **Precautions and monitoring effects**
   a. The major side effect is agranulocytosis, which may be fatal. Thus, patients taking clozapine must be routinely monitored by blood counts at intervals established by the physician but usually as often as once a week. This has contributed to the relatively high annual cost for providing this drug to individual patients.
   b. Other possible side effects are seizures, hypotension, fatigue, sedation, nausea, and vomiting.

STUDY QUESTIONS

Directions: Each of the numbered items or incomplete statements in this section is followed by answers or by completions of the statement. Select the **one** lettered answer or completion that is **best** in each case.

1. All of the following statements concerning antipsychotic agents are true EXCEPT

(A) studies have proven chlorpromazine to be the most effective antipsychotic agent
(B) patients who have responded to a particular drug in the past are likely to respond to retreatment with that same drug
(C) the major differences among antipsychotic drugs are their side effects
(D) any given patient may or may not respond to any given antipsychotic drug
(E) newly diagnosed, young patients tend to respond to drugs better than older chronic schizophrenic patients

2. The four A's that Bleuler used to characterize schizophrenia include all of the following EXCEPT

(A) anxiety
(B) ambivalence
(C) association defect
(D) autism
(E) alteration of affect

3. Which of the following is an example of delusion?

(A) Hearing strange voices
(B) Seeing someone who is not really there
(C) The feeling that ants are crawling all over the body
(D) The lack of any emotional response to any situation
(E) The belief that an advertisement on television is speaking directly to the individual with a secret message

4. Most antipsychotic agents except clozapine are potent blockers of which neurotransmitters?

(A) Acetylcholine
(B) Dopamine
(C) Calcium
(D) Zinc
(E) Norepinephrine

5. The earliest movement disorder to appear during neuroleptic therapy is

(A) pseudoparkinsonism
(B) dystonia
(C) tardive dyskinesia
(D) akathisia
(E) resting tumor

6. Specific therapy for an acute extrapyramidal reaction to chlorpromazine is

(A) physostigmine
(B) diphenhydramine
(C) bethanechol
(D) propranolol
(E) metoclopramide

1-A 4-B
2-A 5-B
3-E 6-B

Questions 7–10

A 35-year-old man was brought to the emergency room because he was swinging at passersby in a shopping mall. He required four-point restraints for acute agitation. No history could be obtained except for the patient declaring that multiple voices were telling him to knock down the people in the mall who were chasing him.

On physical examination, the patient was extremely agitated and uncooperative. Blood pressure was 120/85, pulse 94, and respirations 16. General examination was superficially unremarkable; neurological examination was grossly nonfocal except for the mental status examination, which revealed elements of hallucinations, delusions of persecution, and multiple loose associations. Local authorities reported that the patient had escaped from a local psychiatric facility and had been missing for 3 days. His previous treatment regimen was chlorpromazine (800 mg daily in divided doses). When compliant with the medication, the patient's symptoms were well controlled.

7. What therapeutic agent could be given to control the patient's present symptoms?

(A) Haloperidol
(B) Clozapine
(C) Lithium
(D) Fluoxetine

8. Which subtype of schizophrenia is the patient likely to have?

(A) Hebephrenic
(B) Catatonic
(C) Paranoid
(D) Residual

9. After initial therapy, the patient develops trismus associated with torticollis. Which of the following agents should be administered to control these reactions?

(A) Haloperidol
(B) Clozapine
(C) Diphenhydramine
(D) Diazepam

10. What is the usual dose of the appropriate agent from question number 7?

(A) 5–10 mg every hour intramuscularly until control of symptoms is achieved
(B) 50–100 mg every hour intramuscularly until control of symptoms is achieved
(C) 5–10 mg orally for a single dose
(D) 50–100 mg for a single dose

Directions: The group of items in this section consists of lettered options followed by a set of numbered items. For each item, select the **one** lettered option that is most closely associated with it. Each lettered option may be selected once, more than once, or not at all.

Questions 11–15

Match the drug with the phrase that most accurately describes it.

(A) Used in depot preparations
(B) Used in the management of neuroleptic malignant syndrome
(C) High doses may cause degenerative pigmentary retinopathy
(D) Counteracts dystonias
(E) Produces minimal sedative effects

11. Thioridazine
12. Benztropine mesylate
13. Dantrolene
14. Molindone
15. Haloperidol

7-A	10-A	13-B
8-C	11-C	14-E
9-C	12-D	15-A

ANSWERS AND EXPLANATIONS

1. The answer is A *[II A, G].*
Those individuals most likely to respond to antipsychotic drugs are young patients. Current evidence suggests that clozapine may be more effective than chlorpromazine. Any given patient may respond to any given antipsychotic drug; however, when selecting a drug to treat a patient with schizophrenia, a past history of success with a particular drug indicates that the patient will probably respond to that drug again. The major differences among antipsychotic drugs are their side effects.

2. The answer is A *[I D 1].*
Bleuler described the four A's of schizophrenia by using the symptoms of association defect, abnormal affect, ambivalence, and autism. Anxiety disorders are a different class of psychological disorders.

3. The answer is E *[I D 2 b].*
A hallucination is an abnormal sensory perception, such as hearing or seeing something that is not there. The lack of an emotional response to any situation is due to an abnormal affect. A delusion is a firmly held but false belief, such as having one's thoughts read or the belief that an advertisement is speaking directly to you with a secret message.

4. The answer is B *[II B].*
The classic neuroleptics block dopamine receptors, but clozapine has only weak dopaminergic action. Clozapine has potent antimuscarinic receptor activity.

5. The answer is B *[II F 2 a].*
In patients given antipsychotic drugs, dystonic reactions have the earliest onset—that is, the risk is highest during the first 24–48 hours of therapy and when the dose is increased. Pseudoparkinsonism, which is characterized in part by a resting tremor, may not begin for weeks to months after initiation of antipsychotic therapy; and tardive dyskinesia is usually not seen for months to years. Akathisia begins within the first few weeks of therapy.

6. The answer is B *[II F 2 a–c].*
Acute extrapyramidal reactions are due to excess cholinergic activity resulting from the blockade of dopamine receptors by the neuroleptic agent. Specific treatment is administration of an agent with anticholinergic activity, such as diphenhydramine.

7–10. The answers are: 7-A *[II D 3 a],* **8-C** *[I F 3],* **9-C** *[II F 2 a],* **10-A** *[II D 3 a].*
Haloperidol can be used effectively for the acute treatment of psychosis. Clozapine is reserved for recalcitrant cases. Lithium is used to treat bipolar disorder, which this patient does not have. Fluoxetine is used to treat depression.

The patient described in the question exhibits the classic features of paranoid schizophrenia, including delusions of grandeur or persecution, during which the patient may become extremely aggressive and violent. Some paranoid schizophrenics may become obsessed with homosexual impulses.

The patient is experiencing a dystonic reaction from the haloperidol; this should be treated with the intravenous administration of an anticholinergic agent such as diphenhydramine. Clozapine would not be an appropriate choice for this acute intervention.

Standard dosing of haloperidol for an acute situation is 5–10 mg intramuscularly every hour until the acute symptoms are controlled, adverse effects occur, or the patient falls asleep.

11–15. The answers are: 11-C *[II F 5 a],* **12-D** *[II F 2 a],* **13-B** *[II F 7],* **14-E** *[Table 48-2],* **15-A** *[II D 4 c].*
Pigmentary retinopathy may be caused by thioridazine when administered in doses over 800 mg/day. Benztropine mesylate has anticholinergic activity and may be used to manage the extrapyramidal side effects associated with antipsychotic therapy. Dantrolene, through its effects on muscles, may be able to control the signs of neuroleptic malignant syndrome. Although sedation is common to all antipsychotic agents, molindone, thiothixene, and most piperazine phenothiazines are associated with a lower incidence of this effect. Two antipsychotic agents are currently available in depot (long-acting) formulations: fluphenazine (as the decanoate or the enanthate) and haloperidol decanoate.

49
Affective Disorders

Helen L. Figge

I. INTRODUCTION

A. Definition. Affective disorders are characterized by disturbances of mood, such as low and depressed states or periods of exhilaration to the point of mania. Affective disorders are considered in two major classifications.

1. **Unipolar disorder.** The patient experiences depressive episodes.
2. **Bipolar disorder.** The patient experiences depressive and manic episodes or, less commonly, manic episodes alone.

B. Incidence. Affective disorders rank as the **most common psychiatric disorders**.

1. **Unipolar disorder.** Estimates indicate that 18%–23% of adult women and 8%–11% of adult men experience at least one major depressive episode. Onset of a major depressive illness may occur at any age but is most common in the late twenties.
2. **Bipolar disorder.** This form of affective disorder is much less common than the unipolar type. Its incidence ranges between 0.4% and 1.2% of the adult population with approximately equal distribution among men and women. Onset generally occurs before age 30.

C. Etiology. Although no consensus has been achieved on precise causes for affective disorders, theorists focus on genetic, biologic, and psychological factors.

1. **Genetic factors**
   - **a.** Research indicates an increased frequency of occurrence in families of patients with affective disorders as compared with the general population.
   - **b.** Studies of monozygotic and dizygotic twins support theories of genetic influence on the development of major affective disorders. However, they also indicate that other factors are involved.
2. **Neurochemical factors**
   - **a.** The **biogenic amine hypothesis** proposes that depression is due to a deficiency of either norepinephrine or serotonin and that mania results from an excess of norepinephrine.
   - **b.** The **permissive hypothesis** states the following:
     - **(1)** Serotonin deficiencies may create a predisposition to a major affective disorder.
     - **(2)** Deficiencies of both serotonin and norepinephrine result in depression.
     - **(3)** A serotonin deficiency accompanied by a norepinephrine excess results in mania.
   - **c.** The **receptor sensitivity theory** proposes that there is an alteration of receptor sensitivity to neurotransmitters; consequently, antidepressants exert their effects by altering receptor sensitivity.
3. **Psychological factors.** Theories proposing a psychological basis for the origin of major depressive episodes abound. For example, one hypothesis suggests that stress or loss may result in an episode of clinical depression, especially if coupled with the patient's inability to cope with the event.

D. Treatment goals

1. To shorten the episode
2. To prevent recurrence

II. CLINICAL EVALUATION

A. General. Diagnosis of an affective disorder requires the following determinations.

1. The mood disturbance (unipolar or bipolar) should be evident.

2. The symptoms should not be superimposed on a schizophrenic disorder.

3. The mood disturbance must not be due to an organic mental disorder or simple bereavement.

B. Unipolar disorders

1. Major depressive illness is characterized by mood depression or loss of interest or pleasure in all or almost all usual activities.

2. The mood disturbance must be prominent and relatively persistent.

3. Differential diagnosis requires that four or more of the following associated signs accompany the mood disturbance for 2 weeks:
a. Appetite loss or increase with a correlative weight change
b. Insomnia or hypersomnia
c. Psychomotor retardation or agitation or both
d. Loss of interest in or gratification from family, sexual activity, work, hobbies, clubs, and other social activities
e. Feelings of worthlessness or guilt
f. Loss of energy; feeling of chronic fatigue or lack of pep
g. Decreased ability to think clearly or concentrate; impaired memory
h. Suicidal thoughts, plans, or attempts; thoughts focusing on death

C. Bipolar disorders

1. A diagnosis of bipolar disorder requires one or more periods in which the predominant mood is elated, expansive, or irritable. The mood must predominate for a distinct period, although it may alternate with depressive periods.

2. The diagnosis of the manic phase also requires that at least three of the following associated symptoms have been significant and persistent during the period (four if the mood is solely irritable):
a. Increase in activity or restlessness
b. Unusual verbosity or rapid or pressured speech
c. Flight of ideas, characterized by rapid changes in subject; racing thoughts, which can compromise coherence
d. Ease of distractibility, in which almost anything can disrupt concentration
e. Inflation of self-esteem, which can reach delusional proportions
f. Decreased need for sleep
g. Impairment of judgment, which may lead to involvement in highly consequential activities such as buying sprees, reckless driving, sexual indiscretions, and flamboyant, intrusive socializing (such as making late-night phone calls or visits)

3. The disorder must be severe enough to interfere with work, relationships, or social activities, or require hospitalization to prevent harmful activities.

III. CLINICAL COURSE

A. Depressive episodes

1. These episodes are usually self-limiting, lasting 6 months or less.

2. With proper and timely therapy, up to 85% of patients who experience depressive episodes may achieve a complete response.

3. The clinical course may be:
a. Limited—to a single episode
b. Recurrent—with two or more episodes separated by intervals of varying lengths (episodes may also occur in clusters)
c. Chronic—in which some symptoms may persist for up to 2 years with asymptomatic periods of less than 2 months

4. The major risk for these patients is suicide.

B. Manic episodes

1. If untreated, manic episodes may last from days to months.
2. Recurrence intervals are unpredictable, but it is not unusual for episodes to occur at 1- to 2-year intervals.
3. The sequence of episodes in bipolar disorder is also unpredictable. Manic episodes are not necessarily followed by depressive periods.

IV. TREATMENT OF UNIPOLAR (DEPRESSIVE) DISORDERS.

Depressive episodes may be managed with pharmacotherapy, psychotherapy, electroconvulsive therapy, or a combination of modalities. This discussion will be limited to pharmacotherapy; specifically, cyclic antidepressants and monoamine oxidase (MAO) inhibitors.

A. Cyclic antidepressants

1. **Types** (classified according to number of rings) **available in the United States***
   a. **One ring.** Bupropion (Wellbutrin)
   b. **Two rings.** Fluoxetine (Prozac)
   c. **Three rings**
      (1) Amitriptyline (Elavil)
      (2) Doxepin (Adapin)
      (3) Imipramine (Tofranil)
      (4) Trimipramine (Surmontil)
      (5) Desipramine (Norpramin)
      (6) Nortriptyline (Pamelor)
      (7) Protriptyline (Vivactil)
   d. **Four rings**
      (1) Amoxapine (Asendin)
      (2) Maprotiline (Ludiomil)
      (3) Trazodone (Desyrel)
2. **Pharmacologic properties**
   a. **Blockade of 5-hydroxytryptamine 1A (5-HT1A) [serotonin] receptors**
      (1) **Highest affinities** shown by trazodone, amitriptyline, amoxapine, doxepin, and nortriptyline
      (2) **Possible clinical consequences.** Ejaculatory disturbances
   b. **Blockade of 5-HT2 (serotonin) receptors**
      (1) **Highest affinities** shown by amoxapine, trazodone, doxepin, amitriptyline, and trimipramine
      (2) **Possible clinical consequences.** Hypotension and alleviation of migraine headaches
   c. **Blockade of norepinephrine uptake**
      (1) **Highest potency** shown by desipramine, protriptyline, nortriptyline, amoxapine, and maprotiline
      (2) **Possible clinical consequences.** Tremors, tachycardia, insomnia, erectile dysfunction, blockade of antihypertensive effects of guanethidine and guanadrel, and augmentation of pressor effects of sympathomimetic amines
   d. **Blockade of serotonin uptake**
      (1) **Highest potency** shown by fluoxetine, imipramine, amitriptyline, trazodone, and nortriptyline
      (2) **Possible clinical consequences.** Gastrointestinal disturbances, dose-dependent increase or decrease in anxiety, sexual dysfunction, extrapyramidal side effects, interactions with L-tryptophan and MAO inhibitors
   e. **Blockade of histamine H_1-receptors**
      (1) **Highest affinities** shown by doxepin, trimipramine, amitriptyline, maprotiline, and nortriptyline
      (2) **Possible clinical consequences.** Potentiation of central depressant drugs, sedation, weight gain, and hypotension
   f. **Blockade of muscarinic receptors**
      (1) **Highest affinities** shown by amitriptyline, protriptyline, trimipramine, doxepin, and imipramine

---

*Clomipramine is not marketed in the United States as an antidepressant and, therefore, is not discussed further.

(2) **Possible clinical consequences.** Blurred vision, dry mouth, sinus tachycardia, constipation, urinary retention, and memory dysfunction

g. **Blockade of α_1-adrenergic receptors**

(1) **Highest affinities** shown by doxepin, trimipramine, amitriptyline, trazodone, and amoxapine

(2) **Possible clinical consequences.** Potentiation of the antihypertensive effects of prazosin and terazosin, postural hypotension, dizziness, and reflex tachycardia

h. **Blockade of α_2-adrenergic receptors**

(1) **Highest affinities** shown by trazodone, trimipramine, amitriptyline, doxepin, and nortriptyline

(2) **Possible clinical consequences.** Blockade of the antihypertensive effects of clonidine, guanabenz, methyldopa, and guanfacine; and priapism

i. **Blockade of dopamine D_2-receptors**

(1) **Highest potency** shown by amoxapine but basically shows weak activity

(2) **Possible clinical consequences.** Extrapyramidal movement disorders, endocrine changes, and sexual dysfunction

j. **Blockade of dopamine uptake**

(1) **Highest potency** shown by bupropion but basically shows weak activity

(2) **Possible clinical consequences.** Improvement of parkinsonism and aggravation of psychosis

3. **Mechanism of action** of cyclic antidepressants remains poorly understood. It may result from a supersensitivity of catecholamine receptors in the presence of low levels of serotonin or possibly neurotransmitter receptor down regulation.

4. **Choice of agent.** All antidepressants are equally effective with similar periods of time for onset of action. The choice of an agent depends on the medical status of the patient (the type of depression), the side effect profile of the drug, and the history of a previous response of the patient or a family member to a particular antidepressant. Recommended agents for specific situations include the following:

a. **Cardiovascular effects**

(1) Congestive heart failure (CHF) or coronary disease: nortriptyline

(2) Conduction defect: maprotiline

(3) Untreated mild hypertension: imipramine

(4) Postural hypotension: bupropion, fluoxetine, and maprotiline

b. **Neurologic effects**

(1) Seizure disorder: MAO inhibitor

(2) Chronic pain syndrome: amitriptyline and doxepin

(3) Migraine headaches: trazodone, doxepin, trimipramine, and amitriptyline

c. **Gastrointestinal effects**

(1) Chronic diarrhea: doxepin, trimipramine, amitriptyline, imipramine, and protriptyline

(2) Chronic constipation: trazodone, bupropion, fluoxetine, amoxapine, maprotiline, and desipramine

(3) Peptic ulcer disease: doxepin, trimipramine, amitriptyline, and imipramine

5. **Administration and dosage**

a. **Initiation of treatment**

(1) The recommended daily dosage ranges for antidepressants are presented in Table 49-1. The high end of these dosage ranges is usually reserved for the severely ill hospitalized patient.

(2) Therapy should be initiated with one-fourth of the target dose. For example, 50 mg of amitriptyline should be administered in divided doses to minimize adverse effects.

(3) The dose may be increased once or twice a week until a response is obtained.

(4) Further increases of 50 mg weekly may be necessary until improvement, toxicity, or the upper end of the dosing range is reached.

(5) After a gradual transition, most of these drugs may be administered in a single daily dose, usually at bedtime.

(6) The elderly and patients with cardiovascular disease require lower initial doses and a slower rate of increase.

(7) **Response rate**

(a) Physiologic symptoms (e.g., sleep disturbances, anorexia, psychomotor disturbance) usually respond within 1 week.

Table 49-1. Daily Antidepressant Doses in Adults*

Agents	Starting Dosage (mg/day)	Usual Daily Dose (mg)	Usual Dosage Range (mg/day)	Therapeutic Serum Levels (ng/ml)
Tricyclics				
Amitriptyline	50	150–200	50–300	80–250†
Nortriptyline	20	75–100	30–125	50–150
Imipramine	50	75–150	50–300	150–250†
Desipramine	50	100–200	50–300	125–300
Protriptyline	10	15–40	10–60	70–260
Doxepin	50	75–150	50–300	150–250†
Trimipramine	50	100–200	50–300	150–250
Others				
Maprotiline	50	100–150	50–225	200–600
Amoxapine	50	200–300	50–400	200–600†
Bupropion	100 b.i.d.	300‡	100–450	Unidentified
Trazodone	50	150–400	50–600	800–1600
Fluoxetine	20	20–80	20–80	Unidentified

*Dosages should be divided initially for all listed drugs, and elderly individuals should be treated with about half of the usual dosage for adults.

†Active metabolites included.

‡Divided dose (100 mg t.i.d.) should be given starting on the fourth day of treatment. No single dose should exceed 150 mg, and the total dose should not exceed 450 mg/day because of the risk of seizures.

(b) Psychosocial symptoms usually respond after 2–4 weeks.

(c) Full response may require about 4 weeks. If there is no response after 4 weeks, serum drug levels should be checked, as discussed in IV A 6 b.

b. Maintenance therapy

(1) Therapy is usually maintained for 6 months after recovery to prevent a relapse.

(2) The maintenance dose is 1/3–1/2 of the dose needed to achieve remission.

(3) After the 6 months, the drug is tapered off over 4–8 weeks.

c. Prophylaxis. A patient with a history of frequent or severe episodes may require prophylactic therapy to prevent future episodes.

6. Precautions and monitoring effects

a. Contraindications

(1) Cyclic antidepressants should be avoided in patients with severely impaired liver function or with cardiac conduction defects.

(2) Coadministration of MAO inhibitors and cyclic antidepressants can result in serious reactions, including hyperpyrexia, seizures, excitation, and death. Such combination therapy is rarely warranted and should be initiated with great caution.

(3) Caution is required with administering these agents to patients with cardiovascular disease, glaucoma, benign prostatic hypertrophy, or a history of seizures or urinary retention.

b. Serum level monitoring

(1) Although therapeutic serum levels have been identified for most antidepressants (see Table 49-1), the correlation between levels and activity is unclear. Therapeutic levels do not guarantee either the desired response or a lack of adverse effects. Patients should, therefore, be evaluated by their response to therapy. Therapeutic plasma concentrations have been firmly established for only imipramine, nortriptyline, and desipramine.

(2) Orders for serum levels should account for active metabolites, as applicable.

(3) Assessment of serum levels provides several major benefits, such as helping in the detection and management of antidepressant overdose [see IV A 6 c (6)].

(4) Serum level monitoring is particularly useful in the **nonresponsive patient**.

(a) A **subtherapeutic or low-end serum level** indicates the need for incremental dosage increases.

(b) A **lower than expected serum level** despite a reasonable dose may reveal patient noncompliance.

(c) An **upper-end serum level** suggests the need to change to a different drug.

(d) **Achieving therapeutic serum levels** without obtaining patient response after 4 weeks suggests the need for re-evaluation of the diagnosis. If the physician is confident of the diagnosis, a change in medications is recommended.

c. **Adverse effects** (Table 49-2)

(1) **Sedative effects,** which may be desirable in a patient with insomnia, are usually undesirable in a patient with psychomotor retardation.

(2) **Anticholinergic effects** include dry mouth, constipation, blurred vision, and urinary retention.

(3) **Cardiac effects**

(a) Orthostatic hypotension is the most common cardiac effect (with an incidence as high as 20%).

(b) Tachycardia of the mild sinus type is common.

(c) Arrhythmias and electrocardiogram (ECG) disturbances

(i) ECG changes may include T-wave flattening or prolongation of the P-R, QRS, or Q-T intervals.

(ii) Tricyclic compounds may interfere with atrioventricular conduction, similar to the effect of quinidine. In the presence of bundle-branch block or atrioventricular block, these effects can be life-threatening. Therefore, these agents should be avoided in patients with conduction defects.

(4) **Neurologic effects**

(a) Most cyclic antidepressants tend to lower the seizure threshold.

(i) Cautious administration is required in patients with a history of seizures.

(ii) Anticonvulsant doses may need to be increased.

(iii) Maprotiline has been associated with an increased risk of seizures at doses exceeding 225 mg/day, even in patients without a history of seizures. To minimize this risk, dosage increases should be gradual.

(iv) Bupropion is also associated with increased seizure risk. Careful dosage administration is required (see Table 49-1).

(b) Neuroleptic effects, most common with amoxapine, may include:

(i) Severe restlessness and agitation (akathisia)

(ii) Tardive dyskinesia

(iii) Dystonias

(iv) Drug-induced parkinsonism

(v) Neuroleptic malignant syndrome (e.g., extrapyramidal signs, changes in blood pressure, altered consciousness, hyperpyrexia), a rare but serious complication

(5) **Dermatologic effects.** Exanthemous rash may erupt in 4%–5% of patients taking maprotiline.

Table 49-2. Incidence of Adverse Effects with Cyclic Antidepressant Use

Agents	Sedation	Anticholinergic Effects	Orthostatic Hypotension	Delay in Conduction or Arrhythmias	Lowered Seizure Threshold
Tricyclics					
Amitriptyline	High	High	High	Yes	Moderate
Nortriptyline	Moderate	Low	Low	Yes	Low
Imipramine	Moderate	Moderate	High	Yes	Moderate
Desipramine	Low	Low	Low	Yes	Low
Protriptyline	Low	Moderate	Low	Yes	Low
Doxepin	High	Moderate	High	Yes	Moderate
Trimipramine	High	High	Moderate	Yes	Moderate
Others					
Maprotiline	Moderate	Low	Moderate	Low	High
Amoxapine	Moderate	Low	Moderate	Low	Moderate
Bupropion	Very low	Very low	Very low	Low	High
Trazodone	High	Very low	Moderate	Low	Low
Fluoxetine	Very low	Very low	Very low	Low	Low

(6) **Overdosage**

(a) **Signs and symptoms** may reflect cardiac, central nervous system (CNS), and anticholinergic effects, including arrhythmias, seizures, coma, confusion, respiratory depression, hyperpyrexia, and bladder or bowel dysfunction.

(b) **Treatment** may initially include emesis or gastric lavage and administration of activated charcoal. Additional measures may include phenytoin or diazepam for seizure control and lidocaine or phenytoin for arrhythmias. Physostigmine may be helpful in certain cases.

(7) **Withdrawal symptoms,** such as nausea, headache, and malaise, can be avoided by withdrawing the drug gradually.

B. Monoamine oxidase (MAO) inhibitors

1. **Mechanism of action.** MAO inhibitors block the usual destruction of neurotransmitters by MAO, thus creating a buildup of biogenic amine levels in the brain. This increase probably underlies the antidepressant effect.

2. **Indications.** MAO inhibitors are reserved for patients who have not responded to cyclic antidepressants (first-line agents) or who cannot tolerate their side effects.

3. **Administration and dosage** (Table 49-3)

a. When changing from a cyclic antidepressant or another MAO inhibitor to a new MAO inhibitor, the first drug should be discontinued for 10 days prior to starting the new MAO inhibitor.

b. MAO inhibitors should be initiated at a low dose, and dosage increments should be made slowly and cautiously.

c. When changing from an MAO inhibitor to a cyclic antidepressant, at least 10 days must pass after stopping the MAO inhibitor before beginning therapy with the cyclic agent to avoid a potentially serious interaction.

d. Therapeutic effects may not occur for 2–3 weeks or longer.

4. **Precautions and monitoring effects**

a. **Contraindications**

(1) MAO inhibitors should not be administered to patients who are debilitated or who have a history of hepatic or renal impairment or cardiovascular or cerebrovascular disease.

(2) Administration is also contraindicated within 7–10 days of surgery that requires general anesthesia or a local anesthetic containing cocaine or sympathomimetic vasoconstrictors.

b. **Adverse effects**

(1) Orthostatic hypotension is common but may be minimized by using smaller incremental dosage increases.

(2) MAO inhibitors derived from hydrazide may cause hepatocellular damage. Although of low incidence, this toxic effect can have serious consequences; therefore, liver function should be monitored after a baseline is established. Administration should be avoided if the patient has a history of hepatic impairment.

(3) Weight gain, sexual dysfunction, and edema may occur.

c. **Overdosage** may be signaled by palpitations, agitation, frequent headaches, hypertension, or severe orthostatic hypotension.

d. **Significant interactions**

(1) **Hypertensive crisis,** the most serious and most likely interaction, results from ingestion of sympathomimetic drugs and foods with a high tyramine content.

Table 49-3. Recommended Daily Doses for Monoamine Oxidase (MAO) Inhibitors

Agents	Brand Name	Usual Daily Dose (mg)
Hydrazides		
Phenelzine	Nardil	60–90
Isocarboxazid	Marplan	10–50
Nonhydrazide		
Tranylcypromine	Parnate	10–60

(a) The patient should be given a list of **foods to avoid,** particularly:
(i) Beer and most wines (except white wine)
(ii) Caviar and herring
(iii) Chicken livers
(iv) Chocolate
(v) Most cheeses (especially blue, cheddar, mozzarella, Parmesan)
(vi) Sausage and other smoked meats

(b) Patients should also be warned not to take any medications—including over-the-counter cold, hay fever, or diet preparations—without first consulting a physician or pharmacist.

(c) Patients should not be given MAO inhibitors if they are unwilling or unable to comply with the restrictions.

(d) **Early signs** of hypertensive crisis may include:
(i) Stiff neck
(ii) Occipital headache
(iii) Nausea and vomiting
(iv) Sweating and flushing
(v) Palpitations

(2) **Coadministration of a cyclic antidepressant and a MAO inhibitor** must be undertaken with extreme caution, if at all [see IV A 6 a (2)].

V. TREATMENT OF BIPOLAR DISORDERS.

Neuroleptic agents, lithium, and psychotherapy may be used to manage bipolar disorders. Antidepressants are administered with lithium to manage the depressive phase of the illness. Use of antidepressants alone is usually avoided because of their tendency to provoke the re-emergence of the manic phase.

A. Neuroleptic agents

1. **Indications.** Neuroleptic agents are used in the acute manic phase to decrease agitation and hyperactivity, the first treatment priority.

2. **Therapeutic effects**

a. Neuroleptics such as chlorpromazine and haloperidol quickly lower the arousal level while not interfering with intellectual processes.

b. Emotional or affective displays are reduced; aggressive and impulsive behavior is diminished.

3. **Administration and dosage**

a. Because lithium efficacy has a delayed onset (see V B 2 a), neuroleptics are used until the lithium can achieve a therapeutic effect.

b. Neuroleptic therapy is usually initiated at the same time as the lithium therapy.

c. Neuroleptics can be tapered off as symptoms improve and serum lithium levels reach therapeutic concentrations [see V B 3 b (3)].

d. The dosage varies with the severity of the patient's symptoms and whether the patient is treated in the hospital or as an outpatient.

(1) The usual starting dose of **chlorpromazine** for a hospitalized patient in the manic phase is 25 mg intramuscularly. Doses of 25–50 mg intramuscularly may be administered hourly if necessary. The dose is gradually increased over the next few days to as much as 400 mg every 4–6 hours if needed.

(2) **Haloperidol** may be initiated at a dose of 2–5 mg intramuscularly in an acutely ill patient. Doses may be repeated hourly as needed.

(3) Oral administration should be employed as soon as the patient is calm.

4. **Precautions and monitoring effects**

a. **Chlorpromazine**

(1) This agent should be used with extreme caution or not at all in patients with cardiovascular disease, glaucoma, benign prostatic hypertrophy, or a history of seizures.

(2) Chlorpromazine has a strong sedative effect while bearing only moderate extrapyramidal effects.

b. **Haloperidol**

(1) Extrapyramidal effects may be seen with haloperidol administration. These effects include parkinsonian symptoms, akathisia, and dystonic reactions.

(2) Coadministration of haloperidol (or a phenothiazine) with lithium may result in an acute encephalopathy. Patients should be carefully monitored while receiving this combination.

(3) Haloperidol tends to have a high incidence of extrapyramidal effects (especially akathisia and dystonias) while having a moderate sedative effect.

c. **General.** These agents should not be withdrawn suddenly unless intolerably severe adverse effects arise.

B. Lithium is the drug of choice for control and prophylaxis of manic episodes.

1. **Mechanism of action.** Although the exact mechanism remains unknown, lithium is thought to:

a. Affect membrane stabilization
b. Inhibit norepinephrine release
c. Accelerate norepinephrine metabolism
d. Increase presynaptic re-uptake of norepinephrine and serotonin
e. Decrease receptor sensitivity

2. **Administration and dosage**

a. **General.** Lithium has a very narrow therapeutic index and a significant lag time (3–5 days, longer in some patients) before the initial therapeutic effect is observable. Therefore, monitoring serum lithium levels and evaluating the patient for signs of toxicity provide the keys to determining and adjusting the dosage regimen.

b. **Oral dosage**

(1) For acute episodes, 900 mg twice a day or 600 mg three times a day are given.
(2) For long-term control, 900–1200 mg/day in 2–3 divided doses are given.

c. **Maintenance therapy**

(1) Once the symptoms have diminished, the dose should be decreased to achieve maintenance serum levels [see V B 3 b (3) (b)].
(2) Manic attacks are usually self-limiting. Unless there is an indication for chronic therapy, lithium may be discontinued after 3–6 months. Long-term therapy is indicated for patients with severe or frequent attacks.

3. **Precautions and monitoring effects**

a. **Contraindications**

(1) Renal, cardiovascular, and thyroid disorders may preclude the use of lithium or necessitate extremely cautious monitoring.
(2) Lithium is contraindicated during the first trimester of pregnancy because it increases the risk of congenital cardiovascular anomalies, particularly valvular malformations.

b. **Serum level monitoring.** To minimize the likelihood of lithium toxicity while assuring adequate dosage, the patient's blood levels should be monitored closely.

(1) Levels should be checked twice a week during the first few weeks of therapy and at least every 2 months thereafter.
(2) The ideal time to check serum levels is 12 hours after the last dose. Drawing the sample in the morning before the first dose of the day is generally most convenient.
(3) Therapeutic serum level ranges are as follows:
(a) **Initial therapy:** 1.0–1.5 mEq/L
(b) **Maintenance therapy:** 0.6–1.2 mEq/L

c. **Laboratory test results** can be affected by lithium intake, including:

(1) Elevations in urinary serum glucose tests
(2) Decreases in serum uric acid levels and serum protein-bound iodine studies
(3) Increased thyroid-stimulating hormone
(4) Decreased thyroxine levels
(5) Increased serum sodium levels, which can increase secondary to diabetes insipidus [see V B 3 e (4) (b)]

d. **Breast feeding** should be avoided by mothers taking lithium because significant concentrations of the drug have been detected in breast milk.

e. **Adverse effects** are generally related to increasing serum concentration levels.

(1) Below 1.5 mEq/L, the effects are usually tolerable or manageable by dividing or reducing the dose. These effects include:
(a) Gastrointestinal distress, such as anorexia, nausea, vomiting, and diarrhea. These may be minimized by taking the drug with food or dividing the dose.

(b) Polyuria and polydipsia
(c) Fine hand tremor
(d) Slight muscle weakness

(2) Effects associated with lithium serum levels between 1.5 and 2.5 mEq/L should be considered early **warning signs of toxicity**. These effects include:
(a) Persistent or recurring gastrointestinal distress
(b) Coarse hand tremor
(c) Hyperirritability
(d) Slurred speech
(e) Confusion or somnolence

(3) Lithium toxicity usually occurs when levels exceed 2.5 mEq/L. This is a potentially fatal medical emergency requiring immediate attention.
(a) Signs and symptoms include:
(i) Increased deep tendon reflexes
(ii) Irregular pulse
(iii) Hypotension
(iv) Seizures
(v) Stupor or coma

(b) Treatment of acute toxicity should include attempts to empty the stomach by emesis or gastric lavage. Supportive treatment should be administered, and diuresis may increase urinary lithium elimination. Hemodialysis may be necessary if serum lithium levels exceed 3 mEq/L or if the patient's condition does not improve or begins to decline.

(4) Some effects occur with ongoing therapy but are unrelated to serum levels. These include:
(a) White blood cell counts may range from 10,000 mm^3 to 15,000 mm^3 (leukocytosis) and may remain elevated throughout therapy.
(b) Patients may develop an inability to concentrate urine, with increased urine output and increased thirst (nephrogenic diabetes insipidus syndrome).
(i) Dosage reduction or specific therapy may be needed if urine output becomes excessive.
(ii) Thyroid function tests and serum electrolytes should be monitored prior to initiating therapy and periodically thereafter to monitor for hypothyroidism and hypernatremia secondary to diabetes insipidus, respectively.
(c) Gain of 10 kg (22 lb) or more may occur.
(d) Clinically evident hypothyroidism or goiter may occur in a few cases.

4. Significant interactions. Lithium interacts with many drugs, only a few of which are discussed below. These interactions either increase lithium levels or increase lithium excretion. Lithium is eliminated through the kidneys by glomerular filtration and competes with sodium for reabsorption in the renal tubules.

a. Thiazide diuretics interfere with sodium reabsorption and, thus, may favor lithium reabsorption, which could lead to lithium toxicity. Care should be given to adjust the dosage of the lithium, and serum levels should be monitored closely. Conversely, lithium doses may need to be increased if the diuretic is discontinued. Furosemide therapy does not present this concern because the increased reabsorption of lithium in the proximal tubule is counteracted by decreased absorption in the loop of Henle.

b. Osmotic diuretics, sodium bicarbonate, and **theophylline** increase lithium excretion, thereby diminishing the therapeutic effect.

STUDY QUESTIONS

Directions: Each of the numbered items or incomplete statements in this section is followed by answers or by completions of the statement. Select the **one** lettered answer or completion that is **best** in each case.

1. All of the following patterns are associated with a bipolar major affective disorder EXCEPT

(A) a history of manic episodes only
(B) a history of depressed episodes only
(C) a history of several depressed episodes and only one manic episode
(D) cycling from manic to depressed episodes with periods of normal mood in between
(E) a history of several manic episodes and only one depressed episode

2. Unipolar affective disorder is characterized by which of the following signs?

(A) Flight of ideas
(B) Unusual verbosity
(C) Poor judgment leading to reckless driving
(D) Loss of interest in the job and family
(E) Ease of distractability

3. As a group, cyclic antidepressants have which of the following characteristics?

(A) They have similar therapeutic efficacy
(B) They have potent anticholinergic activity
(C) They lack histamine H_1 blocking activity
(D) They prevent the synthesis of neurotransmitters
(E) They have nearly identical side effect profiles

4. Therapeutic serum lithium levels during initiation of therapy are defined as

(A) 0.4–0.8 mEq/L
(B) 1.0–1.5 mEq/L
(C) 0.6–1.0 μg/L
(D) 0.8–1.0 mg/L
(E) 1.2–1.6 μg/L

5. Which of the following relatively mild adverse effects is associated with initiation of lithium therapy?

(A) Blurred vision
(B) Dystonic reactions
(C) Fine hand tremor
(D) Pseudoparkinsonism
(E) Tinnitus

6. Foods high in tyramine such as pickled herring and most cheeses (especially blue, cheddar, Parmesan) should be avoided by patients who are taking

(A) doxepin
(B) phenelzine
(C) maprotiline
(D) alprazolam
(E) trazodone

7. Which of the following drugs prescribed for control of a major affective disorder is associated with an almost immediate onset of activity?

(A) Lithium carbonate
(B) Protriptyline
(C) Tranylcypromine
(D) Chlorpromazine
(E) Isocarboxazid

8. Under the biogenic amine hypothesis, mania is thought to be due to

(A) an excess of epinephrine activity
(B) an excess of norepinephrine activity
(C) an excess of dopamine activity
(D) a deficiency of epinephrine activity
(E) a deficiency of dopamine activity

1-B 4-B 7-D
2-D 5-C 8-B
3-A 6-B

Questions 9–13

A 28-year-old woman presents with complaints of suicidal ideation. She has lost interest in her usual activities and because of poor appetite, she has lost approximately 15 pounds over the last 6 months. She complains of severe insomnia. She has a poorly formulated suicide plan but states that she would not carry out the plan. There is no history of previous suicide attempts. Her past medical history is unremarkable except for a normal pregnancy at age 23 years (full term, viable infant).

On physical examination, she appears mildly agitated. Blood pressure is 110/70 with a pulse of 72 and respirations 12; she is afebrile. The general examination is unremarkable. Heart, lungs, abdomen, and neurologic examinations are normal. Routine laboratory studies including an electrocardiogram are within normal limits. The patient was prescribed amitriptyline.

9. Which feature of amitriptyline makes it a reasonable therapeutic choice for this patient?

(A) The patient has a bipolar disorder, and amitriptyline is effective in this disorder
(B) The sedative properties of amitriptyline might prove beneficial
(C) Amitriptyline lacks significant H_1 blocking activity
(D) Amitriptyline does not cause any cardiac side effects

10. All of the following symptoms are potential anticholinergic side effects of amitriptyline EXCEPT

(A) blurred vision
(B) constipation
(C) sinus bradycardia
(D) urinary retention

11. What is an appropriate starting dose of amitriptyline?

(A) 50 mg/day
(B) 150 mg/day
(C) 200 mg/day
(D) 250 mg/day

12. How long will it take for the amitriptyline to be fully therapeutically effective?

(A) 1 week
(B) 2 weeks
(C) 1 month
(D) 3 months

13. The patient's husband brings her back to the emergency room and states that the patient has taken an overdose of the amitriptyline. All of the following choices are appropriate EXCEPT

(A) obtain an electrocardiogram
(B) obtain a toxic screen with a tricyclic level included
(C) gastric lavage
(D) observe patient only; no laboratory work would be needed because the drug is not toxic

---

9-B
10-C
11-A
12-C
13-D

ANSWERS AND EXPLANATIONS

1. The answer is B *[I A 2; II C 1, 2].*
Bipolar depression is characterized by periods of depression and mania, or mania alone. Therefore, someone with a history of depressed episodes only would not fit the definition of a bipolar disorder.

2. The answer is D *[II B 3 d].*
Loss of interest in the job or family is a common sign of a unipolar affective disorder. Flight of ideas, unusual verbosity, poor judgment that could lead to reckless driving, and ease of distractability are all signs of the manic phase of a bipolar affective disorder.

3. The answer is A *[IV A 2, 4].*
The cyclic antidepressants all have equivalent therapeutic efficacy when given at the appropriate dose. Each drug has its own unique side effect profile. Several of the drugs are potent antihistamines (e.g., doxepin, amitriptyline). While some of the drugs have potent anticholinergic activity, others are nearly devoid of this activity (e.g., bupropion, trazodone, fluoxetine). Cyclic antidepressants block the re-uptake of neurotransmitters but do not block neurotransmitter synthesis.

4. The answer is B *[V B 3 b (3) (a)].*
Therapeutic serum lithium levels during initiation of lithium therapy range from 1.0–1.5 mEq/L. During maintenance therapy, the therapeutic serum level range is 0.6–1.2 mEq/L. It is important to monitor serum levels because lithium, like digoxin, has a narrow range between therapeutic and toxic doses. During the first weeks of therapy, serum levels are checked several times a week until the levels have stabilized. During maintenance therapy, serum lithium levels are checked at least once every 2 months.

5. The answer is C *[V B 3 e].*
The relatively mild adverse effects associated with lithium therapy consist of gastrointestinal disturbances, polyuria, and polydipsia, muscle weakness, and fine hand tremor. Pseudoparkinsonism and dystonic reactions do not occur with lithium therapy; tinnitus and blurred vision are not signs of lithium toxicity.

6. The answer is B *[IV B 4 d (1) (a)].*
Foods high in tyramine should be avoided in patients who are taking monoamine oxidase (MAO) inhibitors such as phenelzine. The enzyme MAO takes part in the oxidative deamination of biogenic amines (e.g., dopamine, norepinephrine, serotonin, tyramine). MAO inhibitors prevent this enzymatic degradation. (This is considered to be the mechanism of their antidepressant effects.) When a person taking a MAO inhibitor eats foods high in tyramine, the tyramine is not degraded in the body. The tyramine can induce the release of stored catecholamines (e.g., norepinephrine), and this may precipitate an episode of severe hypertension. Doxepin, maprotiline, alprazolam, and trazodone are not MAO inhibitors.

7. The answer is D *[IV A 5 a (7), B 3 d; V A 2 a, 3 a].*
Protriptyline is a tricyclic antidepressant. Full response may require about 4 weeks. Tranylcypromine and isocarboxazid are monoamine oxidase (MAO) inhibitors. The onset of antidepressant effects may be delayed for 2–3 weeks. Lithium carbonate has a delayed onset and may take up to 2 weeks for maximum effectiveness. Chlorpromazine is the only agent listed in the question that has an immediate onset of activity.

8. The answer is B *[I C 2 a].*
Under the biogenic amine hypothesis, depression is thought to be due to a deficiency of serotonin or norepinephrine activity, and mania is thought to be due to an excess of norepinephrine activity.

9–13. The answers are: 9-B *[IV A 6 c (1)],* **10-C** *[IV A 6 c (3) (b)],* **11-A** *[IV A 5 a (2)],* **12-C** *[IV A 5 a (7)],* **13-D** *[IV A 6 c (6)].*
The patient described in the question does not have a bipolar disorder. Amitriptyline is a potent H_1 blocker, and its sedating properties might be beneficial for this patient. Amitriptyline can cause cardiac side effects such as arrhythmias.

Blurred vision, constipation, and urinary retention are anticholinergic side effects. Sinus tachycardia, not sinus bradycardia, is an anticholinergic effect.

An appropriate starting dose of amitriptyline is 50 mg/day (in divided doses); this should be titrated up to the target dose.

Physiologic symptoms usually respond in 1 week, and psychosocial symptoms usually respond after 2–4 weeks. However, full therapeutic effectiveness usually requires about 4 weeks.

Tricyclic overdose is potentially fatal. Treatment may initially include emesis and gastric lavage and administration of activated charcoal. An electrocardiogram and a toxic screen are routine emergency room evaluation tools.

50
Asthma and Chronic Obstructive Pulmonary Disease

Louise Glassner Cohen

I. ASTHMA

A. Definition. Asthma is a condition of tracheobronchial hyperreactivity to various stimuli, leading to episodic bronchospasms and reversible airway obstruction. This narrowing of the airway changes spontaneously or as a result of therapy.

B. Classification. Previous classifications for asthma (i.e., intrinsic, extrinsic) are no longer used. It is now recognized that patients respond to a variety of stimuli. An allergic component can be demonstrated in 35%–55% of asthmatics. Also, 70%–90% of all asthmatics experience exercise–induced asthma. The degree of airway hyperreactivity is dependent on whether the asthmatic is in remission.

C. Incidence. Asthma affects approximately 10–20 million Americans. (These numbers depend on the definition of asthma used.) It has been estimated that 5% of adults and 7%–10% of children suffer from asthma.

1. In about half the cases, the disorder arises before age 10; approximately 33% of the remaining cases are diagnosed before age 40.
2. Up to age 30, asthma is more prevalent in males; after age 30, men and women are equally affected.
3. Up to 50% of cases of childhood asthma resolve by adulthood.

D. Etiology

1. **Precipitating factors** of an acute asthma attack include:
   - **a.** Allergens (e.g., pollen, dust, animal dander)
   - **b.** Upper respiratory tract infection (e.g., rhinovirus, influenza)
   - **c.** Exercise
   - **d.** Emotions (e.g., anxiety, stress, laughter)
   - **e.** Occupational exposure to such agents as gasoline fumes and fresh paint
   - **f.** Environmental exposure to cold air, sulfur dioxide, and cigarette smoke
   - **g.** **Drugs.** Two different mechanisms can trigger drug-related asthma.
     - **(1)** **Hypersensitivity reaction** due to drugs (e.g., aspirin, ibuprofen, penicillin, products containing tartrazine) with release of bronchoactive mediators
     - **(2)** **Extension of pharmacologic effect** may develop with such drugs as β-adrenergic blockers and bethanechol.
2. The **mechanism of bronchial hyperreactivity** has not been determined; however, several theories are suggested:
   - **a.** Increased airway inflammation: This is due to altered cellular response and increased levels of mediators, which increase airway hyperresponsiveness.
   - **b.** β-Adrenergic defect producing β-blockade: This theory is based on the principle that β-blockers alter respiratory function. This has not been proven in asthmatic patients.
   - **c.** Increased cholinergic response: Asthmatic patients seem to be more responsive to bronchoconstriction after inhalation of cholinergic agents. This has not been proven.
   - **d.** Increased sensitivity of mast cells in asthmatic patients: Asthmatics may be more sensitive to the triggers that cause mast cell degranulation.

E. Pathophysiology

1. **Allergic stimuli** produce a biphasic response that has been linked to the inflammatory process.
   a. **Early asthmatic response**
      (1) There is an immediate response to an allergen with a peak effect at 10–30 minutes and a duration of 1.5–3.0 hours.
      (2) The allergen reacts with immunoglobulin E (IgE), which is attached to mast cells, causing release of mediators (see I E 4).
      (3) The asthmatic response can be inhibited by premedication with β_2-adrenergic agents, cromolyn sodium, or glucocorticoids (when given for the proper duration).
      (4) The response can be reversed by the administration of β_2-adrenergic agents.
   b. **Late asthmatic response**
      (1) A late asthmatic response is seen in about 50% of asthmatic patients following an acute response. The response begins 3–4 hours after the early response and reaches a peak effect after 8–12 hours. The duration of the response may last several days. Bronchial hyperreactivity may last several weeks.
      (2) Mediators involved in the late response may include those released from mast cells, including eosinophil chemotactic factor, neutrophil chemotactic factor, and basophil chemotactic factor. Platelet-activating factor (PAF) and leukotrienes are released from eosinophils.
      (3) Mediators cause an influx of inflammatory cells including eosinophils, macrophages, neutrophils, and lymphocytes with release of additional mediators.
      (4) This response can be prevented by administration of cromolyn sodium and corticosteroids. β-adrenergic agents have no effect on this response.
2. **Nonallergic stimuli,** such as exercise, methacholine, or cold air, produce acute bronchospasm that lasts about 1 hour and is not followed by a late asthmatic response. These stimuli may cause bronchoconstriction, using some of the inflammatory mediators, but the process is still controversial.
3. **Acute asthma attacks** are characterized by a response that triggers airway obstruction.
   a. In response to a precipitating factor, mediators from mast cells cause bronchial smooth muscle to become spasmodic, leading to bronchoconstriction, which triggers blood vessel engorgement and infiltration of inflammatory cells (neutrophils).
   b. Mucous glands and **goblet cells,** the mucus-secreting cells of the respiratory tract epithelium, become edematous, which leads to increased mucus production, further narrowing the airway.
   c. Airway obstruction reduces ventilation to some lung regions; this, in turn, causes a **ventilation/perfusion (V/Q) imbalance** that leads to hypoxemia. This is reflected by a reduction in the partial pressure of arterial oxygen (PaO_2) more frequently in a moderate to severe attack.
   d. In the early stages, hyperventilation results in a decrease in the partial pressure of arterial carbon dioxide ($PaCO_2$). If the asthma attack progresses and the airways remain narrowed, respiratory muscles suffer fatigue.
   e. **Respiratory acidosis** develops if hypoxemia worsens and the patient's respiratory rate is not maintained; then the $PaCO_2$ level begins to increase.
   f. Peak expiratory flow rate (PEFR) and forced expiratory volume (1 second) [FEV_1] may drop in the early stages of an acute asthma attack. As the attack worsens, FEV_1 decreases, resulting in **air trapping** and **lung hyperinflation**.
4. **Immunopathologic events.** The adrenergic and cholinergic responses in asthma are governed by immunologic, environmental, and physical stimuli.
   a. After exposure to an asthma "trigger," mediators are released from the mast cells, alveolar macrophages, and eosinophils. The mediators that are released [e.g., histamine, heparin, prostaglandin D_2 (PGD_2), leukotrienes, chymotrypsin/trypsin] cause the early asthmatic response.
   b. Additional mediators (e.g., eosinophil chemotactic factor, neutrophil chemotactic factor, basophil chemotactic factor, PAF, others) are responsible for the late asthmatic response.
      (1) Some of these mediators may be released in response to nonallergic stimuli, but this is still controversial.
      (2) These mediators are responsible for bronchoconstriction, airway edema, and mucus production (Figure 50-1). Bronchial hyperresponsiveness may also be induced by these mediators and may last up to 4 weeks after the initial asthma attack, increasing sensitivity to stimuli.

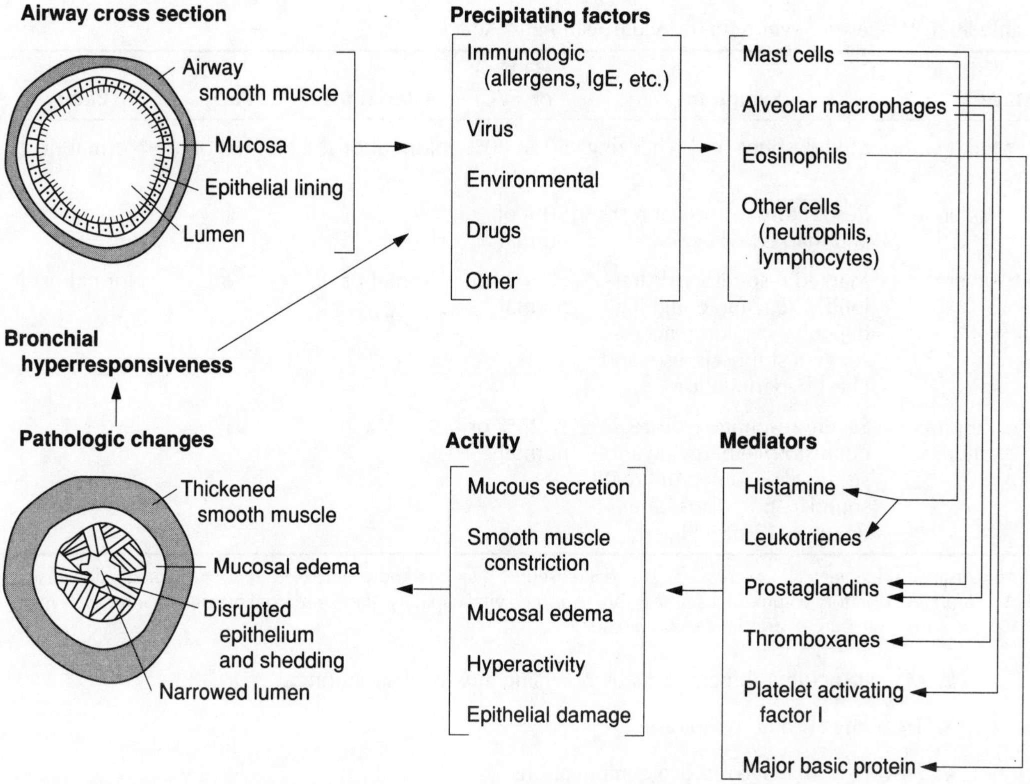

Figure 50-1. Diagrammatic representation of the pathophysiology of asthma.

F. Clinical evaluation

1. Physical findings

a. An acute attack, which may have a sudden or gradual onset, produces respiratory distress and wheezing of a variable degree, depending on the severity of the attack (Table 50-1).

b. Other common findings include chest tightness, cough, tachypnea, tachycardia, accessory muscle use, and pulsus paradoxus.

c. Between acute asthma attacks, the patient may be asymptomatic. Physical findings are dependent on the severity of the disease.

2. Diagnostic test results

a. Blood analysis typically shows a slightly elevated white blood cell count during an acute attack; eosinophilia also may be present.

b. Sputum analysis may reveal Curschmann's spirals (mucous casts of the small airways), eosinophils, Charcot-Leyden crystals (products of eosinophil breakdown), Creola bodies (clumps of epithelial cells), and bacteria (if there is an infection).

c. Arterial blood gas measurements help gauge the severity of the asthma attack (see Table 50-1).

d. Pulmonary function tests help determine the degree of airway obstruction and gas exchange impairment. During an acute asthma attack, FEV_1 decreases while residual volume (RV) and functional residual volume (FRV) increase. Total lung capacity (TLC) may be elevated. Changes in the PEFR correlate well with FEV_1 and may be used to evaluate lung function.

e. An **electrocardiogram (ECG)** may show sinus tachycardia.

f. Chest x-ray is useful in detecting an accompanying pneumothorax or pneumonia.

g. Allergy skin tests may identify allergens that trigger asthma. (Skin tests should not be done during an acute attack.)

G. Treatment objectives

1. Identify and eliminate causative agents, thus reducing the incidence of acute asthma attacks

Table 50-1. Stages of Severity of an Acute Asthmatic Attack

Stage	Symptoms	FEV_1 or FVC	Arterial pH	Pa_{O_2}	Pa_{CO_2}
I: Mild	Mild dyspnea and wheezing	50%–80% of normal	Normal or ↑	Normal or ↓	Normal or ↓
II: Moderate	Respiratory distress at rest and marked wheezing	50% of normal	↑	↓	↓
III: Severe	Marked respiratory distress, loud wheezing, coughing, difficulty speaking, accessory chest muscle use, and chest hyperinflation	< 50% of normal	Normal or ↓	↓	Normal or ↑
IV: Respiratory failure	Severe respiratory distress, confusion, lethargy, cyanosis, disappearance of breath sounds, and pulsus paradoxus > 12 mm Hg	< 25% of normal	↓ ↓	↓	↑ ↑

Arrows indicate changes: ↑ = increased; ↓ = decreased; ↑ ↑ = markedly increased; ↓ ↓ = markedly decreased. FEV_1 = forced expiratory volume in 1 second; FVC = forced vital capacity; Pa_{O_2} = partial pressure of arterial oxygen; Pa_{CO_2} = partial pressure of arterial carbon dioxide.

2. Manage acute asthma attacks by reversing airway obstruction

3. Treat any chronic symptoms

4. Prevent or manage disease complications

5. Teach the patient about the disease state, proper use of medication, and possible side effects, thereby improving compliance and promoting preventive measures

H. Therapy

1. **Management of acute asthma.** A stepped approach is used with suggested administration in the order discussed below. The role of theophylline is controversial.
   a. **β-Adrenergic agents** (e.g., isoproterenol, epinephrine, metaproterenol, terbutaline) usually are given first (Table 50-2).
      (1) **Therapeutic effects.** Among their various effects, these agents (also called **sympathomimetics**) relieve bronchoconstriction and, thus, help reverse an acute asthma attack.
      (2) **Mechanism of action.** β-Adrenergic agonists stimulate β_2-receptors, activating adenyl cyclase, which increases intracellular production of cyclic adenosine monophosphate (cAMP). This produces relaxation of smooth muscle (bronchial relaxation), stabilization of mast cell membranes, and stimulation of skeletal muscles (tremor). Additional effects include gluconeogenesis, insulin secretion, and activation of Na^+, K^+–adenosine triphosphatase (ATPase). β-Adrenergic agents differ in their affinity for the β_1- and β_2-receptors. Agents with β_1 effects can cause cardiotoxicity.
      (3) **Administration and dosage.** Whenever possible, these agents are given to asthmatics via a nebulizer or a metered dose inhaler (MDI) because of their longer duration and fewer side effects when compared to the other dosage forms. In an emergency situation, a motorized nebulizer is preferred. This route has been shown to be as effective as parenteral agents in severe acute asthma. Agents can also be administered to patients on mechanical ventilation by insertion of the MDI into the respiratory circuit. For chronic therapy, they are administered orally only to patients who cannot use aerosols with spacer devices properly. For dosage information, see Table 50-2.
      (4) **Precautions and monitoring effects**
         (a) These drugs should be used cautiously in patients with a history of arrhythmias, coronary artery disease, hypertension, or diabetes.
         (b) Tremor, nervousness, headache, dizziness, weakness, and insomnia are common central nervous system (CNS) effects of β-adrenergic agents.

(c) Palpitations and tachycardia occur. Pulse rate should be monitored closely in patients receiving any of the β-adrenergics.

(d) Excessive use of β_2-adrenergics with some β_1 effects (e.g., metaproterenol) may lead to paradoxical bronchiolar constriction or cardiac arrest.

(e) Epinephrine and isoproterenol in repeated doses may cause myocardial ischemia and arrhythmias.

(f) **Drug tolerance** can occur with inhaled or oral β-adrenergic agents. Suggested mechanisms include:

(i) A decrease in the number of active β-receptors due to movement of receptors from the cell surface into the cell (**down regulation**)

(ii) A decreased sensitivity in the β-receptors to stimuli making them unable to activate adenyl cyclase. The clinical significance of this effect is unclear in patients taking normal doses of β-adrenergic agents. Patients may only become tolerant to the extrapulmonary effects and not to the bronchodilation. Tolerance is signaled by an increase in the requirement for β-adrenergic agents when they are used on a regular schedule. This effect can be reversed by adding oral or aerosol corticosteroids to the regimen.

(5) **Significant interactions**

(a) Concomitant use of β-adrenergic agents with **monoamine oxidase (MAO) inhibitors** with ephedrine or terbutaline may lead to severe hypertension. In addition, combinations of β-agonists (i.e., epinephrine) and **tricyclic antidepressants** or **methyldopa** may result in an increased pressor response.

(b) **β-Adrenergic blockers** (e.g., propranolol) block the bronchodilatory and cardiostimulating effects of β-adrenergic agents.

(c) β-Adrenergic agents should not be combined with other **sympathomimetic agents** because of additive cardiovascular effects. Vasoconstrictive and pressor effects of epinephrine are antagonized by α-adrenergic blocking agents (e.g., phentolamine).

b. **Theophylline compounds.** These spasmolytic agents can be administered if β-adrenergics fail to control an acute asthma attack. Whether or not theophylline should be used and the order in which it is used in acute asthma is controversial.

(1) **Therapeutic effects.** Among their various effects, these drugs relax bronchial smooth muscle, reduce mucus secretions, enhance mucociliary transport, and improve diaphragmatic contractility.

(2) **Mechanism of action.** Inhibition of the enzyme phosphodiesterase, resulting in an increase of cAMP, occurs only at toxic concentrations. Other suggested mechanisms include alteration of intracellular calcium and increased binding of cAMP to its binding protein. Adenosine antagonism and inhibited production of contractile prostaglandins have also been proposed.

(3) **Administration and dosage**

(a) **Intravenous therapy.** Theophylline and aminophylline both are available.

(i) **Theophylline.** The usual loading dose for adults and children is 5–6 mg/kg based on lean body weight, administered over 30 minutes. Loading doses for obese patients (i.e., weight greater than 20% over standard weight per insurance tables) should be based on total body weight. If the patient is currently on theophylline and the serum concentration is unknown, one-half the loading dose is given.

(ii) **Aminophylline.** Aminophylline contains 80% theophylline. Dosage for aminophylline is, therefore, approximately 1.2 times that of theophylline.

(b) **Maintenance dose** is administered by continuous infusion and is adjusted by monitoring theophylline serum levels (Table 50-3). Maintenance dosage for obese patients should be based on lean body weight.

(c) **Oral therapy**

(i) Oral loading doses of theophylline and aminophylline can be given when the situation is not an emergency. The initial dose of theophylline for adults and children over age 1 year is the lesser of 400 mg/day or 16 mg/kg/day. The dose can be titrated slowly upward and the serum level monitored until a therapeutic level is obtained. The maximum dose varies with age, from 24 mg/kg/day for children aged 1–9 years, to 16 mg/kg/day for adults.

Table 50-2. β-Adrenergic Agents Used in the Treatment of Asthma

Agent	Acute Severe		Chronic		Site of Action	Duration of Action	Comments
	Pediatric	Adult	Pediatric	Adult			
Isoproterenol							
INH: 1:200 (5 mg/ml)	NCR	NCR	NCR	NCR	β_1-receptors + + + β_2-receptors + + + +	1–2 hours (inhalation) 1–2 hours (intravenous)	It has a short duration of action and is less selective. Tolerance develops quickly.
MDI various	NCR	NCR	NCR	NCR			
Epinephrine							
SQ: 1:1000 (1 mg/ml)	0.01 mg q 20 minutes up to 3 doses (maximum 0.3 mg)	0.2–0.5 mg q 20 minutes up to 3 doses	NCR	NCR	β_1-receptors + + + β_2-receptors + + +	1–4 hours (subcutaneous)	Additional doses are not recommended.
SQ (sustained): 1:200 (Susphrine) (5 mg/ml)	0.025 mg/kg q 6–10 hours (maximum 0.75 mg)	0.5–1.5 mg q 6–10 hours	NCR	NCR		. . .	It has a longer duration than epinephrine.
Isoetharine							
NEB: 1% (10 mg/ml)	0.1–0.2 mg/kg q 2–4 hours	2.5–10 mg q 2–4 hours	NCR	NCR	β_1-receptors + + β_2-receptors + + +	1–3 hours (inhalation)	More selective agents with longer durations of action are preferred.
MDI (0.34 mg/spray)	NCR	NCR	NCR	NCR			
Metaproterenol							
NEB: 5% (15 mg/0.3 ml)	0.25–0.5 mg/kg q 1–2 hours*	10–15 mg q 1–2 hours*	0.25–0.5 mg/kg q 4–6 hours (maximum 15 mg)	10–15 mg q 4–6 hours	β_1-receptors + + β_2-receptors + + +	3–5 hours (inhalation) 4 hours (oral)	. . .
MDI (0.65 mg/puff)	2 puffs q 1–2 hours*	3 puffs q 1–2 hours*	1–2 puffs q 4 hours	1–3 puffs q 4 hours			

Oral	NCR	NCR	0.3–0.5 mg/kg q 4–6 hours; increase by 0.25 mg/kg as tolerated	20 mg q 4–6 hours			
Terbutaline							
SQ (1 mg/ml)	0.005–0.01 mg/kg q 2–6 hours (maximum 0.25 mg)	0.25–0.5 mg q 2–6 hours	NCR	NCR	β_1-receptors + β_2-receptors + + + +	1.5–4 hours (subcutaneous) 6–8 hours (inhalation)	SQ product used in NEB is not FDA approved.
MDI (0.25 mg/puff)	2 puffs q 20 minutes for 3 doses*	3 puffs q 20 minutes for 3 doses*	1–2 puffs q 4–6 hours	1–3 puffs q 4–6 hours			
Oral	NCR	NCR	0.05–0.1 mg/kg q 6–8 hours	2.5–5 mg q 6–8 hours		4–8 hours (oral)	
Albuterol							
INH: 0.5% (5 mg/ml)	0.05–0.15 mg/kg q 20 minutes for 3 doses (maximum 5 mg)*	2.5–5 mg q 20 minutes for 3 doses*	0.05–0.15 mg/kg q 4–8 hours	2.5–5 mg q 4–8 hours	β_1-receptors + β_2-receptors + + + +	6–8 hours (inhalation) 4–6 hours (oral)	. . .
MDI 0.09 mg/puff	2 puffs q 20 minutes for 3 doses*	3 puffs q 20 minutes for 3 doses	1–2 puffs q 4–6 hours	2–3 puffs q 4–6 hours			
Oral	NCR	NCR	0.1 mg/kg q 6 hours	2–4 mg q 6–8 hours			
Bitolterol MDI 0.37 mg/puff	NCR	NCR	1–2 puffs q 4–6 hours	2–3 puffs q 4–6 hours	β_1-receptors + β_2-receptors + + + +	6–7 hours (inhalation)	. . .
Pirbuterol MDI 0.2 mg/puff	NCR	NCR	1–2 puffs q 4–6 hours	2–3 puffs q 4–6 hours	β_1-receptors + β_2-receptors + + + +	6–8 hours (inhalation)	. . .

FDA = Food and Drug Administration; INH = inhalation; MDI = metered dose inhaler; NCR = not currently recommended; NEB = solution for nebulizer; SQ = subcutaneous.

*Current recommendations may not be FDA approved.

Table 50-3. Theophylline Maintenance Doses

Age and Circumstance	Infusion Rate (mg/kg/hr)
Young child (1–9 years old)	0.8
Older child (9–16 years old)	0.7
Adult (older than 16 years)	0.4
Adult smoker	0.7
Adult with cardiac decompensation, cor pulmonale, liver dysfunction, or a combination of these	0.2

(ii) Other theophylline "salts" are available; dosing is based on theophylline content. These products claim fewer side effects but are comparable when used in equivalent doses (Table 50-4).

(iii) Sustained-release forms of theophylline are available to increase the dosing interval and improve compliance. The products can vary in their time to peak concentration (see Table 50-4).

(4) Precautions and monitoring effects

(a) These drugs are contraindicated in patients with hypersensitivity to xanthine compounds and in those with a history of arrhythmias.

(b) Cautious use is indicated in patients with peptic ulcer disease, gout, coronary artery disease, and diabetes mellitus.

(c) These agents may cause such adverse CNS effects as dizziness, restlessness, insomnia, and convulsions.

(d) Palpitations and sinus tachycardia have been reported, even in the therapeutic dosage range.

(e) Adverse gastrointestinal effects include nausea, vomiting, and anorexia. These effects should be carefully differentiated from theophylline toxicity, which can occur with serum levels over 20 μg/ml.

(f) Because individuals metabolize theophylline compounds at different rates, serum drug levels should be monitored to ensure a level in the therapeutic range (10–20 μg/ml). Levels should be monitored at steady-state (about 4–5 half-lives of drug). During infusion therapy, levels can be measured at 32–40 hours after the start or change in infusion. During oral therapy, a trough level is taken before the dose is given after the first 1½–2 days. Peak serum levels should be monitored in patients with rapid theophylline elimination to avoid transient adverse effects.

(g) These drugs may potentiate cardiac glycosides and increase toxic potential.

(h) Drug clearance may be altered by various factors, including significant drug interactions (Table 50-5).

Table 50-4. Selection of Theophylline Products

Salt	Theophylline Content (%)	Equivalent Dose (mg)
Theophylline anhydrous	100	100
Theophylline monohydrate	91	110
Aminophylline anhydrous	86	116
Aminophylline dihydrate	79	127
Oxtriphylline	64	156
Theophylline sodium glycinate	46	217
Formulation	**Time to Peak**	**Dosing Interval**
Uncoated tablets	1–2 hours	q 6 hours
Oral liquids	1–2 hours	q 6 hours
Sustained-release		
Capsule	3–6 hours	q 8 hours
Tablet	4–10 hours	q 12 hours
Capsule	11–15 hours	q 24 hours

Table 50-5. Factors That Alter Theophylline Clearance

Factors that increase clearance (causing a reduced serum drug level)
Age < 16
Fever
Smoking
Concurrent use of carbamazepine, isoproterenol, phenobarbital, phenytoin, and rifampin
Factors that decrease clearance (causing an increased serum drug level)
Advanced age
Cor pulmonale
Congestive heart failure
Liver failure
Pneumonia
Concurrent use of allopurinol, cimetidine, erythromycin, oral contraceptives, propranolol, troleandomycin, ciprofloxacin, ofloxacin, norfloxacin, enoxacin, and clarithromycin

c. Corticosteroids (e.g., beclomethasone, betamethasone, hydrocortisone, prednisone) may be given if bronchoconstriction fails to respond to β-adrenergics or theophylline compounds.

(1) Therapeutic effects. When used to treat asthma, corticosteroids suppress the inflammatory response.

(2) Mechanism of action. Multiple mechanisms of action include:

(a) Decreased inflammatory cell activation, recruitment, and infiltration

(b) Decreased metabolites of arachidonic acid (e.g., prostaglandins, leukotrienes)

(c) Increased synthesis of proteins that enhances the β-adrenergic response

(d) Decreased mucus production

(e) Prevention of increased vascular permeability

(3) Administration and dosage. A lag time may occur with the onset of these agents because they lack direct bronchodilatory effects on smooth muscle and must be administered with other agents. After administration of intravenous, oral, or inhaled agents, some patients may show improvement of pulmonary function tests in 1–3 hours with a maximum effect in 6–9 hours.

(a) There is no significant difference in the clinical efficacy of the corticosteroid products. The agent should have the following properties: good glucocorticoid activity, minimal mineralocorticoid activity, short-to-intermediate duration of action. The route of administration is determined by the condition of the patient.

(b) Intravenous corticosteroids are administered when the patient cannot use the oral route during a severe acute asthma attack. The duration of therapy is short but may be continued as oral therapy if symptoms persist; the dose is then rapidly tapered. Hydrocortisone and methylprednisolone are the most commonly used agents. Dosing is controversial and is determined by the severity of the attack and current corticosteroid used by the patient.

(c) Beclomethasone, dexamethasone, flunisolide, triamcinolone, and budesonide are available in aerosol form, which is preferred because of the lower incidence of adverse effects. These agents should not be used as primary therapy for a severe acute attack but are useful with other therapies for chronic management (Table 50-6).

(d) Prednisone (1 mg/kg/day) and prednisolone are the preferred oral agents. They can be administered in "short bursts" to improve recovery during an acute exacerbation.

(4) Precautions and monitoring effects

(a) Corticosteroids should be used cautiously in elderly and pediatric patients and in those with diabetes mellitus, hypothyroidism, peptic ulcers or other gastrointestinal diseases, chronic infections, Cushing's syndrome, myasthenia gravis, and psychotic tendencies.

(b) Patients receiving daily or alternate-day oral corticosteroid therapy, using the smallest effective dose, should be monitored closely for adverse systemic effects (Table 50-7).

Table 50-6. Aerosol Corticosteroids

Agent	MDI Dose Delivered	Recommended Dosage Adults	Pediatric
Dexamethasone sodium phosphate	84 μg/puff	3 puffs 3–4 times daily (maximum 12)	2 puffs 3–4 times daily (maximum 8)
Beclomethasone dipropionate	42 μg/puff	2 puffs 3–4 times daily (maximum 20)	1–2 puffs 3–4 times daily (maximum 10)
Triamcinalone acetonide	100 μg/puff	2 puffs 3–4 times daily (maximum 16)	1–2 puffs 3–4 times daily (maximum 12)
Flunisolide	250 μg/puff	2 puffs 2 times daily (maximum 8)	2 puffs 2 times daily (maximum 4)

MDI = metered dose inhaler.

(c) Inhaled steroids may cause such local effects as dry mouth, hoarseness, and fungal infection of the mouth and throat (spacer devices reduce these adverse effects) and rare systemic side effects.

(d) **Significant interactions**

(i) Concurrent use of **hepatic microsomal enzyme inducers** (e.g., rifampin, barbiturates, hydantoins) cause enhanced corticosteroid metabolism, reducing therapeutic efficacy.

(ii) Concurrent use of **estrogens, oral contraceptives, ketoconazole, macrolide antibiotics** (e.g., erythromycin, clarithromycin) may decrease corticosteroid metabolism.

(iii) **Cyclosporine** may decrease plasma clearance of some corticosteroids (i.e., methylprednisone), and these agents may increase the plasma concentration of cyclosporine.

(iv) Administration of **potassium-depleting diuretics** (e.g., thiazides, furosemide, ethacrynic acid) or other potassium-depleting drugs (e.g., amphotericin) with corticosteroids cause enhanced hypokalemia. Serum potassium should be closely monitored, especially in patients on **digitalis glycosides**.

(v) Corticosteroids can decrease the serum concentrations of **isoniazid** and **salicylates** when the agents are used concurrently.

d. **Other agents** used in the treatment of acute asthma include the following:

(1) **Anticholinergics** (also called cholinergic blocking agents). These drugs may cause bronchodilation by inhibiting acetylcholine stimulation of efferent vagal pathways, reducing intrinsic vagal tone to bronchial smooth muscle. Bronchoconstriction due to

Table 50-7. Systemic Effects of Corticosteroid Therapy

Effect	Clinical Manifestations	Intervention/Prevention
Appetite stimulation	Weight gain	Reduction in caloric intake
Fluid and sodium retention	Edema	Reduction in sodium intake
Hyperacidity	Esophagitis, gastritis	Antacids, histamine$_2$-receptor antagonists (e.g., ranitidine)
Hypertension	Headache, cerebrovascular accident	Blood pressure monitoring
Psychosis	Disruptive behavior	Tranquilizers
Increased intraocular pressure	Glaucoma	Ophthalmologic evaluation
Hypokalemia	Muscle weakness	Potassium replacement therapy
Increased gluconeogenesis	Hyperglycemia	Adjustment of dietary, insulin, or oral hypoglycemic therapy

mediator release may be partially mediated through cholinergic stimulation. This effect may vary from patient to patient. During an acute attack, anticholinergics may be synergistic when combined with β-adrenergic agonists and should be used only as second-line therapy in selected patients.

(a) **Aerosolized atropine** usage has decreased due to the high incidence of adverse effects and lack of demonstrated efficacy in studies.

(b) **Ipratropium bromide** can be given to patients with acute and chronic asthma poorly controlled by β-adrenergics alone. The nebulized form is more effective in acute attacks but is not available at this time in the United States. The dose for maintenance therapy is two to four inhalations every 6 hours.

(2) **Antihistamines. Terfenadine** and **astemizole** compete with histamine for histamine$_1$-receptor sites on effector cells and, thus, help prevent the histamine-mediated responses that influence asthma. However, their use in asthma requires further study. These agents are useful for patients with allergic rhinitis.

(3) **Calcium channel blockers** (e.g., verapamil, nifedipine). Theoretically, these agents may have therapeutic effects in asthma. In vitro, these agents cause relaxation of smooth muscle by inhibition of calcium influx. This has not been proved in clinical studies, however, and further investigation is needed.

(4) **Antibiotics** are administered if the patient has a known or suspected bacterial infection as suggested by yellow, green, or brown sputum.

e. **Non-pharmacologic treatment**

(1) **Humidified oxygen** is administered to all patients with severe, acute asthma to reverse hypoxemia. The fraction of inspired oxygen (FIO_2) administered is based on the patient's arterial blood gas status; generally 1–3 L/min are given via Venturi mask or nasal cannula.

(2) **Intravenous fluids and electrolytes** may be required if the patient is dehydrated.

2. **Management of chronic asthma.** A stepped approach to manage chronic asthma is used as well, but the order is dependent on whether the symptoms are intermediate, seasonal, or chronic. The goal of therapy is to decrease the morbidity and mortality of asthma by early treatment of the increasing severity of symptoms.

a. **Intermittent asthma** is caused by a response to specific stimuli and is managed with medications only as the episodic symptoms occur.

b. **Seasonal asthma** occurs when symptoms are limited to a particular season of the year (i.e., spring, summer) and become more frequent than intermittent asthma. Agents should be administered as needed throughout the rest of the year, then as prophylactic therapy during the season of increased symptoms.

c. **Chronic asthma** occurs when the symptoms are frequent and require long-term prophylactic therapy. Medications are added in a stepped approach until symptoms are under control.

(1) **β-Adrenergic agonists** by inhalation are used alone for mild-to-moderate episodes. They also can be used for chronic prophylaxis in patients with frequent symptoms. Proper use of the MDI, with or without a spacing device, increases the efficacy of these agents. Spacer devices, especially when used in very young and elderly individuals, increase the amount of drug delivered to the lung twofold.

(2) **Corticosteroids** are used in combination with other agents for the treatment of moderate-to-severe chronic asthma.

(a) Inhaled corticosteroids are used for moderate episodes or as chronic prophylaxis. This route is the least likely to cause adverse reactions (see Table 50-6).

(b) Short course oral therapy ("burst" therapy) is used when the intermittent episodes are severe. Prednisone (or equivalent) is given in high doses (40–80 mg/day in adults; 1–2 mg/kg/day in children) for up to 5–10 days, then rapidly tapered. Improvement in the PEFR is used to monitor therapy.

(c) Chronic oral steroids are used after the failure of other medications to relieve chronic symptoms. Agents should be given in the lowest possible dose to avoid serious complications.

(3) **Cromolyn sodium** is used adjunctively to treat mild, moderate, or severe chronic asthma; it sometimes helps reduce the amount of corticosteroid needed. When used prophylactically, it may prevent exercise-induced asthma and seasonal asthma. It has no value in the treatment of an acute asthma attack. Initial improvement is within 1–2 weeks; the maximum effect may take longer.

(a) **Therapeutic effect.** Cromolyn suppresses allergen-induced bronchospasm. When used as maintenance therapy for asthma, it suppresses nonspecific bronchial hyperreactivity.

(b) **Mechanism of action.** Cromolyn acts locally on the lung mucosa, inhibiting the degranulation of sensitized mast cells by prevention of calcium influx that takes place after exposure to specific antigens. It also suppresses the release of histamine and other mediators from mast cells, thereby decreasing the stimulus for bronchospasm.

(c) **Administration and dosage.** Cromolyn is available as 20-mg capsules whose contents are inhaled via a special turboinhaler, as a nebulizer solution (20 mg/2 ml), and as a MDI, providing 0.8 mg per inhalation.

(i) As adjunctive therapy for severe chronic asthma, a 20-mg capsule is given for inhalation four times a day; or the solution is sprayed via nebulizer into each nostril three to six times a day; or two sprays of the MDI are used four times a day.

(ii) To prevent asthma attacks, cromolyn is used 10–15 minutes before exposure to the triggering factor (e.g., pollen).

(d) **Precautions and monitoring effects**

(i) Cromolyn is not intended for use during an acute asthma attack or status asthmaticus.

(ii) Generally, this drug is well tolerated; occasionally, the inhaled form causes paradoxical bronchospasm, wheezing, and coughing, as well as nasal congestion and dryness of the throat and trachea. There are fewer side effects with the MDI.

(iii) Rarely, laryngeal edema, urticaria, or anaphylaxis occurs.

(4) **Theophylline** may be added to the regimen when therapy with other inhaled agents has been maximized. Because of the availability of sustained-release products, this agent is most beneficial in patients with early morning symptoms. Monitoring serum levels, adverse reactions, and concomitant drug use is essential for long-term therapy.

(5) **Anticholinergic agents,** especially **ipratropium bromide,** are effective bronchodilators and may be added instead of theophylline or when theophylline has failed.

(6) **Spacer devices** are used with MDIs to increase the amount of drug delivered to the lung and decrease oropharyngeal disposition. These devices are indicated in pediatric and geriatric patients where coordination is a problem. Devices vary in structure and efficacy.

(a) **Holding chamber** (e.g., Aerochamber, Inhal-Aid, Inspirease)

(b) **Tube spacer** (e.g., Brethancer)

I. Complications of asthma

1. **Status asthmaticus.** This life-threatening condition occurs when a prolonged asthma attack fails to respond to normal treatment.

a. **Physical findings** include altered consciousness, cyanosis (even with oxygen therapy), and pulsus paradoxus (> 12 mm Hg).

b. **Standard therapy** for status asthmaticus involves oxygen, intravenous fluids and electrolytes, inhaled β-adrenergics, subcutaneous β-adrenergics, and corticosteroids. In some cases, intravenous aminophylline is added.

c. **Aggressive therapy** is warranted if standard therapy fails.

(1) If the patient has respiratory acidosis, **tracheal intubation** and **mechanical ventilation** are necessary.

(2) If the patient does not respond adequately to these measures, any of the following steps may be taken in addition to mechanical ventilation.

(a) **Sedatives** (e.g., morphine, diazepam) may be administered.

(b) **Skeletal muscle paralysis** may be induced via **pancuronium** administration.

(c) **General anesthesia** may be induced via a bronchodilating anesthetic (e.g., halothane).

(d) Segmental bronchial lavage may be performed to remove the mucous plugs blocking the airway.

2. **Pneumothorax.** This condition is characterized by accumulation of air in the pleural space, as sometimes occurs during an acute asthma attack.

a. **Physical findings** include sudden sharp chest pain, dyspnea, tachypnea, hypotension, diaphoresis, pallor, and anxiety.

b. Therapy includes placing the patient in Fowler's position, oxygen therapy, aspiration of pleural air via a chest tube, and analgesics.

3. Atelectasis. This disorder, which inhibits gas exchange during respiration, may occur if bronchiolar obstruction causes collapse of lung tissue. In asthmatics, atelectasis usually involves the right middle lobe but sometimes affects the entire lung.

a. Physical findings include diminished breath sounds, mediastinal shift toward the affected side, worsening dyspnea, anxiety, and cyanosis.

b. Therapy includes incentive spirometry, postural drainage, chest percussion, coughing and deep breathing exercises, and bronchodilators. Bronchoscopy may be necessary to remove secretions.

II. CHRONIC OBSTRUCTIVE PULMONARY DISEASE

A. Definitions. Chronic obstructive pulmonary disease (COPD) is a general term for conditions characterized by chronic, progressive lower airway obstruction, causing reduced pulmonary inspiratory and expiratory capacity. The two major forms of COPD—**chronic bronchitis** and **emphysema**—frequently coexist.

1. Chronic bronchitis. In this disorder, excessive mucus production by the tracheobronchial tree results in airway obstruction due to edema and bronchial inflammation. Bronchitis is considered chronic when the patient has a cough producing more than 30 ml of sputum in 24 hours for at least 3 months of the year for 2 consecutive years.

2. Emphysema. This condition is marked by permanent alveolar enlargement distal to the terminal bronchioles and destructive changes of the alveolar walls.

B. Incidence. Approximately 7.5 million Americans have COPD. More common in men than women, COPD affects about 20% of older men. However, due to the increased number of women smokers, the incidence of emphysema in women is rising.

C. Etiology. Various factors have been implicated in the development of COPD.

1. Cigarette smoking. The major causative factor, smoking predisposes an individual to COPD by impairing ciliary action and macrophage function and by causing airway inflammation, increased mucous secretion, alveolar wall destruction, and peribronchiolar fibrosis.

2. Other etiologic factors include exposure to irritants such as sulfur dioxide (as in polluted air), noxious gases, and organic or inorganic dusts; a history of childhood respiratory infections; familial and hereditary factors (e.g., α_1-antitrypsin deficiency); and allergy.

D. Pathophysiology

1. Chronic bronchitis

a. Respiratory tissue inflammation (as from smoking) results in vasodilation, congestion, mucosal edema, and goblet cell hypertrophy. These events trigger goblet cells to produce excessive amounts of mucus.

b. Changes in tissue include increased smooth muscle, cartilage atrophy, infiltration of neutrophils and other cells, and impairment of cilia.

c. Chronic bronchitis, due to lung impairment, predisposes patients to **lung infections,** both viral and bacterial, which further **destroy small bronchioles**.

d. As the disease progresses:

(1) Airways are blocked by thick, tenacious mucus secretions, which triggers a productive cough.

(2) As the **airways degenerate,** overall gas exchange is impaired, causing **exertional dyspnea**.

(3) Hypoxemia results from V/Q imbalance and is reflected in an increasing $Pa{CO_2}$ and hypercapnia.

(4) Sustained hypercapnia desensitizes the brain's respiratory control center and central chemoreceptors. As a result, compensatory action to correct hypoxemia and hypercapnia (i.e., a respiratory rate increase) does not occur.

2. Emphysema

a. Anatomical changes destroy lung elasticity.

(1) **Inflammation** and **excessive mucous secretion** (as from long-standing chronic bronchitis) cause **air trapping in the alveoli**. This contributes to breakdown of the bronchioles, alveolar walls, and connective tissue.
(2) As clusters of alveoli merge, the number of alveoli diminishes, leading to increased space available for air trapping.
(3) Destruction of alveolar walls causes collapse of small airways on exhalation and disruption of the pulmonary capillary beds.
(4) These changes result in **V/Q abnormalities;** blood is shunted away from destroyed areas to maintain a constant V/Q ratio, unlike the case in chronic bronchitis.
(5) **Hypercapnia** and **respiratory acidosis** may develop, causing desensitization of brain centers to hypercapnia. When this occurs, hypoxemia serves as the stimulus for breathing.

b. **Specific lung regions** in which characteristic anatomical changes of emphysema occur
(1) In **centrilobular emphysema,** associated with chronic bronchitis, the upper lung portions are affected. Typically, bronchioles, but not alveoli, become dilated and merge.
(2) In **panlobular emphysema,** all lung segments are involved. The alveoli enlarge and atrophy, and the pulmonary vascular bed is destroyed. This form of emphysema is associated with α_1-antitrypsin deficiency.
(3) In **paraseptal emphysema,** the lung periphery adjacent to fibrotic regions is the site of alveolar distention and alveolar wall destruction.

E. Clinical evaluation

1. Physical findings

a. **Predominant chronic bronchitis** typically has an insidious onset after age 45.
(1) **A chronic productive cough** is the **hallmark** of chronic bronchitis. It occurs first in winter, then progresses to year-round. It is usually worse in the morning.
(2) **Exertional dyspnea,** the most common presenting symptom, is progressive. However, the severity of this symptom does not reflect the severity of the disease.
(3) Other common findings include obesity, rhonchi and wheezes on auscultation, cyanosis, prolonged expiration, and a normal respiratory rate. As the disease progresses, the following are also common: jugular venous distention, peripheral edema, hepatomegaly, and cardiomegaly.

b. **Predominant emphysema** has an insidious onset and symptoms occur after age 55.
(1) The **cough** is chronic but less productive than in chronic bronchitis.
(2) **Exertional dyspnea** is progressive, constant, and severe.
(3) Other common findings include weight loss, tachypnea, pursed-lip breathing, prolonged expiration, accessory chest muscle use, hyperresonance on percussion, diaphragmatic excursion, and diminished breath sounds.

c. Patients may have elements and physical findings from each of these diseases simultaneously.

2. Diagnostic test results

a. **Chronic bronchitis**
(1) **Blood analysis** usually reveals an increased hematocrit value and sometimes shows an elevated erythrocyte level. With bacterial infection, the white blood cell count may be elevated.
(2) **Sputum inspection** reveals thick purulent or mucopurulent sputum tinged yellow, white, green, or gray; the color change is diagnostic of infection. Microscopic analysis may detect neutrophils and microorganisms.
(3) **Arterial blood gas studies** may show a markedly decreased Pa_{O_2} level (45–60 mmHg) [hypoxemia] and a Pa_{CO_2} level that is normal (50–60 mmHg) or elevated (hypercapnia).
(4) **Pulmonary function tests** may be normal in early disease stages. Later, they show an increased RV, a decreased vital capacity (VC) and FEV, and normal diffusing capacity and static lung compliance.
(5) **Chest x-ray** typically identifies lung hyperinflation and increased bronchovascular markings.
(6) An **ECG** may reveal right ventricular hypertrophy and changes consistent with cor pulmonale.

b. **Emphysema**
(1) **Blood analysis** may indicate an increased hemoglobin value in late disease stages; it also may show a decreased α_1-antitrypsin level.

(2) **Sputum inspection** reveals scanty sputum that is clear or mucoid. Infections are less frequent than in chronic bronchitis.

(3) **Arterial blood gas studies** typically indicate a reduced or normal Pa_{O_2} (65–75 mm Hg) level and, in late disease stages, an increased Pa_{CO_2} level (35–40 mm Hg).

(4) **Pulmonary function tests** show normal or increased static lung compliance, reduced diffusing capacity, and increased TLC and RV.

(5) **Chest x-ray** usually reveals bullae, blebs, a flattened diaphragm, lung hyperinflation, vertical heart, enlarged anteroposterior chest diameter, decreased vascular markings in the lung periphery, and a large retrosternal air space.

F. Treatment objectives

1. Relieve symptoms and, thus, enable the patient to carry on normal daily activities
2. Improve pulmonary function
3. Control life-threatening disease exacerbations
4. Prevent complications
5. Teach the patient about the disease and the use of medications and, thus, improve therapeutic compliance

G. Therapy

1. **Drug therapy.** β-Adrenergic agents and anticholinergic drugs are the most commonly used agents. Corticosteroids are beneficial when an allergic component has been demonstrated. Methylxanthines are added when the response to other agents is inadequate.

a. **β-Adrenergic agents** (see I H 1 a; Table 50-2) are effective in relieving dyspnea due to airway obstruction. Response is not as significant as in asthmatic patients. These agents may also increase mucociliary clearance by stimulating ciliary activity.

(1) β-Adrenergic agents are administered via aerosol (e.g., MDI with or without a spacer or a nebulizer) unless the patient cannot use the drug properly, then an oral agent is used.

(2) Agents in this class should not be used in combination. An adequate dose of a single agent provides peak bronchodilation.

(3) Prolonged use of high doses of β-adrenergic agents may lead to drug tolerance.

b. **Ipratropium bromide and atropine.** These agents produce bronchodilation by competitively inhibiting cholinergic receptors. Some studies have shown an increased response to these agents in COPD when they are combined with β-adrenergics.

(1) **Ipratropium bromide** is three to five times more potent and has fewer side effects than atropine. It is administered through two inhalations, four times daily. The degree of bronchodilation may be comparable to inhaled β-adrenergic agonists.

(2) **Atropine** is administered by diluting 0.025 mg/kg to 0.05 mg/kg in 2–4 ml of normal saline and placing it in a nebulizer for spraying every 6 hours. Side effects include dry mouth, tachycardia, and urinary retention.

c. **Corticosteroids** (see I H 1 c, Table 50-7) play a less prominent role in COPD than in asthma.

(1) These agents may be added to the drug regimen after maximal β-adrenergic therapy.

(2) Candidates for corticosteroid therapy should have a history of positive response to bronchodilator therapy (as evidenced by an FEV_1 increase of more than 15%–20%) and frequent disease exacerbations accompanied by wheezing.

(3) Corticosteroids may be given via aerosol to minimize adverse effects.

(4) Acute exacerbations can be treated intravenously with methylprednisolone, 0.5–1.0 mg/kg every 6 hours for 72 hours, then tapered off.

(5) For oral use, these agents are administered in a dosage of 20–40 mg/day for the first 2–4 weeks, then titrated to the lowest effective dosage.

d. **Theophylline compounds** (see I H 1 b; Table 50-4) typically are added to the drug regimen after a trial of β-adrenergics.

(1) In COPD, these drugs increase mucociliary clearance, stimulate the respiratory drive, enhance diaphragmatic contractility, and improve the ventricular ejection fraction.

(2) A trial of 1–2 months, with the serum drug level maintained at 10–20 μg/ml, is needed to assess therapeutic efficacy. An increase in FEV_1 by more than 15%–20% indicates a positive response.

(3) Serum drug levels should be monitored closely in patients with congestive heart failure (CHF) or cor pulmonale.

e. **Antibiotics** are used only to treat a documented infection or to prevent infection in high-risk patients. Therapy should be initiated rapidly when patients observe an increase in the amount of sputum or a change in the viscosity or color.
   (1) The most common infecting organisms are *Mycoplasma pneumoniae, Streptococcus pneumoniae, Haemophilus influenzae,* and *Moraxella catarrhalis.*
   (2) Antibiotics commonly used (for 7–10 days) in COPD include:
      (a) Ampicillin (500 mg given four times a day)
      (b) Amoxicillin (500 mg given three times a day)
      (c) Erythromycin (500 mg given four times a day)
      (d) Tetracycline (250–500 mg given four times a day)
      (e) Trimethoprim (80 mg) and sulfamethoxazole (400 mg) given as a combination product twice daily
   (3) Alternative agents for resistant organisms
      (a) Amoxicillin/clavulanate (250 mg given three times a day)
      (b) Cefuroxime axetil (250 mg given two times a day)
      (c) Cefixime (460 mg daily)
      (d) Cefaclor (250 mg three times a day)

2. **Other measures.** Depending on individual patient needs, COPD therapy also may include the following:
   a. **Fluid administration** helps to liquefy secretions; water is a good expectorant.
   b. **Mucolytics** (e.g., acetylcysteine); their use is controversial due to side effects.
   c. **Expectorants** (e.g., potassium iodide, ammonium chloride) promote mucus removal but with some side effects.
   d. **Oxygen therapy** (administered at a low flow rate) reverses hypoxemia. Patients with severe COPD may require oxygen for at least 15 hr/day, administered at a flow rate of 2 L/min.
   e. **Chest physiotherapy** loosens secretions, helps re-expand the lungs, and increases the efficacy of respiratory muscle use. Techniques used include postural drainage, chest percussion and vibration, and coughing and deep breathing.
   f. **Physical rehabilitation** improves the patient's exercise tolerance. A rehabilitation program usually includes exercises that improve diaphragmatic and abdominal muscle tone.
   g. **Vaccines** (e.g., influenza virus, pneumococcal, and *H. influenzae* type b polysaccharide vaccines) may be administered to prevent infection.

H. **Complications of COPD.** Patients with COPD have an increased risk for developing several life-threatening complications.

1. **Pulmonary hypertension.** With decreased pulmonary vascular bed space (due to lung congestion), pulmonary arterial pressure increases. In some cases, pressure rises high enough to cause **cor pulmonale** (right ventricular hypertrophy) with consequent heart failure.

2. **Acute respiratory failure.** In advanced stages of emphysema, the brain's respiratory center may become seriously compromised, leading to poor cerebral oxygenation and an increased $PaCO_2$ level. Hypoxia and respiratory acidosis may ensue. If the condition progresses, respiratory failure occurs.

3. **Infection.** In chronic bronchitis, trapping of excessive mucus, air, and bacteria in the tracheobronchial tree sets the stage for infection. In addition, impairment of coughing and deep breathing, which normally cleanse the lungs, leads to respiratory cilia destruction. Once an infection sets in, reinfection can easily occur.

STUDY QUESTIONS

Directions: Each of the numbered items or incomplete statements in this section is followed by answers or by completions of the statement. Select the **one** lettered answer or completion that is **best** in each case.

1. The symptoms of allergin-mediated asthma result from

(A) increased release of mediators from mast cells
(B) increased adrenergic responsiveness of the airways
(C) increased vascular permeability of bronchial tissue
(D) decreased calcium influx into the mast cell
(E) decreased prostaglandin production

2. Acute exacerbations of asthma can be triggered by all of the following EXCEPT

(A) bacterial or viral pneumonia
(B) hypersensitivity reaction to penicillin
(C) discontinuation of asthma medication
(D) hot, dry weather
(E) stressful emotional events

3. The selection of an oral theophylline product depends primarily on

(A) the percentage of theophylline content of the product
(B) preexisting disease states (e.g., gout, peptic ulcer disease)
(C) theophylline half-life
(D) concurrent asthma medication
(E) age of the patient

4. In the emergency room, the preferred first-line therapy for asthma is

(A) theophylline
(B) a β-agonist
(C) a corticosteroid
(D) cromolyn sodium
(E) an antihistamine

5. The primary goals of asthma therapy include all of the following EXCEPT

(A) treatment of secondary complications
(B) management of acute attacks
(C) chronic symptom management
(D) prevention of acute exacerbations
(E) prevention of lung tissue destruction

6. In the treatment of chronic obstructive pulmonary disease (COPD), corticosteroids

(A) are more effective than in the treatment of asthma
(B) are more beneficial when used alone
(C) produce more side effects when used in the aerosol form
(D) should have the dosage titrated upward until side effects are seen
(E) should be used for at least 2 weeks before efficacy is assessed

---

1-A 4-B
2-D 5-E
3-A 6-E

Directions: The item below contains three suggested answers of which **one or more** is correct. Choose the answer

A if **I only** is correct
B if **III only** is correct
C if **I and II** are correct
D if **II and III** are correct
E if **I, II, and III** are correct

7. The disease process of chronic bronchitis is characterized by

I. the destruction of central and peripheral portions of the acinus
II. an increased number of mucous glands and goblet cells
III. edema and inflammation of the bronchioles

Directions: The item in this section consists of lettered options followed by a set of numbered items. For each item, select the **one** lettered option that is most closely associated with it. Each lettered option may be selected once, more than once, or not at all.

Questions 8–10

Match the description with the appropriate agent.

(A) Cimetidine
(B) Albuterol
(C) Ipratropium bromide
(D) Epinephrine
(E) Atropine

8. Decreases theophylline clearance

9. Has anticholinergic activity with few side effects

10. Has high β_2-adrenergic selectivity

7-D
8-A
9-C
10-B

ANSWERS AND EXPLANATIONS

1. The answer is A *[I E 4; Figure 50-1].*
In asthma, airborne antigen binds to the mast cell, activating the immunoglobulin E (IgE)-mediated process. Mediators (e.g., histamine, leukotrienes, prostaglandins) are then released, causing bronchoconstriction and tissue edema.

2. The answer is D *[I D 1; Figure 50-1].*
Exacerbations of asthma can be triggered by allergens, respiratory infections, occupational stimuli (e.g., fumes from gasoline or paint), emotions, and environmental factors. Studies have shown that cold air can cause release of mast cell mediators by an undetermined mechanism. Hot, dry air does not cause this release.

3. The answer is A *[I H 1 b; Table 50-4].*
Theophylline or aminophylline products vary in their percentage of active drug, or theophylline content, and in the type of preparation. Sustained-release products decrease the absorption rate and do not alter theophylline half-life.

4. The answer is B *[I H 1 a (3)].*
In an emergency situation, the most rapidly acting agent is used first. Selection of the route of administration depends on the severity of the attack. An inhaled β-agonist administered in a nebulizer or administered as a subcutaneous agent is the most appropriate first-line therapy.

5. The answer is E *[I E, G; II D].*
Asthma is a reversible narrowing of airways in response to specific stimuli. Mast cells release mediators, which trigger bronchoconstriction. After an acute attack, in most cases, symptoms are minimal, and pathologic changes are not permanent. Unlike asthma, chronic obstructive pulmonary disease (COPD) does cause progressive airway destruction, chronic bronchitis by excessive mucus production and other changes, and emphysema by destruction of the acinus.

6. The answer is E *[II G 1 c].*
In chronic obstructive pulmonary disease (COPD), corticosteroids are used in addition to β-adrenergic agents and theophylline compounds after maximal therapy with these agents. Corticosteroids may be used in aerosol form to minimize side effects. If given orally, dosage is reduced after 2–4 weeks of therapy to the lowest effective dosage. Since the onset of benefit is unknown, an adequate trial of therapy (at least 2–4 weeks) is needed.

7. The answer is D (II, III) *[II D 1 a, c, 2].*
Chronic bronchitis is characterized by an increase in the number of mucous and goblet cells due to bronchial irritation.This results in increased mucus production. Other changes include edema and inflammation of the bronchioles and changes in smooth muscle and cartilage. Emphysema is a permanent destruction of the central and peripheral portions of the acinus distal to the bronchioles. In this disease, adequate oxygen reaches the alveolar duct, but there is inadequate blood perfusion.

8–10. The answers are: 8-A *[Table 50-5],* **9-C** *[II G 1 b (1)]* , **10-B** *[Table 50-2].*
Cimetidine, a histamine$_2$-receptor antagonist, decreases theophylline clearance by inhibiting hepatic microsomal mixed-function oxidase metabolism. Theophylline clearance can be decreased by 40% during the first 24 hours of concurrent therapy. Anticholinergic agents such as atropine and ipratropium bromide produce bronchodilation by competitively inhibiting cholinergic receptors. The disadvantages of atropine include dry mouth, tachycardia, and urinary retention. Ipratropium bromide is three to five times more potent than atropine and does not have these side effects. Albuterol is one of the most β_2-selective adrenergic agents available. Other such agents include terbutaline, bitolterol, and pirbuterol. Agents with β_2-selectivity dilate bronchioles without causing side effects related to β_1-stimulation (e.g., increased heart rate).

51 Rheumatoid Arthritis

Larry N. Swanson

I. INTRODUCTION

A. Definition. Rheumatoid arthritis is a chronic, systemic, inflammatory condition that is most apparent in its synovial joint involvement. Inflammation may extend to extra-articular sites such as tendons and organ structures.

B. Classification. Patients are said to have rheumatoid arthritis if they have satisfied at least four of the following criteria. The first four criteria must be present for at least 6 weeks.

1. **Morning stiffness** must be present in and around the joints lasting at least 1 hour before maximal improvement.
2. **Three joint areas** (at least) must have **soft-tissue swelling** or **fluid** observed by a physician. The possible joint areas are right or left **proximal interphalangeal (PIP) joint, metacarpophalangeal (MCP) joint, wrist, elbow, knee, ankle,** and **metatarsophalangeal (MTP) joint**.
3. **One joint area (at least) in the hand joints** (i.e., a wrist, MCP, PIP) **must be swollen** and observed by a physician.
4. **Symmetric arthritis.** There must be simultaneous involvement of the same joint areas on both sides of the body.
5. **Subcutaneous nodules (rheumatoid nodules)** over bony prominences, over extensor surfaces, or in juxta-articular regions must be observed by a physician.
6. **Abnormal amounts of serum rheumatoid factor** must be demonstrated by any method that has been positive in less than 5% of normal control subjects.
7. **Radiologic changes** typical of rheumatoid arthritis, including erosions or unequivocal bony decalcification localized to or most marked adjacent to the involved joints, must be present on hand and wrist x-rays.

C. Incidence. Rheumatoid arthritis is more common in women than in men, occurring with a female to male ratio of between 2:1 and 3:1. The condition occurs in approximately 1%–3% of the general adult population with the peak onset between the ages of 30 and 50 years.

D. Etiology. The cause of this disease remains unknown; however, the following factors may play a role:

1. A specific human leukocyte antigen (HLA-DR4) may be involved. When patients with this antigen are exposed to certain environmental factors, an inappropriate immune response occurs, which results in chronic inflammation.
2. Some infectious agent may be involved in precipitating rheumatoid arthritis in patients genetically predisposed.
3. Although no specific agent has been identified, for many years investigators have noted the occurrence of polyarthritis in association with microbial organisms, including bacteria (i.e., Lyme disease).

E. Pathogenesis

1. The initial event inciting synovial inflammation (the earliest synovial response) is unknown. Vasodilation, edema, sensation of heat, and loss of function result. Synovial fluid production increases with a resultant accumulation of an effusion. If untreated, the synovitis of rheumatoid arthritis becomes self-perpetuating and chronic. The synovium becomes thickened and boggy.

2. Inward overgrowth of the enlarged synovium across the surface of the articular cartilage results in the formation of **pannus** (an exuberant synovial thickening). The inflammatory reaction at the cartilage–pannus junction may eventually result in:
   a. Articular cartilage degradation
   b. Loss of adjacent bone
   c. Characteristic marginal erosions, which are observable on x-ray

3. The effect of degradation of cartilage is bone rubbing against bone in the joint, producing bony crepitus and pain.

F. Clinical manifestations

1. Usually, rheumatoid arthritis presents as **symmetric synovitis** affecting similar joints bilaterally. Occasionally, the disease may present as arthritis in only one joint or in an asymmetric pattern affecting a few joints. Over time, however, the arthritis assumes a symmetric pattern.

2. **Frank joint inflammation in a previously healthy individual** is a common presentation.

3. **A rapidly progressive arthritis affecting many joints,** accompanied by organ system involvement, is an uncommon presentation.

4. **Organ system involvement without clinically evident joint inflammation** is a very uncommon presentation.

G. Clinical course

1. Rheumatoid arthritis often follows one of the following patterns:
   a. **Sporadic.** This is the most common course; it is distinguished by periods of spontaneous remission and has the most favorable prognosis.
   b. **Gradual and steady.** A gradual but steady and persistent progression of joint inflammation is furthered by periodic debilitating flares. These flares are accompanied by severe polyarticular pain, marked synovial inflammation, joint effusion, stiffness, low-grade fever, and extreme exhaustion.
   c. **Malignant.** This course is less common but more rapid and aggressive. It is characterized by severe, multiple joint synovitis, rheumatoid nodules, weight loss, and very high titers of rheumatoid factor. Complications are common and include involvement of the skin (e.g., vasculitis), eyes (e.g., scleritis, corneal ulcers), lungs (e.g., pleural effusions, nodules, interstitial fibrosis), heart (e.g., pericarditis), blood (e.g., anemia, thrombocytosis), and nervous system (e.g., neuropathies).

2. Very early symptoms may be vague and lack evidence of synovial inflammation. The presenting complaints may include variable aching, multiple joint pain, and fatigue. Over months, the synovitis gradually evolves, usually in the feet and hands.
   a. Early involvement occurs most often in the hands, with swelling, warmth, and tenderness affecting mainly the PIP and MCP joints.
   b. Although hand and foot involvement is the most common initial presentation, synovitis can be prominent in the large joints of the knee, ankle, and elbow, as well as in the intervertebral and temporomandibular joints.

3. The hallmark of rheumatoid arthritis is maximal pain and stiffness upon awakening; this so-called morning gel typically lasts for more than 30 minutes and may persist for hours.

4. Rheumatoid arthritis is a progressive disease, which may result in irreversible joint deformities, such as:
   a. Ulnar deviation of fingers
   b. Swan-neck deformity
   c. Boutonniére deformities of PIP joints

H. Clinical evaluation

1. A thorough **joint system evaluation** with documentation of the swelling, synovial thickening, tenderness, pain, and reduced range of motion in peripheral joints is mandatory.

2. **Presence of rheumatoid nodules** (i.e., firm, round, rubbery masses that are pathognomonic for rheumatoid arthritis) are found in about 20% of patients. These nodules are most commonly located in subcutaneous tissues at sites prone to external pressure (e.g., the elbow), but they may affect other organs.

3. **X-rays** of involved joints may reveal only soft-tissue swelling initially. If inflammation is entrenched, the films may reveal juxta-articular osteoporosis, symmetrical joint space narrowing, and erosions near the joint capsular attachments.

4. **Laboratory findings**
   a. **Rheumatoid factors** (i.e., a heterogeneous group of antibodies produced in most patients with rheumatoid arthritis) are detectable through various serologic techniques and are present in about 80% of patients. The most commonly found rheumatoid factors are **immunoglobulin G (IgG)** and **immunoglobulin M (IgM)**. Patients with rheumatoid arthritis who are seropositive for rheumatoid factors generally follow a more serious disease course then those who are seronegative.
   b. **Erythrocyte sedimentation rate** may be increased, reflecting the inflammatory response.
   c. **Normochromic, normocytic anemia** may be seen (anemia of chronic disease).

I. Treatment objectives

1. To provide pain relief
2. To reduce or suppress inflammation
3. To avoid, minimize, or eliminate adverse effects resulting from therapy
4. To preserve or restore joint function
5. To maintain the patient's life-style

J. Monitoring parameters. Selected parameters are used to assess disease activity and drug response to rheumatoid arthritis. These parameters may include:

1. Duration of morning stiffness
2. Number of painful and tender joints
3. Number of swollen joints
4. Range of joint motion
5. PIP joint circumference
6. Time to onset of fatigue
7. Time to walk 50 feet
8. The erythrocyte sedimentation rate

II. THERAPY.

THERAPY. The treatment of rheumatoid arthritis combines two approaches: mechanical and pharmacologic. Mechanical therapy includes a balanced program of rest and exercise. The pharmacologic component now includes both symptomatic and disease-modifying therapy, which usually requires a combination of agents (Figures 51-1 and 51-2).

A. Mechanical therapy. The patient is educated in a balanced daily program of exercise and rest.

1. Initially, the joints are rested.
2. Exercises are then introduced to strengthen muscles and increase the range of motion without undue joint strain.
3. Alignment of the joints in a position of function is ensured during sleep through use of specially designed lightweight splints.
4. Complete immobilization is avoided.

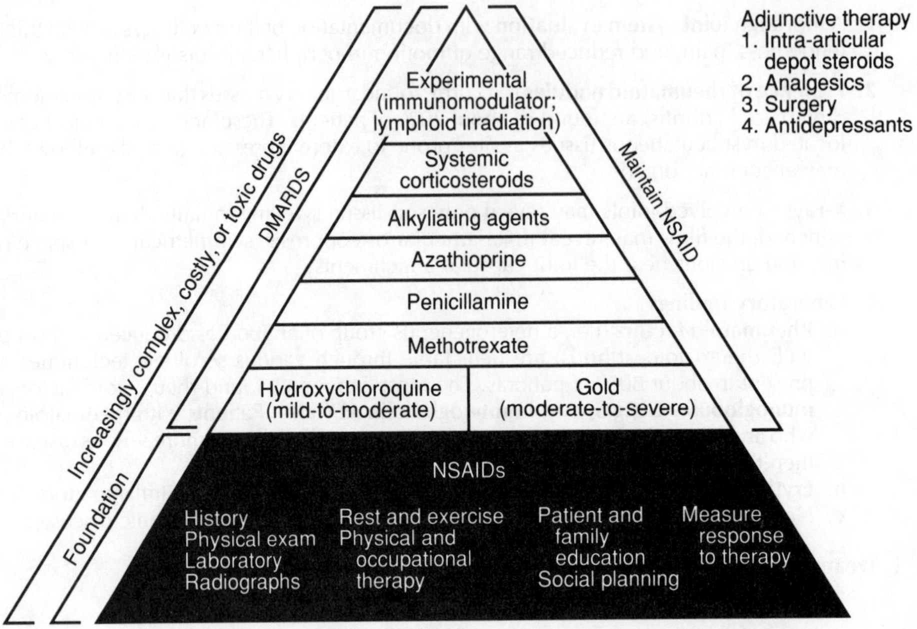

Figure 51-1. The pyramid approach to rheumatoid arthritis. The base of the pyramid comprises the standard therapy that all patients receive. The top of the pyramid comprises an increasingly complex, costly, or toxic regimen. Adjunctive therapy is given at any time during the disease. NSAIDs = nonsteroidal anti-inflammatory drugs; DMARDs = disease modifying anitrheumatic drugs. (Reprinted with permission from Gall EP: Update on drug treatments for rheumatoid arthritis. *Drug Therapy* 23(2):28, 1991.)

5. When preventive measures fail, surgery to improve function of the hands and knees is sometimes beneficial.

B. Symptomatic pharmacologic therapy. The choice of aspirin or **aspirin-like agents** is usually empirical because patients' responses vary widely. Further decisions on the drug regimen should be based on the therapeutic effect after 2–3 weeks. However, an inadequate response to one drug in this group may not reflect a patient's response to another. Furthermore, adverse effects or toxicity may override an adequate therapeutic response.

1. **Aspirin** is the first-line agent, administered initially as an analgesic, then in higher doses as an anti-inflammatory agent. Aspirin is as effective as any other nonsteroidal anti-inflammatory drug (NSAID) and is much less expensive.
   a. **Mechanism of action.** In common with other NSAIDs, aspirin appears to work, at least in part, by inhibiting prostaglandin synthesis and release.
   b. **Dosage.** The usual total dose is 3.6–5.4 g daily.
   c. **Precautions and monitoring effects**
      (1) Aspirin interferes with platelet function and can cause serious bleeding; this effect may persist for 4–7 days after the drug has been discontinued.
      (2) Tinnitus and, rarely, hepatitis or renal damage can occur with high-dose aspirin therapy.
      (3) The intolerable gastrointestinal effects experienced by some patients may be avoided by using an enteric-coated agent.

2. **Other NSAIDs (e.g., ibuprofen, naproxen, sulindac, piroxicam, indomethacin, others).** Many patients tolerate effective doses of the NSAIDs better than high-dose aspirin therapy. However, the newer drugs are much more expensive. No clinical evidence has proven that any one of these drugs is consistently more effective than another, but research shows that a patient who does not respond to one NSAID may respond to another. By trial and error, patients may need to try three or four of these agents. Generally, a 2–3-week trial of an adequate dose is required to identify treatment success or failure.
   a. **Mechanism of action** (see II B 1 a)

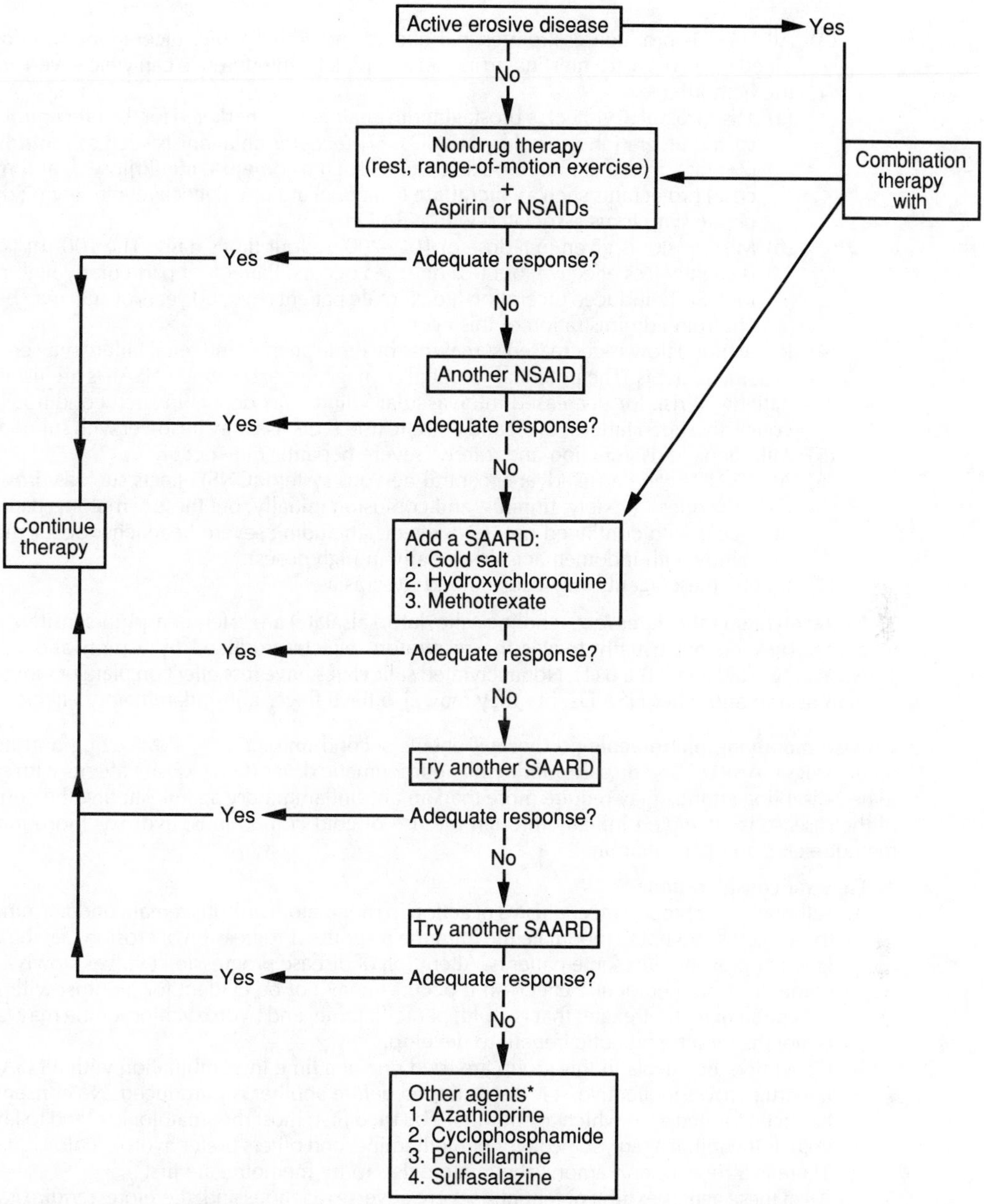

Figure 51-2. Algorithm for the treatment of rheumatoid arthritis. Corticosteroids may be necessary for patients with severe inflammatory disease in any of these phases to enable patients to be more functional while awaiting the beneficial effects of therapy or treatment failure. *NSAIDs* = nonsteroidal anti-inflammatory drugs; *SAARDs* = slow-acting antirheumatic drugs. (Reprinted with permission from DiPiro JT, Talbert RL, Hayes PE, et al: *Pharmacotherapy: A Pathophysiologic Approach,* 2nd ed. Norwalk, CT, Appleton & Lange, 1993, p 1321.)

b. Precautions and monitoring effects. The NSAIDs differ somewhat in adverse effects with none demonstrably safer in all patients. However, phenylbutazone and indomethacin are considered second-line agents that are usually avoided because of an association with aplastic anemia (phenylbutazone) and CNS effects (indomethacin).

(1) NSAIDs should be avoided in asthmatic patients sensitive to aspirin because they may trigger bronchospasm and respiratory failure.

(2) All NSAIDs interfere with platelet function and prolong bleeding time. However, unlike the effect with aspirin, this effect is quickly reversible with discontinuation of the drug.

(3) All NSAIDs produce gastrointestinal effects, including peptic ulceration. The combined effect of gastrointestinal irritation and platelet interference can yield severe gastric hemorrhage.

(a) **Misoprostol** (Cytotec), a prostaglandin analogue, is marketed for the prevention of gastric ulceration caused by NSAIDs. H_2-receptor antagonists such as **ranitidine** (Zantac), hydrogen ion blocking agents such as **omeprazole** (Prilosec), and mucosal protectants such as **sucralfate** (Carafate) are often effective in relieving dyspeptic symptoms associated with NSAID use.

(b) Misoprostol is given in a dose of 100–200 μg four times daily. The 100-μg dose is slightly less effective, but less diarrhea occurs. Patients at particularly high risk for NSAID-induced ulceration (i.e., female patients over 60 years of age) may benefit from administration of this agent.

(4) Renal blood flow is decreased somewhat by these agents, and renal failure may ensue in some patients. The potential for renal damage increases when NSAIDs are used in patients at risk for decreased intravascular volume, as occurs in such conditions as congestive heart failure (CHF) and diuretic use. (This risk may be lower with sulindac.)

(5) Mild hepatic dysfunction and, rarely, severe hepatitis may occur.

(6) All NSAIDs can cause adverse central nervous system (CNS) effects such as drowsiness, dizziness, anxiety, tinnitus, and confusion initially, but these symptoms usually disappear with continued use. CNS effects, including severe headache, occur more frequently with indomethacin (especially in high doses).

(7) Rarely, these agents may cause blood dyscrasias.

3. **Nonacetylated salicylates** (e.g., choline salicylate, salsalate) are safer for aspirin-sensitive patients. They do not usually trigger the respiratory effects produced by aspirin and other NSAIDs, as stated in II B 2 b (1). Nonacetylated salicylates have less effect on platelet function than aspirin and other NSAIDs, but they may also have fewer anti-inflammatory effects.

C. **Disease-modifying pharmacologic therapy** entails second-line agents—slow-acting antirheumatic drugs (SAARDs) and disease-modifying antirheumatic drugs (DMARDs). Patients with sustained disabling arthritis may require more than an anti-inflammatory agent. Altering the course of the disease is attempted initially through the use of gold compounds, hydroxychloroquine, methotrexate, and penicillamine.

1. **General considerations**

a. Although their precise mechanisms of action in rheumatoid arthritis remain undetermined, these agents attempt to modulate the immune response. Progression of erosion may be delayed or prevented in some patients. Alteration of disease progression evolves slowly and gradually, and therapeutic effect—if it occurs—may not be evident for months, with the exception of methotrexate; that is, gold, penicillamine, and hydroxychloroquine may take 6 months for a therapeutic benefit to develop.

b. Generally, the agents in this group are tried one at a time in combination with a NSAID. If a drug proves ineffective, it is discontinued before another is introduced. No consensus has been formed as to which agent should be tried first; most rheumatologists tend to favor gold as the initial agent, some favor penicillamine, and others prefer hydroxychloroquine. There is a recent trend among rheumatologists to try methotrexate first.

c. All of these agents exhibit potentially severe adverse reactions and, therefore, require careful monitoring of patients.

d. Some clinicians now begin the second-line drugs early in the course of the disease because prolonged prior use of NSAIDs often has not prevented deformity and joint destruction.

2. **Gold compounds** may be administered in oral or intramuscular form. Gold has been used for several years and may be effective in delaying or preventing progression of joint erosion in some patients, although one recent report questioned its ability to change the course of the disease.

a. **Intramuscular agents** [e.g., **gold sodium thiomalate** (Myochrysine) and **aurothioglucose** (Solganal)]. These agents are considered equally effective.

(1) **Administration and dosage.** Initially, a test dose of 10 mg is administered, followed by 25 mg once a week for 2 weeks, and then 50 mg in weekly intervals for up to 20 weeks. Once there is a therapeutic effect, treatment intervals are lengthened to every 2 weeks, then every 3 weeks, and finally to regular monthly administration. Patients who respond should remain at least on monthly therapy; if therapy is discontinued, arthritic symptoms may recur and may not be controlled when gold is restarted.

(2) **Precautions and monitoring effects.**

(a) The most common **side effects** are proteinuria and rash.

(i) Some clinicians obtain a complete blood count (CBC) and urinalysis before each injection or every other injection to detect drug-related decreases in blood counts or the presence of proteinuria.

(ii) Pruritus usually precedes stomatitis and a diffuse rash, which can progress to generalized exfoliation; therefore, the drug should be discontinued when pruritus occurs. Lower-dose therapy may be tried later if pruritus does occur.

(b) Leukopenia, thrombocytopenia, and aplastic anemia have been reported.

(c) Anaphylaxis, angioneurotic edema, glossitis, and interstitial pneumonitis can also occur.

(d) Aurothioglucose (fat-soluble) may be safer than gold sodium thiomalate (water-soluble), which is more likely to cause vasodilation and nitritoid reactions. These reactions are rare and usually mild, but hypotension, syncope, and myocardial infarction have been reported.

b. Oral agents. Auranofin (Ridaura) may be slightly less toxic, but slightly less effective, than other forms of gold.

(1) **Administration and dosage.** The initial regimen for auranofin consists of 3 mg twice a day or 6 mg once a day for 6 months. If there is no response, the dosage is increased to 3 mg three times daily (9 mg/day). If there is still no response after 3 more months, auranofin should be discontinued.

(2) **Precautions and monitoring effects.** Common, reversible side effects include diarrhea, abdominal pain, rash, stomatitis, and proteinuria. Oral gold causes less mucocutaneous, bone marrow, and renal toxicity than injectable gold but more diarrhea and other gastrointestinal reactions.

3. Methotrexate (Rheumatrex) is a folic acid antagonist that has been used as an antineoplastic agent. Some rheumatologists now consider it a first-line drug for rheumatoid arthritis.

a. Administration and dosage. Initially, the weekly regimen should consist of 5–10 mg. (Taking divided doses at 12-hour intervals is not more effective or safer than a single weekly dose.) This can be increased slowly—at 3–6-week intervals—to 15–20 mg a week.

b. Precautions and monitoring effects

(1) Aspirin (and possibly other NSAIDs) may increase the toxicity of methotrexate by slowing its rate of excretion.

(2) Adverse effects associated with methotrexate include gastrointestinal effects (e.g., anorexia, nausea, vomiting, abdominal cramps, gastrointestinal ulceration, bleeding), bone marrow suppression, hepatic toxicity, and allergic pneumonitis. Because the drug is used in lower doses than those for chemotherapy, the serious side effects are not usually seen.

(3) Monitoring should include baseline and follow-up CBCs, platelet counts, and monthly renal and liver function profiles.

4. Penicillamine (Depen). The effectiveness of this agent as an anti-inflammatory may result from its effect on the altered immune response.

a. Administration and dosage. Penicillamine should be given on an empty stomach because food decreases absorption. Initially, 125–250 mg should be administered once daily. Then the dosage should be increased (by the same amount) at 1–3-month intervals until an effective daily dose has been achieved (usually, 750 mg/day; rarely, 1000–1500 mg/day). The dosing motto for this drug is "go low—go slow."

b. Precautions and monitoring effects. Penicillamine has a high incidence of toxic effects, which limits its usefulness.

(1) Adverse effects (usually reversible) include rash, fever, hematuria, proteinuria, dysgeusia, and aphthous ulcers.

(2) Of more serious consequence are potential hematologic effects such as leukopenia, thrombocytopenia, and aplastic anemia.

(3) Autoimmune conditions such as systemic lupus erythematosus (SLE), Goodpasture's syndrome, and pemphigus have occurred.

5. Hydroxychloroquine (Plaquenil)

a. Administration and dosage. Hydroxychloroquine should be given in dosages of 400 mg/day (200 mg twice a day maximum) or 6.5 mg/kg/day, whichever is less. It may be reduced to 200 mg/day.

b. Precautions and monitoring effects

(1) Hydroxychloroquine can cause severe and sometimes irreversible adverse effects on the eyes, skin, CNS, and bone marrow, but these are rare with recommended doses.

(2) An ophthalmologist should check for loss of visual acuity every 3–6 months. Toxicity can generally be avoided if the drug is discontinued promptly at the first signs of retinal toxicity.

(3) This retinopathy, the most common side effect of hydroxychloroquine, results from deposition of the drug in a melanin layer of the cones. Symptoms include blurred vision, scotomata, and halos, and early damage may occur without warning. Mild defects in accommodation and convergence or corneal deposits are common and reversible.

6. Sulfasalazine (Azulfidine) recently has been shown to be useful in the treatment of rheumatoid arthritis.

a. Indications

(1) In a limited number of trials, sulfasalazine has been shown to be as effective as injectable gold and penicillamine and with fewer side effects.

(2) Sulfasalazine may be more effective than hydroxychloroquine in preventing the progression of joint damage.

b. Administration and dosage. The usual starting dose of sulfasalazine is 0.5 g twice daily, increased in increments of 0.5 g weekly to a maintenance dose of 2–3 g daily taken in two or three divided doses.

c. Precautions and monitoring effects. Common side effects include gastrointestinal disturbances and rash. Serious reactions such as blood dyscrasias and hepatitis are rare, but monitoring by liver function tests and CBCs is recommended every 2–3 weeks during the first 3 months of treatment and less frequently thereafter.

7. Azathioprine (Imuran) is a purine analogue immunosuppressive drug. It is generally used after other agents have failed.

a. Administration and dosage. Initially, 50–100 mg (about 1 mg/kg) should be given once or twice daily. After 6–8 weeks and then every 4 weeks, the doses can be increased by 0.5 mg/kg/day up to a maximum of 2.5 mg/kg/day. A maintenance regimen should use the lowest effective dose. The dosage should be reduced in patients with renal dysfunction.

b. Precautions and monitoring effects

(1) Adverse effects include nausea, vomiting, abdominal pain, hepatitis, and reversible bone marrow depression.

(2) Increased risk of carcinoma and severe infections are potential effects.

(3) A CBC and liver function profile should be obtained every 2–4 weeks as the dosage is increased.

8. Cyclophosphamide (Cytoxan) has been used primarily as an antineoplastic agent but may be used in refractory rheumatoid arthritis. However, cyclophosphamide is significantly more toxic than other immunosuppressive agents.

a. Administration and dosage. The usual initial dose in 1.5–3.0 mg/kg/day.

b. Precautions and monitoring effects. Serious toxic effects include bone marrow depression, hemorrhagic cystitis, sterility, alopecia, and malignant diseases (e.g., bladder cancer).

9. Chlorambucil and **cyclosporin A** are relatively toxic but may play a role in treating refractory rheumatoid arthritis.

D. Corticosteroids

1. General considerations. In severe, progressive rheumatoid arthritis, prednisone may afford some degree of control, but corticosteroids are usually recognized as agents of last resort. They occasionally may be used:

a. For acute flare-ups of the disease

b. During the interim before the therapeutic effects of slow-acting drugs are observed

c. In elderly patients as alternatives to the risks of second-line agents

d. In patients who cannot tolerate NSAIDs

e. For patients with significant systemic manifestations of rheumatoid arthritis

2. Administration and dosage

a. Oral prednisone in a dose of 5–10 mg/day may benefit some patients. Because adverse effects are related to dose and duration, an effort must be made to keep the dose as low as possible.

b. If painful symptoms are restricted to one or a few acutely inflamed joints, intra-articular injections may provide relief.

3. Precautions and monitoring effects. Long-term administration may produce gastrointestinal bleeding, poor wound healing, myopathy, cataracts, hyperglycemia, hypertension, and osteoporosis.

III. POSSIBLE NEW APPROACHES

A. Over the past decade, sequential monotherapy (pyramid approach) for rheumatoid arthritis has been challenged by the recognition of the need for early and more aggressive treatment. However, controversy exists concerning appropriate therapeutic approaches.

B. The toxicity of the NSAIDs and a greater awareness of the bleak prospects for many patients with rheumatoid arthritis have led to new therapeutic strategies.

1. Combination therapy. Combinations of SAARDs are popular alternatives to sequential monotherapy, the rationale being that they may achieve greater efficacy without a corresponding increase in toxicity, since each drug has different anti-inflammatory mechanisms.

2. Step-down bridge approach

a. Prednisone is administered for 1 month. Patients who fail to respond adequately then receive a combination of antimalarials, oral gold, parenteral gold, and methotrexate. Other SAARDs may be substituted. After 3 months of multiple-drug therapy, the dosages are tapered in the hope that the antimalarials alone will control the disease.

b. The step-down bridge approach attempts to control early inflammation before joint damage occurs, to shorten the duration of treatment with potentially toxic drugs, and to achieve a simpler and less expensive program than that provided by the conventional pyramid.

3. Sawtooth strategy. This approach advocates the use of SAARDs early in the course of rheumatoid arthritis and then the serial substitution of new agents throughout the disease course as the drugs that are being used lose their therapeutic benefit.

STUDY QUESTIONS

Directions: Each of the numbered items or incomplete statements in this section is followed by answers or by completions of the statement. Select the **one** lettered answer or completion that is **best** in each case.

1. A 50-year-old woman is admitted to the hospital with a chief complaint of bilateral swelling of her knees for 3 days, early morning stiffness, and lethargy. She is not responding to 650 mg of aspirin three times daily. The patient is an obese white woman who states that her ability to move about has slowly regressed due to the stiffness and swelling. She has also noticed a progressive swelling of the hands and wrists. A diagnosis of rheumatoid arthritis is made. Initial suggestion for drug therapy of this patient is

(A) hydroxychloroquine, 200 mg daily
(B) steroid injections into all swollen joints
(C) aspirin, 975 mg four times a day
(D) penicillamine, 250 mg four times a day
(E) gold injections, 50 mg intravenously once weekly

2. Which of the following agents and dosage regimens is the best choice of treatment for a patient with rheumatoid arthritis who is considered sensitive to aspirin?

(A) Ibuprofen, 800 mg three times per day
(B) Acetaminophen, 650 mg every 4 hours
(C) Gold injections, 25 mg intramuscularly once a week
(D) Azathioprine, 75 mg per day
(E) Cyclophosphamide, 100 mg per day

3. Which of the following statements best describes the usual course of rheumatoid arthritis?

(A) It is an acute exacerbation of joint pain treated with short-term anti-inflammatory therapy
(B) It is a chronic disease characterized by acute changes within nonsynovial joints
(C) It is an acute disease that is characterized by rapid synovial changes due to inflammation
(D) It is a chronic disease characterized by acute exacerbations followed by remissions, with consequences associated with chronic inflammatory changes
(E) It is a joint disease characterized by a marked loss of calcium from the bones and a resultant thinning of the bones

Directions: Each group of items in this section consists of lettered options followed by a set of numbered items. For each item, select the **one** lettered option that is most closely associated with it. Each lettered option may be selected once, more than once, or not at all.

Questions 4–8

Match the drug characteristic with the appropriate agent.

(A) Corticosteroids
(B) Ibuprofen
(C) Aspirin
(D) Auranofin
(E) Penicillamine

4. Persistent platelet function effect
5. Oral form of gold
6. Given on an empty stomach
7. May be used intra-articularly
8. May cause drowsiness

1-C	4-C	7-A
2-C	5-D	8-B
3-D	6-E	

Questions 9–13

Match the phrase below with the appropriate agent used to treat rheumatoid arthritis.

(A) Phenylbutazone
(B) Aspirin
(C) Hydroxychloroquine
(D) Methotrexate
(E) Cyclophosphamide

9. May cause hemorrhagic cystitis
10. Should be avoided in the treatment of rheumatoid arthritis (because of aplastic anemia)
11. Enteric-coated form may be useful in treating some patients
12. Aspirin may slow this drug's rate of excretion
13. Vision should be monitored every 3–6 months

9-E
10-A
11-B
12-D
13-C

ANSWERS AND EXPLANATIONS

1. The answer is C *[II B 1].*
Unless there are contraindications to the use of salicylates, aspirin administered in anti-inflammatory doses is the agent of choice for initial treatment of the patient with rheumatoid arthritis. The patient in the question has only been taking analgesic doses of aspirin; that is, 650 mg three times a day (1950 mg/day). Parenteral gold preparations are given by intramuscular injection, not intravenously.

2. The answer is C *[II B 2 b (1), C 2 a (1)].*
Patients with nasal polyps, hay fever, or asthma have an increased incidence of aspirin hypersensitivity. In these patients, aspirin administration may result in rhinorrhea, bronchospasm, or anaphylaxis. Patients who are intolerant of aspirin may also show a cross-sensitivity to ibuprofen and other nonsteroidal anti-inflammatory drugs (NSAIDs). Acetaminophen may provide some analgesic effect but has essentially no anti-inflammatory properties and, therefore, would not be a good choice for a patient with rheumatoid arthritis. If available, a nonacetylated salicylate may be given. Many rheumatologists use gold injections (10 mg as a test dose and 25–50 mg at weekly intervals) as the next most appropriate agent. Azathioprine and cyclophosphamide usually are reserved for later therapy.

3. The answer is D *[I A, G].*
Rheumatoid arthritis is a chronic disease that most often follows a sporadic course of acute exacerbations of synovial inflammation followed by remissions, with eventual joint manifestations of chronic inflammation.

4–8. The answers are: 4-C *[II B 1 c (1)],* **5-D** *[II C 2 b],* **6-E** *[II C 4 a],* **7-A** *[II D 2 b],* **8-B** *[II B 2 b (6)].*
Both aspirin and other NSAIDs interfere with platelet function; with aspirin, the effect may persist for 4–7 days after the drug has been discontinued, whereas platelet function usually returns quickly to normal after stopping other NSAID therapy. Most gold preparations are given by intramuscular injection, but auranofin is given orally. Penicillamine is given on an empty stomach because food decreases its absorption. Intra-articular injection of a corticosteroid is helpful when painful symptoms are restricted to one or a few joints. Ibuprofen, like other NSAIDs, may cause drowsiness and other central nervous system (CNS) effects, but these usually subside with continued use.

9–13. The answers are: 9-E *[II C 8 b],* **10-A** *[II B 2 b],* **11-B** *[II B 1 c (3)],* **12-D** *[II C 3 b (1)],* **13-C** *[II C 5 b (2)].*
Cyclophosphamide is significantly more toxic than other immunosuppressive agents; one of its serious side effects is hemorrhagic cystitis. Phenylbutazone should not be selected for long-term treatment of rheumatoid arthritis because of its association with aplastic anemia. There are many other less toxic NSAIDs that can be used. Many patients taking high doses of aspirin cannot tolerate regular aspirin but can take the enteric-coated form. Aspirin administration may slow the excretion of methotrexate; this can increase the latter drug's toxicity. Because hydroxychloroquine can cause ophthalmic adverse effects, patients receiving this drug should have their vision checked at least every 6 months.

52
Hyperuricemia and Gout

Larry N. Swanson

I. INTRODUCTION

A. Definitions

1. **Hyperuricemia** refers to a serum uric acid level that is elevated more than 2 standard deviations above the population mean. In most laboratories, the upper limit of normal is 7 mg/dl (uricase methods). However, the level varies with the laboratory method used; the upper limit of normal is about 1 mg/dl lower for women than for men.
   a. **Uricase methods** are specific for uric acid and are not subject to interference by drugs.
   b. **Phosphotungstic acid (colorimetric) methods** are nonspecific for uric acid; they are subject to interference (false elevation) by drugs.
2. **Gout** is a disease that is characterized by recurrent acute attacks of urate crystal-induced arthritis. It may include **tophi**—deposits of monosodium urate—in and around the joints and cartilage and in the kidneys, as well as uric acid nephrolithiasis.

B. Incidence

1. Gout affects approximately 0.2%–1.5% of the population in the United States.
2. Most gout victims are men (approximately 95% of cases); most women with the disease are postmenopausal.
3. The mean age at disease onset is 47 years.
4. The risk of developing gout increases as the serum uric acid level rises. Virtually all gout patients have a serum uric acid level above 7 mg/dl.
5. Recent research shows that among patients with a serum uric acid level above 9 mg/dl, the cumulative incidence of gout reached 22% after 5 years.
6. Gout has a familial tendency; 10%–60% of cases occur in family members of patients with the disease.
7. Obesity, heavy alcohol consumption, and certain other life-style factors increase the chances of developing gout.

C. Uric acid production and excretion

1. An end product of **purine metabolism,** uric acid is produced from both dietary and endogenous sources. Its formation results from the conversion of adenine and guanine moieties of nucleoproteins and nucleotides (Figure 52-1).
2. **Xanthine oxidase** catalyzes the reaction that occurs as the final step in the degradation of purines to uric acid.
3. The body ultimately excretes uric acid via the kidneys (300–600 mg/day; two-thirds of total uric acid) and via the gastrointestinal tract (100–300 mg/day; one-third of the total uric acid).
4. Uric acid has no known biologic function.
5. The body has a total uric acid content of 1.0–1.2 g; the daily turnover rate is approximately 600–800 mg.

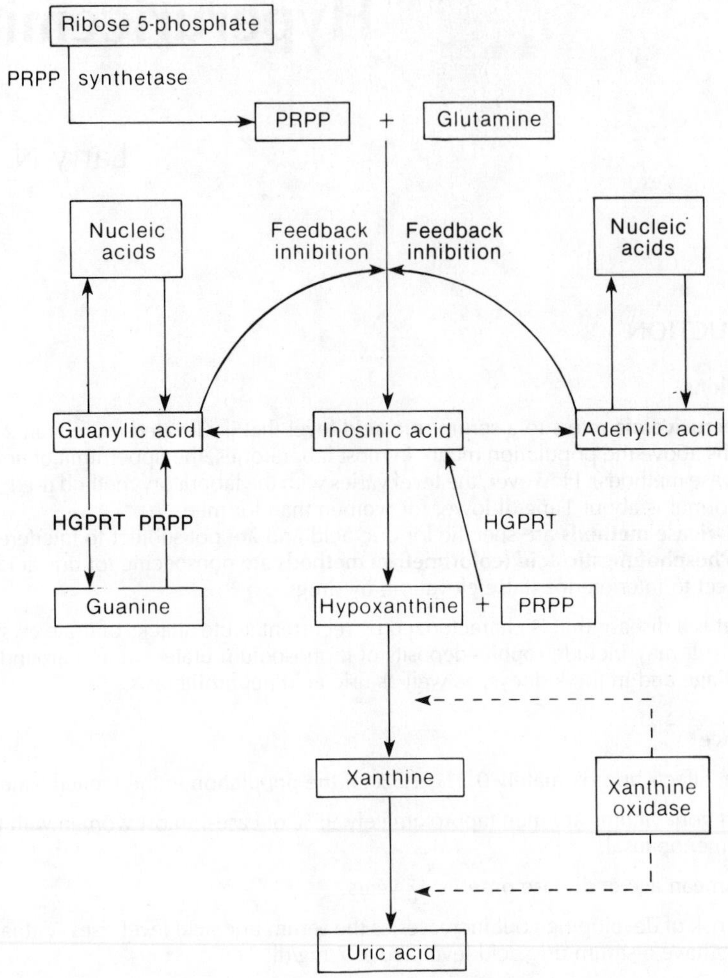

Figure 52-1. Uric acid formation. *PRPP* = phosphoribosyl-1-pyrophosphate; *HGPRT* = hypoxanthine–guanine phosphoribosyltransferase. (Redrawn with permission from DiPiro J, Talbert R, Hayes P, et al: *Pharmacotherapy—A Pathophysiologic Approach.* East Norwalk, CT, Appleton & Lange, 1993, p 1344.)

6. At a pH of 4.0–5.0 (i.e., in urine), uric acid exists as a poorly soluble free acid; at physiologic pH, it exists primarily as **monosodium urate salt.**

7. Uric acid filtration, reabsorption, and secretion sites are shown in Figure 52-2.

D. Etiology. Hyperuricemia and gout may be primary or secondary.

1. Primary hyperuricemia and gout apparently result from an innate **defect in purine metabolism or uric acid excretion**. The exact cause of the defect usually is unknown.

a. Hyperuricemia may result from **uric acid overproduction, impaired renal clearance of uric acid,** or a combination of these.

b. Some patients with primary hyperuricemia and gout have a known enzymatic defect, such as hypoxanthine–guanine phosphoribosyltransferase (HGPRT) deficiency or phosphoribosyl-1-pyrophosphate (PRPP) synthetase excess (see Figure 52-1).

c. Principally for therapeutic purposes, patients with primary hyperuricemia and gout can be classified as **overproducers** or **underexcretors** of uric acid.

(1) Overproducers (about 10% of patients) synthesize abnormally large amounts of uric acid and excrete excessive amounts—more than 800–1000 mg daily on an unrestricted diet or more than 600 mg daily on a purine-restricted diet. They generally have a markedly increased miscible urate pool (greater than 2.5 g).

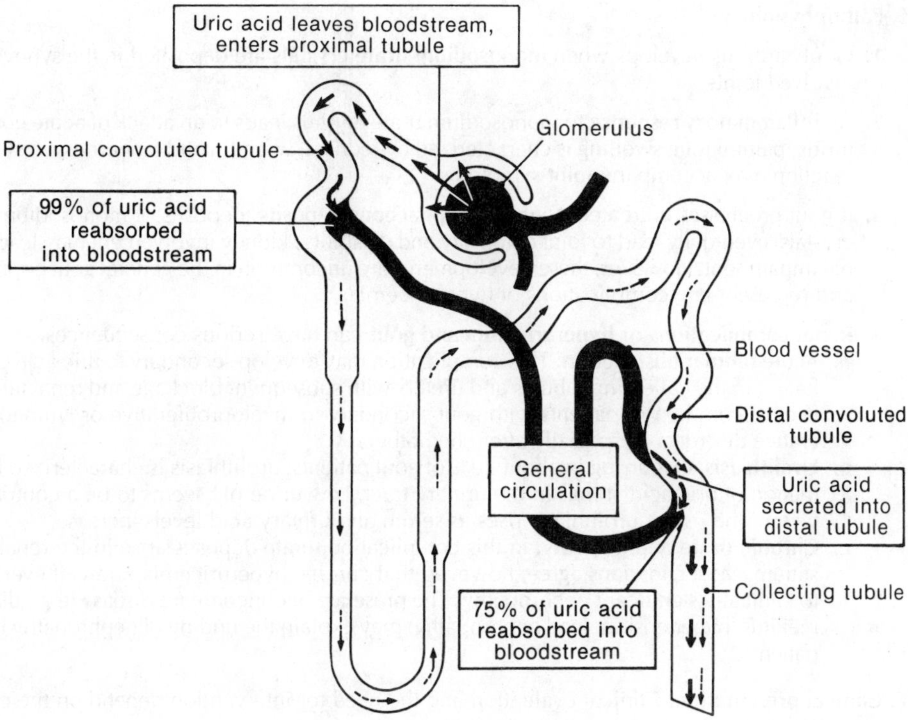

Figure 52-2. Uric acid filtration, reabsorption, and secretion sites. At the glomerulus, uric acid is filtered and enters the proximal tubule. Here, approximately 99% of uric acid is reabsorbed into the bloodstream. At the distal tubule, uric acid is secreted; subsequently, about 75% of the amount secreted is reabsorbed. Therefore, almost all urinary uric acid is excreted at the distal tubule.

(2) **Underexcretors** (about 90% of patients) generally produce normal or nearly normal amounts of uric acid but excrete less than 600 mg daily on a purine-restricted diet. They generally have only a slightly increased miscible urate pool. Some underexcretors also are overproducers.

2. **Secondary hyperuricemia and gout** develop during the course of another disease or as a result of drug therapy.
   a. **Hematologic causes** of hyperuricemia and gout (associated with increased nucleic acid turnover and breakdown to uric acid)
      (1) Lymphoproliferative disorders
      (2) Myeloproliferative disorders
      (3) Certain hemolytic anemias and hemoglobinopathies
   b. **Chronic renal failure.** In this condition, reduced renal clearance of uric acid can lead to hyperuricemia.
   c. **Drug-induced disease**
      (1) **Aspirin** and **other salicylates** inhibit tubular secretion of uric acid when given in low doses (e.g., less than 2 g/day of aspirin). At high doses, they frequently cause uricosuria.
      (2) **Cytotoxic drugs** increase uric acid concentrations by enhancing nucleic acid turnover and excretion.
      (3) **Diuretics** (except spironolactone) may cause hyperuricemia; most likely, this occurs via volume depletion, which, in turn, increases proximal tubular reabsorption, or via impaired tubular secretion of uric acid.
      (4) **Ethambutol** and **nicotinic acid** increase uric acid concentrations by competing with urate for tubular secretion sites, thereby decreasing uric acid excretion.
      (5) **Cyclosporine** decreases renal urate clearance.
      (6) **Heavy alcohol consumption.** By forming lactate, which competes for urate for tubular secretion sites, alcohol overuse reduces uric acid excretion.
   d. **Miscellaneous disorders.** Diabetic ketoacidosis, psoriasis, and chronic lead poisoning are examples of conditions that may cause hyperuricemia.

E. Pathophysiology

1. Gouty arthritis develops when **monosodium urate crystals** are deposited in the synovium of involved joints.

2. An **inflammatory response** to monosodium urate crystals leads to an attack of acute gouty arthritis; painful joint swelling is characterized by redness, warmth, and tenderness. A systemic reaction may accompany joint symptoms.

3. If gout progresses untreated, **tophi,** or **tophaceous deposits** (deposits of monosodium urate crystals) eventually lead to joint deformity and disability; kidney involvement may lead to renal impairment. However, these developments are uncommon in the general gout population and represent late complications of hyperuricemia.

4. **Renal complications of hyperuricemia and gout** can have serious consequences.
   a. **Acute tubular obstruction.** This complication may develop secondary to uric acid precipitation in the collecting tubules and ureters with subsequent blockage and renal failure. It is most common in patients with gout secondary to myeloproliferative or lymphoproliferative disorders—especially after chemotherapy.
   b. **Urolithiasis.** Occurring in about 20% of gout patients, urolithiasis is characterized by formation of uric acid stones in the urinary tract. Low urine pH seems to be a contributing factor. The risk of urolithiasis rises as serum and urinary acid levels increase.
   c. **Chronic urate nephropathy.** In this complication, urate deposits arise in the renal interstitium. Most clinicians agree, however, that chronic hyperuricemia rarely, if ever, leads to clinically significant nephropathy. The presence of concomitant disease (e.g., diabetes mellitus, hypertension, lead nephropathy) may explain the finding of nephropathy in gout patients.

F. Clinical presentation. Clinical evaluation and the need for intervention depend on the clinical presentation.

1. **Asymptomatic hyperuricemia**

2. **Acute gouty arthritis**

3. **Intercritical gout**

4. **Chronic tophaceous gout**

II. ASYMPTOMATIC HYPERURICEMIA is characterized by an elevated serum uric acid level but has no signs or symptoms of deposition disease (arthritis, tophi, or urolithiasis).

A. Clinical presentation. No definitive evidence indicates that asymptomatic hyperuricemia is harmful. Clinicians cannot predict which asymptomatic patients will develop gout symptoms or hyperuricemia-related complications. However, the risk of symptom development and complications increases as the serum uric acid level rises.

B. Therapy. Although some asymptomatic patients may receive drug therapy, most do not require treatment. However, any secondary causes of hyperuricemia should be minimized or reversed, if possible.

1. **Drug therapy** to reduce serum uric acid level is controversial. Some physicians believe that the risk of adverse drug effects and the expense and inconvenience of long-term therapy outweigh the benefits. However, in patients with sustained and marked hyperuricemia, urate-lowering drugs may be given (see IV C 2).

2. **Supportive interventions** may include maintenance of adequate urine output (to prevent uric acid stone formation), avoidance of high purine foods, and regular medical appointments to monitor the serum uric acid level and check for clinical evidence of deposition disease.

III. ACUTE GOUTY ARTHRITIS. This clinical presentation of gout is characterized by **painful arthritic attacks** of sudden onset.

A. Pathogenesis. Monosodium urate crystals form in articular tissues; this process sets off an inflammatory reaction. Trauma, exposure to cold, or another triggering event may be involved in the development of the acute attack.

B. Signs and symptoms

1. The **initial attack** comes on abruptly, usually at night or in the early morning as synovial fluid is reabsorbed, with severe, progressively worsening arthritic pain, generally involving only one or a few joints.
   a. The affected joints typically become hot, swollen, and extremely tender. Seventeenth-century British physician Thomas Sydenham described his personal experience with gout this way: "Now it is a violent stretching and tearing of the ligaments—now it is a gnawing pain and now a pressure and tightening. So exquisite and lively . . . is the feeling of the part affected, that it cannot bear the weight of bedclothes nor the jar of a person walking in the room."*
   b. The most common site of the initial attack is the first metatarsophalangeal joint; an attack there is known as **podagra**. Other sites that may be affected include the instep, ankle, heel, knee, wrist, elbow, and fingers.
2. The first few untreated attacks typically last 3–14 days. Later attacks may affect more joints and take several weeks to resolve.
3. During recovery, as edema subsides, local desquamation and pruritus may occur.
4. **Systemic symptoms** during an acute attack may include fever, chills, and malaise.

C. Diagnostic criteria

1. **Definitive diagnosis** of gouty arthritis can be made by **demonstration of monosodium urate crystals in the synovial fluid of affected joints**. These needle-shaped crystals are termed negatively birefringent when viewed through a polarized light microscope.
2. **Serum analysis** usually reveals an above-normal uric acid level; however, this finding is not specific for acute gout. Other common serum findings include leukocytosis and a moderately elevated erythrocyte sedimentation rate.
3. A **dramatic therapeutic response to colchicine** may be helpful in establishing the diagnosis, but this is not absolute because other causes of acute arthritis may respond as well.
4. Because uric acid crystals may not be found in the affected joints of all acute gout patients, a **probable diagnosis** of acute gouty arthritis can be made using the criteria developed by the American College of Rheumatology. The presence of a minimum of six of the following 11 criteria warrants a suggestive diagnosis:
   a. Development of maximum inflammation within 1 day
   b. More than one arthritis attack
   c. Oligoarthritis attack (limited to a few joints)
   d. Painful or swollen first metatarsophalangeal joint
   e. Exquisite pain involving joint
   f. Unilateral attack involving the first metatarsophalangeal joint
   g. Redness over the affected joint
   h. Tophus
   i. Asymptomatic swelling in one joint
   j. Hyperuricemia
   k. Complete termination of the acute attack

D. Treatment goals

1. To relieve pain and inflammation
2. To terminate the acute attack
3. To restore normal function to the affected joints

E. Therapy

1. **General therapeutic principles**
   a. The affected joint (or joints) should be immobilized.
   b. Anti-inflammatory drug therapy should begin immediately. For maximal therapeutic effectiveness, these drugs should be kept on hand so that the patient may begin therapy as soon as a subsequent attack begins.

*Latham RG (trans): *The Works of Thomas Sydenham,* vol. II. London, Sydenham Society, 1850.

c. Urate-lowering drugs should not be given until the acute attack is controlled as they may prolong the attack by causing a change in uric acid equilibrium.

2. **Specific drugs.** Any of the following agents may be used:

a. **Colchicine.** The traditional drug of choice for relieving pain and inflammation and ending the acute attack, colchicine is most effective when initiated 12–36 hours after symptoms begin (the period of maximal leukocyte migration). Approximately 75%–90% of patients respond to the drug when it is given for an acute attack.

(1) **Mechanism of action.** Colchicine apparently impairs leukocyte migration to inflamed areas and disrupts urate deposition and the subsequent inflammatory response.

(2) **Dosage and administration**

(a) **Oral regimen**

(i) During the **initial attack,** 0.5-mg or 0.6-mg tablets of colchicine are given every hour (or up to 1.2 mg every 2 hours) until a response occurs, a total not exceeding 5–7 mg is administered, or intolerable gastrointestinal distress (e.g., nausea, vomiting, diarrhea) develops.

(ii) Patients typically respond within 12–24 hours after therapy begins. Complete relief usually occurs in 1–3 days.

(iii) During **subsequent attacks,** patients may receive half of the total dose administered for the initial attack, then receive the remaining half as 0.5 mg every hour.

(b) **Intravenous regimen.** This route is rarely used now.

(i) A single dose of 2 mg usually is given in 30 ml of normal saline solution and infused slowly over 5 minutes. If needed, another injection may be given in 6–8 hours. Patients should not receive more than 4 mg per episode. Because it causes tissue irritation, colchicine should never be given intramuscularly or subcutaneously.

(ii) Intravenous administration may relieve acute gouty arthritis more rapidly than oral administration. However, severe toxicity may occur without warning because the early signs of toxicity (e.g., gastrointestinal hypermobility) may not occur.

(3) **Precautions and monitoring effects**

(a) **Gastrointestinal distress** (e.g., nausea, abdominal cramps, diarrhea) occurs in up to 80% of patients receiving oral colchicine. This dosage form should be avoided in patients with peptic ulcer disease and other gastrointestinal disorders.

(b) **Local extravasation** (causing local pain and necrosis) can occur with administration of intravenous colchicine. This risk can be reduced by use of a secure intravenous line.

(c) **Colchicine therapy** may cause bone marrow depression. This rare effect develops mainly in patients who receive excessive doses or who have underlying renal or hepatic disease. Excessively high acute doses (especially given intravenously) or long-term therapy may result in neurologic, renal, hepatic, or other toxicity.

b. **Nonsteroidal anti-inflammatory drugs (NSAIDs)**

(1) **Indications.** Some physicians consider these drugs the agents of choice, especially the newer NSAIDs. These drugs may be preferred when treatment is delayed significantly after symptom onset or when the patient cannot tolerate the adverse gastrointestinal effects of colchicine. Patients typically respond 6–24 hours after therapy begins; symptoms usually resolve completely within 3–5 days.

(a) **Indomethacin** is usually given in a dose of 50 mg three times a day for 2 days, then a gradual tapering of the dose over the next few days.

(b) **Other NSAIDs,** such as **fenoprofen, ibuprofen, naproxen, sulindac,** and **piroxicam** also have been used successfully in the treatment of acute gout.

(c) **Phenylbutazone** has a well-established efficacy; however, it is now used less frequently because of the development of newer and safer NSAIDs.

(2) **Precautions and monitoring effects**

(a) **Adverse effects of indomethacin** usually are dose-related. Occurring in 10%–60% of patients, these effects may warrant drug discontinuation. They primarily include gastrointestinal complaints of nausea and abdominal discomfort and central nervous system (CNS) effects of headaches and dizziness. Indomethacin should be taken with food or milk to minimize gastric mucosal irritation.

(b) **Adverse effects of phenylbutazone** include sodium and fluid retention; consequently, this drug should be avoided in patients with borderline cardiac reserves or overt congestive heart failure (CHF). Gastrointestinal distress (e.g., nausea, abdominal discomfort, peptic ulceration) also may occur. Rarely, blood dyscrasias (e.g., aplastic anemia, agranulocytosis) develop; they are most common in elderly patients and in those receiving the drug for long periods. To avoid these potential toxicities, phenylbutazone therapy should not exceed 1 week.

(c) **Precautions.** NSAIDs, in general, require cautious use in patients with a history of hypertension, CHF, peptic ulcer disease, or mild-to-moderate renal failure.

F. Adrenocorticotropic hormone (ACTH) and **corticosteroids** are reserved for refractory cases. Relapse has been considered a reason to avoid these agents, but recent evidence does not support this contention.

IV. INTERCRITICAL GOUT is the symptom-free period after the first attack. This phase may be interrupted by the recurrence of acute attacks.

A. Onset of subsequent attacks varies. In most patients, the second attack occurs within 1 year of the first, but in some it may be delayed for 5–10 years. A small percentage of patients never experience a second attack. If hyperuricemia is insufficiently treated, subsequent attacks may become progressively longer and more severe and may involve more than one joint.

B. Treatment goals

1. To reduce the frequency and severity of recurrent attacks.
2. To minimize urate deposition in body tissues, thereby preventing progression to chronic tophaceous gout

C. Therapy

1. **Conservative intervention** is indicated for patients with infrequent attacks, a serum uric acid level that is not too elevated (i.e., < 12 mg/dl), no tophi, and no evidence of renal disease or uric acid stones. Such intervention includes the following measures:
   a. **Restriction of alcohol consumption** and **dietary purine** (e.g., organ meats, anchovies) helps reduce uric acid concentrations.
   b. **High-volume fluid intake** and **increased urinary output** (at least 2 L/day) improve uric acid excretion and minimize renal urate precipitation.
   c. **Weight reduction** (in obese patients) sometimes reduces the serum uric acid level slightly; however, "crash diets" should be avoided.
   d. **Colchicine therapy** helps prevent gouty arthritis attacks. This drug may be given in the usual dose of 0.5–1.5 mg/day. (However, some patients require as little as 0.5 mg two or three times weekly.) Patients who cannot tolerate colchicine may receive indomethacin or another NSAID in low doses instead.
2. **Urate-reducing drug therapy.** The goal of such therapy is to reduce the serum uric acid level below 6 mg/dl. Urate-reducing drugs include uricosurics, which increase renal uric acid and excretion, and the xanthine oxidase inhibitor, allopurinol, which reduces uric acid production.
   a. **Indications** for urate-reducing therapy include the following:
      (1) Frequent gouty arthritis attacks despite conservative intervention
      (2) Chronic joint changes with tophi
      (3) Uric acid nephrolithiasis
   b. **Specific drugs**
      (1) **Uricosurics** include **probenecid** and **sulfinpyrazone**. They are the preferred agents for underexcretors. Long-term uricosuric therapy reduces the incidence of gouty arthritis attacks, prevents formation of new tophi, and helps resolve existing tophi.
         (a) **Mechanism of action.** Probenecid and sulfinpyrazone block uric acid reabsorption at the proximal convoluted tubule, thereby increasing the rate of uric acid excretion (see Figure 52-2).
         (b) **Indications.** Uricosurics generally are used to reduce hyperuricemia in patients who excrete less than 600 mg of uric acid per day.

(c) **Dosage and administration**

(i) **Probenecid** is given initially in two daily oral doses of 250 mg for 1 week, then increased to 500 mg twice daily every 1–2 weeks until the serum uric acid level drops below 6 mg/dl. Most patients respond to a dose of 1.5 g/day or less.

(ii) **Sulfinpyrazone** is given initially in two daily oral doses of 50 mg, then increased by 100 mg weekly. Most patients respond to a dose of 200 mg/day or less.

(d) **Precautions and monitoring effects**

(i) Uricosurics are **contraindicated** in patients with urinary tract stones.

(ii) These drugs generally are ineffective in patients with creatinine clearances below 30 ml/min.

(iii) **Aspirin** and **other salicylates** antagonize the action of uricosurics.

(iv) Uricosuric therapy should not be initiated during an acute gout attack. During the first 6–12 months of therapy, these drugs may increase the frequency, severity, and duration of acute attacks (by changing the equilibrium of body urate). Therefore, some clinicians administer prophylactic colchicine concomitantly during the early months of uricosuric therapy.

(v) Patients should maintain a high fluid intake (at least 2 L/day) and a high urine output during uricosuric therapy to decrease renal urate precipitation.

(vi) **Probenecid** is well tolerated by most patients, but it occasionally causes adverse effects, such as gastrointestinal distress (8%). In rare cases, hypersensitivity reactions (5%) occur.

(vii) **Sulfinpyrazone** causes gastrointestinal distress in 10%–15% of patients. Hypersensitivity reactions occur rarely. Sulfinpyrazone reduces platelet adhesiveness and may cause blood dyscrasias; periodic blood counts should be done.

(2) The only **xanthine oxidase inhibitor** available is **allopurinol**.

(a) **Mechanism of action.** Allopurinol and its long-acting metabolite, oxypurinol, block the final steps in uric acid synthesis by inhibiting xanthine oxidase, an enzyme that converts xanthine to uric acid. The drug, thus, reduces the serum uric acid level while increasing the renal excretion of the more soluble oxypurine precursors; this, in turn, decreases the risk of uric acid stones and nephropathy.

(b) **Indications.** Allopurinol is considered by many to be the drug of choice for lowering uric acid levels because it is effective in both underexcretors and overproducers, but it is specifically the preferred urate-reducing agent for patients in the following categories:

(i) Patients who are clearly overproducers (overexcretors) of uric acid

(ii) Patients with recurrent tophaceous deposits or uric acid stones

(iii) Patients with renal impairment (but dose needs to be decreased)

(c) **Dosage and administration.** Allopurinol is given initially in a daily dose of 100–300 mg (preferably as a single dose), then increased in weekly increments if needed. Some patients may need 600–800 mg/day to control hyperuricemia. Typically, the uric acid level starts to fall after 1–2 days with a maximal effect for a given dose in 7–10 days.

(d) **Precautions and monitoring effects.** Allopurinol is generally well tolerated, but serious adverse effects are not uncommon.

(i) Hypersensitivity reactions have been reported.

(ii) Minor skin rashes may occur.

(iii) A life-threatening hypersensitivity/toxicity syndrome occurs rarely. This syndrome may include one or all of the following: vasculitis, rash (usually toxic epidermal necrolysis), eosinophilia, hepatic damage, and progressive renal failure. Accumulation of oxypurinol may be involved; therefore, doses of allopurinol must be decreased with decreased renal function.

(iv) Allopurinol may induce more frequent acute gout attacks. This risk can be minimized by administration of low doses and concurrent colchicine therapy.

(v) Patients receiving concurrent ampicillin have an increased risk of developing a rash.

V. CHRONIC TOPHACEOUS GOUT. This rare clinical presentation may develop if hyperuricemia and gout remain untreated for many years.

A. Pathogenesis. Persistent hyperuricemia leads to the development of tophi in the synovia, olecranon bursae, and various periarticular locations. Eventually, articular cartilage may be destroyed, resulting in joint deformities, bone erosions, deposition of tophi within tissues, and renal disease.

B. Clinical evaluation

1. Patients may develop large subcutaneous tophi in the pinna of the external ear (the classic site) as well as in other locations.
2. Typically, the urate pool is many times the normal size.

C. Therapy. Allopurinol and probenecid may be given in combination to treat severe cases.

STUDY QUESTIONS

Directions: Each of the numbered items or incomplete statements in this section is followed by answers or by completions of the statement. Select the **one** lettered answer or completion that is **best** in each case.

1. All of the following statements concerning an acute gouty attack are correct EXCEPT

(A) the diagnosis of gout is assured by a good therapeutic response to colchicine because no other form of arthritis responds to this drug
(B) to be assured of the diagnosis, monosodium urate crystals must be identified in the synovial fluid of the affected joint
(C) attacks frequently occur in the middle of the night
(D) an untreated attack may last up to 2 weeks
(E) the first attack usually involves only one joint, most frequently the big toe (first metatarsophalangeal joint)

2. A 42-year-old obese man has been diagnosed as having gout. He has had three acute attacks this year, and his uric acid level is presently 11.5 mg/dl (upper limit of normal is 7 mg/dl). He has no other diseases. Rational treatment of this patient during the interval period between gouty attacks might include any of the following EXCEPT

(A) acetaminophen or aspirin 650 mg as needed for joint pain
(B) probenecid
(C) colchicine
(D) allopurinol
(E) a decrease in caloric intake

3. A 45-year-old man is admitted to the hospital with the diagnosis of an acute attack of gout. His serum uric acid is 10.5 mg/dl (normal 3–7 mg/dl). Which of the following would be the most effective initial treatment plan?

(A) Before treating this patient, immobilize the affected joint and obtain a 24-hour urinary uric acid level to determine which drug, either allopurinol or probenecid, would be the best agent to initiate therapy
(B) Begin oral colchicine 0.6 mg every hour until relief is obtained, gastrointestinal distress occurs, or a maximum of 7 mg has been taken; also, begin probenecid 250 mg twice a day concurrently.
(C) Administer oral indomethacin 50 mg three times a day for 2 days, then gradually taper the dose over the next few days
(D) Administer oral phenylbutazone 200 mg every 6 hours for 3 days, then give 100 mg three times a day for an additional 4 months
(E) Give colchicine 0.5 mg intramuscularly followed by 1 mg intravenously piggyback every 12 hours for 2 weeks

---

1-A
2-A
3-C

Directions: The question below contains three suggested answers of which **one or more** is correct. Choose the answer

A if **I only** is correct
B if **III only** is correct
C if **I and II** are correct
D if **II and III** are correct
E if **I, II, and III** are correct

4. Allopurinol is recommended rather than probenecid in the treatment of hyperuricemia in which of the following situations?

I. When the patient has several large tophi on the elbows and knees
II. When the patient has an estimated creatinine clearance of 15 ml/min
III. When the patient has leukemia and there is concern regarding renal precipitation of urate

4-E

ANSWERS AND EXPLANATIONS

1. The answer is A *[III B 1, 2, C 1, 3].*
Other forms of acute arthritis may respond to colchicine, so that the diagnosis of gout cannot be established unequivocally by a good response to this agent. A definitive diagnosis requires the presence of urate crystals in the affected joint, although the presence of other symptoms or laboratory findings may suggest a probable diagnosis of gout.

2. The answer is A *[I D 2 c (1); III E 2 a; IV C 1, 2 b].*
Aspirin in doses less than 2 g/day can inhibit uric acid secretion. Weight reduction, allopurinol, or probenecid to lower the serum uric acid levels, and prophylactic colchicine are all appropriate interventions in the interval phase to reduce the incidence of acute gouty attacks.

3. The answer is C *[III E 1 c, 2 a, b (1) (a); IV C 2 b (1) (d)].*
The most effective initial plan in treating an acute attack of gout is to administer indomethacin orally, giving 50 mg three times a day for 2–3 days, then gradually tapering the dosage over the next few days. Even though joint immobilization is an appropriate initial step, drugs for pain relief should be administered as soon as possible. Uric acid modification therapy (allopurinol or probenecid) should not be initiated until the acute attack is under control. Initiating therapy with probenecid at this point may prolong the acute attack. Phenylbutazone should not be used for longer than 1 week. Colchicine should never be given intramuscularly because it causes tissue irritation.

4. The answer is E (all) *[IV C 2 b (1) (d) (ii), (2) (b)].*
In the treatment of hyperuricemia, allopurinol is indicated rather than probenecid when large tophi are present, when the creatinine clearance is less than 25 ml/min (probenecid would be ineffective, but allopurinol dosage would have to be decreased), when the patient is an overproducer of uric acid, and when there is a need to prevent the formation of large amounts of uric acid (e.g., when conditions like leukemia are present).

53
Peptic Ulcer Disease

Paul F. Souney
S. James Matthews

I. INTRODUCTION

A. Definition. Peptic ulcer disease refers to a group of disorders characterized by circumscribed lesions of the mucosa of the upper gastrointestinal tract (especially the stomach and duodenum). The lesions occur in regions exposed to gastric juices.

B. Manifestations

1. **Duodenal ulcers** almost always develop in the duodenal bulb (the first few centimeters of the duodenum). A few, however, arise between the bulb and the ampulla.
2. **Gastric ulcers** form most commonly in the antrum or at the antral–fundal junction.
3. **Less common forms of peptic ulcer disease**
   a. **Stress ulcers** result from serious trauma or illness, major burns, or ongoing sepsis. The most common site of stress ulcer formation is the proximal portion of the stomach.
   b. **Zollinger-Ellison syndrome** is a severe form of peptic ulcer disease in which intractable ulcers are accompanied by extreme gastric hyperacidity and at least one gastrinoma (a non-beta islet cell tumor of the pancreas or another site).
   c. **Stomal ulcers** (also called marginal ulcers) may arise at the anastomosis or immediately distal to it in the small intestine in patients who have undergone ulcer surgery and have experienced subsequent ulcer recurrence after a symptom-free period.
   d. **Drug-associated ulcers** occur in patients who chronically ingest substances that damage the gastric mucosa, such as nonsteroidal anti-inflammatory drugs (NSAIDs).

C. Epidemiology

1. **Incidence.** Peptic ulcer disease is the most common disorder of the upper gastrointestinal tract.
   a. **Duodenal ulcers** affect roughly 4%–10% of the United States population; **gastric ulcers** occur in approximately 0.03%–0.05% of the population.
   b. Nearly 80% of peptic ulcers are duodenal; the others are gastric ulcers.
   c. Most duodenal ulcers appear in people between the ages 20 and 50 years; onset of gastric ulcers usually occurs between the ages 45 and 55 years.
   d. Duodenal ulcers are twice as common in men as in women; gastric ulcers affect men and women equally.
   e. Approximately 10%–20% of gastric ulcer patients also have a concurrent duodenal ulcer.
2. **Hospitalization**
   a. Hospitalization rates in the United States for peptic ulcers have been declining; they dropped from 25.2 per 10,000 in 1965 to 16.5 per 10,000 in 1981. This reflects a decrease in hospitalization for uncomplicated cases due to increased outpatient diagnosis and treatment.
   b. There has been little or no decrease in duodenal ulcer perforations and only a slight decrease in hemorrhages.
3. **Mortality**
   a. The mortality rate for gastric ulcers declined between 1962 and 1979 from 3.5 per 100,000 to 1.1 per 100,000.
   b. For duodenal ulcer, the mortality rate declined from 3.1 per 100,000 to 0.9 per 100,000.
4. **Costs.** The direct costs of peptic ulcers, such as hospital care, professional charges and drugs, are $1.2 billion per year, while indirect costs for lost work time are at least $1.5 billion per year.

D. Description

1. Ulcer size varies. The average duodenal ulcer typically has a diameter of less than 1 cm; most gastric ulcers are somewhat larger (1–2.5 cm in diameter).
2. Most ulcers are sharply demarcated and have a round, oval, or elliptical shape.
3. The mucosa surrounding the ulcer typically is inflamed and edematous.
4. Ulcers penetrate the **muscularis propria** and, in some cases, extend into the serosa or even into the pancreas.
5. Fibrous tissue, granulation tissue, and necrotic debris form the ulcer base. During ulcer healing, a scar forms as epithelium from the edges covers the ulcer surface.
6. Nearly all duodenal ulcers are benign; up to 10% of gastric ulcers are malignant.

E. Etiology. The precise cause of peptic ulcer disease has not been defined. However, certain factors are known to increase the risk of developing the disease.

1. **Genetic factors**
   a. Ulcers are at least twice as common in siblings of ulcer patients as in the general population.
   b. People with blood type O have an above-normal incidence of duodenal ulcers; those with blood type A have a higher incidence of gastric ulcers.
2. **Smoking.** Smokers have an increased risk of developing peptic ulcer disease. In addition, cigarette smoking delays ulcer healing and increases the risk and rapidity of relapse after the ulcer heals. Nicotine decreases biliary and pancreatic bicarbonate secretion. Smoking also accelerates the emptying of stomach acid into the duodenum.
3. **Nonsteroidal anti-inflammatory drugs (NSAIDs).** When ingested chronically, aspirin, indomethacin, and other NSAIDs promote gastric ulcer formation.
   a. These drugs may injure the gastric mucosa by allowing back-diffusion of hydrogen ions into the mucosa.
   b. NSAIDs also inhibit the synthesis of prostaglandins, substances with a cytoprotective effect on the mucosa.
4. **Alcohol.** A known mucosal irritant, alcohol causes marked irritation of the gastric mucosa if ingested in large quantities.
5. **Coffee.** Both regular and decaffeinated coffee contain peptides that stimulate release of gastrin, a hormone that triggers the flow of gastric juice. However, a direct link between coffee and peptic ulcer disease has not been proven.
6. **Corticosteroids.** According to a recent study, these drugs double the risk (1.8 versus 0.8) of ulcer development. Corticosteroid-induced ulcers have a high incidence of perforation and hemorrhage. To complicate matters, these drugs may mask ulcer symptoms.
7. **Associated disorders.** Peptic ulcer disease is more common in patients with hyperparathyroidism, emphysema, rheumatoid arthritis, and alcoholic cirrhosis.
8. **Advanced age.** Degeneration of the pylorus permits bile reflux into the stomach, creating an environment that favors ulcer formation.
9. ***Helicobacter pylori*** (formerly *Campylobacter pylori*). This bacterial organism has been linked with some cases of duodenal ulcers and gastritis.
   a. This bacterium is found infrequently in people below the age of 20 but is present in most patients over 50 years of age.
   b. In some studies, almost all patients with peptic ulcer disease who did not use NSAIDs and were not hypersecretors had *H. pylori.*
   c. Initial studies have shown that antibiotics and antiulcer drugs markedly reduce relapse rates.
   d. Patients most commonly are treated with bismuth and metronidazole plus amoxicillin or tetracycline.
10. **Psychological factors.** Once assigned key rolls in the pathogenesis of peptic ulcer disease, stress and personality type now are viewed as relatively minor influences.

F. Pathophysiology. Ulcers develop when an imbalance exists between factors that protect the gastric mucosa and factors that promote mucosal corrosion.

1. **Protective factors**
   a. Normally, the mucosa secretes a thick mucus that serves as a barrier between luminal acid and epithelial cells. This barrier slows the inward movement of hydrogen ions and allows their neutralization by bicarbonate ions in fluids secreted by the stomach and duodenum.
   b. Alkaline and neutral pancreatic biliary juices also help buffer acid entering the duodenum from the stomach.
   c. An **intact mucosal barrier** prevents back-diffusion of gastric acids into mucosal cells. It also has the capacity to stimulate local blood flow, which brings nutrients and other substances to the area and removes toxic substances (e.g., hydrogen ions). Mucosal integrity also promotes cell growth and repair after local trauma.
2. **Corrosive factors.** Peptic ulcer disease reflects the inability of the gastric mucosa to resist corrosion by irritants, such as pepsin, hydrochloric acid (HCl), and other gastric secretions.
   a. **Exposure to gastric acid and pepsin** is necessary for ulcer development.
   b. **Disrupted mucosal barrier integrity** allows gastric acids to diffuse from the lumen back into mucosal cells, where they cause injury.
3. **Physiologic defects associated with peptic ulcer disease.** Researchers have identified various physiologic defects in patients with duodenal and gastric ulcers.
   a. **Duodenal ulcer patients** may have the following defects:
      (1) Increased capacity for gastric acid secretion
         (a) Some duodenal ulcer patients have up to twice the normal number of parietal cells (which produce HCl).
         (b) Nearly 70% of duodenal ulcer patients have elevated serum levels of **pepsinogen I** and a corresponding increase in pepsin-secreting capacity.
      (2) Increased parietal cell responsiveness to gastrin
      (3) Above-normal postprandial gastrin secretion
      (4) Defective inhibition of gastrin release at low pH, possibly leading to failure to suppress postprandial acid secretion
      (5) Above-normal rate of gastric emptying, resulting in delivery of a greater acid load to the duodenum
   b. **Gastric ulcer patients** typically exhibit the following characteristics:
      (1) Deficient gastric mucosal resistance, direct mucosal injury, or both
      (2) Elevated serum gastrin levels (in acid hyposecretors)
      (3) Decreased pyloric pressure at rest and in response to acid or fat in the duodenum
      (4) Delayed gastric emptying
      (5) Increased reflux of bile and other duodenal contents
      (6) Subnormal mucosal levels of prostaglandins (these levels normalize once the ulcer heals)

G. **Clinical presentation.** Signs and symptoms of peptic ulcer disease vary with the patient's age and the location of the lesion. Only about 50% of patients experience classic ulcer symptoms. The remainder are asymptomatic or report vague or atypical symptoms.

1. **Pain.** Patients typically describe heartburn or a gnawing, burning, aching, or cramp-like pain. Some report abdominal soreness or hunger sensations. It is unclear whether peptic ulcer pain results from chemical stimulation or from spasm.
   a. **Duodenal ulcer pain** usually is restricted to a small, midepigastric area near the xiphoid. Pain may radiate below the costal margins into the back or the right shoulder. Pain from a duodenal ulcer frequently awakens the patient between midnight and 2 A.M.; it is almost never present before breakfast.
   b. **Gastric ulcer pain** is less localized. It may be referred to the left subcostal region. Gastric ulcer rarely produces nocturnal pain.
   c. **Food** usually relieves duodenal ulcer pain but may cause gastric ulcer pain. This finding may explain why duodenal ulcer patients tend to gain weight, whereas gastric ulcer patients may lose weight. Pain characteristically occurs 90 minutes to 3 hours after meals in duodenal ulcer patients, while pain in gastric ulcer patients is usually present 45–60 minutes after a meal.
2. **Nausea and vomiting** may occur with either ulcer type.
3. **Disease course.** Both duodenal gastric ulcers tend to be chronic with spontaneous remissions and exacerbations. Within a year of the initial symptoms, most patients experience a relapse.
   a. In many cases, relapse is seasonal, occurring more often in the spring and autumn.

b. Prophylactic drug therapy usually is not recommended because of the risk of side effects. However, if relapses are frequent or severe, prophylactic drug therapy is instituted.

H. Clinical evaluation

1. Physical findings. Patients with peptic ulcer disease may exhibit superficial and deep epigastric tenderness and voluntary muscle guarding. With duodenal ulcer, patients also may show unilateral spasm over the duodenal bulb. Gastric ulcer patients may have weight loss.

2. Diagnostic test results

a. Blood tests may show hypochromic anemia.

b. Stool tests may detect occult blood if the ulcer is chronic.

c. Gastric secretion tests may reveal hypersecretion of HCl in duodenal ulcer patients and normal or subnormal HCl secretion in gastric ulcer patients.

d. Upper gastrointestinal series (barium x-ray) reveals the ulcer crater in up to 80% of cases. Duodenal bulb deformity suggests a duodenal ulcer.

e. Upper gastrointestinal endoscopy, the most specific test, may be done if barium x-ray yields inconclusive results. This procedure confirms an ulcer in at least 95% of cases and may detect ulcers not demonstrable by radiography.

f. Biopsy may be necessary to determine whether a gastric ulcer is malignant.

I. Treatment objectives

1. Relieve pain and other ulcer symptoms and promote ulcer healing

2. Prevent complications of peptic ulcer disease

3. Minimize recurrence

4. Maintain adequate nutrition

5. Teach the patient about the disease to improve therapeutic compliance

II. THERAPY

A. Drug therapy. Peptic ulcer patients usually are treated with antacids, histamine$_2$ (H_2)-receptor antagonists, or both; other drugs are added as necessary. Drug regimens that suppress nocturnal acid secretion are found to result in the highest duodenal ulcer healing rates. Drug therapy typically provides prompt symptomatic relief and promotes ulcer healing within 4–6 weeks.

1. Antacids. These compounds, which neutralize gastric acid, are used to treat ulcer pain and heal the ulcer. Studies show antacids and H_2-receptor antagonists to be equally effective. Antacids are available as **magnesium, aluminum, calcium,** or **sodium salts**. The most widely used antacids are mixtures of aluminum hydroxide and magnesium hydroxide (Table 53-1). Duodenal ulcers rarely occur in the absence of acid or when the hourly maximum acid output is less than 10 mEq. Peptic activity decreases as acidity decreases; experimental ulcer formation is inhibited by antacids; and acid-reducing operations cure ulcers.

a. Mechanism of action and therapeutic effects. Antacids reduce the concentration and total load of acid in the gastric contents. By increasing gastric pH, they also inhibit pepsin activity. In addition, they strengthen the gastric mucosal barrier.

b. Choice of agent

(1) Nonsystemic antacids (e.g., magnesium or aluminum substances) are preferred to systemic antacids (e.g., sodium bicarbonate) for intensive ulcer therapy because they avoid the risk of alkalosis.

(2) Liquid antacid forms have a greater buffering capacity than tablets. However, tablets are more convenient to carry. With either dosage form, the size and frequency of doses may limit patient compliance.

(3) Antacid mixtures (e.g., aluminum hydroxide with magnesium hydroxide) provide more even, sustained action than single-agent antacids and permit a lower dosage of each compound. In addition, compounds in a mixture may interact so as to negate each other's untoward effects. For instance, the constipating effect of aluminum hydroxide may counter the diarrhea that magnesium hydroxide frequently produces.

(4) Calcium carbonate usually is avoided because it causes acid rebound, may delay pain relief and ulcer healing, and induces constipation. Another potential adverse effect of

Table 53-1. Comparison of Antacids at a Dose of 140 mEq/hr

Brand Name	Neutralizing Capacity (mEq H^+/ml antacid)	Therapeutic Dose (140 mEq) (ml or no. of tablets)	Composition	Sodium Ion Content (mg/day)
Liquids (Concentrated)				
Maalox TC	4.2	33	$Al(OH)_3$ $Mg(OH)_3$	55
Titralac	4.2	33	$CaCO_3$ Glycerine	508
Delcid	4.1	34	$Al(OH)_3$ $Mg(OH)_3$	71
Mylanta II	3.6	39	$Al(OH)_3$ $Mg(OH)_3$ Simethicone	60
Liquids (Regular)				
Camalox	3.2	44	$Al(OH)_3$ $Mg(OH)_3$ $CaCO_3$	154
Gelusil II	3.0	47	$Al(OH)_3$ $Mg(OH)_3$ Simethicone	86
Maalox Plus	2.3	61	$Al(OH)_3$ $Mg(OH)_3$ Simethicone	214
Gelusil	2.2	64	$Al(OH)_3$ $Mg(OH)_3$ Simethicone	63
Riopan Plus	1.8	78	$Al(OH)_3$ $Mg(OH)_3$ Simethicone	76
Amphojel	1.4	100	$Al(OH)_3$	980
Tablets				
Camalox	16.7	8	$Al(OH)_3$ $Mg(OH)_3$	84
Mylanta II	11.0	13	$Al(OH)_3$ $Mg(OH)_3$ Simethicone	126
Tums	10.5	13	$CaCO_3$ $Al(OH)_3$ $Mg(OH)_3$	246
Riopan Plus	10.0	14	$Al(OH)_3$ $Mg(OH)_3$ Simethicone	29
Titralac	9.5	9.5	$CaCO_3$ Glycerine	32
Rolaids	6.9	6.9	$Al_2(CO_3)_3$	7420
Maalox Plus	5.7	5.7	$Al(OH)_3$ $Mg(OH)_3$ Simethicone	245
Amphojel	2.0	2.0	$Al(OH)_3$	3430

Reprinted from Sleisenger MH, Fordtran JS (eds): *Gastrointestinal Disease: Pathophysiology, Diagnosis and Management*. Philadelphia, WB Saunders, 1983, p 718.

this compound is hypercalcemia; the risk is increased if calcium carbonate is taken with milk or another alkaline substance. The milk-alkali syndrome (i.e., hypercalcemia, alkalosis, azotemia, nephrocalcinosis) may also occur.

c. Administration and dosage

(1) Antacids differ greatly in acid-neutralizing capacity (ANC), defined as the number of milliequivalents (mEq) of a 1 N solution of HCl that can be brought to a pH of 3.5 in 15 minutes. With most duodenal ulcer patients, about 50 mEq/hr of available antacid is needed for ongoing neutralization of gastric contents. Therefore, the required dosage depends on the ANC of the specific antacid.

(2) In the fasting state, antacids have only a transient intragastric buffering effect (15–20 minutes). When ingested 1 hour after a meal, they have a much more prolonged effect, about 3–4 hours; therefore, they should optimally be taken 1 and 3 hours after meals and before sleep. Consequently, the typical antacid regimen calls for doses 1–3 hours after meals and at bedtime.

(3) Dosage

(a) Because the ANC of antacid products varies widely, no standard dosage can be given in terms of milliliters of suspension or number of tablets. However, patients with duodenal ulcers generally require individual dosages of 80–160 mEq of ANC (equivalent to 30–60 ml of Mylanta or Maalox). Thus, the total daily dosage may be as much as 420 ml of Mylanta or Maalox if the standard seven-times–daily dosing regimen is used. Because of the large doses and the need for frequent administration, compliance with antacid treatment regimens has been low.

(b) Antacid therapy usually continues for 6–8 weeks.

d. Precautions and monitoring effects

(1) Calcium carbonate and magnesium-containing antacids should be used cautiously in patients with severe renal disease.

(2) Sodium bicarbonate is contraindicated in patients with hypertension, congestive heart failure (CHF), severe renal disease, and edema. It should not be used for ulcer therapy.

(3) All antacids should be used cautiously in elderly patients (especially those with decreased gastrointestinal motility) and renally impaired patients.

(4) Aluminum-containing antacids should be used cautiously in patients who suffer from dehydration or intestinal obstruction.

(5) The combination of calcium carbonate with an alkaline substance (e.g., sodium bicarbonate) and milk may cause the milk-alkali syndrome.

(6) Low-sodium antacids obviate the problem of fluid retention in hypertension and heart disease.

(7) Chronic administration of calcium carbonate–containing antacids should be avoided because of hypercalcemia and calcium ion stimulation of acid secretion.

(8) Aluminum or magnesium toxicity is unlikely in patients with normal renal function. The encephalopathy of tissue deposition of aluminum only occurs in dialysis patients receiving aluminum hydroxide for control of hyperphosphatemia. Chronic use of magnesium-containing antacids is not advisable in patients with renal insufficiency.

(9) Constipation can occur in patients using calcium carbonate and aluminum-containing antacids.

(10) Diarrhea is a common adverse effect of magnesium-containing antacids. If diarrhea occurs, the patient may alternate the antacid mixture with aluminum hydroxide.

(11) Hypophosphatemia and osteomalacia can occur with long-term use of aluminum hydroxide, but they can also occur with short-term use in severely malnourished patients, such as alcoholics.

e. Significant interactions. Because antacids alter gastric pH and affect absorption of ingested substances, they have a high potential for drug interactions. To ensure consistent absorption and therapeutic efficacy, orally administered drugs should be given 30–60 minutes before antacids.

(1) Antacids bind with **tetracycline,** inhibiting its absorption and reducing its therapeutic efficacy.

(2) Antacids may destroy the coating of **enteric-coated drugs,** leading to premature drug dissolution in the stomach.

(3) Antacids may interfere with the absorption of many drugs, including **cimetidine, ranitidine, digoxin, isoniazid, anticholinergics, iron products,** and **phenothiazines** [see II A 2 e (3)].

(4) Antacids may reduce the therapeutic effects of **sucralfate** (see II A 3 d).

2. **H_2-receptor antagonists.** These relatively new drugs may be preferred to other antiulcer agents because of their convenience and lack of effect on gastrointestinal motility.
   a. **Mechanism of action and therapeutic effects.** H_2-receptor antagonists (Table 53-2) competitively inhibit the action of histamine at parietal cell receptor sites, reducing the volume and hydrogen ion concentration of gastric acid secretions (Figure 53-1). They accelerate the healing of most ulcers.
   b. **Choice of agent. Cimetidine, ranitidine, famotidine** or **nizatidine** may be administered to treat peptic ulcers or hypersecretory states (e.g., Zollinger-Ellison syndrome).
      (1) **Cimetidine,** the first H_2-receptor antagonist approved for clinical use, reduces gastric acid secretion by about 50% (at a total daily dosage of 1000 mg).
      (2) **Ranitidine,** a more potent drug, causes a 70% reduction in gastric acid secretion (at a total daily dosage of 300 mg).
      (3) **Famotidine** is the most potent H_2-receptor antagonist. After a 40-mg dose, mean nocturnal gastric acid secretion is reduced by 94% for up to 10 hours.
      (4) **Nizatidine,** the newest H_2-receptor, may be used to treat and prevent recurrence of duodenal ulcers; it appears to be similar to ranitidine, but its clinical place in therapy has not been thoroughly elucidated.
   c. **Administration and dosage**
      (1) **Cimetidine** usually is administered orally in a dosage of 300 mg four times daily (with meals and at bedtime) for up to 8 weeks.
         (a) Alternatively, duodenal ulcer patients may receive 400 mg twice daily or 800 mg at bedtime. An 800-mg bedtime dose is also effective in treating gastric ulcers.
         (b) Hospitalized patients may receive parenteral doses of 300 mg intravenously every 6 hours.
         (c) For duodenal ulcer prophylaxis, 400 mg may be given orally at bedtime. (However, in 20%–40% of patients, the ulcer recurs despite cimetidine prophylaxis.
      (2) **Ranitidine** usually is given orally in a dosage of 150 mg twice daily. Duodenal ulcer patients may receive 300 mg at bedtime, alternatively. Therapy continues for up to 8 weeks.
         (a) Hospitalized patients may receive ranitidine by the intravenous or intramuscular route (50 mg every 6–8 hours).
         (b) Prophylactic therapy may be administered to reduce the risk of ulcer recurrence. The approved prophylactic dosage is 150 mg at bedtime.
      (3) **Famotidine** administered to duodenal ulcer patients, is given in an oral dosage of 40 mg at bedtime for acute therapy for a maximum of 8 weeks. For prophylactic therapy, the dosage is 20 mg at bedtime.

Table 53-2. Histamine H_2-Receptor Antagonists

	Cimetidine (Tagamet)	**Ranitidine (Zantac)**	**Famotidine (Pepcid)**	**Nizatidine (Axid)**
Ring structure	Imidazole	Furan	Thiazole	Thiazole
Relative potency	1	4–10	4–10	20–50
Evening dose (mg)				
Active ulcer	800	300	40	300
Maintenance	400	150	20	150
Bioavailability (F)	60%–70%	50%–60%	40%–45%	90%–100%
Peak time (t_{max}) (hr)	1–3	1–3	1–3.5	0.5–3
Volume of distribution (L/kg)	1	1.4	1.1–1.4	0.8–1.6
Protein binding	20%	15%	15%–22%	32%–35%
Renal elimination	60%–75%	30% oral 70% intravenous	65%–70%	65%–75%
Half-life (hr)				
Normal	2	2–3	2.5–4	1.6
Anuric	4–5	4–10	20+	6–8/5
Clearance (L/h)	30–48	46	19–29	40–60

Reprinted from Hurwitz A: Clinical pharmacology of agents for the treatment of acid-related disorders. In *Peptic Ulcer Disease and Other Acid-Related Disorders.* Edited by Zakim D, Dannenberg AJ. New York, Academic Research Associates, 1991, p 343.

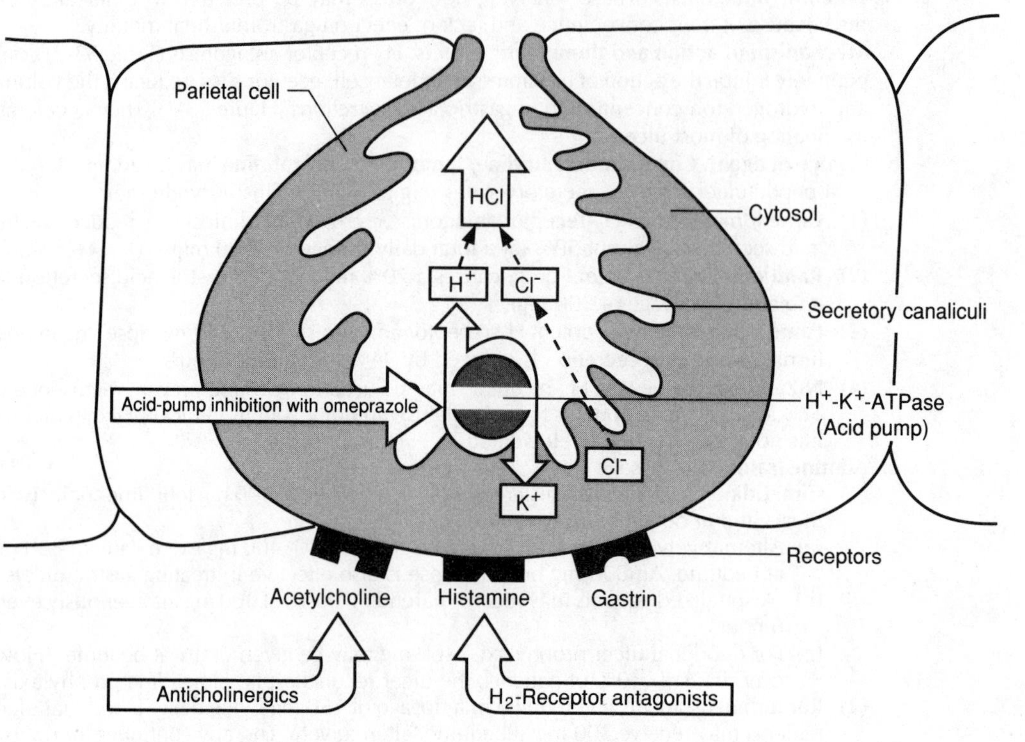

Figure 53-1. Schematic representation of parietal cell depicting sites of drug action.

(a) Hospitalized patients may receive an intravenous injection of 20 mg every 12 hours.

(b) As with cimetidine and ranitidine, the ulcer may recur after drug discontinuation.

(4) **Nizatidine,** for the treatment of duodenal ulcers, is given orally in a dosage of 300 mg once daily at bedtime or 150 mg twice daily for up to 8 weeks. For prophylactic therapy, the dosage is 150 mg at bedtime.

d. Precautions and monitoring effects

(1) Ranitidine must be used cautiously in patients with hepatic impairment. Hepatotoxicity is unusual and occurs most often during intravenous administration. Cimetidine has also been associated with hepatotoxicity.

(2) Cimetidine may cause such hematologic disorders as thrombocytopenia, agranulocytosis, and aplastic anemia.

(3) All of these agents may cause headache and dizziness. Cimetidine additionally may lead to confusion, especially in patients over age 60 years or if the dosage is not adjusted for patients with decreased kidney or liver function.

(4) Cimetidine has a weak androgenic effect, possibly resulting in male gynecomastia and impotence.

(5) Cimetidine and ranitidine rarely can cause bradycardia, which is reversible on discontinuation of therapy.

e. Significant interactions

(1) Cimetidine binds the cytochrome P-450 system of the liver and, thus, may interfere with the metabolism of such drugs as **phenytoin, theophylline, phenobarbital, lidocaine, warfarin, imipramine, diazepam,** and **propranolol**.

(2) Cimetidine decreases hepatic blood flow, possibly resulting in reduced clearance of **propranolol** and **lidocaine.**

(3) **Antacids** impair absorption of cimetidine and ranitidine and should be given 1 hour apart from these drugs.

(4) Cimetidine inhibits the excretion of procainamide by competing with the drug for the renal proximal tubular secretion site.

3. Sucralfate. This mucosal protectant is a nonabsorbable disaccharide containing sucrose and aluminum.

a. Mechanism of action and therapeutic effects. Sucralfate adheres to the base of the ulcer crater, forming a protective barrier against gastric acids and bile salts.

(1) Sucralfate's ulcer-healing efficacy compares favorably to that of the H_2-receptor antagonists.

(2) Duodenal ulcers respond better than gastric ulcers to sucralfate therapy.

b. Administration and dosage

(1) An oral agent, sucralfate usually is given in a dosage of 1 g four times daily (1 hour before meals) and at bedtime. Unless radiography or endoscopy documents earlier ulcer healing, therapy continues for 4–8 weeks.

(2) Continued sucralfate therapy after remission postpones ulcer relapse more effectively than does cimetidine therapy.

(3) There is no evidence that combining sucralfate with H_2-receptor antagonists improves healing or reduces recurrence rates.

c. Precautions and monitoring effects. Constipation is the most common adverse effect of sucralfate.

d. Significant interactions

(1) Antacids may reduce mucosal binding of sucralfate, decreasing its therapeutic efficacy and, thus, should be given 30–60 minutes apart from sucralfate if used in combination ulcer therapy.

(2) Sucralfate may interfere with the absorption of orally administered **digoxin, tetracycline, phenytoin, iron, ciprofloxacin,** and **cimetidine** if doses are given simultaneously.

4. Gastrointestinal anticholinergics (e.g., belladonna leaf, atropine, propantheline) sometimes are used as adjunctive agents for relief of refractory duodenal ulcer pain. However, these agents have no proven value in ulcer healing.

a. Mechanism of action. Anticholinergics decrease basal and stimulated gastric acid and pepsin secretion.

(1) Given in combination with antacids, anticholinergics delay gastric emptying, thereby prolonging antacid retention. They are most effective when taken at night and in large doses.

(2) Anticholinergics occasionally are used in patients who do not respond to H_2-receptor antagonists alone.

b. Administration and dosage

(1) Taken 30 minutes before food, anticholinergics inhibit meal-stimulated acid secretion by 30%–50% with a duration of 4–5 hours.

(2) An optimal effective dose varies from patient to patient.

c. Precautions and monitoring effects

(1) All anticholinergics have side effects to varying degrees, such as dry mouth, blurred vision, tachycardia, urinary retention, and constipation.

(2) These drugs are contraindicated in patients with gastric ulcers because they prolong gastric emptying. They also are contraindicated in patients with narrow-angle glaucoma and urinary retention.

5. Prostaglandins may prove valuable in ulcer therapy. These agents suppress gastric acid secretion and may guard the gastric mucosa against damage from NSAIDs. **Misoprostol** has been approved for use in the prevention of gastric ulcers caused by NSAIDs.

a. Mechanism of action. Misoprostol has both antisecretory (inhibiting gastric acid secretion) and mucosal protective properties. NSAIDs inhibit prostaglandin synthesis, and a deficiency of prostaglandin within the gastric mucosa may lead to diminishing bicarbonate and mucus secretion, contributing to the mucosal damage caused by NSAIDs. Misoprostol increases bicarbonate and mucus production at doses of 200 μg and above—doses that can also be antisecretory. Misoprostol also maintains mucosal blood flow.

b. Administration and dosage

(1) Misoprostol is indicated for the prevention of NSAID-induced gastric ulcers in patients at high risk for complications from gastric ulcers (e.g., patients over 60 years of age, patients with concomitant debilitating disease, patients with a history of ulcers).

(2) Misoprostol has not been shown to prevent duodenal ulcers in patients taking NSAIDs.

(3) The recommended adult dose is 200 μg four times daily with food; it must be taken for the duration of NSAID therapy; if this dose cannot be tolerated, 100 μg four times daily can be used.
(4) Adjustment of dosage in renally impaired patients is not routinely needed.

c. **Precautions and monitoring effects**
(1) Misoprostol is contraindicated, because of its abortifacient property, in women who are pregnant. Patients must be advised of the abortifacient property and warned not to give the drug to others.
(2) Misoprostol should not be used in women with childbearing potential unless the patient requires NSAID therapy and is at high risk of complications from gastric ulcers associated with use of the NSAIDs or is at high risk of developing gastric ulceration. In such patients, misoprostol may be prescribed if the patient:
(a) Is capable of complying with effective contraceptive measures
(b) Has received both oral and written warnings of the hazards of misoprostol, the risk of possible contraception failure, and the danger to other women of childbearing potential should the drug be taken by mistake
(c) Had a negative serum pregnancy test within 2 weeks prior to beginning therapy
(d) Will begin misoprostol only on the second or third day of the next normal menstrual period
(3) The most frequent adverse effects are diarrhea (14%–40%) and abdominal pain (13%–20%). Diarrhea is dose-related, usually develops early in the course (> 2 weeks), and is often self-limiting. Discontinuation of misoprostol is necessary in about 2% of patients. Administration with food minimizes the diarrhea.

d. **Significant interactions.** None has been reported.

6. **Omeprazole** is the first antisecretory agent in this new therapeutic class, the acid pump inhibitors.

a. **Mechanism of action and therapeutic effects.** The gastric proton pump H^+, K^+-ATPase has a sulfhydryl group near the potassium-binding site on the luminal side of the canalicular membrane. Omeprazole sulfenamide (the active form) forms a stable disulfide bond with this specific sulfhydryl, thereby inactivating the ATPase and shutting off acid secretion.
(1) Because of the potency and marked reduction in gastric acidity, omeprazole is more rapidly effective than other approved agents in treating peptic ulcer disease (i.e., it tends to control symptoms and heal ulcers more rapidly than any other antiulcer drugs).
(2) Omeprazole has resulted in significant improvement in patients with pathologic hypersecretory conditions (e.g., Zollinger-Ellison syndrome) and gastroesophageal reflux disease (GERD) compared to H_2-receptor antagonists.

b. **Administration and dosage**
(1) Omeprazole is more potent than H_2-blockers. In the usual dose (20–40 mg/day), it inhibits over 90% of 24-hour acid secretion in most patients, infrequently producing achlorhydria.
(2) **Recommended adult dosages**
(a) Severe erosive esophagitis or GERD is initially treated with 20 mg once daily for 4–8 weeks.
(b) Pathologic hypersecretory conditions require an initial dose of 60 mg once a day (up to 120 mg three times daily have been used). Daily doses greater than 80 mg should be administered as divided doses.
(c) Duodenal ulcer requires 20 mg daily. Most patients heal within 4 weeks.
(3) Omeprazole is a delayed-release capsule and should be taken before eating. It can be used concomitantly with antacids. It should not be opened, chewed, or crushed.
(4) No dosing adjustments are necessary in patients with impaired renal or hepatic function or in the elderly.

c. **Precautions and monitoring effects**
(1) Headache, diarrhea, abdominal pain, nausea and vomiting, and flatulence have been reported in more than 1% of patients.
(2) Fever, fatigue, malaise, elevated liver enzymes, dizziness, vertigo, skin rash, and itching have been reported in less than 1% of patients.
(3) In long-term (2 year) rat studies, omeprazole produced a dose-related increase in gastric carcinoid tumors. This is believed to be related to the hypergastrinemia produced by the inhibition of acid secretion. This effect has not been observed in other animal species or in humans. Gastric carcinoids have also been induced by the administration

of H_2-receptor blockade or fundectomy, supporting the role of gastrin. Some patients with Zollinger-Ellison syndrome have been treated continuously with omeprazole for more than 5 years without evidence of dysplasia or gastric carcinoid development. Long-term studies are ongoing.

d. Significant interactions

(1) Omeprazole interferes with the hepatic microsomal enzyme metabolism (cytochrome P-450) of **diazepam, warfarin,** and **phenytoin**.

(2) Although metabolized by the cytochrome P-450 enzyme system, no evidence of an interaction with **theophylline** and **propranolol** to date exists.

(3) Since gastric pH plays a role in the bioavailability of **ketoconazole, ampicillin esters,** and **iron salts,** prolonged gastric acid inhibition with omeprazole may decrease the absorption of these agents.

(4) Antacids may be used concomitantly with omeprazole.

(5) Increased **cyclosporin** levels have been reported after omeprazole administration.

7. Bismuth compounds (investigational). Colloidal bismuth subcitrate (CBS, tripotassium dicitratobismuthate, TDB)

a. Mechanism of action. CBS blocks pepsin activity, binds mucus to retard hydrogen back-diffusion, stimulates prostaglandin synthesis, and suppresses *H. pylori*.

b. Administration and dosage

(1) CBS has been used since 1971 to treat gastric and duodenal ulcers. Efficacy rates are as follows:

(a) Duodenal ulcer: 80% were healed at 4 weeks and 95% at 8 weeks.

(b) Gastric ulcer: 68% were healed at 4 weeks and 81% at 8 weeks.

(2) After healing by CBS, mucosal morphology is described as more normal in appearance than after H_2-blocker therapy; recurrence rates are also lower.

(3) CBS precipitates at about pH 3.5, binding to ulcer craters. Animal studies have shown that this binding is unique to CBS among the bismuth compounds studies and does not occur with bismuth subsalicylate (Pepto-Bismol).

(4) The recommended dose is two tablets twice daily (480 mg/day).

(5) Subsalicylate with amoxicillin and metronidazole may be used to treat *H. pylori* but not ulcers.

c. Precautions and monitoring effects

(1) Headache, abdominal pain, diarrhea, rash, and dark stool are a few of the adverse effects.

(2) Absorbed bismuth has caused encephalopathy (not CBS).

(3) Salicylism with tinnitus may result from high doses of bismuth subsalicylate.

8. Sedatives are useful adjuncts in promoting rest for highly anxious ulcer patients.

B. Other therapeutic measures

1. Modification of diet and social habits

a. Previously emphasized in ulcer therapy, strict dietary limitations now are considered largely unnecessary.

(1) Bland or milk-based diets formerly were recommended; however, research indicates that these diets do not speed ulcer healing. In fact, most experts now advise ulcer patients to **avoid milk** because recent studies show that milk increases gastric acid secretion. Also, because milk leaves the stomach quickly, it lacks an extended buffering action.

(2) Small, frequent meals, also previously recommended, can worsen ulcer pain by causing acid rebound 2–4 hours after eating.

b. Current dietary guidelines emphasize avoidance of foods and beverages known to exacerbate gastric discomfort or to promote acid secretion. This category typically includes coffee, caffeinated beverages, and alcohol.

c. Smoking. Patients who smoke should be encouraged to quit because smoking markedly slows ulcer healing, even during optimal ulcer therapy.

d. NSAIDs should be avoided by ulcer patients.

2. Surgery. An ulcer patient who develops complications may require surgery—sometimes on an emergency basis (see III). Incapacitating recurrent ulcers also may warrant surgery.

a. Types of surgical procedures for ulcer disease include antrectomy and truncal vagotomy (Billroth I procedure), partial gastrectomy and truncal vagotomy (Billroth II procedure), highly selective (proximal gastric) vagotomy, and total gastrectomy (the treatment of choice for Zollinger-Ellison syndrome that is unresponsive to medical management).

b. A **vagotomy** severs a branch of the vagus nerve, thereby decreasing HCl secretion. An **antrectomy,** by removing the antrum, eliminates some acid-secreting mucosa as well as the major source of gastrin.

III. COMPLICATIONS.

Complications of peptic ulcer disease cause approximately 7000 deaths in the United States annually.

A. Hemorrhage. This life-threatening condition develops from widespread gastric mucosal irritation or ulceration with acute bleeding.

1. Clinical features. The patient may vomit fresh blood or a coffee-ground–like substance. Other signs include passage of bloody or tarry stools, diaphoresis, and syncope. With major blood loss, manifestations of **hypovolemic shock** may appear: The pulse rate may exceed 110 or systolic blood pressure may drop below 100.

2. Management

a. Patient stabilization, bleeding cessation, and measures to prevent further bleeding are crucial.

(1) Airway, breathing, and circulation must be ensured.

(2) Intravenous crystalloids and colloids (e.g., Hetastarch) should be infused as needed.

(3) The patient's electrolyte status must be monitored and any imbalances corrected promptly.

b. Gastric lavage may be performed via a nasogastric or orogastric tube; iced saline solution is instilled until the aspirate returns free of blood.

c. Vasoconstrictors, antacids, or H_2-receptor antagonists may be administered. Vasopressin, an agent that causes contraction of gastrointestinal smooth muscle, may be given to constrict vessels and control bleeding.

d. Emergency surgery usually is indicated if the patient does not respond to medical management.

B. Perforation. Penetration of a peptic ulcer through the gastric or duodenal wall results in this acute emergency. Perforation most commonly occurs with ulcers located in the anterior duodenal wall.

1. Clinical features. Sudden acute upper abdominal pain, rigidity, guarding, rebound tenderness, and absent or diminished bowel sounds are typical manifestations. Several hours after onset, symptoms may abate somewhat; this apparent remission is dangerously misleading because peritonitis and shock may ensue.

2. Management. Emergency surgery is almost always necessary.

C. Obstruction. Inflammatory edema, spasm, and scarring may lead to obstruction of the duodenal or gastric outlet. The pylorus and proximal duodenum are the most common obstruction sites.

1. Clinical features. Typical patient complaints include postprandial vomiting or bloating, appetite and weight loss, and abdominal distention. Tympany and a succussion splash may be audible on physical examination. Gastric aspiration after an overnight fast typically yields more than 200 ml of food residue or clear fluid contents. (Gastric cancer must be ruled out as the cause of obstruction.)

2. Management

a. Conservative measures (as in routine ulcer therapy) are indicated in most cases of obstruction.

b. Patients with marked obstruction may require **continuous gastric suction** with careful monitoring of fluid and electrolyte status. A **saline load test** may be performed after 72 hours of continuous suction to test the degree of residual obstruction.

c. If less than 200 ml of gastric contents are aspirated, liquid feedings can begin. **Aspiration** is performed at least daily for the next few days to monitor for retention and to guide dietary modifications as the patient progresses to a full regular diet.

d. Surgery is indicated if medial management fails.

D. Postsurgical complications

1. **Dumping syndrome.** Affecting about 10% of patients who have undergone partial gastrectomy, this disorder is characterized by rapid gastric emptying.
   a. **Causes.** The mechanism underlying dumping syndrome is poorly defined. However, intestinal exposure to hypertonic chyme may play a key role by triggering rapid shifts of fluid from the plasma to the intestinal lumen.
   b. **Clinical features.** The patient may experience weakness, dizziness, anxiety, tachycardia, flushing, sweating, abdominal cramps, nausea, vomiting, and diarrhea.
      (1) Manifestations may develop 15–30 minutes after a meal (**early dumping syndrome**) or 90–120 minutes after a meal (**late dumping syndrome**).
      (2) Reactive hypoglycemia may partly account for some cases of late dumping syndrome.
   c. **Management.** The patient usually is advised to eat six small meals of high protein and fat content and low carbohydrate content. Fluids should be ingested 1 hour before or after a meal but never with a meal. **Anticholinergics** may be given to slow food passage into the intestine.

2. **Other postsurgical complications** include reflux gastritis, afferent blind loop syndrome, stomal ulceration, diarrhea, malabsorption, early satiety, and iron deficiency anemia.

E. Refractory ulcers. Ulcers that fail to heal on a prolonged course of drug treatment should not be confused with ulcers that recur after therapy is stopped. It is difficult to predict which patients will have a refractory ulcer.

1. **Differential diagnosis.** Any compliant patient who continues to have dyspeptic symptoms after 8 weeks of therapy should have gastroscopy and biopsy to exclude rare causes of ulceration in the duodenum, such as Crohn's disease, tuberculosis, lymphoma, pulmonary or secondary carcinoma, and cytomegalovirus (CMV) infection in immunodeficient patients. Fasting plasma gastrin concentration should be measured to exclude the Zollinger-Ellison syndrome.
2. **Treatment.** In the absence of clinical trials, the options are speculative:
   a. Increase the dose of the H_2-receptor antagonist.
   b. Begin omeprazole therapy.
   c. Select an antibiotic regimen appropriate for *H. pylori* eradication.
   d. Combine therapy with the H_2-receptor antagonist
      (1) Use the anticholinergic propantheline bromide, 15 mg ½ hour before meals and at bedtime; glycopyrrolate, 1–2 mg ½ hour before meals and at bedtime; and oxyphencyclimine, 10 mg twice a day. There is a greater decrease in intragastric acidity with both types of drugs combined.
      (2) Use anticholinergics, H_2-receptor antagonists, and antacids.
   e. Perform surgery.

F. Maintenance regimens

1. Despite healing after withdrawal of therapy, 70% of ulcers recur in 1 year, and 90% in 2 years.
2. Candidates for long-term maintenance therapy include patients with serious concomitant diseases; four relapses per year; or a combination of risk factors, producing a more severe natural history of peptic disease (e.g., old age, male sex, a long history of aspirin or NSAID use, heavy alcohol intake, cigarette smoking, a history of peptic ulcer disease in an immediate relative, high maximal acid output, and a history of ulcer complications).
3. Continuous maintenance should be considered to reduce persistent symptoms or to prevent ulcer relapse and related complications.
4. Intermittent treatment is preferred for patients with uncomplicated, infrequent recurrences (< 2 per year) who are nonsmokers.

STUDY QUESTIONS

Directions: Each of the numbered items or incomplete statements in this section is followed by answers or by completions of the statement. Select the **one** lettered answer or completion that is **best** in each case.

1. Which of the following organisms has been implicated as a possible cause of chronic gastritis and peptic ulcer disease?

(A) *Campylobacter jejuni*
(B) *Escherichia coli*
(C) *Helicobacter pylori*
(D) *Calymmatobacterium granulomatis*
(E) *Giardia lamblia*

2. All of the following statements concerning antacid therapy used in the treatment of duodenal or gastric ulcers are correct EXCEPT

(A) antacids may be used to heal the ulcer but are ineffective in controlling ulcer pain
(B) antacids neutralize acid and decrease the activity of pepsin
(C) if used alone for ulcer therapy, antacids should be administered 1 hour and 3 hours after meals and at bedtime
(D) if diarrhea occurs, the patient may alternate the antacid product with aluminum hydroxide
(E) calcium carbonate should be avoided because it causes acid rebound and induces constipation

3. As part of a comprehensive management strategy to treat peptic ulcer disease, patients should be encouraged to do all of the following EXCEPT

(A) decrease caffeine ingestion
(B) eat only bland foods
(C) stop smoking
(D) avoid alcohol
(E) avoid the use of milk as a treatment modality

4. A gastric ulcer patient requires close follow-up to document complete ulcer healing because

(A) perforation into the intestine is common
(B) spontaneous healing of the ulcer may occur in 30%–50% of cases
(C) there is the risk of the ulcer being cancerous
(D) symptoms tend to be chronic and recur
(E) weight loss may be severe in gastric ulcer patients

Directions: Each item below contains three suggested answers of which **one or more** is correct. Choose the answer

A if **I only** is correct
B if **III only** is correct
C if **I and II** are correct
D if **II and III** are correct
E if **I, II, and III** are correct

5. Correct statements concerning cigarette smoking and ulcer disease include which of the following?

I. Smoking delays healing of gastric and duodenal ulcers
II. Nicotine decreases biliary and pancreatic bicarbonate secretion
III. Smoking accelerates the emptying of stomach acid into the duodenum

6. When administered at the same time, antacids can decrease the therapeutic efficacy of which of the following drugs?

I. Sucralfate
II. Ranitidine
III. Cimetidine

1-C 4-C
2-A 5-E
3-B 6-E

Directions: The group of items in this section consists of lettered options followed by a set of numbered items. For each item, select the **one** lettered option that is most closely associated with it. Each lettered option may be selected once, more than once, or not at all.

Questions 7–11

For each effect, select the agent that is most likely associated with it.

(A) Sodium bicarbonate
(B) Aluminum hydroxide
(C) Calcium carbonate
(D) Magnesium hydroxide
(E) Propantheline

7. May cause diarrhea
8. Cannot be used by patients with heart failure
9. Use with milk and an alkaline substance can cause milk-alkali syndrome
10. May cause dry mouth
11. Can be alternated with an antacid mixture to control diarrhea

---

7-D
8-A
9-C
10-E
11-B

ANSWERS AND EXPLANATIONS

1. The answer is C *[I E 9].*
Helicobacter pylori commonly is found in patients with peptic ulcer disease and always in association with chronic gastritis. Elimination of the organism has resulted in healing of the gastritis and the duodenal ulcer. More data, however, are needed before a definitive cause-and-effect relationship can be established.

2. The answer is A *[II A 1].*
Antacids have been shown to heal peptic ulcers, and their main use in modern therapy is to control ulcer pain. Antacids should be taken 1 hour and 3 hours after meals because the meal prolongs the acid-buffering effect of the antacid. If diarrhea becomes a problem with antacid use, an aluminum hydroxide product can be alternated with the antacid mixture; this takes advantage of the constipating property of aluminum. Since calcium carbonate causes acid rebound and constipation, its use should be avoided.

3. The answer is B *[II B 1 a (1)].*
Bland food diets are no longer recommended in the treatment of ulcer disease because research indicates that bland or milk-based diets do not accelerate ulcer healing. Studies show that patients can eat almost anything; however, they should avoid foods that aggravate their ulcer symptoms.

4. The answer is C *[I D 6].*
Five percent to ten percent of gastric ulcers may be due to cancer. The ulcer may respond to therapy; however, failure of the ulcer to decrease satisfactorily in size and to heal with therapy may suggest cancer. Close follow-up is necessary to document complete ulcer healing.

5. The answer is E (all) *[I E 2; II B 1 c].*
Clinical studies have shown that smoking increases susceptibility to ulcer disease, impairs spontaneous and drug-induced healing, and increases the risk and rapidity of recurrence of the ulcer. These findings may result in part from nicotine's ability to decrease biliary and pancreatic bicarbonate secretion, thus decreasing the body's ability to neutralize acid in the duodenum. Also, the accelerated emptying of stomach acid into the duodenum may predispose to duodenal ulcer and may decrease healing rates.

6. The answer is E (all) *[II A 1 e (3), 3 d].*
The mean peak blood concentration of cimetidine and the area under the 4-hour cimetidine blood concentration curve were both reduced significantly when cimetidine was administered at the same time as an antacid. The absorption of ranitidine is also reduced when it is taken concurrently with an aluminum-magnesium hydroxide antacid mixture. To avoid this interaction, the antacid should be administered 1 hour before or 2 hours after the administration of cimetidine or ranitidine. Antacids may reduce mucosal binding of sucralfate, decreasing its therapeutic efficacy. Antacids should, therefore, be given 30–60 minutes before or after sucralfate.

7–11. The answers are: 7-D *[II A 1 b (3)],* **8-A** *[II A 1 d (2)],* **9-C** *[II A 1 d (5)],* **10-E** *[II A 4 c (1)],* **11-B** *[II A 1 b (3)].*
Magnesium-containing products tend to cause diarrhea, possibly due to the ability of magnesium to stimulate the secretion of bile acids by the gallbladder. Because of its sodium content, sodium bicarbonate is contraindicated in patients with congestive heart failure (CHF), hypertension, severe renal disease, and edema. Sodium bicarbonate is no longer used in peptic ulcer therapy. In addition to causing acid rebound, calcium carbonate, if taken with milk and an alkaline substance for long periods, may cause the milk-alkali syndrome. It also may cause adverse effects such as hypercalcemia, alkalosis, azotemia, and nephrocalcinosis. Propantheline, like other anticholinergic agents, may cause dry mouth, blurred vision, urinary retention, and constipation. These agents are sometimes used as adjuncts to relieve duodenal ulcer pain. They are contraindicated in gastric ulcer because they delay gastric emptying. Aluminum hydroxide is constipating and can be alternated with the patient's current antacid when that antacid product is causing diarrhea.

54
Diabetes Mellitus

Helen L. Figge

I. INTRODUCTION

A. Definition. Diabetes mellitus (DM) refers to a group of disorders characterized by absent or deficient insulin secretion or peripheral insulin resistance, resulting in hyperglycemia and impaired metabolism.

B. Classification. DM occurs in two major forms.

1. **Type I: Insulin-dependent DM** (IDDM, formerly known as juvenile-onset or ketosis-prone diabetes)
   a. This form is most common in children and in adults up to age 30 years but may occur at any age.
   b. Type I diabetics are predisposed to **ketoacidosis**—accumulation of ketone bodies in body tissues and fluids.
   c. Disease onset is sudden.
   d. Beta cells, insulin-producing cells of the pancreatic islets of Langerhans, are destroyed, causing **absolute insulin deficiency**.
   e. All type I diabetics require insulin replacement therapy.

2. **Type II: Non–insulin-dependent DM** (formerly called adult-onset diabetes; may be insulin requiring)
   a. Most type II diabetics are over 40 years and obese.
   b. Disease onset typically is gradual.
   c. In most cases, type II DM is characterized by **insensitivity to insulin in the target tissues, deficient response of pancreatic beta cells to glucose,** or both.
   d. Because some insulin is secreted, ketoacidosis is prevented.
   e. Only a minority of type II diabetics require insulin replacement therapy.

C. Incidence. In the United States, DM affects an estimated 1%–5% of the population. Type I DM accounts for approximately 10% of cases; type II, for about 90% of cases.

D. Etiology. Various factors are thought to contribute to the development of DM.

1. **Type I DM.** Genetic predisposition, environmental factors, and autoimmunity have been proposed.
   a. **Genetics.** Certain genetic markers in the human leukocyte antigen (HLA) system have been strongly linked with type I DM. In addition, many patients have a family history of the disease; that is, 50% of individuals having an identical twin with type I DM also are diabetics.
   b. **Environment.** Viruses (e.g., rubella) and toxic chemicals are among the environmental factors that researchers believe may affect the pancreas and cause beta cell destruction in individuals who are genetically predisposed to DM.
   c. **Autoimmunity.** An autoimmune component is suggested by the presence of antibodies to islet-cell antigens in most new-onset type I diabetics. Much evidence has accumulated to support the autoimmune hypothesis. Both humoral and cell-mediated abnormalities have been described. An abnormal immune response could cause the body to destroy beta cells because it has misidentified them as foreign.

2. **Type II DM.** Genetic factors and a beta cell or peripheral site defect have been implicated.
   a. **Genetics.** Nearly all identical twins of patients with type II DM also have the disease. A high percentage of other type II diabetics have a strong family history of the disease.

b. A **beta cell defect** is postulated to cause abnormalities in insulin secretion resulting in a relative deficiency of insulin.

c. A **peripheral site defect** is postulated to lead to insulin resistance—tissue insensitivity to the action of insulin. This condition is thought to result from a post-receptor defect.

3. **Secondary diabetes** may arise from such conditions as endocrine disorders (e.g., Cushing's syndrome), pregnancy, pancreatic disease, and use of drugs that antagonize insulin (e.g., thiazide diuretics, adrenocorticosteroids).

E. Pathophysiology. In untreated type I and type II DM, the disease follows a typical progression.

1. Without adequate insulin, which stimulates glucose transports across cell membranes, glucose transport to most cells diminishes. Also, the conversion of glucose to glycogen diminishes. As a result, glucose is trapped in the bloodstream and **hyperglycemia** occurs. Some glucose also spills into the urine.

2. Hyperglycemia leads to **osmotic diuresis** and subsequent **dehydration** and **electrolyte abnormalities.**

3. In type I DM, without insulin to stimulate glucose uptake, cells must use protein and fat as energy sources.
   a. Fat is broken down into **free fatty acids** and **glycerol**.
   b. In the liver, free fatty acids are further broken down into **ketone bodies**.
   c. Breakdown is so rapid that excessive ketone bodies spill into the bloodstream. (In type II DM, however, the presence of some insulin prevents ketonemia.)
   d. Increased amounts of glycerol, another by-product of fat metabolism, worsen hyperglycemia.

F. Clinical evaluation

1. **Physical findings.** Type I DM has an abrupt onset and, in some cases, an acute presentation. With type II DM, symptoms develop gradually; some patients are asymptomatic or have only mild symptoms.
   a. Classic signs and symptoms of untreated DM include polydipsia (excessive thirst), polyuria (excessive urination), and polyphagia (excessive hunger). Other common findings are dry, itchy skin; frequent skin and vaginal infections; and visual disturbances.
   b. In addition to the above, the type I diabetic may present with fatigue, weakness, and unintentional weight loss, with or without signs and symptoms of ketoacidosis (see III A 1).
   c. The type II diabetic may present with hyperosmolar coma.
   d. Symptom severity and onset help differentiate type I and type II DM.
   e. Long-standing DM causes typical progressive changes in the retina, kidneys, nervous system, cardiovascular system, and integumentary system. For physical findings reflecting these changes, see III B.

2. **Laboratory findings**
   a. The diagnosis of DM is confirmed by a **fasting blood glucose level of 140 mg/dl or more** on at least two occasions.
   b. If the fasting blood glucose level is normal (below 140 mg/dl) but the patient has suggestive signs and symptoms, an **oral glucose tolerance test (OGTT)** should be done.
      (1) Glucose (75 g), dissolved in 300 ml of water, is given after a 12-hour fast.
      (2) A blood glucose level of 200 mg/dl or more at 2 hours and in at least one earlier sample after the glucose dose is administered confirms DM.
   c. A **random blood glucose level of 200 mg/dl** or more also confirms DM.
   d. Reversible factors that promote hyperglycemia (e.g., increased calorie intake, pregnancy, certain medications) should be ruled out before a diagnosis of DM is established.

G. Treatment objectives

1. To maintain optimal health, thus permitting a productive life

2. To equalize the supply of and demand for insulin to prevent symptomatic hyperglycemia and hypoglycemia

3. To avoid acute disease complications (e.g., ketosis)

4. To prevent or minimize complications of long-standing disease

5. To teach the patient about the disease and ensure therapeutic compliance

II. THERAPY. Diet, drug therapy, exercise, glucose monitoring, patient education, and self-care are crucial in the management of DM.

A. Diet. All diabetics must eat a well-balanced diet to regulate blood glucose. **Type I diabetics must eat at properly spaced intervals. Type II diabetics**—most of whom are obese—should follow a **weight-reduction diet** (increased weight is associated with more pronounced hyperglycemia). Dietary therapy alone is sufficient to control hyperglycemia in many type II patients.

1. Intake of **carbohydrates, proteins,** and **fats** should be regulated, with carbohydrates accounting for 45%–50% of total caloric intake, proteins accounting for 15%–20%, and fats accounting for 35%–40%.
2. **Refined** and **simple sugars** should be avoided.
3. High intake of **fiber** (e.g., bran, beans, fruits, vegetables) seems to improve blood glucose control.
4. **Cholesterol** intake is limited to less than 300 mg/day.
5. The **food exchange system** increases flexibility in meal planning. This system lists equivalent carbohydrate, protein, and fat values for foods in six basic groups.
6. The **glycemic index,** another meal planning aid, categorizes carbohydrates according to the blood glucose level they produce after ingestion; the lower the level, the lower a given carbohydrate's glycemic index. Although this system may allow diabetics to select carbohydrates more carefully, researchers debate its value because the glycemic index of carbohydrates may change when they are consumed along with proteins or fats.
7. Factors that change the blood glucose level (e.g., stress, exercise) necessitate dietary adjustment. For example, before vigorous exercise, the diabetic should consume 30–40 g of a complex carbohydrate, plus protein.

B. Drug therapy. Insulin and sulfonylureas are used in the treatment of DM.

1. Insulin

a. Indications. Insulin replacement therapy is indicated for all type I diabetics and for type II diabetics whose hyperglycemia does not respond to dietary or sulfonylurea therapy.

b. Mechanism of action. Insulin lowers the blood glucose level by increasing glucose transport across cell membranes, enhancing glucose conversion to glycogen, inhibiting release of free fatty acids from adipose tissue, and inhibiting lipolysis and glycogenolysis.

c. Choice of agent

(1) Source. Commercial insulin is derived from three principle sources: beef, pork, and biosynthetic human insulin (produced by recombinant DNA techniques). Use of human insulin in newly diagnosed type I diabetics is preferred because of its reduced antigenicity.

(2) Concentration. Most insulins come in a concentration of 100 units/ml (U100), dispensed in 10-ml vials.

(a) Concentrated insulin preparations (U500) are available for patients with insulin resistance.

(b) Children and adults needing small insulin quantities may use U40 insulin.

(3) Preparations

(a) Three major types of insulin differ in onset and duration of action (Table 54-1).

(i) Fast-acting insulin products include **regular** and **semilente insulin** (insulin zinc suspension).

(ii) Intermediate-acting insulin products include **lente** and **NPH** (isophane insulin suspension).

(iii) Long-acting insulin products include **PZI** (protamine zinc insulin) and **ultralente** (extended insulin zinc suspension).

(b) Insulin mixtures. Some diabetics need a mixture of insulin types (e.g., a rapid-acting insulin to control morning hyperglycemia and an intermediate-acting insulin to control later hyperglycemia).

(i) Insulin may be mixed by the patient or bought in a premixed form (e.g., Novolin 70/30, consisting of 70% NPH insulin and 30% regular insulin).

(ii) Insulins mixed together should be of the same concentration.

d. Administration and dosage. For routine use, insulin is administered by **subcutaneous injection**.

Table 54-1. Major Characteristics of Insulin Preparations

Preparation	Onset of Action (Hours)	Peak Effect (Hours)	Duration of Action (Hours)
Fast-acting insulins			
Regular	0.25–1	2–6	4–12
Semilente	0.5–1	3–6	8–16
Intermediate-acting insulins			
Lente	1–4	6–16	12–28
NPH	1.5–4	6–16	12–24
Long-acting insulins			
PZI	3–8	14–24	24–48
Ultralente	4	18–24	36

NPH = isophane insulin suspension; PZI = protamine zinc insulin.

(1) The subcutaneous injection site should be rotated to avoid lipohypertrophy and fibrosis. However, to prevent variations in drug absorption, injections should be given within the same region (e.g., the abdomen).

(2) Patients with acute hyperglycemia or ketoacidosis may require intravenous administration with regular insulin (insulin injection).

(3) **Insulin pump.** This delivery method, which provides tighter glycemic control, is indicated for selected diabetics who need long-term insulin therapy, who have widely fluctuating blood glucose levels, or whose life-styles preclude regular meals. However, there is a risk of developing serious hypoglycemia when using a pump.

(a) The **closed-loop pump** senses and responds to changing blood glucose levels. Through a subcutaneous needle in the thigh or abdominal wall, the pump administers appropriate amounts of insulin continuously. Because it requires blood aspiration, it can be used only in a hospital setting.

(b) The **open-loop pump** does not have a glucose sensor. It infuses insulin in small continuous doses and in large doses that the patient releases when appropriate (e.g., before meals).

e. Precautions and monitoring effects

(1) Improper insulin therapy may induce **hypoglycemia,** especially in patients with unpredictable changes in insulin requirements. Other causes of hypoglycemia include meal skipping, vigorous exercise, and accidental insulin overdose.

(a) To reverse insulin hypoglycemia in an **unresponsive patient,** glucose may be injected intravenously or honey or a glucose product (e.g., Glutose) may be inserted into the patient's buccal pouch. In addition, glucagon may be given subcutaneously, intramuscularly, or intravenously at a dose of 0.5–1 unit (0.5–1 mg).

(b) A **conscious patient** may be given a food or a beverage containing a simple, fast-acting carbohydrate (e.g., candy, fruit juice) to raise the blood glucose level. Patients should be counseled not to use diet beverages to treat a reaction.

(2) Two types of **insulin reactions** may occur—reactions with **adrenergic symptoms** (e.g., diaphoresis, tachycardia) or reactions with **neuroglycopenia** (e.g., confusion, irritability, loss of consciousness, weakness).

(a) Patients with adrenergic symptoms are usually aware of the fact that they are having a reaction.

(b) Patients with neuroglycopenia may have hypoglycemic unawareness and are at risk for loss of consciousness and seizures. These patients should never be tightly controlled.

(3) Local or systemic **insulin allergy** may occur, particularly after the first dose. Manifestations include allergic urticaria, anaphylaxis, and angioedema.

(4) **Lipoatrophy** (subcutaneous fat loss triggered by an immune reaction) may occur at the injection site. Pure insulin forms have reduced the incidence of this adverse reaction.

(5) **Lipohypertrophy** and **fibrosis** may develop in patients who do not rotate injection sites.

(6) **Insulin resistance** is defined as the need for more than 200 units/day of insulin (in the absence of ketoacidosis). This condition may result from obesity, infection, glucocorticoid excess, or a high concentration of circulating immunoglobulin G (IgG) anti-insulin antibodies.

(a) Nearly all patients receiving insulin develop such antibodies; however, in cases of insulin resistance, serum insulin-binding capacity usually exceeds 30 units/L.

(b) The condition may resolve spontaneously. In some cases, though, it necessitates a switch to a less antigenic insulin (e.g., to pork or human insulin), use of multiple injections of regular insulin rather than an intermediate-acting product, or prednisone therapy (60 mg/day) to suppress the immune response.

(7) Too much insulin can cause the **Somogyi effect** (insulin rebound syndrome). In this syndrome, nocturnal hypoglycemia stimulates a surge of counterregulatory hormones, triggering morning hyperglycemia.

(8) Various factors may change a diabetic's insulin requirements. Regular glucose self-monitoring is needed to evaluate changing insulin requirements and therapeutic efficacy (see II D, E).

(a) Infection, weight gain, puberty, inactivity, hyperthyroidism, and Cushing's disease tend to increase insulin needs.

(b) Renal failure, adrenal insufficiency, malabsorption, hypopituitarism, weight loss, and increased exercise tend to reduce insulin needs.

(9) PZI and regular insulin must not be mixed together in the same syringe.

f. Significant interactions

(1) A decreased response to insulin may occur when **corticosteroids, nicotinic acid,** or **thiazide diuretics** are administered concomitantly.

(2) Hypoglycemic effects may increase, leading to prolonged hypoglycemia, with concomitant use of insulin and **monoamine oxidase (MAO) inhibitors, β-blockers, salicylates, oxytetracycline, fenfluramine,** alcohol, **sulfonylureas,** or **pentamidine**.

2. **Sulfonylureas (oral hypoglycemics)** are used to control hyperglycemia in selected type II diabetics.

a. Indications. These drugs help to reduce blood glucose levels in type II DM that does not respond to diet alone. Because the action of sulfonylureas seems to depend on functioning beta cells, these drugs should never be used in type I diabetics.

b. Mechanism of action. As an acute action, sulfonylureas stimulate beta cell tissue to secrete insulin. In the long-term, these drugs appear to reduce cellular insulin resistance.

c. Choice of agent. First-generation sulfonylureas include **acetohexamide, chlorpropamide, tolbutamide,** and **tolazamide**. **Second-generation agents,** considerably more potent, include **glipizide** and **glyburide**. The most clinically significant difference among sulfonylureas is duration of action (Table 54-2).

(1) **Tolbutamide,** with the shortest duration, is administered mainly to elderly type II diabetics for whom hypoglycemia is a more serious complication.

(2) **Acetohexamide, tolazamide, glipizide,** and **glyburide** have intermediate durations of action. (The duration of acetohexamide is prolonged in renal disease.)

(3) **Chlorpropamide** has the longest duration of action and poses a risk to patients with

Table 54-2. Dosages and Other Characteristics of Sulfonylureas

Agent	Usual Daily Dosage (mg)	Number of Daily Doses	Duration of Action (Hours)	Activity of Hepatic Metabolites
First-generation agents				
Acetohexamide	250–1500	1–2	12–18	Two and a half times more active than original
Chlorpropamide	100–500	1	60	Active
Tolazamide	100–1000	1–2	12–14	Three inactive, three weak
Tolbutamide	500–3000	2–3	6–12	Inactive
Second-generation agents				
Glipizide	2.5–40	1–2	24	Inactive
Glyburide	1.25–20	1–2	24	Mostly inactive

renal or hepatic impairment. It also causes more severe and frequent side effects (including hypoglycemia and hyponatremia) than the other sulfonylureas.

d. **Administration and dosage** (see Table 54-2)

e. **Precautions and monitoring effects**

(1) Sulfonylureas are contraindicated in patients without functioning beta cells, children, pregnant and lactating women, and patients with allergy to sulfa agents. They also are contraindicated during stressful conditions that increase the risk of hyper- or hypoglycemia.

(2) These agents should not be used in patients with severe renal or hepatic impairment.

(3) Sulfonylurea therapy has been associated with a possible increased risk of cardiovascular mortality and morbidity.

(4) Hypoglycemia and alcohol intolerance may occur during sulfonylurea therapy. Alcohol tolerance is less common with second-generation agents.

(5) Sulfonylureas should not be discontinued without a physician's approval.

(6) Untoward reactions to sulfonylureas include gastrointestinal disturbances (e.g., nausea, gastric discomfort, vomiting, constipation), tachycardia, headache, skin rash, and hematologic problems (e.g., agranulocytosis, pancytopenia, hemolytic anemia).

(7) Sulfonylureas pose a risk of cholestatic jaundice.

(8) Sulfonylurea therapy has a relatively **high failure rate** (25%–40%).

(a) **Primary therapeutic failure.** The agent fails to control hyperglycemia within the first 4 weeks after initiation.

(b) **Secondary therapeutic failure.** The drug controls hyperglycemia initially but fails to maintain control. Approximately 5%–30% of initial responders experience secondary therapeutic failure. There is generally no reason to continue sulfonylurea therapy once insulin therapy has been initiated in such patients.

f. **Significant interactions**

(1) Prolonged hypoglycemia and masking of hypoglycemia symptoms may occur with concomitant use of **β-blockers** and **clonidine.**

(2) **Alcohol, salicylates, nonsteroidal anti-inflammatory drugs (NSAIDs), methyldopa, chloramphenicol, warfarin, MAO inhibitors, probenecid,** and **ranitidine** may intensify the hypoglycemic effects of sulfonylureas.

(3) A decreased hypoglycemic response may occur with concomitant use of **corticosteroids, aminophylline, bleomycin, thiazide diuretics, ethacrynic acid, levodopa, rifampin, phenytoin,** and **oral contraceptives**.

C. **Exercise.** A carefully planned and religiously followed exercise program enhances glucose uptake to cells, thereby reducing the blood glucose level. Patients with severe retinopathy must consult an ophthalmologist prior to exercise initiation.

1. **Aerobic exercise** (e.g., swimming, walking, running) has a desirable hypoglycemic effect because it uses glucose as fuel; aerobic exercise also promotes cardiovascular health.

2. **Anaerobic exercise** (e.g., weight-lifting) should be avoided by diabetics because it induces stress that leads to increased blood glucose levels. Also, anaerobic exercise may cause deleterious cardiovascular effects (e.g., increased blood pressure).

D. **Glucose monitoring.** Frequent measurement of the blood glucose level is a key aspect of DM therapy. It helps determine therapeutic efficacy, guides and refines any adjustments to drug therapy, and, when performed by the patient at home, permits better understanding of the glycemic effects of specific foods.

1. **Urine glucose testing** is generally no longer recommended; it has been replaced by blood glucose testing.

2. **Blood glucose testing.** This type of testing is generally indicated for all diabetics. Blood glucose tests are more reliable than urine glucose tests.

a. Some patients (especially type I diabetics) need to measure their blood glucose level several times daily—typically before or after meals.

b. Well-controlled type II diabetics may require monitoring once or twice a week.

c. **Test methods and products**

(1) **Reagent strips** (e.g., Chemstrip bG, Dextrostix, Visidex II) are visual tests in which a blood droplet is applied to the test strip.

(2) **Glucose meters** (multiple brands) are more accurate and convenient to use than reagent strips because they give a numerical blood glucose value.

(3) The **hemoglobin A_{1c} test** (also known as the **glycohemoglobin** or **glycosylated hemoglobin test**) shows long-term glycemic control and serves as an index of therapeutic efficacy or compliance.

(a) A hemoglobin variant produced by glycosylation or hemoglobin A, hemoglobin A_{1c} is more abundant in diabetics than nondiabetics.

(b) The hemoglobin A_{1c} level reflects the average blood glucose level over the preceding 6–8 weeks.

(c) A hemoglobin A_{1c} level of 7.5% or lower indicates good glycemic control; a level of 9.0% or higher reflects poor control.

(d) Patients with underlying hemoglobinopathies will have anomalous values.

3. Urine ketone monitoring should be performed if blood sugars are high or if the patient is acutely ill.

E. Patient education and self-care. Patient education about the disease and patient participation in medical care are important aspects of DM management.

1. **Patient education** improves understanding of the disease, thereby promoting compliance with dietary, drug, and exercise regimens and glucose self-monitoring. Patients also must be taught how to prevent, recognize, and treat hypoglycemia and hyperglycemia.

2. **Self-care measures** are necessary to avoid the potentially dire consequences of trauma and skin abrasions, resulting from disease complications, such as neuropathy and peripheral vascular compromise.

   a. The patient must inspect the skin daily for abrasions, pain, or swelling, and see a physician promptly for treatment. Injuries should be covered immediately with sterile gauze.
   b. Even minor trauma, especially to the legs and feet, should be avoided.
   c. Daily foot cleansing should be performed using only soap and water (with a thermometer to check water temperature if the patient has neuropathy-induced sensation loss). Skin should be dried gently and vegetable oil applied.
   d. Corns and calluses should be removed by a podiatrist.
   e. Only properly fitting, low-heeled shoes should be worn.
   f. Routine ophthalmology follow-up is essential for all diabetics.

F. Pancreas and islet cell transplantation. These experimental procedures may be performed to treat some cases of DM.

G. Disease management in pregnancy. Approximately 2%–3% of pregnant women with no history of DM develop diabetes or impaired glucose tolerance—presumably from the increased insulin requirements of pregnancy.

1. DM in pregnancy carries an increased risk of neonatal morbidity.

2. Tight glycemic control is especially important during pregnancy to avoid neonatal complications. Continuous insulin infusion (via an insulin pump) or multiple insulin injections may be required.

3. Sulfonylureas are contraindicated in pregnant women.

4. Weight reduction is not recommended because this could compromise fetal development.

5. Some experts advise induction of labor or cesarean section at 37–38 weeks gestation.

6. Glucose tolerance usually normalizes within a few weeks after delivery.

III. COMPLICATIONS

A. Acute complications. Life-threatening complications of DM include diabetic ketoacidosis and hyperglycemic hyperosmolar nonketotic coma. Hypoglycemia, another acute complication, usually stems from drug therapy [see II B 1 e (1)].

1. **Diabetic ketoacidosis (DKA).** Usually affecting only type I diabetics, this disorder typically arises after a short period (hours or days) of deteriorating glycemic control. Hyperglycemia and ketonemia trigger osmotic diuresis, electrolyte loss, hypovolemia, and metabolic acidosis. DKA is often the presenting disorder in children with previously undiagnosed type I DM.
   a. **Precipitating factors** include stress, infection, exercise, excessive alcohol consumption, improper insulin therapy, and dietary noncompliance—conditions that lead to an absence or deficiency of insulin.
   b. **Physical findings** include Kussmaul's respirations, acetone breath odor, dehydration, dry skin, poor skin turgor, reduced level of consciousness (ranging from confusion to coma), and abdominal pain. Without treatment, death ensues.
   c. **Laboratory findings** include elevated levels of blood glucose and ketone bodies (e.g., acetone, acetoacetate), low arterial pH and carbon dioxide partial pressure (P_{CO_2}) values, and abnormal serum electrolyte values.
   d. **Therapy** involves fluid, intravenous insulin by continuous infusion, and electrolyte replacement.

2. **Hyperglycemic hyperosmolar nonketotic coma (HHNC),** which occurs in type II diabetics, has a higher mortality rate than DKA.
   a. **Precipitating factors** include various illnesses and conditions that increase insulin requirements [e.g., severe burns, gastrointestinal bleeding, central nervous system (CNS) injury, acute myocardial infarction].
      (1) Use of certain drugs (e.g., steroids, glucagon, thiazide diuretics, cimetidine, propranolol) also can trigger HHNC.
      (2) Such medical procedures as intravenous hyperalimentation and peritoneal dialysis increase the risk of HHNC.
   b. **Physical findings** include polyuria, polydipsia, dehydration, hypotension, rapid respirations, abdominal discomfort, nausea, vomiting, tachycardia, palpitations, focal neurologic signs, and reduced level of consciousness.
   c. **Laboratory findings** include an extremely elevated blood glucose level (800 mg/dl or higher) and a serum osmolarity of 280 mOsm/kg or more.
   d. **Therapy** involves fluid, insulin, and electrolyte replacement.

B. Chronic complications. DM is associated with a high risk for a number of chronic illnesses.

1. **Cardiovascular disease**
   a. Atherosclerosis and peripheral vascular disease are more severe and more common in diabetics than in nondiabetics; also, disease onset typically is earlier.
   b. Microvascular changes, characterized by thickening of the capillary basement membrane, may lead to retinopathy and skin changes.
   c. Diabetics with insulin resistance have a higher incidence of hypertension than nondiabetics.

2. **Ocular complications**
   a. Premature cataracts are most common in diabetics with severe chronic hyperglycemia.
   b. Diabetic retinopathy, a consequence of microvascular changes, affects approximately 50% of diabetics within 10 years of disease onset.
      (1) This syndrome is the leading cause of new blindness in the United States.
      (2) Retinal microaneurysm, the earliest sign of retinopathy, may progress to punctate hemorrhage, exudation, and proliferative retinopathy.
      (3) Retinal detachment, secondary glaucoma, and vision loss may ensue.

3. **Diabetic nephropathy,** another manifestation of microvascular pathology, ultimately may lead to renal insufficiency or failure.
   a. Diabetic nephropathy is characterized by proteinuria, microalbuminuria, glomerular lesions, and renal arteriosclerosis.
   b. Diabetics account for approximately 25% of patients with end-stage renal failure.

4. **Diabetic neuropathies** typically involve both the autonomic and peripheral nervous systems.
   a. Gastric atony, incontinence, diarrhea, and impotence reflect autonomic involvement.
   b. Peripheral neuropathy may give rise to impaired perception of pain and temperature (particularly in the lower extremities).
   c. Ischemia may cause skeletal muscle atrophy and motor abnormalities.

5. **Skin and mucous membrane complications** stem from vascular changes and neuropathy.
   a. Diabetics have an increased risk for infection, such as *Candida* infections of the skin and vagina. Erythema commonly develops beneath the breasts and between fingers; eruptive xanthomas occur most often in long-standing, poorly controlled DM.
   b. Atrophic lesions (round painless lesions) and diabetic dermopathy (reddish-brown papular spots) are common, especially on the lower extremities.
   c. An ulcerating necrotic lesion called **necrobiosis lipoidica diabeticorum** may develop on the anterior leg surface or the dorsum of the ankle.
   d. Injury, infection, neuropathy, vascular disease, or ischemia may lead to gangrene, which is 20 times more common in diabetics than nondiabetics.

STUDY QUESTIONS

Directions: Each of the numbered items or incomplete statements in this section is followed by answers or by completions of the statement. Select the **one** lettered answer or completion that is **best** in each case.

1. Current criteria used in the diagnosis of diabetes mellitus (DM) include all of the following symptoms EXCEPT

(A) fasting hyperglycemia
(B) polyuria
(C) polydipsia
(D) tinnitis
(E) weight loss

2. The most useful glucose test employed in monitoring diabetes mellitus (DM) therapy is

(A) urine monitoring
(B) blood monitoring
(C) renal function monitoring
(D) cardiovascular monitoring
(E) vascular monitoring

3. Which of the following statements concerning insulin replacement therapy is most likely true?

(A) Most commercial insulin products vary little with respect to time, course, and duration of hypoglycemic activity
(B) Regular insulins cannot be mixed with NPH (iosphane insulin suspension)
(C) Regular insulin cannot be given intravenously
(D) Cutting down on carbohydrate consumption is a necessity for all diabetic patients
(E) Insulin therapy does not have to be monitored closely

4. A mass of adipose tissue that develops at the injection site is usually due to the patient's neglect in rotating the insulin injection site. This is known as

(A) lipoatrophy
(B) hypertrophic degenerative adiposity
(C) lipohypertrophy
(D) atrophic skin lesion
(E) dermatitis

5. Sulfonylureas are a primary mode of therapy in the treatment of

(A) insulin-dependent (type I) diabetes mellitus (IDDM) patients
(B) diabetic patients experiencing severe hepatic or renal dysfunction
(C) diabetic pregnant women
(D) patients with diabetic ketoacidosis
(E) non–insulin-dependent (type II) DM patients

6. Patients taking chlorpropamide should avoid products containing

(A) acetaminophen
(B) ethanol
(C) vitamin A
(D) penicillins
(E) milk products

7. The standard recommended dose of glyburide is

(A) 0.5–2 mg/day
(B) 1.25–20 mg/day
(C) 50–100 mg/day
(D) 200 mg/day
(E) 200–1000 mg/day

1-D
2-B
3-D
4-C
5-E
6-B
7-B

Questions 8–12

A 20-year-old previously healthy man presents to the emergency room with a 2-week history of polyuria, polydipsia, and a 20-lb unintentional weight loss. He complains of weakness, fatigue, nausea, and abdominal pain. Physical examination reveals dry, parched mucous membranes. Blood pressure is 110/70 and pulse is 90 supine; blood pressure is 90/60, and pulse is 120 upright. Temperature is 100°F (axillary); respiratory rate is 24. General examination of the heart and lungs is unremarkable. No retinopathy is present. The abdomen is soft with mild tenderness but no rebound. Laboratory values are as follows:

Blood glucose	420 mg/dl
Sodium (Na)	130 mEq/L
Potassium (K)	3.7 mEq/L
Chloride (Cl)	97 mEq/L
Bicarbonate (HCO^{-3})	10 mEq/L
Arterial blood gas	7.20 (pH)
Urinalysis	3+ glucose and 3+ ketones
Chest x-ray	Unremarkable
Abdominal x-ray (KUB)	Unremarkable

8. What is the most likely diagnosis in this patient?

(A) Type II diabetes mellitus (DM) with hyperosmolar state
(B) Type I DM with diabetic ketoacidosis
(C) Type II DM without hyperosmolar state
(D) Type I DM without diabetic ketoacidosis

9. Initial appropriate therapy includes

(A) intravenous fluids and a sulfonylurea agent
(B) intravenous fluids alone
(C) intravenous fluids, 10 units of subcutaneous regular insulin, and discharge to home
(D) intravenous fluids, intravenous regular insulin by continuous drip at 6 units/hr, and hospital admission

10. After the acute illness has resolved, what further therapy would be appropriate?

(A) None, observe only
(B) Start a second-generation sulfonylurea
(C) Daily administration of a regimen of NPH (isophane insulin suspension) and regular insulin plus dietary modification
(D) Dietary modification alone

11. Appropriate follow-up of the patient once discharged to home includes all of the following EXCEPT

(A) periodic monitoring of hemoglobin A_{1c} levels
(B) periodic ophthalmologic examinations
(C) home glucose monitoring with a glucose meter
(D) weight loss diet and an attempt to wean from insulin

12. The patient is at risk for developing all of the following complications EXCEPT

(A) hypoglycemia
(B) coronary artery disease
(C) retinopathy
(D) nonketotic hyperglycemic hyperosmolar state

8-B
9-D
10-C
11-D
12-D

ANSWERS AND EXPLANATIONS

1. The answer is D *[I E, F 1 a].*
Frequent urination (polyuria), thirst (polydipsia), and weight loss are all common signs of diabetes. When these symptoms are present, it is necessary to have a fasting blood glucose level drawn to determine a diabetic state. A fasting blood glucose level of greater than or equal to 140 mg/dl on more than one occasion is diagnostic of a diabetic state.

2. The answer is B *[II D 1, 2].*
Blood glucose monitoring is the most useful form of monitoring glucose levels. Urine monitoring provides only gross estimates of the current status and cannot rule out hypoglycemia. Renal function and cardiovascular functions provide evidence of long-standing disease and are not useful for monitoring daily progress.

3. The answer is D *[II A 1, B 1 c (3) (a)].*
Many commercial insulin preparations vary with respect to duration of activity and time for peak plasma level. Regular insulin can be mixed with NPH (isophane insulin suspension) and can be given intravenously. All insulin therapies should be monitored closely and on a daily basis. Careful regulation of carbohydrate intake is very important for all diabetic patients—carbohydrate consumption plays a major role in the balance of glucose metabolism and antagonizes the effects of insulin therapy.

4. The answer is C *[II B 1 e (5)].*
Lipohypertrophy consists of masses of adipose tissue that develop at the injection site, usually in patients who do not rotate the injection sites properly. The masses gradually disappear if injection in these sites is avoided.

5. The answer is E *[II B 2 a].*
Sulfonylureas should not be used as primary therapy in insulin-dependent (type I) diabetes mellitus (IDDM) patients, in those who have severe hepatic or renal dysfunction, or in those patients who are pregnant. Diabetic ketoacidosis (DKA) should never be treated with sulfonylureas; this condition must be treated with insulin, fluids, and electrolyte replacement. However, sulfonylureas help to reduce blood glucose levels in type II DM that does not respond to diet alone.

6. The answer is B *[II B 2 c (3), e (4), f (2)].*
Acute ingestion of ethanol (alcohol) by patients who are taking any antidiabetic agent carries the risk of severe hypoglycemia especially due to the potential hypoglycemic effects of ethanol (especially if consumed in the fasting state).

7. The answer is B *[II B 2 c; Table 54-2].*
The standard recommended dose of glyburide is 1.25–20 mg/day. Doses greater than 20 mg are not recommended by the manufacturer. Patients may be started on a low dose (e.g., 1.25 mg/day) and titrated up to an effective oral dose, as clinically indicated.

8–12. The answers are: 8-B *[I F 1]*, **9-D** *[II B 1 d (2)]*, **10-C** *[II A, B 1 a, 2 a]*, **11-D** *[II D 2 c (2), (3)]*, **12-D** *[III A 2].*
Type I diabetes mellitus (DM) with diabetic ketoacidosis (DKA) is the most likely diagnosis in the patient described in the question. The patient presented with high blood sugar, weight loss, acidosis, and positive urine ketones (high level). This is a typical presentation of DKA.

Type I DM always requires insulin therapy; it can never be left untreated or treated with diet or liquids alone and can never be treated with sulfonylurea agents. DKA requires hospitalization and should be treated with an insulin drip until the acidosis clears. Patients with DKA are dehydrated and must be given intravenous fluids.

All diabetic patients should be followed with periodic hemoglobin A_{1c} measurements and ophthalmologic examination annually. Home glucose monitoring is the optimal way to follow a patient's level of control. Weight loss and an attempt to wean from insulin are appropriate only for type II DM. Type I diabetics cannot be weaned from insulin therapy.

Hypoglycemia is a possible complication of insulin therapy. All diabetics are at risk for coronary artery disease and retinopathy. Nonketotic hyperglycemic hyperosmolar coma is typically a complication of type II DM.

55
Thyroid Disease

John E. Janosik

I. PHYSIOLOGY

A. Thyroid hormone regulation

1. The thyroid gland synthesizes, stores, and secretes hormones that are important to growth and development and the metabolic rate. These hormones are **thyroxine (T_4)** and **triiodothyronine (T_3)**.
2. The thyroid gland also secretes **calcitonin,** which reduces blood calcium ion concentration.
3. Thyroid hormone secretion and transport are controlled by **thyroid-stimulating hormone (thyrotropin; TSH)**. TSH is released by the anterior pituitary gland, which is triggered by **thyrotropin-releasing hormone (TRH),** secreted from the hypothalamus.
   - a. The process produces increased levels of thyroid hormone (circulating free T_4 and free T_3), which, in turn, signals the pituitary to stop releasing TSH (**negative feedback**).
   - b. Conversely, low blood levels of free hormone trigger pituitary release of TSH, which stimulates the thyroid gland to secrete T_4 and T_3 until free hormone levels return to normal. At this point, the pituitary gland ceases to release TSH, which completes the feedback loop (Figure 55-1.)
   - c. This homeostatic mechanism attempts to maintain the level of circulating thyroid hormone within a very narrow range.

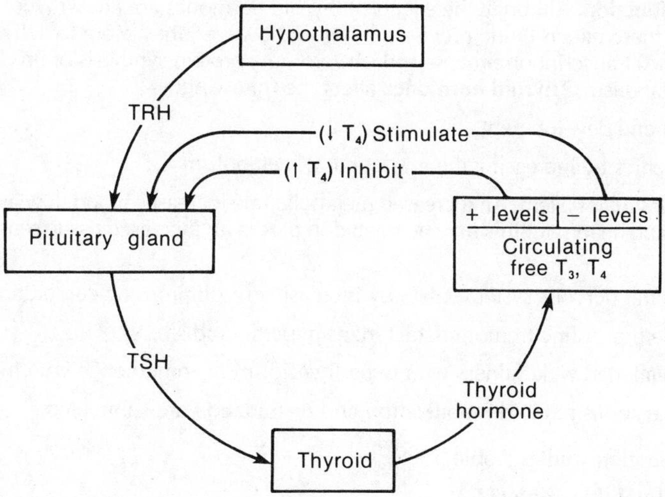

Figure 55-1. Thyroid hormone regulation loop. This carefully balanced hormone regulation system uses both positive (stimulating) and negative (inhibiting) feedback to maintain homeostasis. Disruption of any of these elements can produce serious consequences, such as myxedema crisis (underavailability of thyroid hormone) or thyroid storm (overabundance of thyroid hormone). *TRH* = thyroid-releasing hormone; *TSH* = thyroid-stimulating hormone; T_4 = thyroxine; T_3 = triiodothyronine.

B. Biosynthesis (Figure 55-2)

1. Essential to synthesis of thyroid hormones is dietary iodine, reduced to **inorganic iodide,** which the thyroid actively extracts from the plasma through iodide trapping (**iodide pump**). Some of this iodide is stored within the colloid; some diffuses into the lumen of thyroid follicles.

2. Iodide is oxidized by peroxidase and bound to tyrosyl residues within the thyroglobulin molecule in a process called **organification.**
   a. The synthesis begins with iodide binding to tyrosine, forming **monoiodotyrosine (MIT).**
   b. MIT then binds another iodide to form **diiodotyrosine (DIT).**
   c. Then, slowly, a coupling reaction binds MIT and DIT, producing $\mathbf{T_3}$ and $\mathbf{T_4}$.

C. Hormone transport

1. After TSH stimulation of the thyroid gland, T_3 and T_4 are cleaved from thyroglobulin and released into the circulation.

2. Once in the circulation, thyroid hormone is transported bound to several plasma proteins, a process that:
   a. Helps to protect the hormone from premature metabolism and excretion
   b. Prolongs its half-life in the circulation
   c. Allows it to reach its site of action

3. Most thyroid hormone is transported by **thyroxine-binding globulin (TBG). Prealbumin** and **albumin** also serve as carriers.

D. Hormone metabolism

1. Peripheral conversion of T_4 to T_3 takes place in the pituitary gland, liver, and kidneys and accounts for about 80% of T_3 generation.

2. Deiodination accounts for most hormone degradation. The major steps in this process are shown in Figure 55-3.

3. Deiodinated hormones are excreted in feces and urine.

4. Minor nondeiodination pathways of metabolism include conjugation with sulfate and glucuronide, deamination, and decarboxylation.

E. Hormone function. Although the effects of thyroid hormones are known, the basic mechanisms producing these effects elude precise definition; however, they seem to activate the messenger RNA (mRNA) transcription process and can promote protein synthesis or (in excessive amounts) protein catabolism. **Thyroid hormones** affect the following:

1. Growth and development

2. Calorigenics by increasing the rate of basal metabolism

3. Cardiovascular system. An increased metabolic rate increases blood flow and, in turn, cardiac output and heart rate; this may be related in part to an increased tissue sensitivity to catecholamines.

4. The central nervous system (CNS) by increasing or diminishing cerebration

5. Musculature. A fine tremor characterizes hyperthyroidism.

6. Sleep. Fatigued wakefulness with hyperthyroidism or somnolence with hypothyroidism.

7. Lipid metabolism. Lipid mobilization and degradation are stimulated.

F. Thyroid function studies (Table 55-1)

1. **Serum total thyroxine ($\mathbf{TT_4}$)**
   a. This test provides the most direct reflection of thyroid function through indicating hormone availability to tissues. Total (free and bound) T_4 is determined by radioimmunoassay, which is sensitive and rapid.
   b. Changes in thyroid globulin concentration, especially TBG, which increases during pregnancy, alter the total concentration of T_4 and may produce a misleading high or low test result.
   c. However, these changes in TBG do not affect the concentration of free T_4. Therefore, to clarify thyroid function, either protein binding (T_3 uptake test) or free T_4 must be measured.

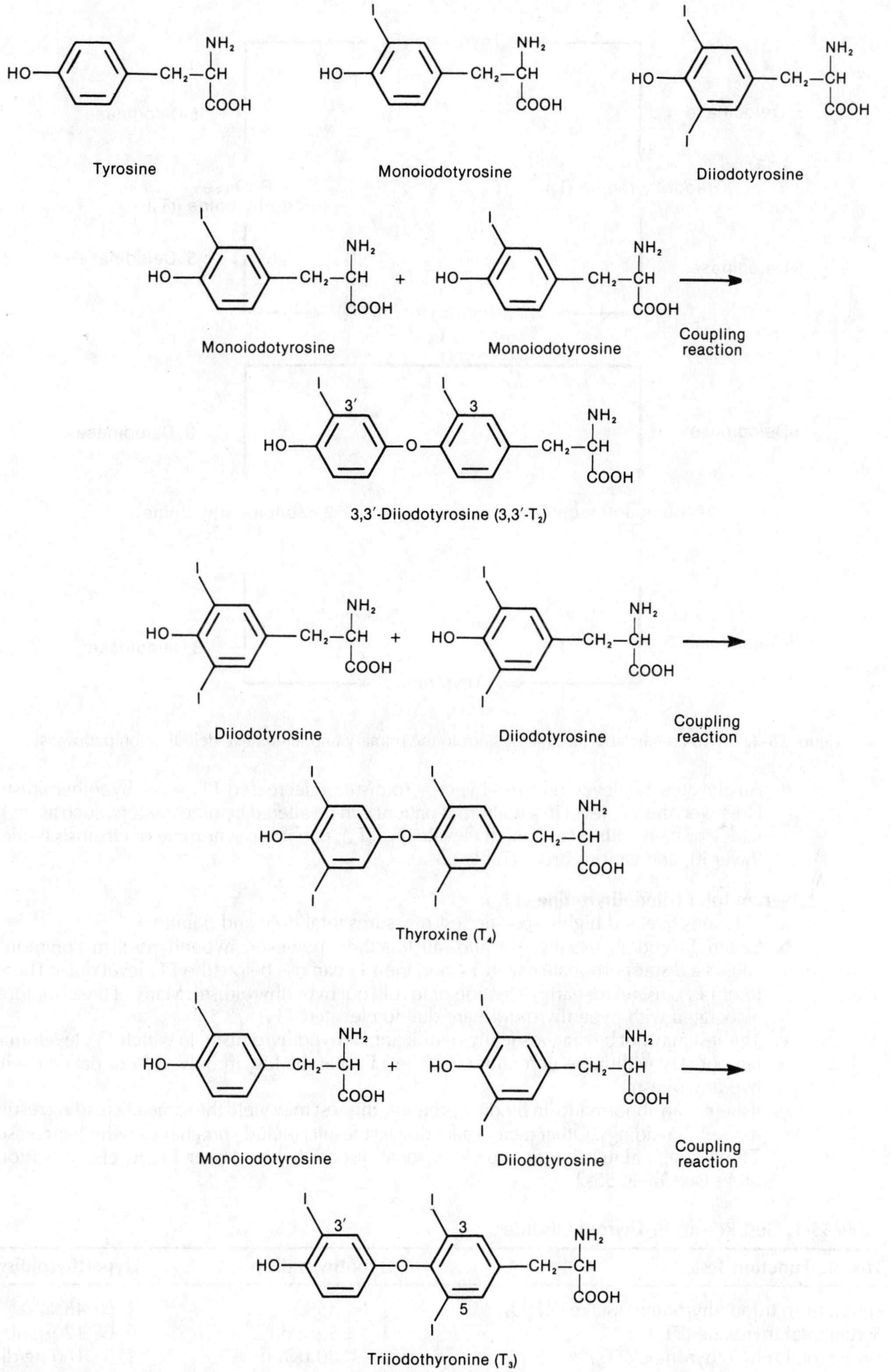

Figure 55-2. Biosynthesis of thyroid hormones. The major products are thyroxine (T_4) and triiodothyronine (T_3). These are formed in the follicle cells of the thyroid gland by iodination of tyrosine residues. Monoiodo- and diiodotyrosine residues are formed first. These then react to form T_3 and T_4.

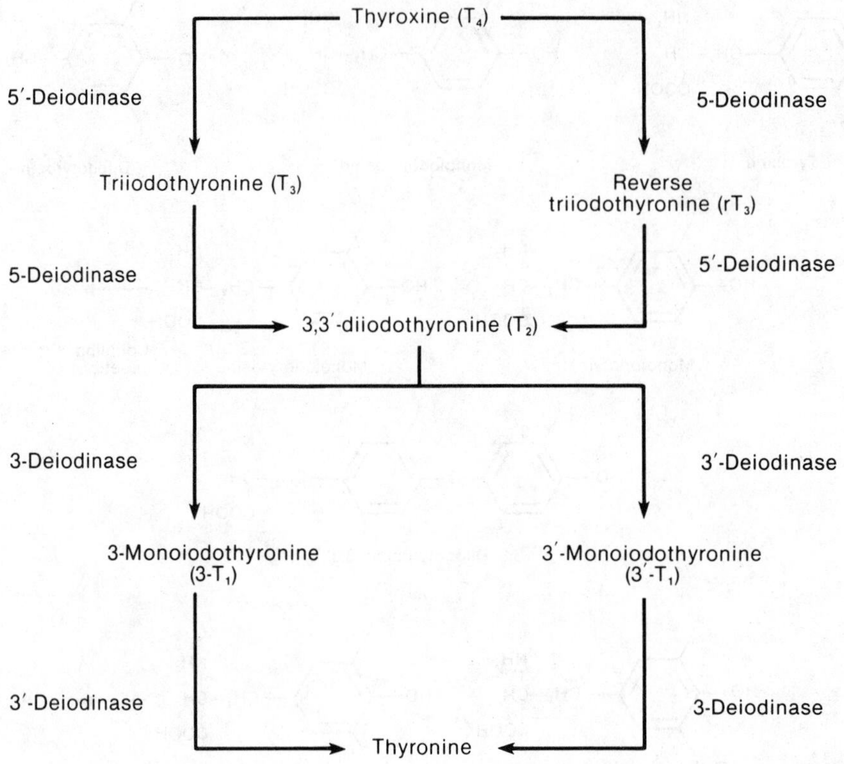

Figure 55-3. Thyroxine metabolism: major steps in the primary and alternative deiodination pathways.

d. An elevated TT_4 level indicates hyperthyroidism; a decreased TT_4 level, hypothyroidism. However, the TT_4 level in a euthyroid patient can be altered by other factors, such as pregnancy or febrile illnesses (which elevate the TT_4), nephrotic syndrome or cirrhosis (which lower it), and various drugs (Table 55-2).

2. Serum total triiodothyronine (TT_3)

a. This sensitive and highly specific test measures total (free and bound) T_3.

b. Serum T_3 and T_4 usually rise and fall together; however, hyperthyroidism commonly causes a disproportionate rise in T_3, and the TT_3 can rise before the TT_4 level does. Therefore, TT_3 is useful for early detection or to rule out hyperthyroidism. Many of the symptoms associated with hyperthyroidism are due to elevated TT_3.

c. This test may not be diagnostically significant for hypothyroidism, in which TT_3 levels may fall but stay within the normal range. The TT_3 may be low in only 50% of patients with hypothyroidism.

d. If there is an abnormality in binding proteins, this test may yield the same misleading results as the TT_4 readings. Other factors affecting test results include pregnancy (which increases TT_3 levels), malnutrition or hepatic or renal disease (which lower TT_3 levels), or various drugs (see Table 55-2).

Table 55-1. Test Results in Thyroid Disorders

Thyroid Function Test	Hypothyroidism	Hyperthyroidism
Serum resin triiodothyronine uptake (RT_3U)	↓ (< 35%)	↑ (> 45%)
Serum total thyroxine (TT_4)	↓ (< 5 μg/dl)	↑ (> 12 μg/dl)
Serum total triiodothyronine (TT_3)	↓ (< 80 ng/dl)	↑ (> 180 ng/dl)
Free thyroxine index (FTI)	↓ (< 5.5)	↑ (< 10.5)
Serum thyrotropin (TSH)	↑ (> 6 μU/ml)	↓ (< 0.5 μU/ml)
Sensitive thyrotropin (TSH) assay	↑ (> 5 μU/ml)	↓ (< 0.2 μU/ml)

↑ = increased levels; ↓ = decreased levels.

3. Resin triiodothyronine uptake (RT_3U)

a. This test clarifies whether abnormal T_4 levels are due to a thyroid disorder or to abnormalities in the binding proteins, because it evaluates the binding capacity of TBG.

b. If an abnormal amount (high or low) of thyroid hormone is present in the blood, the RT_3U results **change in the same direction** as the altered level—elevated in hyperthyroidism; decreased in hypothyroidism.

c. However, if abnormalities in binding proteins underlie the abnormal levels of TT_4, TT_3, or both, the RT_3U results **change in the opposite direction**—decreasing as TBG increases; increasing as TBG decreases.

d. Various drugs can cause spurious changes in the RT_3U (see Table 55-2).

4. Serum thyrotropin (TSH) and sensitive TSH assays

a. Serum TSH assay

(1) This test is the most sensitive test for detecting the hypothyroid state because the hypothalamic–pituitary axis compensates very quickly for even slight decreases in circulating free hormone by releasing more TSH. The TSH levels may be elevated even before low circulating levels of TT_4 are detectable by diagnostic testing.

(2) Serum TSH is not a reliable test for hyperthyroidism (in which TSH is suppressed) because low levels and low-normal levels of TSH may be indistinguishable with the current technology.

(3) Effects of drugs on the serum TSH are shown in Table 55-2.

b. Sensitive TSH assay

(1) The sensitive TSH assay uses immunoradiometric methodology or other new methods of analysis instead of the older radioimmunoassay techniques and demonstrates greater sensitivity in the detection of thyroid disease than older tests.

(2) This assay is usually more expensive and more commonly used to monitor patients receiving replacement therapy to control overtreatment. (Overtreatment can lead to excessive bone demineralization.)

5. Free thyroxine index (FTI)

a. This is not a separate test but rather an estimation of the free T_4 level through a mathematical interpretation of the relationship between RT_3U and serum T_4 levels:

$$\text{FTI} = \frac{TT_4 \times RT_3U}{\text{mean serum } RT_3U}$$

b. FTI values are elevated in hyperthyroidism or when TBG is low and decreased in hypothyroidism or when TBG is elevated.

c. Effects of drugs on FTI are shown in Table 55-2.

G. Strategies and cost considerations for testing

1. The most frequently used and least expensive tests for screening are the TT_4 and the RT_3U, which are used to calculate the FTI. A serum TSH assay may also be used but at an additional cost.

2. Thyroid disease screening for the otherwise generally healthy population is not cost-effective based on the rate of detection and cost associated with massive screening.

3. The most appropriate target population for screening includes elderly patients hospitalized for exacerbations of chronic diseases or who are coincidentally diagnosed with a chronic disease [e.g., congestive heart failure (CHF), rheumatoid arthritis], mental status changes, or psychosocial problems.

4. The American Thyroid Association recommends a FTI and a sensitive TSH assay as the primary laboratory tests to diagnose thyroid disease. The sensitive TSH assay is useful in detecting patients at risk of receiving an excess amount of thyroxine as replacement therapy.

II. HYPOTHYROIDISM. The inability of the thyroid gland to supply sufficient thyroid hormone results in varying degrees of hypothyroidism from mild, clinically insignificant forms to the life-threatening extreme, myxedema coma.

A. Classification

1. Primary hypothyroidism is due to:

a. Gland destruction or dysfunction caused by disease or medical therapies (e.g., radiation, surgical procedures)

Table 55-2. Effects of Drugs on Thyroid Function Tests

Drug	Serum T_4	Resin T_3 Uptake	Free Thyroxine Index (FTI)	Serum T_3	Serum TSH	Comment
p-Aminosalicylic acid (PAS)	↓	(nd)	↓	(nd)	↑ *	Antithyroid effect, rarely, with long-term use
Aminoglutethimide (*Cytadren*)	↓	(nd)	(nd)	(nd)	↑	
Anabolic steroids and androgens	↓	↑	0	↓ *	(nd)	Decreased serum TBG
Antithyroid drugs: Propylthiouracil (PTU) or methimazole (*Tapazole*)	↓	↓	↓	↓	0 or ↑	TSH may increase if patient becomes hypothyroid
Asparaginase (*Elspar*)	↓	↑	(nd)	↓ *	↑ *	Decreased serum TBG
Barbiturates	↓ [a]	(nd)	↓	(nd)	(nd)	Stimulates T_4 metabolism
Contraceptives, oral	↑	↓	0	↑	0	TBG usually increased
Corticosteroids	0 or ↓	0 or ↑	0 or ↓	↓	↓	Usual doses decrease TBG; high doses may increase TBG
Danazol (*Danocrine*)	↓	↑	0[b]	↓	0 or ↓	Decreased serum TBG
Estrogens	↑	↓	0	↑	0	Increased serum TBG
Ethionamide (*Trecator*)	↓	(nd)	↓ *	(nd)	↑ *	Antithyroid effect
Fluorouracil (*Adrucil*)	↑	↓	(nd)	↑	0	Patients clinically euthyroid; TBG increased
Heparin, intravenous	↑ [c]	0 or ↑	↑ *	0	(nd)	FTI is increased with some measures
Hypoglycemics (sulfonylureas)	0[d]	0[d]	0[d]	(nd)	(nd)	
Iodides, inorganic	0	0	0	(nd)	(nd)	
Iodides, organic	0	0	0	(nd)	(nd)	
Levodopa and levodopa–carbidopa (*Sinemet*)	0	0	0	0	↓ [e]	
Levothyroxine (*Levothroid*)	↑ (s)[f,g]	↑ or 0 or ↓ [f,g]	0 or ↑ [f,g]	↑ or 0[f,g]	↑ or 0[f]	
Liothyronine (*Cytomel*)	↓ [f]	0 or ↓ [f]	↓ [f]	↑ or ↓ [f,g]	0[f]	
Liotrix (*Thyrolar*)	0[f] or ↓ (s)	0[f]	0[f]	0[f,g]	0[f]	
Lithium carbonate (*Eskalith*)	0 or ↓	0 or ↓	0 or ↓	0 or ↓	0 or ↑	
Methadone (*Dolophine*)	↑ (s)	↓	0	↑	0	Increased serum TBG
Mitotane (*Lysodren*)	↓	0	0*	(nd)	(nd)	
Nitroprusside (*Nipride*)	↓	(nd)	(nd)	(nd)	(nd)	Clinical hypothyroidism
Oxyphenbutazone (*Oxalid*) and phenylbutazone (*Butazolidin*)	0 or ↓	↑	↓	(nd)	↑ *	May compete with T_4 for TBG binding. Rarely, overt hypothyroidism and goiter may occur

Perphenazine (*Trilafon*)	↑	↓	↓	↑	0*	
Phenytoin (*Dilantin*)	↓	0 or ↑ (s)	0 or ↓ (s)	↓	0	Stimulates T_4 metabolism and may compete with T_4 for TBG binding
Propranolol (*Inderal*)	0 or ↑ [h]	0[i]	(nd)	↓ [j]	0	
Resorcinol (excessive topical use)	↓	↓	↓	↓	↑	
Salicylates (large doses)	↓	↑ (s)	↓ *	↓	0*	Compete with T_4 for TBG binding

↑ = increased; ↓ = decreased; 0 = no effect; (s) = slight effect; (nd) = no data (Adapted from *The Medical Letter* 23:31, 1981).

*Effect deduced rather than based on reported clinical evidence.

[a] Patients requiring thyroid replacement therapy have decreased serum thyroxine when barbiturates are given.

[b] Free thyroxine index may increase slightly but usually remains in the normal range.

[c] T_4 assay by competitive protein binding is spuriously increased, but T_4-RIA is probably not affected. Free thyroxine measured by dialysis may be increased.

[d] May occasionally decrease serum T_4 and increase resin T_3 uptake.

[e] Slight decrease in euthyroid patients; but in long-standing hypothyroid patients, levodopa considerably decreases the elevated TSH.

[f] In a patient on adequate doses for thyroid replacement.

[g] Increased T_4, FTI, and T_3 tend to return to normal after several months of therapy with levothyroxine. After liothyronine, T_3 may be elevated 2 hours after a dose and depressed 24 hours after a dose.

[h] Increased T_4 levels are reported in one study, but not in others.

[i] With short-term propranolol in hyperthyroid patients.

[j] In euthyroid subjects, the decreased serum T_3 returns to normal with continued propranolol therapy.

b. Failure of the gland to develop or congenital incompetence (i.e., **cretinism**)

2. **Secondary hypothyroidism** is due to a pituitary disorder that inhibits TSH secretion. The thyroid gland is normal but lacks appropriate stimulation by TSH.

3. **Tertiary hypothyroidism** refers to a condition in which the pituitary–thyroid axis is intact, but the hypothalamus lacks the ability to secrete TRH to stimulate the pituitary.

B. Causes

1. **Hashimoto's thyroiditis,** which is a chronic lymphocytic thyroiditis that is considered to be an autoimmune disorder

2. **Treatment of hyperthyroidism,** such as radioactive iodine therapy, subtotal thyroidectomy, or administration of antithyroid agents

3. **Surgical excision**

4. **Goiter** (enlargement of the thyroid gland)
   a. **Endemic goiter** results from inadequate intake of dietary iodine. This is common in regions with iodine-depleted soil and in areas of endemic malnutrition.
   b. **Sporadic goiter** can follow ingestion of certain drugs or foods containing **progoitrin** (L-5-vinyl-2-thio-oxazolidone), which is inactive and converted by hydrolysis to goitrin. Goitrins inhibit oxidation of iodine to iodide and prevent iodide from binding to thyroglobulin, thereby decreasing thyroid hormone production. Progoitrin has been isolated in cabbage, kale, peanuts, brussels sprouts, mustard, rutabaga, kohlrabi, spinach, cauliflower, and horseradish. **Goitrogenic drugs** include propylthiouracil (PTU), iodides, phenylbutazone, cobalt, and lithium.
   c. **Less common causes** include acute (usually traumatic) and subacute thyroiditis, nodules, nodular goiter, and thyroid cancer.

C. Signs and symptoms

1. Early clinical features tend to be somewhat vague: lethargy, fatigue, forgetfulness, sensitivity to cold, unexplained weight gain, and constipation.

2. Progressively, the characteristic features of myxedema emerge: dry, flaky, inelastic skin; coarse hair; slowed speech and thought; hoarseness; puffy face, hands, and feet; eyelid droop; hearing loss; menorrhagia; decreased libido; slow return of deep tendon reflexes (especially in the Achilles tendon). If untreated, myxedema coma will develop.

D. Laboratory findings (see Table 55-1)

E. Treatment goal is replacement therapy using oral agents (Table 55-3).

F. Therapeutic agents

1. **Desiccated thyroid preparations**
   a. Once the agent of choice, desiccated thyroid has fallen out of favor since standardized synthetic levothyroxine preparations have become available.
   b. Dessicated thyroid preparations are not considered bioequivalent; they have evidenced varying amounts of active substances. Although they met established *United States Pharmacopeia (USP)* criteria for iodine content, variation in activity was noted. The content assay, while specific for iodine, was unable to specify the ratio of T_3 to T_4, and this ratio varies with animal source. Porcine gland preparations have a higher T_3 to T_4 ratio than those from ovine or bovine sources.

2. **Fixed ratio (liotrix) preparations.** In an effort to standardize the T_3:T_4 ratio, substances that mimic glandular content were developed. However, the T_3 component proved unnecessary (because T_4 is metabolized to T_3) and even disadvantageous because of T_3-induced adverse effects (e.g., tremor, headache, palpitations, diarrhea).

3. **Levothyroxine**
   a. Predictable results and lack of T_3-induced side effects have made levothyroxine the agent of choice.
   b. The two major brands of levothyroxine preparations (Levothroid, Synthroid) have been compared for bioequivalency and were shown to be equivalent in patients with hypothyroidism.
   c. The usual adult maintenance dose is 100–200 μg/day.

Table 55-3. Thyroid Replacement Preparations

Preparation	Trade Names	Advantage	Disadvantage	Comments	Source
Dessicated thyroid	Thyroid USP Enseals Thyroid Strong Armour Thyroid Thyrar	Low cost	Some preparations have unpredictable results Inconsistent T_3:T_4 ratio T_3 increases adverse effects	Contains T_3 Some brands are standardized by iodine content*	Porcine, bovine, or ovine thyroid glands
Liothyronine	Cytomel	Predictable results Useful for myxedema crisis	Lacks T_4	Usually reserved for myxedema crisis	Synthetic
Liotrix	Thyrolar	Standardized formulation	T_3 increases adverse effects Expensive	Fixed T_3:T_4 ratio of 1:4 Metabolism of T_4 to T_3 renders T_3 component unnecessary	Synthetic
Levothyroxine	Levothroid Synthroid	Predictable results Intravenous preparation available	Expensive	Agent of choice Does not contain T_3 All preparations are not interchangeable	Synthetic

*Iodine content, as well as T_3:T_4 ratio, varies with species.

T_3 = triiodothyronine; T_4 = thyroxine.

G. Precautions and monitoring effects

1. Adult patients with a history of cardiac disease and elderly patients should begin therapy with lower doses (e.g., 25 μg/day of levothyroxine). After 2–4 weeks, the dose should be increased gradually to an individually adjusted maintenance dose (usually less than 100 μg daily).
2. Patients should be observed on initiation of therapy for possible **cardiac complications,** such as angina, palpitations, or arrhythmias.
3. **Serum thyroid levels** should be monitored, particularly T_4, TSH, and RT_3U levels, as well as the FTI. Tests should be carried out on a monthly basis until a maintenance dose is determined. Thereafter, one or two tests per year are adequate.
4. Levothyroxine administration, especially long-term therapy, can induce **thyrotoxicosis;** T_4 levels can rise even though the dosage remains unchanged.
5. **Accelerated bone loss** has been associated with over treatment. Patients receiving replacement therapy with low TSH values may have lower bone mineral density since excess hormone accelerates the rate of remodeling (rate of resorption > rate of formation) and may contribute to an increased incidence of nontraumatic fracture.
6. **Drug interactions. Cholestyramine,** a bile acid sequestrant, can contribute to a decrease in **thyroxine** bioavailability when administered concomitantly. Cholestyramine should be administered at least 6 hours after oral thyroxine to reduce the potential for this clinically significant drug interaction.

H. Myxedema coma is a life-threatening complication with a high mortality rate.

1. It is most common in elderly patients with preexisting, although usually undiagnosed, hypothyroidism.
2. **Precipitating factors** include alcohol, sedative, or narcotic use; overuse of antithyroid agents; abrupt discontinuation of thyroid hormone therapy; infection; exposure to cold temperatures; and iatrogenic insult due to radiation therapy or thyroid surgery.
3. The patient usually declines from profound lethargy to coma, hypothermia, and a significant decrease in respiratory rate, potentially leading to respiratory failure as the crisis progresses. Hypometabolism produces a fluid and electrolyte imbalance that leads to fluid retention and hyponatremia. Cardiac effects include decreased heart rate and contractility, decreasing cardiac output.
4. **Treatment** consists of rapid restoration of T_3 and T_4 levels to normal.
   - **a.** A loading dose of levothyroxine 400–500 μg is given as an intravenous bolus. Liothyronine, 25 μg, is then given orally every 6 hours.
   - **b.** Treatment is continued until improvement is noted. Afterwards, liothyronine is discontinued and levothyroxine is changed to the oral preparation. A maintenance dose is then determined (see II G).

III. HYPERTHYROIDISM is the overabundance of thyroid hormone. **Thyrotoxicosis** is the general term applied to overactivity of the thyroid gland.

A. Graves' disease (diffuse toxic goiter)

1. The most common form of hyperthyroidism, Graves' disease occurs primarily, but not exclusively, in young women.
2. The basis of this disease is an **autoimmune disorder** in which antibodies bind to and activate TSH receptors, resulting in the overproduction of thyroid hormone.
   - **a.** These antibodies are termed **long-acting thyroid stimulators (LATS)** because their duration of action extends beyond that of TSH. As TSH is only mimicked, not overabundant, neither testing for TSH nor attempts to influence it are productive.
   - **b.** Antibody titers are often elevated in patients with Graves' disease.
3. **Signs and symptoms** characteristic of Graves' disease include:
   - **a.** Diffusely enlarged nontender goiter
   - **b.** Nervousness, irritability, anxiety, insomnia

c. Heat intolerance and profuse sweating
d. Weight loss despite increased appetite
e. Tremor, muscle weakness
f. Palpitations and tachycardia
g. Exophthalmos, stare, and lid lag (slow upper lid closing)
h. Diarrhea
i. Thrill or bruit over the thyroid
j. Periorbital edema

B. Plummer's disease (toxic nodular goiter)

1. This **form of thyrotoxicosis** is less common than Graves' disease. Its underlying cause remains unknown, but its incidence is highest in patients over 50 years of age, and it usually arises from a long-standing nontoxic goiter.

2. The thyrotoxicosis is a result of one or more adenomatous nodules autonomously secreting excessive thyroid hormone, which suppresses the rest of the gland. Scanning confirms the diagnosis if it indicates that activity and iodine uptake are confined to the nodular mass unless TSH is introduced.

3. **Signs and symptoms** are essentially the same as for Graves' disease except that one or more nodular masses are found, rather than diffuse glandular enlargement, and ophthalmopathy is usually absent. Cardiac abnormalities (e.g., CHF, tachyarrhythmias) are commonly seen with Plummer's disease.

C. Less common forms of hyperthyroidism

1. **Jodbasedow phenomenon** is an overproduction of thyroid hormone following a sudden, large increase in iodine ingestion—through either a sudden reversal of an iodine-deficient diet or the introduction of iodide or iodine in contrast agents or drugs, such as the antiarrhythmic agent amiodarone.

2. **Factitious hyperthyroidism** occurs with abusive ingestion of thyroid replacement agents, usually in a misguided effort to lose weight. Diagnosis is aided by the absence of glandular swelling and of exophthalmos and the lack of autoimmune activity found in Graves' disease.

D. Laboratory findings (see Table 55-1)

E. Treatment goal. Symptomatic relief is provided until definitive treatment can be effected.

F. Therapeutic agents

1. **β-Adrenergic blocking agents—propranolol**
   a. Propranolol reduces some of the peripheral manifestations (e.g., tachycardia, sweating, severe tremor, nervousness) of hyperthyroidism.
   b. In addition to providing symptomatic relief, propranolol inhibits the peripheral conversion of T_4 to T_3.

2. **Antithyroid agents—propylthiouracil (PTU) and methimazole**
   a. Action. These agents may help attain remission through direct interference with thyroid hormone synthesis. Both agents inhibit iodide oxidation and iodotyrosyl coupling. In addition, PTU (but not methimazole) diminishes peripheral deiodination of T_4 to T_3.
   b. Therapeutic uses of these drugs include:
      (1) Definitive treatment in which remission is achieved
      (2) Adjunctive therapy with radioactive iodine until the radiation takes effect
      (3) Preoperative preparation to establish and maintain a euthyroid state until definitive surgery can be performed
   c. Dosages
      (1) Propylthiouracil
         (a) For adults, the initial dose is 300–450 mg/day in three divided doses (i.e., 100–150 mg every 8 hours). Adult patients with severe disease may require as much as 600–1200 mg/day initially.
         (b) The initial dose is continued for about 2 months; then a maintenance dose of 100–150 mg/day is given, as a single dose or divided into two doses.
         (c) Maintenance therapy is continued for approximately 1 year, then gradually discontinued over 1–2 months while the patient is monitored for signs of recurrent

hyperthyroidism. The patient may remain in remission for several years. A recurrent episode of hyperthyroidism is most likely to occur within 3–6 months of drug discontinuation.

(d) If hyperthyroidism recurs after drug therapy is stopped, the agent should be restarted and alternative therapy should be considered (e.g., thyroid gland ablation or removal).

(2) Methimazole

(a) The initial dose range is 5–60 mg/day in three divided doses, depending on disease severity. After 2 months of therapy, a maintenance dose of 5–30 mg/day is initiated.

(b) Maintenance therapy is continued for approximately 1 year at which time the drug is gradually discontinued, usually over 1–2 months.

d. Precautions and monitoring effects

(1) Serum thyroid levels and the FTI should be monitored for a return to normal.

(2) Goiter size should decrease with reduced hormone output.

(3) The incidence of **adverse effects** is less than 1% with PTU and less than 3% with methimazole. The adverse effects are similar for the two agents.

(a) The most bothersome are dermatologic reactions (e.g., rash, urticaria, pruritus, hair loss, skin pigmentation). Others include headache, drowsiness, paresthesia, nausea, vomiting, vertigo, neuritis, loss of taste, arthralgia, and myalgia.

(b) Severe adverse effects—agranulocytosis, granulocytopenia, thrombocytopenia, drug fever, hepatitis, and hypoprothrombinemia—occur less frequently. Patients receiving methimazole who are over 40 years old and are receiving doses above 40 mg/day are at increased risk of developing agranulocytosis. Patients receiving PTU who are over 40 years old are at increased risk of developing agranulocytosis, but no dose association has been established.

3. Radioactive iodine (RAI)

a. Action. The thyroid gland picks up the radioactive element iodine-131 (^{131}I) as it would regular iodine. The radioactivity subsequently destroys some of the cells that would otherwise concentrate iodine and produce T_4, thus decreasing thyroid hormone production.

b. Advantages

(1) High cure rate—almost 100% for patients with Graves' disease and only slightly less for patients with Plummer's disease

(2) Avoids surgical risks—such as adverse reaction to anesthetics, hypoparathyroidism, nerve palsy, bleeding, and hoarseness

(3) Less expensive—avoids cost of hospitalization

c. Disadvantages

(1) Risk of delayed hypothyroidism

(2) Slight, though undocumented, risk of genetic damage

(3) Multiple doses, which may be required, may delay therapeutic efficacy for a long period (many months or a year)

d. Dosage. A dose of 80–100 mCi of ^{131}I per estimated gram of thyroid gland is recommended. Some protocols use lower dosages, but these may be less effective, requiring retreatment. When the dose is higher, there is a potential risk that hypothyroidism will develop.

e. Precautions and monitoring effects

(1) Radioiodine therapy is generally reserved for patients past the childbearing years because effects on future offspring are not known.

(2) Response to ^{131}I is hard to gauge, and patients must be monitored early for recurrence of hyperthyroidism, and later for hypothyroidism, which may develop even 20 years or more after therapy.

4. Subtotal thyroidectomy. Partial removal of the thyroid gland may be indicated if drug therapy fails or radioactive iodine is undesirable. This is a difficult procedure, but the success rate is high and the cure rapid. Risks include those mentioned in III F 3 b (2), precipitating thyroid storm, and permanent postoperative hypothyroidism. The risk of inducing thyroid storm can be minimized by obtaining a euthyroid state through use of antithyroid agents or propranolol (see III F 1).

G. Complications

1. Hypothyroidism may occur iatrogenically or, it has been proposed, as a natural sequel to Graves' disease.

2. **Thyroid storm (thyrotoxic crisis)** is a sudden exacerbation of hyperthyroidism caused by rapid release (leakage) of thyroid hormone. It is invariably fatal if not treated rapidly. In this crisis, unchecked hypermetabolism leads ultimately to dehydration, shock, and death.
   a. **Precipitating factors** include thyroid trauma or surgery, RAI therapy, infection, and sudden discontinuation of antithyroid therapy.
   b. **Characteristics.** It is characterized by a TT_4 level of 25–30 μg/dl, rapidly rising fever, tachycardia disproportionate to the fever, and unexplained, pronounced restlessness and tremor.
   c. **Treatment**
      (1) PTU, in doses of 150–250 mg orally every 6 hours, is the preferred agent, since PTU blocks peripheral deiodination of T_4 to T_3, while methimazole does not. However, if necessary, methimazole, 15 mg orally every 6 hours, can be used instead.
      (2) Propranolol, in doses of 20–200 mg orally every 6 hours or 1–3 mg intravenously every 4–6 hours, should be administered unless contraindicated (e.g., because the patient has CHF).
      (3) Potassium iodide, in doses of 50–100 mg every 12 hours, is given (after PTU) to minimize intrathyroidal iodine uptake.
      (4) Other supportive therapy includes rehydration, cooling, antibiotics, rest, and sedation.

STUDY QUESTIONS

Directions: Each of the numbered items or incomplete statements in this section is followed by answers or by completions of the statement. Select the **one** lettered answer or completion that is **best** in each case.

1. What is the correct formula to use for calculating the free thyroxine index (FTI)?

(A) $T_4 \times RT_3U$/mean serum RT_3U
(B) $T_4 \times T_3$/mean serum RT_3U
(C) $T_3 \times RT_3U$/mean serum RT_3U
(D) $T_4 \times RT_3U \times$ mean serum RT_3U
(E) $T_3 \times RT_3U \times$ mean serum RT_3U

2. What precursor besides dietary iodine is required for thyroxine biosynthesis?

(A) Triiodothyronine (T_3)
(B) Threonine
(C) Tyrosine
(D) Thyrotropin (TSH)
(E) Thyroxine-binding globulin (TBG)

3. All of the following conditions are causes of hyperthyroidism EXCEPT

(A) Graves' disease
(B) Hashimoto's thyroiditis
(C) toxic multinodular goiter
(D) triiodothyronine toxicosis
(E) Plummer's disease

4. Which of the following preparations is used to attain remission of thyrotoxicosis?

(A) Propranolol
(B) Liotrix
(C) Levothyroxine
(D) Propylthiouracil
(E) Desiccated thyroid

5. The thyroid gland normally secretes which of the following substances into the serum?

(A) Thyrotropin-releasing hormone (TRH)
(B) Thyrotropin (TSH)
(C) Diiodothyronine (DIT)
(D) Thyroglobulin
(E) Thyroxine (T_4)

6. All of the following conditions are causes of hypothyroidism EXCEPT

(A) endemic goiter
(B) surgical excision
(C) Hashimoto's thyroiditis
(D) goitrin-induced iodine deficiency
(E) Graves' disease

7. Common tests to monitor patients receiving replacement therapy for hypothyroidism include all of the following EXCEPT

(A) thyrotropin (TSH) stimulation test
(B) sensitive TSH assay
(C) free thyroxine index (FTI)
(D) triiodothyronine resin uptake (RT_3U)
(E) total thyroxine (TT_4)

8. Which of the following pairs of preparations has been most studied for bioequivalency?

(A) Euthroid—Thyrolar
(B) Thyroglobulin—Proloid
(C) Levothroid—Synthroid
(D) Cytomel—Synthroid
(E) Desiccated thyroid—Armour thyroid

9. The inhibition of pituitary thyrotropin secretion is controlled by which of the following?

(A) Free thyroxine (T_4)
(B) Thyroid-releasing hormone (TRH)
(C) Free thyroxine index (FTI)
(D) Reverse triiodothyronine (rT_3)
(E) Total thyroxine (TT_4)

10. Which of the following agents has been shown to interact with oral thyroxine (T_4) replacement therapy?

(A) Propylthiouracil
(B) Cholestyramine
(C) Thyrotropin
(D) Levothyroxine
(E) Lovastatin

1-A	4-D	7-A	10-B
2-C	5-E	8-C	
3-B	6-E	9-A	

11. What laboratory tests are currently recommended by the American Thyroid Association to diagnose thyroid disease?

(A) Triiodothyronine resin uptake (RT_3U) and total thyroxine (TT_4)
(B) Thyrotropin (TSH) and free thyroxine index (FTI)
(C) Total thyroxine (TT_4) and sensitive TSH assay
(D) Free T_4 and sensitive TSH assay
(E) Free T_4 and RT_3U

12. What patient population should be screened for thyroid disease?

(A) Hospitalized patients
(B) Elderly patients with chronic disease
(C) Elderly hospitalized patients
(D) College students
(E) Women over 20 years old

11-D
12-B

ANSWERS AND EXPLANATIONS

1. The answer is A *[I F 5].*
The free thyroxine index (FTI) is a mathematical interpretation of the relationship between the resin triiodothyronine uptake (RT_3U) and serum thyroxine (T_4) levels, compared to the mean population value for RT_3U. The FTI is calculated using reported values for total thyroxine (TT_4) and RT_3U. The normal FTI value in euthyroid patients is 5.5–12.

2. The answer is C *[I B].*
Biosynthesis of thyroid hormones begins with iodide binding to tyrosine which forms monoiodotyrosine (MIT). Monoiodotyrosine binds another iodide atom to form diiodotyrosine (DIT). Once MIT and DIT are formed, a coupling reaction occurs, which produces triiodothyronine (T_3), thyroxine (T_4), reverse triiodothyronine (rT_3), and other byproducts.

3. The answer is B *[II B 1; III A, B]*
Hashimoto's thyroiditis (chronic lymphocytic thyroiditis) is a cause of hypothyroidism. The incidence of Hashimoto's thyroiditis is 1%–2%, and it increases with age. It is more common in women than in men and in whites than in blacks. There may be a familial tendency. Patients with Hashimoto's thyroiditis have elevated titers of antibodies to thyroglobulin: A titer of greater than 1:32 is seen in over 85% of patients. Two variants of Hashimoto's thyroiditis have been described: gland fibrosis and idiopathic thyroid atrophy, which is most likely an extension of Hashimoto's thyroiditis.

4. The answer is D *[III F 1, 2].*
In hyperthyroid patients, remission of thyrotoxicosis is achieved with propylthiouracil (PTU) by two mechanisms: (1) interference of iodination of the tyrosyl residues, ultimately reducing production of thyroxine (T_4); (2) inhibition of peripheral conversion of T_4 to triiodothyronine (T_3). Propranolol is commonly used as an adjunct to PTU for symptomatic management of hyperthyroidism.

5. The answer is E *[I A 1].*
The major compounds secreted by the thyroid gland, after its stimulation by thyrotropin, are triiodothyronine (T_3) and thyroxine (T_4). Once released from the thyroid, T_3 and T_4 are transported by plasma proteins, namely thyroxine-binding globulin (TBG), thyroxine-binding prealbumin, and albumin.

6. The answer is E *[II B; III A 1].*
Graves' disease (diffuse toxic goiter) is the most common form of hyperthyroidism. It occurs most often in women in the third and fourth decades of life. There is a genetic and familial predisposition. The etiology is linked to an autoimmune reaction between immunoglobulin G (IgG) and the thyroid.

7. The answer is A *[II F 4 a].*
The thyrotropin (TSH) stimulation test measures thyroid tissue response to exogenous TSH. It is not commonly used to monitor thyroid replacement therapy. It may be useful in the initial diagnosis of hypothyroidism.

8. The answer is C *[II F 3 b].*
Many brands of levothyroxine are currently available. Both generic and trade-name preparations have been studied with an emphasis on Levothroid and Synthroid. The importance of bioequivalency becomes apparent when patients have received different brands of levothyroxine and have exhibited changes in therapeutic response to equivalent replacement doses.

9. The answer is A *[I A 3 a].*
An increase in the blood level of thyroid hormone [circulating free thyroxine (T_4) and free triiodothyronine (T_3)] signals the pituitary to stop releasing thyroid-stimulating hormone (thyrotropin; TSH). The free fraction of T_4 is available to bind at the pituitary receptors.

10. The answer is B *[II G 6].*
Euthyroid patients receiving oral replacement therapy have become hypothyroid after concomitant administration of bile acid sequestrant therapy. It appears that bioavailability is reduced as a result of administering these agents at close dosing intervals. It is recommended that at least 6 hours pass before administration of a bile acid sequestrant. It would be preferable to select another nonbile acid sequestrant when clinically possible.

11. The answer is D *[I G 4].*
The free thyroxine (free-T_4) and the sensitive thyrotropin (TSH) assay should only be used for the diagnosis of patients most likely to have thyroid disease based on clinical presentation, relative risk (e.g., age, sex, family history) not for population screening. The sensitive TSH assay is also useful to monitor replacement therapy and to minimize overtreatment and the corresponding risk of accelerated bone loss.

12. The answer is B *[I G 3].*
Cost verses benefit is critical to the decision of choosing to screen entire populations. Since the frequency of detection has been proven to be higher in elderly patients (2%–5%) with chronic disease, the relative minor costs associated to obtain resin triiodothyronine uptake (RT_3U) and serum total thyroxine (TT_4) to calculate a free thyroxine index (FTI) are worth the cost. A serum thyrotropin (TSH) assay can be reserved for patients with an abnormal FTI. Another consideration is to use the sensitive TSH assay for diagnosis in place of the serum TSH assay at a higher cost but without the necessity of retesting. If patients admitted to the hospital for an acute illness were screened but the results are misleading, they may be prescribed inappropriate therapy since acute illness may be associated with the temporary effects causing abnormal test results.

56
Renal Failure

Andrew L. Wilson

I. ACUTE RENAL FAILURE

A. Definition. Acute renal failure (ARF) is the sudden, potentially reversible interruption of kidney function, resulting in retention of nitrogenous waste products in body fluids.

B. Classification and etiology. ARF is classified according to its cause.

1. **Prerenal ARF** stems from impaired renal perfusion, which may result from:
   a. Reduced arterial blood volume (e.g., hemorrhage, vomiting, diarrhea, other gastrointestinal fluid loss)
   b. Urinary losses from excessive diuresis
   c. Decreased cardiac output [e.g., from congestive heart failure (CHF) or pericardial tamponade]
   d. Renal vascular obstruction (e.g., stenosis)
   e. Severe hypotension

2. **Intrarenal ARF (intrinsic or parenchymal ARF)** reflects structural kidney damage brought on by any of the following conditions:
   a. **Acute tubular necrosis (ATN),** the leading cause of ARF, may be associated with the following:
      (1) It may arise from exposure to nephrotoxic aminoglycosides, anesthetics, pesticides, organic metals, and radiopaque contrast materials.
      (2) It may stem from ischemic injury (e.g., surgery, circulatory collapse, severe hypotension).
      (3) It may be associated with pigment (e.g., hemolysis, myoglobinuria).
   b. Acute glomerulonephritis
   c. Tubular obstruction, as from hemolytic reactions or uric acid crystals
   d. Acute inflammation (e.g., acute tubulointerstitial nephritis, papillary necrosis)
   e. Renal vasculitis
   f. Malignant hypertension
   g. Radiation nephritis

3. **Postrenal ARF** results from obstruction of urine flow anywhere along the urinary tract. Causes of postrenal ARF include:
   a. Ureteral obstruction, as from calculi, uric acid crystals, or thrombi
   b. Bladder obstruction, as from calculi, thrombi, tumors, or infection
   c. Urethral obstruction, as from strictures, tumors, or prostatic hypertrophy
   d. Extrinsic obstruction, as from hematoma, inflammatory bowel disease, or accidental surgical ligation

C. Pathophysiology. ARF progresses in three phases.

1. **Initiating phase**
   a. The initiating phase is defined as the time between the renal insult, and the point at which extrarenal factors no longer reverse the damage caused by the obstruction or other cause of ARF. This phase may not be well defined clinically and may escape notice or diagnosis.
   b. Urine output may drop markedly to 400 ml/day or less (**oliguria**). In some patients, urine output falls below 100 ml/day (**anuria**). Oliguria may last only hours or as long as 4–6 weeks. However, it has been shown that 40%–50% of ARF patients are not oliguric or anuric.

c. Nitrogenous waste products accumulate in the blood.

(1) **Azotemia** reflects urea accumulation due to impaired glomerular filtration and concentrating capacity.

(2) Serum creatinine, sulfate, phosphate, and organic acid levels climb rapidly.

d. The serum sodium concentration falls below normal from intracellular fluid shifting and dilution.

e. **Hyperkalemia** occurs if potassium intake is not restricted or body potassium is not removed. Without treatment, hyperkalemia may lead to neuromuscular depression and paralysis, impaired cardiac conduction, arrhythmias, respiratory muscle paralysis, cardiac arrest, and ultimately death.

2. Maintenance phase

a. This phase begins when urine output rises above 500 ml/day—typically, after several days of oliguria. A rise in urine output or a "diuretic response" may not be seen in nonoliguric patients.

b. Urine output rises in increments of several milliliters to 300–500 ml/day. Urine output may double from day to day in the initial recovery period.

c. Azotemia and associated laboratory findings may persist until urine output reaches 1000–2000 ml/day.

d. The maintenance phase carries a risk of fluid and electrolyte abnormalities, gastrointestinal bleeding, infection, and respiratory failure.

3. Recovery phase. During the recovery phase, renal function gradually returns to normal. Most recovered renal function appears in the first 2 weeks; however, recovery of renal function may continue for a year. Residual impairment may persist indefinitely.

D. Clinical evaluation

1. Physical findings. Initially, ARF causes azotemia and, in 50%–60% of cases, oliguria. Later, electrolyte abnormalities and other severe systemic effects occur.

a. **Urine output** typically is **low,** from 20 to 500 ml/day. Complete anuria is rare.

b. **Signs and symptoms of hyperkalemia,** resulting from reduced potassium excretion by impaired kidneys, include:

(1) Neuromuscular depression (e.g., paresthesias, muscle weakness, paralysis)

(2) Diarrhea and abdominal distention

(3) Slow or irregular pulse

(4) Electrocardiographic changes with potential cardiac arrest

c. **Uremia,** caused by excessive nitrogenous waste retention, leads to nausea, vomiting, diarrhea, edema, confusion, fatigue, neuromuscular irritability, and coma.

d. **Metabolic acidosis,** a common complication of ARF, is evidenced by:

(1) Deterioration of mental status, obtundation, coma, and lethargy

(2) Depressed cardiac contractility and decreased vascular resistance, leading to hypotension, pulmonary edema, and ventricular fibrillation

(3) Nausea and vomiting

(4) Respiratory abnormalities (e.g., hyperventilation, Kussmaul's respiration)

e. **Hyperphosphatemia** arises from decreased phosphate excretion.

(1) As serum phosphate rises, hypocalcemia results from the formation of insoluble calcium phosphate complexes.

(2) The signs and symptoms relate to resultant hypocalcemia and metastatic soft tissue calcification.

(3) Manifestations of hypocalcemia include the following:

(a) Neuromuscular irritability, cramps, spasms, and tetany

(b) Hypotension

(c) Soft-tissue calcification

(d) Mental status changes (e.g., confusion, mood changes, loss of intellect and memory)

(e) Hyperactive deep tendon reflexes and Trousseau's and Chvostek's signs

(f) Abdominal cramps

(g) Stridor and dyspnea

f. **Hyponatremia** results from dilution and intracellular fluid shifts during the diuretic phase of ARF. Physical findings include lethargy, weakness, seizures, cognitive impairment, and possible reduction in level of consciousness.

g. Intravascular volume depletion, suggesting **prerenal failure,** may cause:
(1) Flat jugular venous pulses when the patient lies supine
(2) Orthostatic changes in blood pressure and pulse
(3) Poor skin turgor and dry mucous membranes

h. Other findings suggesting **prerenal failure** include:
(1) An abdominal bruit, possibly indicating renal artery stenosis
(2) Increased paradoxus, suggesting pericardial tamponade
(3) Increased jugular venous pressure, pulmonary rales, and a third heart sound, signaling CHF

i. Postrenal failure caused by obstructed urinary flow may manifest itself in:
(1) A suprapubic or flank mass
(2) Bladder distention
(3) Costovertebral angle tenderness
(4) Prostate enlargement

2. Diagnostic test results

a. Urinalysis, includes an examination of sediment; identification of proteins, glucose, ketones, blood, and nitrites; and measurement of urinary pH and urine specific gravity (concentration) or osmolality (dilution). Prior administration of fluids, diuretics, and changes in urinary pH may confound accurate diagnosis, using urinalysis.

(1) Urinary sediment examination
(a) Few casts and formed elements are found in prerenal ARF.
(b) Pigmented cellular casts and renal tubular epithelial cells appear with ATN.
(c) Red blood cell and white blood cell casts generally reflect inflammatory disease.
(d) Large numbers of broad white cell casts suggest chronic renal failure (CRF).

(2) The presence of blood in the urine (**hematuria**) or proteins (**proteinuria**) indicates renal dysfunction.
(3) Urine specific gravity ranges from 1.010 to 1.016 in ARF.
(4) Urine osmolality typically rises in prerenal ARF.

b. Measurement of urine sodium and creatinine levels can help classify ARF.
(1) In prerenal ARF, the urine creatinine level increases, and urine sodium level decreases.
(2) In intrarenal ARF resulting from ATN, the urine creatinine level drops, and the urine sodium level rises.

c. Creatinine clearance, an index of the **glomerular filtration rate (GFR),** allows estimation of the number of functioning nephrons; decreased creatinine clearance indicates renal dysfunction.

d. Blood chemistry provides an index of renal excretory function and body chemistry status. Findings typical of ARF include:
(1) Increased blood urea nitrogen (BUN)
(2) Increased serum creatinine
(3) Possible increase in hemoglobin and hematocrit values
(4) Abnormal serum electrolyte values
(a) Serum potassium level above 5 mEq/L
(b) Serum phosphate level above 2.6 mEq/L (4.8 mg/dl)
(c) Serum calcium level below 4 mEq/L (8.5 mg/dl), reflecting hypocalcemia. The serum calcium level must be correlated with the serum albumin level. Each rise or fall of 1 g/dl of serum albumin beyond its normal range is responsible for a corresponding increase or decrease in serum calcium of approximately 0.8 mg/dl. A below normal serum albumin level may result in a deceptively low serum calcium level.
(d) Serum sodium level below 135 mEq/L, reflecting hyponatremia
(5) Abnormal arterial blood gas values [pH below 7.35, bicarbonate concentration (HCO_3^-) below 22], reflecting metabolic acidosis

e. Renal failure index (RFI) is the ratio of urine sodium concentration to the urine-to-serum creatinine ratio. The RFI helps determine the etiology of ARF. Typically, the RFI is less than 1 in prerenal ARF or acute glomerulonephritis (a cause of intrarenal ARF). The RFI is greater than 2 in postrenal ARF and in other intrarenal causes of ARF.

f. Electrocardiography (ECG) may show evidence of hyperkalemia—that is, tall, peaked T waves; widening QRS complexes; prolonged PR interval, progressing to decreased amplitude and disappearing P waves; and, ultimately, ventricular fibrillation and cardiac arrest.

g. **Radiographic findings**
   (1) **Ultrasound** may detect upper urinary tract obstruction.
   (2) **Kidney, ureter, or bladder radiography** may reveal:
      (a) Urinary tract calculi
      (b) Enlarged kidneys, suggesting ATN
      (c) Asymmetrical kidneys, suggesting unilateral renal artery disease, ureteral obstruction, or chronic pyelonephritis
   (3) **Radionuclide scan** may reveal:
      (a) Bilateral differences in renal perfusion, suggesting serious renal disease
      (b) Bilateral differences in dye excretion, suggesting parenchymal disease or obstruction as the cause of ARF
      (c) Diffuse, slow, dense radionuclide uptake, suggesting ATN
      (d) Patchy or absent radionuclide uptake, possibly indicating severe, acute glomerulonephritis
   (4) **Computerized tomography (CT) scan** may provide better visualization of an obstruction.

h. **Renal biopsy** may be performed in selected patients when other test results are inconclusive.

E. Treatment objectives

1. Correct reversible causes of ARF; preventing or minimizing further renal damage or complications.
   a. Discontinue nephrotoxic drugs; remove other nephrotoxins through dialysis or gastric lavage for poisonings.
   b. Treat underlying infection.
   c. Remove any urinary tract obstructions.

2. Correct and maintain proper fluid and electrolyte balance. Match fluid, electrolyte, and nitrogen intakes to urine output.

3. Treat body chemistry alterations, especially hyperkalemia and metabolic acidosis when present. Treatment may include renal dialysis.

4. Improve urine output.

5. Treat systemic manifestations of ARF.

F. Therapy

1. **Conservative management** alone may suffice in uncomplicated ARF.
   a. **Fluid management**
      (1) Fluid intake should match fluid losses. Sensible losses (i.e., urine, stool, tube drainage) and insensible losses (i.e., skin, respiratory tract) should be included in fluid balance calculations.
      (2) Volume overload should minimize the risk of hypertension and CHF.
      (3) The patient should be weighed daily to determine fluid volume status.
   b. **Dietary measures**
      (1) Because catabolism accompanies renal failure, the patient should receive a high-calorie, low-protein diet. Such a diet helps to:
         (a) Reduce renal work load by decreasing production of end products of protein catabolism that the kidneys cannot excrete
         (b) Prevent ketoacidosis
         (c) Alleviate manifestations of uremia (e.g., nausea, vomiting, confusion, fatigue)
      (2) If edema or hypertension is present, sodium intake should be restricted.
      (3) Potassium intake must be limited in most patients.

2. **Management of body chemistry alterations**
   a. **Treatment of hyperkalemia**
      (1) **Dialysis** may be used to treat acute, life-threatening hyperkalemia (see II F 7 for a discussion of this procedure).
      (2) **Calcium chloride**
         (a) **Mechanism of action and therapeutic effects.** Calcium chloride or calcium gluconate replaces and maintains body calcium, counteracting the cardiac effects of acute hyperkalemia.

(b) **Administration and dosage.** When used to reverse hyperkalemia-induced cardiotoxicity, calcium chloride is given intravenously, as 5–10 ml of a 10% solution (1.4 mEq Ca^{2+}/ml) administered over 2 minutes. Doses of up to 20 ml of a 10% solution are safe when given slowly. The initial dose may be followed by another 10–20 ml of a 10% solution placed in a larger fluid volume and administered slowly.

(c) **Precautions and monitoring effects**

(i) Intravenous calcium is contraindicated in patients with ventricular fibrillation or renal calculi.

(ii) The infusion rate should not exceed 0.5 ml/min. Patients should remain recumbent for about 15 minutes after infusion.

(iii) The ECG should be monitored during calcium gluconate therapy.

(iv) Calcium gluconate should not be mixed with solutions containing sodium bicarbonate because this can lead to precipitation.

(v) Adverse effects include tingling sensations and renal calculus formation.

(d) **Significant interactions.** Calcium may cause increased digitalis toxicity when administered concurrently with **digitalis** preparations.

(3) **Sodium bicarbonate** may be given on an emergency measure for severe hyperkalemia or metabolic acidosis.

(a) **Mechanism of action and therapeutic effect.** Intravenous sodium bicarbonate restores bicarbonate that the renal tubules cannot reabsorb from the glomerular filtrate and increases arterial pH. This results in a shift of potassium into cells and reduces serum potassium.

(b) **Onset of action** is 15–30 minutes.

(c) **Administration and dosage**

(i) Sodium bicarbonate is administered intravenously.

(ii) The dosage is calculated as follows:

$$[50\% \text{ of body weight (kg)}] \times [\text{desired arterial bicarbonate } (HCO_3^-) - \text{actual } HCO_3^-]$$

(d) **Precautions and monitoring effects**

(i) To avoid sodium and fluid overload, sodium bicarbonate must be given cautiously. Half of the patient's bicarbonate deficit is replaced over the first 12 hours of therapy.

(ii) Sodium bicarbonate may precipitate calcium salts in intravenous solutions and should not be mixed in the same infusion fluid.

(iii) Arterial blood gas values and serum electrolyte levels should be monitored closely during sodium bicarbonate therapy.

(4) **Regular insulin with dextrose**

(a) **Mechanism of action and therapeutic effect.** The combination of insulin with dextrose deposits potassium with glycogen in the liver, reducing the serum potassium.

(b) **Onset of action** is 15–30 minutes.

(c) **Administration and dosage.** Regular insulin (20–30 U in 200–300 ml of 20% dextrose) is administered intravenously over 30 minutes.

(d) **Precautions and monitoring effects**

(i) The serum glucose level should be monitored during therapy.

(ii) The patient should be assessed for signs and symptoms of fluid overload.

(5) **Sodium polystyrene sulfonate (SPS)**

(a) **Mechanism of action.** SPS is a potassium-removing resin that exchanges sodium ions for potassium ions in the intestine (1 g of SPS exchanges 0.5–1 mEq/L of potassium). The SPS is distributed throughout the intestines and excreted in the feces.

(b) **Therapeutic effect.** Administered as an adjunctive treatment for hyperkalemia, SPS reduces potassium levels in the serum and other body fluids.

(c) **Onset of action** of orally administered SPS is 2 hours; effects are seen in 1 hour when SPS is administered as a retention enema.

(d) **Administration and dosage**

(i) SPS is usually administered orally, although it may be given through a nasogastric tube. The oral dose is 15–30 g in a suspension of 70% sorbitol, administered every 4–6 hours until the desired therapeutic effect is achieved.

(ii) When oral or nasogastric administration is not possible due to nausea, vomiting, or paralytic ileus, SPS may be given by retention enema. The rectal dose is 30–50 g in 100 ml of sorbitol as a warm emulsion, administered deep into the sigmoid colon every 6 hours. Administration may be done with a rubber tube that is taped in place or via a Foley catheter with a balloon inflated distal to the anal sphincter.

(e) Precautions and monitoring effects

(i) The patient's serum electrolyte levels should be monitored closely during SPS therapy. Sodium, chloride, bicarbonate and pH should be monitored in addition to potassium.

(ii) SPS therapy usually continues until the serum potassium level drops to between 4 and 5 mEq/L.

(iii) The patient should be assessed regularly for signs of potassium depletion, including irritability, confusion, cardiac arrhythmias, ECG changes, and muscle weakness.

(iv) SPS exchanges sodium for potassium, so sodium overload may occur during therapy.

(v) For oral administration, SPS should be mixed only with water or sorbitol. Orange juice, which has a high potassium content, should not be used because it decreases the effectiveness of the SPS. For rectal administration, SPS should be mixed only with water and sorbitol, never with mineral oil.

(vi) Adverse effects of SPS include constipation, fecal impaction with rectal administration, nausea, vomiting, and diarrhea.

(vii) SPS should not be used as the sole agent in the treatment of severe hyperkalemia; other agents or therapies should be used in conjunction with this agent.

(f) Significant interactions. Magnesium hydroxide and other nonabsorbable cation-donating laxatives and antacids may decrease the effectiveness of potassium exchange by SPS and may cause systemic alkalosis.

b. Treatment of metabolic acidosis. Sodium bicarbonate may be given if the arterial pH is below 7.35. See I F 2 a (3) for a discussion of this drug.

c. Treatment of hyperphosphatemia

(1) Dialysis may be used to treat acute, life-threatening hyperphosphatemia accompanied by acute hypocalcemia (see II F 7).

(2) Aluminum hydroxide (an aluminum-containing antacid)

(a) Mechanism of action and therapeutic effect. Aluminum binds excess phosphate in the intestine, thereby reducing phosphate concentration.

(b) Onset of action is 6–12 hours.

(c) Administration and dosage. Aluminum hydroxide is administered orally as a tablet or suspension. For the treatment of hyperphosphatemia, 0.5–2 or 15–30 ml of suspension are administered three or four times daily with meals.

(d) Precautions and monitoring effects

(i) Aluminum hydroxide may cause constipation and anorexia.

(ii) Serum phosphate levels should be monitored because aluminum hydroxide can cause phosphate depletion.

(iii) Aluminum hydroxide can cause calcium resorption and bone demineralization.

(3) Calcium carbonate may be given instead of aluminum hydroxide to treat hyperphosphatemia.

d. Treatment of hypocalcemia. Immediate treatment is necessary if the patient has severe hypocalcemia, as evidenced by tetany.

(1) Calcium gluconate [See I F 2 a (2) for a discussion of this drug in the treatment of hyperkalemia.]

(a) Mechanism of action and therapeutic effect. This drug replaces and maintains body calcium, raising the serum calcium level immediately.

(b) Administration and dosage. When used to reverse hypocalcemia, calcium gluconate is administered intravenously in a dosage of 1–2 g over a period of 10 minutes, followed by a slow infusion (over 6–8 hours) of an additional 1 g.

(c) Precautions and monitoring effects and significant interactions [see I F 2 a (2) (c), (d)]

(2) Oral calcium salts. Calcium carbonate, chloride, gluconate, or lactate may be given by mouth when oral intake is permitted or if the patient has relatively mild hypocalcemia. The usual adult dose is 4–6 g/day given in three or four divided doses.

e. Treatment of hyponatremia

(1) Moderate or asymptomatic hyponatremia may require only **fluid restriction**.

(2) Sodium chloride may be given for severe symptomatic hyponatremia (i.e., a serum sodium level below 120 mEq/L).

(a) Mechanism of action and therapeutic effect. Sodium chloride replaces and maintains sodium and chloride concentration, thereby increasing extracellular tonicity.

(b) Administration and dosage

(i) A 3% or 5% sodium chloride solution may be administered by slow intravenous infusion. The amount of solution needed is calculated from the following equation:

(Normal serum sodium level − actual serum sodium level) × total body water

(ii) Typically, 400 ml or less are administered.

(c) Precautions and monitoring effects

(i) Hypertonic sodium chloride must be administered very slowly to avoid circulatory overload, pulmonary edema, or central pontine myelinolysis.

(ii) Serum electrolyte levels must be monitored frequently during therapy.

(iii) Excessive infusion may cause hypernatremia and other serious electrolyte abnormalities and may worsen existing acidosis.

3. Management of systemic manifestations

a. Treatment of fluid overload and edema. As water and sodium accumulate in extracellular fluid during ARF, fluid overload and edema may occur. **Diuretics** and dopamine may be given to reduce fluid volume excess and edema. Treatment should be initiated as soon as possible after oliguria begins. **Mannitol** or a **loop diuretic** may be used; thiazide diuretics are avoided in renal failure because they are ineffective when creatinine clearance is less than 25 ml/min, and they may worsen the patient's clinical status.

(1) Step 1: Loop (high-ceiling) diuretics. These agents include **furosemide, bumetanide,** and **ethacrynic acid.** Loop diuretics are more potent and faster-acting than thiazide diuretics.

(a) Mechanism of action and therapeutic effects. Loop diuretics inhibit sodium and chloride reabsorption at the loop of Henle, promoting water excretion.

(b) Onset of action for an oral dose is 1 hour; it is several minutes for an intravenous dose. Duration of action for an oral dose is 6–8 hours; it is 2–3 hours for an intravenous dose.

(c) Administration and dosage

(i) Furosemide, the most commonly used loop diuretic, usually is administered intravenously in patients with ARF to hasten the therapeutic effect. The dose is titrated to the patient's needs; the usual initial dose is 1–1.5 mg/kg. If the first dose does not produce a urine output of 10–15 ml within 20–30 minutes, a dose of 2–3 mg/kg is administered; if the desired response still does not occur, a dose of 3–6 mg/kg is administered 20–30 minutes after the second dose.

(ii) Bumetanide may be given to patients who are unresponsive or allergic to furosemide. The usual dose, administered intravenously or intramuscularly in the treatment of ARF, is 0.5–1 mg/day; however, some patients may require up to 20 mg/day. A second or third dose may be given at intervals of 2–3 hours. When bumetanide is given orally, the dose is 0.5–2 mg/day, repeated up to two times, if necessary, at intervals of 2–3 hours.

(iii) Ethacrynic acid is less commonly used to treat ARF because ototoxicity (sometimes irreversible) is associated with its use. It may be given intravenously (slowly over several minutes) in a dose of 50–100 mg. The usual oral dose is 50–200 mg/day; some patients may require up to 200 mg twice daily.

(d) Precautions and monitoring effects

(i) Loop diuretics must be used cautiously because they may cause orthostatic hypotension, fluid and electrolyte abnormalities, including volume depletion and dehydration, hypocalcemia, hypokalemia, hypochloremia, hyponatremia, hypomagnesemia, and transient ototoxicity, especially with rapid intravenous injection.

(ii) Serum electrolyte levels should be monitored frequently and the patient assessed regularly for signs and symptoms of electrolyte abnormalities.

(iii) Blood pressure and pulse rate should be assessed during diuretic therapy.

(iv) Gastrointestinal reactions, include abdominal pain and discomfort, diarrhea (with furosemide and ethacrynic acid), and nausea (with bumetanide).

(v) Blood glucose levels should be monitored in diabetic patients receiving loop diuretics because these agents may cause hyperglycemia and impaired glucose tolerance.

(vi) Patients who are allergic to sulfonamides may be hypersensitive to bumetanide and furosemide.

(vii) Furosemide and ethacrynic acid may cause agranulocytosis.

(e) Significant interactions

(i) **Aminoglycoside antibiotics** may potentiate ototoxicity when administered with any loop diuretic.

(ii) **Indomethacin** may hamper the diuretic response to furosemide and bumetanide; **probenecid** may hamper the diuretic response to bumetanide.

(iii) Ethacrynic acid may potentiate the anticoagulant effects of **warfarin**.

(iv) Sweating and flushing may occur when chloral hydrate is administered to patients receiving intravenous furosemide.

(2) Step 2: Mannitol, an osmotic diuretic, is a nonreabsorbable polysaccharide.

(a) Mechanism of action and therapeutic effect. Mannitol increases the osmotic pressure of the glomerular filtrate; fluid from interstitial spaces is drawn into blood vessels expanding plasma volume and maintaining or increasing the urine flow. This drug may be given to prevent ARF in high-risk patients, such as those undergoing surgery or suffering from severe trauma or hemolytic transfusion reactions.

(b) Onset of action is 15–30 minutes. Duration of action is 3–4 hours.

(c) Administration and dosage. Mannitol is available in solutions, ranging from 5% to 25%. For the treatment of oliguric ARF or the prevention of ARF, the usual initial dose is 12.5–25 g, administered intravenously; the maximum daily dose is 100 g, administered intravenously. The exact concentration of the solution is determined by the patient's fluid requirements.

(d) Precautions and monitoring effects

(i) Mannitol is contraindicated in patients with anuria, pulmonary edema or congestion, severe dehydration, and intracranial hemorrhage (except during craniotomy).

(ii) Mannitol may cause or worsen pulmonary edema and circulatory overload. If signs and symptoms of these problems develop, the infusion should be stopped.

(iii) Other adverse effects of mannitol include fluid and electrolyte abnormalities, water intoxication, headache, confusion, blurred vision, thirst, nausea, and vomiting.

(iv) Vital signs, urine output, daily weight, cardiopulmonary status, and serum and urine sodium and potassium levels should be monitored during mannitol therapy.

(v) Mannitol solutions with undissolved crystals should not be administered.

(3) Step 3: Dopamine. This vasopressor, an immediate metabolic precursor of epinephrine and norepinephrine, is a potent sympathomimetic agent.

(a) Mechanism of action and therapeutic effect. Given at doses between 1–5 mcg/kg/min, dopamine dilates mesenteric and renal blood vessels, which leads to enhanced renal blood flow, increased GFR, sodium excretion, and urine output. Dopamine has been used as a means to prevent as well as treat ARF.

(b) Administration and dosage. Dopamine is given intravenously in doses of 1–5 mcg/kg/min. The dose is titrated to the desired response.

(c) Precautions and monitoring effects

(i) Doses greater than 10 mcg/kg/min stimulate α-receptors and produce peripheral vasoconstriction, raising systemic blood pressure. Doses over 20 mcg/kg/min may decrease renal blood flow as α-receptor stimulation overwhelms the dopaminergic vasodilation.

(ii) Dopamine may cause hypotension, tachycardia, arrhythmias, palpitations, anginal pain, ECG abnormalities, and vasoconstriction. These signs and symptoms may warrant slowing of the infusion rate.

(iii) Adverse gastrointestinal effects include nausea and vomiting.

(iv) Extravasation may result in necrosis and tissue sloughing.

(v) Dopamine must be used cautiously in patients receiving monoamine oxidase (MAO) inhibitors.

(vi) During the infusion, the patient's blood pressure, pulse, cardiac function, urine output, and extremity temperature and color should be assessed.

(d) Significant interactions

(i) **Phenytoin** may cause reduced blood pressure.

(ii) **Ergot alkaloids** can lead to dangerously elevated blood pressure.

b. Treatment of other systemic manifestations. ARF typically causes hematologic, gastrointestinal, and skin disturbances. (See II F 5 for a discussion of the management of these problems.)

4. **Dialysis.** Hemodialysis or peritoneal dialysis may be necessary in ARF patients who develop anuria; acute fluid overload; severe hyperkalemia, metabolic acidosis, or hyperphosphatemia; GFR below 5 ml/min; BUN level above 100 mg/dl; or serum creatinine level above 10 mg/dl. For a discussion of dialysis, see II F 7.

II. CHRONIC RENAL FAILURE

A. Definition. Chronic renal failure (CRF) is the progressive, irreversible deterioration of renal function. Usually resulting from long-standing disease, it sometimes derives from ARF that does not respond to treatment.

B. Classification and pathophysiology

1. CRF typically progresses slowly through mild impairment to end-stage renal disease with a total loss of kidney function.
   a. **Mild-to-moderate CRF,** is characterized by decreased renal reserve (GFR of 20–70 ml/min). Despite some loss of renal function at lower GFR, homeostasis is preserved.
   b. **Severe CRF,** where GFR is 5–10 ml/min, is characterized by some clinical evidence of renal failure. At this stage, slight azotemia occurs. Renal reserve has decreased so that the patient may have some trouble maintaining fluid and electrolyte status under stress. This is particularly true when cardiac function is also compromised.
   c. **End-stage renal disease,** when GFR is below 5 ml/min, is characterized by frank uremia. Fluid and electrolyte imbalances develop, azotemia worsens, and systemic manifestations appear.
2. As CRF progresses, nephron destruction worsens, leading to deterioration in the kidneys' filtration, reabsorption, and endocrine functions.
3. Renal function typically does not diminish until about 75% of kidney tissue is damaged. Ultimately, the kidneys become shrunken, fibrotic masses.

C. Etiology. Minor causes of CRF in adults include:

1. Diabetic nephropathy
2. Hypertension
3. Glomerulonephritis
4. Polycystic kidney disease
5. Long-standing vascular disease (e.g., renal artery stenosis)
6. Long-standing obstructive uropathy (e.g., renal calculi)
7. Exposure to nephrotoxic agents

D. Clinical evaluation

1. **Physical findings.** Signs and symptoms, which vary widely, do not appear until renal insufficiency progresses to renal failure.
   a. **Metabolic abnormalities** include loss of the ability to maintain sodium, potassium, and water homeostasis, leading to hyponatremia or hypernatremia, based on relative sodium or water intake. Hyperkalemia is uncommon until end-stage disease. Fluid overload, edema and CHF may become a problem unless fluid intake is closely managed. As renal

failure progresses, the inability to excrete acid and maintain buffer capacity lead to metabolic acidosis. (See I D 1 b, d, g, h for specific findings associated with metabolic abnormalities.)

b. **Neurologic manifestations** include short attention span, loss of memory, and listlessness. As CRF progresses, these advance to confusion, stupor, seizures, and coma. Neuromuscular findings include peripheral neuropathy; pain, itching, and a burning sensation, particularly in the feet and legs. If dialysis is not started after these abnormalities occur, motor involvement begins, including loss of deep tendon reflexes, weakness, and finally, quadriplegia.

c. **Cardiovascular problems** include arterial hypertension, peripheral edema, CHF, and pulmonary edema. Pericarditis is now increasingly infrequent as a result of early dialysis.

d. **Gastrointestinal manifestations** include nausea, vomiting, constipation, stomatitis, and an unpleasant taste in the mouth. CRF patients have an increased incidence of ulcers, pancreatitis, and diverticulosis.

e. **Respiratory problems** include dyspnea when CHF is present, pulmonary edema, pleuritic pain, and uremic pleuritis.

f. **Integumentary findings** typically include pale yellowish, dry, scaly skin; severe itching; uremic frost; ecchymoses; purpura; and brittle nails and hair.

g. **Musculoskeletal changes** range from muscle and bone pain to pathologic fractures and calcifications in the brain, heart, eyes, joints, and vessels.

h. **Hematologic disturbances** include anemia. The signs and symptoms of anemia arise from lack of erythropoietin and reduced life span of red blood cells and include:

(1) Pallor of the skin, nail beds, palms, conjunctivae, and mucosa
(2) Abnormal bruising or ecchymoses
(3) Dyspnea and angina pectoris
(4) Extreme fatigue

2. **Diagnostic test results**

a. **Creatinine clearance** may range from 0 to 70 ml/min, reflecting renal impairment.

b. **Blood tests** typically show:

(1) Elevated BUN and serum creatinine levels
(2) Reduced arterial pH and bicarbonate concentration
(3) Reduced serum calcium level
(4) Increased serum potassium and phosphate levels
(5) Possible reduction in the serum sodium level
(6) Normochromic, normocytic anemia (hematocrit 20%–30%)

c. **Urinalysis** may reveal glycosuria, proteinuria, erythrocytes, leukocytes, and casts. Specific gravity is fixed at 1.010.

d. **Radiographic findings.** Kidney, ureter, and bladder radiography, intravenous pyelography, renal scan, renal arteriography, and nephrotomography may be performed. Typically, these tests reveal small kidneys (less than 8 cm in length).

E. Treatment objectives

1. Improve patient comfort and prolong life.
2. Treat systemic manifestations of CRF.
3. Correct body chemistry abnormalities.

F. Therapy. Management of the CRF patient is generally conservative. Dietary measures and fluid restriction relieve some symptoms of CRF and may increase patient comfort and prolong life until dialysis or renal transplantation is required or available. (See I F 1 a, b for a discussion of these measures.)

1. **Treatment of edema and CHF. Digitalis preparations** and **diuretics** may be given to manage edema and CHF and to increase urine output.

a. **Digitalis preparations.** These agents include **digoxin, digitoxin, digitalis leaf, and deslanoside**. See Chapter 44 for a discussion of these drugs.

b. **Diuretics.** An osmotic diuretic, a loop diuretic, or a thiazide-like diuretic may be given.

(1) **Osmotic and loop diuretics.** See I F 3 a (1), (2) for information on the use of these drugs in renal failure.

(2) **Thiazide-like diuretics. Metolazone** is the most commonly used diuretic in CRF.

(a) **Mechanism of action and therapeutic effect.** Metolazone reduces the body's fluid and sodium volume by increasing sodium reabsorption in the ascending limb of the loop of Henle, thereby increasing urinary excretion of fluid and sodium.

(b) Administration and dosage. Metolazone is given orally in doses of 5–20 mg/day; the dose is titrated to the patient's needs. Furosemide and metolazone act synergistically. Combination use is common.

(c) Precautions and monitoring effects

(i) Metolazone should not be given to patients with hypersensitivity to sulfonamide derivatives, including thiazides.

(ii) To avoid nocturia, the daily dose should be given in the morning.

(iii) Metolazone may cause hematologic reactions, such as agranulocytosis, aplastic anemia, and thrombocytopenia.

(iv) Fluid volume depletion, hypokalemia, hyperuricemia, hyperglycemia, and impaired glucose tolerance may occur during metolazone therapy.

(v) Metolazone may cause hypersensitivity reactions, including vasculitis and pneumonitis.

(d) Significant interactions

(i) Diazoxide may potentiate the antihypertensive, hyperglycemic, and hyperuricemic effects of metolazone.

(ii) Colestipol and **cholestyramine** decrease the absorption of metolazone.

2. Treatment of hypertension. Antihypertensive agents may be needed if blood pressure becomes dangerously high as a result of edema and the high renin levels that occur in CRF. Antihypertensive therapy should be initiated in the lowest effective dose and titrated according to the patient's needs.

a. Angiotensin-converting enzyme (ACE) inhibitors–captopril, enalapril, lisinopril—are widely used to treat CRF because they help preserve renal function and typically cause fewer adverse effects than other antihypertensive agents. (See Chapter 43 for a discussion of ACE inhibitors.)

b. β-adrenergic blockers, including **propranolol** and **atenolol,** reduce blood pressure through various mechanisms. (For a discussion of these agents, see Chapter 43.)

c. Other antihypertensive agents are sometimes used in the treatment of CRF, including α-adrenergic drugs, **clonidine, methyldopa,** and vasodilators, such as **hydralazine**. (See Chapter 43, for information on these drugs.)

3. Treatment of hyperphosphatemia involves administration of a phosphate binder such as aluminum hydroxide or calcium carbonate (see I F 2 c).

4. Treatment of hypocalcemia

a. Oral calcium salts [see I F 2 d (2)]

b. Vitamin D

(1) Mechanism of action and therapeutic effect. Vitamin D promotes intestinal calcium and phosphate absorption and utilization and, thus increases the serum calcium concentration.

(2) Choice of agent. For the treatment of hypocalcemia in CRF and other renal disorders, **calcitriol** (vitamin D_2, the active form of vitamin D) is the preferred vitamin D supplement because of its greater efficacy and relatively short duration of action. Other single-entity preparations include dihydrotachysterol, ergocalciferol, and calcifediol.

(3) Administration and dosage. Calcitriol is given orally; the dose is titrated to the patient's needs (0.5–1 mcg/day may be effective).

(4) Precautions and monitoring effects

(a) Vitamin D administration may be dangerous in patients with renal failure and must be used with extreme caution.

(b) Vitamin D toxicity may cause a wide range of signs and symptoms, including headache, dizziness, ataxia, convulsions, psychosis, soft-tissue calcification, conjunctivitis, photophobia, tinnitus, nausea, diarrhea, pruritus, and muscle and bone pain.

(c) Vitamin D has a narrow therapeutic index, necessitating frequent measurement of BUN and serum and urine calcium and potassium levels.

(d) Because hyperphosphatemia generally accompanies hypocalcemia in renal failure, dietary phosphate should be given during vitamin D therapy to prevent calcification and deterioration in renal function. [See I F 2 c (2) for information on aluminum hydroxide, a binding agent.]

5. Treatment of other systemic manifestations of CRF

a. Treatment of anemia includes administration of iron (e.g., ferrous sulfate), folate supplements, and erythropoietin.

(1) Severe anemia may warrant infusion of fresh frozen packed cells or washed packed cells.

(2) To increase red blood cell production, androgens may be given.

(3) Erythropoietin stimulates the production of red cell progenitors and the production of hemoglobin. It also accelerates the release of reticulocytes from the bone marrow.

(a) An initial dose of erythropoietin is 50–100 U/kg intravenously or subcutaneously three times a week. The dose may be adjusted upward to elicit the desired response.

(b) Erythropoietin works best in patients with a hematocrit below 30%. During the initial treatment, the hematocrit increases 1%–3.5% in a 2-week period. The target hematocrit is 33%–35%. Maintenance doses are titrated based on hematocrit after this level is reached.

(c) Erythropoietin therapy should be temporarily stopped if hematocrit exceeds 36%. Additional side effects include hypertension in up to 25% of patients. Headache and malaise have been reported.

(d) The effects of erythropoietin are dependent on a ready supply of iron for hemoglobin synthesis. Patients who do not respond should have iron stores checked. This includes serum iron, total iron-binding capacity, transferrin saturation, and serum ferritin. Iron supplementation should be increased as indicated.

b. Treatment of gastrointestinal disturbances

(1) Antiemetics help control nausea and vomiting.

(2) Cimetidine may be given to relieve gastric irritation.

(3) Docusate sodium or methylcellulose may be used to prevent constipation.

(4) Enemas may be given to remove blood from the gastrointestinal tract.

c. Treatment of skin problems. An antipruritic agent, such as diphenhydramine, may be used to alleviate itching.

6. Management of body chemistry abnormalities (see I F 2)

7. Dialysis. When CRF progresses to end-stage renal disease and no longer responds to conservative measures, long-term dialysis or renal transplantation is necessary to prolong life.

a. Hemodialysis is the preferred dialysis method for patients with a reduced peritoneal membrane, hypercatabolism, or acute hyperkalemia.

(1) This technique involves shunting of the patient's blood through a dialysis membrane-containing unit for diffusion, osmosis, and ultrafiltration. The blood is then returned to the patient's circulation.

(2) Vascular access may be obtained via an arteriovenous fistula or an external shunt.

(3) The procedure takes only 3–8 hours: Most patients need only two or three treatments a week. With proper training, patients can perform hemodialysis at home.

(4) The patient receives heparin during hemodialysis to prevent clotting.

(5) Various complications may arise, including hemorrhage, hepatitis, anemia, septicemia, cardiovascular problems, air embolism, rapid shifts in fluid and electrolyte balance, itching, nausea, vomiting, headache, seizures, and aluminum osteodystrophy.

b. Peritoneal dialysis is the preferred dialysis method for patients with bleeding disorders and cardiovascular disease.

(1) The peritoneum is used as a semipermeable membrane. A plastic catheter inserted into the peritoneum provides access for the dialysate, which draws excess fluids, wastes, and electrolytes across the peritoneal membrane periodically by osmosis and diffusion.

(2) Peritoneal dialysis can be carried out in three different modes.

(a) **Intermittent peritoneal dialysis** is an automatic cycling mode lasting 8–10 hours, performed three times a week. This mode allows nighttime treatment and is appropriate for working patients.

(b) **Continuous ambulatory peritoneal dialysis** is performed daily for 24 hours with four exchanges daily. The patient can remain active during the treatment.

(c) **Continuous cyclic peritoneal dialysis** may be used if the other two modes fail to improve creatinine clearance. Dialysis takes place at night; the last exchange is retained in the peritoneal cavity during the day, then drained that evening.

(3) **Advantages** of peritoneal dialysis include a lack of serious complications, retention of

normal fluid and electrolyte balance, simplicity, reduced cost, patient independence, and a reduced need (or no need) for heparin administration.

(4) Complications of peritoneal dialysis include hyperglycemia, constipation, and inflammation or infection at the catheter site. Also this method carries a high risk of peritonitis.

8. Renal transplantation. This surgical procedure allows some patients with end-stage renal disease to live normal and—in many cases—longer lives.

a. Histocompatibility must be tested to minimize the risk of transplant rejection and failure. Human leukocyte antigen (HLA) type, mixed lymphocyte reactivity, and blood group types are determined to assess histocompatibility.

b. Renal transplant material may be obtained from a living donor or a cadaver

c. Three types of graft rejection can occur.

(1) Hyperacute (immediate) rejection results in graft loss within minutes to hours after transplantation.

(a) Acute urine flow cessation and bluish or mottled kidney discoloration are intraoperative signs of hyperacute rejection.

(b) Postoperative manifestations include kidney enlargement fever, anuria, local pain, sodium retention, and hypertension.

(c) Treatment for hyperacute rejection is immediate nephrectomy.

(2) Acute rejection may occur 4–60 days after transplantation

(3) Chronic rejection occurs more than 60 days after transplantation.

(a) Signs and symptoms include low-grade fever, increased proteinuria, azotemia, hypertension, oliguria, weight gain, and edema.

(b) Treatment may include alkylating agents, cyclosporine, antilymphocyte globulin, and corticosteroids. In some cases, nephrectomy is necessary.

d. Complications of renal transplantation include:

(1) Infection, diabetes, hepatitis, and leukopenia, resulting from immunosuppressive therapy

(2) Hypertension, resulting from various causes

(3) Cancer (e.g., lymphoma, cutaneous malignancies, head and neck cancer, leukemia, and colon cancer)

(4) Pancreatitis and mental and emotional disorders (e.g., suicidal tendencies, severe depression, brought on by steroid therapy)

STUDY QUESTIONS

Directions: Each of the numbered items or incomplete statements in this section is followed by answers or by completions of the statement. Select the **one** lettered answer or completion that is **best** in each case.

Questions 1–5

A 52-year-old white man has on prior physical examinations demonstrated mild-to-moderate hypertension, which has been controlled with captopril, weight loss, and exercise. His history is negative for diabetes mellitus and heart disease. On the present visit, he complains of dizziness, loss of energy, shortness of breath upon exertion, decreased frequency of urination, edema of the lower extremities, and increased bruising. Physical examination shows a pale, well-nourished man with dry scaly skin, some bruising and ecchymoses, moderate edema of the feet and ankles, and a standing blood pressure of 160/90. His laboratory examination shows a blood urea nitrogen (BUN) of 40 mg/100 ml, a serum creatinine of 3.5 mg/100 ml, a serum calcium of 5.3 mg/ml, a serum potassium of 6.8 mEq/L, and a hematocrit of 25. Serum iron, total iron-binding capacity, transferrin saturation, and serum ferritin are normal. Microscopic and chemical urinalyses reveal only mild proteinuria, and a specific gravity of 1.010.

1. The history, symptoms, and laboratory values best suggest which of the following problems?

(A) Acute renal failure, resulting from a nephrotoxic drug (captopril)
(B) Acute renal failure, resulting from ureteral obstruction by uric acid crystals
(C) Prerenal acute renal failure, resulting from excessive fluid loss
(D) Chronic renal failure, resulting from hypertension or an unknown cause

2. Treatment of the patient's fluid retention and edema should begin with all of the following EXCEPT

(A) restriction of fluid intake
(B) therapy with either furosemide or metolazone
(C) treatment of hypertension using a β-blocker or angiotensin-converting enzyme (ACE) inhibitor
(D) digitalis glycosides if congestive heart failure (CHF) is present
(E) Hemodialysis

3. The most likely cause of the anemia seen in this patient is

(A) substantial blood loss in the urine
(B) vitamin B_{12} deficiency
(C) iron deficiency
(D) decreased red cell life span and a deficiency of erythropoietin

4. This patient's symptoms seem to have appeared with no prior indicator other than his history of hypertension. Hypertension is

(A) a major cause of chronic renal failure
(B) a major cause of acute renal failure
(C) a major cause of both chronic and acute renal failure
(D) only seen after kidney damage leads to a buildup of fluid in a renal-failure patient

5. Peritoneal dialysis or hemodialysis should be considered to treat this patient's renal failure

(A) as soon as possible to prevent further complications, resulting from decreased kidney function
(B) only when renal function has decreased to a point where fluid and electrolyte status cannot be maintained using conservative measures
(C) on an intermittent basis as the situation demands
(D) only if the patient is a kidney transplant candidate

6. Hyperkalemia is a common finding in both acute and chronic renal failure. Methods used to treat hyperkalemia include all of the following EXCEPT

(A) sodium polystyrene sulfonate (SPS) administered orally or rectally
(B) insulin and dextrose infusions
(C) loop diuretics or metolazone to improve urine output
(D) acute dialysis in life-threatening situations
(E) aluminum hydroxide antacids administered orally

1-D
2-E
3-D
4-A
5-B
6-E

7. Life-threatening cardiac arrhythmias due to hyperkalemia should be treated with

(A) calcium chloride or calcium gluconate intravenously
(B) digoxin or other digitalis preparations
(C) loop diuretics to eliminate potassium rapidly
(D) sodium polystyrene sulfonate (SPS)

8. Aluminum hydroxide is used to treat hyperphosphatemia associated with renal failure. Chronic use of aluminum hydroxide may cause all of the following EXCEPT

(A) phosphate depletion
(B) calcium resorption and bone demineralization
(C) anorexia and constipation
(D) fluid retention

9. The diuretic of choice for the initial treatment of a patient with either acute or chronic renal failure (ARF, CRF) whose creatinine clearance is below 25 ml/min is

(A) hydrochlorothiazide
(B) bumetanide
(C) furosemide
(D) ethacrynic acid

10. Erythropoietin is commonly used to treat the anemia associated with chronic renal failure (CRF) The effectiveness of erythropoietin treatment is limited by

(A) a patient's allergy to erythropoietin
(B) depletion of iron stores, requiring parenteral supplementation
(C) the ineffectiveness of erythropoietin as 30% of patients do not respond
(D) the anemia of CRF is not due to a lack of erythropoietin, so erythropoietin will not ameliorate

---

7-A
8-D
9-C
10-B

ANSWERS AND EXPLANATIONS

1–5. The answers are: 1-D *[II D 1]*, **2-E** *[II F 1, 2]*, **3-D** *[II D 1 h]*, **4-A** *[II C 2]*, **5-B** *[II F 7]*.
The fluid and electrolyte status of the patient described in the question combined with urine specific gravity, lack of crystals or casts in the urine, and the complaint of fatigue suggest chronic renal failure, arising either from hypertension or an unknown cause. The patient has not been exposed to any nephrotoxic drug, nor does his blood pressure or fluid status suggest a prerenal cause.

All of these measures are indicated as initial therapy for the treatment of edema and fluid retention due to chronic renal failure except hemodialysis, which should be reserved until more conservative measures are tried.

There is no evidence of frank blood loss. The decreased hematocrit and the clinical signs indicate that the chronic anemia of chronic renal failure (CRF), due to the shortened red blood cell life span and decreased erythropoietin (EPO), is the cause.

Systemic, long-standing high blood pressure is the second most common cause of CRF. Only malignant hypertension can cause acute renal failure (ARF), and it is not common. High blood pressure is common after substantial renal damage has occurred in both CRF and ARF, but it does not occur as the first or only manifestation.

Dialysis should be considered when the patient's renal function has decreased to a point at which conservative measures are ineffective. Peritoneal dialysis and hemodialysis have associated complications and morbidity, so intermittent or early use of these therapies is not indicated. Patients can be maintained on dialysis for extended periods, so eligibility for transplantation is not required.

6. The answer is E *[I F 2 a]*.
All of the therapies listed in the question may be used to treat hyperkalemia except aluminum hydroxide, which is used to bind phosphate. Dialysis is reserved for only the most severe cases where the cardiac effects of increased potassium are life-threatening.

7. The answer is A *[I F 2 a (2)]*.
Intravenous calcium chloride or gluconate is used to treat potassium-induced arrhythmias. Digoxin is not indicated. Loop diuretics and sodium polystyrene sulfonate (SPS) do not have a signficant effect on potassium in a short period to treat a life-threatening arrhythmia. SPS and loop diuretics, along with dialysis, may be considered to remove potassium in the short term, preventing the recurrence of arrhythmias.

8. The answer is D *[I F 2 c (2)]*.
Common effects of the sustained use of aluminum-containing antacids include phosphate depletion, calcium resorption, bone demineralization, anorexia, and constipation. Fluid retention does not result from the use of antacids containing aluminum hydroxide.

9. The answer is C *[I F 3 a (1) (c)]*.
Furosemide is the diuretic of choice for the initial treatment of a patient with either acute or chronic renal failure (ARF, CRF) whose creatinine clearance is below 25 ml/min. A thiazide diuretic will have little effect at a creatinine clearance below 25 ml/min. Both bumetanide and ethacrynic acid are appropriate only if the patient is allergic to furosemide or if repeated doses of furosemide are ineffective.

10. The answer is B *[II F 5 a]*.
Erythropoietin is widely used and highly effective to treat the anemia associated with chronic renal failure (CRF). Few reports of patients refractory to erythropoietin therapy have appeared in the medical literature. However, the depletion of iron stores will not allow the formation of red blood cells even in the presence of erythropoietin. All CRF patients receiving erythropoietin require some iron supplementation, and most require parenteral iron to achieve sufficient supplies to continue developing hemoglobin over the term of their illness.

57
Principles of Cancer Chemotherapy

Lisa P. Shopper

I. PRINCIPLES OF ONCOLOGY. The term **cancer** refers to a heterogeneous group of diseases.

A. Characteristics of cancer cells. Tumors arise from a single abnormal cell, which continues to divide indefinitely. The lack of normal growth controls, the ability to invade local tissues, and the ability to spread, or **metastasize,** are characteristics of cancer cells; these properties contrast with normal cell lines.

B. Incidence. Cancer is the second leading cause of death in the United States. Approximately 30% of *all* people develop cancer at some point in their lives. Not all cancer patients die of their disease; some forms of cancer are considered curable if detected and treated early.

C. Etiology. A number of factors have been implicated in the etiology of cancer, the most common of which are listed below.

1. **Viruses,** including Epstein-Barr virus (EBV), hepatitis B virus (HBV), and herpes simplex virus type 2 (HSV-2)
2. **Environmental and occupational exposures,** such as ionizing and ultraviolet radiation and exposure to chemicals, including vinyl chloride, polychlorinated biphenyls (PCBs), and asbestos
3. **Life-style factors,** such as high-fat, low-fiber diets and tobacco and ethyl alcohol use
4. **Medications,** including alkylating agents and diethylstilbestrol
5. **Genetic factors**

D. Detection and diagnosis are critical for the appropriate treatment of cancer.

1. **Warning signals of cancer** have been outlined by the American Cancer Society.
   a. Change in bowel or bladder habits
   b. A sore that does not heal
   c. Unusual bleeding or discharge
   d. Thickening or lump in the breast or elsewhere
   e. Indigestion or difficulty swallowing
   f. Obvious change in a wart or mole
   g. Nagging cough or hoarseness
2. **Guidelines to screen routinely for the presence of cancer or cancerous cells,** are also published by the American Cancer Society, and recommend that *all* Americans, with or without any of the warning signals, be screened according to these guidelines (Table 57-1). It is also imperative that a yearly physical examination be performed.
3. **Tumor markers** are biochemical indicators of the presence of neoplastic proliferation detected in serum, plasma, or other bodily fluids. These tumor markers may be used either as initial screening tests or to reveal further information after abnormal test results. Elevated levels of these markers are not definitive for the presence of cancer; false-positive results do occur. Some commonly seen tumor markers include:
   a. Carcinoembryonic antigen (CEA)
   b. Alpha-fetoprotein (AFP)
   c. Prostate-specific antigen (PSA)
4. **Tumor biopsy.** The definitive test for the presence of cancerous cells is a surgical biopsy and pathologic examination of the biopsy specimen.

Table 57-1. Summary of American Cancer Society Recommendations for the Early Detection of Cancer in Asymptomatic Persons at Average Risk

Examination	Sex	Age	Periodicity
Sigmoidoscopy	M and F	50 and older	Every 3–5 years
Stool blood test	M and F	50 and older	Every year
Digital rectal examination	M and F	40 and older	Every year
Pap test and pelvic examination	F	Women who are sexually active or are 18 or older	Every year; after 3 or more satisfactory, consecutive, normal annual examinations, the Pap test may be performed less frequently at the discretion of the physician
Endometrial tissue sample	F	At menopause; women at high risk*	At menopause
Breast self-examination*	F	20 and older	Every month
Clinical breast examination	F	20–39 40 and older	Every 3 years Every year
Mammography	F	40–49 50 and over	Every 1–2 years Every year
Health counseling†	M and F	20–40	Every 3 years
Cancer checkup‡	M and F	40 and older	Every year

Reprinted from Holleb AI, et al (eds): *American Cancer Society Textbook of Clinical Oncology*. Atlanta, American Cancer Society, 1991.

*History of infertility, obesity, failure to ovulate, abnormal uterine bleeding, or estrogen therapy.

†To include counseling about tobacco control, sun exposure, diet and nutrition, risk factors, sexual practices, and environmental and other occupational exposures.

‡To include examination for cancers of the thyroid, testicles, prostate, ovaries, lymph nodes, oral cavity, and skin.

5. **Imaging studies,** such as x-rays, computerized tomography (CT scans), or magnetic resonance imaging (MRI), may be used to aid in the diagnosis or location of a suspected tumor.

6. **Other commonly used laboratory tests** include complete blood counts (CBCs) and blood chemistries, which may increase or decrease the likelihood of a specific cancer.

E. Staging. Two different systems are widely employed for the staging of neoplasms.

1. **TNM classification**
   a. **T** indicates tumor size and is classified from 1 to 4 with 1 indicating the smallest tumor.
   b. **N** indicates the presence and extent of nodal involvement and is scaled from 0 to 4 with 0 indicating no nodal involvement and 4 indicating extensive involvement.
   c. **M** indicates the presence or absence of distant metastases and can be classified as only 0 or 1, indicating whether or not distant spread is detected.
   d. **$T_2N_1M_0$,** thus, indicates a moderate-size tumor with limited nodal disease and no distant metastases.

2. **AJC staging** was developed by the American Joint Committee on Staging. This method denotes cancers as stages 0 through IV. The high numbers indicate large tumors with extensive nodal involvement; generally the high numbers also indicate a worse prognosis.

F. Survival depends on the tumor type and extent of disease.

1. Four of ten patients survive more than 5 years. While some of these patients continue to be free of all detectable disease, not all patients who survive are cured. Oncologists prefer to use the term **complete response** or **remission** to indicate a patient with no evidence of disease after treatment; this is *not* a synonym for cure. For some slow-growing tumors, these disease-free periods may extend for 10–15 years after the initial remission. However, a number of patients who have achieved complete remission may have a relapse, possibly even dying of their cancer.

2. With the strides made in cancer research and treatment recently, more tumors are considered treatable than ever before.

II. CELL LIFE CYCLE.

Knowledge of the cell life cycle and cell cycle kinetics is essential to the understanding of combination chemotherapy in the treatment of cancer. Drugs are given in sequence and at specific times in part to account for the cell life cycle of the cancer and at which point the drugs act within the cycle (Figure 57-1).

A. Phases of the cell cycle

1. **M phase,** or **mitosis** is a process in which two daughter cells are produced. Mitosis is subdivided into specific phases (i.e., **prophase, metaphase, anaphase,** and **telophase**).
2. **G_1 phase,** or the **postmitotic gap,** is where RNA and protein synthesis occur.
3. **S phase** (follows G_1) is where DNA synthesis takes place. It is in the S phase that most antineoplastic agents exert their effects.
4. **G_2 phase,** or the **premitotic** or **postsynthetic gap** is the phase in which the nucleus is organized for mitosis.
5. **G_0 phase,** or **resting phase** is not actually part of the cell cycle. The cells that are in G_0 are not committed to division and are not actively undergoing metabolic functions. Therefore, they are least affected by antineoplastic agents. Cells in the resting phase may re-enter the cell cycle; some chemotherapeutic regimens are designed to enhance this re-entry by killing a large number of actively dividing cells. This process is called **recruitment**.

B. Cell growth kinetics.

A number of terms are important to describe cell growth kinetics.

1. **Cell growth fraction** is the *proportion* of cells in the cell cycle dividing or preparing to divide. As the tumor enlarges, the cell growth fraction decreases, since a larger proportion of cells may not be able to obtain adequate nutrients and blood supply for replication.

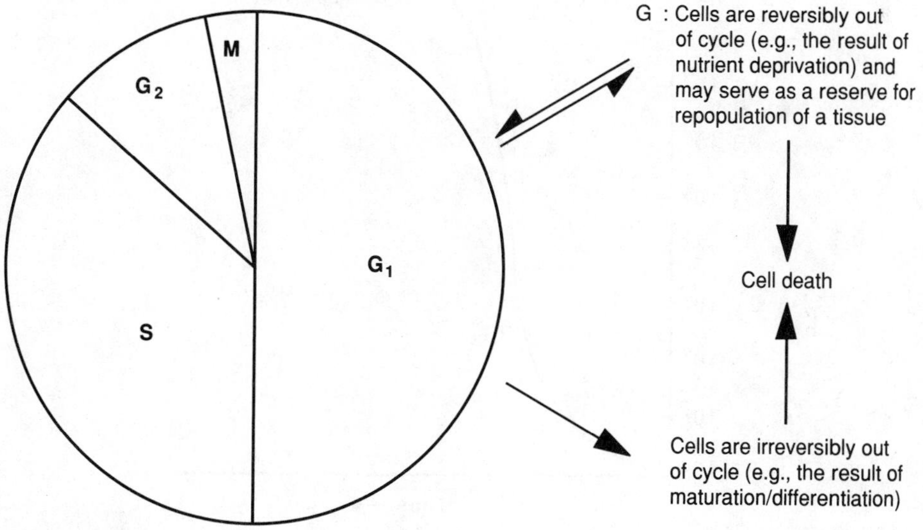

Figure 57-1. Diagrammatic representation of the cell growth cycle, emphasizing the relationship between proliferating cell populations. (Reprinted from Holleb AI, et al (eds): *American Cancer Society Textbook of Clinical Oncology*. Atlanta, American Cancer Society, 1991.)

2. **Cell cycle time** is the average time for a cell that has just completed mitosis to grow and again divide and again pass through mitosis. Cell cycle time is specific for each individual tumor.
3. **Tumor doubling time** is the time for malignant cells to double the tumor size. As the tumor gets larger in size, the doubling time gets longer.
4. The **gompertzian growth curve** (Figure 57-2) illustrates these kinetic concepts.

C. **Tumor cell burden.** Because of the large number of cells required to produce clinical symptoms (greater than 10^9 cells), the tumor cell burden (i.e., number of tumor cells in the body) far exceeds clinically apparent disease. It is, therefore, necessary to kill not only the cells that can be measured, but also the large number of microscopic tumor cells throughout the body. This is accomplished through repeated dosing of chemotherapy regimens designed to kill a certain *fraction of the cells.* This **cell kill hypothesis** assumes that a given drug concentration applied for a defined time interval kills a constant fraction of the cell population, independent of the number of cells. Figure 57-3 illustrates this hypothesis.

D. **Classification of antineoplastic agents** is based on their effects on cell cycle kinetics. A specific antineoplastic drug may logically be combined with agents working in different areas of the cell cycle to produce a maximum cell kill or to recruit cells into the cycle. A cell cycle classification of commonly used antineoplastic agents is listed below.

1. **Cell cycle phase-specific drugs** are most active against cells that are in a specific phase of the cycle. For example:
   - **a.** G_1 phase: L-asparaginase and prednisone
   - **b.** S phase: cytarabine, methotrexate, 6-thioguanine, and hydroxyurea
   - **c.** G_2 phase: bleomycin and etoposide
   - **d.** M phase: vincristine and vinblastine

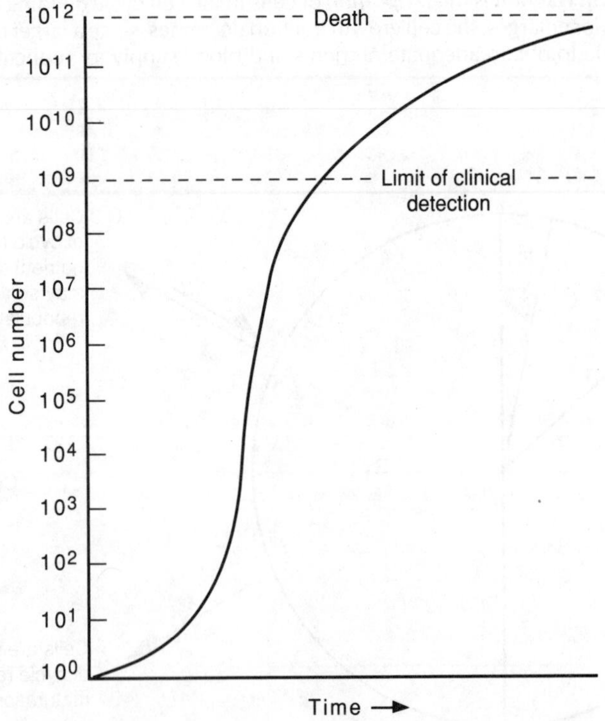

Figure 57-2. The gompertzian growth curve. During the early stages of its development a tumor's growth is exponential. But as a tumor enlarges, the growth slows. By the time a tumor becomes large enough to cause symptoms and be clinically detectable, the majority of its growth has already occurred and is no longer exponential. (Reprinted from Holleb AI, et al (eds): *American Cancer Society Textbook of Clinical Oncology*. Atlanta, American Cancer Society, 1991.)

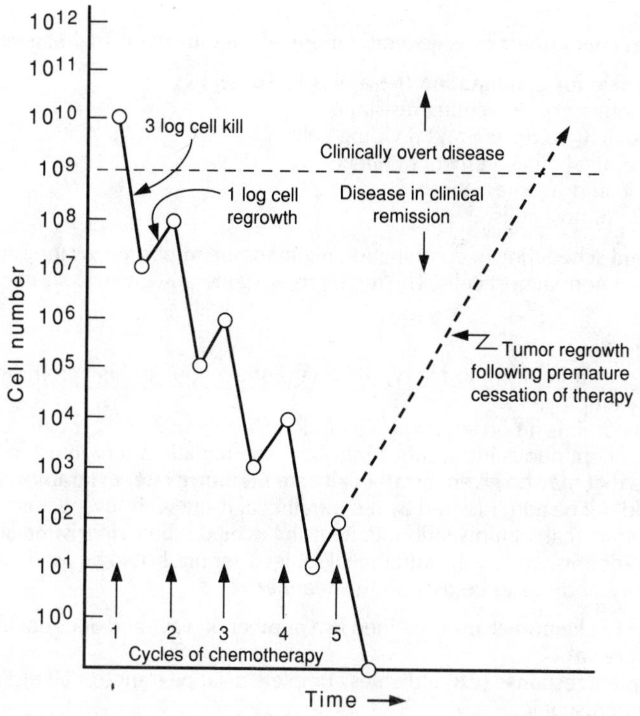

Figure 57-3. Relationship between tumor cell survival and chemotherapy administration. The exponential relationship between chemotherapy drug dose and tumor cell survival dictates that a constant proportion, not number, of tumor cells is killed with each cycle of treatment. In this example each cycle of drug administration results in 99.9% (3 log) cell kill, and 1 log of cell regrowth occurs between cycles. The broken line indicates what would occur if the last cycle of therapy was omitted: Despite complete clinical remission of disease, the tumor would ultimately recur. (Reprinted from Holleb AI, et al (eds): *American Cancer Society Textbook of Clinical Oncology.* Atlanta, American Cancer Society, 1991.)

2. **Cell cycle–specific drugs (phase-nonspecific)** are effective while cells are actually in cycle but are not dependent on the cell being in a particular phase. Examples of phase-nonspecific antineoplastic agents include alkylating agents, antitumor antibiotics, and cisplatin.

3. **Cell cycle–nonspecific agents** are effective whether cancer cells are in cycle or resting; examples include nitrosoureas, mechlorethamine, and radiation.

III. CHEMOTHERAPY

A. Objectives. A number of different objectives exist when cancer patients undergo antineoplastic drug therapy.

1. A **cure** may be sought, with aggressive therapy for a prolonged period of time to eradicate all disease. For leukemias, this curative approach may consist of **remission induction,** attempting the maximal tumor cell kill, followed by **maintenance therapy** to eradicate all clinically undetectable disease and to lower the tumor cell burden below 10^3, where host immunologic defenses may keep the cancer cells in control.

2. If the goal is **palliation,** antineoplastic drugs may be given to control symptoms or decrease tumor size. Palliative therapy is usually given when complete eradication of the tumor is considered unlikely or the patient refuses aggressive chemotherapy.

3. **Adjuvant chemotherapy** is given after more definitive therapy, such as surgery, to eliminate any remaining disease; this is given with a curative intent.

4. **Neoadjuvant chemotherapy** is given prior to more definitive therapy to decrease the tumor burden and eliminate microscopic disease.

B. Combination chemotherapy is generally more efficacious than single-agent therapy.

1. The **rationale for combination therapy** is listed below.
   a. Overcoming or preventing resistance
   b. Cytotoxicity to resting and dividing cells
   c. Biochemical enhancement of effect
   d. Beneficial drug interactions
   e. Rescue of host cells

2. **Dosing and scheduling** of combination regimens are important, as they are designed to allow recovery of normal host cells. The regimens are generally given as short courses of therapy in cycles.

3. **Administration**
   a. Routes of administration vary, although intravenous bolus administration is most commonly employed.
   b. Other administration techniques include oral, subcutaneous, intrathecal, and intra-arterial routes; continuous intravenous infusion; and hepatic artery infusions.
   c. Drugs that may be given **intrathecally** are **methotrexate, cytarabine,** and **thiotepa;** drugs should not be administered by the intrathecal route without specific information supporting intrathecal administration. Patients have died when **vincristine** and other drugs have been administered by the intrathecal route. Caution should be used in the preparation and delivery of drugs to be used in this manner.

4. **Response to chemotherapy** is defined in a number of ways and does not always correlate with patient survival.
   a. **Complete response (CR)** indicates complete disappearance of all disease—clinical, gross, and microscopic.
   b. **Partial response (PR)** indicates a greater than 50% reduction in tumor size, lasting a reasonable period of time; some evidence of disease remains after therapy.
   c. **Response rate (RR)** is defined as CR plus PR.
   d. **Progression or no response** after therapy is defined by a greater than 25% increase in tumor size or the appearance of new lesions.

IV. CLASSIFICATION OF ANTINEOPLASTIC AGENTS

A. Alkylating agents were the first group of antineoplastic agents. The prototype of this class is **mechlorethamine,** or **nitrogen mustard,** which was researched as a chemical warfare agent. Alkylating agents cause cross-linking and abnormal base-pairing of DNA strands, which inhibits replication of the DNA; this mechanism is known as **alkylation**. The subclassifications of alkylating agents are listed below by chemical class; examples of each class are noted.

1. **Nitrogen mustards:** mechlorethamine (NH_2 nitrogen mustard), cyclophosphamide, melphalan (phenylalanine mustard), chlorambucil, and ifosfamide

2. **Ethylenimine derivatives:** thiotepa (triethylene thiophosphoramide)

3. **Alkyl sulfonates:** busulfan

4. **Nitrosoureas:** lomustine (CCNU), carmustine (BCNU), streptozocin, and semustine (methyl CCNU)

5. **Triazenes:** dacarbazine (DTIC)

B. Antitumor antibiotics are obtained from organisms of *Streptomyces* species. They consist of a sugar moiety and a ring structure known as a chromophore. Antitumor antibiotics act by either **alkylation** or **intercalation**. Intercalation is the process by which the chromophore slides between the DNA base pairs, and the DNA is anchored to the sugar moiety of the drug. The drugs then inhibit DNA synthesis. Examples of antitumor antibiotics and their synonyms are listed below.

1. **Anthracyclines:** daunorubicin (daunomycin), doxorubicin (adriamycin, hydroxydaunorubicin), epirubicin (epidoxorubicin), mitoxantrone, and idarubicin

2. **Other agents:** mitomycin C, plicamycin (mithramycin), bleomycin, dactinomycin (actinomycin D), and 2′-deoxycoformycin (pentostatin)

C. Antimetabolites are structural analogues of naturally occurring metabolites. They inhibit DNA synthesis by acting as false substitutions in the production of nucleic acids. The classes of antimetabolites are listed below.

1. **Folic acid analogues (folate antagonists):** methotrexate (MTX) and trimetrexate (TMTX)
2. *Pyrimidine analogues* (pyrimidine antagonists): 5-fluorouracil (5-FU), cytosine arabinoside (cytarabine Ara C), 5-azacytidine, and floxuridine (FUDR)
3. **Purine analogues (purine antagonists):** 6-mercaptopurine (6-MP) and 6-thioguanine (6-TG)

D. Plant alkaloids are derived from plants. The **vinca alkaloids** arrest mitosis at metaphase; the **podophyllotoxins** inhibit an enzyme called topoisomerase II, which is necessary for DNA production.

1. **Vinca alkaloids:** vincristine, vinblastine, and vindesine
2. **Podophyllotoxins:** etoposide (VP-16) and teniposide (VM-26)

E. Miscellaneous agents are categorized because their mechanism of action is either unknown or cannot be appropriately classified in any of the above categories.

1. **Hormones** are a class of heterogenous compounds that have varying effects on cells. Below is a list of some of the most commonly used agents in cancer chemotherapy.
   a. **Corticosteroids:** prednisone
   b. **Estrogens:** diethylstilbestrod (DES) and ethinyl estradiol
   c. **Progestins:** medroxyprogesterone and megestrol
   d. **Antiestrogens:** tamoxifen
   e. **Antiandrogens:** flutamide
   f. **Antiadrenals:** aminoglutethimide and ketoconazole
   g. **Androgens:** testosterone and fluoxymesterone
   h. **Gonadotropin hormone-releasing analogues:** leuprolide and goserelin
   i. **Estrogen/nitrogen mustard:** estramustine
2. **Platinum coordination complexes** [e.g., carboplatin (CBDCA), cisplatin], **substituted ureas** (e.g., hydroxyurea), procarbazine, and altretamine (e.g., hexamethylmelamine) act similarly to alkylating agents.
3. **L-Asparaginase** is an enzyme that works by preventing protein synthesis in cells requiring asparagine. The drug is available in two formulations: The *Escherichia coli* is the commerically available formulation, and the L-asparaginase derived from *Erwinia carotovora* is available only from the National Cancer Institute; it is reserved for patients who cannot tolerate the commercially available formulation due to anaphylactic reactions.
4. **Biologic response modifiers** alter or enhance the host's immunologic response to the tumor. Examples are listed below.
   a. **Monoclonal antibodies** (investigational)
   b. **Colony-stimulating factors (CSF):** (filgrastim (G-CSF), sargramostim (GM-CSF), and erythropoietin (EPO)
   c. **Interleukins**
   d. **Interferons:** alpha, beta, and gamma
   e. **Bacille Calmette-Guérin** (BCG)
   f. **Levamisole**

V. TOXICITIES OF ANTINEOPLASTIC AGENTS.

Antineoplastic agents are most toxic to the rapidly proliferating host cells. The tissues most commonly affected are those of the mucous membranes, skin, hair, gastrointestinal tract, and bone marrow. Of these, bone marrow toxicity is the most potentially fatal to the patient.

A. Bone marrow suppression is the most dose-limiting side effect of cancer chemotherapy.

1. **Complications**
   a. While all cell lines may be affected, a significant decrease in the white blood cells (**neutropenia**) predisposes the patient to serious infection.
   b. Platelet production may also be decreased, (**thrombocytopenia**), which can lead to bleeding and may require platelet transfusions and supportive therapy.

c. **Anemias** secondary to the antineoplastic agents are not as common as the other bone marrow toxicities, owing to the long circulating half-life of red blood cells (i.e., about 120 days).

2. **Time course.** The **onset of the myelosuppression** is generally 7–10 days. The lowest point of the neutrophil count, called the **nadir,** is usually reached in 10–14 days; recovery generally occurs in 2–3 weeks.

3. **Drugs that cause severe myelosuppression** include **cytarabine, carmustine, lomustine, mechlorethamine, dactinomycin, mitomycin C,** and **busulfan**. Only a few antineoplastic agents are not myelosuppressive; these include **vincristine, cisplatin,** and **bleomycin.**

B. Alopecia is the loss of hair commonly observed in chemotherapy patients.

1. Hair loss may be sporadic or complete; patients may wish to wear a wig during this period. Measures to prevent hair loss, such as ice caps worn during chemotherapy administration, are not universally effective.

2. **Drugs that cause alopecia** include **doxorubicin, daunorubicin, cyclophosphamide, vincristine,** and **mechlorethamine.**

C. Gastrointestinal toxicities are observed with chemotherapy administration.

1. **Nausea and vomiting** are the most limiting toxicities from the patient's point of view.
   a. Severe vomiting can lead to dehydration, esophageal tears, electrolyte imbalances, and discontinuation of cancer chemotherapy.
   b. The nausea and vomiting may be acute, delayed, or anticipatory in nature. It is, therefore, best to administer antiemetic agents prophylactically with chemotherapy agents of relatively high emetic potential.
   c. Table 57-2 lists commonly used antineoplastic agents and their relative emetic potential. It is important to understand that emesis is a function of the drug, route of administration, schedule, and dose of that chemotherapy.

2. **Stomatitis** is a generalized inflammation of the oral mucosa or other areas of the gastrointestinal tract. It occurs because of the rapid turnover of mucosal membrane cells.
   a. **Signs and symptoms** include erythema, generalized pain of the mucosal membranes, dryness of the mouth, burning or tingling of the lips, ulcerations, and bleeding.
   b. **Drugs that cause stomatitis** are **L-asparaginase, bleomycin, cytarabine, plicamycin, cyclophosphamide, chlorambucil, dacarbazine, daunorubucin, doxorubicin, vinblastine,** and **vincristine.**
   c. **Time course.** Stomatitis usually appears from 2–5 days after the offending agent is administered and may last from 1–2 weeks
   d. **Consequences** of stomatitis include infection of the ulcerated area, inability to eat, pain requiring narcotic analgesic therapy, and a decrease in chemotherapy dose or schedule.

Table 57-2. Relative Emetic Potential of Antineoplastic Drugs

High (> 90%)	**Moderately High** (60%–90%)	**Moderate** (30%–60%)	**Moderately Low** (10%–30%)	**Low** (< 10%)
Cisplatin	Semustine	5-Fluorouracil	Bleomycin	Busulfan
Dacarbazine	Carmustine	Doxorubicin	Hydroxyurea	Chlorambucil
Mechlorethamine	Lomustine	Daunorubicin	Melphalan	6-Thioguanine
Streptozocin	Cyclophosphamide	L-Asparaginase	Etoposide	Vincristine
Cytarabine*	Dactinomycin	Mitomycin	Cytarabine‡	Estrogens
	Plicamycin	5-Azacitidine	6-Mercaptopurine	Progestins
	Procarbazine	Altretamine	Methotrexate‡	Corticosteroids
	Methotrexate†	Carboplatin	Thiotepa	Androgens
		Vinblastine		
		Ifosfamide		
		Mitoxantrone		

Adapted from Tortorice PV, O'Connell MB: Management of chemotherapy induced nausea and vomiting. *Pharmacotherapy* 10 (2): 130, 1990.

*High-dose therapy (> 500 mg/m²)

†High-dose therapy (> 200 mg/m²)

‡Standard or low-dose therapy

3. Other gastrointestinal toxicities are **anorexia, diarrhea,** and **taste alterations.**

D. **Chills and fever** may be observed after administration of chemotherapy agents. This fever is generally differentiated from that of infection by its temporal relationship to chemotherapy administration. The chills and fevers usually do not require treatment. **Drugs most commonly associated with this syndrome** include **L-asparaginase, bleomycin, cytarabine, plicamycin, cyclophosphamide, chlorambucil, dacarbazine, daunorubicin, doxorubicin, vinblastine,** and **vincristine.**

E. **Pulmonary toxicity** is a potentially fatal toxicity and is seen most commonly with bleomycin.

1. **Signs and symptoms** of this syndrome are respiratory insufficiency, dyspnea, cough, and fever. It appears to be related to the dose of bleomycin; other risk factors include prior chest irradiation and oxygen therapy.
2. **Other drugs associated with pulmonary toxicities** include **busulfan, carmustine, chlorambucil, cyclophosphamide,** and **melphalan.**

F. **Cardiac toxicity** may manifest as an acute or chronic syndrome.

1. The acute changes that have been observed are primarily electrocardiographic (ECG) abnormalities, whereas the chronic syndrome is generally a diffuse chronic heart failure (CHF).
2. **Drugs that cause cardiotoxicity** are **doxorubicin, daunorubicin,** and **cyclophosphamide.** It has been associated with high cumulative doses (doxorubicin $\geq$ 550 mg/m^2) and prior chest irradiation.

G. **Anaphylaxis** has been most commmonly seen with **asparaginase, cisplatin, bleomycin,** and other antitumor antibiotics. Test doses *do not* preclude possible anaphylaxis. An anaphylactic kit or crash cart should be readily available when these agents are administered.

H. **Neurotoxicity** may occur with systemic or intrathecal chemotherapy.

1. **Vincristine** is associated with autonomic and peripheral neuropathies; patients may experience gait disturbances, tingling of hands and feet, and loss of deep tendon reflex.
2. High-dose **cytarabine** produces a cerebellar toxicity with loss of hand–eye coordination and possible coma.
3. Anarachnoiditis may be observed after intrathecal administration of **methotrexate** or **cytarabine.**

I. **Local necrosis. Vesicant drugs,** such as **dactinomycin, daunorubicin, doxorubicin, epirubicin, mechlorethamine, mitomycin C, plicamycin, vincristine,** and **vinblastine,** produce local necrosis when extravasated during administration.

1. Most **extravasations** with these agents produce an immediate reaction of pain and burning on administration; a delayed syndrome may occur hours or weeks later. Significant tissue injury, such as ulceration and necrosis, may ensue.
2. While definitive treatment of extravasations remains controversial for most agents, ice packs are recommended immediately and two to four times daily thereafter; heat should be applied to extravasations caused by vinca alkaloids. The efficacy of antidotes (other than sodium thiosulfate for mechlorethamine extravasation) is debatable.

J. **Hemorrhagic cystitis** is a **bladder toxicity** that is most commonly observed after administration of **cyclophosphamide** or **ifosfamide.** It is due to a metabolite, acrolein, having prolonged contact with bladder membranes. It may be prevented by aggressive hydration, frequent urination, or the concomitant administration of the uroprotectant drug mesna.

K. **Renal toxicity** may also be observed, resulting in tubular necrosis. This is manifested by an increase in serum creatinine and blood urea nitrogen (BUN); renal failure may ensue. Nephrotoxicity is most commonly observed after **cisplatin, methotrexate, plicamycin, ifosfamide,** and **streptozocin.**

L. **Hepatotoxicity** may be manifested by increased results on liver function tests, jaundice, or hepatitis. It is most commonly seen with **cyclophosphamide, mercaptopurine, cytarabine,** and **L-asparaginase.**

M. Secondary malignancies are most commonly seen with **alkylating agents** and **diethylstilbestrol**. These may be leukemias, lymphomas, or solid tumors. The secondary malignancies usually occur 5–10 years after chemotherapy or radiation.

VI. OTHER THERAPEUTIC MODALITIES

A. Surgery remains an important tool in the diagnosis and treatment of malignancies, despite continued progress with antineoplastic drugs and radiation therapy. Surgery may be **diagnostic** (e.g., biopsy, exploratory laparotomy, "second-look" surgeries) or **therapeutic** (e.g., tumor debulking or removal). It is frequently used in conjunction with chemotherapy, radiation therapy, or both.

B. Radiation therapy targets high doses of radiation specifically to tumor tissues. Radiation may be used alone but is more commonly used in combination with surgery or chemotherapy. Adverse reactions may include stomatitis, alopecia, nausea, vomiting, and diarrhea; possible long-term sequelae are secondary malignancies.

STUDY QUESTIONS

Directions: Each of the numbered items or incomplete statements in this section is followed by answers or by completions of the statement. Select the **one** lettered answer or completion that is **best** in each case.

1. The granulocyte nadir associated with antineoplastic agents generally occurs

(A) during administration of therapy
(B) 1–2 days after therapy
(C) 10–14 days after therapy
(D) 1 month after therapy
(E) immediately prior to the next chemotherapy course

2. Stomatitis is characterized by all of the following signs and symptoms EXCEPT

(A) headache
(B) erythema
(C) sore throat
(D) ulcerations
(E) dryness of mouth

3. All of the following antineoplastic agents can be used for intrathecal administration EXCEPT

(A) methotrexate
(B) cytarabine
(C) thiotepa
(D) vincristine

4. Rationales for the use of combination chemotherapy include all of the following EXCEPT

(A) overcoming or preventing resistance
(B) biochemical enhancement of antineoplastic effect
(C) additive activity without additive adverse effects
(D) maximal suppression of granulopoiesis
(E) cytotoxicity to resting and dividing cells

1-C
2-A
3-D
4-D

ANSWERS AND EXPLANATIONS

1. The answer is C *[V A 2].*
Bone marrow suppression, particularly of the white blood cells or granulocytes, usually is at the lowest point 10–14 days after chemotherapy administration. Some agents, such as the nitrosoureas, have delayed and prolonged bone marrow suppression, but these drugs are the exceptions.

2. The answer is A *[V C 2].*
Stomatitis, or mucositis, is an inflammation of the mucous membranes, particularly the oral mucosa. While the symptoms are generally limited to the mouth and throat, stomatitis may affect any part of the gastrointestinal tract, potentially causing diarrhea and anal fissures.

3. The answer is D *[III B 3 c].*
Intrathecally administered vincristine usually causes death. All syringes of vincristine should be labeled "for intravenous use only."

4. The answer is D *[III B 1].*
Combination chemotherapy has been developed to have maximal cytotoxicity with minimal toxicity. The drugs are scheduled such that maximal cell kill is achieved, while allowing normal cells to replicate. If possible, antineoplastic agents with different spectrums of toxicity are chosen to be given at the same time.

58
Pain

David R. Platt

I. INTRODUCTION

A. Definition

1. **Pain** is an unpleasant sensory and emotional experience that is usually associated with structural or tissue damage. It is a subjective, individual experience that has physical, psychological, and social determinants. There is no objective measurement of pain.
2. **Acute pain** occurs following tissue injury, such as trauma or surgery. The pain is usually self-limiting, decreasing with time as the injury heals. It is described as a linear process with a beginning and an end. Increased autonomic nervous system activity often accompanies acute pain, causing tachycardia, tachypnea, hypertension, diaphoresis, and mydriasis. Increased anxiety may also occur.
3. **Chronic pain** is pain that lasts more than several months. **Chronic nonmalignant pain** is a complication of acute injury where the healing process does not occur as expected. The pain is constant and consumes the patient's existence. It does not improve with time and is described as a cyclic process (vicious cycle). Compared to acute pain, there is no longer autonomic nervous system stimulation so the patient may not "appear" in pain. Instead the patient may be depressed, suffer insomnia, weight loss, sexual dysfunction, and may not be able to cope with the normal activities of daily living, including family and job-related activities.
4. **Chronic cancer pain** occurs in 60%–90% of patients with cancer. Its characteristics are similar to those of chronic nonmalignant pain. In addition to depression; fear, anger, and agony may be prominent occurrences. The etiology of chronic cancer pain can be related to the tumor, cancer therapy, or be idiosyncratic. Tumor causes of pain include bone metastasis, compression of nerve structures, occlusion of blood vessels, obstruction of bowel, or infiltration of soft tissue.
5. **Breakthrough pain** is the intermittent, transitory increase in pain that occurs at a greater intensity over baseline chronic pain. It may have temporal characteristics, precipitating factors, and predictability.

B. Principles of management

1. **Comprehensive pain assessment** should determine the characteristics of the patient's pain complaint, clinical status, and pain management history.
   - **a.** Assessment of the pain complaint should include location, quality, provocative factors, temporal qualities, severity, and pain history.
   - **b.** Assessment of clinical status should include the extent of underlying trauma or disease. Also, the patient's physical, psychological, and social conditions should be determined.
   - **c.** Assessment of pain management history includes drug allergies, analgesic response, onset, duration, and side effects.
2. **Appropriate pain management targets** should be established.
   - **a.** The primary pain management goal is to improve patient comfort.
   - **b.** For acute pain management, improved comfort can aid the healing and rehabilitation process.
   - **c.** For chronic pain, the specific objectives are to break the pain cycle (i.e., erase pain memory) and minimize breakthrough pain.
   - **d.** Other targets for chronic pain management include improvement of general well-being, sleep, outlook, self-esteem, activities of daily living, support, and mobility.

3. **Individualized pain management regimens** should be determined and initiated promptly.
   a. The optimal analgesic regimen, including dose, dosing interval, and mode of administration, should be selected.
   b. Additional pharmacologic adjuncts and nonpharmacologic therapies should be added if needed.
   c. The most common regimens for acute pain include intermittent (as needed) dosing, patient controlled analgesia (PCA), or epidural infusions with narcotic or non-narcotic agents.
   d. Although the practice is controversial, narcotic use is usually minimized or avoided for chronic nonmalignant pain. Non-narcotic analgesics and nonpharmacologic management are usually maximized.
   e. For chronic cancer pain, an individualized around-the-clock analgesic regimen is established, using a long-acting analgesic. An intermittent, as-needed regimen for breakthrough pain, using a short-acting analgesic, is also determined.

4. **Monitoring the pain management regimen and re-assessment of the patient's pain** should occur on a continuous, timely basis. Any changes in analgesic, dose, dosing interval, or method of administration should be carried out immediately.

II. ANALGESICS

A. **Non-narcotic analgesics** include aspirin, other salicylates, acetaminophen, and nonsteroidal anti-inflammatory drugs (NSAIDs) (Table 58-1). Aspirin products, acetaminophen, and low-dose ibuprofen (200 mg) are available for use without a prescription.

1. **Mechanism of action.** The non-narcotic analgesics act peripherally. Salicylates and NSAIDs are prostaglandin inhibitors and prevent peripheral nociception by vasoactive substances such as prostaglandins and bradykinins. The exact mechanism of action of acetaminophen is not known.

Table 58-1. Some Commonly Used Nonnarcotic Analgesics

Drug	Average Dose (mg)	Dosing Interval (hr)	Maximum Daily Adult Dose (mg)
Acetaminophen	500–1000	4–6	4000
Salicylates			
Aspirin	500–1000	4–6	4000
Choline magnesium trisalicylate	1000–1500	12	2000–3000
Diflunisal	1000 (load)		
	500 (maintenance)	8–12	1500
Nonsteroidal anti-inflammatory drugs (NSAIDs)			
Propionic acids			
Ibuprofen	200–400	4–6	2400
Naproxen	500 (load)		
	250 (maintenance)	6–8	1250
Naproxen sodium	550 (load)		
	275 (maintenance)	6–8	1375
Fenoprofen	200	4–6	800
Ketoprofen	25–50	6–8	300
Indoleacetic acid			
Indomethacin	25	8–12	100
Anthranilic acid			
Mefenamic acid	500 (load)		
	250 (maintenance)	6	1500
Pyranocarboxylic acid			
Etodolac	200–400	6–8	1200
Pyrrolopyrrole			
Ketorolac*	30–60 (load)		
	15–30 (maintenance)	6	120

* Administered intramuscularly.

2. Therapeutic effects

a. The non-narcotic analgesics have several effects in common. These effects distinguish them from narcotic analgesics.

(1) They are antipyretic.

(2) They are anti-inflammatory (except acetaminophen).

(3) There is a ceiling effect to the analgesia.

(4) They do not cause tolerance.

(5) They do not cause physical or psychological dependence.

b. The efficacy of non-narcotics is compared to aspirin. Most are comparable to aspirin; however several NSAIDs have shown a superior effect to 650 mg of aspirin.

(1) Diflunisal (500 mg)

(2) Ibuprofen (200–400 mg)

(3) Naproxen sodium (550 mg)

(4) Ketoprofen (25–50 mg)

3. Clinical use

a. Generally, the **non-narcotic analgesics are used orally to manage mild-to-moderate pain.**

(1) They are particularly suited for acute pain of skeletal muscle (orthopedic) or oral (dental) origin.

(2) They are used in chronic malignant pain and can have an additive effect with narcotic analgesics.

(3) They may also be effective in managing pain due to bone metastases.

b. The NSAID, ketorolac, is administered intramuscularly and is useful in moderate-to-severe pain, especially in cases where narcotics are undesirable (e.g., with drug addicts, excessive narcotic sedation, respiratory depression).

c. Patients may vary in their response and tolerance to non-narcotics analgesics. If a patient does not respond to the maximum therapeutic dose, then an alternate NSAID should be tried. Likewise, if a patient experiences side effects with one drug, then another agent should be tried.

d. Several drugs (e.g, diflunisal, choline magnesium trisalicylate, naproxen) have long half-lives and, therefore, may be administered less frequently.

e. The cost of non-narcotic analgesics is highly variable and should be considered when an agent is selected.

4. Adverse effects

a. Gastrointestinal effects. Most non-narcotic analgesics cause gastrointestinal symptoms secondary to prostaglandin inhibition. At normal doses, acetaminophen and choline magnesium trisalicylate produce minimal gastrointestinal upset.

(1) The most common gastrointestinal symptom is dyspepsia, but ulceration, bleeding, or perforation can occur.

(2) Patients most predisposed to severe gastrointestinal effects include the elderly, patients with a history of ulcers or chronic disease, and those who smoke or use alcohol.

(3) To minimize gastrointestinal effects, the lowest possible analgesic dose should be used. Aspirin, available as enteric-coated products, may minimize gastrointestinal upset. Combination therapy with a gastrointestinal "protectant" (e.g., antacid, H_2-antagonist, sucralfate, misoprostol) may be needed.

(4) Even in normal doses, acetaminophen can cause hepatotoxicity in patients with liver disease or chronic alcoholism.

b. Hematologic effects. Most non-narcotic analgesics inhibit platelet aggregation. The effect is produced by reversible inhibition of prostaglandin synthetase. Aspirin is an irreversible inhibitor. Acetaminophen and choline magnesium trisalicylate lack antiplatelet effects.

(1) The effect of the NSAIDs correlates to the presence of an effective serum concentration.

(2) Use of anticoagulants (e.g., heparin, warfarin) is relatively contraindicated in combination with aspirin or NSAIDs.

c. Renal effects. NSAIDs can produce renal dysfunction.

(1) The mechanism of NSAID-induced renal dysfunction includes prostaglandin inhibition, interstitial nephritis, impaired renin secretion, and enhanced tubular water/sodium reabsorption.

(2) Many risk factors have been implicated including congestive heart failure (CHF), chronic renal failure (CRF), cirrhosis, dehydration, diuretic use, and atherosclerotic disease in elderly patients.

(3) The renal dysfunction is commonly manifested as abrupt onset oliguria with sodium/water retention. The effect reverses after discontinuation of the NSAID.

d. Miscellaneous effects

(1) Some patients exhibit acute hypersensitivity reactions to aspirin. Manifestations include either a rhinitis or asthma presentation or a true allergic reaction (e.g., urticaria, wheals, hypotension, shock, syncope). A cross-sensitivity to other NSAIDs may develop.

(2) Some NSAIDs produce central nervous system (CNS) effects, including impaired mentation and attention deficit disorder.

5. Drug interactions. Salicylates have two clinically significant drug interactions.

a. Oral anticoagulants. Aspirin should be avoided in anticoagulated patients. Aspirin inhibits platelet function and can cause gastric mucosal damage. This significantly increases the risk of bleeding in anticoagulated patients. Also, doses of more than 3 g/day of aspirin produce hypoprothrombinemia. Choline magnesium trisalicylate or acetaminophen should be used if a non-narcotic is needed in an anticoagulated patient.

b. Methotrexate. Salicylates may enhance the toxicity of methotrexate. The primary mechanism is blockage of methotrexate renal tubular secretion by salicylates. The resultant methotrexate toxicity has been reported as pancytopenia or hepatotoxicity. Salicylates should be avoided in patients receiving methotrexate.

B. Narcotic analgesics include the opiate agonists (Table 58-2). There is also a group of mixed agonist–antagonist drugs (Table 58-3). Because of their abuse potential, opiates are classified as controlled drugs and are placed in schedules II or III. Special regulations control their prescribing.

1. Mechanism of action

a. Endogenous opiates afford the body self-pain relieving mechanisms. These endogenous peptides include the endorphins, enkephalins, and dynorphins.

b. Exogenous opiates are classified as agonists (stimulate opiate receptors), antagonists (displace agonists from opiate receptors), and mixed opiates (agonist–antagonist or partial agonist actions).

c. Opiate receptors are located in the brain and spinal cord. Several types of opiate receptors have been identified, including mu, kappa, delta, sigma, and epsilon.

d. Stimulation of mu receptors produce the characteristic narcotic (morphine-like) effects:

(1) Analgesia
(2) Miosis
(3) Euphoria
(4) Respiratory depression
(5) Sedation
(6) Physical dependence
(7) Bradycardia

e. The specific mechanism (central and spinal) of opiate agonism is alteration of the effects of nociceptive neurotransmitters, possibly norepinephrine or serotonin.

Table 58-2. Some Commonly Used Opiate Agonists

Drug	Equivalent Dose (mg)* Parenteral	Equivalent Dose (mg)* Oral	Duration of Effect (hr)
Codeine	75	130	3–4
Oxycodone	. . .	20–30	3–4
Morphine	10	20–30 (chronic dosing) 60 (single dose)	4–6†
Hydromorphone	1.5	7.5	3–4
Levorphanol	2	4	4–8
Meperidine	100	400	2–3
Methadone	10	20	6–8
Fentanyl	0.1	. . .	1–2‡

*These drugs produce analgesia equivalent to 10 mg intramuscular morphine.
†Controlled-release morphine has a duration of effect of about 8–12 hours.
‡Transdermal fentanyl has a duration of effect of about 72 hours.

Table 58-3. Mixed Agonist–Antagonists

Drug	Equivalent Dose (mg)*	Duration of Effect (hr)
Partial agonist		
Buprenorphine	0.4 (intramuscular)	6–8
Mixed agonists–antagonists		
Pentazocine	60 (intramuscular)	3–6
	180 (oral)	3–6
Nalbuphine	10 (intramuscular)	3–6
Butorphanol	2 (intramuscular)	3–4
Dezocine	10 (intramuscular)	3–4

*These drugs produce analgesia equivalent to 10 mg intramuscular morphine.

2. Clinical use

a. Narcotics are used for the management of moderate-to-severe pain (acute or chronic pain) of somatic or visceral origin.

b. The use of narcotics should be individualized for each patient. The optimal analgesic dose varies from patient to patient. Each analgesic regimen should be titrated by increasing the dose up to the appearance of limiting adverse effects. Changing to another analgesic should only occur after an adequate therapeutic trial.

c. The appropriate route of administration should be selected for each patient.

(1) Oral administration is the preferred route, especially for patients with chronic, stable pain.

(2) Intramuscular, subcutaneous administrations is very commonly used in the postoperative period. Fluctuations in absorption may occur, especially in elderly or cachectic patients.

(3) Intravenous bolus administration has the most rapid, predictable onset of effect.

(4) Intravenous infusion is used to titrate pain relief rapidly, especially in patients with unstable chronic pain. Morphine is most commonly used, often with supplemental intravenous bolus doses for breakthrough pain. A mechanical infusion device is necessary.

(5) Intravenous patient-controlled analgesia (PCA) is most often used for acute postoperative pain. It produces prompt analgesia with minimal side-effects because small doses (e.g., 1–2 mg morphine) are delivered at frequent intervals (e.g., every 10 minutes). It allows patient control of pain management. Morphine and meperidine are the most commonly used agents. A mechanical infusion device and properly trained patient and staff are necessary.

(6) Epidural and intrathecal administration is used for acute postoperative pain and early management of chronic cancer pain.

(a) Low opiate doses stimulate spinal opiate receptors and reduce the amount of narcotic reaching the brain. This results in delayed or minimal effects such as sedation, nausea, and respiratory depression. The opiate distribution that causes such effects is dependent on site of spinal injection, water solubility of the opiate, and the volume infused. For example, after lumbar administration of a more water-soluble opiate (morphine), severe respiratory depression can be observed 12–24 hours after initial dosing.

(b) Local side effects of intraspinal opiate administration are itching and urinary retention. Depending on the opiate used and the type of pain being treated, intermittent doses or continuous infusions (via a mechanical infusion device) can be employed (Tables 58-4 and 58-5).

(c) Sometimes local anesthetics (e.g., bupivicaine, lidocaine) are administered with the opiate for additive analgesic effect.

(7) Rectal administration is an alternative for patients unable to take oral narcotics. Generally, poor absorption results in a variable analgesic response. It is an unacceptable route of administration for many patients.

(8) Transdermal administration is an alternative for patients with chronic pain who are unable to take oral narcotics. A controlled-release patch is available for fentanyl. Slow-onset requires additional analgesia while starting treatment. The duration of analgesia is 72 hours per patch. A slow reduction of effect follows removal of the patch and requires 24–36 hours of monitoring.

Table 58-4. Epidurally Administered Narcotics (Intermittent Dosing)

Drug	Usual Dose (mg)	Onset of Action (min)	Time to Peak Effect (min)	Duration of Action (hr)
Morphine	5–10	25	60	12–24
Fentanyl	0.1	5–10	20	6
Meperidine	50–100	5–10	15–30	7
Hydromorphone	1	10–15	20	12
Buprenorphine	0.3	30	40–60	8–9

d. Patients who have chronic pain or acute pain that is constant throughout the day should receive regularly scheduled (around-the-clock) doses of narcotics.

(1) Long-acting opiates (e.g., controlled-release morphine, methadone) are preferable.

(2) A supplement given as needed may be necessary to manage breakthrough pain, for which short-acting opiates (e.g., immediate-release morphine, hydromorphone) are preferable. If frequent supplements are required, then the around-the-clock regimen should be adjusted based on morphine equivalents (see Table 58-2).

e. Although the analgesia and side effects of opiates are qualitatively similar, individual patients may respond differently. Analgesic selection is based on:

(1) Patient's past analgesia experience

(2) Need for a rapid onset of effect

(3) Preference for a long (or short) duration of action

(4) Preference for a particular mode of delivery

(5) Preference for a particular dosage form

(a) Controlled-release morphine for a long duration of action (8–12 hours) may be preferable to opiates with long half-lives (e.g., methadone, levorphanol), which can accumulate and cause overdose symptoms (e.g., respiratory depression).

(b) Transdermal fentanyl can be used for patients who are unable to swallow.

(c) Rectal suppositories can be used for patients who are unable to swallow. They are available for morphine, hydromorphone, and oxymorphone.

(d) Concentrated hydromorphone injection (10 mg/ml) can be used for cachectic patients who require subcutaneous injections and in patients whose injection volumes must be minimized.

(6) Individual sensitivity to side effects, especially nausea, euphoria, sedation, and respiratory depression

(a) Partial agonists or mixed agonist–antagonists may be preferable for acute pain management in patients at risk for respiratory depression secondary to opiate agonists. They should not be used in patients who have received chronic doses of opiates because withdrawal symptoms will occur.

(b) Epidural administration may be preferable for critically ill patients at risk for respiratory depression secondary to systemic narcotic administration.

3. Adverse effects. All narcotics can produce a variety of side effects that range from bothersome to life-threatening.

a. Constipation occurs as a result of decreased intestinal tone and peristalsis. There is a patient variability, but generally most patients experience constipation after several days of therapy. Constipation may be more bothersome with certain types of opiates (e.g., codeine). It may occur sooner and be more problematic in hospitalized or bedridden patients or in patients who have received anesthesia or drugs with anticholinergic effects. Prophylaxis with a laxative/stool softener combination (e.g., bisacodyl/docusate) and dietary counseling are warranted in patients who need chronic opiate therapy.

Table 58-5. Epidurally Administered Narcotics (Continuous Infusion)

Drug	Initial Bolus Dose (mg)	Infusion Concentration (mg/ml)	Infusion Rate (mg/hr)
Morphine	2	0.05–0.25	0.2–1.5
Fentanyl	0.05–0.1	0.005–0.025	0.02–0.15
Meperidine	50–100	10–20	5–20
Hydromorphone	0.5—1	0.02–0.05	0.15–0.3

b. Nausea/vomiting occurs due to central stimulation of the chemoreceptor trigger zone. It is more problematic with one-time or intermittent parenteral dosing for acute pain. Occasionally, patients require concomitant therapy with an antiemetic (e.g., hydroxyzine, prochlorperazine); however these agents may add to the sedative effects of opiates.

c. Sedation is a dose-related effect but sometimes is enhanced by concomitant use of other drugs with sedating effects (e.g., benzodiazepines, antiemetics). Most chronic pain patients become tolerant to this effect, but occasionally the addition of a CNS stimulant, such as dextroamphetamine or methylphenidate, is needed. Patients starting therapy with narcotics should be warned about driving or operating machinery. Sedation may be a sign of excessive dosing or accumulation. However, sedation should not be confused with physiologic sleep in patients who have pain control difficulties. Patients in pain often develop insomnia. When pain is brought under control by appropriate narcotic titration, the patient initially may sleep for several hours.

d. Respiratory depression is the most serious adverse effect accompanying narcotic overdose. Respiratory depression may be a sign of a excessive dose, accumulation of long half-lived opiates (e.g., methadone, levorphanol), or accumulation of active morphine metabolites in renal failure patients.

(1) Respiratory rate should be carefully monitored in patients receiving intravenous or epidural opiates, in neonates, in elderly patients, and in patients receiving other drugs that cause respiratory depression.

(2) The opiate antagonist, naloxone, is administered intravenously to reverse life-threatening respiratory depression. Use of naloxone in an opiate-dependent patient (e.g., a chronic cancer pain patient) can precipitate opiate withdrawal.

e. Anticholinergic effects, such as dry mouth and urinary retention, can be bothersome for some patients.

f. Hypersensitivity reactions, such as itching due to histamine release, can occur secondary to opiate use, particularly with epidural or intrathecal administration. Wheals sometimes occur at the site of morphine injection. These reactions do not represent true allergy.

g. CNS excitation, such as myoclonus and other seizure-like activity, can be produced with the use of meperidine in renal failure. These symptoms have also been observed in patients with normal renal functions who receive high doses of meperidine (e.g., more than 800 mg/day of intramuscular meperidine). The accumulation of the metabolite normeperidine is the cause.

4. Drug Interactions

a. Narcotics have additive CNS depressant effects when used in combination with other drugs that also are CNS depressants. (e.g., alcohol, anesthetics, antidepressants, antihistamines, barbiturates, benzodiazepines, phenothiazines).

b. Narcotics, especially meperidine, can cause severe reactions such as excitation, sweating, rigidity, and hypertension in patients receiving monoamine oxidase (MAO). Meperidine should be avoided and other narcotics started at lower doses in patients on MAO inhibitors.

5. Tolerance means that increasing doses of opiate are needed to maintain analgesia. This is usually observed as a decreasing duration of analgesia in chronic pain patients. The addition of a NSAID may help delay or provide adequate analgesia in tolerant patients.

6. Dependence. The use of opiates for chronic pain results in physical dependence, such that the abrupt discontinuation of the opiate results in the development of withdrawal symptoms.

a. Withdrawal symptoms include anxiety, irritability, insomnia, chills, salivation, rhinorrhea, diaphoresis, nausea, vomiting, gastrointestinal cramping, and piloerection.

(1) The appearance and intensity of withdrawal symptoms vary according to the half-life of the opiate. For example, the withdrawal symptoms after discontinuation of chronic methadone may take several days to develop and be less intense as compared to withdrawal from morphine (shorter half-life).

(2) The development of tolerance may be associated with withdrawal symptoms.

(3) The use of naloxone in a patient receiving chronic opiate therapy produces acute withdrawal.

b. The development of physical dependence seen in chronic pain patients is not the same as psychological dependence or addiction. Also, the "drug seeking" behavior observed in many acute pain patients (i.e, postoperative pain) is not a sign of addiction, but rather a need for adequate pain relief. The analgesic needs of this type of patient should be reassessed and usually necessitates increasing the dose of opiate, changing to a longer duration drug, changing to a PCA, or adding an analgesic adjunct.

C. Analgesic adjuncts. Other classes of drugs affect nonopiate pain pathways and may be useful in certain types of pain (e.g., neurogenic pain). They are often used with other analgesics and some may help manage narcotic side-effects (Table 58-6).

D. Nonpharmacologic pain management. Other therapeutic modalities for pain management include cognitive behavioral interventions and physical methods. These modalities are appropriate for interested patients, patients experiencing anxiety with their pain, patients who have incomplete relief from analgesic therapy, and patients who need to avoid or reduce analgesic use (e.g., those with chronic nonmalignant pain).

1. **Cognitive behavioral interventions** include education/instruction, simple relaxation, biofeedback, and hypnosis.
2. **Physical methods** include heat and cold applications, massage, exercise, rest, immobilization, and transelectrode neurostimulation (TENS).

Table 58-6. Analgesic Adjuncts

Class	Drugs	Indications
Tricyclic antidepressants	Amitriptyline Desipramine Doxepin Imipramine	Neurogenic pain; chronic pain complicated by depression or insomnia
Anticonvulsants	Carbamazepine Clonazepam Phenytoin Valproate	Lancinating neurogenic pain (e.g., trigeminal neuralgia, phantom limb pain, post-trauma neurogenic pain)
Neuroleptics	Fluphenazine Haloperidol Prochlorperazine	Refractory neurogenic pain; pain complicated by delirium or nausea (prochlorperazine)
Corticosteroid	Dexamethasone	Pain from neural infiltration
Antihistamine	Hydroxyzine	Pain complicated by anxiety or nausea
Benzodiazepines	Alprazolam Lorazepam	Pain complicated by anxiety or muscle spasm
Amphetamines	Dextroamphetamine Methylphenidate	For excessive opiate-induced sedation in chronic pain patients

STUDY QUESTIONS

Directions: Each of the numbered items or incomplete statements in this section is followed by answers or by completions of the statement. Select the **one** lettered answer or completion that is **best** in each case.

1. An emaciated 69-year-old man with advanced inoperable throat cancer is hospitalized for pain management. He is receiving a morphine solution (40 mg orally) every 3 hours for pain. He complains of dysphagia and about the frequency with which he must take morphine. An appropriate analgesic alternative for this patient would be

(A) changing to a controlled-release oral morphine
(B) increasing the dose of the oral morphine solution
(C) changing to intramuscular methadone
(D) changing to transdermal fentanyl
(E) decreasing the frequency of oral morphine administration

Questions 2 and 3

A 52-year-old woman with a diagnosis of ovarian cancer presents with complaints of pain. Her pain was reasonably well controlled with two capsules of oxycodone every 4 hours until 2 weeks ago at which point she was hospitalized for pain control. She was placed on meperidine (75 mg) every 3 hours but still complained about pain. Her meperidine dosage was increased to 100 mg every 2 hours.

2. At the dosage of meperidine, the patient is likely to experience

(A) excellent pain relief
(B) respiratory depression
(C) worsening renal function
(D) myoclonic seizures
(E) excessive sedation

3. An appropriate next step in this patient's therapy would be to

(A) add a nonsteroidal anti-inflammatory drug (NSAID)
(B) discontinue the meperidine and convert her to a controlled-release oral morphine
(C) continue the present meperidine dosage because she will eventually get relief
(D) decrease the meperidine dose to avoid side effects
(E) consider hypnosis or relaxation techniques

4. A 20-year-old victim of a motor vehicle accident is 3 days post surgery for orthopedic and internal injuries. He has been in severe pain on a regimen of intramuscular morphine (5–10 mg) every 4 hours as needed for pain. A pain consultant starts the patient with a 20-mg intravenous morphine loading dose and then begins a continuous intravenous morphine infusion with as needed morphine boosters. Two hours after this regimen is started, the patient is asleep. The nurse is concerned and calls the physician. The physician should

(A) call for a psychiatric consult
(B) administer naloxone
(C) examine the patient and reconfirm the dosage and monitoring parameters
(D) add an injectable nonsteroidal anti-inflammatory drug (NSAID)
(E) add an amphetamine

5. Potential adverse effects associated with aspirin include all of the following EXCEPT

(A) gastrointestinal ulceration
(B) renal dysfunction
(C) enhanced methotrexate toxicity
(D) cardiac arrhythmias
(E) hypersensitivity asthma

1-D
2-D
3-B
4-C
5-D

6. All of the following facts are true about nonsteroidal anti-inflammatory drugs (NSAIDs) EXCEPT

(A) they are antipyretic
(B) there is a ceiling effect to their analgesia
(C) they can cause tolerance
(D) they do not cause dependence
(E) they are anti-inflammatory

7. Which of the following narcotics has the longest duration of effect?

(A) Methadone
(B) Controlled-release morphine
(C) Levorphanol
(D) Transdermal fentanyl
(E) Dihydromorphone

Directions: The item below contains three suggested answers of which **one or more** is correct. Choose the answer

A if **I only** is correct
B if **III only** is correct
C if **I and II** are correct
D if **II and III** are correct
E if **I, II, and III** are correct

8. Agents that are safe to use in a patient with bleeding problems include

I. choline magnesium trisalicylate
II. acetaminophen
III. ketorolac

6-C
7-D
8-C

ANSWERS AND EXPLANATIONS

1. The answer is D *[II B 2 c (8)].*
Patients with throat cancer often cannot take oral analgesics. The patient described in the question is also having pain difficulties with an every 3 hour regimen. Transdermal fentanyl is a good alternative because, after titration, excellent analgesia can be produced without using oral or parenteral agents. Also, the frequency of analgesic use may be decreased once titration has occurred.

2 and 3. The answers are: 2-D *[II B 3 g],* **3-B** *[II B 2 c (1), d (1)].*
Myoclonic seizures can occur after frequent, high-dose meperidine due to the accumulation of the metabolite, normeperidine.

Both oxycodone and meperidine have short durations of effect. In a chronic pain patient, an around-the-clock regimen, using a controlled-release oral morphine, would be an appropriate alternative. With titration, the patient should have good pain relief with an every 8–12 hour regimen.

4. The answer is C *[II B 3 c].*
A patient suffering from pain cannot sleep properly. Once the pain is adequately controlled, the patient may sleep initially for many hours. This usually is not oversedation due to the narcotic. These patients should be monitored closely (e.g., respiratory rate), and other sedating drugs eliminated. Usually, no other intervention is needed.

5. The answer is D *[II A 4].*
Aspirin has several adverse effects and drug interactions. However, cardiac arrhythmias are not induced by aspirin.

6. The answer is C *[II A 2].*
Unlike the opiates, nonsteroidal anti-inflammatory drug (NSAID) use is not associated with the development of tolerance.

7. The answer is D *[Table 58-2].*
Transdermal fentanyl is a controlled-release dosage form that is effective for a 72-hour period. All of the other drugs listed in the question are effective for periods of 1–8 hours.

8. The answer is C (I,II) *[II A 4 b].*
Unlike aspirin and nonsteroidal anti-inflammatory drugs (NSAIDs), acetaminophen and choline magnesium trisalicylate lack antiplatelet effects. Therefore, they are safe to use for patients with bleeding problems.

59
Nutrition and the Hospitalized Patient

Robert A. Quercia
Kevin P. Keating

I. NUTRITIONAL PROBLEMS IN HOSPITALIZED PATIENTS

A. Incidence. It has been estimated that up to 75% of patients undergo a deterioration of nutritional status while in the hospital.

B. Definitions

1. **Malnutrition** is a pathologic state, resulting from a relative or absolute deficiency or excess of one or more essential nutrients.

2. **Marasmus** is a chronic disease that develops over months or years as a result of a deficiency in total caloric intake. Depletion of fat stores and skeletal protein occurs to meet metabolic needs. Marasmic patients are generally not hypermetabolic and are able to preserve their visceral protein compartment as determined by measurements of serum albumin, prealbumin, and transferrin.
   - **a.** Marasmus is a well-adapted form of malnutrition, and despite a cachectic appearance, immunocompetence, wound healing and the ability to handle short-term stress are generally well preserved.
   - **b.** Nutritional support in these patients should be initiated cautiously since aggressive repletion can result in severe metabolic disturbances, such as hypokalemia and hypophosphatemia.

3. **Kwashiorkor** is an acute process that can develop within weeks and is associated with visceral protein depletion and impaired immune function. It is due to poor protein intake with adequate to slightly inadequate caloric intake; thus, patients usually appear well nourished. A hypermetabolic state (e.g., trauma, infection) combined with protein deprivation can rapidly develop into a severe kwashiorkor malnutrition characterized by hypoalbuminemia, edema, and impaired cellular immune function.
   - **a.** In hospitalized patients, the development of kwashiorkor has been implicated in poor wound healing, gastrointestinal bleeding, and sepsis.
   - **b.** Aggressive nutritional support to replete protein stores and decrease morbidity and mortality is indicated when the diagnosis of kwashiorkor is made.

4. **Mixed marasmic kwashiorkor** is a severe form of protein–calorie malnutrition that usually develops when a marasmic patient is subjected to an acute hypermetabolic stress, such as trauma, surgery, or infection.
   - **a.** This condition results in depletion of fat stores, skeletal muscle protein, and visceral protein.
   - **b.** Because of the marked immune dysfunction that develops in this state, vigorous nutritional support is indicated.

II. NUTRITIONAL ASSESSMENT AND METABOLIC REQUIREMENTS

A. Nutritional assessment. The two most commonly used tools for nutritional assessment are discussed below.

1. **Subjective global assessment** (SGA) relies heavily on the patient's history.
   - **a.** SGA takes into account:
     - **(1)** Recent weight change

(2) Diet history
(3) Type and length of symptoms impacting on nutritional status (e.g., nausea, vomiting, diarrhea)
(4) Functional status
(5) Metabolic demands of the current disease process
(6) Gross physical signs
(a) Status of subcutaneous fat
(b) Evidence of muscle wasting
(c) The presence or absence of edema and ascites

b. Patients are then classified as being well nourished or moderately or severely malnourished.

2. Prognostic nutritional index (PNI) is derived from a formula that attempts to quantify a patient's risk of developing complications based on a variety of markers of nutritional status.

a. Serum markers (i.e., albumin, transferrin) are indicators of visceral protein status.

b. Anthropomorphic measurement (i.e., triceps skin fold thickness) is an indicator of subcutaneous fat stores.

c. Delayed hypersensitivity reaction is an indicator of immune competence.

B. Metabolic requirements

1. Energy requirements are determined as **nonprotein calories (NPC)**. It is important to avoid excess calories to minimize complications of nutrient delivery and to optimize nutrient metabolism. Energy requirements can be determined by the following three methods:

a. Indirect calorimetry or measured energy expenditure (MEE) is the most accurate method of determining caloric requirements. Oxygen consumption and carbon dioxide production are measured directly. Energy expenditure is related directly to oxygen consumption and is calculated from these measurements.

b. Estimated energy expenditure (EEE) first requires the calculation of the **basal energy expenditure (BEE)** from the **Harris-Benedict equation;** the BEE is then multiplied by appropriate stress and activity factors.

(1) Men. BEE = 66.5 + 13.8 wt (kg) + [5 × ht (cm)] − [6.8 × age (years)]
(2) Women. BEE = 655 + 9.6 wt (kg) + [1.8 x ht (cm)] − [4.7 x age (years)]
(3) **Stress factors:** uncomplicated surgery 1.00–1.05, peritonitis 1.05–1.25, and sepsis or multiple trauma 1.25–1.5
(4) **Activity factors:** bed rest 0.95–1.10 and ambulation 1.10–1.30

c. Simple nomogram. The least accurate method of estimating caloric requirements, it is based on the patient's weight in kilograms. It is useful when the other methods cannot be used. Patients with mild-to-moderate degrees of stress require approximately 25–30 kcal/kg/day, while the severely stressed patient (e.g., a patient with major burns) may require as much as 35 kcal/kg/day.

2. Protein (nitrogen) requirements can be determined by a number of techniques, but nitrogen balance determinations and nomograms appear to be the most practical.

a. Nitrogen balance techniques. The practitioner determines the patient's nitrogen output and develops a nutritional support program in which the protein administered results in a nitrogen input that exceeds losses.

(1) Nitrogen balance = 24-hour nitrogen intake − 24-hour nitrogen output.
(2) A 24-hour nitrogen intake = 24-hour total protein intake, divided by 6.25 (approximately 16% of protein is comprised of nitrogen).
(3) A 24-hour nitrogen output = [24-hour urine urea nitrogen (UUN) x 1.25] + 2, where 1.25 accounts for nonurea urine nitrogen losses (e.g., ammonia, creatinine) and 2 accounts for nonurine nitrogen losses (e.g., skin, feces).
(4) A positive nitrogen balance of 3–6 g is the goal.
(5) This method cannot be used in renally impaired patients.

b. Nomogram method. This method estimates protein needs based on lean body weight. Protein requirements are 1.5–2.0 g protein/kg/day for hospitalized patients.

c. Nonprotein calorie to nitrogen (NPC:N) ratio. A NPC:N ratio of 125–150:1 has been generally recommended for the mildly to moderately stressed patient to achieve optimal nitrogen retention and protein synthesis. In the severely stressed patient, a lower ratio (100:1) may be more effective.

3. **Essential fatty acids**
   a. **Linoleic acid** cannot be synthesized by humans. It is a primary component of cell membranes and is required for prostaglandin synthesis.
   b. Deficiency states are characterized by diarrhea, dermatitis, and hair loss.
   c. The currently available lipid emulsions have a high linoleic acid content.
   d. Providing 4%–7% of a patient's caloric requirements as linoleic acid from lipid emulsion prevents the development of essential fatty acid deficiency.

4. **Vitamins** are essential for proper substrate metabolism. Accepted daily allowances for oral administration have been established, but there is less of a consensus on recommendations for intravenous administration.
   a. **Vitamin A** (fat soluble). Normal stores can last up to a year but are rapidly depleted by stress. Vitamin A has essential functions in vision, growth, and reproduction. Recommended oral intake is 2500–5000 IU/day. Intravenous requirements are 2800–8000 IU/day secondary to binding of the intravenous form to glass and plastic.
   b. **Vitamin D** (fat soluble). In conjunction with parathormone and calcitonin, vitamin D helps to regulate calcium and phosphorous homeostasis. Recommended intake is 100–400 IU/day. Intravenous requirements are 200–400 IU/day.
   c. **Vitamin E** (fat soluble) appears to function as an antioxidant, inhibiting the oxidation of free unsaturated fatty acids. Recommended daily oral allowances are 12–15 IU/day. Suggested intravenous requirements are 2.1–60 IU/day. The presence of polyunsaturated fatty acids increases the requirement for vitamin E, a fact that needs to be taken into account with the use of lipid system parenteral nutrition (PN).
   d. **Vitamin K** (fat soluble) plays an essential role in the synthesis of clotting factors. The suggested oral intake is 0.7–2.0 mg/day.
   e. **Vitamin B_1 (thiamine)** [water soluble] functions as a coenzyme in the phosphogluconate pathway and as a structural component of nervous system membranes. The development of its deficiency state (i.e., acute pernicious beriberi with high output cardiac failure) is well described in patients on PN receiving inadequate thiamine replacement. A prolonged deficiency state can cause Wernicke's encephalopathy. Recommended doses are 0.5 mg/1000 oral calories/day and 3–21 mg/day on PN.
   f. **Vitamin B_2 (riboflavin)** [water soluble] functions as a coenzyme in oxidative phosphorylation. Essentially, no intracellular stores are maintained. Oral requirements are 1.3–1.7 mg/day. Intravenous requirements are 3.6–7.5 mg/day.
   g. **Vitamin B_3 (niacin)** [water soluble] functions as a coenzyme in oxidative phosphorylation and biosynthetic pathways. Pellagra is the well-described deficiency state. Oral requirements are 14.5–19.8 mg/day. Intravenous requirements are 40–140 mg/day.
   h. **Vitamin B_5 (pantothenic acid)** [water soluble]. The functional form of vitamin B_5 is coenzyme A, which is essential to all acylation reactions. Oral requirements are 5–10 mg/day. Intravenous requirements are 10–29 mg/day.
   i. **Vitamin B_6 (pyridoxine)** [water soluble] functions as a coenzyme in a variety of enzymatic pathways. Deficiency states are accentuated by some medications, including isoniazid, penicillamine, and cycloserine. Oral requirements are 1.5–2.0 mg/day. Intravenous requirements are 4.0–6.3 mg/day.
   j. **Vitamin B_7 (biotin)** [water soluble] functions in carboxylation reactions. It is synthesized by intestinal flora; therefore, deficiency states are rare. Intravenous requirements are 60 μg/day.
   k. **Vitamin B_9 (folic acid)** [water soluble] is involved in a variety of biosynthetic reactions and amino acid conversions. Stores usually last 3–6 months; however, rapid depletion is seen with metabolic stress. Deficiency of vitamin B_{12} causes deficiency in folate. A megaloblastic anemia is classic in the deficiency state. Oral requirements are 200–400 μg/day. Intravenous requirements are 0.4–1.0 mg/day.
   l. **Vitamin B_{12} (cyanocobalamin)** [water soluble] has a variety of metabolic and biosynthetic functions. Because of large stores, deficiency states can take years to develop. Megaloblastic (pernicious) anemia is one manifestation of deficiency. Oral requirements are 2–3 μg/day. Intravenous requirements are 5.0–15 μg/day.
   m. **Vitamin C (ascorbic acid)** [water soluble] has a variety of metabolic and biosynthetic functions, including collagen synthesis. Body stores are minimal. A deficiency state results in the clinical syndrome of scurvy. No specific requirement has been recommended. Recommended oral intake is 30–45 mg/day. Intravenous requirements are 100–500 mg/day.

5. **Trace mineral deficiency** may develop during PN because of reduced intake, increased use, decreased plasma binding, or increased excretion.
   a. **Iron** is necessary for hemoglobin and myoglobin production and is a necessary cofactor in a variety of enzymatic reactions. Deficiency is classically demonstrated by a hypochromic, microcytic anemia as well as by the development of immune deficiency. Oral requirements are 16–18 mg/day. Intravenous requirements are 0.5–1.0 mg/day.
   b. **Zinc** is necessary for DNA and RNA synthesis and is a necessary cofactor in a variety of enzymatic reactions. Zinc deficiency results in impaired wound healing, growth retardation, hair loss, dermatitis, diarrhea, anorexia, and glucose intolerance. Patients at high risk for developing zinc deficiency are those with long-term steroid therapy, malabsorption syndromes, fistulas, sepsis, and major surgery. Oral requirements are 10–15 mg/day. Intravenous requirements are 2.5–4.0 mg/day.
   c. **Copper** is necessary for heme synthesis, electron transport, and wound healing. Deficiency that develops during PN usually manifests as anemia, leukopenia, and neutropenia. Oral requirements are 30 μg/kg/day. Intravenous requirements are 20 μg/kg/day (0.5–1.5 mg/day).
   d. **Manganese** is involved in protein synthesis and possibly glucose use. Oral requirements are 0.7–22 mg/day. Intravenous requirements are 2–10 μg/kg/day (0.1–0.8 mg/day).
   e. **Selenium** is important in antioxidant reactions. Deficiency during PN has been associated with muscle pain and cardiomyopathy. Intravenous requirements are 20–40 μg/day.
   f. **Iodine** is a component of the thyroid hormones. Deficiency manifests as a goiter. Recommended intake is 1 μg/kg/day.
   g. **Chromium** is important in glucose use and potentiates the effect of insulin. Signs of deficiency include hyperglycemia and abnormal glucose tolerance. Oral requirements are 70–80 μg/day. Intravenous requirements are 0.14–0.2 μg/kg/day (10–15 μg/day).
   h. **Molybdenum** is essential to xanthine oxidase. Oral requirements are 2.0 μg/kg/day.

III. METHODS OF SUPPORT

A. **Parenteral nutrition** (PN) is also called **total parenteral nutrition** (TPN) and **hyperalimentation**. It is used to meet the patient's nutritional requirements when this cannot be accomplished by the enteral route.

1. **Indications.** When the enteral route cannot be used because of dysfunction or disease states (e.g., acute pancreatitis, inflammatory bowel disease, complete bowel obstruction), PN is instituted.

2. **Initiation of PN** should be undertaken within 1–3 days in moderately to severely malnourished patients when the inadequacy of enteral support is anticipated for more than 5–7 days. In healthy or mildly malnourished patients, PN should be initiated within 5–7 days if enteral support has not been initiated.

3. **Routes of administration**
   a. **Central venous route** is used with hypertonic PN formulations (i.e., dextrose concentrations greater than 10%). Most commonly, dextrose concentrations of 25% are used centrally, and the osmolarity exceeds 2000 mOsm/L. Such highly osmolar solutions must be infused into a large diameter central vein (e.g., superior vena cava) where they are rapidly diluted by high flow rates.
   b. **Peripheral venous route** can be used when the dextrose concentration is 10% or less. However, solutions with 10% dextrose, amino acids, electrolytes, and trace minerals have a resulting osmolarity of 900–1000 mOsm/L. The hypertonicity of this solution can result in phlebitis and frequent intravenous site changes. Peripheral PN is better tolerated with a dextrose concentration of 5% administered concurrently with a lipid emulsion.

4. **NPC sources**
   a. **Dextrose monohydrate** is the form of dextrose used for parenteral administration. It yields 3.4 kcal/g. It is the component in PN formulas that contributes the most to osmolarity. It is available commercially in concentrations up to 70%.
   b. **Intravenous lipids** are commercially available as 10% or 20% emulsions derived from soybean oil (Intralipid) or a combination of soybean oil and safflower oil (Liposyn II).
      (1) Both the 10% and 20% emulsions are isotonic (280 and 340 mOsm/L) and can be administered via the peripheral vein with a low incidence of phlebitis; they provide 1.1 and 2.0 kcal/cc, respectively.

(2) Lipid emulsions can be given as part of the daily NPC requirement or 2–3 times per week to prevent essential fatty acid deficiency. Both types of lipid emulsion contain particles of 0.4–0.5 μm, which prevents the use of 0.22 μm bacterial retention filters.

5. Protein (nitrogen) source. Synthetic crystalline amino acids are currently used as the nitrogen source in PN formulations.

a. They are available commercially in concentrations of 3.5%, 5.5%, 7%, 8.5%, 10%, 11.4%, and 15%.

b. They yield 4 kcal/g.

c. These solutions generally contain a mixture of free essential and nonessential L-amino acids.

d. Specialized amino acid formulations are available for specific disease states.

6. Systems of PN

a. Glucose system PN

(1) Definitions. The glucose system PN is a parenteral formulation in which dextrose is used exclusively as the NPC source. Nitrogen is provided as crystalline amino acids. Electrolytes, vitamins, and trace minerals are added to the formulation as needed.

(2) Administration. The glucose system PN formulations usually have dextrose concentrations of 25% or greater and must be administered by the central venous route. They are also referred to as two-in-one formulations since the dextrose and amino acids are usually mixed in one container with electrolytes, vitamins, and trace minerals.

(a) Because of the high dextrose concentration, initial administration should be at low hourly rates (e.g., 50 cc/hr) and increased gradually over 24 hours to avoid hyperglycemia (> 200 mg/dl).

(b) To avoid reactive hypoglycemia (< 70 mg/dl), discontinuation should be gradual over 24 hours.

(c) Lipid emulsions should be administered for **essential fatty acid replacement** in a dose that provides 4%–7% of required calories as linoleic acid. This can be accomplished by the administration of 250 ml of 20% or 500 ml of 10% emulsion, two to three times per week.

b. Lipid system PN

(1) Definition. The lipid system PN is a parenteral formulation in which lipid is administered daily to provide a substantial proportion of the NPC. Nitrogen is provided as crystalline amino acids. Electrolytes, vitamins, and trace minerals are added to the formulation as needed.

(2) Administration. The lipid system PN is administered peripherally when the dextrose concentration is less than or equal to 10% and centrally when the dextrose concentration is more than 10%.

(a) Piggyback method. The solution with amino acids, dextrose, electrolytes, trace minerals, and vitamins is infused concurrently with a separate bottle of lipid emulsion through a Y site on the intravenous administration set.

(b) Total nutrient admixture method (TNA, three-in-one, all-in-one). Lipids, amino acids, dextrose, electrolytes, trace minerals, and vitamins are mixed in one container and administered by the central or peripheral route, depending on dextrose concentration.

(i) Advantages include simplification of administration and decreased training time for home PN patients.

(ii) Disadvantages include the inability to inspect for particulate matter in the opaque admixture, the inability to use 0.22 μm bacterial retention filters, and stability problems.

(c) Lipid dosage

(i) Lipid calories should not exceed 60% of total daily calories, including protein calories.

(ii) Maximum dosage of lipids for adults is 2.5 g/kg/day.

(iii) Baseline and weekly serum triglycerides must be monitored in patients on lipid system PN.

(3) Adverse effects of lipids are uncommon. The most frequent adverse effects include fever, chills, sensation of warmth, chest pain, back pain, vomiting, and urticaria (overall incidence < 1%). Severe hypoxemia has been reported with rapid infusion of lipid emulsion.

7. **Additives**
   a. **Electrolytes.** PN formulations must include adequate amounts of sodium, magnesium, calcium, chloride, potassium, phosphorous, and acetate. The intracellular "anabolic" electrolytes—potassium, magnesium, and phosphate—are essential for protein synthesis. Requirements vary widely, depending on a patient's fluid and electrolyte losses; renal, hepatic, and endocrine status; acid–base balance; metabolic rate; and type of PN formula used. The electrolyte composition of the PN formula must be adjusted to meet the needs of the individual patient.
   b. **Vitamins and trace minerals.** Vitamins are usually added to PN solutions in the form of commercially available multivitamin preparations containing the recommended daily allowances. Because of stability problems, these preparations usually consist of two vials or a dual chamber vial. One vial or chamber contains vitamins A, D, E, B_1, B_2, B_3, B_5, B_6, and C. The second vial or chamber contains vitamins B_{12}, biotin, and folic acid. Trace minerals may be added individually or as a commercially available multielement preparation. Precise requirements for trace minerals have yet to be determined.
   c. **Insulin** may be required for patients receiving PN formulations (especially glucose system PN) to maintain blood glucose levels less than 200 mg/dl. If insulin is required, it is best provided by the addition of an appropriate amount of regular insulin to the PN formulation at the time of admixture. Although a small amount of insulin (5–10 units per bag) may be adsorbed to the container and tubing, such losses can be overcome by appropriate titration of the dose. The addition of insulin to the PN formulation has the advantage of changes in the rate of PN infusion being automatically accompanied by appropriate changes in the rate of insulin infusion.
   d. **Miscellaneous drugs.** A number of medications have been successfully admixed with PN formulations for continuous infusion. The H_2-receptor antagonists are the most common drugs used in this way. The routine addition of medications to PN formulations remains controversial because of:
      (1) Questions of stability over the wide range of PN component concentrations
      (2) Possible therapeutic inadequacy or toxicity secondary to PN rate changes and loss of peak and trough levels
      (3) Increased potential for waste with dose changes

8. **Complications** with the use of PN can be serious and potentially life-threatening but can be avoided by careful management. Complications can be divided into mechanical, infectious, and metabolic.
   a. **Mechanical complications** generally relate to the central venous catheter or its placement and include pneumothorax, catheter occlusion, and venous thrombosis.
   b. **Infectious complications** are also related to the central venous catheter. This line-related sepsis is secondary to multiple catheter manipulations, contamination during insertion, or contamination during routine maintenance.
   c. **Metabolic complications** are the most numerous. These commonly include: hyperglycemia, hypoglycemia, hypokalemia, hypomagnesemia, hypophosphatemia, metabolic acidosis, respiratory acidosis, prerenal azotemia, and zinc deficiency.

B. Enteral nutrition (EN). Use of the gastrointestinal tract to achieve total nutritional support or partial support in combination with the parenteral route should be attempted whenever possible in the face of inadequate oral intake. Theoretic advantages include maintenance of normal digestion, absorption, and gut mucosal barrier function.

1. **Contraindications** to EN include complete intestinal obstruction, high output intestinal fistulas, severe acute pancreatitis, severe acute inflammatory bowel disease, and severe diarrhea.

2. **Routes of administration.** Tube feedings can be administered via nasogastric, nasoduodenal, nasojejunal, gastrostomy, and jejunostomy tubes.

3. **EN formulations** can be classified as being standard (complete) or modular.
   a. **Standard formulas** generally contain carbohydrates, fats, vitamins, trace minerals, and a nitrogen source. They are further classified according to their nitrogen source.
      (1) **Monomeric formulas** contain crystalline amino acids as their nitrogen source. They are usually marketed commercially for specific indications (e.g., ileus, pancreatitis, hepatic coma).

(2) **Short-chain peptide formulas** contain di- and tripeptides from hydrolyzed protein or de novo synthesis as their nitrogen source. They are currently marketed for the metabolically stressed patient.

(3) **Polymeric formulas** contain either intact proteins or protein hydrolysates as their nitrogen source. Most patients can be managed with these formulas.

b. **Modular formulas** consist of separate modules of specific nutrients that can be combined or administered separately. They are used for supplemental use or to custom-design an EN formula to meet a specific clinical situation.

(1) **Carbohydrate modules** differ in the type of carbohydrate present (e.g., polysaccharides, disaccharides, monosaccharides).

(2) **Protein modules** contain either intact protein, hydrolyzed protein, or crystalline amino acids.

(3) **Fat modules** contain either long-chain triglycerides (LCT) prepared from vegetable oils or medium-chain triglycerides (MCT) prepared from coconut oil. MCT are more water soluble and more easily absorbed than LCT. (Bypassing the intestinal lacteal and lymphatic system, MCT are transported directly to the portal system.) MCT are, however, relatively expensive and contain no essential fatty acids.

4. **Complications.** The two most common complications of EN are diarrhea and improper tube placement.

a. **Diarrhea** in patients receiving EN is usually secondary to concomitant administration of medication (e.g., antibiotics). Infectious etiologies should be eliminated (e.g., *Clostridium difficile*), after which antidiarrheal medications may be beneficial. Reducing the rate or concentration may also be effective.

b. **A feeding tube improperly placed** into the tracheo-bronchial tree can have disastrous implications. Tube feedings should never be initiated without radiologic verification of tube position.

IV. MONITORING SUPPORT

A. **Parenteral nutrition (PN).** In addition to appropriate general medical and nursing care, patients receiving PN initially require daily and weekly laboratory monitoring to assess nutritional progress and metabolic status.

1. **Electrolytes**

a. **Potassium, sodium, and chloride** should be determined daily initially. Potassium is used intracellularly; thus, hypokalemia is not an uncommon finding.

b. **Calcium, magnesium, and phosphate** are primarily intracellular electrolytes, serum levels of which become depleted during protein synthesis. Serum levels generally do not fall as rapidly as potassium; therefore, monitoring two to three times a week is recommended initially until the patient is stabilized, then weekly thereafter

c. **Bicarbonate** should be monitored to assess acid–base balance. Hyperchloremic metabolic acidosis may develop in patients on PN. This imbalance can be corrected by providing the potassium and sodium as acetate (converted to bicarbonate in the serum) rather than as the chloride salt. After initial correction, provision of one-half the sodium and potassium requirements as the acetate salt and one-half as the chloride salt may be beneficial.

2. **Serum glucose** should be monitored daily, especially in central glucose systems. Maintaining a blood glucose concentration between 100–200 mg/dl is generally recommended.

3. **Weights** obtained on a daily or every other day basis track optimum lean body weight gain of 1/4–1/2 lb/day. Weight gain in excess of 1/2 lb/day generally indicates fluid overload or fat deposition.

4. **Visceral proteins** (e.g., albumin, prealbumin, transferrin) are important indicators of the adequacy of nutritional support.

a. **Albumin** is useful in the initial assessment of nutritional status, but its long half-life (18–21 days) limits its utility as a short-term marker of nutritional repletion.

b. **Prealbumin** has a short half-life (2–3 days) and is a more sensitive and early indicator of the adequacy of nutritional support. Its serum value is falsely elevated in renal failure.

c. **Transferrin** has an intermediate half-life (7–10 days), which makes weekly monitoring useful. Transferrin may be falsely elevated in iron-deficiency states.

5. **Serum creatinine and blood urea nitrogen (BUN)** should be obtained at least weekly. Evidence of renal impairment may require modification of the PN formula. Elevation of the BUN in the absence of renal impairment may be secondary to the PN formula (e.g., excess nitrogen, low NPC:N ratio) and appropriate adjustments need to be made.

6. **Liver function tests** [aspartate aminotransferase (AST), alanine aminotransferase (ALT), alkaline phosphatase, lactate dehydrogenase (LDH), bilirubin] require weekly monitoring because of potential toxicity from the PN formulation (i.e., fatty infiltration of the liver). Abnormal liver function studies may necessitate changes in the PN formulation.

7. **Serum triglycerides** should be measured for a baseline and weekly thereafter for patients on lipid system PN. It is not necessary to monitor triglycerides on a weekly basis for patients receiving lipids two to three times per week for essential fatty acid replacement.

8. **Twenty-four hour UUN** should be obtained weekly to determine nitrogen balance for patients in whom nitrogen requirements are uncertain. These are usually highly stressed, severely ill, or injured patients in an intensive care unit (ICU) setting.

9. **Serum iron** levels should be obtained weekly to determine deficiency and to allow appropriate interpretation of serum transferrin levels.

B. **Enteral nutrition** (EN) generally requires less intense laboratory monitoring. Specific laboratory guidelines for monitoring EN support varies from institution to institution.

V. DISEASE-SPECIFIC SUPPORT

A. **Nutritional support for renal failure.** The goal of nutritional support in acute renal failure (ARF) is to meet the patient's NPC requirements while minimizing volume, protein load, and potential electrolyte imbalance.

1. **PN formulations** used in ARF are low-nitrogen, high-caloric density formulas (e.g., 2% amino acid/47% dextrose), resulting in NPC:N ratios of approximately 500:1.

2. **Commercial renal failure formulations,** (e.g., Nephramine, RenAmin, Aminosyn RF), containing primarily essential amino acids, have shown no clinical advantage over less expensive, low-concentration standard amino acid formulations.

3. **Standard glucose system formulation** (4.25% amino acid/25% dextrose) can generally be used in renal failure patients who are being dialyzed on a regular basis. This can provide adequate protein to attain positive nitrogen balance, which is not possible with renal failure PN.

4. **Monitoring transferrin** is a more sensitive and accurate visceral protein marker compared to albumin and prealbumin for assessing nutritional progress in these patients.

5. **Enteral formulations** that are low in nitrogen and calorie dense (1.7–2.0 NPC/ml) are available for patients with renal failure.

B. **Nutritional support for hepatic failure.** Patients with hepatic failure have altered protein metabolism, resulting in decreased serum levels of branched-chain amino acids (i.e., leucine, isoleucine, valine) and increased levels of aromatic amino acids (i.e., phenylalanine, tyrosine, tryptophan), methionine, and glutamine. A similar amino acid profile can exist in the cerebrospinal fluid (CSF) and is thought to contribute to hepatic encephalopathy. Fluid and electrolyte disturbances are frequently associated with hepatic failure as well.

1. **PN formulations** enriched in branched-chain amino acids (36%) and low in aromatic amino acids (e.g., Hepatamine) improve mental status in patients with altered serum amino acid profiles and hepatic encephalopathy. However, studies have not demonstrated definitive clinical differences in morbidity and mortality with these expensive formulations compared to standard formulas.

2. **Adequate NPC** with a 20–40 g/day protein load (e.g., 2% amino acid/25% dextrose) is an alternative approach to the use of hepatic failure amino acid formulations. Protein load can be slowly liberalized as long as mental status does not deteriorate.

3. **EN formulations** (e.g., Hepatic-Aid II) enriched with branched-chain amino acids and low in aromatic amino acids are commercially available for patients with hepatic failure.

C. Nutritional support for respiratory failure. The type and amount of substrate administered as NPC can have an impact upon a patient's ventilatory status. Overfeeding results in lipogenesis, which produces eight times the amount of carbon dioxide produced by glycolysis. This increased carbon dioxide load requires an increase in minute ventilation or respiratory acidosis ensues. Even in the presence of appropriate amounts of NPC administered as carbohydrate, the carbon dioxide load generated by glycolysis may be excessive for the patient with underlying pulmonary dysfunction [e.g., chronic obstructive pulmonary disease (COPD)].

1. **PN lipid system formulations** (e.g., 4.25% amino acid/15% dextrose with daily lipid emulsion) where the lipid component constitutes 40%–50% of the total NPC may be beneficial in reducing the ventilatory demands in respiratory failure patients because lipolysis generates less carbon dioxide than glycolysis.
2. **EN formulations** containing similar amounts of fat can be prepared from standard EN formulas with the use of lipid modules (i.e., MCT oil, corn oil). More expensive commercial pulmonary formulas are also available.

D. Nutritional support for cardiac failure. The goal in these patients is to meet metabolic needs while restricting fluid and sodium intake.

1. **PN formulations** that provide protein and calories in as high a concentration as possible is the goal of nutritional therapy. This can be accomplished with both central glucose or lipid system PN formulations (e.g., 5% amino acid/35% dextrose; 7% amino acid/21% dextrose/20% lipid emulsion).
2. **Serum electrolyte monitoring and adjustment** are imperative in cardiac failure patients receiving PN, especially when potent diuretics are used concurrently.
3. **EN formulations** with high nutrient density are available for oral supplementation or tube feedings. Infusion of enteral tube feedings should begin at 1/3–1/2 strength with a gradual increase in concentration, while maintaining a slow infusion rate (30–50 cc/hr) to avoid rapid increases in fluid load, cardiac output, heart rate, and myocardial oxygen consumption.

E. Nutritional support in pancreatitis. Severe acute pancreatitis is a hypercatabolic state that without nutritional support renders the patient a poor surgical candidate and at increased risk of infection. The goal of nutritional support in severe acute pancreatitis is to "rest" the pancreas by limiting exocrine stimulation while providing adequate nutrition.

1. **PN** is generally favored over EN to achieve this goal in the early phases of pancreatitis. Lipid system PN has been shown to be safe and effective when administered to these patients, provided there is no concurrent hyperlipidemia; in fact, it may be valuable in the patient with recalcitrant hyperglycemia.
2. **EN,** using chemically defined (elemental), low-fat formulas administered into the jejunum, results in minimal pancreatic stimulation and has been used safely in these patients.

VI. TECHNICAL ASPECTS OF PARENTERAL NUTRITION (PN) PREPARATIONS

A. PN formula preparation is performed **aseptically** in the pharmacy under a laminar flow hood that filters the air, removing airborne particles and microorganisms.

B. Compatibility of the various components of PN formulations is determined by a number of factors, including their concentration, solution pH, temperature, and the order of admixture. The most common compatibility concern regards the addition of calcium and phosphate salts to PN solutions.

C. Following admixture of the various components, the PN solution should be **visually inspected** for precipitate or particulate matter. After labeling and final checking, the PN solution should be refrigerated until delivery to the nursing unit.

D. A statistically valid, continuous **sterility testing program** should be an essential component of quality control in preparing PN solutions.

VII. HOME PARENTERAL NUTRITION (HPN). HPN has become a widely accepted and useful technique for provision of complete nutritional requirements in the home setting. When used appropriately, this modality benefits the patient medically and psychologically with a decreased cost to the health care system.

A. Indications for HPN include short bowel syndrome, severe inflammatory bowel disease, radiation enteritis, enterocutaneous fistulae, and selected malignancies.

B. Candidate selection requires a multidisciplinary approach to determine if the patient and family can assume the responsibility and training needed for safe and successful HPN.

C. Administration. HPN is infused through a central venous silastic catheter (e.g., Hickman, Broviac), which allows for prolonged PN with low clotting and infection rates. The PN solution is generally infused over a 12–15-hour period at night. This type of **cycling program** allows the patient to be free from the infusion pump during the day, allowing for a more normal life-style.

D. Clinical monitoring and follow-up are done periodically, depending on the needs of the individual patient. Long-term HPN patients are generally seen by the physician on a monthly basis after initial stabilization.

VIII. MISCELLANEOUS AGENTS

A. Glutamine. This amino acid is a component of some EN formulations. Glutamine is known to be used as a fuel source by enterocytes. It also may have trophic effects on the gut mucosa. Whether the free form of this amino acid is necessary is controversial. Because of its instability, glutamine is not present in currently available PN amino acid solutions.

B. Omega 3 polyunsaturated fatty acids are derived from fish oils and are currently found in some EN formulations. They have been shown experimentally to enhance immune responses. They are not found in the currently available lipid emulsions used for PN.

C. Arginine. This amino acid has been shown experimentally to enhance immune responsiveness. Specialized EN formulations enriched with free arginine are available commercially.

D. Soluble fiber is present in some commercially available EN formulas. It is fermented by normal large intestinal flora to short-chain fatty acids that are used by colonocytes as a fuel source. These short-chain fatty acids also seem to have a trophic effect on the large intestinal mucosa.

STUDY QUESTIONS

Directions: Each of the numbered items or incomplete statements in this section is followed by answers or by completions of the statement. Select the **one** lettered answer or completion that is **best** in each case.

1. A hospitalized patient with low visceral proteins (albumin, 1.9; transferrin, 90), normal somatic proteins, and normal body weight is

(A) suffering from severe marasmic malnutrition
(B) at low risk for hospital-acquired infection and other complications
(C) suffering from severe kwashiorkor malnutrition
(D) suffering from mixed marasmic kwashiorkor
(E) suffering from chronic malnutrition

2. Which of the following methods would be the most accurate in assessing the calorie requirements of a critically ill patient in the intensive care unit (ICU)?

(A) Estimated energy expenditure (EEE)
(B) Nomogram
(C) Measured energy expenditure (MEE)
(D) Prognostic nutritional index (PNI)
(E) Nitrogen balance

3. Which of the following statements concerning parenteral nutrition (PN) is true?

(A) It is indicated after 7 days for patients with severe malnutrition who are unable to meet their needs by the enteral route
(B) It is indicated within 5–7 days for patients who are well nourished on admission but unable to meet their needs by the enteral route
(C) It should never be administered to patients who can take any food by mouth
(D) It is contraindicated for use in the home setting
(E) It is more effective than enteral nutrition (EN)

4. Which of the following statements concerning glucose system parenteral nutrition (PN) is true?

(A) It requires central venous administration
(B) It should be discontinued without tapering
(C) It requires the daily administration of lipid emulsion
(D) It cannot provide adequate calories for the highly stressed patient
(E) It requires daily serum triglyceride monitoring

5. Which of the following statements regarding the monitoring of patients on nutritional support is true?

(A) Albumin is the best marker to follow short-term nutritional progress
(B) Prealbumin is the best marker to follow in patients with renal failure
(C) Transferrin is falsely decreased in iron-deficiency states
(D) Optimal lean body weight gain is 1/4–1/2 lb/day
(E) Optimal positive nitrogen balance is greater than 8–10 g of nitrogen a day

6. A patient in acute renal failure (ARF) not on regular dialysis would benefit most from which of the following parenteral nutrition (PN) programs?

(A) 4.25% amino acid/25% dextrose
(B) 7% amino acid/21% dextrose/20% lipid emulsion
(C) 2% amino acid/47% dextrose
(D) 2% amino acid/5% dextrose
(E) 2% amino acid/25% dextrose

7. Which amino acid solution would be best tolerated in patients with liver disease and encephalopathy?

(A) Low–branched-chain, high-aromatic amino acid solution
(B) Essential amino acid solution
(C) Low-aromatic, high–branched-chain amino acid solution
(D) Glutamine-enriched amino acid solution
(E) Methionine- and cysteine-enriched amino acid solution

1-C	4-A	7-C
2-C	5-D	
3-B	6-C	

Questions 8–10

A 57-year-old man involved in a motor vehicle accident sustains severe chest and abdominal injuries. After resuscitation, he is brought to the operating room where he undergoes a splenectomy, partial hepatectomy, segmental small bowel resection, and insertion of a feeding jejunostomy. He is in the intensive care unit (ICU) and on a ventilator. The attending surgeon would like him started on tube feedings beginning on the first postoperative day. His prior history is significant for tobacco abuse and moderate emphysema. He is 175 cm tall and weighs 100 kg. The indirect calorimeter is currently unavailable to ascertain his energy requirements.

8. The best estimate of this patient's nonprotein calorie (NPC) needs would be

(A) 2900–3400 NPC
(B) 2400–2900 NPC
(C) 1900–2400 NPC
(D) 1400–1900 NPC
(E) 900–1400 NPC

Six days after initiating enteral support, the patient develops a small bowel fistula at the site of his small bowel anastomosis. His 24-hour urine urea nitrogen (UUN) is 15. He is switched to parenteral nutrition (PN) using Aminosyn 4.25% (6.7 g of nitrogen per liter).

9. To meet the patient's previously calculated needs and put him in positive nitrogen balance, this patient would require

(A) 47% dextrose/4.25% amino acid at 150 cc/hr
(B) 25% dextrose/4.25% amino acid at 150 cc/hr
(C) 47% dextrose/4.25% amino acid at 135 cc/hr
(D) 25% dextrose/4.25% amino acid at 135 cc/hr
(E) 47% dextrose/4.25% amino acid at 75 cc/hr

10. Concerned about a persistent respiratory acidosis and a high minute ventilation, the physician obtains a measured energy expenditure (MEE), which indicates that the patient is not being overfed. He switches the patient to lipid system PN. The order calls for a 15% dextrose/4.25% amino acid/insulin/cimetidine formulation at 135 cc/hr with 500 cc of 20% lipid emulsion per day. The physician is concerned about the order because

(A) the resultant NPC:N ratio is unacceptable
(B) the cimetidine is incompatible with the insulin in the formulation
(C) the lipid administration is excessive
(D) lipid system PN is contraindicated in patients on mechanical ventilation
(E) none of the above

8-B
9-D
10-E

ANSWERS AND EXPLANATIONS

1. The answer is C *[I B 3].*
Kwashiorkor is an acute process that can develop within weeks. It is associated with visceral protein depletion and impaired immune function.

2. The answer is C *[II B 1 a].*
Measured energy expenditure (MEE) is the most accurate method of determining caloric requirements. It is especially beneficial in severely ill patients in whom stress factors are variable.

3. The answer is B *[III A 2].*
Parenteral nutrition (PN) should be initiated within 5–7 days in healthy or mildly malnourished patients if enteral support is inadequate. In moderately to severely malnourished patients, PN should be undertaken within 1–3 days if enteral support is inadequate.

4. The answer is A *[III A 6 a (2)].*
Glucose system parenteral nutrition (PN) formulations usually have a dextrose concentration of 25% or greater and must be administered by the central venous route. These highly osmolar solutions (2000 mOsm/L) are rapidly diluted by high flow rates in large diameter central veins.

5. The answer is D *[IV A 3].*
Weights obtained on a daily or every other day basis are used to track the optimal lean body weight gain of 1/4–1/2 lb/day. Weight gain in excess of this amount generally indicates fluid overload or fat deposition.

6. The answer is C *[V A 1].*
Parenteral nutrition (PN) formulations for use in acute renal failure (ARF) are high-caloric density, low-nitrogen formulas that can meet caloric requirements in a small volume and with a small protein load. They are used until renal failure resolves or dialysis is undertaken.

7. The answer is C *[V B 1].*
Parenteral nutrition (PN) formulations enriched in branched chain amino acids and low in aromatic amino acids have been shown to improve mental status in hepatic failure patients with altered serum amino acid profiles and encephalopathy.

8–10. The answers are: 8-B *[II B 1 b],* **9-D** *[II B 2 a],* **10-E** *[II B 2 c; III A 4, 6 b, 7 d; V C].*
Use of the Harris-Benedict equation to determine basal energy expenditure (BEE) and multiplying that by a stress factor of 1.25–1.50 for multiple trauma is the most accurate way of determining this patient's nonprotein calorie (NPC) needs in the absence of indirect calorimetry.

A mixture of 25% dextrose/4.25% amino acid at 135 cc/hr yields 2754 NPC and 22 g of nitrogen (N) [3.24 L/day; 850 NPC/L; 6.7 g N/L]. The patient's 24-hour urine urea nitrogen (UUN) was 15 g N. Nitrogen in − nitrogen out = nitrogen balance. Thus, 22 g N − [(15 g N × 1.25) + 2 g N] = + 1 g N.

The nonprotein calories to nitrogen (NPC:N) ratio is an acceptable 122:1. Cimetidine can be added to the parenteral nutrition (PN) to run as a continuous infusion. This patient is receiving 1 g fat/kg/day (31% of total calories as lipid). Lipid system PN is sometimes beneficial in patients with underlying pulmonary disease.

Appendix A: Prescription Dispensing Information and Metrology

Prescriptions

PARTS OF A PRESCRIPTION

A prescription is an order for medication issued by a physician, dentist, veterinarian, or other properly licensed medical practitioner (prescriber) to be filled by a pharmacist and used by the patient. Medication orders are similar to prescriptions but are intended for patients in an institutional setting.

A prescription generally contains the following information:

1. Name, address, and age of the patient
2. Date on which the prescription was written
3. Superscription symbol, or ℞, meaning "take thou" or "recipe"
4. Inscription, the name and amount of medication prescribed
5. Subscription, the dispensing and compounding instructions to the pharmacist
6. Signa or Sig, the directions to the patient
7. Signature of the prescriber
8. Name, address, and telephone number of the prescriber
9. Drug Enforcement Agency (DEA) registry number for controlled substances
10. Refill information

The following is an example of a prescription for a common generic drug:

Noel Legraphs, M.D.
3917 Wellspring Lane
Boston, MA 02115

(617) 123-4567 Date: 2/05/93

Name: John Smith Age: 28
Address: Brookline, MA 02146

℞

Penicillin VK 250 mg

Disp. tabs #40

Sig: One tablet q.i.d. × 10 days

____________________ M.D.
DEA #

Refills 1

The following is an example of a prescription that requires extemporaneous compounding:

Noel Legraphs, M.D.
3917 Wellspring Lane
Boston, MA 02115

(617) 123-4567 Date: 2/05/93

Name: John Smith Age: 28
Address: Brookline, MA 02146

℞

Codeine phosphate 0.24 g
Ammonium chloride 7.2 g
Phenergan expectorant
qs ad 120.0 ml

M. et ft syrup

Sig: One tsp q 4 to 6 hr prn cough

____________________ M.D.
DEA #

Refills 0

THE PRESCRIPTION LABEL

The prescription label should provide accurate and specific information to the patient for identification and use of the medication so that proper compliance by the patient may be attained. A prescription label usually contains the following information:

1. Pharmacy name and address
2. Prescription number
3. Date on which the prescription was dispensed
4. Name of the physician
5. Name of the patient
6. Directions for use of the medication
7. Name of the medication, including potency and quantity. A compounded prescription containing more than two ingredients generally does not have all the ingredients labeled.
8. Initials of the pharmacist
9. Expiration date or beyond-use date of the medication
10. Appropriate auxiliary or cautionary labels, as needed
11. For generic medication, the manufacturer's name or abbreviation

Additional information may be included on the label according to local state law.

MEYERS	**102 MAIN ST. EVERYWHERE, PA**
711942870	**03/22/93**
JOHN SMITH	**N. LEGRAPHS, M.D.**

TAKE 1 TABLET 4 TIMES A DAY FOR 10 DAYS

0040TB REFILLS 0

PENICILLIN VK 250MG TABL
UNITE POTENCY EXP 03/94

FINISH ALL THIS MEDICATION
TAKE ON EMPTY STOMACH

AUXILIARY LABELS

Auxiliary, or cautionary, labels should attract the patient's attention and should contain special additional information regarding the use of and the precautions and/or storage conditions for the medication. Generally, auxiliary labels should use positive statements, such as "For the ear," as opposed to negative statements, such as "Not to be swallowed." If appropriate, auxiliary labels in Spanish or other languages may be helpful for the patient.

An auxiliary label for suspensions and emulsions might read "Shake well"; for heat-sensitive materials such as insulin, "Keep in refrigerator"; for topical ointments and creams, "For external use only." A positive statement indicates exactly where the product is to be instilled or applied (e.g., "For the ear"). Warnings concerning alcohol consumption, exposure to sunlight, and possible discoloration of urine or feces may also appear on labels.

Metrology

METRIC, APOTHECARY, AND AVOIRDUPOIS SYSTEMS

Metric system

1. Basic units

Mass	=	g or gram
Length	=	m or meter
Volume	=	L or liter
		1 cc (cubic centimeter) of water is approximately equal to 1 mL and weighs 1 g.

2. Prefixes

kilo-	10^3 or 1000 times the basic unit
hekto-	10^2 or 100 times the basic unit
deka-	10 or 10 times the basic unit
deci-	10^{-1} or 0.1 times the basic unit
centi-	10^{-2} or 0.01 times the basic unit
milli-	10^{-3} or 0.001 times the basic unit
micro-	10^{-6} or one-millionth of the basic unit
nano-	10^{-9} or one-billionth of the basic unit
pico-	10^{-12} or one-trillionth of the basic unit

Examples of these prefixes include milligram (mg), which equals one-thousandth of a gram, and deciliter (dL), which equals 100 mL or 0.1 L.

Apothecary system

1. Volume (fluids or liquid)

60 minims (♏)	=	1 fluidrachm or fluidram (f ʒ) or (ʒ)
8 fluidrachms (480 minims)	=	1 fluid ounce (f ℥ or ℥)
16 fluidounces	=	1 pint (pt or 0)
2 pints (32 fluidounces)	=	1 quart (qt)
4 quarts (8 pints)	=	1 gallon (gal or C)

2. Mass (weight)

20 grains (gr)	=	1 scruple (℈)
3 scruples (60 grains)	=	1 drachm or dram (ʒ)
8 drachms (480 grains)	=	1 ounce (℥)
12 ounces (5760 grains)	=	1 pound (lb)

Avoirdupois system

1. Volume

1 fluidrachm	=	60 min.
1 fluid ounce	=	8 fl. dr.
	=	480 min.
1 pint	=	16 fl. oz.
	=	7680 min.
1 quart	=	2 pt.
	=	32 fl. oz.
1 gallon	=	4 qt.
	=	128 fl. oz.

2. Mass (weight)

The *grain* is common to both the apothecary and avoirdupois systems.

437.5 grains (gr)	=	1 ounce (oz)
16 ounces (7000 grains)	=	1 pound (lb)

CONVERSION

Exact equivalents

Exact equivalents are used for the conversion of specific quantities in pharmaceutical formulas and prescription compounding.

1. Length

1 meter (m)	=	39.37 in.
1 inch (in)	=	2.54 cm.

2. Volume

1 mL	=	16.23 minims (♏)
1 ♏	=	0.06 mL
1 f ʒ	=	3.69 mL
1 f ℥	=	29.57 mL
1 pt	=	473 mL
1 gal (U.S.)	=	3785 mL

3. Mass

1 g	=	15.432 gr
1 kg	=	2.20 lb (avoir.)
1 gr	=	0.065 g or 65 mg
1 oz (avoir.)	=	28.35 g
1 ℥ (apoth.)	=	31.1 g
1 lb (avoir.)	=	454 g
1 lb (apoth.)	=	373.2 g

4. Other equivalents

1 oz (avoir.)	=	437.5 gr
1 ℥ (apoth.)	=	480 gr
1 gal (U.S.)	=	128 fl ℥
1 fl ℥ (water)	=	455 gr
1 gr (apoth.)	=	1 gr (avoir.)

Approximate equivalents

Approximate equivalents may be used by physicians in prescribing the dose quantities using the metric and apothecary systems of weights and measures, respectively.

Household units are often used to inform the patient of the size of the dose. In view of the almost universal practice of employing the *teaspoon* ordinarily available in the household for the administration of medicine, the teaspoon may be regarded to represent 5 mL. When accurate measurement of a liquid dose is required, the USP recommends that a calibrated oral syringe or dropper is used.

1 fluid dram	=	1 teaspoonful
	=	5 mL
4 fluidounces	=	120 mL
8 fluidounces	=	1 cup
	=	240 mL
1 grain	=	65 mg
1 kg	=	2.2 pounds (lbs)

Common Abbreviations

There is considerable variation in the use of capitalization, italicization, and punctuation in abbreviations. The forms of abbreviation in this list are those most often encountered by pharmacists.

A, aa., or $\overline{aa}$	of each
a.c.	before meals
ad	to, up to
a.d.	right ear
ad lib.	at pleasure, freely
a.m.	morning
amp.	ampule
ante	before
aq.	water
a.s.	left ear
asa	aspirin
a.u.	each ear, both ears
b.i.d.	twice a day
BP	British Pharmacopoeia
BSA	body surface area
c. or $\bar{c}$	with
cap. or caps.	capsule
cp	chest pain
D.A.W.	dispense as written
cc or cc.	cubic centimeter
comp.	compound, compounded
dil.	dilute
D.C., dc, or disc.	discontinue
disp.	dispense
div.	divide, to be divided
dl or dL	deciliter
d.t.d.	give of such doses
DW	distilled water
D_5W	dextrose 5% in water
elix.	elixir
e.m.p.	as directed
et	and
ex aq.	in water
fl or fld	fluid
fl oz	fluid ounce
ft.	make
g or Gm	gram
gal.	gallon
GI	gastrointestinal
gr or gr.	grain
gtt or gtt.	drop, drops
H	hypodermic
h. or hr.	hour
h.s.	at bedtime
IM	intramuscular
inj.	injection
IV	intravenous
IVP	intravenous push
IVPB	intravenous piggyback
K	potassium
l or L	liter
lb.	pound
M	mix
m^2 or M^2	square meter
mcg, mcg., or μg	microgram
mEq	milliequivalent
mg or mg.	milligram
ml. or mL	milliliter
μl or μL	microliter
♏	minim
N&V	nausea and vomiting
Na	sodium
N.F.	National Formulary
No.	number
noct.	night, in the night
non rep.	do not repeat
NPO	nothing by mouth
N.S., NS, or N/S	normal saline
½ NS	half strength normal saline
O	pint
o.d.	right eye, every day
o.l. or o.s.	left eye
OTC	over the counter
o.u.	each eye, both eyes
o_2	both eyes
oz.	ounce
p.c.	after meals
PDR	*Physicians' Desk Reference*
p.m.	afternoon; evening
p.o.	by mouth
Ppt	precipitated
pr	for the rectum
prn or p.r.n.	as needed
pt.	pint
pulv.	powder
pv	for vaginal use
q.	every
q.d.	every day
q.h.	every hour
q. 4 hr.	every four hours
q.i.d.	four times a day
q.o.d.	every other day

q.s.	a sufficient quantity
q.s. ad	a sufficient quantity to make
R	rectal
R.L. or R/L	Ringer's lactate
℞	prescription
s. or s̄	without
Sig.	write on label
sol.	solution
S.O.B.	shortness of breath
s.o.s.	if there is need (once only)
ss. or s̄s̄	one half
stat.	immediately
subc, subq, or s.c.	subcutaneously
sup. or supp	suppository
susp.	suspension
syr.	syrup
tab.	tablet
tal.	such, such a one
tal. dos.	such doses
tbsp. or T	tablespoonful
t.i.d.	three times a day
tr. or tinct.	tincture
tsp. or t.	teaspoonful
TT	tablet triturates
U or u.	unit
u.d. or ut dict.	as directed
ung.	ointment
U.S.P. or USP	United States Pharmacopoeia
w/v	weight/volume

Appendix B: Common Prescription Drugs

How to crack the *Orange Book* drug codes*

Drug product selection can be a complicated matter. The Food and Drug Administration (FDA) publishes a guide entitled *Approved Drug Products with Therapeutic Equivalence Evaluations* to help you choose alternatives to prescribed drugs, but pharmacists often find the material difficult to decipher. So, here is a simplified explanation of what is going on.

More commonly known as the *Orange Book,* the compilation offers a detailed description (pared-down definitions appear below) of each of the two-letter drug ratings. It also provides a listing of all approved products and their equivalency ratings if they are multiple-source drugs.

The first letter of the rating—either an "A" or a "B"—is most pertinent to you. Products receiving an "A" rating are considered by the FDA to be "therapeutically equivalent" to other "pharmaceutically equivalent products." That means, among other things, that the product is deemed bioequivalent to something else containing identical amounts of the same active ingredient manufactured in the same dosage form.

A "B" rating, on the other hand, is a signal that, for one reason or another, the FDA has not judged that product to be bioequivalent. That does not, however, mean that the product has been deemed inequivalent or that it will not work. It may, for instance, simply be that nobody has ever performed the necessary bioequivalence testing.

The second letter of the code gives you a bit more information. In many cases, it refers to product category. Each drug type has its own subset of rules. For instance, a label of "AT" refers to a topical considered to be therapeutically equivalent to another product with the same active ingredient in the same strength and dosage form.

Or take a "BS" rating. The "S," or second letter, tells you the drug has been stamped inequivalent because of "drug standard deficiencies." In other words, the standards used to judge a particular product's equivalency are not up to doing the job.

The "BX" rating indicates that a product is not bioequivalent ("B") because the agency did not have enough data to prove that a product was equivalent ("X"). There are probably fewer than 100 drugs that fall into this category.

Finally, pharmacists will find that an estimated 20% of drugs on today's market receive no rating at all and thus do not appear in the *Orange Book*. Such products were in existence before 1938 and have received a "grandfathered" FDA approval. They predate the approval process and are simply assumed to be safe and effective because they have been in use for so long (e.g., digoxin tablets and phenobarbital).

If a prescription is written generically, you can essentially choose whatever appropriate product you wish to use. Although you have to look to your state's laws when it comes to a substitutable prescription for a brand-name product, keep in mind that you are guaranteed therapeutic equivalence only with an "A" rated product.

WHAT THEY MEAN

The following codes and descriptions are taken from the Food and Drug Administration's (FDA's) *Approved Drug Products with Therapeutic Equivalence Evaluations,* also known as the *Orange Book*.

AA: Products not presenting bioequivalence problems in conventional dosage forms
AB: Products meeting necessary bioequivalence requirements
AN: Solutions and powders for aerosolization
AO: Injectable oil solutions
AP: Injectable aqueous solutions
AT: Topical products
BC: Controlled-release tablets, capsules, and injectables
BD: Active ingredients and dosage forms with documented bioequivalence problems
BE: Enteric-coated oral dosage forms
BN: Products in aerosol–nebulizer drug-delivery systems
BP: Active ingredients and dosage forms with potential bioequivalence problems
BR: Suppositories or enemas for systemic use
BS: Products having drug standard deficiencies
BT: Topical products with bioequivalence issues
BX: Insufficient data

*Reprinted from *1993 Red Book.* Montvale, NJ, Medical Economics Inc., 1993.

Generic Drugs

Generic Name	Brand Name	Company	Category
Acetaminophen/codeine*	Tylenol/Codeine	McNeil	Non-opioid/opioid analgesic
Acyclovir	Zovirax	Burroughs Wellcome	Antiviral
Albuterol*	Ventolin Aerosol	Allen & Hanburys (Glaxo)	Beta-2 adrenergic bronchodilator
	Proventil Aerosol	Schering	Beta-2 adrenergic bronchodilator
Allopurinol*	Zyloprim	Burroughs Wellcome	Xanthine oxidase inhibitor (reduces uric acid)
Alprazolam	Xanax	Upjohn	Benzodiazepine, anti-anxiety
Amiloride HCl/hydrochlorothiazide*	Moduretic	Merck Sharp & Dohme	Diuretic/antihypertensive
Amitriptyline hydrochloride*	Elavil	Merck Sharp & Dohme	Tricyclic antidepressant
Amoxicillin*	Trimox	Squibb	Penicillin antibiotic
	Polymox	Bristol	Penicillin antibiotic
	Amoxil	SmithKline Beecham	Penicillin antibiotic
	Wymox	Wyeth-Ayerst	Penicillin antibiotic
Amoxicillin/clavulanate potassium	Augmentin	SmithKline Beecham	Penicillin antibiotic/beta lactamase inhibitor
Ampicillin*	Totacillin	SmithKline Beecham	Penicillin antibiotic
	Amcill	Warner Chilcott	Penicillin antibiotic
	Omnipen	Wyeth-Ayerst	Penicillin antibiotic
Atenolol*	Tenormin	ICI Pharma	Beta adrenergic blocker
Atenolol/chlorthalidone	Tenoretic	ICI Pharma	Beta adrenergic blocker/diuretic
Azatadine maleate/pseudoephedrine sulfate	Trinalin	Schering	Antihistamine/decongestant
Betaxolol hydrochloride	Betoptic	Alcon	Cardioselective beta-1 adrenergic receptor blocking agent (ophthalmic)
Bumetanide	Bumex	Roche	Loop diuretic
Buspirone hydrochloride	BuSpar	Mead Johnson	Anxiolytic
Butalbital/acetaminophen/caffeine*	Fioricet	Sandoz	Sedative/analgesic
Butalbital/aspirin/caffeine*	Fiorinal	Sandoz	Sedative/analgesic
Butalbital/aspirin/caffeine/codeine	Fiorinal/Codeine	Sandoz	Sedative/analgesic
Captopril	Capoten	Squibb	Angiotensin converting enzyme (ACE) inhibitor/antihypertensive
Carbamazepine*	Tegretol	Basel	Anticonvulsant
Carbidopa/levodopa	Sinemet	Merck Sharp & Dohme	Aromatic amino acid decarboxylase inhibitor/antihypertensive
Cefaclor	Ceclor	Lilly	Cephalosporin antibiotic

Cefadroxil monohydrate	Duricef	Mead Johnson	Cephalosporin antibiotic
Cefuroxime axetil	Ceftin	Allen & Hanburys (Glaxo)	Cephalosporin antibiotic
Cephalexin	Keftab	Dista	Cephalosporin antibiotic
Cephalexin*	Keflex	Dista	Cephalosporin antibiotic
Chlorpheniramine maleate d-pseudoephedrine HCl	Deconamine	Berlex	Antihistamine/decongestant
Chlorpropamide*	Diabinese	Pfizer	Oral hypoglycemic
Chlorthalidone*	Hygroton	Rhone-Poulenc	Diuretic/antihypertensive
Chlorzoxazone*	Parafon Forte DSC	McNeil	Skeletal muscle relaxant
Cimetidine	Tagamet	SmithKline Beecham	Histamine H_2 receptor antagonist
Ciprofloxacin	Cipro	Miles	Fluoroquinolone
Clemastine fumarate/ phenylpropanolamine hydrochloride	Tavist-D	Sandoz	Antihistamine/nasal decongestant
Clindamycin phosphate	Cleocin T	Upjohn	Antibiotic (topical)
Clonidine hydrochloride*	Catapres	Boehringer Ingelheim	Antihypertensive
Clorazepate dipotassium*	Tranxene	Abbott	Benzodiazepine
Clotrimazole	Lotrimin	Schering	Antifungal
	Gyne-Lotrimin	Schering	Antifungal
Clotrimazole/betamethasone	Lotrisone	Schering	Antifungal/corticosteroid topical cream
Codeine phosphate/iodinated glycerol*	Tussi-Organidin	Wallace	Antitussive/mucolytic expectorant
Codeine phosphate/iodinated glycerol/dextromethorphan*	Tussi-Organidin DM	Wallace	Antitussive/mucolytic expectorant
Conjugated estrogens	Premarin Oral	Wyeth-Ayerst	Estrogenic agent
Cromolyn sodium	Intal	Fisons	Mast cell stabilizer/antiallergy
	Nasalcrom	FIsons	Mast cell stabilizer/antiallergic nasal solution
Crystalline warfarin sodium	Coumadin Oral	Du Pont	Oral anticoagulant
Cyclobenzaprine hydrochloride*	Flexeril	Merck Sharp & Dohme	Muscle relaxant
Desipramine hydrochloride*	Norpramin	Marion Merrell Dow	Tricyclic antidepressant
Desoximetasone*	Topicort	Hoechst-Roussel	Corticosteroid (topical)
Diazepam*	Valium	Roche	Benzodiazepine
Diclofenac	Voltaren	Geigy	Nonsteroidal anti-inflammatory agent (NSAID)
Dicyclomine hydrochloride*	Bentyl	Marion Merrell Dow	Antispasmodic-irritable bowel syndrome
Diflunisal	Dolobid	Merck Sharp & Dohme	Nonsteroidal anti-inflammatory agent (NSAID)
Digoxin*	Lanoxin	Burroughs Wellcome	Cardiac glycoside
Diltiazem hydrochloride*	Cardizem	Marion Merrell Dow	Calcium ion influx inhibitor
Diphenoxylate HCl/atropine sulfate*	Lomotil	Searle	Antispasmodic/anticholinergic (antidiarrheal combination)

*Generic product available.

Continued on next page

Generic Drugs—*Continued*

Generic Name	Brand Name	Company	Category
Dipivefrin hydrochloride (dipvalyl epinephrine)	Propine	Allergan	Antiglaucoma
Dipyridamole*	Persantine	Boehringer Ingelheim	Coronary vasodilator
Doxepin hydrochloride*	Sinequan	Roerig	Psychotropic/antianxiety
Enalapril maleate	Vasotec	Merck Sharp & Dohme	Angiotensin converting enzyme (ACE) inhibitor/antihypertensive
Erythromycin ethylsuccinate*	E.E.S.	Abbott	Macrolide antibiotic
	Erythrocin	Abbott	Macrolide antibiotic
Erythromycin ethylsuccinate/ sulfisoxazole acetyl*	Pediazole	Ross	Antibiotic combination (otitis media)
Erythromycin stearate*	Erythrocin stearate	Abbott	Macrolide antibiotic
Erythromycin*	PCE	Abbott	Macrolide antibiotic (enteric coated particles)
	Ery-Tab	Abbott	Macrolide antibiotic (delayed release, enteric coated tablet)
	E-Mycin	Boots	Macrolide antibiotic (enteric coated)
	ERYC	Parke-Davis	Macrolide antibiotic (delayed release)
	E-Mycin 333	Boots	Macrolide antibiotic
Extended phenytoin sodium	Dilantin Sodium	Parke-Davis	Antiepileptic
Famotidine	Pepcid	Merck Sharp & Dohme	H_2 antagonist
Fenoprofen calcium*	Nalfon	Dista	Nonsteroidal anti-inflammatory drug (NSAID)
Flunisolide	Nasalide	Syntex	Topical anti-inflammatory steroid (nasal solution)
Fluocinonide*	Lidex	Syntex	Corticosteroid topical cream
Fluoxetine hydrochloride	Prozac	Dista	Antidepressant
Flurazepam hydrochloride*	Dalmane	Roche	Benzodiazepine
Flurbiprofen	Ansaid	Upjohn	Nonsteroidal anti-inflammatory agent (NSAID)
Flutamide	Eulexin	Schering	Androgen blocker
Furosemide*	Lasix Oral	Hoechst-Roussel	Diuretic
Gemfibrozil	Lopid	Parke-Davis	Lipid regulating agent
Glipizide	Glucotrol	Roerig	Oral hypoglycemic
Glyburide	DiaBeta	Hoechst-Roussel	Oral hypoglycemic
Glyburide	Micronase	Upjohn	Oral hypoglycemic
Haloperidol*	Haldol	McNeil	Major tranquilizer/psychotropic
Hydrochlorothiazide*	HydroDIURIL	Merck Sharp & Dohme	Diuretic/antihypertensive
Hydrocodone bitartrate*	Vicodin	Knoll	Opioid analgesic

Hydrocodone polistirex/ phenyltoloxamine polistirex	Tussionex	Pennwalt	Narcotic antitussive/antihistamine (Pennkinetic extended release suspension)
Hydrocortisone combination suppository*	Anusol-HC	Parke-Davis	Hydrocortisone combination hemorrhoidal rectal suppository
Hydroxyzine hydrochloride*	Atarax	Roerig	Antianxiety/antihistamine
Ibuprofen*	Motrin	Upjohn	Nonsteroidal anti-inflammatory agent (NSAID)
	Rufen	Boots	Nonsteroidal anti-inflammatory agent (NSAID)
Indapamide	Lozol	Rhone-Poulenc	Antihypertensive/diuretic
Indomethacin*	Indocin SR	Merck Sharp & Dohme	Nonsteroidal anti-inflammatory agent (NSAID), sustained release
Indomethacin*	Indocin	Merck Sharp & Dohme	Nonsteroidal anti-inflammatory agent (NSAID)
Ipratropium bromide	Atrovent	Boehringer Ingelheim	Anticholinergic bronchodilator
Isophane	Iletin I NPH	Lilly	Insulin (beef-pork)
Isophane NPH insulin	Humulin N	Lilly	Insulin (human)
Isosorbide dinitrate*	Isordil	Wyeth-Ayerst	Coronary vasodilator
Ketoconazole	Nizoral	Janssen	Antifungal
Labetalol hydrochloride	Normodyne	Key	Adrenergic blocker/antihypertensive
Levonorgestrel/ethinyl estradiol	Triphasil-28	Wyeth-Ayerst	Combination oral contraceptive
Levothyroxine sodium*	Synthroid	Boots	Thyroid hormone
Lisinopril	Prinivil	Merck Sharp & Dohme	ACE inhibitor
Lisinopril	Zestril	Stuart	ACE inhibitor
Loperamide hydrochloride	Imodium	McNeil	Antidiarrheal
Lorazepam*	Ativan	Wyeth-Ayerst	Benzodiazepine
Lovastatin	Mevacor	Merck Sharp & Dohme	Antilipidemic
Meclizine hydrochloride*	Antivert	Roerig	Antihistamine
Medroxyprogesterone acetate*	Provera	Upjohn	Progestational agent
Metaproterenol sulfate*	Alupent Aerosol	Boehringer Ingelheim	Beta adrenergic bronchodilator
	Alupent Syrup	Boehringer Ingelheim	Beta adrenergic bronchodilator
Methyldopate hydrochloride*	Aldomet	Merck Sharp & Dohme	Antihypertensive
Methyldopa/hydrochlorothiazide*	Aldoril	Merck Sharp & Dohme	Antihypertensive/diuretic
Methylphenidate hydrochloride*	Ritalin	CIBA	Mild central nervous system stimulant
Methylprednisolone*	Medrol Oral	Upjohn	Glucocorticoid
Metoclopramide hydrochloride*	Reglan	Robins	Upper GI (gastrointestinal) tract motility stimulator
Metoprolol tartrate	Lopressor	Geigy	Beta adrenergic blocker
Miconazole nitrate	Monistat Dual-Pak	Ortho	Antifungal vaginal suppository and cream with applicator
	Monistat-7	Ortho	Antifungal vaginal suppository
Minocycline hydrochloride*	Minocin	Lederle	Tetracycline antibiotic

*Generic product available.

Continued on next page

Generic Drugs—*Continued*

Generic Name	Brand Name	Company	Category
Multivitamin and fluoride supplement	Poly-Vi-Flor	Mead Johnson	Multivitamin and fluoride supplement drops
Multivitamin/multimineral combination	Stuartnatal 1 + 1	Stuart	Multivitamin/multimineral pre- or postnatal supplement
Nadolol	Corgard	Princeton	Beta adrenergic blocker
Naproxen	Naprosyn	Syntex	Nonsteroidal anti-inflammatory agent (NSAID)
Naproxen sodium	Anaprox	Syntex	Nonsteroidal anti-inflammatory agent (NSAID/analgesic)
Nicotine polacrilex	Nicorette	Marion Merrell Dow	Nicotine gum
Nifedipine*	Procardia	Pfizer	Calcium ion channel blocker
Nitrofurantoin macrocrystals	Macrodantin	Norwich Eaton	Antibacterial
Nitroglycerin*	Nitrostat	Parke-Davis	Coronary vasodilator/anti-anginal agent
	Nitro-Bid	Marion Merrell Dow	Coronary vasodilator
	Transderm-Nitro	CIBA	Coronary vasodilator/anti-anginal agent
	Nitro-Dur II	Key	Coronary vasodilator (transdermal)
Nizatidine	Axid	Lilly	H_2 antagonist
Norethindrone/ethinyl estradiol*	Ortho-Novum 7/7/7-28	Ortho	Combination oral contraceptive
	Ortho-Novum 1/35-21	Ortho	Combination oral contraceptive
	Ortho-Novum 1/35-28	Ortho	Combination oral contraceptive
	Ortho-Novum 7/7/7-21	Ortho	Combination oral contraceptive
	Ovcon	Mead Johnson	Combination oral contraceptive
	Tri-Norinyl	Syntex	Combination oral contraceptive
Norethindrone/mestranol*	Ortho-Novum 1/50-28	Ortho	Combination oral contraceptive
	Ortho-Novum 1/50-21	Ortho	Combination oral contraceptive
Norgestrel/ethinyl estradiol*	Lo/Ovral-28	Wyeth-Ayerst	Combination oral contraceptive
	Lo/Ovral-21	Wyeth-Ayerst	Combination oral contraceptive
Nortriptyline hydrochloride	Pamelor	Sandoz	Antidepressant
Omeprazole	Prilosec	Merck Sharp & Dohme	ACE inhibitor
Oxazepam*	Serax	Wyeth-Ayerst	Benzodiazepine
Oxycodone/acetaminophen*	Tylox	McNeil	Opioid/non-opioid analgesic
	Percocet-5	Du Pont	Opioid/non-opioid analgesic
Oxycodone/aspirin*	Percodan	Du Pont	Opioid/non-opioid analgesic
Penicillin VK (potassium)*	Veetids	Apothecon	Penicillin antibiotic
	V-Cillin K	Lilly	Penicillin antibiotic
	Pen-Vee K	Wyeth-Ayerst	Penicillin antibiotic
	LEDERCILLIN VK	Lederle	Penicillin antibiotic

	Beepen-VK	SmithKline Beecham	Penicillin antibiotic
	Betapen-VK	Bristol	Penicillin antibiotic
Pentazocine HCl/naloxone HCl	Talwin-Nx	Winthrop	Strong analgesic/narcotic antagonist
Pentoxifylline	Trental	Hoechst-Roussel	Improves blood flow in chronic occlusive artery disease
Perphenazine/amitriptyline*	Triavil	Merck Sharp & Dohme	Antipsychotic/antidepressant
Phenobarbital*	Phenobarbital	Lilly	Barbiturate
Phenobarbital/belladonna alkaloids*	Donnatal	Robins	Barbiturate/belladonna alkaloids (hydroscyamine sulfate; atropine sulfate; scopolamine hydrobromide anticholinergic)
Phenylephrine/chlorpheniramine tannates	Rynatan	Wallace	Nasal decongestant/antihistamine combination
Phenylpropanolamine hydrochloride combination	Naldecon	Bristol	Nasal decongestant/antihistamine combination (phenylpropanolamine HCl/phenylephrine HCl/phenyltoloxamine)
Phenylpropanolamine hydrochloride/guaifenesin*	Entex LA	Norwich Eaton	Decongestant/expectorant (long acting)
Piroxicam	Feldene	Pfizer	Nonsteroidal anti-inflammatory agent (NSAID)
Polymyxin B/neomycin/hydrocortisone*	Cortisporin Otic	Burroughs Wellcome	Antibiotic/corticosteroid combination
Potassium chloride*	Slow-K	CIBA	Potassium supplement
	Klotrix	Mead Johnson	Potassium supplement
	Micro-K 10	Robins	Potassium supplement
	K-Tab	Abbott	Potassium supplement
	Micro-K	Robins	Potassium supplement
Prazepam	Centrax	Parke-Davis	Benzodiazepine
Prazosin hydrochloride*	Minipress	Pfizer	Antihypertensive
Prednisone*	Deltasone	Upjohn	Corticosteroid
	Orasone	Solvay	Corticosteroid
Prednisone acetate/sodium sulfacetamide	Bleph-10	Allergan	Corticosteroid/antibiotic (ophthalmic)
Prochlorperazine*	Compazine	SmithKline Beecham	Phenothiazine antinauseant
Promethazine HCl/codeine phosphate*	Phenergan/codeine	Wyeth-Ayerst	Phenothiazine antihistamine/opioid analgesic-antitussive
Promethazine hydrochloride*	Phenergan	Wyeth-Ayerst	Phenothiazine/antihistamine
Propoxyphene napsylate/acetaminophen*	Darvocet-N-100	Lilly	Analgesic
Propranolol hydrochloride	Inderal LA	Wyeth-Ayerst	Beta adrenergic blocker
Propranolol hydrochloride*	Inderal	Wyeth-Ayerst	Beta adrenergic blocker
Ranitidine hydrochloride	Zantac	Glaxo	Histamine H_2 receptor antagonist
Sucralfate	Carafate	Marion Merrell Dow	Anti-ulcer

*Generic product available.

Continued on next page

Generic Drugs—*Continued*

Generic Name	Brand Name	Company	Category
Sulindac*	Clinoril	Merck Sharp & Dohme	Nonsteroidal anti-inflammatory agent (NSAID)
Temazepam*	Restoril	Sandoz	Benzodiazepine
Terbutaline sulfate	Brethine	Geigy	Beta adrenergic bronchodilator
Terfenadine	Seldane	Merrell Dow	Antihistamine
Tetracycline hydrochloride*	Sumycin	Squibb	Tetracycline antibiotic
	Achromycin V	Lederle	Tetracycline antibiotic
Theophylline anhydrous*	Theo-Dur	Key	Bronchodilator
	Slo-bid	Rhone-Poulenc	Bronchodilator (timed release)
Thiothixene hydrochloride*	Navane	Roerig	Psychotropic
Thioridazine hydrochloride*	Mellaril	Sandoz	Phenothiazine psychotropic
Timolal maleate	Timoptic	Merck Sharp & Dohme	Intraocular pressure lowering agent in glaucoma treatment
Tobramycin	Tobrex	Alcon	Aminoglycoside antibiotic (ophthalmic)
Tolmetin sodium	Tolectin DS	McNeil	Nonsteroidal anti-inflammatory agent (NSAID)
Trazodone hydrochloride*	Desyrel	Mead Johnson	Antidepressant
Tretinoin	Retin-A Acne	Ortho	Retinoic acid (vitamin A) topical
Triamterene/hydrochlorothiazide	Maxzide	Lederle	Diuretic/antihypertensive
Triamterene/hydrochlorothiazide*	Dyazide	SmithKline Beecham	Diuretic/antihypertensive
Triazolam	Halcion	Upjohn	Triazolbenzodiazepine, hypnotic
Trimethoprim/sulfamethoxazole*	Bactrim DS	Roche	Antifolate/antibacterial (double strength)
	Septra DS	Burroughs Wellcome	Antifolate/antibacterial (double strength)
	Septra	Burroughs Wellcome	Antifolate/antibacterial
Verapamil hydrochloride	Calan SR	Searle	Slow channel calcium blocker (sustained release)
Verapamil hydrochloride*	Calan	Searle	Slow channel calcium blocker

*Generic product available.

Brand Drugs

Brand Drugs—*Continued*

Brand Name	Generic Name	Company	Category
Achromycin V	Tetracycline hydrochloride*	Lederle	Tetracycline antibiotic
Aldomet	Methyldopate hydrochloride*	Merck Sharp & Dohme	Antihypertensive
Aldoril	Methyldopa/hydrochlorothiazide	Merck Sharp & Dohme	Antihypertensive/diuretic
Alupent Aerosol	Metaproterenol sulfate*	Boehringer Ingelheim	Beta adrenergic bronchodilator
Alupent Syrup	Metaproterenol sulfate*	Boehringer Ingelheim	Beta adrenergic bronchodilator
Amcill	Ampicillin*	Warner Chilcott	Penicillin antibiotic
Amoxil	Amoxicillin*	SmithKline Beecham	Penicillin antibiotic
Anaprox	Naproxen sodium	Syntex	Nonsteroidal anti-inflammatory agent (NSAID)/analgesic
Antivert	Meclizine hydrochloride*	Roerig	Antihistamine
Anusol-HC	Hydrocortisone combination suppository	Parke-Davis	Hydrocortisone combination hemorrhoidal rectal suppository
Atarax	Hydroxyzine hydrochloride*	Roerig	Antianxiety/antihistamine
Ativan	Lorazepam	Wyeth-Ayerst	Benzodiazepine
Atrovent	Ipratropium bromide	Boehringer Ingelheim	Anticholinergic bronchodilator
Augmentin	Amoxicillin/clavulanate potassium	SmithKline Beecham	Penicillin antibiotic/beta lactamase inhibitor
Bactrim DS	Trimethoprim/sulfamethoxazole	Roche	Antifolate/antibacterial (double strength)
Beepen-VK	Penicillin VK (potassium)*	SmithKline Beecham	Penicillin antibiotic
Bentyl	Dicyclomine hydrochloride	Lakeside	Antispasmodic-irritable bowel syndrome
Betapen-VK	Penicillin VK (potassium)*	Bristol	Penicillin antibiotic
Betoptic	Betaxolol hydrochloride	Alcon	Cardioselective beta-1 adrenergic receptor blocking agent (ophthalmic)
Bleph-10	Prednisone acetate/sodium sulfacetamide	Allergan	Corticosteroid/antibiotic (ophthalmic)
Brethine	Terbutaline sulfate	Geigy	Beta adrenergic bronchodilator
Bumex	Bumetanide	Roche	Loop diuretic
BuSpar	Buspirone hydrochloride	Mead Johnson	Anxiolytic
Calan	Verapamil hydrochloride*	Searle	Slow channel calcium blocker
Calan SR	Verapamil hydrochloride	Searle	Slow channel calcium blocker (sustained release)
Capoten	Captopril	Squibb	Angiotensin converting enzyme (ACE) inhibitor/antihypertensive
Carafate	Sucralfate	Marion Merrell Dow	Anti-ulcer
Cardizem	Diltiazem hydrochloride	Marion Merrell Dow	Calcium ion influx inhibitor
Catapres	Clonidine hydrochloride	Boehringer Ingelheim	Antihypertensive
Ceclor	Cefaclor	Lilly	Cephalosporin antibiotic

*Generic product available.

Continued on next page

Brand Drugs—*Continued*

Brand Name	Generic Name	Company	Category
Ceftin	Cefuroxime axetil	Allen & Hanburys (Glaxo)	Cephalosporin antibiotic
Centrax	Prazepam	Parke-Davis	Benzodiazepine
Cleocin T	Clindamycin phosphate	Upjohn	Antibiotic (topical)
Clinoril	Sulindac	Merck Sharp & Dohme	Nonsteroidal anti-inflammatory agent (NSAID)
Compazine	Prochlorperazine	SmithKline Beecham	Phenothiazine antinauseant
Corgard	Nadolol	Princeton	Beta adrenergic blocker
Cortisporin Otic	Polymyxin B/neomycin/hydrocortisone	Burroughs Wellcome	Antibiotic/corticosteroid combination
Coumadin Oral	Crystalline warfarin sodium	Du Pont	Oral anticoagulant
Dalmane	Flurazepam hydrochloride	Roche	Benzodiazepine
Darvocet-N-100	Propoxyphene napsylate/acetaminophen	Lilly	Analgesic
Deconamine	Chlorpheniramine maleate/ d-pseudoephedrine HCl	Berlex	Antihistamine/decongestant
Deltasone	Prednisone*	Upjohn	Corticosteroid
Desyrel	Trazodone hydrochloride	Mead Johnson	Antidepressant
DiaBeta	Glyburide	Hoechst-Roussel	Oral hypoglycemic
Diabinese	Chlorpropamide	Pfizer	Oral hypoglycemic
Dilantin Sodium	Extended phenytoin sodium	Parke-Davis	Antiepileptic
Dolobid	Diflunisal	Merck Sharp & Dohme	Nonsteroidal anti-inflammatory agent (NSAID)
Donnatal	Phenobarbital/belladonna alkaloids	Robins	Barbiturate/belladonna alkaloids (hydroscyamine sulfate; atropine sulfate; scopolamine hydrobromide anticholinergic)
Duricef	Cefadroxil monohydrate	Mead Johnson	Cephalosporin antibiotic
Dyazide	Triamterene/hydrochlorothiazide*	SmithKline Beecham	Diuretic/antihypertensive
Elavil	Amitriptyline hydrochloride*	Merck Sharp & Dohme	Tricyclic antidepressant
Entex LA	Phenylpropanolamine HCl/guaifenesin	Norwich Eaton	Decongestant/expectorant (long acting)
ERYC	Erythromycin*	Parke-Davis	Macrolide antibiotic (delayed release)
Erythrocin	Erythromycin ethylsuccinate*	Abbott	Macrolide antibiotic
Erythrocin stearate	Erythromycin stearate*	Abbott	Macrolide antibiotic
Ery-Tab	Erythromycin*	Abbott	Macrolide antibiotic delayed release (enteric coated tablet)
E-Mycin	Erythromycin*	Upjohn	Macrolide antibiotic (enteric coated)
E-Mycin 333	Erythromycin*	Upjohn	Macrolide antibiotic
E.E.S.	Erythromycin ethylsuccinate*	Abbott	Macrolide antibiotic
Feldene	Piroxicam	Pfizer	Nonsteroidal anti-inflammatory agent (NSAID)
Fioricet	Butalbital/acetaminophen/caffeine	Sandoz	Sedative/analgesic
Fiorinal	Butalbital/aspirin/caffeine	Sandoz	Sedative/analgesic

Fiorinal/Codeine	Butalbital/aspirin/caffeine/codeine	Sandoz	Sedative/analgesic
Flexeril	Cyclobenzaprine hydrochloride	Merck Sharp & Dohme	Muscle relaxant
Glucotrol	Glipizide	Roerig	Oral hypoglycemic
Gyne-Lotrimin	Clotrimazole*	Schering	Antifungal
Halcion	Triazolam	Upjohn	Triazolbenzodiazepine, hypnotic
Haldol	Haloperidol	McNeil	Major tranquilizer/psychotropic
Humulin N	Isophane NPH insulin	Lilly	Insulin (human)
HydroDIURIL	Hydrochlorothiazide*	Merck Sharp & Dohme	Diuretic/antihypertensive
Hygroton	Chlorthalidone*	Rhone-Poulenc	Diuretic/antihypertensive
Iletin I NPH	Isophane	Lilly	Insulin (beef-pork)
Imodium	Loperamide hydrochloride	Janssen	Antidiarrheal
Inderal	Propranolol hydrochloride*	Wyeth-Ayerst	Beta adrenergic blocker
Inderal LA	Propranolol hydrochloride	Wyeth-Ayerst	Beta adrenergic blocker
Indocin	Indomethacin*	Merck Sharp & Dohme	Nonsteroidal anti-inflammatory agent (NSAID)
Indocin SR	Indomethacin	Merck Sharp & Dohme	Nonsteroidal anti-inflammatory agent (NSAID), sustained release
Intal	Cromolyn sodium	Fisons	Mast cell stabilizer/antiallergy
Isordil	Isorbide dinitrate*	Wyeth-Ayerst	Coronary vasodilator
Keflex	Cephalexin*	Dista	Cephalosporin antibiotic
Keftab	Cephalexin	Dista	Cephalosporin antibiotic
Klotrix	Potassium chloride*	Mead Johnson	Potassium supplement
K-Tab	Potassium chloride*	Abbott	Potassium supplement
Lanoxin	Digoxin*	Burroughs Wellcome	Cardiac glycoside
Lasix Oral	Furosemide*	Hoechst-Roussel	Diuretic
LEDERCILLIN VK	Penicillin VK (potassium)*	Lederle	Penicillin antibiotic
Lidex	Fluocinonide	Syntex	Corticosteroid topical cream
Lomotil	Diphenoxylate HCl/atropine sulfate	Searle	Antispasmodic/anticholinergic (antidiarrheal combination)
Lopid	Gemfibrozil	Parke-Davis	Lipid regulating agent
Lopressor	Metoprolol tartrate	Geigy	Beta adrenergic blocker
Lotrimin	Clotrimazole	Schering	Antifungal
Lotrisone	Clotrimazole/betamethasone	Schering	Antifungal/corticosteroid topical cream
Lozol	Indapamide	Rhone-Poulenc	Antihypertensive/diuretic
Lo/Ovral-21	Norgestrel/ethinyl estradiol*	Wyeth-Ayerst	Combination oral contraceptive
Lo/Ovral-28	Norgestrel/ethinyl estradiol*	Wyeth-Ayerst	Combination oral contraceptive
Macrodantin	Nitrofurantoin macrocrystals	Norwich Eaton	Antibacterial
Maxzide	Triamterene/hydrochlorothiazide	Lederle	Diuretic/antihypertensive
Medrol Oral	Methylprednisolone	Upjohn	Glucocorticoid
Mellaril	Thioridazine hydrochloride*	Sandoz	Phenothiazine psychotropic

*Generic product available.

Continued on next page

Brand Drugs—*Continued*

Brand Name	Generic Name	Company	Category
Micronase	Glyburide	Upjohn	Oral hypoglycemic
Micro-K	Potassium chloride*	Robins	Potassium supplement
Micro-K 10	Potassium chloride*	Robins	Potassium supplement
Minipress	Prazosin hydrochloride	Pfizer	Antihypertensive
Minocin	Minocycline hydrochloride	Lederle	Tetracycline antibiotic
Moduretic	Amiloride HCl/hydrochlorothiazide	Merck Sharp & Dohme	Diuretic/antihypertensive
Monistat Dual-Pak	Miconazole nitrate	Ortho	Antifungal vaginal suppository and cream with applicator
Monistat-7	Miconazole nitrate	Ortho	Antifungal vaginal suppository
Motrin	Ibuprofen*	Upjohn	Nonsteroidal anti-inflammatory agent (NSAID)
Naldecon	Phenylpropanolamine HCl combination	Bristol	Nasal decongestant/antihistamine combination (phenylpropanolamine HCl/phenylephrine HCl/phenyltoloxamine citrate/chlorpheniramine maleate)
Nalfon	Fenoprofen calcium	Dista	Nonsteroidal anti-inflammatory agent (NSAID)
Naprosyn	Naproxen	Syntex	Nonsteroidal anti-inflammatory agent (NSAID)
Nasalcrom	Cromolyn sodium*	Fisons	Mast cell stabilizer/antiallergic nasal solution
Nasalide	Flunisolide	Syntex	Topical anti-inflammatory steroid (nasal solution)
Navane	Thiothixene hydrochloride	Roerig	Psychotropic
Nicorette	Nicotine polacrilex	Marion Merrell Dow	Nicotine gum
Nitrostat	Nitroglycerin	Parke-Davis	Coronary vasodilator/anti-anginal agent
Nitro-Bid	Nitroglycerin	Marion	Coronary vasodilator
Nitro-Dur II	Nitroglycerin	Key	Coronary vasodilator (transdermal)
Nizoral	Ketoconazole	Janssen	Antifungal
Normodyne	Labetalol hydrochloride	Key	Adrenergic blocker/antihypertensive
Norpramin	Desipramine hydrochloride*	Marion Merrell Dow	Tricyclic antidepressant
Omnipen	Ampicillin*	Wyeth-Ayerst	Penicillin antibiotic
Orasone	Prednisone*	Solvay	Corticosteroid
Ortho-Novum 1/35-21	Norethindrone/ethinyl estradiol*	Ortho	Combination oral contraceptive
Ortho-Novum 1/35-28	Norethindrone/ethinyl estradiol*	Ortho	Combination oral contraceptive
Ortho-Novum 1/50-21	Norethindrone/mestranol*	Ortho	Combination oral contraceptive
Ortho-Novum 1/50-28	Norethindrone/mestranol*	Ortho	Combination oral contraceptive
Ortho-Novum 7/7/7-21	Norethindrone/ethinyl estradiol*	Ortho	Combination oral contraceptive
Ortho-Novum 7/7/7-28	Norethindrone/ethinyl estradiol*	Ortho	Combination oral contraceptive
Ovcon	Norethindrone/ethinyl estradiol*	Mead Johnson	Combination oral contraceptive

Pamelor	Nortriptyline hydrochloride	Sandoz	Antidepressant
Parafon Forte DSC	Chlorzoxazone	McNeil	Skeletal muscle relaxant
PCE	Erythromycin*	Abbott	Macrolide antibiotic (enteric coated particles)
Pediazole	Erythromycin ethylsuccinate/ sulfisoxazole acetyl	Ross	Antibiotic combination (otitis media)
Pen-Vee K	Penicillin VK (potassium)*	Wyeth-Ayerst	Penicillin antibiotic
Percocet-5	Oxycodone/acetaminophen*	Du Pont	Opioid/non-opioid analgesic
Percodan	Oxycodone/aspirin*	Du Pont	Opioid/non-opioid analgesic
Persantine	Dipyridamole*	Boehringer Ingelheim	Coronary vasodilator
Phenergan	Promethazine hydrochloride	Wyeth-Ayerst	Phenothiazine/antihistamine
Phenergan/codeine	Promethazine HCl/codeine phosphate	Wyeth-Ayerst	Phenothiazine antihistamine/opioid analgesic-antitussive
Phenobarbital	Phenobarbital*	Lilly	Barbiturate
Polymox	Amoxicillin*	Bristol	Penicillin antibiotic
Poly-Vi-Flor	Multivitamin and fluoride supplement	Mead Johnson	Multivitamin and fluoride supplement drops
Premarin Oral	Conjugated estrogens	Wyeth-Ayerst	Estrogenic agent
Procardia	Nifedipine	Pfizer	Calcium ion channel blocker
Propine	Dipivefrin HCl (dipvalyl epinephrine)	Allergan	Antiglaucoma
Proventil Aerosol	Albuterol	Schering	Beta-2 adrenergic bronchodilator
Provera	Medroxyprogesterone acetate	Upjohn	Progestational agent
Prozac	Fluoxetine hydrochloride	Dista	Antidepressant
Reglan	Metoclopramide hydrochloride*	Robins	Upper GI (gastrointestinal) tract motility stimulator
Restoril	Temazepam	Sandoz	Benzodiazepine
Retin-A Acne	Tretinoin	Ortho	Retinoic acid (vitamin A) topical
Ritalin	Methylphenidate hydrochloride	CIBA	Mild central nervous system stimulant
Rufen	Ibuprofen*	Boots-Flint	Nonsteroidal anti-inflammatory agent (NSAID)
Rynatan	Phenylephrine/chlorpheniramine/ pyrilamine tannates	Wallace	Nasal decongestant/antihistamine combination
Seldane	Terfenadine	Marion Merrell Dow	Antihistamine
Septra	Trimethoprim/sulfamethoxazole*	Burroughs Wellcome	Antifolate/antibacterial
Septra DS	Trimethoprim/sulfamethoxazole	Burroughs Wellcome	Antifolate/antibacterial (double strength)
Serax	Oxazepam	Wyeth-Ayerst	Benzodiazepine
Sinemet	Carbidopa/levodopa	Merck Sharp & Dohme	Aromatic amino acid decarboxylase inhibitor/ antihypertensive
Sinequan	Doxepin hydrochloride	Roerig	Psychotropic/antianxiety
Slow-K	Potassium chloride*	Summit	Potassium supplement
Slo-bid	Theophylline anhydrous*	Rhone-Poulenc	Bronchodilator (timed release)
Stuartnatal 1 + 1	Multivitamin/multimineral combination	Stuart	Multivitamin/multimineral pre- or postnatal supplement

*Generic product available.

Continued on next page

Brand Drugs—*Continued*

Brand Name	Generic Name	Company	Category
Sumycin	Tetracycline hydrochloride*	Squibb	Tetracycline antibiotic
Synthroid	Levothyroxine sodium +	Boots-Flint	Thyroid hormone
Tagamet	Cimetidine	SmithKline Beecham	Histamine H_2 receptor antagonist
Talwin Nx	Pentazocine HCl/naloxone HCl	Winthrop	Strong analgesic/narcotic antagonist
Tavist-D	Clemastine fumarate/ phenylpropanolamine HCl	Sandoz	Antihistamine/nasal decongestant
Tegretol	Carbamazepine	Geigy	Anticonvulsant
Tenoretic	Atenolol/chlorthalidone	ICI Pharma	Beta adrenergic blocker/diuretic
Tenormin	Atenolol	ICI Pharma	Beta adrenergic blocker
Theo-Dur	Theophylline anhydrous*	Key	Bronchodilator
Timoptic	Timolal maleate	Merck Sharp & Dohme	Intraocular pressure lowering agent in glaucoma treatment
Tobrex	Tobramycin	Alcon	Aminoglycoside antibiotic (ophthalmic)
Tolectin DS	Tolmetin sodium	McNeil	Nonsteroidal anti-inflammatory agent (NSAID)
Topicort	Desoximetasone	Hoechst-Roussel	Corticosteroid (topical)
Totacillin	Ampicillin*	SmithKline Beecham	Penicillin antibiotic
Transderm-Nitro	Nitroglycerin	CIBA	Coronary vasodilator/anti-anginal agent
Tranxene	Clorazepate dipotassium	Abbott	Benzodiazepine
Trental	Pentoxifylline	Hoechst-Roussel	Improves blood flow in chronic occlusive artery disease
Triavil	Perphenazine/amitriptyline	Merck Sharp & Dohme	Antipsychotic/antidepressant
Trimox	Amoxicillin*	Squibb	Penicillin antibiotic
Trinalin	Azatadine maleate/pseudoephedrine sulfate	Schering	Antihistamine/decongestant
Triphasil-28	Levonorgestrel/ethinyl estradiol	Wyeth-Ayerst	Combination oral contraceptive
Tri-Norinyl	Norethindrone/ethinyl estradiol*	Syntex	Combination oral contraceptive
Tussionex	Hydrocodone polistirex/ phenyltoxamine polistirex	Pennwalt	Narcotic antitussive/antihistamine (Pennkinetic extended release suspension)
Tussi-Organidin	Codeine phosphate/iodinated glycerol	Wallace	Antitussive/mucolytic expectorant
Tussi-Organidin DM	Codeine phosphate/iodinated glycerol/ dextromethorphan	Wallace	Antitussive/mucolytic expectorant
Tylenol/Codeine	Acetaminophen/codeine*	McNeil	Non-opioid/opioid analgesic
Tylox	Oxycodone/acetaminophen	McNeil	Opioid/non-opioid analgesic
Valium	Diazepam*	Roche	Benzodiazepine

Vasotec	Enalapril maleate	Merck Sharp & Dohme	Angiotensin coverting enzyme (ACE) inhibitor/ antihypertensive
Veetids	Penicillin VK (potassium)*	Squibb	Penicillin antibiotic
Ventolin Aerosol	Albuterol	Allen & Hanburys (Glaxo)	Beta-2 adrenergic bronchodilator
Vicodin	Hydrocodone bitartrate	Knoll	Opioid analgesic
V-Cillin K	Penicillin VK (potassium)*	Lilly	Penicillin antibiotic
Wymox	Amoxicillin*	Wyeth-Ayerst	Penicillin antibiotic
Xanax	Alprazolam	Upjohn	Benzodiazepine, anti-anxiety
Zantac	Ranitidine hydrochloride	Glaxo	Histamine H_2 receptor antagonist
Zovirax	Acyclovir	Burroughs Wellcome	Antiviral
Zyloprim	Allopurinol	Burroughs Wellcome	Xanthine oxidase inhibitor (reduces uric acid)

*Generic product available.

Drug Product Abbreviations and Dosage Forms

Drug Product	Example	Company	Description/Comment
Caplet	Advil Caplet	Whitehall	Ibuprofen in a capsule-shaped compressed tablet (caplet)
Chronotab	Disophrol Chronotab	Schering	Dexbrompheniramine maleate/pseudoephedrine sulfate controlled release tablet
CR	Norspace CR	Searle	Disopyramide phosphate (controlled release) capsule
Depo	Depo-Medrol	Upjohn	Sterile methylprednisolone acetate suspension
Dispertabs	PCE	Abbott	Erythromycin enteric coated particles in a tablet
Dividose	Desyrel	Mead Johnson	Trazodone in a bisected/trisected tablet
Dospan	Tenuate Dospan	Marion Merrell Dow	Diethylproprion hydrochloride controlled release tablet
DS	Septra DS	Burroughs Wellcome	Trimethoprim/Sulfamethoxazole (Double Strength)
Dura-tab	Quinaglute	Berlex	Quinidine gluconate sustained release tablet
Enduret	Preludin Enduret	Boehringer-Ingelheim	Phenmetrazine hydrochloride prolonged action tablets
Enseal	DES Enseals	Lilly	Enteric coated
Extencaps	Micro-K Extencaps	Robins	Microencapsulated potassium chloride controlled release capsule
Extentab	Dimetane Extentabs	Robins	Brompheniramine maleate extended (controlled) release tablets
Filmtab	Erythrocin Stearate Filmtab	Abbott	Erythromycin stearate film coated compressed tablet
Forte	Thiosulfil Forte	Wyeth-Ayerst	Higher dose (0.5 g) sulfamethizole (Forte = stronger)
GITS	Procardia XL	Pfizer	Nifedipine gastrointestinal therapeutic system
Gradumet	Desoxyn Gradumet	Abbott Pharmaceuticals	Methamphetamine hydrochloride sustained release tablet
Gyrocap	Slo-Bid Gyrocaps	Rhone-Poulenc	Theophylline anhydrous controlled release capsule
Infatab	Dilantin Infatabs	Parke-Davis	Phenytoin tablets, USP
Kapseals	Dilantin Kapseals	Parke-Davis	Extended phenytoin sodium capsule (Kapseal = sealed hard gelatin capsule)
LA	Inderal LA	Wyeth-Ayerst	Propranolol hydrochloride (long acting) capsule
Ocumeter	Timoptic	Merck Sharp & Dohme	Ophthalmic drop dispenser
Oros	Acutrim	CIBA Geigy	Phenylpropanolamine HCl controlled release osmotic tablet
Pennkinetic	Tussionex	Pennwalt	Hydrocodone polistirex/chlorpheniramine polistirex extended release ion exchange suspension
Perles	Tessalon Perles	Du Pont	Benzonatate in a soft gelatin capsule (Perle)
Plateau Caps	Nitro-Bid Plateau Caps	Marion Merrell Dow	Nitroglycerin controlled release capsules
Progestasert	Progestasert	Alza	Intrauterine progesterone contraceptive system
Pulvule	Darvon Compound	Lilly	Propoxyphene hydrochloride/aspirin/caffeine capsule (Pulvule)
Repetabs	Polaramine Repetabs	Schering	Dexchlorpheniramine maleate repeat action tablets
RTU	Flagyl I.V. RTU	Searle	Metronidazole injection ready-to-use (RTU)
SA	Sudafed SA	Burroughs Wellcome	Pseudoephedrine hydrochloride sustained release (sustained action) tablet

Sequels	Ferro-Sequels	Lederle	Ferrous (iron) fumarate sustained release capsule
Softab	Bucladin-S	Stuart	Buclizine chewable tablet
Spansule	Dexedrine Spansule	SmithKline Beecham	Dextroamphetamine sulfate controlled release capsule
Spinhaler	Intal Inhaler	Fisons	Cromolyn sodium inhalation aerosol for delivery of powder from capsule
Sprinkle	Theo-Dur Sprinkle	Key	Microencapsulated theophylline granules contained in capsule which may be swallowed whole or sprinkled on food
SR	Elixophyllin SR	Berlex	(Sustained release) theophylline
Tabloid	Empirin Aspirin tablets	Burroughs Wellcome	Compressed tablet (Tabloid) containing 325 mg aspirin
Tembids	Isordil Tembids capsules	Wyeth-Ayerst	Isosorbide dinitrate controlled release capsule
Tempules	Nicobid Tempules	Rhone-Poulenc	Niacin timed release capsule
Ten-tab	Tepanil Ten-tab	3M Riker Laboratories	Diethylpropion hydrochloride sustained release tablets
Timesule	Isoclor Timesule	Fisons	Chlorpheniramine maleate/pseudoephedrine sulfate controlled release capsule
Tubex	Closed injection system	Wyeth-Ayerst	Injection system for delivering premeasured doses of medication
-Dur	Theo-Dur	Key	Theophylline anhydrous sustained release

Drugs That Should Not Be Crushed

Pharmacists may encounter patients who, for one reason or another, cannot swallow tablets or capsules. When an alternative liquid formulation is not available, pulverizing the solid dosage form before administration may serve as a quick, safe solution to the problem.

But not all pharmaceutical products may be crushed before administration. Controlled-release formulations can deliver dangerous immediate doses of their active ingredients if the integrity of the delivery system is destroyed. And enteric-coated products must remain intact in order to prevent their dissolution in the stomach.

Listed below are controlled-release and enteric-coated products that should not be crushed or chewed.

In general, capsules containing sustained-release or enteric-coated particles may be opened and their contents administered on a spoonful of soft food. Instruct patients not to chew the particles, though. (Patients should, in fact, be discouraged from chewing any medication unless it is specifically formulated for that purpose.)

This list should not be considered all-inclusive. Generic and alternate brands of some products may exist. Tablets intended for sublingual or buccal administration (not included in this list) should also be administered only as intended, in an intact form.

Controlled-release = cr **Enteric-coated = ec**

Actifed 12-Hour capsules	Burroughs Wellcome	cr
Acutrim tablets	Ciba	cr
Adipost capsules	Ascher	cr
Aerolate SR	Fleming	cr
Aerolate JR	Fleming	cr
Aerolate III	Fleming	cr
Afrinol Repetab tablets	Schering-Plough	cr
Aller-Chlor capsules	Rugby	cr
Allerest 12-Hour capsules	Pharmacraft	cr
Ammonium Chloride Enseals tablets	Lilly	ec
APF Arthritis Pain Formula tablets	Whitehall	ec
Artane Sequels	Lederle	cr
ASA Enseals	Lilly	ec
Atrohist Sprinkle tablets	Adams	cr
Atrohist L.A. tablets	Adams	cr
Azulfidine EN-tab tablets	Pharmacia	ec
Belladenal-S tablets	Sandoz	cr
Bellergal-S tablets	Sandoz	cr
Bisacodyl tablets	various	ec
Bontril Slow-Release capsules	Carnrick	cr
Bromfed capsules	Muro	cr
Bromfed-PD capsules	Muro	cr
Bromphen tablets	Schein	cr
Bromphen TD tablets	Schein	cr
Bromphen Compound TD tablets	Schein	cr
Carter's Little Pills	Carter	ec
Cerespan capsules	Rorer	cr
Chexit tablets	Sandoz	cr
Choledyl tablets	Parke-Davis	ec
Choledyl SA tablets	Parke-Davis	cr
ChlorTrimeton Repetab tablets	Schering-Plough	cr
ChlorTrimeton Decongestant Repetab tablets	Schering-Plough	cr
Codimal L.A. capsules	Central	cr
Codimal L.A. Half capsules	Central	cr
Comhist LA capsules	Norwich Eaton	cr
Compazine Spansule capsules	SKF	cr
Congess SR capsules	Fleming	cr
Congess JR capsules	Fleming	cr
Constant-T tablets	Geigy	cr
Contac 12 Hour capsules	SKF	cr
Contac Maximum Strength caplets	SKF	cr
Control capsules	Thompson	cr
Cotazym-S capsules	Organon	ec
Cystospaz-M capsules	Webcon	cr
Dallergy-Jr capsules	Laser	cr
Deconamine SR capsules	Berlex	cr
Deconsal LA tablets	Adams	cr
Deconsal Sprinkle capsules	Adams	cr
Dehist capsules	Forest	cr
Depakote tablets	Abbott	ec
Desoxyn Gradumet tablets	Abbott	cr
Dexatrim capsules	Thompson	cr
Dexedrine Spansule capsules	SKF	cr
Diamox Sequel capsules	Lederle	cr
Diethylstilbestrol Enseal tablets	Lilly	ec
Dilatrate-SR capsules	Reed & Carnick	cr
Dimetane Extentab tablets	Robins	cr
Dimetapp Extentab tablets	Robins	cr
Disobrom tablets	Geneva	cr
Disophrol Chronotab tablets	Schering	cr
Donnatal Extentab tablets	Robins	cr
Donnazyme tablets	Robins	cr
Drixoral tablets	Schering-Plough	cr
Drize capsules	Ascher	cr
Dulcolax tablets	Ciba	ec
Duotrate capsules	JMI	cr

Controlled-release = cr **Enteric-coated = ec**

Duraquin tablets	Parke-Davis	cr
Easprin tablets	Parke-Davis	ec
Ecotrin tablets	SKF	ec
Ecotrin Maximum Strength	SKF	ec
Eight-hour Bayer caplets	Sterling Health	cr
Elixophyllin SR capsules	Forest	cr
E-Mycin tablets	Upjohn	ec
Entex-LA tablets	Norwich Eaton	cr
Entozyme tablets	Robins	cr
ERYC capsules	Parke-Davis	ec
Ery-Tab tablets	Abbott	ec
Eskalith-CR tablets	SKF	cr
Extendryl JR capsules	Fleming	cr
Extendryl SR capsules	Fleming	cr
Fedahist Gyrocaps capsules	Kremers Urban	cr
Fedahist Timecaps	Kremers Urban	cr
Feosol capsules	SKF	ec
Fergon capsules	Winthrop-Breon	ec
Ferralyn Lanacap capsules	Lannett	cr
Fero-Grad-500 tablets	Abbott	cr
Fero-Gradumet tablets	Abbott	cr
Ferro-Sequel capsules	Lederle	cr
Ferrous Sulfate Enseal tablets	Lilly	ec
Festal II tablets	Hoechst	ec
Genabid capsules	Goldline	cr
Guaifed capsules	Muro	cr
Hispril Spansule capsules	SKF	cr
Histafed-LA capsules	Geriatric	cr
Histaspan-D capsules	Rorer	cr
Histaspan-Plus capsules	Rorer	cr
Humibid LA tablets	Adams	cr
Humibid Sprinkle	Adams	cr
Iberet-500 tablets	Abbott	cr
Iberet-Folic-500 tablets	Abbott	cr
Ilotycin tablets	Dista	ec
Inderal LA capsules	Wyeth-Ayerst	cr
Inderide LA capsules	Wyeth-Ayerst	cr
Indocin-SR capsules	MSD	cr
Iso-Bid capsules	Geriatric	cr
Isoclor Timesule capsules	Ciba	cr
Isordil Tembid capsules	Wyeth-Ayerst	cr
Isordil Tembid tablets	Wyeth-Ayerst	cr
Kaon-CL tablets	Adria	cr
Kaon-CL-10 tablets	Adria	cr
K-Dur 10 tablets	Key	cr
K-Dur 20 tablets	Key	cr
K-Tab tablets	Abbott	cr
Klor-Con 8/Klor-Con 10 tablets	Upsher-Smith	cr
Klotrix tablets	Mead Johnson	cr
Levsinex Timecap capsules	Kremers Urban	cr
Levsinex with Pb Timecap capsules	Kremers Urban	cr
Lithobid tablets	Ciba	cr
Mandameth tablets	Major	ec
Measurin tablets	Winthrop-Breon	cr
Meprospan capsules	Wallace	cr
Mestinon Timespan tablets	ICN	cr
Micro-K Extencap capsules	Robins	cr
MS Contin tablets	Purdue Frederick	cr
Naldecon tablets	Bristol	cr
Niac capsules	Forest	cr
Nico-400	JMI	cr
Nicobid Tempule capsules	Rorer	cr
Nitro-Bid Plateau Cap capsules	Marion	cr
NItrocine Timecaps	Schwarz	cr
Nitroglyn capsules	Kenwood	cr
Nitrospan capsules	Rorer	cr
Nitrostat-SR capsules	Parke-Davis	cr
Nolamine tablets	Carnrick	cr
Nolex LA	Carnrick	cr
Norflex tablets	Riker	cr
Norpace-CR capsules	Searle	cr
Novafed capsules	Lakeside	cr
Novafed-A capsules	Lakeside	cr
Ornade Spansule capsules	SKF	cr
Pabalate tablets	Robins	ec
Pabalate-SF tablets	Robins	ec
Pancrease capsules	McNeil	ec
Pancrease MT capsules	McNeil	ec
Pancreatin Enseals Triple Strength tablets	Lilly	ec
Pavabid Plateau Cap capsules	Marion	cr
PBR/12 capsules	Scott-Alison	cr
PBZ-SR tablets	Geigy	cr
PCE tablets	Abbott	cr
Pentol SA tablets and capsules	Major	cr
Peritrate-SA tablets	Parke-Davis	cr
Phenetron Compound tablets	Lannett	ec
Phyllocontin tablets	Purdue Frederick	cr
Polaramine Repetab tablets	Schering	cr
Poly-Histine-D capsules	Bock	cr
Potassium Chloride Enseal tablets	Lilly	ec
Potassium Iodide Enseal tablets	Lilly	ec
Prelu-2 capsules	Boehringer Ingelheim	cr
Preludin Enduret tablets	Boehringer Ingelheim	cr
Procan-SR tablets	Parke-Davis	cr
Promine-SR tablets	Major	cr
Pronestyl-SR tablets	Squibb	cr
Quibron Bidcaps capsules	Mead Johnson	cr
Quibron-T/SR tablets	Mead Johnson	cr
Quinaglute Dura-Tab tablets	Berlex	cr
Quinatime tablets	CMC	cr
Quinidex Extentab tablets	Robins	cr
Respbid tablets	Boehringer Ingelheim	cr
Ritalin-SR tablets	Ciba	cr
Robimycin Robitab tablets	Robins	ec
Rondec-TR tablets	Ross	cr
Roxanol-SR tablets	Roxane	cr
Ru-Tuss tablets	Boots	cr
Ru-Tuss II capsules	Boots	cr

Controlled-release = cr **Enteric-coated = ec**

Sinemet CR	DuPont	cr
Singlet tablets	Lakeside	cr
Slo-bid Gyrocaps capsules	Rorer	cr
Slo-Phyllin Gyrocaps capsules	Rorer	cr
Slow-Fe tablets	Ciba	cr
Slow-K tablets	Ciba	cr
Sodium Chloride Enseal tablets	Lilly	ec
Sodium Salicylate Enseal tablets	Lilly	ec
Somophyllin-CRT capsules	Fisons	cr
Sorbitrate-SA tablets	Stuart	cr
Span-FF capsules	MetroMed	cr
Span-Niacin-150 tablets	Scrip	cr
Sudafed 12 Hour capsules	Burroughs Wellcome	cr
Sustaire tablets	Pfipharmecs	cr
Tamine SR tablets	Geneva	cr
Tavist-D tablets	Sandoz	cr
Tedral-SA tablets	Parke-Davis	cr
Teldrin Spansule capsules	SKF	cr
Temaril Spansule capsules	Herbert	cr
Ten-K tablets	Geigy	cr
Tenuate Dospan tablets	Lakeside	cr
Tepanil Ten-tab tablets	Riker	cr
Theo-24 capsules	Searle	cr
Theobid Duracap capsules	Glaxo	cr
Theobid Jr Duracap capsules	Glaxo	cr
Theoclear-LA capsules	Central	cr
Theochron tablets	Forest	cr
Theo-Dur tablets	Key	cr
Theo-Dur Sprinkle capsules	Key	cr
Theolair-SR tablets	Riker	cr
Theospan-SR capsules	Laser	cr
Theo-Time capsules	Major	cr
Theovent capsules	Schering	cr
Thorazine Spansule capsules	SKF	cr
Thyroid-Enseal tablets	Lilly	ec
Tranxene-SD tablets	Abbott	cr
Triaminic-12 tablets	Sandoz	cr
Triaminic TR tablets	Dorsey	cr
Trilafon Repetab tablets	Schering	cr
Trinalin Repetab tablets	Schering	cr
Trental tablets	Hoechst	cr
Tussagesic tablets	Sandoz	cr
Tuss-Ornade Spansule capsules	SKF	cr
Uniphyl tablets	Purdue Frederick	cr
Uracel 5 tablets	Vortech	ec
Valrelease capsules	Roche	cr
Verin tablets	Hauck	cr
Voltaren tablets	Ciba-Geigy	ec
Zorprin tablets	Boots	cr

Sugar-Free Products

Listed below, by therapeutic category, is a selection of drug products that contain no sugar. When recommending these products to diabetic patients, keep in mind that many may contain sorbitol, alcohol, or other sources of carbohydrates. Always check product labeling for a current listing of inactive ingredients.

ANALGESICS

Bufferin AF Nite Time	Bristol-Myers
Children's Myapap Elixir	My-K
Children's Panadol Drops	Sterling Health
Children's Panadol Liquid	Sterling Health
Children's Panadol Tablets, Chewable	Sterling Health
Dolanex Elixir	Lannett
Extra Strength Tylenol PM	McNeil
Methadone HCl Intensol	Roxane
Myapap Drops	My-K
St. Joseph Aspirin-Free Liquid	Plough
St. Joseph Aspirin-Free Drops	Plough
Tempra Tablets, Chewable	Mead Johnson

ANTACIDS/ANTIFLATULENTS

Alamag Suspension	Goldline
Aluminum Hydroxide Concentrated Suspension	Roxane
Aludrox Suspension	Wyeth-Ayerst
Calglycine Tablets	Rugby
Camalox Suspension	Rorer
Citrocarbonate Granules	Upjohn
Di-Gel Liquid	Plough
Dimacid	Otis Clapp
Eno Powder	SmithKline Beecham
Gaviscon Liquid	Marion
Gelusil Liquid	Parke-Davis
Gelusil II Suspension	Parke-Davis
Gelusil-M Suspension	Parke-Davis
Kolantyl Gel	Lakeside
Maalox Suspension	Rorer
Maalox Plus, Extra Strength Suspension	Rorer
Maalox Therapeutic Concentrate	Rorer
Magnesia and Alumina Oral Suspension USP	various
Mallamint Tablets, Chewable	Mallard
Marblen Suspension	Fleming
Marblen Tablets	Fleming
Milk of Magnesia USP	various
Mylanta Liquid	Stuart
Mylanta II Liquid	Stuart
Mylicon Drops	Stuart
Nephrox Suspension	Fleming
Pepto-Bismol Liquid	Procter & Gamble

Pepto-Bismol Tablets	Procter & Gamble
Riopan Suspension	Whitehall
Riopan Plus Suspension	Whitehall
Titracid Tablets	Trimen
Titralac Plus Liquid	3M
Titralac Tablets	3M
WinGel Liquid	Winthrop
WinGel Tablets	Winthrop

ANTIASTHMATIC/RESPIRATORY AGENTS

Aerolate Liquid	Fleming
Elixophyllin Elixir	Forest
Elixophyllin-GG Liquid	Forest
Lufyllin Elixir	Wallace
Metaprel Syrup	Sandoz
Mucomyst Solution	Mead Johnson
Mudrane-GG Elixir	Poythress
Organidin Solution	Wallace
Slo-Phyllin 80 Syrup	Rorer
Theo-Organidin Elixir	Wallace

ANTICONVULSANTS

Mysoline Suspension	Wyeth-Ayerst

ANTIDIARRHEALS

Diasorb Liquid	Columbia Labs
Kaolin with Pectin Suspension	various
Konsyl Powder	Lafayette
Lomotil Liquid	Searle
Paregoric USP	various
Pepto-Bismol Liquid	Procter & Gamble

ANTIHISTAMINES/DECONGESTANTS

Dimetane Decongestant Elixir	Robins
Dimetapp Elixir	Robins
Hay-Febrol Liquid	Scot-Tussin
Naldecon Pediatric Drops	Bristol
Naldecon Pediatric Syrup	Bristol
Naldecon Syrup	Bristol
Novahistine Elixir	Lakeside
Phenergan Syrup	Wyeth-Ayerst
Phenergan Fortis Syrup	Wyeth-Ayerst
Ryna Liquid	Wallace
Tavist Syrup	Sandoz
Trind Liquid	Mead Johnson

ANTI-INFECTIVE AGENTS

Augmentin Suspension	Beecham
Furadantin Suspension	Norwich Eaton
Furoxone Suspension	Norwich Eaton
Humatin	Parke-Davis
Mandelamine Suspension Forte	Parke-Davis
Minocin Suspension	Lederle
NegGram Suspension	Winthrop-Breon

ANTIMANIC AGENTS

Cibalith-S Syrup	Ciba
Lithium Citrate Syrup	Roxane

BLOOD MODIFIERS/IRON PREPARATIONS

Amicar Syrup	Lederle
Geritol Complete Tablets	Beecham
Geritonic Liquid	Geriatric
Iberet Liquid	Abbott
Incremin with Iron Syrup	Lederle
Kovitonic Liquid	Freeda
Niferex Elixir	Central
Nu-Iron Elixir	Mayrand
Vita-Plus H Liquid	Scot-Tussin

CORTICOSTEROIDS

Decadron Elixir	MSD
Dexamethasone Solution	Roxane
Dexamethasone Intensol Solution	Roxane
Pediapred Oral Liquid	Fisons

COUGH/COLD PREPARATIONS

Anatuss Syrup	Mayrand
Cerose-DM	Wyeth-Ayerst
Chlorgest HD	Great Southern
Codagest Expectorant	Great Southern
Codiclear DH Syrup	Central
Codimal-DM Syrup	Central
Colrex Expectorant	Reid-Rowell
Comtrex, Day-Night	Bristol-Myers
Conex with Codeine Syrup	Forest
Contac Jr. Liquid	SKF
Decorel Forte	Medique
Dexafed Cough Syrup	Hauck
Dimetane-DC Cough Syrup	Robins
Dimetane-DX Cough Syrup	Robins
Elixir Terpin Hydrate with Codeine	various
Entuss Expectorant Syrup	Hauck
Fedahist Expectorant Syrup	Kremers Urban
Fedahist Expectorant Pediatric Drops	Kremers Urban
Histafed Pediatric Liquid	Geriatric
Hycomine Syrup	DuPont
Hycomine Pediatric Syrup	DuPont
Lanatuss Expectorant	Lannett
Naldecon-DX Adult Liquid	Bristol
Naldecon-DX Pediatric Drops	Bristol
Naldecon-EX Syrup	Bristol
Non-Drowsy Comtrex	Bristol-Myers
Organidin Solution	Wallace
Potassium Iodide Solution	various
Robitussin-CF Liquid	Robins
Robitussin Night Relief Liquid	Robins
Ryna Liquid	Wallace
Ryna-C Liquid	Wallace
Ryna-CX Liquid	Wallace
Scot-Tussin DM Cough Chasers	Scot-Tussin
S-T Decongestant Liquid	Scot-Tussin
S-T Forte SF Liquid	Scot-Tussin
Scot-Tussin Expectorant	Scot-Tussin
Scot-Tussin DM Syrup	Scot-Tussin
Silexin Cough Syrup	Clapp
Tolu-Sed Cough Syrup	Scherer
Tolu-Sed DM Elixir	Scherer
Trind-DM Liquid	Mead Johnson
Tussar SF Syrup	Rorer
Tussi-Organidin Liquid	Wallace
Tussionex Extended-Release Suspension	Pennwalt

Tussirex Sugar-Free Liquid	Scot-Tussin
Tuss-Ornade Liquid	SKF

GASTROINTESTINAL DRUGS

Dipentum	Kabi
Paregoric	various
Reglan Syrup	Robins
Tagamet Liquid	SKF

LAXATIVES

Agoral Marshmallow Emulsion	Parke-Davis
Agoral Plain Emulsion	Parke-Davis
Agoral Raspberry Emulsion	Parke-Davis
Cascara Sagrada Fluid Extract	various
Castor Oil	various
Colace Liquid	Mead Johnson
Disonate Liquid	Lannett
Doxinate Solution	Hoechst
Emulsoil	Paddock
Fiberall Powder	Ciba
Haley's M-O	Winthrop
Hydrocil Instant Powder	Reid-Rowell
Kondremul Plain Emulsion	Ciba
Konsyl Powder	Lafayette
Magnesium Citrate Solution	various
Metamucil Sugar Free Powder	Procter & Gamble
Metamucil Instant Mix, lemon-lime or orange	Procter & Gamble
Milk of Magnesia Suspension	various
Milkinol Emulsion	Schwarz
Mineral Oil	various
Neoloid Liquid	Lederle
Nu-LYTELY	Braintree

MISCELLANEOUS

Artane Elixir	Lederle
Bicitra Solution	Willen
Colestid	Upjohn
Duvoid	Roberts
Digoxin Elixir	Roxane
Lipomul Liquid	Upjohn
Nicorette Chewing Gum	Merrell Dow
Polycitra-K Solution	Willen
Polycitra-LC Solution	Willen

POTASSIUM SUPPLEMENTS

Cena-K Solution	Century
K-G Elixir	Geneva
Kaochlor-Eff Tablets for Solution	Adria
Kaochlor-S-F Solution	Adria
Kaon Elixir	Adria
Kaon-Cl 20% Solution	Adria
Kay Ciel Elixir	Forest
Kay Ciel Powder	Forest
Klor-Con Powder	Upsher-Smith
Klor-Con/25 Powder	Upsher-Smith
Klor-Con/EF Tablets	Upsher-Smith
Klorvess Effervescent Granules	Sandoz
Klorvess Tablets for Solution	Sandoz
Kolyum Powder	Pennwalt
Kolyum Solution	Pennwalt
Potasalan Liquid	Lannett
Potassium Chloride Oral Solution USP	various
Potassium Gluconate Elixir NF	various
Rum-K Solution	Fleming
Tri-K Liquid	Century

PSYCHOTROPICS/SEDATIVES

Butabarbital Elixir	various
Butisol Elixir	Wallace
Haldol Concentrate	McNeil
Loxitane C Drops	Lederle
Permitil Concentrate Solution	Schering
Serentil Concentrate Solution	Boehringer Ingelheim
Thorazine Concentrate Solution	SKF

TOPICAL ORAL PREPARATIONS

Anbesol Gel	Whitehall
Anbesol Liquid	Whitehall
Babee Teething Lotion	Pfeiffer
Baby Orajel	Commerce
Chloraseptic Mouthwash/Gargle	Vicks
Moi-Stir Solution	Kingswood
Mycinettes Lozenges	Pfeiffer
N'ice Lozenges	Beecham
Orabase with Benzocaine	Colgate-Hoyt
Orabase-O	Colgate-Hoyt
Orabase Plain	Colgate-Hoyt
Orajel Brace-Aid Gel	Commerce
Orajel/d Gel	Commerce
Orajel Mouth-Aid Gel	Commerce
Peroxyl Gel	Colgate-Hoyt
Peroxyl Mouthrinse	Colgate-Hoyt
Rid-A-Pain Drops	Pfieffer
Rid-A-Pain Gel	Pfeiffer
Salivart Solution	Westport
Sucrets Maximum Strength Mouthwash/Gargle	Beecham
Tanac Liquid	Commerce
Tanac Stick	Commerce
Tanac Roll-On Liquid	Commerce
Xero-Lube Solution	Scherer

VITAMINS/MINERALS

Aquasol A Capsules	Astra
Bugs Bunny Chewable Tablets	Miles
Bugs Bunny Plus Iron Chewable Tabs	Miles
Bugs Bunny with Extra C Chewable Tabs	Miles
Bugs Bunny Plus Minerals Chewable Tabs	Miles
Calciferol Drops	Kremers Urban
Caltrate 600 Tablets	Lederle
Cod Liver Oil	various
Decagen Tablets	Goldline
DHT Solution	Roxane
DHT Intensol Solution	Roxane
Flintstones Complete Chewable Tablets	Miles
Flintstones Plus Iron Chewable Tablets	Miles
Flintstones with extra C Chewable Tablets	Miles

Fluorinse	Oral-B
Gel-Kam	Scherer
Incremin with Iron Liquid	Lederle
Karidium Drops	Lorvic
Karidium Tablets	Lorvic
Karigel	Lorvic
Karigel-N	Lorvic
Luride Drops	Colgate-Hoyt
Luride Lozi-tabs	Colgate/Hoyt
Luride-SF Lozi-tabs	Colgate/Hoyt
Luride 0.25 Lozi-tabs	Colgate/Hoyt
Luride 0.5 Lozi-tabs	Colgate-Hoyt
Oyst-Cal 500 Tablets	Goldline
Pediaflor Drops	Ross
Phos-Flur Rinse	Colgate/Hoyt
Phos-Flur Rinse/supplement	Colgate/Hoyt
Point-Two Mouthrinse	Colgate/Hoyt
Poly-Vi-Flor Drops	Mead Johnson
Poly-Vi-Sol Infant Drops	Mead Johnson
Poly-Vi-Sol with Iron Drops	Mead Johnson
Posture Tablets	Wyeth-Ayerst
Spider-Man Children's Chewable Vitamin Tablets	Nature's Bounty
Spider-Man Plus Iron Tablets	Nature's Bounty
Stop Gel	Oral-B
Theragran Jr. Children's Chewable Tablets	Squibb
Tri-Vi-Flor Drops	Mead Johnson
Tri-Vi-Flor with Iron Drops	Mead Johnson
Tri-Vi-Sol Drops	Mead Johnson
Tri-Vi-Sol with Iron Drops	Mead Johnson
Vi-Daylin Drops	Ross
Vi-Daylin ADC Drops	Ross
Vi-Daylin/F Drops	Ross
Vi-Daylin/F ADC Drops	Ross
Vi-Daylin plus Iron Drops	Ross
Vi-Daylin plus Iron ADC Drops	Ross
Vitalize SF Liquid	Scot-Tussin

Table B-1. Food and Drug Administration Pregnancy Categories

Pregnancy Category*	Definition†
A	Adequate studies in pregnant women have not demonstrated a risk to the fetus in the first trimester of pregnancy, and there is no evidence of risk in later trimesters.
B	Animal studies have not demonstrated a risk to the fetus, but there are no adequate studies in pregnant women; or animal studies have shown an adverse effect, but adequate studies in pregnant women have not demonstrated a risk to the fetus during the first trimester of pregnancy, and there is no evidence of risk in later trimesters.
C	Animal studies have shown an adverse effect on the fetus, but there are no adequate studies in humans; the benefits from the use of the drug in pregnant women may be acceptable despite its potential risks; or there are no animal studies and no adequate studies in humans.
D	There is evidence of human fetal risk, but the potential benefits from the use of the drug in pregnant women may be acceptable despite its potential risks.
E	Studies in animals and humans, adverse reaction reports, or both have demonstrated fetal abnormalities; the risk of use in pregnant women clearly outweighs any possible benefit.‡

Reprinted from *Drug Facts and Comparisons.* St. Louis, Lippincott, January, 1993.

*The Food and Drug Administration (FDA) has established five categories to indicate a systemically absorbed drug's potential for causing birth defects. The key differentiation among the categories rests upon the degree (reliability) of documentation and the risk:benefit ratio. Pregnancy (category X) is particularly notable in that if any data exist that may implicate a drug as a teratogen and if the risk:benefit ratio is clearly negative, the drug is contraindicated during pregnancy.

†The use of any medication requires a risk versus benefit assessment. Pregnancy is one of the most perplexing of the factors that complicate this assessment.

‡Regardless of the pregnancy category or presumed safety, no drug should be administered during pregnancy unless it is clearly needed.

Appendix C: Pharmacy Schools and Organizations

Colleges and Schools of Pharmacy

UNITED STATES

Although all schools listed have accredited first professional degree programs, not all PharmD programs have been accredited by the American Council on Pharmaceutical Education. The accreditation status of programs can be obtained by contacting the ACPE, 311 West Superior, Chicago, Illinois 60610, (312) 664-3575.

Alabama

School of Pharmacy
Auburn University
Alabama, 36849-5501
205/844-4740

School of Pharmacy
Samford University
800 Lakeshore Drive
Birmingham, Alabama 35229
205/870-2820

Arizona

College of Pharmacy
The University of Arizona
Tucson, Arizona 85721
602/626-1427

Arkansas

College of Pharmacy
University of Arkansas for Medical Sciences
4301 West Markham—Slot 522
Little Rock, Arkansas 72205-7122
501/686-5557

California

School of Pharmacy
University of California S-926
San Francisco, California 94143-0446
415/476-1225

School of Pharmacy
University of the Pacific
3601 Pacific Avenue
Stockton, California 95211
209/946-2561

School of Pharmacy
University of Southern California
1985 Zonal Avenue
Los Angeles, California 90033-1086
213/224-7501

Colorado

School of Pharmacy
University of Colorado
Box 297
Boulder, Colorado 80309-0297
303/492-6278

Connecticut

School of Pharmacy
The University of Connecticut
Box U-92
372 Fairfield Road
Storrs, Connecticut 06269-2092
203/486-2129

District of Columbia

College of Pharmacy and Pharmacal Sciences
Howard University
2300 4th Street, N.W.
Washington, DC 20059
202/636-6530

Florida

College of Pharmacy and Pharmaceutical Sciences
Florida Agricultural and Mechanical University
P.O. Box 367
Tallahassee, Florida 32307
904/599-3578

Southeastern College of Pharmaceutical Sciences
1750 N.E. 168th Street
N. Miami Beach, Florida 33162-3097
305/949-4000

College of Pharmacy
University of Florida
Box J-484
Health Science Center
Gainesville, Florida 32610
904/392-9713

Georgia

Southern School of Pharmacy
Mercer University
3001 Mercer University Drive
Atlanta, Georgia 30341
404/986-3300

College of Pharmacy
The University of Georgia
Athens, Georgia 30602
404/542-1911

Idaho

College of Pharmacy
Idaho State University
Pocatello, Idaho 83209-0009
208/236-2175

Illinois

College of Pharmacy
University of Illinois at Chicago
833 South Wood St., Box 6998
M/C 874
Chicago, Illinois 60680-6998
312/996-7240

Indiana

College of Pharmacy
Butler University
46th & Sunset Avenue
Indianapolis, Indiana 46208
317/283-9322

School of Pharmacy and Pharmacal Sciences
Purdue University
West Lafayette, Indiana 47907-0708
317/494-1357

Iowa

College of Pharmacy
Drake University
28th & Forest
Des Moines, Iowa 50311
515/271-2172

College of Pharmacy
The University of Iowa
Iowa City, Iowa 52242
319/335-8794

Kansas

School of Pharmacy
University of Kansas
2056 Malott
Lawrence, Kansas 66045-2500
913/864-3591

Kentucky

College of Pharmacy
University of Kentucky
Rose Street—Pharmacy Building
Lexington, Kentucky 40536-0082
606/257-2738

Louisiana

School of Pharmacy
Northeast Louisiana University
700 University Avenue
Monroe, Louisiana 71209-0470
318/342-2180

College of Pharmacy
Xavier University of Louisiana
7235 Palmetto Street
New Orleans, Louisiana 70125
504/483-7424

Maryland

School of Pharmacy
University of Maryland
20 North Pine Street
Baltimore, Maryland 21201-1180
301/328-7650

Massachusetts

Massachusetts College of Pharmacy and Allied Health Sciences
179 Longwood Avenue
Boston, Massachusetts 02115
617/732-2800

College of Pharmacy and Allied Health Professions
Northeastern University
360 Huntington Avenue
Boston, Massachusetts 02115
617/437-3321

Michigan

School of Pharmacy
Ferris State University
901 South State Street
Big Rapids, Michigan 49307
616/592-2254

College of Pharmacy
The University of Michigan
Ann Arbor, Michigan 48109-1065
313/764-7312

College of Pharmacy and Allied Health Professions
Wayne State University
105 Shapero Hall
Detroit, Michigan 48202-3489
313/577-1574

Minnesota

College of Pharmacy
University of Minnesota
5-130 Health Sciences Unit F
308 Harvard Street, S.E.
Minneapolis, Minnesota 55455-0343
612/624-1900

Mississippi

School of Pharmacy
The University of Mississippi
University, Mississippi 38677-9814
601/232-7265

Missouri

St. Louis College of Pharmacy
4588 Parkview Place
St. Louis, Missouri 63110-1088
314/367-8700

School of Pharmacy
University of Missouri—Kansas City
5005 Rockhill Road
Kansas City, Missouri 64110
816/276-1607

Montana

School of Pharmacy and Allied Health Sciences
University of Montana
Missoula, Montana 59812
406/243-4621

Nebraska

School of Pharmacy and Allied Health Professions
Creighton University
California at 24th Street
Omaha, Nebraska 68178
402/280-2950

College of Pharmacy
University of Nebraska
42nd & Dewey Avenue
Omaha, Nebraska 68105-1065
402/559-4333

New Jersey

College of Pharmacy
Rutgers University
The State University of New Jersey
Post Office Box 789
Piscataway, New Jersey 08855-0789
201/932-2666

New Mexico

College of Pharmacy
University of New Mexico
Albuquerque, New Mexico 87131
505/277-2461

New York

Arnold & Marie Schwartz College of Pharmacy and Health Sciences
Long Island University
75 DeKalb Ave. at University Plaza
Brooklyn, New York 11201
718/403-1060

College of Pharmacy and Allied Health Professions
St. John's University
Grand Central and Utopia Parkways
Jamaica, New York 11439
718/990-6161

School of Pharmacy
State University of New York at Buffalo
C126 Cooke-Hochstetter Complex
Buffalo, New York 14260
716/636-2823

Albany College of Pharmacy
Union University
106 New Scotland
Albany, New York 12208
518/445-7211

North Carolina

School of Pharmacy
Campbell University
Post Office Box 1090
Buies Creek, North Carolina 27506
919/893-4111

School of Pharmacy
University of North Carolina
Beard Hall #7360
Chapel Hill, North Carolina 27599-7360
919/966-1121

North Dakota

College of Pharmacy
North Dakota State University
Fargo, North Dakota 58105
701/237-7456

Ohio

College of Pharmacy and Allied Health Sciences
Ohio Northern University
Ada, Ohio 45810
419/772-2275

College of Pharmacy
The Ohio State University
500 West 12th Avenue
Columbus, Ohio 43210-1291
614/292-2266

College of Pharmacy
University of Cincinnati-Medical Center
Mail Location #4
Cincinnati, Ohio 45267
513/558-3784

College of Pharmacy
The University of Toledo
2801 West Bancroft Street
Toledo, Ohio 43606
419/537-2019

Oklahoma

School of Pharmacy
Southwestern Oklahoma State University
100 Campus Drive
Weatherford, Oklahoma 73096
405/774-3105

College of Pharmacy
University of Oklahoma
P.O. Box 26901
Oklahoma City, Oklahoma 73190-5040
405/271-6484

Oregon

College of Pharmacy
Oregon State University
Corvallis, Oregon 97331-3507
503/737-3424

Pennsylvania

School of Pharmacy
Duquesne University
Pittsburgh, Pennsylvania 15282
412/434-6380

School of Pharmacy
Philadelphia College of Pharmacy and Science
Woodland Avenue at 43rd Street
Philadelphia, Pennsylvania 19104
215/596-8800

School of Pharmacy
Temple University
3307 North Broad Street
Philadelphia, Pennsylvania 19140
215/221-4990

School of Pharmacy
University of Pittsburgh
1103 Salk Hall
Pittsburgh, Pennsylvania 15261
412/648-8579

Puerto Rico

College of Pharmacy
University of Puerto Rico
GPO Box 5067
San Juan, Puerto Rico 00936-5067
809/758-2525 (ext) 5400

Rhode Island

College of Pharmacy
University of Rhode Island
Kingston, Rhode Island 02881-0809
401/792-2761

South Carolina

College of Pharmacy
Medical University of South Carolina
171 Ashley Avenue
Charleston, South Carolina 29425-2301
803/792-3115

College of Pharmacy
University of South Carolina
Columbia, South Carolina 29208
803/777-4151

South Dakota

College of Pharmacy
South Dakota State University
Box 2202C
Brookings, South Dakota 57007-0197
605/688-6197

Tennessee

College of Pharmacy
University of Tennessee
874 Union Avenue
Memphis, Tennessee 38163
901/528-6036

Texas

School of Pharmacy
Texas Southern University
3100 Cleburne
Houston, Texas 77004
713/527-7164

College of Pharmacy
University of Houston
4800 Calhoun
Houston, Texas 77204-5511
713/749-4106

College of Pharmacy
University of Texas at Austin
Austin, Texas 78712-1074
512/471-1737

Utah

College of Pharmacy
University of Utah
Salt Lake City, Utah 84112
801/581-6731

Virginia

School of Pharmacy
Virginia Commonwealth University
MCV Campus—Box 581
410 North 12th Street
Richmond, Virginia 23298-0581
804/786-7346

Washington

School of Pharmacy
University of Washington
T-341 Health Science Center, SC-69
Seattle, Washington 98195
206/543-2030

College of Pharmacy
Washington State University
Pullman, Washington 99164-6510
509/335-8664

West Virginia

School of Pharmacy
West Virginia University
Morgantown, West Virginia 26506
304/293-5101

Wisconsin

School of Pharmacy
University of Wisconsin-Madison
425 North Charter Street
Madison, Wisconsin 53706
608/262-1416

Wyoming

School of Pharmacy
University of Wyoming
P.O. Box 3375
Laramie, Wyoming 82071-3375
307/766-6120

Canada

Faculty of Pharmacy and Pharmaceutical Sciences
The University of Alberta
Edmonton, Alberta
T6G 2N8 Canada

Faculty of Pharmaceutical Sciences
University of British Columbia
2146 East Mall
Vancouver, B.C.
V6T 1W5

College of Pharmacy
Dalhousie University
5968 College Street
Halifax, Nova Scotia
B3H 3J5 Canada

Ecole De Pharmacie
University Laval
Quebec (Quebec)
G1K 7P4 Canada

The Faculty of Pharmacy
The University of Manitoba
Winnipeg, Manitoba
R3T 2N2 Canada

Memorial University of Newfoundland
Health Science Complex
St. John's, Newfoundland
A1B 3B6 Canada

Faculty of Pharmacy
University of Montreal
C.P. 6128 Succursale A
Montreal, Quebec
H3C 3J7 Canada

College of Pharmacy
University of Saskatchewan
Saskatoon, Saskatchewan
S7N 0W0 Canada

Faculty of Pharmacy
University of Toronto
Toronto, Ontario
M5S 1A1 Canada

Philippines

University of the Philippines
Padre Faura, Manila
Philippines

Malaysia

School of Pharmaceutical Sciences
University Sains Malaysia
Minden, Penang 11800
Malaysia 011-04-888333

Pharmacy Acronyms and Abbreviations

The following are the most commonly used acronyms and abbreviations in pharmacy and licensure:

AACP American Association of Colleges of Pharmacy
ACA American College of Apothecaries
ACPE American Council of Pharmaceutical Education
AFPE American Foundation on Pharmaceutical Education
AIHP American Institute of the History of Pharmacy
APhA American Pharmaceutical Association
ASCP American Society of Consultant Pharmacists
ASHP American Society of Hospital Pharmacists
ASP American Society of Pharmacognosy

ASPL	American Society of Pharmacy Law
CLEAR	The National Clearinghouse on Licensure, Enforcement & Regulation
CPSC	Consumer Product Safety Commission
DEA	Drug Enforcement Administration
DWA	Drug Wholesalers Association, Inc.
FAHRB	Federation of Association of Health Regulatory Boards
FDA	Food & Drug Administration
HHS	Department of Health and Human Services
NABP	National Association of Boards of Pharmacy
NABPF	National Association of Boards of Pharmacy Foundation
NABPLEX	National Association of Boards of Pharmacy Licensure Examination
NACDS	National Association of Chain Drug Stores
NAPM	National Association of Pharmaceutical Manufacturers
NARD	National Association of Retail Druggists
NCPIE	National Council on Patient Information and Education
NCPDP	National Council on Third Party Prescription Drug Programs
NDTC	National Drug Trade Conference
NPC	National Pharmaceutical Council
PA	The Proprietary Association
PMA	Pharmaceutical Manufacturers Association
USP	United States Pharmacopeial Convention, Inc.

The following are abbreviations used internally by NABP:

ACE	Advisory Committee on Examinations
ACT	American College Testing
BVC	Bureau of Voluntary Compliance
CBL	Committee on Constitution and Bylaws
CCE	Committee on Continuing Education
CIP	Committee on Institutional Pharmacy
CIT	Committee on Internship Training
CLL	Committee on Law Enforcement/Legislation Executive Committee
FDLE	Federal Drug Law Examination
FPGEC	Foreign Pharmacy Graduate Examination Commission
FPGEC-SC	Foreign Pharmacy Graduate Examination Commission Steering Committee
FPGEE	Foreign Pharmacy Graduate Equivalency Examination
NRC	NABPLEX Review Committee
NSC	NABPLEX Steering Committee
UTD	Uniform Testing Date

Pharmacy Organizations

American Association of Colleges of Pharmacy
1426 Prince Street
Alexandria, VA 22314
(703) 739-2330

American College of Apothecaries
205 Daingerfield Road
Alexandria, VA 22314
(703) 684-8603

American College of Clinical Pharmacy
3101 Broadway, Suite 380
Kansas City, MO 64111
(816) 531-2177

American Foundation for Pharmaceutical Education
618 Somerset Street
P.O. Box 7126
North Plainfield, NJ 07060
(908) 561-8077

American Institute of the History of Pharmacy
c/o Pharmacy Building
University of Wisconsin
Madison, WI 53706
(608) 262-5378

American Pharmaceutical Association
2215 Constitution Avenue NW
Washington, DC 20037
(202) 628-4410

American Society of Consultant Pharmacists
1321 Duke Street
Alexandria, VA 22314
(703) 739-1300

American Society of Hospital Pharmacists
7272 Wisconsin Avenue
Bethesda, MD 20814
(301) 657-3000

American Society of Pharmacognosy
College of Pharmacy
University of Utah
Salt Lake City, UT 84112

American Society for Pharmacy Law
P.O. Box 2184
Vienna, VA 22183

Association of Pharmacy Technicians
10123 Alliance Road, Suite 130
P.O. Box 42696
Cincinnati, OH 45242
(513) 793-3555

The Drug Chemical and Allied Trades Assn., Inc.
2 Roosevelt Avenue, Suite 301
Syosset, NY 11791
(718) 229-8891

Food and Drug Law Institute
1000 Vermont Avenue NW, Suite 1200
Washington, DC 20005
(202) 371-1420

Generic Pharmaceutical Industry Association
200 Madison Avenue, Suite 2404
New York, NY 10016
(212) 683-1881

Metropolitan Pharmaceutical Secretaries Association
P.O. Box 8194
St. Louis, MO 63156
(314) 531-6929

National Association of Boards of Pharmacy
700 Busse Highway
Park Ridge, IL 60068
(312) 698-6227

National Association of Chain Drug Stores
413 N. Lee Street
P.O. Box 1417-D49
Alexandria, VA 22313
(703) 549-3001

National Association of Pharmaceutical Manufacturers
747 Third Avenue
New York, NY 10017
(212) 838-3720

National Association of Retail Druggists
20 Daingerfield Road
Alexandria, VA 22314
(703) 683-8200

National Catholic Pharmacists Guild of U.S.
1012 Surrey Hills Drive
St. Louis, MO 63117
(314) 645-0085

National Council on Patient Information and Education
666 11th Street NW, Suite 810
Washington, DC 20001
(202) 466-6711

National Council of State Pharmaceutical Assn. Executives
P.O. Box 151
Chapel Hill, NC 27514
(317) 634-4968

National Institutes of Health
Building 10, Room 1S-257
Bethesda, MD 20205
(301) 496-4363

National Pharmaceutical Association
1288 Rt. 73
Mount Laurel, NJ 08054
(609) 722-0902

National Pharmaceutical Council
1894 Preston White Drive
Reston, VA 22091
(703) 620-6390

National Pharmaceutical Foundation
P.O. Box 5439, Takoma Park Station
Washington, DC 20912
(202) 829-5008

National Wholesale Druggists Association
P.O. Box 238
Alexandria, VA 22313
(703) 684-6400

Parenteral Drug Association, Inc.
7500 Old Georgetown Road
Bethesda, MD 20814
(301) 986-0293

Pharmaceutical Manufacturers Association
1100 15th Street NW
Washington, DC 20005
(202) 835-3400

The Proprietary Association
1150 Connecticut Avenue NW, Suite 1200
Washington, DC 20036
(202) 429-9260

State Pharmaceutical Editorial Association
223 W. Jackson, Suite 1000
Chicago, IL 60606
(312) 939-7663

U.S. Adopted Names (USAN)
American Medical Association
515 N. State Street
Chicago, IL 60610
(312) 464-4045

U.S. Navy
Defense Medical Standardization Board
Fort Detrick
Frederick, MD 21701-5013
(301) 663-7387

U.S. Pharmacopeial Convention, Inc.
12601 Twinbrook Parkway
Rockville, MD 20852
(301) 881-0666

U.S. Public Health Service
CA2, 5600 Fishers Lane
Parklawn Building, Room 9-05
Rockville, MD 20857
(301) 443-1993

Veterans Administration
810 Vermont Avenue NW
Washington, DC 20420
(202) 233-3277

State Boards of Pharmacy

Alabama	Jerry Moore, 1 Perimeter Park South, Suite 425 S., Birmingham 35243
Alaska	Laura Murphy, PO Box 110806, Juneau 99811-0806
Arkansas	Lester Hosto, 320 W. Capitol, Suite 802, Little Rock 72201, (501) 324-9200
California	Patricia Harris, 400 R St., Suite 4070, Sacramento 95814
Colorado	David L. Simmons, 1560 Broadway, Suite 1310, Denver 80202-5146
Connecticut	Sharon Milton-Wilhelm, 165 Capitol Ave., Room G1-A, Hartford 06106
Delaware	Bonnie Wallner, P.O. Box 637, Cooper Building, Room 205, Dover 19903
Florida	John Taylor, 1940 N. Monroe St., Tallahassee 32399-0775
Georgia	Gregg W. Schuder, 166 Pryor St. SW, Atlanta 30303
Hawaii	Charlene Kaninau, P.O. Box 3469, Honolulu 96801
Idaho	R.K. Markuson, 280 N. Eighth St., Suite 204, Boise 83720
Illinois	Ed Duffy, 100 W. Randolph St., Suite 9-300, Chicago 60601
Indiana	Tim Nation, 402 West Washington, Room 041, Indianapolis 46204
Iowa	Lloyd K. Jessen, 1209 East Ct., Executive Hills West, Des Moines 50319
Kansas	Tom Hitchcock, 900 Jackson, Room 513, Topeka 66612
Kentucky	Richard L. Ross, 1228 U.S. Hwy, 127 S., Frankfort 40601
Louisiana	Howard B. Bolton, 5615 Corporate Blvd., Suite 8E, Baton Rouge 70808
Maine	Douglas Libby, Commission of Pharmacy, State House Station #35, Augusta 04333
Maryland	Roslyn Scheer, 4201 Patterson Ave., Baltimore 21215
Massachusetts	Harold R. Partamian, 100 Cambridge St., Room 1514, Boston 02202

Michigan	Cathy Seyka, 611 W. Ottawa St., P.O. Box 30018, Lansing 48909
Minnesota	David E. Holmstrom, 2700 University Ave. W., #107, St. Paul 55114
Mississippi	Harold Stringer, 2310 Hwy, 80 W., C and F Plaza Suite D, Jackson 39204
Missouri	Kevin E. Kinkade, P.O. Box 25, Jefferson City 65102
Montana	Warren R. Amole, Jr., 510 First Avenue N., Suite 100, Great Falls 59401
Nebraska	Katherine Brown, Box 95007, 301 Centennial Mall S., Lincoln 68509
Nevada	Keith W. Macdonald, 1201 Terminal Way, Suite 212, Reno 89502-3257
New Hampshire	Paul G. Boisseau, 57 Regional Drive, Concord 03301
New Jersey	H. Lee Gladstein, 124 Halsey St., Newark 07102
New Mexico	Richard Thompson, 1650 University Boulevard NE, Suite 400 B, Albuquerque 87102
New York	Cultural Education Center, Room 3035, Albany, 12230
North Carolina	David R. Work, P.O. Box 459, 602H Jones Ferry Rd., Carrboro 27510
North Dakota	William J. Grosz, P.O. Box 1354, Bismarck 58501
Ohio	Franklin Z. Wickham, 77 High St., 17th Floor, Columbus 43266-0320
Oklahoma	Bryan H. Potter, 4545 N. Lincoln Blvd., Suite 112, Oklahoma City 73105
Oregon	Ruth Vandever, 800 N.E. Oregon St. #9, Portland 97232
Pennsylvania	Frank Wiercinski, PO Box 2649, Harrisburg 17105
Puerto Rico	Irza Torres Aguiar, Call Box 10200, Santurce 00908
Rhode Island	Mario Casinelli, Three Capitol Hill, Room 304, Providence 02908-5097
South Carolina	C. Douglas Chavous, 1026 Sumter St., Room 209, P.O. Box 11927, Columbia 29211
South Dakota	Gallen Jordre, Box 518, Pierre 57501
Tennessee	J. Floyd Ferrell Jr., 500 James Robertson Parkway, Nashville 37243-1149
Texas	Fred S. Brinkley, Jr., 8505 Cross Park Dr., Suite 110, Austin 78754
Utah	David E. Robinson, 160 East 300 S., P.O. Box 45805, Salt Lake City 84145-0805
Vermont	John R. Low, Office of Professional Services, 109 State St., Montpelier 05609-1106
Virginia	Scottie Milley, 1601 Rolling Hills Dr., Richmond 23230
Washington	Donald H. Williams, 1300 Quince St. S.E., Mail Stop 7863, Olympia 98504-7863
West Virginia	Sam Kapourales, 236 Capitol St., Charleston 25301
Wisconsin	Patrick Brantz, PO Box 8935, 1400 E. Washington Ave., Madison 53708
Wyoming	Marilynn H. Mitchell, 1720 S. Poplar St., Suite 5, Casper 82601

Directors and Addresses for State Pharmacy Associations

Alabama	Mitchel C. Rothholz, R.Ph., 1211 Carmichael Way, Montgomery 36106-3672 (205) 271-4222
Alaska	William F. Davnie, 13121 Biscayne Circle, Anchorage 99516 (907) 563-8880
Arizona	State Pharmacy Association, 1845 E. Southern Ave., Tempe 85282-5831 (602) 838-3385
Arkansas	Norman F. Canterbury, 417 S. Victory, Little Rock 72201 (501) 372-5250
California	Robert Marshall, 1112 I St., Suite 300, Sacramento 95814 (916) 444-7811
Colorado	S. Thomas Gray, 770 Grant St., #244, Denver 80203-3517 (303) 861-0328
Connecticut	Daniel C. Leone, 35 Cold Spring Rd., Suite 125, Rocky Hill 06067 (203) 563-4619
Delaware	Maryanne Uricheck, R.Ph., Executive Director, 707 Philadelphia Pike, Wilmington 19809 (302) 762-6019
District of Columbia	John Smith, T.N.C., Executive Director, 6406 Georgia Ave. N.W., Suite 202, Washington 20012 (202) 829-1515
Florida	C. Rod Presnell, 610 N. Adams St., Tallahassee 32301 (904) 222-2400
Georgia	Larry L. Braden, R.Ph., P.O. Box 95527, Atlanta 30347 (404) 231-5074
Hawaii	Edmund E. Ehlke, H.Ph.A, P.O. Box 1198, Honolulu 96807 (808) 595-3708
Idaho	JoAn Condie, 1365 N. Orchard, Suite 316, Boise 83706 (208) 376-2273

Illinois	Mark A. Pilkington, 223 W Jackson Blvd., Suite 1000, Chicago 60606 (312) 939-7300
Indiana	Lawrence J. Sage, 156 E. Market St., Suite 900, Indianapolis 46204 (317) 634-4968
Iowa	Thomas R. Temple, 8515 Douglas, Suite 16, Des Moines 50322 (515) 270-0713
Kansas	Robert R. Williams, 1308 W. 10th St., Topeka 66604 (913) 232-0439
Kentucky	Robert L. Barnett, Jr., 1228 U.S. Hwy. 127 S., Frankfort 40601 (502) 227-2303
Louisiana	Patricia M. Willford, 5800 One Perkins Place, Bldg. 7B, Baton Rouge 70808 (504) 767-7115
Maine	Stanley Stewart, R.Ph., P.O. Box 817, Bangor 04402 (207) 947-0885
Maryland	David Miller, 650 W. Lombard St., Baltimore 21201 (410) 727-0746
Massachusetts	Jeffrey J. Burgoyne, 111 Speen St., Ste 305, Framingham 01701 (508) 875-1774
Michigan	Larry D. Wagenknecht, 815 N. Washington Ave., Lansing 48906 (517) 484-1466
Minnesota	William E. Bond, Court International-North, 2550 University Ave. W., Suite 320N, St. Paul 55114 (612) 644-3566, (800) 451-8349 (non-metro MN)
Mississippi	Phylliss M. Moret, R.Ph., 341 Edgewood Terrace Dr., Jackson 39206-6299 (601) 981-0416
Missouri	George L. Oestreich, 410 Madison Ave., Jefferson City 65101 (314) 638-7522
Montana	Bonnie Tippy, P.O. Box 4718, Helena 59604 (406) 449-3843
Nebraska	Tom R. Dolan, R.Ph., 6221 S. 58th St., Suite A, Lincoln 68516 (402) 420-1500
Nevada	Karen Peska, 3660 Baker Lane, Reno 89509 (702) 826-3981
New Hampshire	Craig R. Merrick, R.Ph., 76 S. State St., Concord 03302 (603) 753-8759
New Jersey	Alvin N. Geser, 120 W. State St., Trenton 08608 (609) 394-5596
New Mexico	R. Dale Tinker, 4800 Zuni SE, Albuquerque 87108 (505) 265-8729
New York	Elizabeth Lasky, Pine West Plaza IV, Washington Ave. Ext., Albany 12205 (518) 869-6595
North Carolina	A. H. Mebane, III, P.O. Box 151, Chapel Hill 27514-0151 (919) 967-2237, (800) 852-7343
North Dakota	Howard C. Anderson, Jr., R.Ph., Executive Secretary/Treasurer, Box 5008, Bismarck 58502 (701) 258-9312
Ohio	Ernest E. Boyd, Pharmacist, Executive Director, 6037 Frantz Rd., Suite 106, Dublin 43017 (614) 798-0037
Oklahoma	John D. Donner, 45 N. E. 52nd St., Box 18731, Oklahoma City 73154 (405) 528-3338
Oregon	Chuck Gress, 1460 State St., Salem 97301-4296 (503) 585-4887
Pennsylvania	Carmen A. DiCello, R.Ph., Executive Director, 508 N. Third St., Harrisburg 17101-1199 (717) 234-6151
Puerto Rico	LCDA Amelia Diaz, G.P.O. Box 360206, San Juan 00936-0206 (809) 753-7157
Rhode Island	Donald H. Fowler, 500 Prospect St., Pawtucket 02860 (401) 725-4141
South Carolina	Robert H. Burnside, Jr., 1405 Calhoun St., Columbia 29201 (803) 254-1065
South Dakota	Galen Jordre, Box 518, Pierre 57501-0518 (605) 224-2338
Tennessee	Tom C. Sharp Jr., 226 Capitol Blvd., Suite 810, Nashville 37219 (615) 256-3023
Texas	Paul F. Davis, P.O. Box 14709, Austin 78761 (512) 836-8350
Utah	C. Neil Jensen, 1062 E. 21st St. S., Suite 212, Salt Lake City 84106 (801) 484-9141
Vermont	James S. Craddock, 109 State St., Montpelier 05609 (802) 229-9455
Virginia	John W. Hasty, R.Ph., 3119 W. Clay St., Richmond 23230 (804) 355-7941
Washington	Raymond A. Olson, 1420 Maple Ave. SW, Suite 101, Renton 98055-3196 (206) 228-7171
West Virginia	Richard D. Stevens, Kanawha Valley Bldg., 300 Capitol St., Suite 1002, Charleston 25301 (304) 344-5302
Wisconsin	Christopher J. Decker, R.Ph., 202 Price Place, Madison 53705 (608) 238-5515
Wyoming	Jerry Palmer, 815 Easy Circle, Box 280, Green River 82935 (307) 875-3334

State Licensure Requirements

All states require candidates for pharmacist licensures to have graduated from an accredited college of pharmacy and to be of good moral character. All states except California use the National Association of Boards of Pharmacy Licensure Examination (NABPLEX). Virtually every state allows students to retake the exam in case of failure. A few states also require students to take the Federal Drug Law Exam or a practical exam. (Contact the appropriate state board about additional examinations.) Some states require full citizenship, and many states require a candidate to be at least 18 years old.

Most states will grant you a license on the basis of your having been licensed in another state. Check with individual state boards for special requirements and fees. There are two states that do not reciprocate licensure at all: Florida and California.

	Internship Requirements		CE Requirements	
State	**Total Hours**	**Postgrad Hours**	**Hours**	**Industry Intern Credit**
Alabama	1,500	400	15/1 yr.	No
Alaska	1,500	160	15/1 yr.	No
Arizona	1,500	None	30/2 yrs.	500 hours
Arkansas	2,000	1,000	15/1 yr.	May be allowed
California	1,500	1,000	30/2 yrs.	Under 600 hours
Colorado	1,800	—	No	Case by case
Connecticut	1,500	None	15/1 yr.	Varies
Delaware	1,500	None	30/2 yrs.	N.A.
District of Columbia	1,500/1,000	None	30/2 yrs.	No
Florida	2,080 (varies)	N.A.	15/1 yr.	Case by case
Georgia	1,500	None	30/2 yrs.	Case by case
Hawaii	2,000	None	No	Yes
Idaho	1,500	None	5/1 yr.	One-half credit
Illinois	400	None	30/2 yrs.	No
Indiana	1,040	520	30/2 yrs.	No
Iowa	1,500	None	30/2 yrs.	May be allowed
Kansas	1,500	None	15/1 yr.	May be allowed
Kentucky	1,500	None	15/1 yr.	400 hours
Louisiana	1,500/1 yr.	500	5/1 yr.	No
Maine	1,500	None	15/1 yr.	May be allowed
Maryland	1,560	None	30/2 yrs.	Yes
Massachusetts	1,500	None	30/2 yrs.	Up to 400 hours
Michigan	1,000	None	30/2 yrs.	Up to 400 hours
Minnesota	1,500	None	30/2 yrs.	Varies
Mississippi	1,500	None	20/2 yrs.	300 hours
Missouri	1,500	None	10/1 yr.	200 hours
Montana	1,500	None	15/1 yr.	May be allowed
Nebraska	1,500	None	30/2 yrs.	May be allowed
Nevada	1,500	None	30/2 yrs	No
New Hampshire	1,500	None	15/1 yr.	May be allowed
New Jersey	1,000	Varies	30/2 yrs.	No
New Mexico	1 yr/1500	None	15/1 yr.	Yes
New York	6 mos	None	No	No
North Carolina	1,500	None	10/1 yr.	Up to 500 hours
North Dakota	1,500	None	30/2 yrs.	400 hours
Ohio	1,500	None	45/3 yrs.	Up to 300 hours
Oklahoma	2,000	None	15/1 yr.	Yes
Oregon	1,500	400	15/1 yr.	Varies
Pennsylvania	1,500	None	30/2 yrs.	Case by case
Puerto Rico	1,500	None	35/3 yrs.	300 hours
Rhode Island	1,500	None	15/1 yr.	One-half credit
South Carolina	1,500	None	15/1 yr.	500 hours max.

State	Internship Requirements		CE Requirements	
	Total Hours	Postgrad Hours	Hours	Industry Intern Credit
South Dakota	1,500	None	12/1 yr.	400 hours
Tennessee	1,500	None	15/1 yr.	Up to 400 hours
Texas	1,500	None	12/1 yr.	Varies
Utah	1,500	None	No	Varies
Vermont	1,500	None	15/1 yr.	Up to 750 hours
Virginia	6 mos	None	No	Yes
Washington	1,500	None	15/1 yr.	300 hours
West Virginia	1,500	None	15/1 yr.	520 hours
Wisconsin	1,500	500	No	500 hours max.
Wyoming	1,500	None	6/1 yr.	500 hours max.

Reprinted from National Association of Boards of Pharmacy: *1992 NABP Survey of Pharmacy Law,* Park Ridge, IL, 1992.

Appendix D: General References

Table D-1. Budgeting for Drug Information Resources

A. Basic Library

References	Update	Cost*
American Hospital Formulary Service (AHFS) Drug Information	Quarterly	$100.00
Drug Facts and Comparisons	Monthly	$150.00
Drug Interaction Facts	Quarterly	$100.00
King's Guide to Parenteral Admixtures	Quarterly	$200.00
Physicians' Desk Reference	Quarterly	$ 50.00
Martindale: The Extra Pharmacopoeia		
First-year expense		$225.00
Subsequent-year expense		$150.00

B. Additional Resources

References	Cost*
Therapeutics	$100.00
Internal medicine	$150.00
Pharmacokinetics	$100.00
Pharmacology	$100.00
Pregnancy/breast-feeding	$ 50.00
OTC drugs	$100.00
Pediatric drug handbook	$ 50.00
Dosing in renal failure	$ 25.00
USP DI (three-volume set)	$150.00
Remington's Pharmaceutical Sciences	$150.00

C. Microfiche Systems

References	Cost*
Iowa Drug Information System	$1300.00
Micromedex	
DRUGDEX Information System	$2700.00
IDENTIDEX Information System	$ 400.00
POISINDEX Information System	$2300.00
Paul deHaen Drug Data Information System	
Drugs in Prospect (DIP)	$1300.00
Drugs in Research (DIR)	$ 800.00
Drugs in Use (DIU)	$1000.00
Adverse Drug Reactions and Interactions Data (ADRID)	

D. CD-ROM Computer Systems

References	Cost*
Physicians' Desk Reference	$ 600.00
Martindale: The Extra Pharmacopoeia	$ 600.00
CCIS System (POISINDEX, DRUGDEX, EMERGINDEX)	
(any one)	$ 4000.00
(any two)	$ 7500.00
(any three)	$10,000.00

E. Major On-Line Vendors

Bibliographic Retrieval Services (BRS)
Dialog Information Services, Inc.
Medlars Management System
PaperChase
System Development Corporation Search Service (SDC)

*Costs are approximate and are based on Spring 1993 figures

Pharmaceutics

Ansel, HC; Popovich, NG: *Pharmaceutical Dosage Forms and Drug Delivery Systems,* 5th ed, Lea & Febiger, Malvern, Pa., 1990

Gennaro, AR: *Remington's Pharmaceutical Sciences,* 18th ed, Mack Publishing, Easton, Pa., 1990

Gibaldi, M: *Biopharmaceutics and Clinical Pharmacokinetics,* 3rd ed, Malvern, Pa., 1984

Lachman, L; Lieberman, HH; Kanig, JL: *The Theory and Practice of Industrial Pharmacy,* 3rd ed, Lea & Febiger, Malvern, Pa., 1986

Martin, A; Swarbrick, J; Cammarata, A: *Physical Pharmacy,* 3rd ed, Lea & Febiger, Malvern, Pa., 1983

Martindale: The Extra Pharmacopeia, 30th ed, The Pharmaceutical Press, London, 1993

Notari, RE: *Biopharmaceutics and Clinical Pharmacokinetics. An Introduction,* 4th ed, Marcel Dekker, Inc., New York, 1987

Rowland, M; Tozer, TN: *Clinical Pharmacokinetics. Concepts and Applications,* 2nd ed, Lea & Febiger, Malvern, PA., 1989

Shargel, L; Yu, ABC: *Applied Biopharmaceutics and Pharmacokinetics,* 2nd ed, Appleton-Century-Crofts, Norwalk, Conn., 1985

Stoklosa, MJ; Ansel, AC: *Pharmaceutical Calculations,* 9th ed, Lea & Febiger, Malvern, Pa., 1991

The United States Pharmacopeia XXII, United States Pharmacopeial Convention, Inc., Rockville, Md., 1990

Professional Pharmacy Practice

AMA Drug Evaluations, American Medical Association, WB Saunders, Philadelphia, 1992

Dukes, MNG; Beeley, L: *Side Effects of Drugs Annual,* Elsevier Science Publishing, New York, 1993

Facts and Comparisons, Facts and Comparisons, Inc., JB Lippincott, St. Louis (published annually)

Handbook of Nonprescription Drugs, 9th ed, American Pharmaceutical Association, Washington, 1990

Hansten, PD; Horn, JR: *Drug Interactions,* 6th ed, Lea & Febiger, Malvern, Pa., 1989

Hassan, WE, Jr: *Hospital Pharmacy,* 5th ed, Lea & Febiger, Malvern, Pa., 1986

McElvoy, GK: *Drug Information,* American Society of Hospital Pharmacists, Bethesda, Md., 1989

Pharmacy Law Digest, Facts and Comparisons, Inc., JB Lippincott, St. Louis, 1988

Physicians' Desk Reference, Medical Economics, Montvale, N.J. (published annually)

Turco, S; King, RE: *Sterile Dosage Forms,* 3rd ed, Lea & Febiger, Malvern, Pa., 1987

United States Pharmacopeia Dispensing Information (three volumes), United States Pharmacopeial Convention, Rockville, Md., 1993

Medicinal Chemistry and Pharmacology

Albert, A: *Selective Toxicity,* 7th ed, Chapman and Hall, New York, 1985

Amdur, MO: *Casarett and Doull's Toxicology. The Basic Science of Poisons,* 4th ed, McGraw-Hill, New York, 1991

Csaky, TZ; Barnes, BA: *Cutting's Handbook of Pharmacology,* 7th ed, Appleton & Lange, Norwalk, Conn., 1984

Foye, WO: *Principles of Medicinal Chemistry,* 3rd ed, Lea & Febiger, Malvern, Pa., 1989

Gibson, GG; Skett, P: *Introduction to Drug Metabolism,* Chapman and Hall, New York, 1986

Gilman, AG; Rall, TW; Nies, AS; Taylor, P; *Goodman and Gilman's The Pharmacological Basis of Therapeutics,* 8th ed, McGraw-Hill, New York, 1990

Jacob, LS: *Pharmacology,* 3rd ed, Harwal Publishing, Malvern, Pa., 1992

Katzung, BG: *Basic and Clinical Pharmacology,* 5th ed, Appleton & Lange, Norwalk, Conn., 1992

Lemke, TL: *Review of Organic Functional Groups: Introduction to Medicinal Organic Chemistry,* 2nd ed, Lea & Febiger, Malvern, Pa., 1988

Nogrady, T: *Medicinal Chemistry,* Oxford University Press, New York, 1988

Pratt, WB; Taylor, P: *Principles of Drug Action: The Basis of Pharmacology,* 3rd ed, Churchill Livingstone, New York, 1990

Clinical Pharmacy

Benet, LZ; Massoud, N; Gambertoglio, JG: *Pharmacokinetic Basic for Drug Treatment,* Raven Press, New York, 1984

Braunwald, E; Isselbacher, KJ; Petersdorf, RG; Martin, JB; Fauci, AS: *Harrison's Principles of Internal Medicine,* 11th ed, McGraw-Hill, New York, 1987

DiPiro, JT; Talbert, RL; Hayes, PE; Yee, PE; Posey, LM: *Pharmacotherapy: A Pathophysiologic Approach,* 2nd ed, Elsevier Science Publishers, New York, 1992

Dorland's Illustrated Medical Dictionary, 27th ed, WB Saunders, Philadelphia, 1988

Evans, WE; Schentag JJ; Jusko, WJ: *Applied Pharmacokinetics: Principles of Therapeutic Drug Monitoring,* 2nd ed, Applied Therapeutics, Spokane, Wash., 1992

Haddad, LM; Winchester, JF: *Clinical Management of Poisoning and Drug Overdose,* WB Saunders, Philadelphia, 1983

Harvey, AM; Johns, RJ; McKusick, VA; Owen, AH, Jr; Ross, RS: *Principles and Practice of Medicine,* 21st ed, Appleton & Lange, Norwalk, Conn., 1984

Herfindal, ET; Gourley, DR: *Clinical Pharmacy and Therapeutics,* 3rd ed, Williams & Wilkins, Baltimore, 1992

Knoben, JE; Anderson, PO: *Handbook of Clinical Drug Data,* 7th ed, Drug Intelligence Publications, Hamilton, Ill., 1993

Krupp, MA; Schroeder, SA; Tierney, LM, Jr: *Current Medical Diagnosis and Treatment,* Appleton & Lange, Norwalk, Conn., 1987

Macklis, RM; Mendelsohn, ME; Mudge, GH: *Manual of Introductory Clinical Medicine,* 2nd ed. Little, Brown, Boston, 1985

Melmon, KL; Morrelli, HF: *Clinical Pharmacology,* McGraw-Hill, New York, 1992

Shirkey, HC: *Pediatric Therapy,* 5th ed, Mosby Year Book, St. Louis, 1975

Stedman's Medical Dictionary, 25th ed, Williams & Wilkins, Baltimore, 1990

Traub, S: *Interpreting Laboratory Data,* American Society of Hospital Pharmacists, Washington, D.C., 1992

Wallach, J: *Interpretation of Diagnostic Tests,* 5th ed, Little, Brown, Boston, 1992

Woodley, M; Whelan, A: *Manual of Medical Therapeutics,* 25th ed, Little, Brown, Boston, 1986

Young, LY; Koda-Kimble, MA: *Applied Therapeutics: The Clinical Use of Drugs,* 5th ed, Applied Therapeutics, Vancouver, Wash., 1992

Miscellaneous Texts

Pediatrics

Benitz, WE; Tatro, DS: *The Pediatric Drug Handbook,* 2nd ed, Mosby Year Book, St. Louis, 1988

Rowe, PC: *The Harriet Lane Handbook,* Mosby Year Book, 12th ed, St. Louis, 1991

Poisoning and Toxicology

Dreisbach, RH: *Handbook of Poisoning,* 12th ed, Lange Medical Books, Seattle, 1987

Ellenhorn, MJ; Barceloux, DG: *Medical Toxicology: Diagnosis and Treatment of Human Poisoning,* Elsevier Science Publishing, 1988

Pregnancy

Folb, D: *Drug Safety in Pregnancy,* Elsevier Science Publishing, New York, 1990

Cloherty, JP; Stark, AR: *Manual of Neonatal Care,* 3rd ed, Little, Brown, Boston, 1991

Oncology

Fischer, DS; Knobf, MT: *The Cancer Chemotherapy Handbook,* 4th ed, Mosby Year Book, St. Louis, 1991

United States Pharmacopeia on Drug Information (USP DI) 3 volume set, 8th ed, United States Pharmacopeial Convention, Inc., Rockville, Md., 1993

Infectious Diseases

Conte, JE: Barriere, SL: *Manual of Antibiotics and Infectious Diseases,* 7th ed, Lea & Febiger, Malvern, PA, 1992

Mandell, GL; Douglas, RG; Bennet, JE: *Principles and Practice of Infectious Diseases,* 3rd ed, Churchill Livingstone, New York, 1990

Sanford, JP: *Guide to Antimicrobial Therapy,* Jay P. Sanford, 1992

Miscellaneous Journals

Pharmacy

American Journal of Hospital Pharmacy

Clinical Pharmacy

Drug Intelligence and Clinical Pharmacy

Hospital Pharmacy

General Medicine Subscriptions

Annals of Internal Medicine

British Medical Journal

New England Journal of Medicine

Journal of the American Medical Association (JAMA)

On-Line Database Vendors

Bibliographic Retrieval Services (BRS) Information Technologies, Latham, N.Y.

Dialog Information Services, Inc., Palo Alto, Calif.

National Library of Medicine Medlars Management System, Bethesda, Md.

PaperChase, Boston, Mass.

System Development Corporation (SDS) Search Service, Santa Monica, Calif.

Surface Area Nomograms
Body Surface Area of Adults and Children[a]

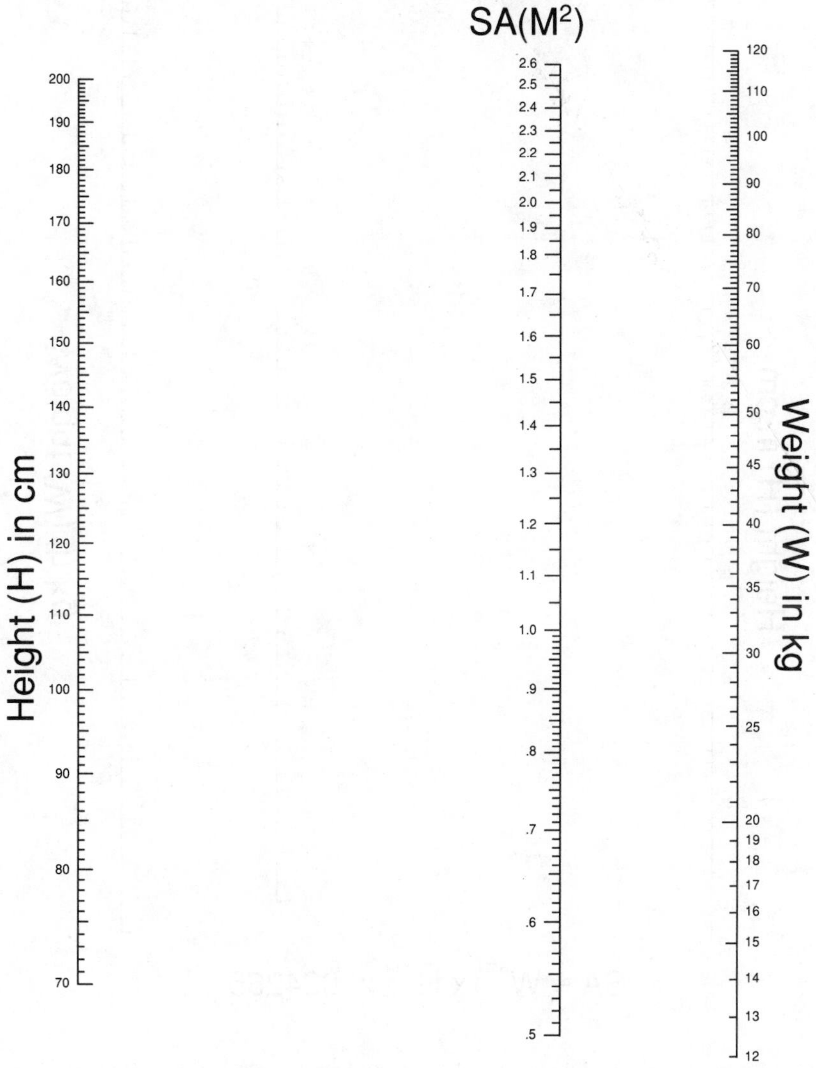

$$SA = W^{.5378} \times H^{.3964} \times .024265$$

Nomogram representing the relationship among height, weight, and surface area in adults and children. To use the nomogram, a ruler is aligned with the height and weight on the two lateral axes. The point at which the center line is intersected gives the corresponding value for surface area. Reprinted with permission.

[a] From Haycock GB, Schwartz GJ, Wisotsky DH: Geometric method for measuring body surface area: a height–weight formula validated in infants, children, and adults. *J. Pediatr,* 93:62–66, 1978.

Body Surface Area of Infants*

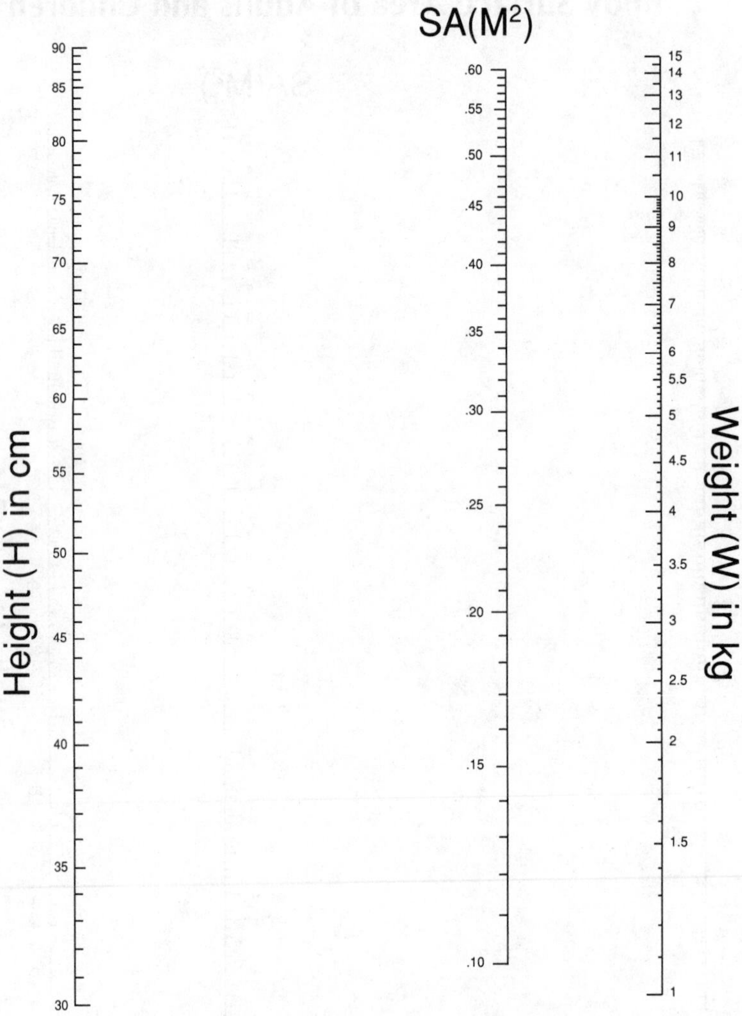

$$SA = W^{.5378} \times H^{.3964} \times .024265$$

Nomogram representing the relationship among height, weight, and surface area in infants. To use the nomogram, a ruler is aligned with the height and weight on the two lateral axes. The point at which the center line is intersected gives the corresponding value for surface area. Reprinted with permission.

*From Haycock GB, Schwartz GJ, Wisotsky DH: Geometric method for measuring body surface area: a height–weight formula validated in infants, children, and adults. *J. Pediatr,* 93:62–66, 1978.

Dietary Considerations

Potassium and Tyramine Content of Foods and Beverages

Potassium Content of Selected Foods, Beverages, and Salt Substitutes*†

Beverages [8 fl ʒ]	mg	mEq
Apple juice, bottled/canned	296	7.6
Apricot juice, nectar, canned	286	7.3
Grape juice, bottled/canned	334	8.5
Grapefruit juice, canned	378	9.7
Milk, whole, 3.5% fat (high in sodium)	351	9.0
Milk, lowfat, 2% fat (high in sodium)	377	9.6
Milk, skim (high in sodium)	406	10.4
Orange juice, fresh	496	12.7
Orange juice, canned	436	11.2
Pineapple juice, canned	334	8.5
Prune juice, canned	706	18.1
Tangerine juice, canned	443	11.3
Tomato juice, canned (high in sodium)	598	15.3
Fruits	**mg**	**mEq**
Apricots, raw, 3 medium	313	8.0
Banana, raw, 1 medium	451	11.5
Cantaloupe, raw, 1 cup pieces	494	12.6
Dates, dried, 10	541	13.8
Figs, dried, 10	1332	34.1
Fruit cocktail, canned, 1 cup	230	5.9
Grapefruit, pink, raw, ½ medium	158	4.0
Orange, navel, raw, 1 medium	250	6.4
Peach, raw, 1 medium	171	4.4
Pear, raw, 1 medium	208	5.3
Pineapple, raw, 1 cup pieces	175	4.5
Prunes, dried, 10	626	16.0
Raisins, seedless, ⅔ cup	751	19.2
Strawberries, raw, 1 cup	247	6.3
Watermelon, raw, 1 cup	186	4.8
Vegetables	**mg**	**mEq**
Avocado, raw, 1 medium (California)	1097	28.1
Avocado, raw, 1 medium (Florida)	1484	38.0
Beans, green lima, cooked, ½ cup	338	8.6
Beans, red kidney, cooked, ½ cup	425	10.9
Broccoli, cooked, ⅔ cup	267	6.8
Brussels sprouts, cooked 6–8 medium	273	7.0
Carrot, raw, 1 large	341	8.7
Corn, yellow, canned, ½ cup	138	3.5
Mushrooms, raw, 10 small	414	10.6
Potato, baked, 1 medium	503	12.9
Spinach, cooked, ½ cup	291	7.4
Squash, winter, baked, ½ cup	461	11.8
Tomato, raw, 1 medium	366	9.4
Salt Substitutes	**mg**	**mEq**
Adolph's, 1 g	485	12.4
Co-Salt, 1 g	469	12.0
Diasal, 1 g	442	11.3
Featherweight K, 1 g	465	11.9
Lite-Salt, 1 g (high in sodium)	293	7.4
Morton, 1 g	504	12.9
Neocurtasal, 1 g	470	12.1
NoSalt (Regular), 1 g	500	12.8
NoSalt (Seasoned), 1 g	266	6.8
Nu-Salt, 1 g	434	11.1
Salfree, 1 g	548	14.1

*Food values adaped from Pennington JAT, Church HN: *Bowes and Church's Food Values of Portions Commonly Used,* 14th ed. Philadelphia, JB Lippincott, 1985.

†Potassium content amounts are approximations. Salt substitute formulations, and hence potassium content, are subject to change by manufacturer. Salt substitute values from: Pearson RE,Fish KH: Potassium content of selected medicines, foods and salt substitutes. *Hosp Pharm* 1971;6:6–9; Sopko JA, Freeman RM: Salt substitutes as a source of potassium. *JAMA* 1977;238:608–10; and product information.

Tyramine Content of Foods and Beverages*†

Alcoholic Beverages	Estimated Levels‡
Beer and ale§	Low
Chartreuse‖	Unknown
Drambuie‖	Unknown
Sherry‖	Low
Wine, red#	Low
Wine, white**	Little or none

Cheese	Estimated Levels‡
American, processed	Low
Blue	Moderate to high
Boursault	Very high
Brick, natural	Moderate to high
Brie	Moderate to high
Camembert	Very high
Cheddar	Very high
Cottage cheese	Little or none
Cream cheese	Little or none
Emmenthaler	Very high
Gruyere	Moderate to high
Mozzarella	Moderate to high
Parmesan	Moderate to high
Romano	Moderate to high
Roquefort	Moderate to high
Stilton	Very high

Fruits	Estimated Levels‡
Bananas	Low
Figs, canned, particularly if overripe	Low to moderate

Meat and Fish	Estimated Levels‡
Beef liver, unrefrigerated, fermented	Moderate
Caviar	High
Chicken, liver, unrefrigerated, fermented	Moderate
Fish, unrefrigerated, fermented	Moderate
Fish, dried	Moderate
Herring, dried, salted	Moderate to high
Herring, pickled, if spoiled	Highest levels found
Sausages, fermented: Bologna, Pepperoni, Salami, Summer sausage	Very high
Other unrefrigerated, fermented meats	Moderate

Vegetables	Estimated Levels‡
Avocado, particularly if overripe	Low to moderate
Broad bean pods	Probably contain dopamine
Fava beans, particularly if overripe	Contain dopamine

Other Foods and Beverages	Estimated Levels‡
Caffeine, very large amounts	A weak pressor agent
Chocolate, very large amounts	Contains phenylethylamine, a weak pressor agent
Yeast extracts such as Marmite††	Very high

*Anon: Monoamine oxidase inhibitors for depression. *Med Lett Drugs Ther* 1980;22:58–60.

†For more detailed information, consult McCabe B, Tsuang MT: Dietary consideration in MAO inhibitor regimens. *J Clin Psychiatry* 1982;43:178–81.

‡The tyramine content of most foods is not entirely predictable. These estimates are taken from isolated reports, some based on small samples. The amount of tyramine in food and beverages could vary with different conditions, different samples, and different manufacturers.

§Fermentation of beer does not ordinarily involve processes that produce tyramine. However, the amount can vary greatly, and some imported beers have caused reactions in patients taking MAO inhibitors. McCabe and Tsuang (footnote †) state that beer is among the most important food restrictions and should be avoided.

‖Some patients have had reactions.

#Fermentation of wine does not ordinarily produce tyramine. However, contamination with other than the usual fermenting organisms and production of appreciable amounts of tyramine has occurred in Chianti and could occur in any red wine.

**White wine is free of tyramine because it is made without the grape pulp and seeds, which may be the source of amino acids in red wine.

††Baked goods do not contain appreciable amounts of tyramine.

Index

NOTE: Page numbers in *italic* denote illustrations; those followed by (t) denote tables; those followed by Q denote questions; and those followed by E denote explanations.

M

N

O